THE PHYSIOLOGIC
BASIS OF SURGERY

FOURTH EDITION

THE PHYSIOLOGIC BASIS OF SURGERY

EDITOR

J. Patrick O'Leary, MD, FACS

Executive Associate Dean of Clinical Affairs
Assistant Vice President Strategic Development
Florida International University Colleage of Medicine
Miami, Florida

CO EDITOR

Arnold Tabuenca, MD, FACS

Professor of Surgery
Loma Linda University Medical Centre
Loma Linda, California

ASSOCIATE EDITOR

Lea Rhea Capote, BGS

Administrative Manager
Department of Cardiovascular and Thoracic Surgery
The University of Texas Southwestern Medical Center at Dallas
Dallas, Texas

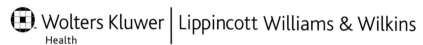

Wolters Kluwer | Lippincott Williams & Wilkins
Health

Philadelphia • Baltimore • New York • London
Buenos Aires • Hong Kong • Sydney • Tokyo

Acquisitions Editor: Brian Brown
Managing Editor: Julia Seto
Project Manager: Nicole Walz
Senior Manufacturing Manager: Ben Rivera
Marketing Manager: Lisa Parry
Design Coordinator: Holly Reid McLaughlin
Cover Designer: Christine Jenny
Production Services: Laserwords Private Limited, Chennai, India

Painting on cover from Royal Cabinet of Paintings
Mauritshuis The Hague
Rembrandt: *The Anatomy Lesson, #146.*

530 Walnut Street
Philadelphia, PA 19106 USA
LWW.com

Library of Congress Cataloging-in-Publication Data

The physiologic basis of surgery / editor, J. Patrick O'Leary ; associate editor, Lea Rhea Capote.—4th ed.
   p. ; cm.
  Includes bibliographical references and index.
  ISBN-13: 978-0-7817-7138-2
  ISBN-10: 0-7817-7138-2
  1. Pathology, Surgical. 2. Surgery—Physiological aspects. I. O'Leary, J. Patrick, 1941- II. Capote, Lea Rhea.
  [DNLM: 1. Surgery. 2. Physiology. WO 102 P5782 2008]
  RD57.P494 2008
  617—dc22
                                                                    2007027642

10 9 8 7 6 5 4 3 2

To all surgery residents past, present, and future.

CONTENTS

CONTRIBUTORS

Wayne L. Backes, PhD Professor/Associate Dean for Research, Department of Pharmacology and Experimental Therapeutics and Stanley S. Scott Cancer Center, Louisiana State University Health Sciences Center, New Orleans, Louisiana

Jody M. Barber, MD Radiologist, Center for Cancer Care at Goshen Health System, Goshen, Indiana

Ann Y. Becker, MD Assistant Professor, Department of Urology, Medical College of Georgia, Augusta, Georgia

Daniel L. Beckles, MD, PhD Chief Resident, Department of Cardiovascular and Thoracic Surgery, University of Texas, Southwestern Medical Center and Affiliated Hospitals, Dallas, Texas

Navin Bedi, MD Radiologist, Center for Cancer Care at Goshen Health System, Goshen, Indiana

Patrick I. Borgen, MD, FACS Director, Department of Breast Surgery, Maimonides Medical Center, Brooklyn, New York

Mary L. Brandt, MD Professor, Michael E. DeBakey Department of Surgery, Division of Pediatric Surgery, Baylor College of Medicine, Houston, Texas

Victor M. Brugh, MD Assistant Professor, Department of Urology, Eastern Virginia Medical School, Virginia Beach, Virginia

L. Michael Brunt, MD Professor, Department of Surgery, Washington University School of Medicine, St. Louis, Missouri; Attending Surgeon, Barnes-Jewish Hospital, St. Louis, Missouri

Lea Rhea Capote Administrative Manager, Cardiovascular and Thoracic Surgery, University Of Texas Southwestern Medical Center, Dallas, Texas

Kent Choi, MD, FACS Associate Professor, Department of Surgery, University of Iowa Carver College of Medicine; Surgical Critical Care Director, Department of Surgery, University of Iowa Hospitals and Clinics, Iowa City, Iowa

Dai H. Chung, MD Associate Professor, Department Of Surgery, University Of Texas Medical Branch, Galveston, Texas

Mark S. Cohen, MD Assistant Professor, Department of Surgery, Department of Pharmacology, Toxicology and Therapeutics, University of Kansas Medical Center; Attending Surgeon, Department of Surgery, University of Kansas Hospital, Kansas City, Missouri

Alan T. Davis, MS, PhD Associate Professor, Department of Surgery, Michigan State University, East Lansing, Michigan; Director, Research Department, Grand Rapids Medical Education and Research Center, Grand Rapids, Michigan

John W. Davis, MD Department of Urology, MD Anderson Cancer Center, Houston, Texas

Kraig S. de Lanzac, MD Assistant Professor of Clinical Anesthesiology-Gratis, Department of Anesthesiology, Louisiana State University Health Sciences Center School of Medicine, New Orleans, Louisiana; Staff Anesthesiologist, Department of Anesthesiology and Perioperative Medical Consultants, LLC, Slidell Memorial Hospital, Slidell, Louisiana

Alexander L. Eastman, MD Chief Resident in General Surgery, Department of Surgery, The University of Texas Southwestern Medical Center; Chief Resident in General Surgery, Department of Surgery Portland, Memorial Hospital, Dallas, Texas

Michael Emmett, MD Chairman, Department of Internal Medicine, Baylor University Medical Center, Dallas, Texas

Gregg R. Eure, MD, FACS Assistant Professor of Urology, Eastern Virginia Medical School, Virginia Beach, Virginia

B. Mark Evers, MD Professor and Robertson-Poth Distinguished Chair in General Surgery, Department of Surgery, The University of Texas Medical Branch, Galveston, Texas

Michael D. Fabrizio, MD Associate Professor, Department of Urology, Eastern Virginia Medical School, Norfolk, Virginia

Andrew Z. Fenves, MD Department of Medicine, Baylor University Medical Center, Dallas, Texas; Director, Division of Nephrology, Baylor University Medical Center, Dallas, Texas

Amin Frotan, MD Resident Physician, Department of Surgery, University of South Alabama, Mobile, Alabama; Housestaff, Department of Surgery, University of South Alabama Medical Center, Mobile, Alabama

Donald E. Fry, MD Professor Emeritus, Department of Surgery, University of New Mexico School of Medicine, Albuquerque, New Mexico

Robert E. Glasgow, MD Assistant Professor, Department of Surgery, University of Utah, Salt Lake City, Utah

Julie Glowacki, PhD Associate Professor, Department of Orthopedic Surgery, Harvard Medical School; Director, Skeletal Biology, Department of Surgery, Brigham and Women's Hospital, Boston, Massachusetts

Richard P. Gonzalez, MD Professor, Chief, Division of Trauma and Critical Care, Department of Surgery, University of South Alabama, Mobile, Alabama

Colin D. Goodier, MD Resident in General Surgery, Department of Surgery, Louisiana State University Health Sciences Center, New Orleans, Louisiana

Seza A. Gulec, MD, FACS Surgical & Nuclear Oncologist, Department of Surgical Oncology, Center For Cancer Care At Goshen Health System, Goshen, Indiana

Subhas Gupta, MD, CM, PhD, FRCSC, FACS Professor and Chairman, Department of Plastic Surgery, Loma Linda University School of Medicine, Loma Linda, California

Keith A. Hansen, MD Professor and Chair, Department of Obstetrics and Gynecology, Sanford School of Medicine, University of South Dakota; Reproductive Endocrinologist, Sanford Women's Health Fertility and Reproductive Endocrinology, Sanford Health, Sioux Falls, South Dakota

Herman A. Heck, Jr., MD, FACS Professor of Clinical Surgery; Interim Chief, Cardiothoracic Surgery, Department of Surgery, Section of Cardiothoracic Surgery, Louisiana State University Health Sciences Center; Clinical Director of Cardiothoracic Surgery, Department Of Surgery, Medical Center of Louisiana at New Orleans University Hospital, New Orleans, Louisiana

Erica N. Hoenie, BS Research Associate, Center for Cancer Care at Goshen Health System, Goshen, Indiana

Jean G. Hollowell, MD Assistant Professor, Department of Urology, Eastern Virginia Medical School, Children's Hospital of the King's Daughters, Norfolk, Virginia

Charles E. Horton, Jr., MD, FAAP Assistant Professor, Department of Urology, Eastern Virginia Medical School, Children's Hospital of the King's Daughters, Norfolk, Virginia

Robert J. Johnson, Jr., MD Neurosurgeon, Baptist Medical Center-Princeton, Birmingham, Alabama

Gerald H. Jordan, MD, FACS, FAAP Professor and Chairman, Department of Urology, Eastern Virginia Medical School; Director, The Devine Center for Genitourinary Reconstruction, Sentara Norfolk General Hospital, Norfolk, Virginia

Peter O. Kwong, MD Assistant Professor, Department of Urology, Eastern Virginia Medical School, Chesapeake, Virginia

W. Thomas Lawrence, MPH, MD Professor and Chief, Section of Plastic Surgery, Kansas University Medical Center, Kansas City, Kansas

Edward A. Levine, MD Associate Professor, Department of Surgery, Wake Forest University School of Medicine; Chief Surgical Oncology Service, Department of Surgery, North Carolina Baptist Hospital, Winston-Salem, North Carolina

Michael G. Levitzky, PhD Professor, Department of Physiology, Louisiana State University School of Medicine, New Orleans, Louisiana

Donald F. Lynch, Jr., MD Professor and Chairman, Department of Urology, Professor of Clinical Obstetrics and Gynecology, Eastern Virginia School Of Medicine, Norfolk, Virginia; Urologic Oncologist, Sentara Hospitals Southside, Norfolk and Virginia Beach, Virginia

Henry J. Mankin, MD Edith M. Ashley Professor, Department of Orthopedic Surgery, Harvard Medical School; Former Chief of Service, Department of Orthopedics, Massachusetts General Hospital, Boston, Massachusetts

Robert G. Martindale, MD, PhD Associate Professor, Department of Surgery, Oregon Health and Science University; Medical Director For Hospital Nutrition Services, Department Of Surgery, Oregon Health and Science University, Portland, Oregon

Kurt A. McCammon, MD Associate Professor, Department of Urology, Eastern Virginia Medical School, Virginia Beach, Virginia

Joseph M. Moerschbaecher, III, PhD Professor, Department of Pharmacology, Louisiana State University Health Sciences Center, New Orleans, Louisiana

Mary Morrogh, MD Breast Service, Department of Surgery, Memorial Sloan-Kettering Cancer Center, New York, New York

Sean J. Mulvihill, MD Professor and Chairman, Department of Surgery, University of Utah, School of Medicine, Salt Lake City, Utah

Martha Meaney Murray, MD Assistant Professor, Department of Orthopedic Surgery, Harvard Medical School; Orthopedic Surgeon, Department of Orthopedic Surgery, Children's Hospital, Boston, Massachusetts

J. Patrick O'Leary Executive Associate Dean of Clinical Affairs, Assistant Vice President Strategic Development, Florida International University College of Medicine, Miami, Florida

Oluyinka O. Olutoye, MBChB, PhD, FACS, FAAP Assistant Professor, Department of Surgery and Pediatrics, Baylor College of Medicine; Codirector, Texas Children's Fetal Center, Houston, Texas

Herbert A. Phelan, MD Assistant Professor, Department of Surgery, University Of South Alabama; Attending Surgeon, Department of Surgery, University of South Alabama Medical Center, Mobile, Alabama

Walter E. Pofahl, II, MD Chief of Staff, Pitt County Memorial Hospital; Associate Professor of Surgery, Chief, Division of Advanced Laparoscopic, Gastrointestinal, and Endocrine Surgery, Department of Surgery, Brody School of Medicine, East Carolina University, Greenville, North Carolina

Archana Rao, MD Nephrology fellow, Baylor University Medical Center, Dallas, Texas

Timothy J. Redden, MD Chief Resident, Department of Urology, Eastern Virginia Medical School, Norfolk, Virginia

Mark E. Reeves, MD, PhD Associate Professor, Residency Program Director, and Cancer Center Director, Department of Surgery and Cancer Center, Loma Linda University; Attending Surgeon, Division of Surgical Oncology, Loma Linda University and Veteran Affairs Medical Centers, Loma Linda, California

James M. Riopelle, MD Professor of Clinical Anesthesiology, Department of Anesthesia, Louisiana State University Health Sciences Center; Staff Anesthesiologist, Department of Anesthesiology, Medical Center of Louisiana at New Orleans, New Orleans, Louisiana

Edwin L. Robey, MD Associate Professor, Department of Urology, Eastern Virginia Medical School, Norfolk, Virginia

Richard J. Rohrer, MD Professor, Department Of Surgery, Tufts University School of Medicine; Chief, Division of Transplant Surgery, Department of Surgery, Tufts-New England Medical Center, Boston, Massachusetts

Ronnie A. Rosenthal, MD, FACS Associate Professor, Department of Surgery, Yale University School of Medicine; Chief, Surgical Service, Veteran Affairs Connecticut Healthcare System, West Haven, Connecticut

Paul F. Schellhammer, MD Professor, Department of Urology, Eastern Virginia Medical School, Norfolk, Virginia

C. William Schwab, II, MD Fellow in Laparoendoscopic Urology, Eastern Virginia Medical School, Norfolk, Virginia

Carol E. H. Scott-Conner, MD, PhD Professor, Department of Surgery, Carver College of Medicine, University of Iowa; Professor, Department of Surgery, University of Iowa Hospitals and Clinics, Iowa City, Iowa

Aryeh Shander, MD, FCCM, FCCP Clinical Professor, Department of Anesthesiology Medicine and Surgery, Mount Sinai School of Medicine, New York, New York; Chief, Department of Anesthesiology, Critical Care Medicine and Hyperbaric Medicine, Englewood Hospital and Medical Center, Englewood, New Jersey

Sarah C. Shaves, MD Vice Chairman, Department of Radiology, Eastern Virginia Medical School, Norfolk, Virginia

Roger D. Smith, MD Chief, Department of Neurosurgery, Ochsner Clinic Foundation, New Orleans, Louisiana

Richard K. Spence, MD Director of Surgical Education, Baptist Health Systems Inc.; Clinical Professor, Department of Surgery, University of Alabama School of Health Related Professions, Birmingham, Alabama

John H. Stewart, IV, MD Assistant Professor, Department of Surgical Oncology, Wake Forest University School of Medicine; Assistant Professor, Department of Surgical Oncology, North Carolina Baptist Hospital, Winston-Salem, North Carolina

Hugo St. Hilaire, MD, DDS Chief Resident in Plastic Surgery, Department of Surgery, Louisiana State University Health Sciences Center, New Orleans, Louisiana

Arnold Tabuenca, MD, FACS Professor, Department of Surgery, Loma Linda University Medical Center, Loma Linda, California; Chairman, Department of Surgery and CMO, Riverside County Regional Medical Center, Moreno Valley, California

Jonathan R. Taylor, MD Chief Resident, Department of Urology, Eastern Virginia Medical School, Norfolk, Virginia

Mack A. Thomas, MD, FACS Clinical Professor of Surgery and Anesthesia, Department of Surgery, Louisiana State University Health Sciences Center; Staff Anesthesiologist, Ochsner Foundation Hospital, New Orleans, Louisiana

Robert L. Tiel, MD Professor, Department of Neurosurgery, University of Mississippi Medical Center, Jackson, Mississippi

Michael A. Wait, MD, FACS Associate Professor, Department of Cardiovascular and Thoracic Surgery, The University of Texas Southwestern Medical Center at Dallas, Dallas, Texas

Le Roy D. Weaver, Jr., MD Radiologist, Center for Cancer Care at Goshen Health System, Goshen, Indiana

Thomas V. Whelan, MD Assistant Clinical Professor, Department of Medicine, Eastern Virginia Medical School, Norfolk, Virginia

M. Whitten Wise, MD Assistant Professor, Department of Surgery, Division of Plastic Surgery, Louisiana State University Health Sciences Center, New Orleans, Louisiana

Minhao Zhou, MD General Surgery Resident, Department of Surgery, Oregon Health and Science University, Portland, Oregon

PREFACE TO THE FIRST EDITION

It is rare that an undertaking as expansive as *The Physiologic Basis of Surgery (PBS)* has a discreet starting point. That is not the case with this project. I remember well walking through the somewhat deserted foyer of the Georgia Trade Center during the week of the American College of Surgeons meeting in Atlanta on my was to the session of the Association of Program Directors in Surgery (APDS). As I approached a particularly long and abandoned hallway (I was about 10 minutes late and the session had already begun), a figure materialized from behind a large column. The figure was Dr. Paul Friedman. He asked if I had a few minutes to spend talking about a project that he and other members of the executive committee of the APDS had been discussing. A word of warning to the wise, if Dr. Friedman ever approaches you with this type of introduction, do not pause, not even for the slightest moment. Tell him that you have some place to be or invent some other hyperbole and leave the area, immediately. I was not that smart and became enthralled with the sound of Paul's voice. I also became excited by the project that he had described and endorsed the concept in its entirety. In my own naïveté, I agreed that the project was large, but I thought that it could be accomplished in 18 months. The project, in fact, has now taken more than $3^1/_2$ years, and the potential for revision, updating, and new types of computer interfaces are staggering.

Although I have always had an interest in basic science and the teaching of basic science to both medical students and housestaff, I do not consider myself a basic scientist. I am a surgeon with an understanding of the laboratory and of scientific method. My selection to head this project still remains an enigma to me.

One of the reasons that I accepted the responsibility was that the concept of a blend between electronic media, standard publishing technology, and the use of tutorials to facilitate adult education had been an area of interest of mine for many years. When Dr. Gene Woltering was still a resident at Vanderbilt University, we had talked of developing another project that would incorporate publishing and electronic media. This project was designed so that not only the surgeons in training but also the surgeons preparing for recertification would be able to have at their fingertips a mechanism for updating current information with recent publications, revisiting older concepts, and then testing themselves using the computer as a tool to gain not only self-assessment but also CME credit. This concept brewed for more than 8 years and was endorsed by a major publishing company. They then contracted with an extremely large corporation who had expressed interest in this area. The project was finally abandoned when industry withdrew financial support as the full extent of the project became apparent.

This *PBS* project could have been a spinoff of the original project, and as Dr. Friedman and I talked, it became apparent that this was an opportunity to at least fulfill a portion of the more global scheme.

In 1989, the American Board of Surgery (ABS) had struggled with the concept of a surgical basic science examination. The board had discussed in great depth the concept of a preliminary examination given during the residency (after the first 2 years of general surgery training) that would deal predominately, if not wholly, with basic science information. This was proposed as a third component of the board certification process. In their memo of April 20, 1989, they provided the APDS with an outline of content that they thought would be appropriate as a backbone of such an examination. That outline, with certain modifications, serves as the chapter headings for the *PBS* text.

The APDS received this notification with a certain amount of concern. The general consensus of the organization was that basic science was an extremely important part of the curriculum and should be emphasized, but there was a problem. At that time, there were about 290 training programs in surgery in the country. Approximately 126 of those programs were associated with a medical school, while the remainder were housed in institutions that did not necessarily have strong ties with a medical school. This meant that the abilities of these latter institutions to generate a basic science curriculum might be compromised. In an attempt to establish a curriculum that crossed the boundaries between university-based and community-based programs, the APDS responded by initiating the process that would result in *The Physiologic Basis of Surgery*.

By late 1989, after careful introspection, the ABS decided to move away from the position that there should be a third phase in the certification process, deciding instead to emphasize basic sciences on their yearly in-training examination. This decision was favorably received by all concerned, as it minimized a host of problems that could have been produced by the change in the certification process.

The concept of the importance of basic science education in surgical training stands on its own merit. It is true that all of the advances in surgery that have occurred are based on basic science principles. It is my opinion that when residents complete their training, they have only begun to accrue the information that they need to be an accomplished surgeon 20 years hence. Residents need to be exposed to and required to learn as much about our current understanding of basic science as is possible. This will allow them the ability to make appropriate judgments about new technology and therapy as these are presented in the future. Nothing could be more dated than surgeons who, at the peak of their clinical careers, are still practicing the dogma imposed on them 20 years earlier when they were surgical residents. Surgeons should be encouraged to question dogma and to accept new information as long as it fits with the basic rules of physiology. Doing something simply because your mentor did it or because you feel comfortable with the particular procedure or therapy should not be enough. Surgeons should critically assess new modalities of treatment, know enough about biostatistics to make informed judgments on the data presented, and endorse or discard studies on their own merit.

The Physiologic Basis of Surgery is an attempt by a group of surgeons to collect information about the basic sciences and present it in an understandable and attractive format. To the best of our ability, this represents an overview of surgery as we practice it today. It is not a complete anthology of all basic information, but an attempt to gather in one place a compendium of facts and concepts, laced with appropriate references and selected readings.

In addition to the standard textbook, this program provides educators with a sizable number of multiple-choice questions (MCQ) that have been collected from the material presented in the text. Although most of the questions are specifically answered in the text, some are answered in the references and in the texts proposed as a part of the selected readings. These questions can be used by program directors for self-study or they may be used to test the material presented in any particular chapter. Another aspect of this pool of questions is that sorting methods have been provided so that the educator can search the pool of questions by organ or organ system. The pool may also be searched by disease process (neoplastic, mechanical, metabolic, immunological, infectious, iatrogenic, anatomic, physiologic, etc.) or by chapter. These tests can be taken electronically and graded in the same way. They may be also printed and used in the hard-copy mode. The program director may choose to give a pretest before the learning experience and then again test the residents with a different set of questions after the chapter has been discussed in whatever mode the program director chooses.

At our institution, we have a basic science conference on a weekly basis. We use *The Physiologic Basis of Surgery* as our outline and deal with a subdivision of the assigned chapter at every session. We either use members of our basic science faculty, our clinical faculty, or our residents as the experts who present the topic. The assigned topic is presented in a 20-minute didactic session. We then open the discussion with a point and counterpoint session, which is followed by an open discussion of the topic. All members of the audience are encouraged to participate. At our institution, the medical students also participate in this forum. We use the MCQ aspect as a self-study aid. Generally, three or four of the residents will work at a computer answering each of the MCQs as it appears on the screen.

The tutorials are arranged somewhat differently. They are patterned after patient management problems, but we have attempted to deal with basic science concepts. A problem is generally presented as a vignette, and then followed by a list of options from which a choice is requested. If the individual chooses an incorrect answer, the explanation for why the answer was incorrect appears on the screen. If the answer chosen was correct, either the word *correct* appears or the word *correct* with a short description of why the answer was true. Each of these tutorials has from two to seven subsets. Although residents will know how many they have answered correctly of the total number of correct answers (they will also find out how many incorrect answers they chose), we have not weighted the answers or attempted to score the tutorials. They are primarily intended to be a self-education portion of the curriculum.

Although the electronic portion of this packet is intriguing and modern by current standards, we are just beginning to use the capability of computer-assisted education in our adult programs. I am sure that our feeble efforts are but a prodrome of more sophisticated interactive programs that will appear in the near future.

The intention of all of this is to produce a rough outline of a basic science curriculum (certainly many creative modifications of the material presented are possible) so that educators may bring to residents in surgery a foundation on which their understanding of basic science may be structured. There are as many ways to use this program as there are intellects who choose to use it.

J. Patrick O'Leary, M.D.

PREFACE TO THE SECOND EDITION

Gratification comes to each individual in slightly different ways. For the teacher there can be no greater sense of achievement than to watch the awakening of understanding in a student as they grasp a new concept or, more importantly, the relationship between two previously known facts. For the editor or the author, the production of the tome is clearly the end product of the work. This product is tangible, has form, substance, occupies space, and has a certain attractiveness to it that is magnified by a sense of ownership or achievement. It is not the tangible product that produces the ultimate long lasting gratification, rather it is seeing the product picked up, read, and incorporated into a life long learning pattern. It is seeing the resident who has spent time delving into the book emerge from the encounter with a fresh understanding and perhaps new knowledge. Nothing in *The Physiologic Basis of Surgery (PBS)* is new. In fact, most every resident in surgery during their medical school experience probably heard these concepts and this rhetoric any number of times. The real purpose of the project was to collapse mountains of information into a reasonable volume that was structured by surgeons in such a way that surgeons-in-training would be able to assimilate those important basic science concepts inherent in the treatment of patients with disease. It was not the purpose of this book to present knowledge for knowledge's sake, but to present salient information that provides the underpinning for an understanding of the patient's disease process. It is only when an understanding of such basic principles reaches a certain critical level that true understanding of disease processes can be attained.

I have heard it said by many residents that spending time on basic science studies is a waste of effort. I contend, however, that it is only when a resident is substantially grounded in basic science that he begins to have a true understanding of disease and is not memorizing a certain litany of arcane signs and symptoms signifying disease.

As discussed in the preface of the first edition, this project was sponsored by the Association of Program Directors in Surgery (APDS) and was in response to a movement in the American Board of Surgery which had hoped to emphasize the basic science curriculum in residency training programs. Although implementation of some of the suggestions by the American Board of Surgery did not occur, the American Board of Surgery In Training Examination (ABSITE) was modified so that basic science topics were emphasized. Because there was no standardized text on the market to serve as a benchmark for residents in training or for the individuals making up the examination, there was a great deal of variability among items in the test, as to how well residents performed on the examination. It would now appear that the *PBS* has demonstrated a substantial penetration into the market with almost as many volumes sold as there are residents currently in categorical positions in the country.

The second edition responds to several criticisms that were couched in a very constructive way by Dr. Francis Moore in his review of the first volume in *The New England Journal of Medicine*, and by Dr. George Higgins, now deceased, in a personal letter. Topics such as shock, fluid and electrolytes, and reproductive physiology have been added. Some chapters have been modified slightly, while other chapters have undergone a near complete revision.

Whenever someone does something for the first time they always silently marvel at their accomplishments. As time passes and experience grows, the individual often begins to realize that although the first foray was a worthy effort, with practice comes refinement and often improvement. So it is with *PBS*. The second edition is an improvement over the first edition in many ways. The most important difference is probably in the computer program that will be a part of the overall package. The multiple choice questions that were included in the first packet have been expanded to include a discussion of each distractor and why the correct answer was chosen by the author. The questions and text are now available together on CD ROM allowing a complete interactive interface for the resident. This will allow a full description of the circumstances surrounding each question. Although this is still a fledgling attempt to use the power of computers to enhance self learning, it is a step in the proper direction.

PREFACE TO THE THIRD EDITION

A long time ago, in a land far away, an idea emerged that it would be a good thing to apply an understanding of the basic sciences to the education of fledgling surgeons.

The purpose of the preface is not to sell the book. One would hope that, by the time the reader got this far into the text, the book would already be their property. The preface does, however, state the philosophy of the author. In this case, it is my contention that a student/resident must have a sound basis in the basic science of medicine to practice surgery at the highest level. This quest for an understanding of basic science is, in fact, a lifelong quest. The basic principles of the science will not change; however, our understanding of these principles will change. From understanding comes innovation in therapeutic intervention, and from therapeutic intervention comes the basis for outcome studies. From outcome studies come the justification for pathways and principles of best practice. It is the achievement of this goal, the principles of best practice that should be the dominating force that directs our management of each of our patients.

In the two previous prefaces, a bit of the history about how this book came to be has been described. The impetus remains the same and the refinements in this version simply emerged from the experiences encountered in the first two publications. The premise that a strong foundation in basic science is paramount to an understanding of clinical disease remains the parapet upon which the entire concept revolves.

I have been impressed and encouraged by the resounding success of this book. As a visiting professor at a substantial number of programs, residents have approached me to comment on the quality and readability of the text. Of course, this has very little to d with my job as editor and all to do with the various authors who have arduously worked to make the tome approachable. For this accomplishment, the authors are solely responsible.

In this edition, a new chapter on geriatrics has been added. This is in response to the aging of our population and the growing imperative that, just as children are not small adults, patients in the advancing throes of age are also different from the prototypic healthy athletic male at age 30. This concept is not exactly new, but it is an aspect of the practice of surgery that has only recently come under scrutiny and been exposed to the critical eye of many sophisticated researchers. In addition to this new chapter, most of the chapters have undergone some revision and five chapters have been almost totally rewritten. At the time of publication of this edition, a companion CD will also be available. Over 1,000 multiple choice questions that relate to specific areas in the text will be available. Each of these queries will have associated with it a commentary, which in a very succinct way, validate the correct answer while explaining why the other potential answers are incorrect. References back to the text will be available for most of the questions. The editors hope that this third edition will provide a springboard for learning surgical basic science in the new millennium.

PREFACE TO THE FOURTH EDITION

It is truly a daunting task to write a preface to a textbook that was conceived many years ago to meet a need that was, in some ways, ethereal. A preface should be a condensation of the purpose for which the tome was created. Most surgeons never have the opportunity to edit a textbook and for those few who do, the creation of the preface is often a singular event. Such is not the case here. The contribution that follows is the fourth edition. In revisiting the previous three prefaces, I was struck by how they became progressively shorter.

The purpose of this book remains as it was in the beginning—to level the playing field in surgical training by gathering together in one place a certain aliquot of the basic information necessary for residents to master, on their way to becoming competent surgeons. It is all about knowledge. But knowledge, presented only for knowledge's sake, suffers from a lack of relevance or, more simply stated, applicability to the learner's needs. Learners, in this circumstance, are all adults exhibiting that collage that characterizes mature individuals as they move from one level of understanding to another.

This thing, knowledge, is a fragile morsel that ages poorly. Knowledge needs to be constantly renewed, to be reinvigorated, and be manicured. The fringes of knowledge need to be continually revisited, reprocessed, and experience their own rebirth. Knowledge is the basis for all performance, especially in the professions. But knowledge is a fickle partner that frequently changes. All professionals, especially those in medicine and, in medicine, especially those in surgery, must massage their database, extracting that which is outdated and replacing it with the new.

It is certainly true that with each passing decade, those things that we had held as immutable first principles have morphed into something else. No bit of information is *sacrosanct* in our current scientific environment. The atom is certainly no longer the primary building block of the universe. There is strong evidence that not all breast cancers behave the same, although histologically they may not be distinguishable one from the other. Without question, healing wounds and neoplastic tumors exert an angiogenic effect and new blood vessels are produced, but the process involved in each may be different. Or, perhaps, it may be the same.

For the learner, understanding flows from a grasp of basic concepts that are then applied to the more sophisticated or complex problem. One's clinical acumen is a compilation of experience, both successes and failures, which in turn is based on an infrastructure of the understanding of basic science that includes cellular physiology, organ system interactions, and pathophysiology. These, in turn, often revert to biochemical relationships that have their origins in the interaction of genes and then in proteomics.

Each adult learns differently but all adult learning has certain things in common. First, there must be perceived "a need to know." For the young surgeons, it would appear that the best way to understand the complex mechanisms at play in sick patients would be to understand the disease processes at the cellular or even at the organelle level. It would follow that when this baseline of understanding has been achieved, it must constantly be updated. As basic science discoveries are subsequently made, the adult learner must modify their knowledge base and thereby facilitate a better understanding of what constitutes proper surgical management.

Surgery is, of course, about the incision, but surgery is much, much more. Once an extensive knowledge base is in place, this knowledge base can be modified and "brought up to snuff" relatively easily. As the knowledge base infrastructure changes, it often brings with it a better understanding of the disease and, with that, a better justification of the classic approach to treatment or perhaps an altogether different way that certain patients should be managed.

To return to the second tenet espoused earlier, every individual adult utilizes some similar and many dissimilar processes to accrue new information. One way that many adults learn is through an active process of interaction with the database such as in case presentations or, in the circumstances of this text, interaction with a sophisticated collection of questions and answers. A bank of questions has been a part of each of the previous editions though considerably underutilized by most readers. Testing one's understanding of complex problems using a tool, such as a bank of questions, facilitates understanding and illuminates areas where further studying might be indicated. In the past, this aspect of the program was relegated to tapes and then CDs, but each was met with the problems inherent in the vehicle. With this edition, the question bank has been expanded and scrubbed. It has been placed in an accessible site on the web for the use of the participants. The use of this modality should facilitate the ease of access and provide immediate feedback to the participants as they work through the question bank of well in excess of 1,250 questions. These queries cover the vast majority of the concepts covered in the text.

Mastery of the book and the items in the question bank does not assure competency in the clinical field of surgery, but it certainly goes a long way to assure educators that an understanding of the basic science principles is present in the learner.

ACKNOWLEDGMENTS

The power and quality of this book is a testament to the superb efforts of the authors gathered together. It depicts their understanding of and dedication to the concepts of basic science and the education of residents which flows through this tome. Again, it was the Association of Program Directors in Surgery (APDS) that hatched the project and got it started. It has been brought to fruition by the efforts of many. It is again true that without the empowering efforts of Mrs. Lea Rhea Capote, who has been the Associate Editor for all four editions, the book would have failed. This particular edition also benefited from the contributions of Dr. Arnold Tabuenca, who has joined as Coeditor and has contributed enormously, especially in the area of the electronic modifications, infrastructure, and the question bank.

CHAPTER 1

Cell Biology

Mark E. Reeves

Our world is populated by an enormous variety of cells. In spite of the diversity in size, shape, and function, cells share many features at a subcellular level, especially when grouped according to their complexity.

The simplest cells are classified as *prokaryotes* and contain few intracellular membranes and no specialized compartments. Members of this class include all bacteria, certain algae, and the pleuropneumonia-like organisms. Their name is derived from the fact that their nuclear material or karyon lacks a discrete membrane, leaving the solitary molecule of double-stranded DNA condensed but not enclosed (Fig. 1.1). Prokaryotes are small (0.1–2.0 μm) and primitive.

By contrast, *eukaryotic* cells have a more developed and complex intracellular organization that allows most of their specialized functions to be performed within membrane-bound compartments or organelles. This compartmentation is accommodated by the larger size of eukaryotic cells

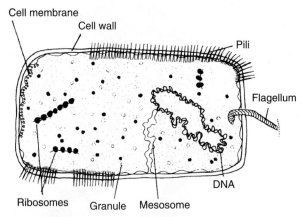

FIGURE 1.1 The generalized prokaryote, represented by a bacterium. Almost all bacteria are surrounded by a cell wall, which is attached to the cell membrane at relatively few points. Either flagella or pili, or both, may extend from the cytoplasm through the wall. Ribosomes, granules of various kinds, and DNA are found in the cytoplasm. (From Dyson RD. *Essentials of cell biology,* 2nd ed. Englewood Cliffs, NJ: Prentice Hall, 1978:12, with permission.)

(5–20 μm). Cells of this class include unicellular protozoa, most algae, and all plant and animal cells (Fig. 1.2). There are more than 250 cell types in the human body, and these cells have grown and differentiated into a highly integrated and complex system of tissues and organs.

In this chapter, we will focus on the relation between structure and function in the cells of the human body and elucidate mechanisms that contribute to their control. Because of recent explosive progress in molecular and cellular biology, this review will only highlight important aspects of these topics.

PLASMA MEMBRANE

General Features

A plasma membrane defines the surface of each cell and effectively separates its internal aqueous environment from the outside world. The most basic function of this barrier is to maintain transmembrane gradients by controlling the passage of small and large molecules. An even more elegant role, however, is to provide a substrate for the various enzyme systems and receptors that, when stimulated, produce cellular responses. Structurally, biologic membranes are composed of approximately equal weights of lipids and proteins; carbohydrates account for a small but extremely important fraction of the total.

Lipids

The lipids in the membrane are typically amphiphilic molecules composed of a hydrophilic polar head and one or two hydrophobic hydrocarbon tails (Fig. 1.3). The three main lipid classes found in membranes are phospholipids, cholesterol, and glycolipids. The most common of these, the phospholipids, are arranged as a bilayer, with their hydrocarbon tails juxtaposed to form a hydrophobic interior domain, whereas their hydrophilic polar head groups face the aqueous environment on either side. The phospholipid molecules exhibit a remarkable degree of lateral and

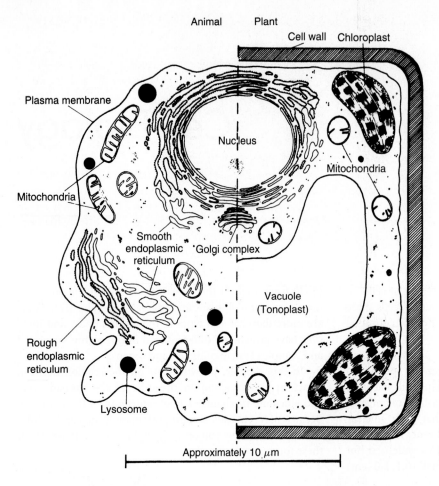

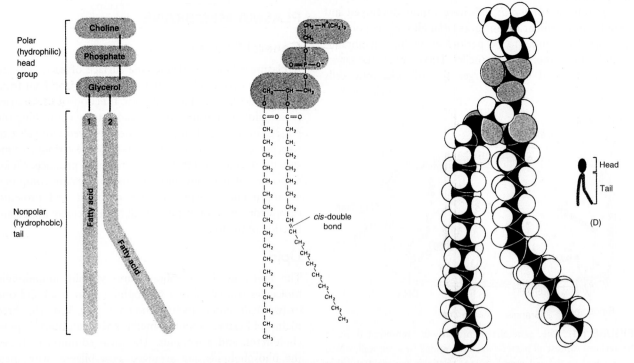

FIGURE 1.2   The generalized eukaryotic cell. The diagram shows organelles of eukaryotic animal and plant cells as revealed by electron microscopy. (From Gennis RB. *Biomembranes: molecular structure, and function.* New York: Springer-Verlag, 1989, with permission.)

FIGURE 1.3   The parts of a phospholipid molecule, phosphatidylcholine, represented (*far left*) schematically, (*middle left*) in formula, (*middle right*) as a space-filling model, and (*far right*) as a symbol. (From Alberts B, Bray D, Lewis J, et al. *Molecular biology of the cell*, 2nd ed. New York: Garland, 1989, with permission.)

rotational movement. This important phenomenon, called *membrane fluidity,* indirectly influences many membrane functions (1).

Large amounts of cholesterol are also present in most eukaryotic membranes, often reaching a molecular ratio as high as 1:1 with phospholipids. Because the smaller cholesterol molecule tends to become packed between adjacent phospholipid molecules, it provides mechanical stability and thereby limits membrane fluidity. Glycolipids generally account for a small fraction of the total lipids in the membrane. Although their function is still uncertain, they do function in cell–cell recognition and modulation of transmembrane signaling.

The basic function of membrane lipids is to provide a permeability barrier for the cell. However, lipids also function as mediators and anchors. Arachidonic acid, a common constituent of membrane phospholipids, is released in response to the local action of phospholipases activated by specific receptors (2). Once released, arachidonate can be oxidized through either the cyclooxygenase or lipoxygenase (LO) pathways. The active metabolites, leukotrienes, prostaglandins, and thromboxanes are critical mediators in a variety of inflammatory disorders (Fig. 1.4).

Another novel class of membrane lipids, the phosphatidylinositols, serve as the sole anchors for a diverse group of cell surface proteins, including alkaline phosphatase, carcinoembryonic antigen, and acetylcholinesterase. This superficial arrangement provides lateral mobility to the bound proteins and allows their rapid release under appropriate circumstances. Phosphatidylinositols are also precursors for inositol-l,4,5-triphosphate (IP$_3$) and diacylglycerol (DAG), which are important in many signaling pathways (see "Receptors and Cell Signaling").

Cells attach to each other to form tissues through specialized zones within the membrane called *junctions.* At *tight junctions,* the plasma membranes of adjacent cells are fused together, totally sealing the intercellular space. This limits movement and maintains the polarity of individual cells by preventing mixing of their different membrane regions. In this manner, for example, the mucosal enzymes of intestinal epithelia remain segregated from their apical surface.

In highly stressed tissues, *anchoring junctions* bolster the normal mechanical support by linking the interior cytoskeletons of individual cells and distributing their tensile strength across many cells. One form, the adherence junction, is characterized by dense bands of amorphous protein that

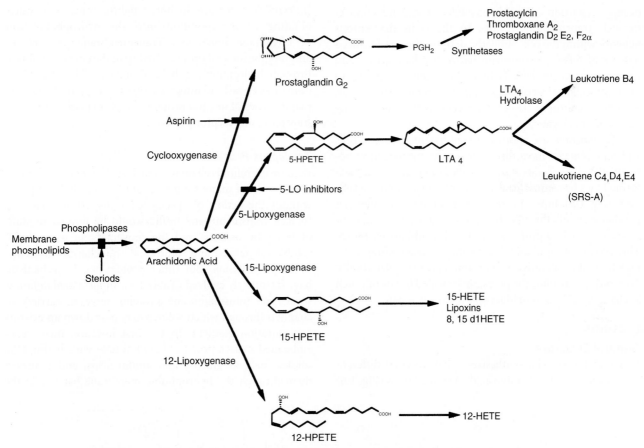

FIGURE 1.4 Arachidonic acid metabolism through the cyclooxygenase and lipoxygenase (*LO*) pathways. Putative sites of action for steroids, aspirin, and 5-LO inhibitors are indicated by *shaded boxes. 15-HETE,* 15-hydroxyeicosatetraenoic acid; *5-HPETE,* 15-hydroperoxyeicosatetraenoic acid; *SRS-A,* slow-reacting substance of anaphylaxis. (From Sigal E. The molecular biology of mammalian arachidonic acid metabolism. *Am J Physiol* 1991;260(4):L13–L28, with permission.)

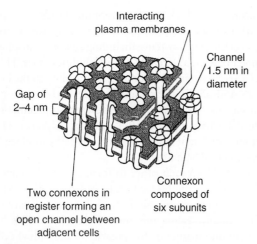

Interacting plasma membranes

Channel 1.5 nm in diameter

Gap of 2–4 nm

Two connexons in register forming an open channel between adjacent cells

Connexon composed of six subunits

FIGURE 1.5   A model of gap junction showing the interacting plasma membranes of two adjacent cells. The apposed lipid bilayers are penetrated by protein assemblies called *connexons*, each of which is formed by six identical protein subunits. Two connexons join across the intercellular gap to form a continuous aqueous channel connecting the two cells. (From Alberts B, Bray D, Lewis J, et al. *Molecular biology of the cell*, 2nd ed. New York: Garland, 1989, with permission.)

occupy a portion of the intercellular space and connect through transmembrane links to the actin filamentous network within the cell. Similarly, desmosomes are localized patches of linker glycoprotein that rivet cells together and then anchor them by attachment proteins connected to their intracellular intermediate filaments. Hemidesmosomes, present in epithelial tissues, rivet cells to their underlying basement membrane.

Gap junctions are another area of fixation between cells and represent the most direct form of communication between them. Specialized pores, called *connexons*, are each formed by a hexagonal arrangement of transmembrane subunits (Fig. 1.5). Ions and small water-soluble molecules can pass between cells through these pores, whereas larger macromolecules, such as proteins and nucleic acids, are excluded. This avenue of rapid and direct solute transfer allows for a high level of cooperative activity among closely related cells. To avoid catastrophe, the pores can be sealed by stimuli such as changing pH, as individual cells approach death.

Proteins

General Structure

A typical human cell synthesizes 3,000 to 6,000 different proteins from only 20 amino acids. Peptide bonds (Fig. 1.6)

link individual amino acids by joining the α-carboxyl group of one to the α-amino group of the other. The resulting polypeptide chain has an amino and a carboxyl terminus along with specific side chains. Protein structure exists at four levels. The *primary structure* is its amino acid sequence, which is genetically determined (Fig. 1.7). The three-dimensional arrangement of amino acids in a specific segment of the protein is its *secondary structure*. Examples of secondary structures are the α-helix and the β-pleated sheet. *Tertiary structure* refers to the complex folding pattern of the overall protein. Lastly, multiple fully folded protein subunits sometimes associate together to form *quaternary structure*. These various structures occur as the result of rapid self-assembly, that is, the form that is finally taken is determined by both the amino acid sequence and the surrounding environment. The three-dimensional structure gives proteins their unique functions and their ability to interact with the diverse range of molecules to which they are exposed.

Most functions specific to the membrane depend on proteins being arranged between adjacent lipids, the "fluid mosaic" pattern (Fig. 1.8). Some proteins (*peripheral proteins*) in this mosaic are attached superficially by loose bonds and can be removed easily. Other proteins (*integral proteins*) are anchored tightly either by covalent bonding or incorporation into the hydrophobic core of membrane lipids (3). Transmembrane proteins are amphiphilic integral proteins that span the entire membrane through hydrophobic α-helix domains. The extracellular domains of nearly all integral proteins are glycosylated. Two major classes of integral proteins are particularly important: transport and receptor proteins.

Transport Proteins

Because the bilipid cell membrane is such an effective barrier, the transfer of many solutes would be drastically impeded without the action of specialized transport mechanisms. In fact, transmembrane traffic would be limited to shifts of water by osmosis and the movement of gases, lipid-soluble substances, and some small, noncharged molecules by *simple diffusion*. But other protein-based mechanisms have fortunately evolved (Table 1.1). In *facilitated diffusion*, specialized transmembrane proteins serve as carriers or channels through which solutes may pass down an existing concentration gradient. In the first instance, membrane-embedded carrier proteins (CPs) couple with hydrophilic solutes, such as glucose and amino acids, and transport them through the hydrophobic membrane barrier. In the

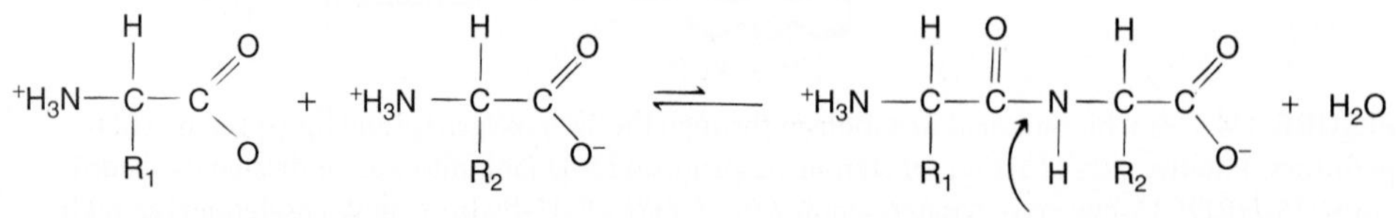

FIGURE 1.6   Formation of a peptide bond. (From Stryer L. *Molecular design of life*. New York: W.H. Freeman and Company, 1988:22, with permission.)

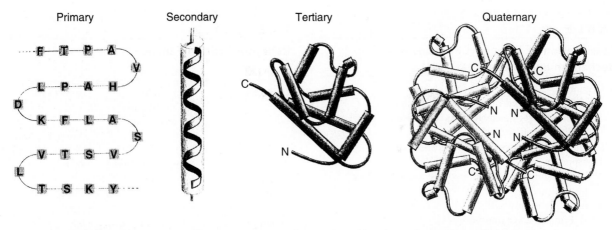

FIGURE 1.7 The levels of protein structure. The amino acid sequence of a protein is called its *primary structure*. Different regions of the sequence form local regular secondary structure, such as an α-helix or a β-pleated sheet. The tertiary structure is formed by packing such structural elements into compact globular domains. The final protein may contain several polypeptide chains arranged in a quaternary structure. Because of tertiary and quaternary structure, amino acids far apart in the sequence can be brought close together in three dimensions to form a functional region, or an active site. (From Branden C, Tooze J. *Introduction to protein structure.* New York: Garland, 1991, with permission.)

second, integral membrane proteins form gated, ion-specific (e.g., Na^+, K^+, and Ca^{2+}) aqueous channels that can open in response to either voltage shifts or neurotransmitter signaling (Fig. 1.9). This allows very rapid ion flow (approximately 10^6/sec) to occur down an existing concentration gradient. Finally, specialized protein pumps provide energy-dependent *active transport* for selected ions (e.g., Ca^{2+}, Na^+/K^+, and H^+) by working against existing concentration gradients.

Receptors and Cell Signaling

Multicellular organisms have evolved an elaborate system of cell–cell communication. Much of this communication depends on proteins. The extracellular information that cells process is provided in the form of humoral or contact-mediated signals (see "Extracellular Structure and Function"). These signals (ligands) bind to specific transmembrane receptor proteins, and this is then transduced

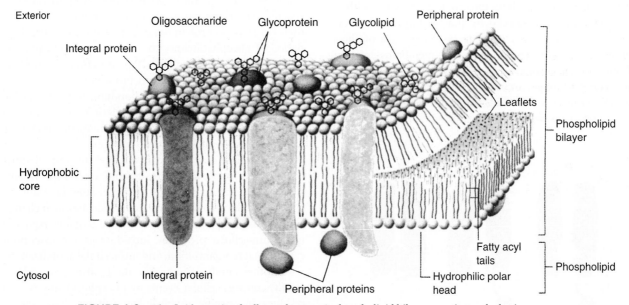

FIGURE 1.8 The fluid mosaic of cell membranes. A phospholipid bilayer constitutes the basic structure, in which the hydrophobic fatty acyl tails form the middle of the bilayer, and the polar hydrophilic head groups line both surfaces. Integral proteins have one or more regions embedded in the lipid bilayer. Peripheral proteins are associated primarily with the membrane by specific protein–protein interaction. Oligosaccharides bind mainly to membrane proteins; however, some bind to lipids, forming glycolipids. (From Darnell JE, Lodish H, Baltimore D. *Molecular cell biology.* Scientific American Books Inc, 1990, with permission of W.H. Freeman and Company.)

TABLE 1.1

Classification of Transport Proteins Based on Mechanism and Energetics

1. Channels
   A. Voltage-regulated channels (e.g., Na^+ channel)
   B. Chemically regulated channels (e.g., nicotine acetylcholine receptor)
   C. Other (unregulated, pressure-sensitive, etc.)
2. Transporters
   A. Passive uniporters (e.g., erythrocyte glucose transporter)
   B. Active transporters
      1. Primary active transporters
         a. Redox coupled (e.g., cytochrome *c* oxidase)
         b. Lig ht coupled (e.g., bacteriorhodopsin)
         c. ATPases (e.g., Na/K-ATPase)
      2. Secondary active transporters
         a. Symporters (e.g., Na^+/glucose symporter)
         b. Antiporters (e.g., cardiac Na^+/Ca^{2+} antitransporter)

Adapted from Gennis RB. *Biomembranes, structure and function.* New York: Springer-Verlag, 1989, with permission.

TABLE 1.2

Receptor Protein Families

Receptor	Morphology	Ligands
G protein	Sevenfold membrane-spanning	Epinephrine
		Norepinephrine
		Peptide Hormones
Protein tyrosine kinase	Single membrane-spanning	EGF
		PDGF
		Insulin
Integrin	Two membrane-spanning subunits	Fibronectin
		Vitronectin
		Fibrinogen
Neurotransmitter spanning	Fourfold membrane-spanning	*n*-Acetylcholine
		GABA

EGF, epidermal growth factor; GABA, γ-aminobutyric acid; *n*-acetylcholine, nicotinic acetylcholine; PDGF, platelet-derived growth factor.

into a cytoplasmic signal that initiates a second messenger cascade within the cell. Therefore, receptor proteins are able to discriminate between various stimuli and send greatly amplified signals to the interior of the cell.

Large families of receptor proteins have been characterized (Table 1.2). The largest of these, the *G protein–linked family,* is a member of the guanosine triphosphatase (GTPase) superfamily, a ubiquitous molecular switch with on and off positions triggered by the binding and hydrolysis of guanosine 5′-triphosphate (GTP) (4). All of the G protein–coupled receptors have seven membrane-spanning domains (Fig. 1.10). Ligands (most peptide hormones, catecholamines, many drugs, and protooncogenes) bind to specific receptors, which are coupled to the heterotrimeric G proteins, causing them to interact with GTP. This results

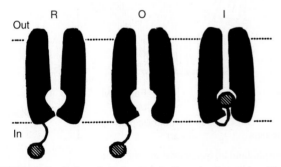

FIGURE 1.9 Ball-and-chain model of inactivation gating. Three gating states of the channel exist: resting (*R*), open (*O*), and inactivated (*I*). The receptor for the inactivation ball becomes exposed on opening of the channel. (From Miller C. 1990: annus mirabilis of potassium channels. *Science* 1991;252:1092. Copyright © 1991 by AAAS. Reprinted with permission.)

in the activation of second messengers or the opening of ion channels. In one such second messenger system, membrane-bound adenyl cyclase is activated, leading to the generation of cyclic adenosine monophosphate (cAMP), which, together with calcium, controls the activity of various protein kinases. These enzymes, in turn, catalyze the phosphorylation of specific cytoplasmic proteins, thereby inducing changes in their behavior. G protein binding may also cause the degradation of phosphatidylinositol, a membrane phospholipid, to inositol-l,4,5-triphosphate (IP_3) and DAG. Cytosolic IP_3 promotes calcium release from intracellular stores, allowing the formation of calcium–calmodulin complexes, which stimulate further protein phosphorylation. DAG stimulates protein kinase C activation, which modulates membrane function and activates gene transcription.

G proteins may also be coupled to ion channels, which open to allow entry of cations once their receptor is activated. In this way, for example, submembrane and cytoplasmic levels of calcium rapidly increase; such changes, along with phosphorylation, are instrumental in regulating most intracellular processes, including gene transcription, cytoskeletal reorganization, and intracellular mobilization.

Another family of receptors, the *protein tyrosine kinase family,* controls cellular events by phosphorylating tyrosine residues in specific intracellular proteins. This induces a conformational change sufficient to initiate a specific intracellular response (Fig. 1.11) (5). This receptor family, most of which is composed of single membrane-spanning polypeptides, includes growth factors such as epidermal growth factor (EGF), platelet-derived growth factor (PDGF) and transforming growth factor-α (TGF-α). The insulin

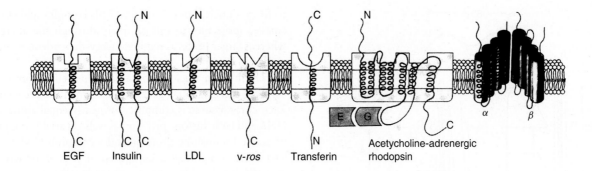

FIGURE 1.10   Topology of receptor structures in the membrane. *E*, effector protein; *G*, G protein; *C*, C-terminus; *N*, N-terminus; *EGF*, epidermal growth factor; *LDL*, low-density lipoprotein. (From Hesch RD. Classification of receptors. *Curr Top Pathol* 1991;83:13–51, with permission of Springer-Verlag.)

receptor is also a member of this family but has a unique dimeric configuration.

A third type of cell membrane receptor is the *nicotinic acetylcholine receptor* (nAchR), which is a neurotransmitter-gated ionic channel. It is structurally unrelated to the muscarinic acetylcholine (Ach) receptors, which belong to the G protein superfamily, but acts together with them to regulate the activity of the peripheral cells innervated by the autonomic nervous system and the cholinergic neurons

of the central nervous system. The nAchR is composed of four different polypeptide chains located around a single ion channel (Fig. 1.12). Ach binds to the receptor, mediating transmission of nerve impulses to muscle at the motor end plate. This receptor family also includes the γ-aminobutyric acid (GABA) and glycine receptor–gated channels.

Finally, the *integrin receptor family* is essential both for the adhesion of cells to extracellular matrix (ECM) proteins and for cell–cell adhesion (6). This provides the cell with

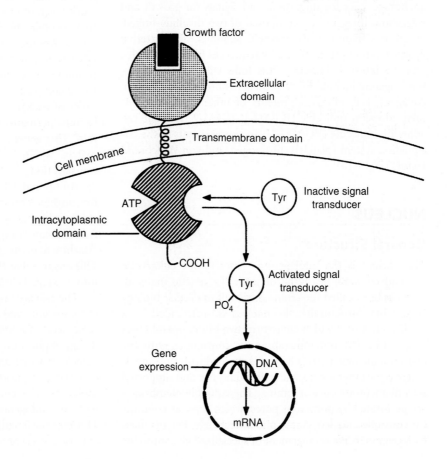

FIGURE 1.11   The protein tyrosine kinase receptor and its molecular cascades. *Tyr*, tyrosine; *ATP*, adenosine triphosphate; *mRNA*, messenger RNA. (From Arbeit J. Molecules, cancer and the surgeon. *Ann Surg* 1990;212:3–13, with permission.)

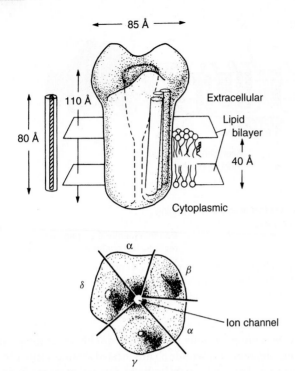

FIGURE 1.12 Schematic representation of the nicotinic acetylcholine receptor, composed of two α units and separate β, γ, and δ units around a central ion channel. (From Williams RC. *Molecular biology in clinical medicine.* New York: Copyright ©1991 by Elsevier Science Publishing Co Inc, 1991, with permission.)

anchorage, cues for migration, and signals for growth and migration. Integrins are composed of two disulfide-linked, membrane-spanning glycoprotein subunits. The external ligand-binding site is formed by sequences from both units, and the internal domain forms links with the cytoskeleton. Ligands include ECM proteins (fibronectin, laminin, collagen), cell adhesion proteins of other cells [intracellular adhesion molecule (ICAM)-1, ICAM-2, vascular cell adhesion molecule (VCAM)-1], and components of the coagulation system (platelets, fibrinogen, and von Willebrand factor) (Fig. 1.13).

NUCLEUS

General Structure

The nucleus is the information center of the eukaryotic cell and contains nearly all of the cell's genetic material. This has been called the *central dogma* of molecular biology (Fig. 1.14). Structurally, the nucleus is surrounded by a nuclear envelope, which consists of two bilipid membranes (Fig. 1.15). The outer membrane is continuous with the endoplasmic reticulum (ER) and is studded with ribosomes, whereas the inner membrane is ribosome-free and supported by a filamentous nuclear lamina. These double membranes are perforated by numerous pores, which serve as conduits for controlled nucleocytoplasmic interchange. Each is filled by a grommet-like arrangement of specialized glycoproteins

to form a nuclear pore complex. This complex allows some smaller molecules to diffuse freely through the apertures, whereas larger proteins require energy-dependent, receptor-mediated transport.

The human nucleus contains 23 paired chromosomes carrying at least 30,000 genes, which constitute the genome. Each chromosome is composed of nearly equal amounts of DNA and basic histone proteins, as well as variable quantities of acidic nonhistone proteins and small amounts of RNA. The DNA component is composed of two, extremely long deoxyribonucleotide polymers coiled together into a double helix (Fig. 1.16). The basic repeating unit of each polymer is a deoxyribose sugar with a phosphate attached at one end and a nitrogenous base attached to the other (Fig. 1.17). These units are linked by phosphodiester bridges between the 5′-hydroxyl of one sugar and the 5′-hydroxyl of the next sugar to form a polar backbone. Two nucleotide chains so formed are held together by hydrogen bonds between either adenine (A) and thymine (T), or guanine (G) and cytosine (C). As a consequence, the base sequence on one chain exactly specifies the sequence of bases on the other.

Each human chromosome, if extended, would measure approximately 40 mm in length. Because all 46 chromosomes need to function within a nucleus that measures approximately 0.006 mm in diameter, the DNA must be densely packed (7). The hierarchy of organization begins with coils of DNA, called *nucleosomes.* (Fig. 1.18). Each nucleosome is formed by the wrapping of approximately 200 base pairs of DNA twice around an octameric core composed of two copies each of four histones: H2A, H2B, H3, and H4. These basic proteins bind tightly with the more acidic DNA segments. Another histone, H1, is associated directly with the DNA as it enters and exits the nucleosome, and appears to promote the coiling of six or more nucleosomes to form larger complexes, called *solenoids.* Finally, in an even higher order of packaging, many chromatin loops of varying sizes become permanently attached to a proteinaceous axial scaffold. This genetic material is further attached to a nuclear matrix, which maintains it in position for replication or transcription.

Additional DNA sequence elements are also required for normal chromosomal function. The *centromere* is a specialized area of constriction present in all chromosomes. A *kinetochore* complex assembles at this site and mediates the attachment of the chromosome to the spindle during mitosis. This ensures that the chromosome is divided longitudinally into two equal chromatids.

The *telomere* is a specialized DNA cap at the end of all chromosomes and consists of simple repeats of nongenomic sequences. Telomeres prevent chromosomal shortening during replication. As outlined in the subsequent text (see "DNA Structure and Synthesis"), DNA polymerases cannot completely replicate the 3′ end of a double-stranded DNA molecule. The enzyme *telomerase*, a reverse transcriptase with an endogenous RNA template, solves this problem. This enzyme lengthens or maintains the length of telomeres with each cycle of replication by adding simple repeats to the

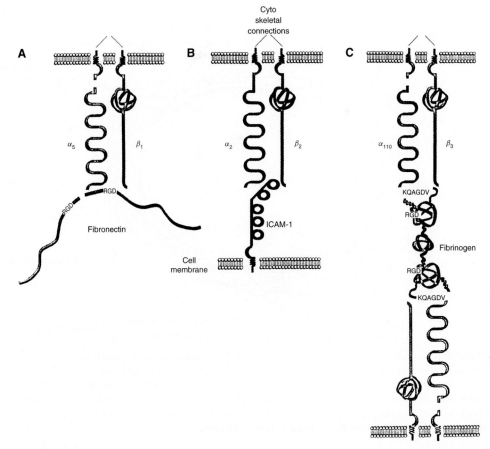

FIGURE 1.13   Integrin structure and interactions depicting three binding modes of various integrins. (From Ruoslahti E. Integrins. *J Clin Invest* 1991;87:1–5, with permission of the American Society for Clinical Investigation.)

3′ end of the DNA using its endogenous RNA as a template (Fig. 1.19). Most somatic human cells lack telomerase, and their telomeres shorten with each cell cycle. This leads to planned death of the cells after a defined number of cell cycles. Many cancer cells, on the other hand, express telomerase. Therefore, they can overcome planned cell death and continue to divide indefinitely.

Chromosomal separation at the time of mitosis is facilitated by the depolymerization of nuclear lamina, condensation of chromatin, and breakdown of the nuclear envelope. These events are associated with phosphorylation of nuclear laminar proteins and histone H1. The structural features of chromosomes are most easily studied during mitosis when they are condensed. At that time, they can be

stained to yield banding patterns that permit karyotyping (Fig. 1.20).

DNA Replication

DNA Structure and Synthesis

DNA is the chemical basis for inheritance. The double helix structure of DNA allows it to be duplicated by the unwinding and use of each chain as a template for copying by complementary base pairing (Fig. 1.21). This results in *semiconservative replication,* in which each new DNA molecule is composed of one old (conserved) and one new strand of DNA. *DNA polymerases* catalyze the polymerization of deoxynucleoside triphosphates into DNA. There are several DNA polymerases, which were

FIGURE 1.14   Established informational relations between DNA, RNA, and protein. (From Singer M, Berg P. *Genes and genomes.* Mill Valley, CA: University Science Books, 1991:36, with permission.)

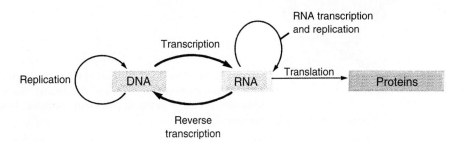

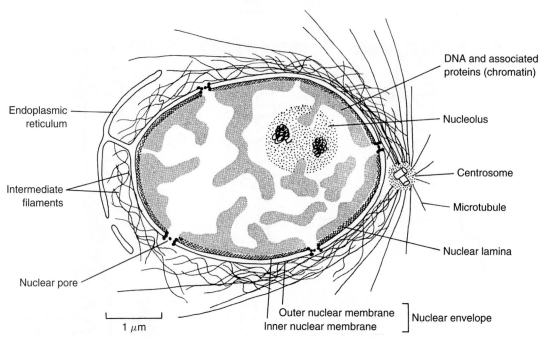

Endoplasmic reticulum

Intermediate filaments

Nuclear pore

DNA and associated proteins (chromatin)

Nucleolus

Centrosome

Microtubule

Nuclear lamina

Outer nuclear membrane
Inner nuclear membrane } Nuclear envelope

1 μm

FIGURE 1.15 Cross-section of a typical cell nucleus. The nuclear envelope consists of two membranes; the outer one is continuous with the endoplasmic reticulum membrane. The lipid bilayers of the inner and outer nuclear membranes are fused at the nuclear pores. Two networks of ropelike intermediate filaments (*wavy lines*) provide mechanical support for the nuclear envelope; the filaments inside the nucleus form a sheetlike nuclear lamina. (From Alberts B, Bray D, Lewis J, et al. *Molecular biology of the cell,* 2nd ed. New York: Garland, 1989, with permission.)

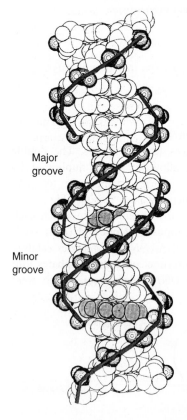

Major groove

Minor groove

Normal DNA

FIGURE 1.16 Space-filling model of the normal right-handed Watson-Crick DNA. Normal DNA has two grooves (one major and one minor). (From Darnell JE, Lodish H, Baltimore D. *Molecular cell biology.* Scientific American Books Inc, 1990, with permission of W.H. Freeman and Company.)

Bases

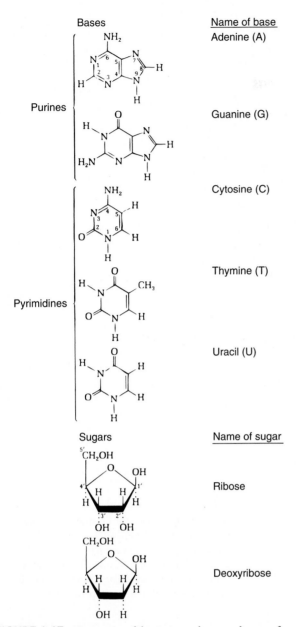

Name of base

Adenine (A)

Purines

Guanine (G)

Cytosine (C)

Pyrimidines

Thymine (T)

Uracil (U)

Sugars

Name of sugar

Ribose

Deoxyribose

FIGURE 1.17 Structures of the common bases and sugars found in nucleic acids. (From Kleinsmith LJ, Kish VM. *Principles of cell biology.* New York: Harper & Row, 1988, with permission of HarperCollins Publishers.)

numbered in order of their discovery rather than in order of their importance. DNA polymerase III catalyzes DNA elongation by nucleotide linkage, whereas gap-filling and repair functions are accomplished by DNA polymerase I. DNA polymerase has other functions. A proofreading function is provided by a 3′ to 5′ exonuclease activity, whereas a 5′ to 3′ exonuclease activity links Okazaki fragments and repairs DNA. These editing functions are part of an elaborate system that is critical for maintaining DNA integrity (8).

The molecular mechanisms of DNA replication are complex, requiring several additional proteins (Fig. 1.22). These include *helicase,* involved in the unwinding step; *primase,* which catalyzes the formation of RNA primers

used to initiate DNA synthesis; and *ligase,* which joins DNA fragments generated by degradation of the RNA primers. Furthermore, because the DNA polymerase can only function in a 5′ to 3′ direction, one strand of DNA is copied by discontinuous synthesis of small DNA fragments (Okazaki fragments) initiated by RNA primers, which are later removed and replaced by DNA (Fig. 1.21).

Cell Cycle

The eukaryotic cell cycle has four phases: G_1, S, G_2, and M (Fig. 1.23). *Interphase*, the time between *mitoses*, is divided into G_1, S, and G_2 phases. During G_1, or first gap, messenger RNA (mRNA) and protein are formed in preparation for *S phase*, during which DNA is synthesized. After S phase, another short gap, called G_2, precedes *mitosis* or the *M phase* in which the nucleus and cell divide. Under certain conditions, cells will go into a resting phase, or G_0, and will reenter the cycle later when conditions are more favorable.

Mitosis is divided into four major stages (Fig. 1.24): *prophase, metaphase, anaphase,* and *telophase.* In *prophase,* the chromatin fibers condense into separate, discrete chromosomes. A pair of *chromatids,* or the individual parts of the chromosomes, are joined by a *centromere.* Upon condensation of the chromosomes, transcription of the DNA slows down and stops. Nucleoli disperse, and the mitotic spindle begins to assemble. Cytoplasmic microtubule-containing structures, called *centrioles,* migrate to opposite sides of the nucleus. Prophase ends as the nuclear envelope breaks down.

In *metaphase,* the nuclear envelope is gone. Spindle microtubules attach to the centromeres of the chromosomes, and the chromosomes migrate toward the equator of the spindle, where they line up adjacent to one another. Centromeres of each chromosome are attached to two sets of microtubules, one from each pole of the centriole-associated spindle. During metaphase, chromosomes can be easily examined microscopically, and karyotypes can be generated based on chromosome size, shape, and staining patterns.

During *anaphase,* the two chromatids separate from each other to generate two independent chromosomes. Each of the newly formed chromosomes migrates to opposite poles of the spindle. When the chromatids attach to the spindle microtubules, their specialized structures known as *kinetochores* attach to the centromere at opposite sides. Therefore, the kinetochore attachment ensures that the chromosomes are sent to opposite poles of the spindle during anaphase.

When the chromosomes arrive at opposite poles of the spindle, this is the start of *telophase.* During this step, the chromosomes unfold and disperse into typical interphase chromatin fibers. The nuclear envelope and nucleoli reappear, and this is followed by *cytokinesis,* or division of the cytoplasm.

Controls

Many proteins are involved in the control of the cell cycle (Table 1.3). Chromosome condensation and folding involves

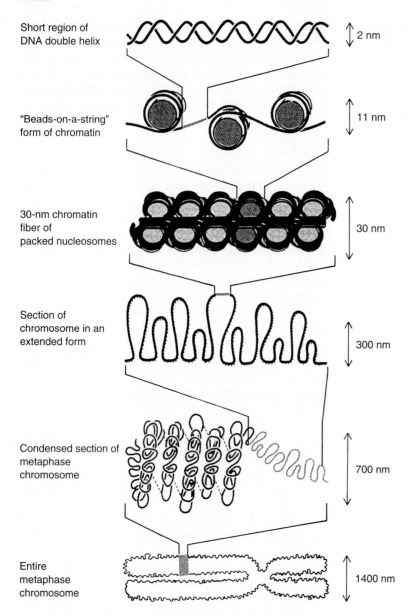

Short region of
DNA double helix

2 nm

"Beads-on-a-string"
form of chromatin

11 nm

30-nm chromatin
fiber of
packed nucleosomes

30 nm

Section of
chromosome in an
extended form

300 nm

Condensed section of
metaphase
chromosome

700 nm

Entire
metaphase
chromosome

1400 nm

FIGURE 1.18 Schematic illustration of some of the many orders of chromatin packing that have been postulated to give rise to the highly condensed metaphase chromosome. (From Alberts B, Bray D, Lewis J, et al. *Molecular biology of the cell,* 2nd ed. New York: Garland, 1989, with permission.)

protein phosphorylation through specific proteins such as maturation-promoting factor (MPF). Cyclins and cyclin-dependent kinases (CDKs) play critical roles in cell cycle regulation. Therefore, complexes between the regulatory cyclin subunits and the catalytic CDK subunits regulate the passage of cells through the cell cycle. In fact, different cyclin/CDK complexes are important in different parts of the cell cycle. (Fig. 1.25). Cyclins are also involved in cell differentiation and embryogenesis.

Cell proliferation is regulated by many factors, including protooncogenes and growth factors (9). Protooncogenes (also called c-*onc*s, referring to the cellular "oncogenes") are normal cell growth and regulatory genes that correspond to a variety of aberrant oncogenes isolated from tumor-causing viruses or cancer cells. Viral oncogenes are called v-*onc*s. Protooncogene-encoded proteins include growth factors, growth factor receptors, GTP-binding proteins, protein kinases, and nuclear proteins (Table 1.4). Changes in cellular

protooncogene sequences or expression can contribute to altered growth control. For example, the protein products of two protooncogenes, *fos* and *jun*, are members of the AP-1 transcription factor family that play a critical role in cell cycle control. Because of this, transcription of *c-jun* and *c-fos* are normally highly regulated (10). However, in cancer cells, mutant forms of *jun* and *fos* may be abnormally regulated, resulting in abnormal cell cycle control, DNA synthesis, and cell proliferation.

Other important molecules in human cancer also play a critical role in the cell cycle. Rb protein is the gene product of the *RB* tumor suppressor gene. Unphosphorylated Rb binds to and inactivates an important set of transcription factors, called *E2Fs*, and this prevents progression through the cell cycle in late G_1. In normal cells, Rb can be phosphorylated by specific cyclin/CDK complexes, resulting in the controlled release of inhibition of E2Fs so that cells can progress into S phase. However, loss-of-function mutations in *RB* result in

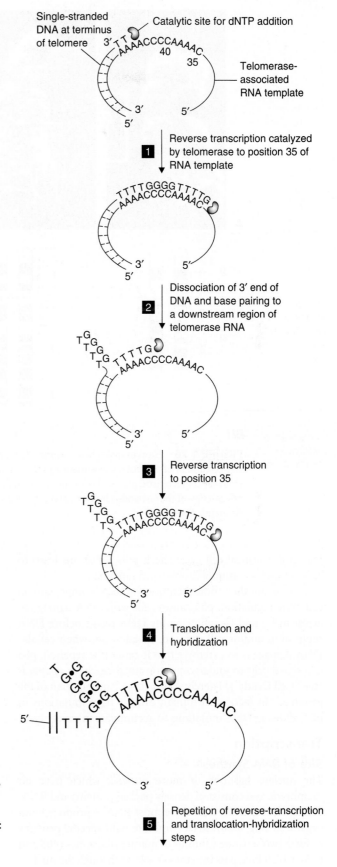

FIGURE 1.19 Mechanism of action of telomerase. The single-stranded 3′ terminus of a telomere is extended by telomerase, counteracting the inability of the DNA replication mechanism to synthesize the extreme terminus of linear DNA. (From Lodish H, Berk A, Matsudaira P, et al. *Molecular cell biology,* 5th ed. New York: W.H. Freeman and Company, 2004, with permission.)

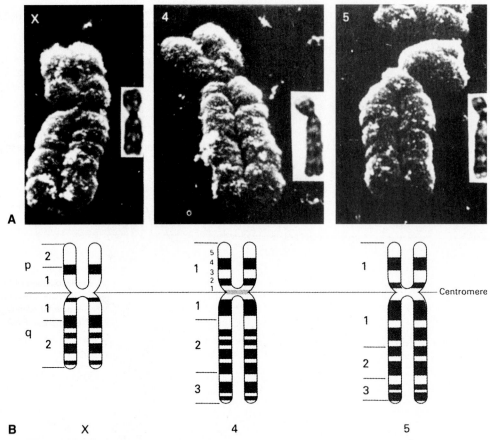

FIGURE 1.20   Human male chromosomes X, 4, and 5 after G-banding. The chromosomes were subjected to brief proteolytic treatment and then stained with Giemsa reagent, producing distinctive bands at characteristic places. (From Harrison CJ, Britch M, Allen TD, et al. Scanning electron microscopy of the G-banded human karyotype. *Exp Cell Res* 1981;134:141–153, with permission of Academic Press.)

loss of this critical cell cycle check point, and this leads to cancers such as retinoblastomas and sarcomas.

p53 is another tumor suppressor that is important in cell cycle regulation. p53 causes cells with DNA damage to arrest in G_1 and G_2, allowing for DNA repair before DNA replication and/or cell division. In addition, when cellular DNA damage is so extensive that it cannot be repaired, p53 can signal cells to undergo programmed death, or *apoptosis* (see "Cell Death"). Thereby, p53 acts as "the guardian of the genome." In fact, most human cancers have mutations in p53, allowing DNA mutations to accumulate in cancer cells.

Transcription

Site of RNA Synthesis

The nucleus has one or more *nucleoli*, which have no membrane and consist of densely packed proteins and RNA. The nucleolus is the site where most RNA is produced and organized (Fig. 1.26). RNA combines with specific proteins to form two separate subunits of mature ribosomes (40S and 60S), which then pass into the cytoplasm through the nuclear pores.

The process of RNA synthesis, or *transcription*, generally resembles DNA synthesis, with two major differences: (i) the base uracil (U) is substituted in RNA for thymine (T) such that U pairs with A, and (ii) transcription is asymmetric because the polymerase selectively copies only one of the two DNA strands; the choice of strands depends on the gene. There are three major types of RNA: ribosomal RNA (rRNA), transfer RNA (tRNA), and mRNA. Each plays an important role in synthesis of cellular proteins, but only mRNA contains the base sequence that codes for the amino acids of the newly synthesized protein. It obtains this through RNA polymerase, which catalyzes the polymerization of ribonucleoside triphosphates into RNA, using DNA as the template.

Eukaryotic mRNA synthesis is more complicated than in prokaryotes because larger precursor molecules called *heterogeneous nuclear RNAs* (hnRNAs) are shortened into mRNA by a process called *splicing* (Fig. 1.27). This is necessary because the protein-coding sequences of RNA (exons) are separated by intervening, noncoding sequences (introns). Splicing is performed by spliceosomes, which contain small nuclear ribonucleoprotein molecules and specialized cellular enzymes that excise introns from hnRNAs to generate mRNAs, which contain only exons.

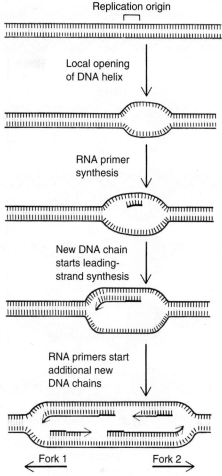

Replication origin

Local opening
of DNA helix

RNA primer
synthesis

New DNA chain
starts leading-
strand synthesis

RNA primers start
additional new
DNA chains

Fork 1   Fork 2

Two complete replication forks are formed,
one moving leftward with leading (top)
and lagging (bottom) strands, and one
moving rightward with leading (bottom)
and lagging (top) strands

FIGURE 1.21   An outline of the processes involved in the initiation of replication forks at replication origins. (From Alberts B, Bray D, Lewis J, et al. *Molecular biology of the cell,* 2nd ed. New York: Garland, 1989, with permission.)

Regulatory Mechanisms

Transcription is highly regulated. The sites on the DNA molecule where the RNA polymerase begins and ends transcription are determined by the base sequence and by the complex tertiary or quaternary structure. Regions of the DNA that precede and follow the protein-coding region are called the upstream and downstream *regulatory regions.* While the details of transcriptional regulation are beyond the scope of this chapter, some general features are important (Table 1.5). A common upstream element in the start-site region for RNA synthesis is the TATA box, so named for its thymine–adenine rich sequences. Other regulatory regions include binding sites for transcription factors, proteins that play key roles in regulating transcription. The complement of transcription factors expressed by a cell ultimately plays a role in determining the specific cell type and its unique properties (11).

Transcription factors can be categorized into three major families based on amino acid homology and protein structure. The *zinc finger* family includes steroid hormones, thyroid hormone, retinoic acid, and vitamin D_3 receptors.

These receptors have a domain that contains zinc atom(s) that bind to multiple amino acids, generating a three-dimensional structure with looped-out "zinc finger" regions, which bind to the major groove of DNA (Fig. 1.28). In the case of steroid receptors, zinc fingers bind to *hormone-responsive elements* (HREs) in DNA. When a hormone binds to this receptor, the receptor–ligand complex is transported to the nucleus and then binds to DNA, thereby activating transcription.

The *helix-turn-helix* family of transcription factors includes the *homeodomain* protein, which is encoded by *homeobox* regions of DNA. It has a 60–amino acid domain that functions as a DNA-binding region and is composed of three α-helices. These proteins play a critical role in development and are expressed temporally in subsets of embryonic cells.

The *leucine zipper* family of transcription factors contains short coils of two parallel α-helices with approximately eight turns per helix. The zipper motif of the protein characteristically occurs as a Y-shaped "scissor-grip" structure within the DNA molecule (Fig. 1.29). Juxtaposed regions of basic amino

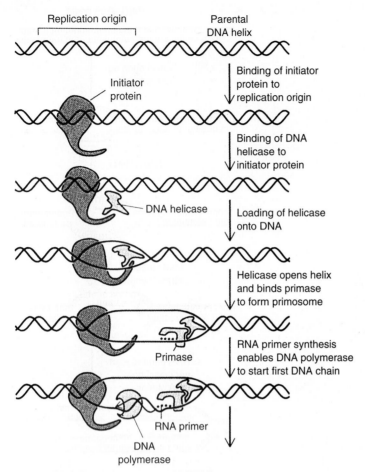

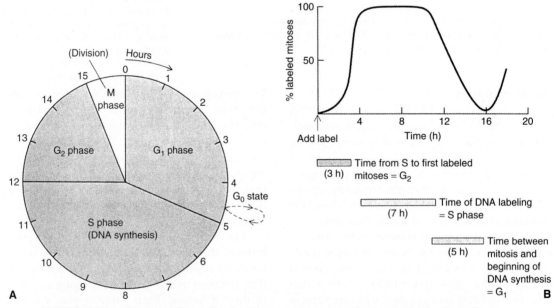

FIGURE 1.22   A simplified outline of the initial steps leading to the formation of replication forks at the *Escherichia coli* and bacteriophage λ replication origins. Discovery of the indicated mechanism required studies *in vitro* that used a mixture of highly purified proteins. Subsequent steps cause the initiation of three more DNA chains by a pathway that is not yet clear. For *E. coli* DNA replication, the initiator protein is the dnaA protein and the primosome is composed of the dnaB (DNA helicase) and dnaG (RNA primase) proteins. (From Alberts B, Bray D, Lewis J, et al. *Molecular biology of the cell*, 2nd ed. New York: Garland, 1989, with permission.)

FIGURE 1.23   The mammalian cell cycle with a generation time of 16 hours. **A:** The three phases spanning the first 15 hours or so—the G_1 (first gap) phase, the S (synthetic) phase, and the G_2 (second gap) phase—make up interphase, during which DNA and other cellular macromolecules are synthesized. The remaining hour is the M (mitotic) phase, during which the cell actually divides. **B:** The phases of the cell cycle were determined by exposing a culture briefly to labeled thymidine, which is incorporated into DNA, and then observing the time of appearance of labeled mitotic cells. (From Darnell JE, Lodish H, and Baltimore D. *Molecular cell biology*. Scientific American Books Inc, 1990, with permission of W.H. Freeman and Company.)

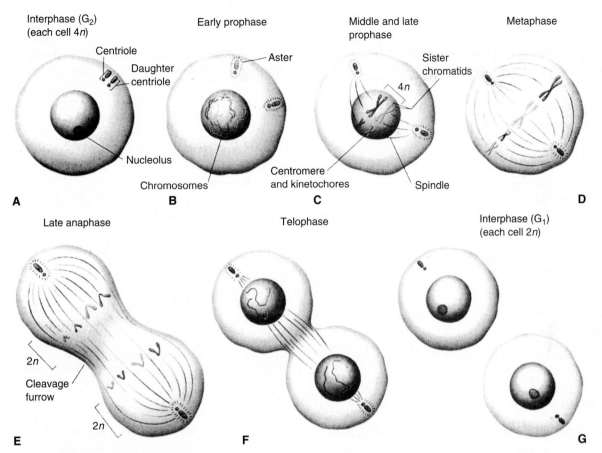

Interphase (G₂)
(each cell 4n)

Early prophase

Middle and late prophase

Metaphase

Centriole

Daughter centriole

Aster

Sister chromatids

4n

Nucleolus

Chromosomes

Centromere and kinetochores

Spindle

A   B   C   D

Late anaphase

Telophase

Interphase (G₁)
(each cell 2n)

2n

Cleavage furrow

2n

E   F   G

FIGURE 1.24   The stages of mitosis and cytokinesis in an animal cell. **A:** Interphase. During the S phase, chromosomal DNA is replicated and bound to protein, but the chromosomes are not seen as distinct structures. The nucleolus is the only nuclear substructure that is visible under the light microscope. **B:** Early prophase. The centrioles begin moving toward opposite poles of the cell; the chromosomes can be seen as long threads. The nuclear membrane begins to disaggregate. **C:** Middle and late prophase. Chromosome condensation is completed; each visible chromosome structure is composed of two chromatids held together at their centromeres. Each chromatid contains one of the two newly replicated daughter DNA molecules. The microtubular spindle begins to radiate from the regions just adjacent to the centrioles, which are moving closer to their poles. Some spindle fibers reach from pole to pole, but most go to chromatids and attach at kinetochores. **D:** Metaphase. The chromosomes move toward the equator of the cell, where they become aligned in the equatorial plane. The sister chromatids have not yet separated. This is the phase in which morphologic studies of chromosomes are usually carried out. **E:** Late anaphase. The two sister chromatids separate into independent chromosomes. Each contains a centromere that is linked by a spindle fiber to the one pole to which it moves. Therefore, one copy of each chromosome is donated to each daughter cell. Simultaneously, the cell and the pole-to-pole spindles elongate. Cytokinesis begins as the cleavage furrow starts to form. **F:** Telophase. New membranes form around the daughter nuclei; the chromosomes uncoil and become less distinct, the nucleolus becomes visible again, and the nuclear membrane forms around each daughter nucleus. Cytokinesis is nearly complete, and the spindle disappears as the microtubules and other fibers depolymerize. Throughout mitosis, the daughter centriole at each pole grows until it is full length. At telophase, the duplication of each of the original centrioles is completed, and a new daughter centriole will be generated during the next interphase. **G:** Interphase. Upon completion of cytokinesis, the cell enters the G₁ phase of the cell cycle and proceeds again through the system. (From Darnell JE, Lodish H, and Baltimore D. *Molecular cell biology.* Scientific American Books Inc, 1990, with permission of W.H. Freeman and Company.)

TABLE 1.3

Functions Proposed for Some of the Known Regulatory Factors Involved in Mitosis

Proposed Function	Factor(s)	Biochemical Mechanism(s)
Promotes mitosis and meiosis	MPF	Ser/Thr protein kinase
Regulatory subunit of MPF	Cyclins	Substrate for kinases
Induces mitotic arrest; stabilizes MPF	CSF	Ser/Thr protein kinase
	Wee-I	Ser/Thr protein kinase
Regulates timing of ser/thr protein kinase	per^{cdc2}	Ser/Thr protein kinase
MPF activation	*mos*	Ser/Thr protein kinase
Catalytic subunit of MPF	Histone H1	DNA-binding protein
Activator of MPF in meiosis	MAP-2	Microtubule-associated protein
In vitro p34^{cdc2} substrate	*src*	Tyrosine protein kinase
In vivo p34^{cdc2} substrate	Lamins	Nuclear matrix structure

cdc, cell-division-cycle gene; CSF, cytostatic factor; MAP, microtubule-associated protein; MPF, maturation-promoting factor.

TABLE 1.4

Some General Classes of Protein Products Encoded by Representative Oncogenes

General Class	Representative Oncogene(s)
Protein kinases	
Tyrosine-specific	*src, yes, fes, abl, neu, fgr*
Tyrosine-specific (EGF receptor fragment)	*erb-B*
Serine–threonine-specific	*raf, mil, mos*
GTP-binding proteins	*ras^H, ras^K, ras^N*
Nuclear binding proteins, affecting	*fos, jun, myc, ski, myb*
DNA replication and transcription	
Growth factors	
PDGF	*sis*
EGF receptor (tyrosine kinase)	*erb-B*
Macrophage colony-stimulatory factor	*fms*
Thyroid hormone receptor	*erb-A*

DNA, deoxyribonucleic acid; EGF, epidermal growth factor; GTP, guanosine 5'-triphosphate; PDGF, platelet-derived growth factor.

can bind, localize, and position DNA sequences so that they are available for transcription of genes for specific cell types or tissues. This control of the three-dimensional DNA conformation confers specificity for transcription factor binding that regulates *cell differentiation*, with the resultant production of unique cell type–specific proteins. Therefore, the nuclear matrix is not simply a structural system but also a functional system that helps organize and coordinate the function of individual cell types.

CYTOPLASM

General Structure and Organelles

The cytoplasm has many components. The soluble fraction, or *cytosol*, consists of approximately 70% water and 20% protein, which produces a viscous gel. In addition, many cells have inclusion bodies to provide storage for metabolic fuels such as glycogen and fat.

The cytoplasm is compartmentalized by membrane-bound organelles, with each type capable of performing its own unique set of functions. One compartment, the *endoplasmic reticulum* (ER), consists of an extensive network of interconnected tube-like structures and flattened cisternae, all formed by a single membrane. The rough ER has attached *ribosomes* (Fig. 1.31). Nucleated cells contain 20,000 to 50,000 ribosomes, the sites of protein synthesis. Those attached to the ER are sites where proteins are synthesized for incorporation into the cell's various membranes or for export outside the cell. Other ribosomes are free in the cytoplasm, where they participate in the synthesis of proteins destined to stay within the cell. The smooth ER,

acids within the protein cause a bipartite DNA-binding domain from each of the basic regions of the dimer. Leucine zipper motifs are found in some eukaryotic transcription factors and nuclear oncogenes (e.g., *jun, fos,* and *myc*) (12).

Gene expression is also regulated by association of DNA with the nuclear matrix (Fig. 1.30). Nuclear matrix proteins

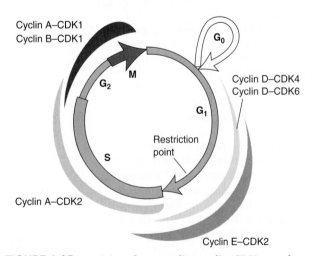

FIGURE 1.25 Activity of mammalian cyclin–CDK complexes through the course of the cell cycle. The width of the bands is proportional to the protein kinase activity of the indicated complexes. (From Lodish H, Berk A, Matsudaira P, et al. *Molecular cell biology*, 5th ed. New York: W.H. Freeman and Company, 2004, with permission.)

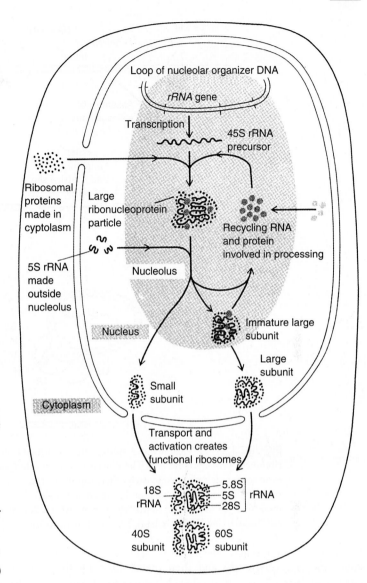

FIGURE 1.26 The function of the nucleolus in ribosome synthesis. The 45S ribosomal RNA (*rRNA*) transcript is packaged in a large ribonucleoprotein particle containing many ribosomal proteins imported from the cytoplasm. Although this particle remains in the nucleolus, selected pieces are discarded as it is processed into immature large and small ribosomal subunits. The two subunits attain their final functional form only as they are transported individually through the nuclear pores into the cytoplasm. (From Alberts B, Bray D, Lewis J, et al. *Molecular biology of the cell*, 2nd ed. New York: Garland, 1989, with permission.)

devoid of ribosomes, serves as the site for many other reactions, including steroid and lipoprotein biosynthesis, xenobiotic detoxification, molecular conjugation, and fatty acid desaturation.

The *Golgi apparatus* is associated closely with, but separate from, the smooth ER. It consists of multiple flat cisternae arranged in stacks and joined by interconnecting tubules. It has three functionally distinct units: the cis, medial, and trans subsections. Newly synthesized lipids and proteins are transported and modified in the Golgi before being released (13).

Lysosomes are membranous, saclike organelles containing a large variety of acidic hydrolases capable of controlled enzymatic degradation of intracellular macromolecules. Lysosomes are important in the autolysis of dead and dying cells and organelles. They also digest the material taken into healthy cells by the process of endocytosis.

Peroxisomes are saccular cytoplasmic organelles which contain a variety of enzymes that can break down smaller molecules such as amino acids, xanthine, and fatty acids,

often producing toxic hydrogen peroxide. Fortunately, this highly reactive molecule is metabolized by the action of catalase, another peroxisomal enzyme, to yield water and oxygen. Peroxisomes may represent primitive, vestigial organelles whose functions have been replaced largely by the mitochondria.

Mitochondria are motile, sausage-shaped organelles with a double membrane enclosing a fluid-filled matrix. Numerous infoldings (cristae) extend from the inner membrane into the central matrix. This results in four specialized compartments with specific functions: the inner and outer membranes, the intermembrane space, and the matrix (Fig. 1.32). Mitochondria produce adenosine 5′-triphosphate (ATP), the universal currency of energy in biologic systems. ATP is generated by the oxidative phosphorylation of energy-rich molecules, such as fats, proteins, and glycogen (Fig. 1.33). When needed, these substrates are transported across the double membrane of the mitochondria as fatty acids and pyruvate (Fig. 1.34). Once in the matrix, both molecules are converted to acetyl

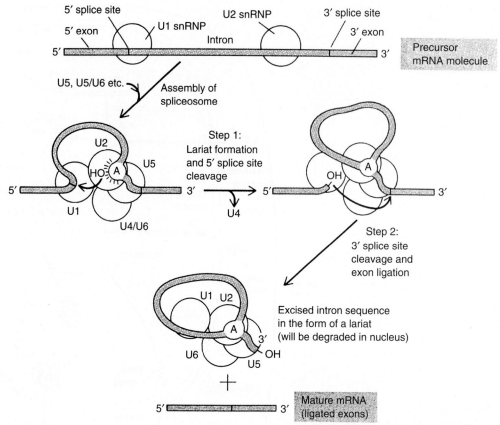

FIGURE 1.27   RNA splicing. A spliceosome is formed from multiple small nuclear ribonucleoproteins (*snRNPs*). The spliceosome then catalyzes splicing in two steps. As a result, the two exon sequences are joined to each other, and the intron sequence is released as a lariat. These splicing reactions occur in the nucleus and generate messenger RNA (*mRNA*) molecules from mRNA precursor molecules. U1 to U6 refer to snRNPs. (From Alberts B, Bray D, Lewis J, et al. *Molecular biology of the cell,* 2nd ed. New York: Garland, 1989, with permission.)

coenzyme A (acetyl-CoA) and then metabolized by the citric acid (Krebs) cycle to produce nicotinamide adenine dinucleotide (NADH) and flavin adenine dinucleotide ($FADH_2$). These are the reducing equivalents that drive oxidative phosphorylation. High-energy electrons from NADH and $FADH_2$ are passed along the electron transport chain, a series of three enzyme complexes embedded in the inner mitochondrial membrane (Fig. 1.35). Protons are pumped out of the matrix at these sites, creating a proton gradient across the inner membrane. Protons can then move passively back into the matrix through the transmembrane protein ATP-synthase, where the energy of their flow is coupled to the synthesis of ATP from adenosine 5'-diphosphate (ADP) and P_i. ATP can then move into the cytoplasm, where its potential energy can be used to perform work. Some of the remaining electrons are transferred to cytochrome *c* oxidase, which catalyzes the reduction of molecular oxygen to two molecules of water.

Mitochondria are probably symbiotic descendants of primitive bacteria. The evidence is compelling: the inner mitochondrial membrane is typical for bacteria. Also, mitochondria have their own genetic material, from 2 to 10 circular DNA molecules per organelle. Only the mother

transmits mitochondrial DNA (mtDNA). Mutations or deletions in mtDNA can cause rare, maternally transmitted diseases, particularly defects of the electron transfer chain and oxidative phosphorylation (14).

Cytoskeleton

The *cytoskeleton* is a complex structural framework composed of three major protein polymers: actin filaments, microtubules, and intermediate filaments. Each polymer is assembled from repeating subunits, which are held together by noncovalent bonds and are modified by regulatory proteins. Cytoskeletal polymers can also interact with at least four families of motor proteins: myosin, kinesin, dynein, and dynamin. These motor proteins produce unidirectional movement along polymers by using ATP or GTP for energy. Together, the structural, accessory, and motor components of the cytoskeleton maintain cellular shape, produce movement inside and outside the cell, and provide anchorage for subcellular organelles.

Actin filaments are linear polymers of globular actin, a contractile protein found in nearly all cells. The three-dimensional structure of filamentous actin is tailored to the functional demands of each specific cell type and

TABLE 1.5

Components of Transcriptional Regulation in Eukaryotes

Factor(s) or Structure(s)	Description
Transcription factors	Site-specific DNA-binding proteins
Zinc fingers	
Helix-turn-helix	
Leucine zippers	
Control module	DNA sequence associated with transcription factor(s); >50 modules are known; therefore large numbers of combinations are possible
Upstream promotor elements	Usually 100–200 base pairs in length and close to site of transcription initiation; includes A–T base pair–rich region known as TATA box
Enhancer elements	Short DNA sequences that enhance transcription; sometimes close to promotor but may be far away(e.g., >20,000 base pairs) or not even in the 5′ region

DNA, deoxyribonucleic acid; TATA, thymine–adenine rich sequences.

is controlled by actin-binding proteins. For example, large actin bundles, or stress fibers, are attached to the adhesion plaques situated immediately adjacent to the plasma membrane. These contacts are then linked with the ECM through integrin-type membrane receptors. Another example is provided by intestinal epithelial cells

(Fig. 1.36). In each brush-border microvillus, tightly aligned bundles of actin extend from the tip of the microvillus to the cell cortex. The specialized binding proteins—villin, fimbrin, and tropomyosin—maintain the microvilli in their most efficient, erect position and provide the structural framework that allows efficient cell function. Another example is that of skeletal and cardiac muscle. Muscle myofibrils have multiple repeating contractile subunits called *sarcomeres*, which are composed of parallel thick myosin filaments alternating with thin actin filaments. Muscle contraction occurs when the thick filaments slide inside of the thin filaments as a result of calcium-dependent molecular interactions between them (Fig. 1.37).

Another component of the cytoskeleton, the *microtubule*, is a cylindrical linear polymer formed by the aggregation of proteins called *tubulins*, which are themselves formed from two different proteins, α- and β-tubulin. Polymerization of tubulins is initiated in the centrosome, which is adjacent to the nucleus and contains two centrioles and γ-tubulin. In most interphase cells, microtubules are oriented along the long axis of the cell between the centrosome and the plasma membrane. Cell division also requires microtubules. During mitosis, centrosomes are replicated, initiating the growth of microtubules that form the mitotic spindle. By attaching to chromosomes at their kinetochores, spindle microtubules precisely segregate the DNA of the dividing cell into two equal parts.

Microtubules also participate in the motility of cilia and flagella. These motile cylinders consist of nine microtubule doublets surrounding two central tubules and enclosed by a membrane. Their characteristic movements occur when adjacent doublets slide longitudinally over one another as a result of conformational changes in the dynein bridges (motors) that link them (Fig. 1.38). In addition, subcellular organelles, such as lysosomes, vesicles, the ER, and the

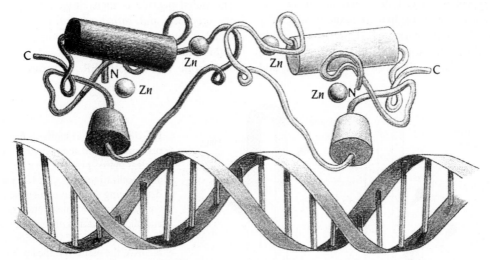

FIGURE 1.28 A hypothetical model of the DNA-binding domain of the glucocorticoid receptor bound to DNA as a dimer. The α-helices of the first zinc finger of each subunit are positioned in successive major grooves on one face of the DNA double helix, whereas the second zinc finger of each subunit is involved in dimer formation. (From Branden C, Tooze J. *Introduction to protein structure.* New York: Garland, 1991, with permission.)

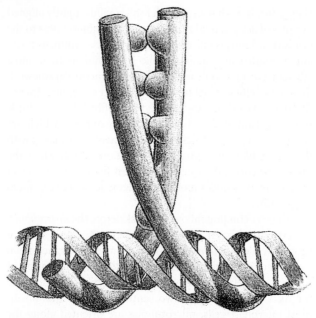

FIGURE 1.29 The scissors-grip model of DNA recognition by the leucine zipper motif. Two DNA-binding domains dimerize through their α-helical leucine zipper region to form a Y-shaped molecule. Each arm of the Y forms a single α-helix that contains the DNA recognition region of the domain and is positioned in the major groove of the DNA molecule. Each of these helices is kinked so that it can follow the path of the major groove. (From Branden C, Tooze J. *Introduction to protein structure.* New York: Garland, 1991, with permission.)

Golgi apparatus, are moved along microtubules by the motor proteins dynein (centrifugal movement) and kinesin (centripetal movement).

The third major component of the cytoskeleton, the *intermediate filament* protein family, is a group of long, ropelike fibrous proteins (Fig. 1.39). There are at least six types of intermediate filaments; five are tissue specific. The cytokeratins type I (acidic) and type II (basic), are found in epithelial cells; vimentin, in mesenchymal tissues; desmin, in muscle; glial fibrillary acidic protein, in glial cells; and

neurofilaments, in neurons. By contrast, the nuclear lamins are present in all cells. As highly organized, dynamic sheets of filaments, they form the nuclear lamina that lines the inside surface of the nuclear envelope. During mitosis, the nuclear envelope and lamina rapidly disassemble and then reassemble.

Proteins—From Translation to Sorting

All proteins are synthesized in the cell cytoplasm where ribosomes serve as the sites for *translation* of mRNA. This is the second stage of the process by which genes encoded in the DNA are synthesized into proteins. Translation is dictated by the *genetic* code in which triplets of mRNA bases, called *codons,* encode a single amino acid (Fig. 1.40). Because there are 4 bases, there are 64 (4^3) different codons, but only 20 amino acids. Three of the codons are stop signals. Because more than one codon may specify the same amino acid (in a pattern in which the first two bases are the same and the third base may vary), the genetic code is referred to as *degenerate.*

The tRNA serves as an adaptor to "read" the mRNA codon and determine which amino acid will be added to the growing protein chain (Fig. 1.41). Each tRNA has a triplet base sequence, an *anticodon,* which is complementary to the mRNA codon and carries a specific amino acid. The tRNA molecules have a three-dimensional "L" shape which ensures that both the bound amino acid and the anticodon loop are accessible for translation.

Newly synthesized proteins are sorted by regulated movement through various intracellular compartments. The ER is the initial assembly point for most membrane or secreted proteins. Protein synthesis actually starts in the cytoplasm on free ribosomes, but is quickly targeted to the ER by a signal peptide at the N-terminus of the new peptide chain. The ribosomal complex docks over a protein-conducting channel, through which the nascent polypeptide chain translocates into the lumen of the ER. The signal peptide is then cleaved, and the new proteins are *processed* and *sorted* according to specific targeting signals contained within them. Some proteins are retained within the ER. Others are enclosed within vesicles that bud from the smooth ER and fuse to the *cis*-Golgi

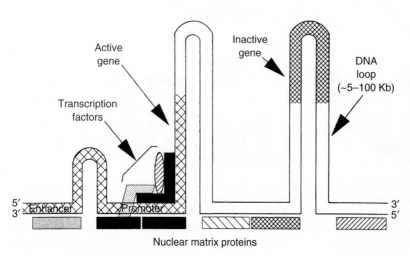

FIGURE 1.30 Hypothesis depicting DNA organization and gene activity. Tissue-specific nuclear matrix proteins are involved in the binding and localization of specific DNA sequences and determining the position of genes in proper configuration for transcription factors to interact and allow activation of gene expression. By controlling the three-dimensional conformation of DNA, the tissue-specific nuclear matrix proteins confer specificity to transcription factor/receptor binding. (From Pienta KJ, Getzenberg RH, Coffey DS. Cell structure and DNA organization. *Crit Rev Eukaryot Gene Expr* 1991;1:355, with permission. Copyright CRC Press Inc., Boca Raton, Florida.)

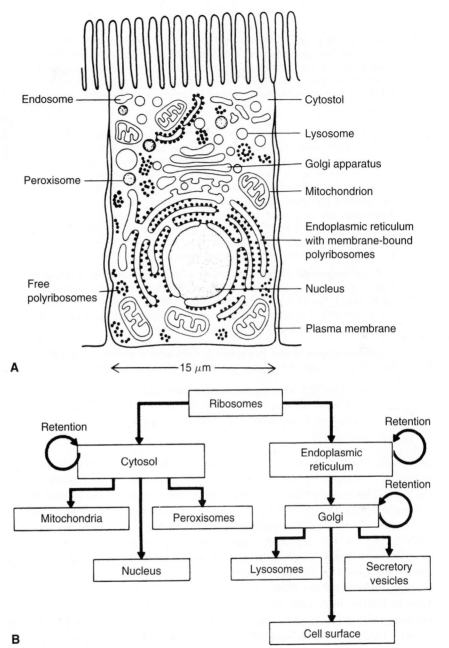

FIGURE 1.31   A: A drawing of an animal cell emphasizing the major intracellular compartments. The cytosol, endoplasmic reticulum, Golgi apparatus, nucleus, mitochondrion, endosome, lysosome, and peroxisome are distinct compartments isolated from the rest of the cell by at least one selectively permeable membrane. **B:** A simplified road map of biosynthetic protein traffic. The signals that direct a given protein's movement through the system, and thereby determine its eventual location in the cell, are contained in its amino acid sequence. The journey begins with the synthesis of a protein on a ribosome and terminates when the final destination is reached. At each intermediate station (*boxes*), a decision is made as to whether to retain the protein or to transport it further. In principle, a signal could be required either for retention or for leaving each of the compartments shown, with the alternative fate being the default pathway (one that requires no signal). (From Alberts B, Bray D, Lewis J, et al. *Molecular biology of the cell,* 2nd ed. New York: Garland, 1989, with permission.)

network. Here posttranslational modification is completed through a series of steps that may include proteolytic cleavage, glycosylation, phosphorylation, and sulfation. The resulting product is released from the *trans*-Golgi after being targeted to its final destination (15). Secretory proteins are either released continuously (constitutive) or stored in granules until an appropriate stimulus is received (regulated). Integral membrane proteins are delivered to specific plasma membrane domains by a transport vesicle that fuses to the inner membrane (Fig. 1.42).

Endocytosis

Cellular traffic is not one-way. Substances on the surface of the cell can be enclosed in membrane-bound vesicles and taken into the cell by the process of *endocytosis*. There

are three types of endocytosis. In *pinocytosis*, solutions are internalized; in *phagocytosis*, particles are ingested. The contents of the early endosomes so formed are generally degraded by fusing with lysosomes, which contain autolytic enzymes. *Receptor-mediated endocytosis* occurs when certain ligands (nutrients, hormones, proteins, and viruses) migrate with their receptor to clathrin-coated pits and are then internalized as coated vesicles. Ligands and receptors commonly dissociate in the endosome, allowing recycling of the receptors to the plasma membrane and routing of the ligands to lysosomes for disposal.

Antigen Processing and Presentation

A specialized form of protein sorting occurs when foreign proteins are processed as antigens by antigen-presenting

Matrix. The matrix contains a highly concentrated mixture of hundreds of enzymes, including those required for the oxidation of pyruvate and fatty acids and for the citric acid cycle. The matrix also contains several identical copies of the mitochondrial DNA genome, special mitochondrial ribosomes, tRNAs, and various enzymes required for expression of the mitochondrial genes.

Inner membrane. The inner membrane is folded into numerous cristae, which greatly increase its total surface area. It contains proteins with three types of functions: (i) those that carry out the oxidation reactions of the respiratory chain, (ii) an enzyme complex called *ATP synthetase* that makes ATP in the matrix, and (iii) specific transport proteins that regulate the passage of metabolites into and out of the matrix. Since an electrochemical gradient that drives the ATP synthetase is established across this membrane by the respiratory chain, it is important that the membrane be impermeable to most small ions.

Outer membrane. Because it contains a large channel-forming protein (called porin), the outer membrane is permeable to all molecules of 10,000 da or less. Other proteins in this membrane include enzymes involved in mitochondrial lipid synthesis and enzymes that convert lipid substrates into forms that are subsequently metabolized in the matrix.

Intermembrane space. This space contains several enzymes that use the ATP passing out of the matrix to phosphorylate other nucleotides.

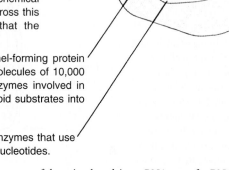

FIGURE 1.32 Structural and functional components of the mitochondrion. *tRNA*, transfer RNA; *ATP*, adenosine triphosphate. (From Alberts B, Bray D, Lewis J, et al. *Molecular biology of the cell,* 2nd ed. New York: Garland, 1989, with permission.)

cells (APCs) such as dendritic cells and macrophages, and presented to another component of the immune system, the T cell (16). In one pathway, a virus or other endogenous antigen is degraded by the action of intracellular proteasomes and transferred to the ER by specialized transport proteins. Once in the ER, the peptide fragments bind to proteins of the class I major histocompatibility complex (MHC). This MHC–peptide complex is carried to the surface of the APC where the MHC molecule "presents" the peptide antigen to T cells, and specific T-cell receptors recognize the MHC–peptide complex. When the T-cell receptor binds to the MHC–peptide complex in the context of other costimulatory molecules on the surface of the APC, this initiates immune response cascades that involve cytokine production and cell stimulation. In a second pathway, exogenous antigens are taken into the cell through endocytosis and are degraded before binding to class II MHC proteins. The resulting MHC–peptide complex is then presented on the cell surface where it can be detected by specific T-cell receptors as described in the preceding text (Fig. 1.43).

EXTRACELLULAR STRUCTURES AND FUNCTION

Extracellular Matrix

Most eukaryotic cells are in contact with a complex scaffolding of insoluble macromolecules collectively termed the *extracellular matrix* (ECM) (Fig. 1.44). The ECM can vary from the basement membrane in epithelial tissues to the ground substance of mesenchymal tissues (17). It not only provides structural support for cells, but also regulates their behavior. Complex tissues may have large amounts of ECM and mesenchymal cells which provide a substrate for attachment and growth of parenchymal cells. An example of this is the epithelium that lines the gut (Fig. 1.45).

The ECM is composed of at least four types of macromolecules: collagens, noncollagenous glycoproteins, proteoglycans, and elastin. The *collagens* are the major constituents of the ECM and are the most abundant proteins in the human body. Collagens are glycoproteins, of which there are at least 15 types. Collagens have unique structural characteristics: they contain triple helical regions, glycine occupies every third amino acid position in the three polypeptide a-chains, and proline and hydroxyproline are frequently present. The fibrillar collagens (Types I, II, III, V, and XI) are mainly found in connective tissue where they are secreted in their inactive procollagen form with long nonhelical extensions at both ends. The terminal propeptides are cleaved, and the collagen molecules self-assemble into fibrils and assume their typical striated appearance, a result of the incomplete overlapping of adjacent molecules (Fig. 1.46). The prototypical Type I collagen is the most common type in mammals. Its architecture is adapted to the needs of the surrounding tissue: a loose weave in skin, a highly oriented aligned structure in tendons, or a tight orthogonal network in bone. Type II collagen is distributed in cartilage and corneal

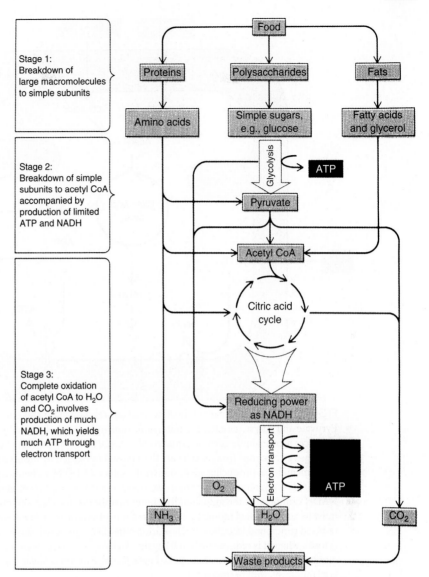

FIGURE 1.33 Simplified diagram of the three stages of catabolism that lead from food to waste products. This series of reactions produces adenosine triphosphate (*ATP*), which is then used to drive biosynthetic reactions and other energy-requiring processes in the cell. *Acetyl-CoA*, acetyl coenzyme A. (From Alberts B, Bray D, Lewis J, et al. *Molecular biology of the cell*, 2nd ed. New York: Garland, 1989, with permission.)

tissue, whereas the nonfibrillar Type IV collagen is present exclusively as a sheetlike mesh in the basement membrane. Many of the remaining types influence tissue properties by combining with Types I and II to form heterotypic fibrils.

The *noncollagenous glycoproteins* are adhesive macromolecules that interact with cells and other ECM components to promote adhesion, migration, proliferation, and gene expression (Fig. 1.47). The best characterized of these, *fibronectin*, is a large dimeric protein which contains separate binding sites for collagen, heparin, fibrin, and specific cell surface receptors. Fibronectin is produced in both a soluble form (serum) and an insoluble form (cellular). Its cell attachment domain contains a specific tripeptide recognition sequence, Arg-Gly-Asp (RGD), which is the sequence recognized by cellular integrin receptors. Fibronectin plays an important role in cell-to-cell attachment, clot stabilization, wound healing, nerve regeneration, and phagocytosis. *Laminin* is a large multidomain glycoprotein that has three polypeptide chains bonded into a cruciform shape. It is located primarily in the basement membrane, where it interacts with many cells (through integrin receptors) and other ECM molecules. It plays an important role in muscle and epithelial differentiation, stimulating neurons to extend new processes, and cancer invasion and metastasis.

Proteoglycans are large molecules composed of a protein core to which are attached side chains of glycosaminoglycans (GAGs). These polysaccharide chains contain repeating disaccharide units in which one of the two residues is an amino sugar. Proteoglycans are classified into major types according to their dominant disaccharide unit: hyaluronate, chondroitin, dermatan, keratan, heparan, and heparin. Because they form bulky hydrated gels, this provides a milieu in which water-soluble molecules can readily diffuse and cells can easily migrate. They also interact with other ECM components to help determine the biomechanical properties of the surrounding tissue, such as the compressibility of cartilage. Their GAG side chains may bind and modulate various growth factors, thereby acting as a reservoir for these and other soluble bioactive molecules.

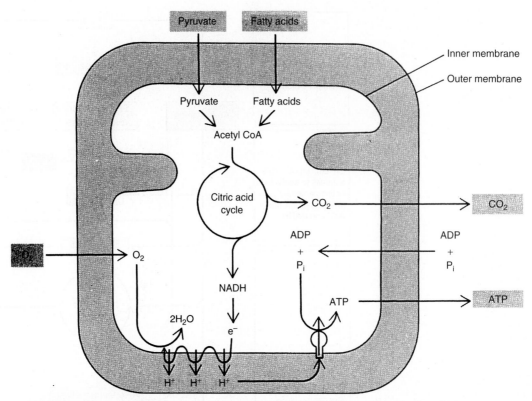

FIGURE 1.34 A summary of the flow of major reactants into and out of the mitochondrion. Pyruvate and fatty acids enter the mitochondrion and are metabolized by the citric acid cycle, which produces nicotinamide adenine dinucleotide (*NADH*). In the process of oxidative phosphorylation, high-energy electrons from NADH are then passed to oxygen by means of the respiratory chain in the inner membrane, producing adenosine triphosphate (*ATP*) by a chemiosmotic mechanism. NADH generated by glycolysis in the cytosol also passes electrons to the respiratory chain (not shown). Because NADH cannot cross the mitochondrial inner membrane, the electron transfer from cytosolic NADH must be accomplished indirectly by means of one of several shuttle systems that transport another reduced compound into the mitochondrion; after being oxidized, this compound is returned to the cytosol, where it is reduced by NADH again. *Acetyl-CoA*, acetyl coenzyme A; *ADP*, adenosine diphosphate. (From Alberts B, Bray D, Lewis J, et al. *Molecular biology of the cell,* 2nd ed. New York: Garland, 1989, with permission.)

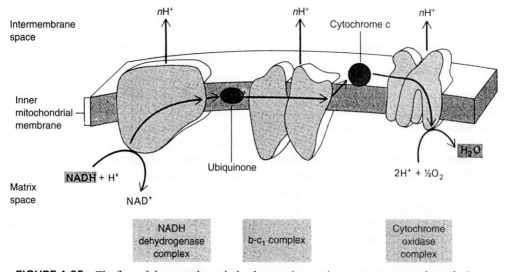

FIGURE 1.35 The flow of electrons through the three major respiratory enzyme complexes during the transfer of two electrons from nicotinamide adenine dinucleotide (*NADH*) to oxygen. Ubiquinone and cytochrome *c* serve as carriers between the complexes. *NAD*, nicotinamide adenine dinucleotide. (From Alberts B, Bray D, Lewis J, et al. *Molecular biology of the cell,* 2nd ed. New York: Garland, 1989, with permission.)

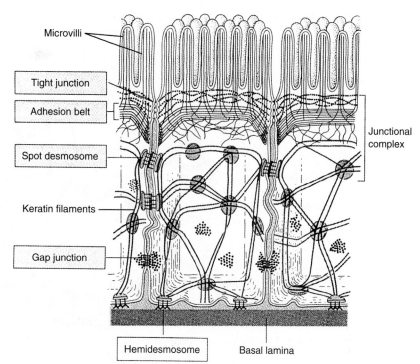

Microvilli

Tight junction

Adhesion belt

Spot desmosome

Keratin filaments

Gap junction

Junctional complex

Hemidesmosome

Basal lamina

FIGURE 1.36 Distribution of the various cell junctions formed by epithelial cells of the small intestine. Bundles of actin microfilaments run down the centers of the microvilli of the intestinal epithelial cell and intersect with a layer of filaments called the *terminal web*. (From Alberts B, Bray D, Lewis J, et al. *Molecular biology of the cell*, 2nd ed. New York: Garland, 1989, with permission.)

FIGURE 1.37 Structure of myocardial cells at the level of light and electron microscopy. **A:** The drawing shows a portion of ventricular myocardium with branching muscle cells enmeshed in collagen. Nuclei are placed centrally, and intercalated discs contain sites for end-to-end attachment of cells. **B:** The drawing shows ultrastructure of portions of two cells in a cutaway view; the arrangement of myofibrils is evident. A network of intermediate filaments, which surrounds the myofibrils like a cage, is periodically anchored to cell membrane plaques at the Z bands and at transverse regions of the intercalated discs. Within the sarcomeres, the contractile units of the muscle, delimited at each end by a Z band, consist of three sets of filaments. Thick filaments primarily containing myosin are located in the A band; thin filaments containing actin, tropomyosin, troponin, and thin elastic filaments of titin extend from each Z band toward the middle of the sarcomere. **C:** The thick and thin filaments interdigitate regularly to form a hexagonal array seen in cross-section. The thin filaments attach periodically along the thick filament. The Z band is a lattice of axial and cross-connecting Z filaments. The ends of the thin filaments from adjacent sarcomeres overlap and interdigitate in a centered tetragonal array and are held together periodically by cross-connecting filaments (four sets are shown here). (From Goldstein MA, Schroetter JP, Michael LH. Role of the Z band in the mechanical properties of the heart. *FASEB J* 1991;5:2167–2174, with permission.)

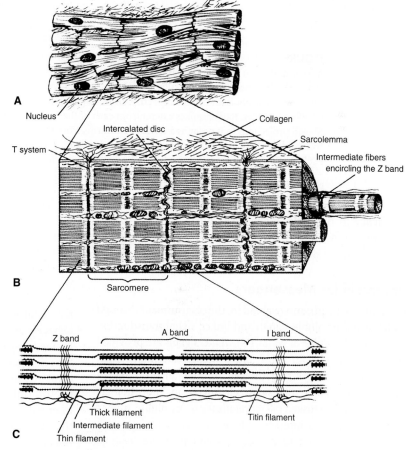

A

Nucleus

Intercalated disc

Collagen

T system

Sarcolemma

Intermediate fibers encircling the Z band

B

Sarcomere

Z band

A band

I band

Thick filament

Intermediate filament

Titin filament

Thin filament

C

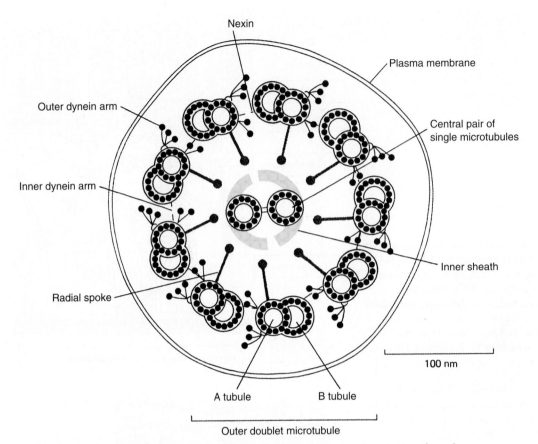

FIGURE 1.38   A cilium shown in cross-section. The various structural projections from the microtubules that occur at regular intervals along the cilium are responsible for ciliary function. Dynein arms, which project from microtubule doublets, interact with adjacent doublets to produce bending upon ATP hydrolysis and removal of cross-links by proteolysis. Nexin links hold adjacent microtubule doublets together. Radial spokes extend from each of the nine outer doublets inward to the central pair. Sheath projections that occur as a series of side arms from the central pair of microtubules regulate the form of the ciliary beat in concert with the radial spokes. (From Alberts B, Bray D, Lewis J, et al. *Molecular biology of the cell,* 2nd ed. New York: Garland, 1989, with permission.)

Elastin is an unfolded hydrophobic protein that provides resiliency to tissue. Its highly cross-linked, random-coiled structure allows it to stretch and relax. It is most prominent in the tissues of skin, blood vessels, and lungs.

Intercellular Messengers

Cells interact with, and respond to, the environment through soluble and insoluble signals and linked signal transduction pathways. *Insoluble* or *contact-mediated signals* are provided by the ECM glycoproteins and proteoglycans that, when linked to the interior of the cell through integrin receptors, can modulate adhesion, cell migration, morphologic changes, and cytoskeletal reorganization. Insoluble matrix proteins may also interact with many local soluble factors to initiate inflammatory responses and promote healing. Cell–cell contact similarly induces extracellular and intracellular changes by the transduction of signals across specific transmembrane receptors. In specialized cells, such as leukocytes, membrane-bound adhesive proteins serve to maintain cell contact and optimize cell–cell interaction.

Soluble signals include cytokines, hormones, neurotransmitters, and other small molecules. These signal molecules bind to cellular receptors, which then activate various intracellular biochemical cascades. They may have only a local effect (paracrine and autocrine) or may act at distant sites to which they are transported by blood (endocrine) (Table 1.6).

Cytokines are nonenzymatic extracellular signaling proteins that generally act locally both to modify cell-specific behavior and to remodel the extracellular architecture. Cytokines may exhibit many different activities depending on the cell types and matrix proteins involved. Specific classes of cytokines include the growth factors, tumor necrosis factors (TNFs), interleukins, and interferons (18). One important example of cytokine function is depicted in the response of the immune system to foreign antigens (Fig. 1.48). Some inflammatory cells and the cytokines they produce are listed in Table 1.7.

Peptide hormones are synthesized by specialized cells in endocrine glands, the central nervous system, and the gastrointestinal tract and either remain in the local environment or are transported in serum to remote sites

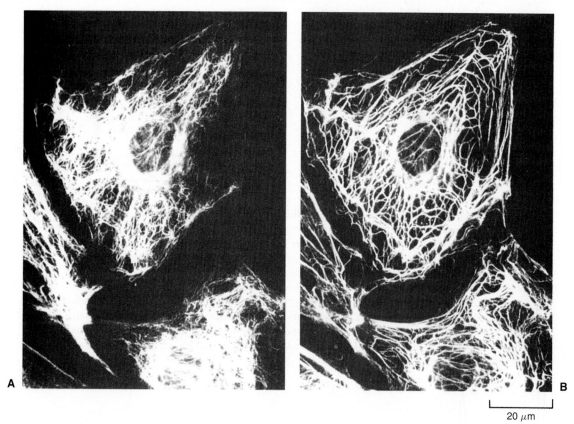

20 μm

FIGURE 1.39   Immunofluorescence micrographs of rat kangaroo epithelial cells (PtK2 cells) in interphase. The cells have been labeled with antibodies to vimentin (**A**) and to keratin (**B**). The cells contain separate arrays of vimentin filaments and keratin filaments, although the two arrays have a similar distribution. (From Alberts B, Bray D, Lewis J, et al. *Molecular biology of the cell,* 2nd ed. New York: Garland, 1989, with permission.)

FIGURE 1.40   The genetic code. Sets of three nucleotides (codons) in a messenger RNA (*mRNA*) molecule are translated into amino acids during protein synthesis according to the rules shown. For example, the codons GUG and GAG are translated into valine and glutamic acid, respectively. Note that those codons with U or C as the second nucleotide tend to specify the more hydrophobic amino acids. (From Alberts B, Bray D, Lewis J, et al. *Molecular biology of the cell,* 2nd ed. New York: Garland, 1989, with permission.)

First position (5′ end)	Second position				Third position (3′ end)
	U	**C**	**A**	**G**	
U	Phe	Ser	Tyr	Cys	U
	Phe	Ser	Tyr	Cys	C
	Leu	Ser	STOP	STOP	A
	Leu	Ser	STOP	Trp	G
C	Leu	Pro	His	Arg	U
	Leu	Pro	His	Arg	C
	Leu	Pro	Gln	Arg	A
	Leu	Pro	Gln	Arg	G
A	Ile	Thr	Asn	Ser	U
	Ile	Thr	Asn	Ser	C
	Ile	Thr	Lys	Arg	A
	Met	Thr	Lys	Arg	G
G	Val	Ala	Asp	Gly	U
	Val	Ala	Asp	Gly	C
	Val	Ala	Glu	Gly	A
	Val	Ala	Glu	Gly	G

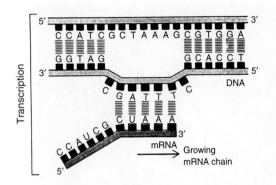

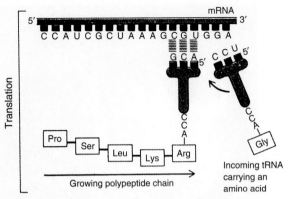

FIGURE 1.41 Information flow in protein synthesis. The nucleotides in a messenger RNA (*mRNA*) molecule are joined together to form a complementary copy of a segment of one strand of DNA. They are then matched three at a time to complementary sets of three nucleotides in the anticodon regions of transfer RNA (*tRNA*) molecules. At the other end of each tRNA molecule, a specific amino acid is held in a high-energy linkage; when matching occurs, this amino acid is added to the end of the growing polypeptide chain. Therefore translation of the mRNA nucleotide sequence into an amino acid sequence depends on complementary base pairing between codons in the mRNA and corresponding tRNA anticodons. In fact, the molecular basis of information transfer in translation is similar to that in DNA replication and transcription. The mRNA is both synthesized and translated starting from its 5' end. (From Alberts B, Bray D, Lewis J, et al. *Molecular biology of the cell,* 2nd ed. New York: Garland, 1989, with permission.)

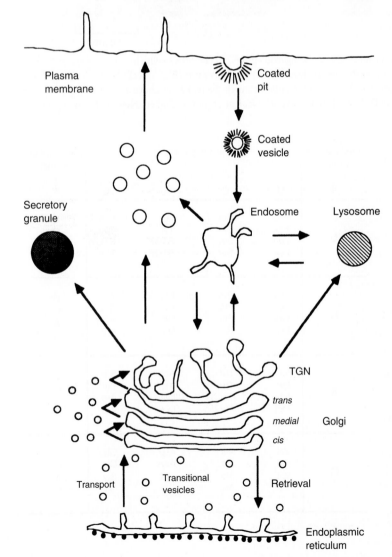

FIGURE 1.42 Sorting and traffic in the central vacuolar system. The organelles within this system include the rough and smooth endoplasmic reticulum; the *cis-*, *medial-*, and *trans*-Golgi; the *trans*-Golgi network (*TGN*), secretory vesicles, secretory granules, the endosomal system, lysosomes, and the plasma membrane. In addition, an unknown variety of transitional and/or transport organelles mediate the communication between these multiple compartments. Each of these organelles possesses characteristic resident membrane proteins that define the unique structure and function of that compartment. (From Klausner RD. Sorting and traffic in the central vacuolar system. *Cell* 1989;57:703, with permission of Cell Press.)

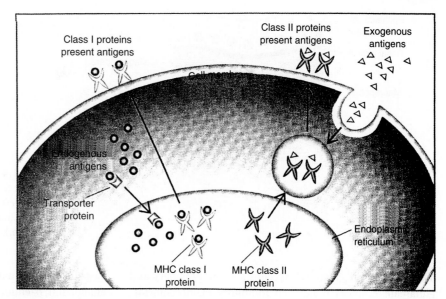

FIGURE 1.43 Pathways for major histocompatibility complex (*MHC*) proteins. MHC proteins, which regulate the immune system, must be linked to antigens to reach the cell surface. The class I proteins, unlike the class II proteins, rely on transporter molecules to bring them antigens. (From Rennie J. *First-class culprit. Sci Am* 1992;266:24. Copyright © 1992 by Scientific American, Inc., with permission.)

where they bind to specific receptors. Many hormones are synthesized initially as inactive precursors and must be modified by proteolytic cleavage and/or chemical binding to become active before being secreted (Fig. 1.49). Negative and positive feedback mechanisms fine-tune the final effects.

Steroid hormones are synthesized from cholesterol and are therefore lipophilic and able to cross cell membranes easily. Together with several other molecular signals such as thyroid hormone, vitamin D_3, and retinoic acid, steroid hormones form complexes with cytoplasmic receptors that

become activated and move into the nucleus to bind to regulatory units on the DNA. This activates the transcription of specific genes, whose products carry out the characteristic effects of these signaling molecules (Fig. 1.50).

Neurotransmitters are released by exocytosis from cells in the nervous system, and bind to one of two different types of receptors. The *channel-linked receptors* abruptly change the conformation of ion channels, allowing specific ions to cross the membrane rapidly and produce a short-lived voltage change in the cell. Excitatory cationic channels

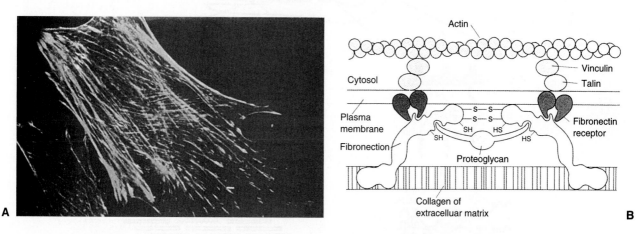

FIGURE 1.44 **A:** Immunofluorescence of a fibroblast showing colocalization of the fibronectin receptor and actin-containing stress fibers. At the ends of the stress fibers, where the cells contact the substratum, there is coincidence of actin and the fibronectin receptor. (From Duband JL, Nuckolls GH, Ishihara A, et al. Fibronectin receptor exhibits high lateral mobility in embryonic locomoting cells but is immobile in focal contacts and fibrillar streaks in stationary cells. *J Cell Biol* 1988;107:1385, with permission of the Rockefeller University Press.) **B:** Model of the connections between actin, fibronectin, and the extracellular matrix at the regions of contact between stationary fibroblasts and the substratum. The two-subunit transmembrane fibronectin receptor binds to fibronectin on its exoplasmic side and talin on its cytoplasmic side. Vinculin binds to talin and probably directly to an actin filament; fibronectin binds to fibrous collagen and to many proteoglycans. (From Darnell JE, Lodish H, Baltimore D. *Molecular cell biology.* Scientific American Books Inc, 1990, with permission of W.H. Freeman and Company.)

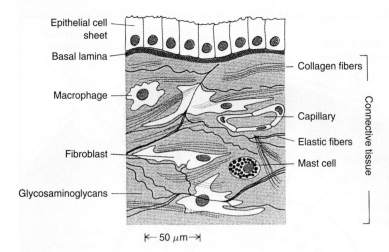

Epithelial cell
sheet

Basal lamina

Macrophage

Fibroblast

Glycosaminoglycans

Collagen fibers

Capillary

Elastic fibers

Mast cell

Connective tissue

|← 50 μm →|

FIGURE 1.45 Cell interactions and cell function. The connective tissue underlying an epithelial cell sheet. (From Alberts B, Bray D, Lewis J, et al. *Molecular biology of the cell,* 2nd ed. New York: Garland, 1989, with permission.)

are primarily linked to Ach receptors in the periphery and glutamate receptors in the brain. Inhibitory, mainly chloride, channels are primarily linked to receptors for GABA and glycine. By contrast, binding of *nonchannel neuroreceptors* activates either G protein or tyrosine kinase pathways, which are slower and more sustained. Included in this group are the monoamines (e.g., epinephrine, norepinephrine, dopamine, serotonin) and certain neuropeptides (e.g.,

vasoactive intestinal peptide, somatostatin, substance P, enkephalin, β-endorphin). Complex interactions of multiple factors are often present, as seen in the regulation of gastric parietal cell secretion (Fig. 1.51).

Nitric oxide (NO) is a critically important small molecule signal. It is synthesized by NO synthase from α-arginine and diffuses from its cell of origin into nearby cells. Once inside the target cell, it binds to the NO receptor, setting off

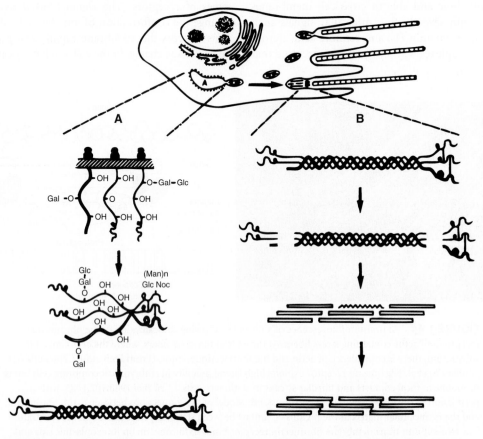

FIGURE 1.46 Fibroblast assembly of collagen fibrils. **A:** Intracellular posttranslational modifications of precursor chains. **B:** Enzymic cleavage of procollagen to collagen, self-assembly of collagen monomers into fibrils, and cross-linking of fibrils. (From Prockop DJ, Kivirikko KI. Heritable diseases of collagen. *N Engl J Med* 1984;311:377, with permission.)

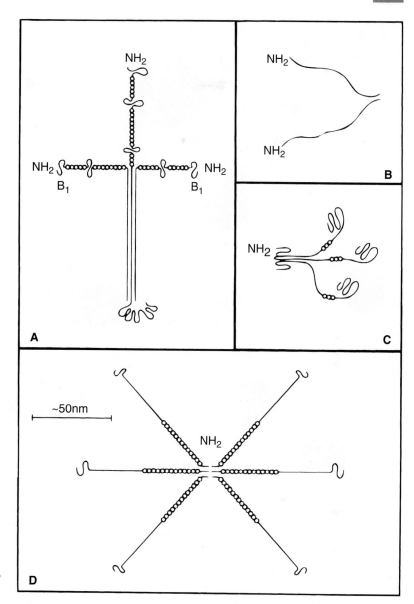

FIGURE 1.47 Schematic drawing of (**A**) laminin, (**B**) fibronectin, (**C**) thrombospondin, and (**D**) tenascin with epidermal growth factor–like domains indicated by circles. The molecules are drawn approximately to scale. (From Engel J. Common structural motifs in proteins of the extracellular matrix. *Curr Opin Cell Biol* 1991;3:782, with permission of Current Science.)

TABLE 1.6

Delivery Pathways of Vertebrate Hormones and Growth Factors

Pathway	Transport of Bioactive Molecules
Endocrine	Hormone-producing cells synthesize and release into circulation
Paracrine	Nonneural cells synthesize factors that are released locally and affect neighboring target cells
Autocrine	Molecules reenter and affect (e.g., stimulation, inhibition) the cells synthesizing the bioactive factors
Neuroendocrine	Neural origin cells synthesize and release molecules into the circulation
Neurocrine	Local release of neurotransmitter or other neural cell molecules into the intercellular space adjacent to a target cell

a cascade mediated by the production of cyclic guanosine monophosphate (cGMP) and the activation of protein kinase G. It is important in processes as diverse as the relaxation of vascular smooth muscle to the induction of irreversible shock in endotoxemia (19).

Matrix Metalloproteinases

The ECM is highly regulated and dynamic. As such, its orderly breakdown is essential to such diverse processes as embryogenesis, organ morphogenesis, wound healing, and tissue resorption and remodeling. ECM degradation is mediated by a family of extracellular zinc–dependent proteinases called *matrix metalloproteinases* (MMPs). More than 20 MMPs have been isolated and characterized. Expression of MMP genes are inducible by a variety of effectors including growth factors, cytokines, physical stresses, and drugs. In turn, MMPs may be downregulated by retinoic acid, glucocorticoids, TGF-β and specific

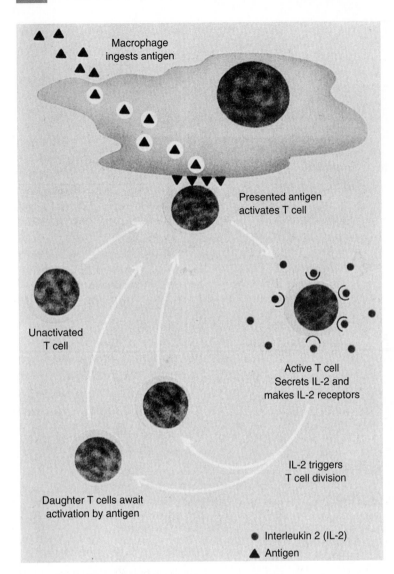

FIGURE 1.48 Proliferation of T cells is controlled by interleukin 2 (*IL-2*) after an antigen, ingested and presented by a macrophage, activates individual T cells. The antigen stimulates the T cells to secrete IL-2 and to make IL-2 receptors. Subsequently, the binding of IL-2 with its receptors signals the T cells to divide, thereby producing pairs of daughter cells that can also be activated by the antigen. In this way, a clone of identical antigen-specific T cells grows until the immune system eliminates the antigen from the body. (From Smith KA. Interleukin-2. *Sci Am* 1990;262:50, with permission.)

TABLE 1.7

Some Inflammatory Cells and Their Important Cytokines

Cell Type	Normal Function	Disease(s)	Cytokines
Basophils	Release of histamine, serotonin	Allergies	IL-8, MIP-1α, MCP-1, MCP-3, RANTES
Eosinophils	Destroying parasites	Asthma	IL-8, MIP-1α, MCP-3, RANTES, eotaxin
Neutrophils	Destroying bacteria	Rheumatoid arthritis, respiratory distress	IL-8, Groα, Groβ, Groγ, ENA-78, others
Monocytes	Phagocytosis of microbes, dead and dying cells	Pneumonia, atherosclerosis	MIP-1α, MIP-1β, MCP-1, MCP-2, MCP-3, others

Table adapted from Gura T. Chemokines take center stage in inflammatory ills. *Science* 1996;272:954–956.

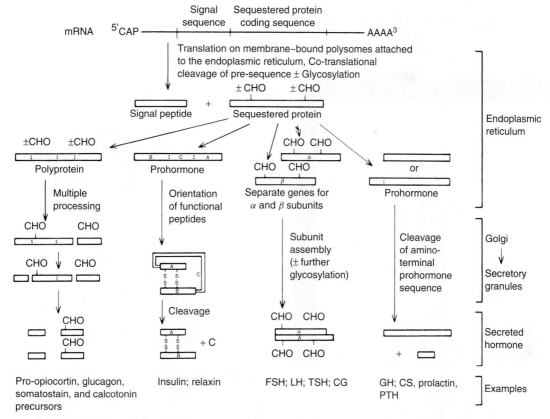

FIGURE 1.49 Several schemes whereby various groups of hormones are assembled from signal and subsequent prohormone products. *mRNA*, messenger RNA; *FSH*, follicle stimulating hormone; *LH*, leutinizing hormone; *TSH*, thyroid stimulating hormone; *CG*, chorionic gonadotropin; *GH*, growth hormone; *CS*, chorionic somatomammotropin; *PTH*, parathyroid hormone. (From Williams RC. *Molecular biology in clinical medicine*. New York: Elsevier Science, 1991, with permission.)

endogenous tissue inhibitors (TIMPs or tissue inhibitors of metalloproteinases).

Recently, MMPs have received more attention because of their putative roles in pathologic processes such as cardiovascular disease, neurologic disease, arthritis, emphysema, and especially cancer (20). MMP genes contain regulatory elements that are highly responsive to oncogenic transcription factors. In addition, evidence suggests that MMPs can promote tumor invasion and metastasis by causing controlled degradation of the basement membrane and other ECM components. Therefore, it is possible that MMP inhibition and/or TIMP stimulation with drugs or other interventions could delay or prevent tumor spread.

CELL DEATH

Cells are not immortal. In multicellular organisms they may die either as the result of an accident (necrosis) or as part of a carefully defined programmed cell death (apoptosis). These two terminal processes are distinct, although areas of overlap can sometimes be observed.

Necrosis represents the cell's response to such injuries as ischemia or irradiation. In this type of death, cells often swell

and burst, releasing their intracellular contents. This results in inflammation and damage to surrounding cells. *Apoptosis*, on the other hand, is a precisely controlled program of cell death. In apoptosis, cells shrink, condense and fragment, forming membrane-bound apoptotic bodies which are typically phagocytosed by surrounding cells. Therefore, cells that die by apoptosis do not release cellular debris, cause inflammation, or damage surrounding cells (Fig. 1.52).

Apoptosis can be activated by at least two different pathways: the extrinsic pathway, and the intrinsic pathway (21). In the extrinsic pathway, ligands (e.g., TNFα, FAS-ligand) bind to "death receptors" (e.g., TNF-R, FAS), which results in the activation of a caspase cascade. Caspases (**C**ysteine **asp**artyl-specific prote**ases**) are intracellular cysteine proteases that cleave proteins after aspartic acid residues. In the intrinsic pathway, the intracellular Bcl-2 family of proteins regulates the release of cytochrome c from the mitochondria. The Bcl-2 family contains pro- and antiapoptotic members. When the relative balance of pro- and antiapoptotic Bcl-2 proteins favors apoptosis, cytochrome c is released from the mitochondria into the cytoplasm where it activates Apaf-1. Active Apaf-1 then activates the caspase cascade.

Whether activated by the extrinsic or intrinsic pathway, the activated caspase cascade sets off a terminal series of events

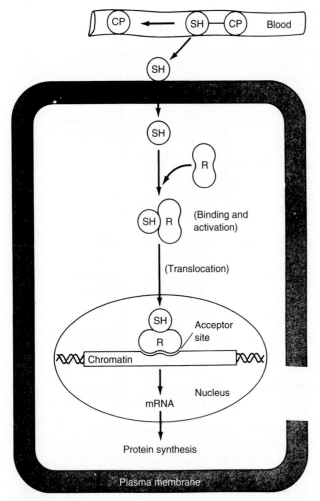

FIGURE 1.50 A general model for the mechanism of action of steroid hormones. The steroid hormone (*SH*) is transported in the blood bound to a carrier protein (*CP*). This complex dissociates and the hormone moves into the cytoplasm, where it binds to a receptor (*R*). This results in activation and translocation of the steroid hormone–receptor complex into the nucleus, where it binds to a specific acceptor site in chromatin, leading to transcription of a specific gene. The resulting messenger RNA (*mRNA*) is translated in the cytoplasm into a polypeptide molecule. This model applies to the action of estradiol as well as to that of other steroid hormones. (From Kleinsmith LJ, Kish VM. *Principles of cell biology.* New York: Harper & Row, 1988, with permission of HarperCollins Publishers.)

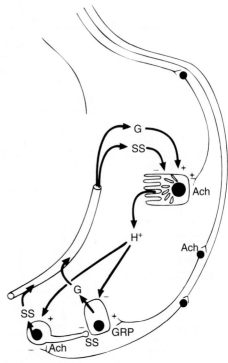

FIGURE 1.51 Regulation of acid secretion is a complex interplay of hormonal, neurocrine, and paracrine influences. Vagal cholinergic stimulation directly causes H$^+$ secretion from the parietal cell and indirectly through release of gastrin from antral G cells. The latter effect is mediated through gastric gastrin-releasing peptide (*GRP*)-containing neurons. The released gastrin acts hormonally to further stimulate acid secretion. Luminal acidification stimulates somatostatin release from d cells. Somatostatin acts in a paracrine manner to inhibit further gastrin release and in both paracrine and endocrine manner to inhibit H$^+$ secretion. *Ach*, acetylcholine; *G*, gastrin; *SS*, somatostatin. (From Debas HT. Neuroendocrine design of the gut. *Am J Surg* 1991;161:246, with permission.)

by cleaving key cellular proteins. Some proteins are activated by caspase cleavage, such as other caspases (further activating the caspase cascade) and protein kinases (further activating downstream death signaling). However, other proteins are destroyed by caspase cleavage, including cytoskeletal and nuclear matrix structural proteins, DNA repair proteins, and inhibitory subunits of endonucleases. The ensuing progression of apoptosis is characterized by a fixed sequence of events that begin when the cell shrinks and loses its external membrane contacts. Cellular budding and fragmentation follow; the resultant apoptotic bodies are then phagocytosed rapidly by macrophages and other neighboring cells.

Apoptosis is a complex process that is still incompletely understood. Obviously, the characterization of genes that are responsible for regulating or modifying cell death promises to have broad applications to such areas as cancer, cardiovascular disease, neurologic disease, developmental biology, and immunology.

APPLICATIONS

Molecular Technology

As with surgery, technical advances in methodology have had a major impact on cellular and molecular research. This new technology has its own nomenclature, as exemplified in Table 1.8. Sophisticated biochemical techniques for nucleic acid purification and analysis include a variety of nucleic acid hybridization methods for which the relatedness of two nucleic acid chains are compared by testing the ability of their bases to form complementary hybrids with one another. Conditions have been defined to generate hydrogen-bonded DNA–DNA, DNA–RNA, or RNA–RNA hybrids.

TABLE 1.8

Glossary of Terms Used in Recombinant DNA Studies

Term	Definition
General terms	
Cleavage maps	Structural maps generated by use of multiple restriction endonucleases to determine arrangements of genomic regions in DNA
Clone	Genetically identical molecule, cell, or organism
DNA probe	DNA labeled radioactively or with chromogen, then hybridized with another nucleic acid to determine sequence relations
Host cell	Cell (prokaryotic or eukaryotic) in which vectors are propagated
Library	Complete set of genomic or cDNA clones from one cell or microbe type; maintained in plasmids or phage
Restriction endonuclease	Enzyme that site-specifically recognizes and cuts in DNA regions with mirror-image sequences (i.e., palindromes of usually four to eight bases)
Vector	Plasmid or virus DNA molecule containing inserted gene or DNA fragment of interest (prokaryotic or eukaryotic)
DNA types	
cDNA	"Complementary" DNA copied from an mRNA molecule
Genomic	Inherited genetic sequence of an organism
Phage	Bacterial virus–derived DNA, commonly used as vector
Plasmid	Extrachromosomal, independently replicating circular DNA molecules
Recombinant	Pieces of DNAs from two or more sources ligated into a single vector
RNA terms	
Cap	Modified bases at 5′ terminus of mRNA
Exon	Regions of RNA that are part of protein-coding sequences
Intron	Regions of RNA removed during splicing
PolyA	Polyadenylated regions at 3′ end of mRNA; important for nuclear transport and mRNA longevity
Reverse transcriptase	Enzyme that copies RNA into cDNA
RNA interference (RNAi)	Inhibition of function of a specific gene by introduction of complementary double-stranded RNA; mediates the degradation of only the specific mRNA encoded by that gene
Splicing	Process by which RNA transcript is cleaved and religated to generate a functional mRNA
Untranslated regions	Regions at the 5′ and 3′ ends of mRNA that do not code for protein but have regulatory functions
Methods	
Blot	Methods used to study macromolecules separated by gel electrophoresis, then transferred onto membrane filters; can be visualized by specific probes and/or staining methods
DNA microarray	A defined set of thousands of different oligonucleotides attached in an array to a solid surface; patterns of gene expression in various cell populations can be simultaneously determined by hybridization of the array with labeled cDNAs from the cell populations
DNA sequencing	Determining the series of bases comprising a sequence
Gel electrophoresis	Biochemical separation of macromolecules based on size and charge
Hybridization	Denaturation of two sources of nucleic acids followed by reassociation and base pairing to assess genetic identity or relatedness
Immunoassays	Immunologic methods in which antibodies are used as tools to measure very low concentrations of biologic agents
Mutagenesis	Induction of mutation; can be random but certain methods can yield site-specific mutagenesis
Northern blot	Transfer and binding of RNAs; allows probing for DNA expression of specific genes
Polymerase chain reaction	Method to enzymatically amplify a specific segment of DNA manymillionfold
Southern blot	Transfer and binding of DNAs; allows probing for presence of specific genes
Western blot	Transfer and binding of proteins; allows comparative protein analyses, augmented with use of protein-specific antibodies to establish identity

cDNA, complementary deoxyribonucleic acid; mRNA, messenger ribonucleic acid.

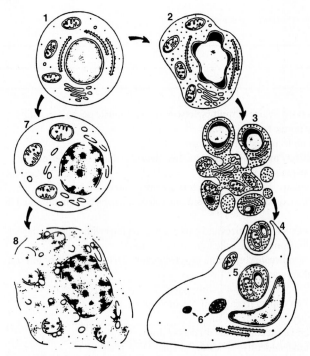

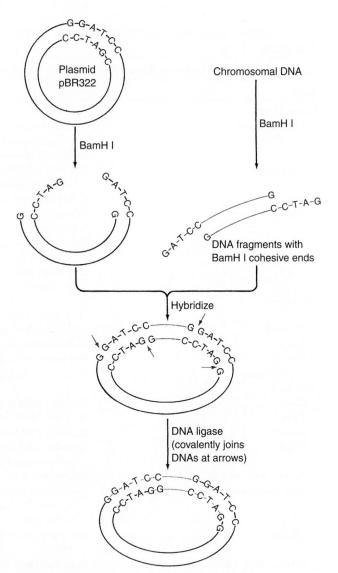

FIGURE 1.52 The sequence of ultrastructural events that take place in apoptosis (*right*) and necrosis (*left*). A normal cell is represented at (*1*). In the early stages of apoptosis (*2*), the chromatin compacts to form sharply delineated masses on the nuclear envelope, the cytoplasm begins to condense, and the nuclear and cellular outlines become mildly convoluted (*3*). Marked convolution of the cell surface occurs with breaking up of the nucleus into discrete, membrane-enclosed fragments, and budding of the cell as a whole to produce membrane-bound apoptotic bodies containing well-preserved organelles. In tissues, these are phagocytosed by adjacent cells (*4*), degraded within lysosomal vacuoles (*5*), and reduced to compact debris within telolysosomes (*6*). There is no inflammation, and unaffected cells close ranks as the apoptotic bodies are phagocytosed. Cell deletion is effected without disruption of overall tissue architecture. The onset of necrosis in irreversibly injured cells (*7*) is characterized by condensation of chromatin, without radical change in its distribution, producing irregular clumps with ill-defined edges. Simultaneously, all cytoplasmic compartments undergo marked swelling, and membranes begin to break down. At a later stage (*8*), the nuclei and organelles disintegrate, but the cells tend to retain their overall configuration until removed by mononuclear phagocytes. (From Kerr JFR. Neglected opportunities in apoptosis research. *Trends Cell Biol* 1995;5:55–57, with permission.)

FIGURE 1.53 The use of restriction enzymes to generate recombinant DNA molecules. This general approach can be used with restriction enzymes that cut the cloning vector in a single location and that also generate suitable fragments of the DNA sample being cloned. (From Kleinsmith LJ, Kish VM. *Principles of cell biology.* New York: Harper & Row, 1988, with permission of HarperCollins Publishers.)

Nucleic acid hybridization, combined with the discovery of restriction-modification endonucleases (*restriction enzymes*), has led to an unprecedented explosion of knowledge on gene organization and expression. Restriction enzymes recognize specific mirror-image, 4- to 8-pair base sequences called *palindromes,* and therefore can be used as "molecular scalpels" to dissect DNA into reproducible sets of fragments according to specific base sequences.

When DNA is cut into fragments by restriction enzymes, these fragments can be used to generate recombinant molecules for structural analyses and other studies (Fig. 1.53).

When locations of enzyme cleavage sites in DNA are compared, a DNA structural map can be created. The exact sequence of each base in the map can also be determined with relative ease by analyzing restriction enzyme-generated fragments using automated DNA sequencing methods. The ability to sequence DNA is an extremely powerful tool, as it also permits predictions of the amino acid sequences of large proteins by using the genetic code and selecting the appropriate reading frame. Because these predictions do not require that the protein be purified, proteins that are difficult to obtain because of a short half-life or limited synthesis can now be easily studied. This information can lead to production of clinically important proteins; examples

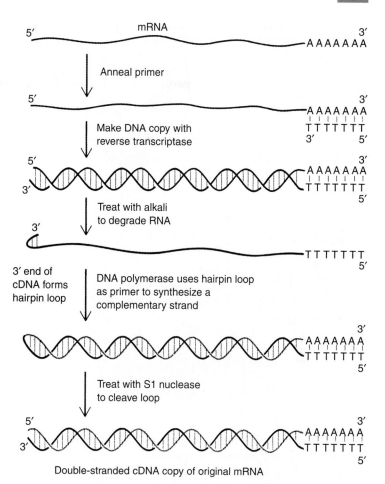

FIGURE 1.54 The synthesis of complementary DNA (*cDNA*). A DNA copy of an messenger RNA (*mRNA*) molecule is produced by the enzyme reverse transcriptase, thereby forming a DNA–RNA hybrid helix. Treating the DNA–RNA hybrid with alkali selectively degrades the RNA strand into nucleotides. The remaining single-stranded cDNA is then copied into double-stranded cDNA by the enzyme DNA polymerase. As indicated, both reverse transcriptase and DNA polymerase require a primer to begin their synthesis. For reverse transcriptase, a small oligonucleotide is used; in this example, oligo(dT) has been annealed with the long poly A tract at the 3′ end of most mRNAs. Note that the double-stranded cDNA molecule produced here lacks cohesive ends. (From Alberts B, Bray D, Lewis J, et al. *Molecular biology of the cell,* 2nd ed. New York: Garland, 1989, with permission.)

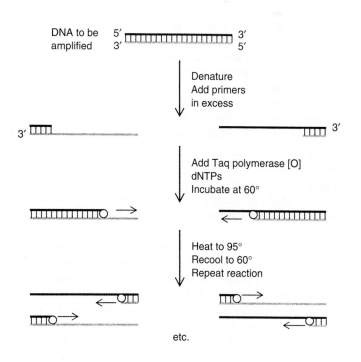

FIGURE 1.55 The polymerase chain reaction. Taq polymerase, a heat-resistant DNA polymerase from *Thermus aquaticus* is used to extend primers between two fixed points on a DNA molecule. All the components for chain elongation (primers, deoxynucleotides, and polymerase) are heat stable. Therefore, multiple heating and cooling cycles cause alternating DNA melting and synthesis. DNA between the two oligonucleotide primers accumulates exponentially. Overnight, it may be amplified as much as a millionfold. *dNTP,* deoxyribonucleotide triphosphate. (From Darnell JE, Lodish H, Baltimore D. *Molecular cell biology.* Scientific American Books Inc, 1990, with permission of W.H. Freeman and Company.)

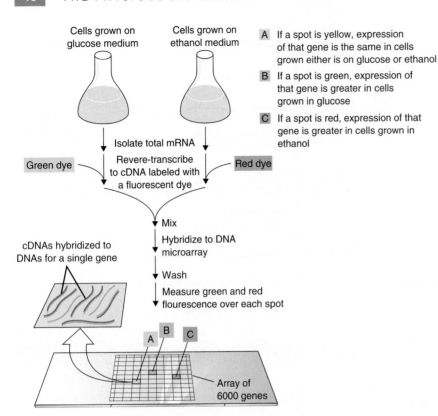

FIGURE 1.56 DNA microarray analysis to determine differences in gene expression. In this example, yeast cells are grown in either glucose or ethanol. Messenger RNA (*mRNA*) is harvested from both cell suspensions, and complementary DNA (*cDNA*) is generated and labeled with a different fluorescent dye, red for the cells grown in ethanol, green for the cells grown in glucose. The cDNAs are mixed and hybridized to a DNA microarray that was created by robotically spotting DNA representing all of the yeast genes onto a glass slide. The ratio of intensities of red and green fluorescence indicates the relative expression of each gene in cells grown in the different media. (From Lodish H, Berk A, Matsudaira P, et al. *Molecular cell biology*, 5th ed. New York: W.H. Freeman and Company, 2004, with permission.)

include vaccine production, immunoassays for diagnostic use, and therapeutic products for injection.

Another important technique is the generation of complementary DNA (cDNA) from mRNA molecules using the enzyme reverse transcriptase (Fig. 1.54). These cDNAs can then be used to prepare genetic *libraries,* which are recombinants between the cDNA molecules and vector DNAs, such as plasmids. Therefore each library will contain the relevant information about mRNAs expressed by specific cells or tissues.

The *polymerase chain reaction* (PCR) technique has revolutionized molecular medicine, and it is responsible for a number of applications, including detection of pathogens, gene cloning, forensics studies, paternity testing, and assessments of genetic mutations or rearrangements (Fig. 1.55). In the PCR technique, unique oligonucleotide primers, which are complementary to flanking regions of opposite DNA strands, are used to amplify a specific DNA segment. The key to this technique is that a heat-resistant DNA polymerase from the bacteria *Thermus aquaticus* (*Taq polymerase*) is used to elongate the DNA between the two flanking primers as the DNA is alternately melted and annealed through multiple heating and cooling cycles. Oligonucleotides are chosen based on the base sequence of the opposite strand flanking regions, each of which must be unique. The power of this procedure is that it can amplify a specific sequence of DNA by millions so that even rare molecular events, limited starting material, and partially degraded DNA can be studied (22).

DNA microarray technology allows the expression of thousands of genes to be measured at the same time. DNA microarrays are created by attaching specific sequences of DNA to a solid surface, and the resulting array is then hybridized with appropriately labeled probes. This concept has many applications. In one such application (Fig 1.56), many thousands of gene sequences approximately 1 kb in size are cloned and amplified using PCR technology. These thousands of genes are then robotically spotted and cross-linked onto a glass slide. Next, the mRNA is separately isolated from experimental and control cells for whom the expression of these genes is to be measured. cDNA is reverse transcribed from the mRNA, and the cDNA from the control cells is labeled with green fluorescent dye while the cDNA from the experimental cells is labeled with red fluorescent dye. The two cDNA solutions are then mixed and hybridized to the microarray matrix containing several thousands of gene spots. Green and red fluorescence is then measured over each of the gene spots using a scanning laser microscope. The relative intensity of green and red fluorescence tells whether the gene represented at each spot is over- or underexpressed in the experimental cells compared with the control cells. Therefore, the expression of many thousands of genes can be measured simultaneously.

The microarray concept of placing biologic materials in compact, defined solid-state arrays can be expanded to many other applications. One application is the determination of signaling pathways by finding transcriptional targets of a given gene product. This is accomplished by comparing the expression profiles of cells that express the gene product with those that do not. Another application is tumor expression profiling, in which expression profiles (a molecular "fingerprint")

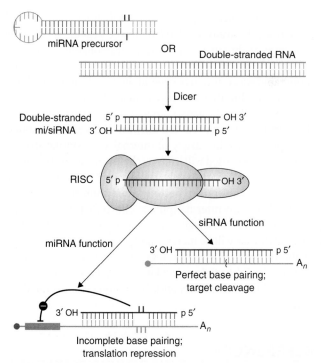

the role of specific mutations in tumorigenesis, and polymorphism analysis. Beyond DNA microarrays, protein microarrays and tissue microarrays offer the next levels of analysis of neoplasia and other disease states (23).

RNA interference (RNAi) is a powerful tool that can be used to silence virtually any gene. RNAi was discovered when control dsRNA was found to powerfully silence genes whose mRNA was complimentary to sequences in the dsRNA. dsRNA is processed to short interfering RNA (siRNA) 21–23 nucleotides in length by a dsRNA-specific endonuclease called *Dicer*. One strand of the siRNA is incorporated into a nuclease complex called *RNA-induced silencing complex* (RISC), which then cleaves the mRNA that is exactly complementary to the siRNA that was incorporated into RISC (Fig 1.57). Thereby, any gene can be silenced by introducing dsRNA that contains the complementary sequence to that gene's mRNA. It is now known that 21–23 nucleotide siRNAs can be incorporated directly into RISC, and also that short hairpin RNAs (shRNA) (which can be introduced through plasmid methods) can be processed by Dicer for incorporation into RISC. Therefore, siRNA or shRNA methods can be used to silence virtually any gene (24).

FIGURE 1.57 Mechanism of RNA interference. Double-stranded RNA is processed by Dicer to form short interfering RNA (*siRNA*). One strand of the siRNA is incorporated into RNA-induced silencing complex (*RISC*), which then degrades the complementary messenger RNA (mRNA). *miRNA*, microRNA. (From Lodish H, Berk A, Matsudaira P, et al. *Molecular cell biology,* 5th ed. New York: W.H. Freeman and Company, 2004, with permission.)

Human Genome Project

A revolutionary step in human cell physiology has been achieved with the sequencing of the entire human genome (25,26). Although the precise number of genes is still undetermined (current estimates range from 26,000 to 120,000), this feat establishes a firm foundation upon which many new tools for diagnostic, therapeutic, and preventive applications will be built. However, knowledge of the DNA structure alone provides an incomplete picture of the human organism. It does not elucidate the quantity, quality, or function of the encoded proteins. Moreover, the expression of proteins can be modified at many points from transcription through posttranslation; most of these steps and their

are obtained from tumors from many different patients. Computer algorithms then determine which of these molecular fingerprints are associated with good or bad patient outcomes. Other applications include the elucidation of the steps in neoplastic progression, determination of

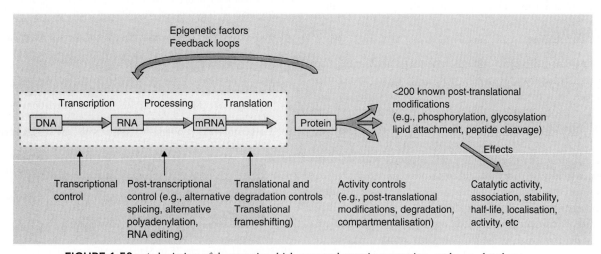

FIGURE 1.58 A depiction of the ways in which gene and protein expression can be regulated or modified from transcription to posttranscription. *mRNA*, messenger RNA. (From Banks RE, Dunn MJ, Hochstrasser DF, et al. Proteomics: new perspectives, new biomedical opportunities. *Lancet* 2000;356:1749–1756, with permission.)

modifiers cannot be determined accurately by a study of nucleic acids alone (Fig. 1.58). Proteomics is an important field that complements genomics by identifying the structure, function, and interactions of the proteins produced by specific genes (27). This information can be used to help define the role of specific proteins in disease processes. Although this approach is likely to be a long-term undertaking, it will almost certainly result in many new and beneficial applications.

Stem Cells

Stem cells, or progenitor cells, are primitive cells with the potential for multilineage differentiation into many cell types. The potential clinical applications for use of these cells are numerous and will influence cell-, gene-, and tissue-based therapeutics. Because many legal and ethical issues surround the use of human stem cells, particularly human embryonic stem cells, care must be taken to assure responsible decision making as it relates to improving the human condition. Early embryonic stem cells have the potential to become any cell type. Other stem cells demonstrate commitment to a specific lineage versus multiple lineages depending on the genetic programming and stage of differentiation of the organism, organ, tissue, or individual cell. The differentiation processes are complex and involve intracellular and extracellular signaling. For example, in the blood system, bone marrow cells may differentiate into the many types of blood cells or into mesenchymal cells (e.g., from smooth muscle, endothelium, cartilage, bone, or fibroblasts.) Depending on the nutritional environment, cytokines, ECM, physical substrate, and other factors, the circulating progenitor cells can repair wounds, heal blood vessels, fight pathogens, and perform many other functions. The complex applications for whole tissue and organ remodeling will become achievable once cell and tissue propagation and differentiation become integrated with bioengineering and surgical skills.

SUMMARY

The proteins within a cell determine its character. The identity of these proteins, as specified by their amino acid sequence, is a direct function of the genetic code. In this way, the code programs the range of properties that can be exhibited by a given cell. Even cell death appears to be encoded by a genetic clock, a phenomenon called *apoptosis*.

Ultimately, the survival of a cell depends on its ability to relate to its environment and to respond appropriately to the stimuli that surround it. The pathways of these responses can be enormously complex and are largely uncharted; they occur in several time frames and at multiple levels of function. Metabolic, muscular, or neurobiologic responses may occur within seconds to minutes, whereas new protein synthesis requires minutes to hours. None of these responses occur in isolation; rather, each is integrated closely with the functions of many other cells, tissues, and organs.

The fundamental processes of cell differentiation and growth are basically controlled by the regulation of gene transcription, but in each instance, numerous environmental cues play a major role. Other functions that require much more rapid execution may depend on cytoplasmic metabolic mechanisms, but they are still modulated by the information contained within the genetic code. Any abnormalities within the genetic code or an inability of the cell to respond appropriately to the variety of internal and external stresses to which it is exposed will lead to cell death, placing the entire organism at risk. Fortunately, these complex and interactive relations will continue to become more comprehensible as a result of the many interdisciplinary efforts that are now under way. Moreover, the diagnosis and treatment of medical and surgical disease will be increasingly predicated on knowledge of the intricacies of cell biology. It is therefore imperative that the disciplines of molecular biology become integrated into our knowledge base, and, by inference, into our daily practice.

REFERENCES

1. Schacter O. Fluidity and function of hepatocyte plasma membranes. *Hepatology* 1984;4:140–151.
2. Sigal E. The molecular biology of mammalian arachidonic acid metabolism. *Am J Physiol* 1991;260:L13–L28.
3. Singer SJ. The structure and insertion of integral proteins in membranes. *Annu Rev Cell Biol* 1990;6:247–296.
4. Uings IJ, Farrow SN. Cell receptors and cell signalling. *J Clin Pathol* 2000;53:295–299.
5. Hunter T. Protein modification: phosphorylation on tyrosine residues. *Curr Opin Cell Biol* 1989;1:1168–1181.
6. Ruoslahti R, Pierschbacher MD. New perspectives in cell adhesion: RGD and integrins. *Science* 1987;283:491–497.
7. Getzenberg RH, Pienta KJ, Ward WS, et al. Nuclear structure and the three-dimensional organization of DNA. *J Cell Biochem* 1991;47:289–299.
8. Radman M, Wagner R. The high fidelity of DNA duplication. *Sci Am* 1988;259:40–46.
9. Freeman RS, Donoghue DJ. Protein kinases and protooncogenes: biochemical regulators of the eukaryotic cell cycle. *Biochemistry* 1991;30:2293–2302.
10. Angel P, Karin M. The role of Jun, Fos and the AP-1 complex in cell-proliferation and transformation. *Biochim Biophys Acta* 1991;1072:129–157.
11. Ptashne M. How eukaryotic transcriptional activators work. *Nature* 1988;334:683–689.
12. McKnight SL. Molecular zippers in gene regulation. *Sci Am* 1991;264:54–64.
13. Featherstone C. Coming to grips with the Golgi. *Science* 1998;282:2172–2174.
14. Harding AE. The other genome. *Br Med J* 1991;303:377–378.
15. Rothman JE, Orci L. Molecular dissection of the secretory pathway. *Nature* 1992;355:409–415.
16. Banchereau J, Steinman RM. Dendritic cells and the control of immunity. *Nature* 1998;392:245–252.
17. Hay ED. Extracellular matrix, cell skeletons, and embryonic development. *Am J Med Genet* 1989;34:14–29.
18. Nagase H, Woessner JF Jr. Matrix metalloproteinases. *J Biol Chem* 1999;274:21491–21494.
19. Curfs JH, Meis JF, Hoogkamp-Korstanje JA. A primer on cytokines: sources, receptors, effects and inducers. *Clin Microbiol Rev* 1997;10:742–780.

20. Snyder SH, Bredt DS. Biological roles of nitric oxide. *Sci Am* 1992;266:68–77.

21. Reed JC. Mechanisms of apoptosis. *Am J Pathol* 2000;157: 1415–1430.

22. Mullis KB. The unusual origin of the polymerase chain reaction. *Sci Am* 1990;262:56–60.

23. Quackenbush J. Microarray analysis and tumor classification. *N Engl J Med* 2006;354:2463–2472.

24. Stevenson M. Therapeutic potential of RNA interference. *N Engl J Med* 2004;351:1772–1777.

25. Venter JC, Adams MD, Myers EW, et al. The sequence of the human genome. *Science* 2001;291:1304–1351.

26. Lander ES, Linton LM, Birren B, et al. Initial sequencing and analysis of the human genome. *Nature* 2001;409:860–921.

27. Pandey A, Mann M. Proteomics to study genes and genomes. *Nature* 2000;405:837–846.

SUGGESTED READINGS

Alberts B, Johnson A, Lewis J, et al. *Molecular biology of the cell*, 4th ed. New York: Garland, 2002.

Branden C, Tooze J. *Introduction to protein structure*, 2nd ed. New York: Garland, 1999.

Gennis RB. *Biomembranes: molecular structure, and function*. New York: Springer-Verlag, 1989.

Hay ED. *Cell biology of extracellular matrix*, 2nd ed. New York: Plenum Publishing, 1991.

Leder P, Clayton DA, Rubenstein E. *Introduction to molecular biology*. New York: Scientific American, 1994.

Lodish H, Berk A, Matsudaira P, et al. *Molecular cell biology*, 5th ed. New York: W.H. Freeman and Company, 2004.

Sambrook J, Russell DW. *Molecular cloning. A laboratory manual*, 3rd ed. Cold Spring Harbor, NY: Cold Spring Harbor Laboratory Press, 2001.

USEFUL LINKS

www.cellsalive.com provides animation, movies, and microscopic images of unicellular life and viruses.

www.cell-biology.com covers cellular topics including components and organelles, communication, division, and common methods used to study cells and issues.

www.mblab.gla.ac.uk/dictionary provides quick access to easily understood and cross-referenced definitions.

www.gwu.edu/~mpb offers graphic representations of all major metabolic pathways, primarily those important to human biochemistry.

CHAPTER 2

Growth and Development

Oluyinka O. Olutoye and Mary L. Brandt

The DNA messages that are brought to an individual and the intrauterine environmental factors that are met by the fertilized egg and developing embryo are critical to the eventual outcome of the pregnancy and the fetus. Although the etiology of human malformations is often difficult to ascertain, it has been estimated that 15% are primarily of genetic origin, 10% result from chromosomal aberrations, 10% are of viral or teratogenic origin, and 65% are of unknown origin (1,2). Only 30% of fertilized eggs result in normal babies (Fig. 2.1) (3). As many as 58% of fertilized eggs fail to implant or are lost before the next menstrual period so that a clinical pregnancy is not established (3,4). Approximately 50% of these losses are caused by chromosomal abnormalities. Pregnancy outcome based on fetal loss and infant death for 92 weeks after conception is shown graphically in Figure 2.2 (5,6). By the 42nd week of gestation, and before birth, there are an estimated 295 deaths per 1,000 conceptions with implantation. Of the 705 live births, approximately 13 infants will have died *in utero* by 92 weeks from conception (6). Most of these deaths are caused by fetal maldevelopment, usually as a result of environmental factors during or after the pregnancy.

Approximately 66% of malformations occur in the first month of gestation, and almost 25% occur during the second month (7). Only an estimated 9% occur after the second month of gestation, emphasizing the critical role early prenatal care can play in a successful outcome. In Figure 2.3, the probable age at which developmental errors arise is shown for 203 different congenital anomalies of concern to the surgeon (1).

GENETICS

An understanding of genetics and embryology provides clinicians a guide to the events in development and those in many disease processes. As our understanding of the genetic events of a human lifetime evolves, it is apparent that this "map" of our existence has a direct bearing on surgical

intervention. Surgery is no longer limited to dissection with the scalpel and scissors but has now entered the realm of molecular "dissection" as well.

To understand the new frontier of molecular surgery, it is important to understand the building blocks of the genome, beginning with DNA. DNA is a polymer composed of a sugar (deoxyribose), nitrogen-containing bases (purines and pyrimidines), and a phosphate. The sequencing of the purine (adenine and guanine) and pyrimidine (thymine and cytosine) bases provides the code for subsequent protein synthesis.

Translation of the DNA code is carried out by messenger RNA (mRNA). Transcription of the DNA into RNA is carried out in the nucleus. The mRNA is then extruded into the cytoplasm where transfer RNA (tRNA) transfers amino acids onto the mRNA template, thereby creating a protein.

DNA sequences that contain codes for proteins (exons) and noncoding sequences (introns) are found in certain locations on the chromosomes called *genes*. In addition to the exons and introns, a gene will also have segments that regulate gene expression, that is, protein synthesis. Each gene is matched with an identical gene on the second chromosome in each chromosome pair. The different gene forms for a specific site are called *alleles*. In each pair of alleles, one is inherited from the mother and one from the father.

There are 46 chromosomes in humans: 22 pairs of autosomes and one pair of sex chromosomes, XX in the female and XY in the male. All of the genetic information required for the maintenance of life and expression of individuality is contained within these chromosomes. Certain disease states are transmitted from the parents with specific patterns of inheritance.

Patterns in Human Genetics
Single-Gene Disorders
Approximately 4,000 disorders in humans have been attributed to single genes. These single-gene disorders follow the classic Mendelian pattern of inheritance (8).

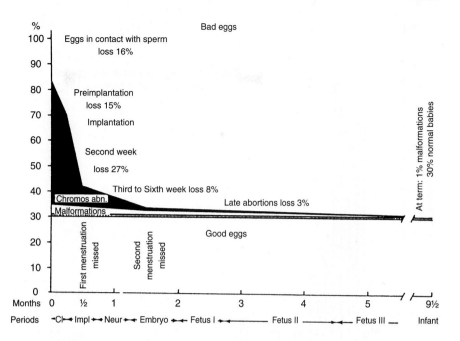

FIGURE 2.1 Graph of postovulatory survival and development in humans. Baselines give age and developmental periods. Under assumed favorable conditions, 30% of eggs develop to normal babies (good eggs); 1% become live born infants with cognitive defects (hatched), of which approximately 1 in 25 have chromosome anomalies; 69% perish (reabsorbed or aborted), and this class (malformations) may be chromosomally normal (white) or anomalous (black). *Cl*, cleavage; *Impl*, implantation; *Neur*, neurula. (From Witschi E. Development and differentiation of the uterus. In: Mark HC, ed. *Prenatal life*. Detroit: Wayne State University Press, 1970.)

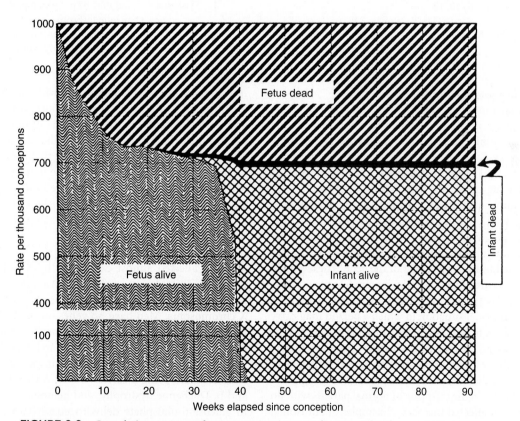

FIGURE 2.2 Cumulative outcome of 1,000 pregnancies according to weeks after conception. By week 44, there will have been 705 live births of which 13 infants have died after having been born alive. The remaining 295 will have died before birth. (From Stickle G. Defective development and reproductive wastage in the United States. *Am J Obstet Gynecol* 1968;100:442–447, with permission.)

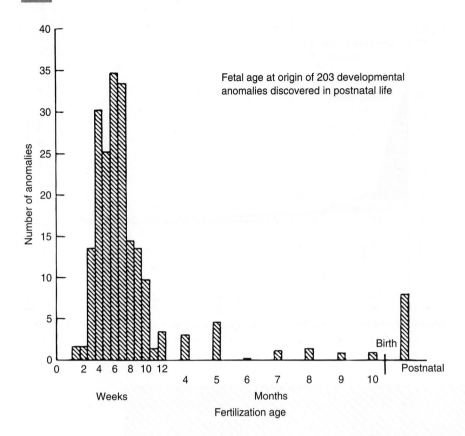

FIGURE 2.3 The probable age at which developmental errors arise to produce 203 of the congenital anomalies discussed in this book. Only anomalies that may be present in postnatal life are included. (From Gray SW, Skandalakis JE. *Embryology for surgeons*. Philadelphia: WB Saunders, 1972, with permission.)

Autosomal Dominant Disorders

An autosomal dominant disorder implies that only one of the two genes in a pair needs to be abnormal for the individual to exhibit characteristics of a disease (9). Because the abnormality is carried on an autosomal chromosome, the sexes are equally affected and the risk of an affected individual having an affected child is one out of two.

Unlike autosomal recessive diseases, a carrier state does not commonly occur in autosomal dominant diseases. That is, a person with the gene for an autosomal dominant disease has the disease, and a person with no evidence of the disease can be assumed not to be a carrier of the gene. These simple Mendelian rules are complicated by incomplete penetrance, variable expressivity, and mutation. Incomplete penetrance describes the unusual situation in which a person may carry the gene but show no signs of the disease and yet can pass the gene and disease to the offspring. Variable expressivity refers to the variability of manifestations among individuals with the same genetic disorder. A mutation describes the appearance of the disease in the offspring of normal parents with no family history of affected members. Examples of autosomal dominant disorders include Ehlers-Danlos syndrome, osteogenesis imperfecta, Marfan syndrome, neurofibromatosis, and achondroplasia (10).

Autosomal Recessive Disorders

Autosomal recessive disorders are manifested only when both genes are abnormal. Men and women are equally affected. Unlike autosomal dominant disorders, which show vertical transmission (affected parent to affected child), autosomal recessive disorders are horizontal, with multiple affected members within the same generation born to normal parents. The normal parents are carriers of the disorder. When two carriers mate, the risk is one in four that the pregnancy will result in an affected child, two in four that the child will be a carrier of the abnormal gene, and one in four that the child will have no abnormal gene and not be a carrier. Examples of autosomal recessive diseases include sickle cell anemia, cystic fibrosis, β-thalassemia, and Tay-Sachs disease.

X-Linked Recessive Disorders

Men are affected almost exclusively by X-linked recessive disorders. This is because women with a mutant gene on one X chromosome will usually have a normal gene on the other X chromosome. Men have no genes on the Y chromosome to match those on the X chromosome. The abnormal gene is transmitted to the male child by a carrier mother. The risk of a male child being affected is one in two, and the risk of a female child being a carrier is one in two. Hemophilia A and B, Duchenne dystrophy, and hemolytic anemia related to glucose-6-phosphate dehydrogenase (G6PD) deficiency are well-known examples of X-linked recessive disorders. Screening tests are available for the detection of the carriers of these disorders.

X-Linked Dominant Disorders

X-linked dominant disorders are very rare. Because an affected man cannot pass an X chromosome to his son, these disorders do not have male-to-male transmission, and because the affected father can pass only an abnormal gene to his daughter, all of his female offspring will be affected. Vitamin-D–resistant rickets and telecanthus-hypospadias syndrome are two examples of an X-linked dominant disorder.

Multifactorial Disorders

Multifactorial disorders refer to familial disorders that cannot be explained by a single mutant gene; such disorders are attributed to the additive effects of multiple genes and environmental factors. Within an affected family, these disorders tend to have an occurrence of 3% to 7%. Parents, siblings, and offspring are all equally likely to be affected. However, the risk increases if more than one family member is affected. Examples of multifactorial disorders include pyloric stenosis, neural tube defects, cleft lip and palate, clubfoot, and congenital hip dislocation.

Chromosomal Abnormalities

The normal number of human chromosomes, 46, is referred to as the *diploid number*. Each gamete has a haploid number, 23. The addition of an extra complete set of chromosomes within a cell is referred to as *polyploidy*. The presence or absence of a single or several chromosomes is referred to as *aneuploidy*. Trisomy, the presence of three chromosomes, is a common example of aneuploidy. Trisomies result from an accident in meiosis during the formation of the gametes—eggs and sperm. The chromosome pair fails to segregate appropriately during meiosis, so that one gamete gets both chromosomes. This is referred to as *nondisjunction*. This gamete then joins with the normal gamete (now a zygote), which is trisomic for the involved chromosome. Because nondisjunction occurs during formation of a single gamete only, future gametes and, therefore, offspring are not likely to be affected. Nondisjunction is more likely to occur in older women. Down syndrome can occur as either nondisjunction (95%) or translocation (5%). In approximately 33% of individuals with Down syndrome because of translocation, one of the parents will have 45 chromosomes with a balanced translocation between a chromosome 21 and 1 of the D- or G-group chromosomes. That parent is at substantial risk of having another child with Down syndrome. The most common example of an internal structural abnormality is a translocation. A translocation refers to a chromosomal abnormality in which part or all of a chromosome becomes attached to another chromosome. Translocations occur as a result of chromosome breakage and recombination.

Although most trisomies result in spontaneous abortion, trisomies 21, 18, and 13 frequently result in live births. Trisomy 21 results in Down syndrome. Trisomies 18 and 13 both have very poor prognoses with severe mental retardation. In the past, only approximately 10% to 20% survive to 1 year of age, but increasing numbers of these children now survive well beyond infancy.

Sex chromosome abnormalities include Turner syndrome (XO) and Klinefelter syndrome (XXY). Turner syndrome is the result of loss of a sex chromosome during early meiotic division in the zygote after fertilization. This results in complex forms of mosaicism in which the individual has two or more populations of cells, each with a different chromosome complement (XO, XX). However, Klinefelter syndrome is thought to be the result of meiotic nondisjunction in one of the parents.

Single Nucleotide Polymorphism

Single nucleotide polymorphism (SNP) is when a single nucleotide in a gene sequence is replaced by another nucleotide (for example TACGTCGA and TACGTTGA). These single nucleotide variations in the DNA sequence account for approximately 90% of all human genetic variation. For a variation to be considered an SNP, it must occur in greater than 1% of the population. Due to variations in human populations, certain SNPs may occur in higher frequency in certain geographic areas or ethnic groups and be rare in others. The nucleotide alterations can occur in the coding or on-coding regions of the DNA. Therefore SNPs may affect gene splicing. SNPs are not thought to affect cell function. Even when the coding sequences are involved in SNPs, due to the redundancy in the genetic code, the amino acid sequence of the protein produced may not necessarily be changed. SNPs are not thought to cause disease, but variations in DNA sequence may affect how an individual develops disease or responds to infectious agents or pharmaceuticals. This has made the study of SNPs an exciting area of biomedical research. For example, Apolipoprotein E (*ApoE*) is a gene linked to Alzheimer disease. Within this gene are two SNPs that can therefore result in three possible alleles: E2, E3, and E4. Each allele differs by one base pair and the protein product differs by one amino acid. Each individual inherits one copy of *ApoE* from the father and one from the mother. Individuals who inherit at least one copy of E4 allele appear to be at greater risk of developing Alzheimer disease, while individuals who inherit the E2 allele appear to be less likely to develop Alzheimer disease. As in most complex diseases, this is not absolute as an individual with two E4 alleles may still not develop the disease while another with two E2 alleles might (11,12).

Recombinant DNA

Bacteria have no immune system and can be infected by foreign DNA from a virus. The method of defense used by bacteria against these attacking viruses is an enzyme called *restriction endonuclease*. This enzyme "cuts" DNA into segments at a specific site (restriction site). More than 200 of these restriction endonucleases have been discovered, and their discovery was the first step in developing the concept of recombinant DNA. DNA fragments, cut by the restriction endonuclease, can be sequenced and, therefore, the protein for which they code can also be sequenced.

Recombinant DNA means, simply, combining DNA from two different organisms. The foreign DNA is attached to a vector and inserted into the genome of the host. In other words, and most commonly, a human gene can be introduced into bacteria. The two vectors used are bacterial plasmids and viral phages. This process allows, at least conceptually, the introduction of a "missing gene" into a genome, for example, the gene for α_1-antitrypsin could be introduced into a patient with α_1-antitrypsin deficiency.

Embryology

An overview of the early stages of development is helpful in understanding the malformations that are of surgical importance. The first 2 weeks, or the time from fertilization to completion of implantation in the uterine wall, is known as the *period of the ovum*. The 3rd to 8th week following conception is considered the embryonic period, and the 8th to the 40th week of gestation is known as the *fetal period*. During the embryonic period, approximately 90% of congenital anomalies occur. Unfortunately, it is difficult to obtain exact dates of conception and it is very difficult to measure the embryo accurately. Although embryologists use more precise and complex methods to estimate embryonic and fetal age, for the interested surgeon embryonic size may be most simply and adequately given as crown–rump length and age from conception, which is estimated as 14 days after the onset of the last menstrual period. Table 2.1 compares the crown–rump length with the number of somites and estimated age from fertilization (1,13–15).

The period of the ovum extends from fertilization until implantation in the wall of the uterus. During this period, fertilization occurs with restoration of the diploid number of chromosomes, determination of chromosomal sex, and the initiation of cleavage. The cells of the zygote arrange in an outer mass to form the trophoblast and an inner mass to

form the embryo proper. By the end of the second week, the zygote, now known as the blastocyst, has become embedded in the endometrial stroma, and a primitive uteroplacental circulation develops. During the second week, the embryo formed from the inner cell mass is known as the *embryoblast*, which differentiates into a bilaminar germ disc. The epiblast cells are contiguous with the cells that surround the amniotic cavity and the hypoblast cells are contiguous with the cells surrounding the primitive yolk sac (Fig. 2.4) (16).

During the third week of gestation, the three germ layers of the embryo are established. The primitive streak appears at the beginning of this week. Cells of the epiblast migrate through the primitive streak forming the three germ layers—ectoderm, mesoderm, and endoderm (Fig. 2.5) (16). Therefore, the three germ layers are derived from the epiblast. The layer of the embryo in contact with the amniotic cavity is the ectoderm and the layer in contact with the yolk sac is the endoderm. Cells of the mesoderm migrate between the ectoderm and endoderm. At the cephalic end of the primitive streak is the primitive pit. Epiblast cells that invaginate in the primitive pit move forward in the midline to form a tubelike process forming the notochordal or head process (Fig. 2.6) (16). The notochord is important for the axial orientation of the embryo and stimulates the development of the overlying ectoderm into neuroectoderm—the precursor of the nervous system.

During the embryonic period, which extends from the third week through the eighth week of development, each of the three germ layers gives rise to specific tissues and organs. The ectodermal germ layer forms the central and peripheral nervous systems, including the sensory epithelium of the ear, nose, and eye. This layer also forms the epidermis, nails, hair, subcutaneous glands, mammary glands, pituitary gland, adrenal medulla, and the enamel of the teeth. Tissues and organs of mesodermal origin include supporting tissues (connective tissue, cartilage, bone, and muscle); blood and lymph cells; heart, blood, and lymph vessels; kidneys, gonads, and their ducts; cortical portion of the adrenal gland; and the spleen. The endoderm forms the epithelial lining of the gastrointestinal, respiratory, and urinary tracts. It also forms the thyroid, parathyroid, liver, and pancreas. The epithelial lining of the tympanic cavity and eustachian tubes are also of endodermal origin.

The fetal period extends from the 9th week until birth, usually at 38 weeks after fertilization or 40 weeks after the onset of the last menstruation. Although the embryonic period is characterized by differentiation of tissues and development of organs, the fetal period is characterized by rapid growth and maturation of tissues and organs. Growth in length is most striking during the third through the fifth months. Weight gain is most prominent during the last 2 months of gestation, when the fetal weight nearly doubles. The proportion of the head to the body also changes rapidly during fetal development (Fig. 2.7) (17). During the fetal period, perinatologists can assess growth and development of the fetus by ultrasound. Intrauterine growth retardation (IUGR) applies to an infant who is at or below the 10th

TABLE 2.1

Age and Size of Embryos

Crown–Rump Length (mm)	No. of Somites	Estimated Age (d)
0.05	—	7–8
0.10	—	7–9
0.15	—	11–15
0.30	—	14–17
0.7	—	19
1.5	—	20
2.0	—	21
2.8	1–4	24
3.3	5–12	27
3.5	13–20	28
4.0	21–24	30
4.3	28–29	31
5.4	30–32	35
6.0	38	35–37
8.0	—	35–38
10.0	—	40
12.0	—	42
14.0	—	44
17.0	—	49
22–250	—	56

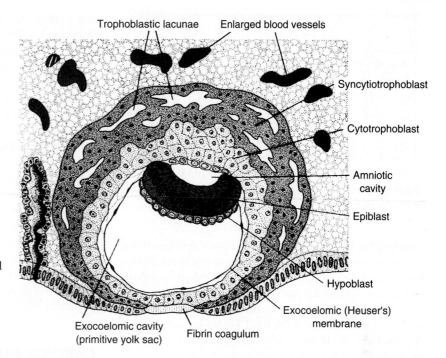

FIGURE 2.4 Drawing of a 9-day human blastocyst. The syncytiotrophoblast shows a large number of lacunae. Note the flat cells that form the exocoelomic membrane. The bilaminar germ disc consists of a layer of columnar epiblast cells and a layer of bucoidal hypoblast cells. The original surface defect is closed by a fibrin coagulum. (From Sadler TW. *Langman's medical embryology*, 8th ed. Philadelphia: Lippincott Williams & Wilkins, 2000, with permission.)

FIGURE 2.5 **A:** Schematic drawing of the dorsal side of a 16-day presomite embryo. The primitive streak and node are clearly visible. (Modified after Streeter.) **B:** Transverse section through the region of the primitive streak (as indicated in **A**), showing the invagination and subsequent lateral migration of the epiblast cells that will form the embryonic mesoderm and endoderm. (From Sadler TW. *Langman's medical embryology*, 8th ed. Philadelphia: Lippincott Williams & Wilkins, 2000, with permission.)

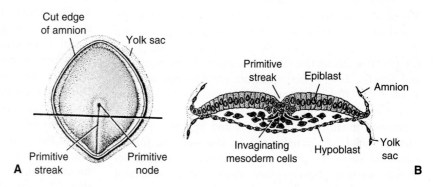

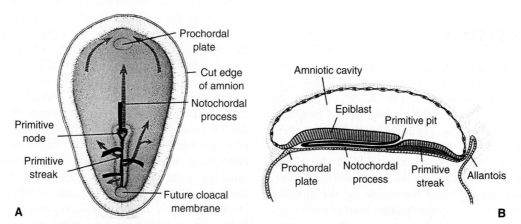

FIGURE 2.6 **A:** Schematic representation of the dorsal side of the germ disc, indicating the movement of surface cells (solid black lines) toward the primitive streak and node and the subsequent migration of cells between the hypoblast and epiblast germ layers (broken lines). **B:** Cephalocaudal midline section through a 16-day embryo. The notochordal process occupies the midline region extending from the prochordal plate to the primitive node. Note the notochordal or central canal in the center of the notochordal process. (From Sadler TW. *Langman's medical embryology*, 8th ed. Philadelphia: Lippincott Williams & Wilkins, 2000, with permission.)

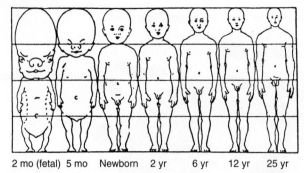

2 mo (fetal) 5 mo Newborn 2 yr 6 yr 12 yr 25 yr

FIGURE 2.7 Illustration of the change in body proportions during the fetal period.

percentile for the expected weight at a given gestational age. This is thought to occur in approximately one in ten babies. Individuals with IUGR will be at increased risk of neurologic deficiencies, congenital malformations, meconium aspiration, hypoglycemia, hypocalcemia, and respiratory distress syndrome. Factors responsible for IUGR babies include chromosomal abnormalities, congenital infections, drug abuse, and poor maternal nutrition and health (18,19).

Congenital malformations are recognized in 2% to 3% of all live births (7,16,20). This number doubles by 1 year of age as other anomalies manifest symptoms and are recognized (21). The factors responsible for these congenital malformations are environmental, chromosomal, and genetic. Environmental factors are now estimated to account for 10% of human malformations (16). These factors include infectious agents, radiation, chemical agents, hormones, nutritional deficiencies, and hypoxia (22–25). Chromosomal and genetic factors also account for an estimated 10% of human malformations. These factors include numeric chromosomal abnormalities, structural chromosomal abnormalities, and gene abnormalities.

IMMUNE SYSTEM

The immune system in the fetus develops from stem cells, which originate in the extraembryonic yolk sac. These cells, after migrating to different sites in the developing fetus, are stimulated to develop into the neutrophils and lymphoid cells of the immune system. The initial lymphoid cells appear in the thymus and elsewhere in the fetus such as the bone marrow and fetal liver. The T cells responsible for the cellular immune response develop under the influence of the thymus. B cells, which are primarily responsible for the humoral immune response, develop chiefly in the bone marrow (26).

At birth, the term *infant* is essentially competent immunologically but suffers from several problems that may increase the risk of sepsis. First, the barriers that prevent entry of bacteria may be compromised. The newborn has very thin, permeable skin, which is easily injured. The newborn ileum may absorb macromolecules, even entire bacteria (27). This may be accentuated even more in the presence of compromised intestine, such as necrotizing enterocolitis. At birth, infants have a high level of maternal immunoglobulin (Ig) G and quickly develop their own IgM and IgA. The premature infant, however, has a delayed ability to manufacture immunoglobulins, with an increased risk of sepsis as a result (27).

Deficiencies in any of the components of the immune system may lead to dramatic clinical presentations with multiple or unusual infections. B-cell deficiencies, or an inability to produce normal immunoglobulins, result in recurrent, invasive infection from pyogenic bacteria. T-cell deficiencies result in a decreased cellular response and, because the T cells are important in regulating the function of the B cells, may also result in defective immunoglobulin production. Examples of these syndromes include severe combined immunodeficiency syndrome (SCIDS), immunodeficiency with ataxia and telangiectasia, Wiskott-Aldrich syndrome (eczema, thrombocytopenia, multiple infections), and DiGeorge syndrome (congenital thymic aplasia, hypoparathyroidism) (28).

CARDIOVASCULAR SYSTEM

Development of the fetal heart begins at approximately the third week of gestation. The mesoderm splits into a somatic dorsal and splanchnic ventral portion. This results in the development of a column that later divides into a series of vesicles. The cranial and medial portions evolve into the pericardial cavity. The ventral portion of the mesoderm contains the neomyocardium or the cardiogenic plate and this then becomes lined with an angioblastic layer, which forms the cardiac tube or endocardium (Fig. 2.8) (29). During the fourth gestational week, the epimyocardium becomes enfolded at a number of sites, developing sulci that will eventually define the chambers of the heart. These include the infundibulotruncal sulcus, the interventricular sulcus, and the atrioventricular (AV) sulcus. These give rise to the truncus arteriosus, the right infundibulum and the right and left ventricles, and the left and right aorta, respectively. During the fifth week of gestation, the heart tube undergoes a rotation forward and to the right with demarcation of the sinus venosus, atrium, ventricles, and truncus arteriosus (1). During the fourth to sixth weeks, the AV canal divides into two channels. The anterior and posterior edges become thickened and fuse to form the endocardial cushions. This results in the division of the AV canal into right and left orifices. Failure of the fusion may result in septal defects or malformation of the AV valves. During this time, the atrial septum (septum primum) also forms and migrates toward the fused endocardial cushion, thereby dividing the atria and closing the foramen primum. Concurrently, the foramen secundum develops in the cranial portion of the septum, thereby maintaining communication between the left and right atria. Following this, a second septum develops to the right of the septum primum. This second septum never develops enough to completely close the foramen secundum and the resulting opening becomes

FIGURE 2.8 Transition from straight cardiac tube to four-chamber heart. **A:** Straight cardiac tube stage with four segments in series. The sinoatrium (*SA*) is destined to become the right atrium (*RA*) and left atrium (*LA*), the primitive ventricle (*V*) is precursor to the left ventricle (*LV*), the bulbus cordis (*BC*) becomes the right ventricle (*RV*), and the truncus arteriosus (*TA*) divides into the aorta (*Ao*) and main pulmonary artery (*PA*). The proximal and distal ends of the tube are fixed. **B:** Differential growth causes the tube to bend toward the right. **C:** The bulboventricular portion of the tube doubles over on itself, so that the right and left ventricles lie side by side. **D:** The right and left atria still connect to the left ventricle by the atrioventricular canal. The atrioventricular canal migrates toward the right, so that it lies over both ventricles. **E:** The anterior and posterior endocardial cushions meet and divide the atrioventricular canal into tricuspid and mitral orifices. (From Kramer TC. The partitioning of the truncus and conus and the formation of the membranous portion of the interventricular septum in the human heart. *Am J Anat* 1942;71;343–370. Copyright ©1942 Kramer; with permission of Wiley-Liss, a division of John Wiley and Sons, Inc.)

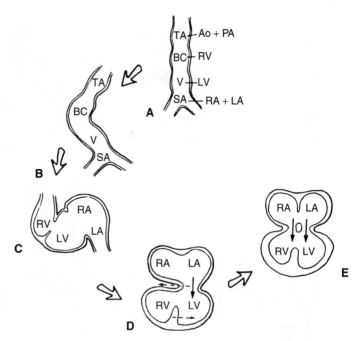

the foramen ovale. The septa and their foramina form a one-way valve allowing flow from right to left but not from left to right. This correlates with fetal circulation in which right atrial pressures are greater than left atrial pressures. This difference is a result of umbilical vein flow from the placenta and a lack of pulmonary venous flow secondary to a patent ductus arteriosus and relative pulmonary arterial constriction due to high pressures in the fluid-filled fetal lungs. At birth, the lungs expand, pulmonary artery pressure decreases, and systemic pressure increases, resulting in a preferential flow to the pulmonary bed. This causes an increase in pulmonary return and left atrial pressure relative to the low systemic venous pressure of the right atrium, which functionally closes the one-way valve (1,30,31). Following functional closure, a fibroplastic hypertrophy of the septum primum occurs, and it adheres to the septum secundum, resulting in an anatomic closure of the flap. Anatomic defects as well as various causes of pulmonary hypertension can result in persistence of the right-to-left shunt through the atria (32). These will be discussed later.

The ventricles also form during this period of fetal growth. Two areas of trabeculation and rapid growth occur proximally and distally in the endocardial tube. The proximal area is ventral and eventually develops into the left ventricle; distally, the trabeculation occurs dorsolaterally and develops into the right ventricle. These two plates grow toward each other to develop into the muscular portion of the interventricular septum. The membranous portion of the septum develops as connective tissue outgrowths from the valvular and truncus ridges as well as from the endocardial cushions. Fusion of the membrane and muscular portions results in closure of the interventricular canal. Failure of this process results in the majority of ventricular septal defects (VSDs).

The pulmonary and aortic trunks develop from ridges that develop in the truncus arteriosus and eventually divide into two separate tubes (1,33). This process starts at approximately the fifth week of gestation. These ridges eventually fuse proximally with the developing interventricular septum. Thickening of endocardial tissue at this site eventually develops into the semilunar valves (Fig. 2.9) (34). Distally, the ridges develop between the fourth and sixth aortic arches, eventually separating these into the systemic and pulmonary outflow, respectively. Appropriate orientation of the truncal separation to the ventricular septum is essential for normal development between the right ventricle and pulmonary artery and the left ventricle and the aorta. Failure of proper orientation results in various types of transposition of the great vessels (32,35).

Fetal Circulation

During fetal development, the pulmonary bed is almost entirely excluded from fetal circulation (Fig. 2.10) (31,36). Studies by Fox and Duara (36,37) suggest that the pulmonary circulation receives only 7% of the cardiac output. Instead, most of the blood is shunted in a right-to-left fashion through the foramen ovale or ductus arteriosus. In general, blood returns to the fetus from the placenta through the umbilical vein. This bypasses the liver through the ductus venosus and flows into the right atrium with the major portion of the flow crossing the foramen ovale and entering the left atrium. The remainder flows into the right ventricle and then to the pulmonary artery. However, because of the high resistance in the pulmonary vascular bed and the low pressure in the systemic bed, the blood bypasses the lung through the ductus arteriosus. Premature closure of the foramen ovale *in utero* is usually fatal. The defect results in a marked increase in right ventricular work and a decrease in flow to the left ventricle, causing it to become hypoplastic. The ductus arteriosus may provide enough systemic flow to maintain the fetus *in utero*,

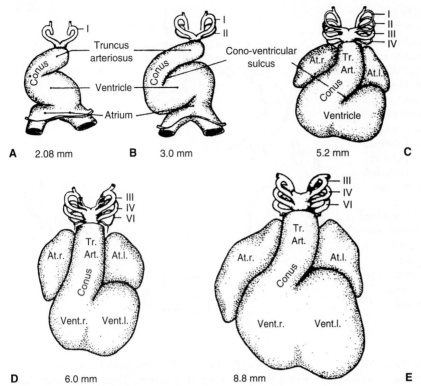

FIGURE 2.9 The developing heart from the cardiac loop. *At.r.*, right atrium; *Tr. Art.*, truncus arteriosus; *At.l.* left atrium; *Vent.r.*, right ventricle; *Vent.l.*, left ventricle.

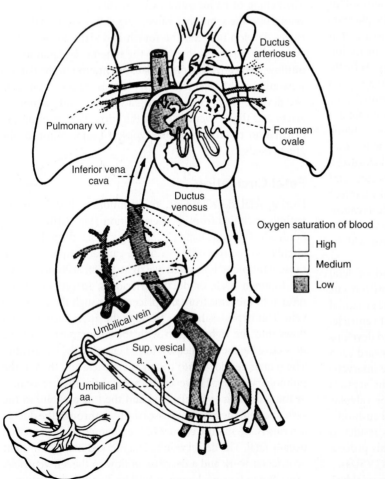

FIGURE 2.10 Normal fetal circulatory pattern. Pulmonary vv., pulmonary veins; sup. vesical a., superior vesical artery; umbilical aa., umbilical artery. (From Krummel TM, Greenfield LJ, Kirkpatrick BV, et al. Alveolar-arterial oxygen gradients vs neonatal pulmonary insufficiency index for prediction of mortality in ECMO candidates. *J Pediatr Surg* 1984;19:380–384, with permission.)

but at birth, cyanosis and left heart failure usually result in death.

Transitional Circulation

With the infant's initial breaths, the lungs expand, resulting in a marked decrease in the pulmonary vascular resistance. This allows for increased flow from the right ventricle into the pulmonary artery and into the pulmonary vascular bed. Concurrently, there is an increase in the systemic vascular pressure, which causes an increase in the left atrial and ventricular pressures. These changes result in decreased flow across the foramen ovale and ductus arteriosus, essentially obliterating the right-to-left shunt. In the initial postnatal period, these changes are not irreversible and alterations in oxygenation, acid–base status, and pulmonary artery pressures can result in a shift back toward fetal circulation. This period is known as the *transitional phase* between fetal and newborn circulation. The hallmarks of this phase are right and left ventricles that are relatively equal in size and musculature. The foramen ovale and ductus arteriosus have not yet fibrosed and remain anatomically patent. Furthermore, the smooth muscle in the pulmonary arterioles is relatively hypertrophied, is reactive, and is very sensitive to changes in blood pH and PaO_2 (30).

Therefore, changes during the first weeks of life that result in hypoxia and acidosis can cause an increase in pulmonary arterial pressures. This is known as *persistent pulmonary hypertension of the newborn* (PPHN). The pulmonary hypertension causes an increase in right-sided heart pressures and can result in right-to-left shunting across the foramen ovale and patent ductus arteriosus, a phenomenon known as *persistent fetal circulation*. Besides hypoxia and acid–base status, the pulmonary vasculature is also affected by prostaglandins. Briefly, PGE_1, PGE_2, and prostacyclin (PGI_2) act as pulmonary vasodilators, whereas the F-series prostaglandins are vasoconstrictors. It is likely that thromboxane also acts as a pulmonary vasoconstrictor. Therefore, in the normal newborn, an increased PaO_2, increased pH, PGE_2, and PGI_2 all work together to decrease pulmonary vascular pressures (31,38,39). PGE_2 also inhibits constriction and closure of the ductus arteriosus and is therefore used in ductus-dependent lesions (e.g., hypoplastic left heart syndrome) to permit blood flow across the ductus arteriosus.

Another issue is primary failure of the ductus to close (patent ductus arteriosus), which can result in a large left-to-right shunt with congestion of the pulmonary bed and evidence of congestive heart failure. This is especially common in the premature infant whose immature lungs, coupled with some degree of persistent pulmonary hypertension, prevent normal closure of the ductus (40). This can be a progressive problem, as hypoxia and acidosis can cause increased pulmonary arterial spasm and increased pulmonary hypertension. Clinically, the patent ductus results in a holosystolic murmur, bounding pulses with a widened pulse pressure, and evidence of congestive heart failure. Treatment is either with indomethacin, which blocks the synthesis of certain prostaglandins that inhibit duct closure,

or with direct surgical ligation (32). The merits of the various techniques are beyond the scope of this discussion.

Neonatal and Infant Circulation

Once the transition has been made from fetal circulation to neonatal circulation, the cardiovascular physiology is in general similar to that of children and adults (Fig. 2.11) (36). Initially, the newborn is relatively hyperdynamic with increased cardiac output. This state presents itself primarily as an increased pulse rate, a decreased blood pressure, and an increased respiratory rate. Figure 2.12 shows normal blood pressures for various age-groups (41–43). It should be noted that the differences are even more extreme in the severely premature infant.

Cyanotic Congenital Heart Disease

Cyanotic congenital heart disease consists of lesions that result in a right-to-left shunt, the bypass of the pulmonary bed, a relative peripheral hypoxia, and varying degrees of cyanosis. These lesions include (i) defects in the development of the truncus arteriosus; (ii) transposition of the great vessels; (iii) persistent truncus arteriosus; (iv) total anomalous pulmonary venous return; (v) a combination of lesions also affecting the endocardial cushion; and (vi) maldevelopment

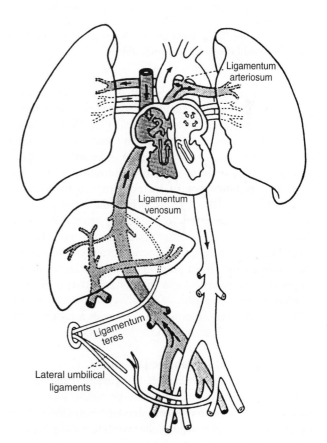

FIGURE 2.11 Normal newborn circulatory pattern. (From Krummel TM, Greenfield LJ, Kirkpatrick BV, et al. Alveolar-arterial oxygen gradients vs neonatal pulmonary insufficiency index for prediction of mortality in ECMO candidates. *J Pediatr Surg* 1984;19:380–384, with permission.)

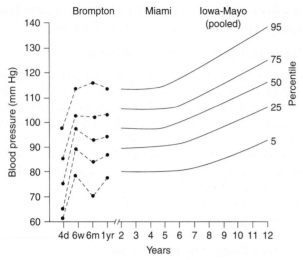

FIGURE 2.12 Percentiles of blood pressure. Infants 4 days to 1 year: percentiles of blood pressure (BP) in awake infants, both sexes pooled (Brompton study). At age 6 weeks, the percentile values were calculated from the 594 boys and 538 girls who were awake at the time of BP measurement. At ages 6 months and 1 year, all infants were awake. At age 4 days, there were only 174 infants awake at the time of BP measurement, and the percentile values were, therefore, taken from these measurements plus the measurements made on the sleeping infants after correction for wakefulness. Children ages 2 to 14 years: percentiles from the values for 29 to 45 boys from the Miami study and 453 to 592 boys from the Muscatine and Rochester studies (Iowa-Mayo pool) as summarized by the Task Force for Blood Pressure Control in Children.

of the AV and/or similar valves, that is, tricuspid atresia, pulmonary atresia with associated hypoplastic right heart, and Fallot tetralogy (right ventricular outflow stenosis; VSD; right ventricular hypertrophy; and dextroposition of the aorta) (32,38). There are a number of surgical procedures that attempt to provide adequate flow to the pulmonary bed for oxygenation and of oxygenated blood to the systemic circulation. These include the Blalock-Taussig surgery (subclavian artery to pulmonary artery), Waterson shunt (ascending aorta to right pulmonary artery), Fontan procedure (right atrium to pulmonary artery), Potts surgery (descending aorta to left pulmonary artery), Glenn surgery (superior vena cava to right pulmonary artery), Blalock-Hanlon surgery [creation of atrial septal defect (ASD)], balloon septostomy (creation of ASD with a catheter and balloon), and total correction of a transposition.

Congestive or Noncyanotic Lesions
Congestive lesions result in a left-to-right shunt and include ASDs, VSDs, and AV canal defects. As previously mentioned, these defects arise from abnormal development of the septa or the endocardial cushion. Surgical correction usually requires simple closure or patching of the defects.

Associated Thoracic Vascular Anomalies
Most of the other major thoracic vascular defects arise from abnormal development of the aortic arch. This includes two

primary categories that are of significance in the neonate: coarctation and vascular ring.

The thoracic aorta arises from pairs of arteries (aortic arches) that migrate from the primitive heart forming laterally around the gut and moving posteriorly and caudad (Fig. 2.13) (33). The vessels fuse on the dorsal surface of the fetus to form a common aorta. During development, there are six pairs of arches that develop and regress at various stages. Initially, there are two dorsal aortae, but eventually they fuse to form a single posterior aorta. The first and second aortic arches regress and become small local arteries. The third arch develops into the internal carotid artery. The right fourth arch usually regresses and the left fourth arch becomes the proper aortic arch, occurring at approximately the eighth week of gestation. The sixth arch fuses with primordial vessels developing off the truncus to form the pulmonary artery. Persistence of the right aortic arch, or various elements, can lead to vascular rings, which can encircle the trachea, esophagus, or both, causing partial airway or gastrointestinal obstruction at birth (1,38,44,45).

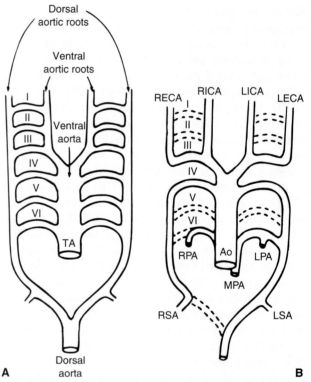

FIGURE 2.13 **A:** Diagram of the aortic arches and dorsal aorta during early fetal stage. **B:** The aorta after transformation into the definitive vascular pattern. The obliterated components are indicated by broken lines. *RECA,* right external carotid artery; *RICA,* right internal carotid artery; *LICA,* left internal carotid artery; *LECA,* left external carotid artery; *RPA,* right pulmonary artery; *MPA,* main pulmonary artery; *LPA,* left pulmonary artery; *RSA,* right subclavian artery; *LSA,* left subclavian artery; *TA,* truncus arteriosis; *Ao,* aorta. (From Congdon ED. Transformation of the aortic-arch system during the development of the human embryo. *Contrib Embryol* 1922;14:47–110, with permission of the Carnegie Institution of Washington.)

Coarctation of the aorta has been classified into two types: (i) infantile—a long, narrow segment proximal to the ductus arteriosus, and (ii) adult—a short, constricted segment, either preductal or postductal (35). Development of coarctation is thought to occur as the result of an imbalance of aortic and pulmonary artery blood flow in the fetus. This may be caused by an inadequate foramen ovale, aortic stenosis, or mitral valve deficiency. Lack of adequate blood flow following birth results in a failure of dilation of the aortic isthmus and a persistence of fetal narrowing or coarctation. Other short-segment coarctations may simply be the result of local atresias and lack of adequate development *in utero*. Treatment consists of either resection with end-to-end anastomosis or graft, or using the subclavian artery as a patch. Spontaneous or surgical closure of a significant ductus arteriosus in a patient with a preductal stenosis can result in substantial distal ischemia. PGE$_2$ is utilized in these patients to keep the ductus open.

PULMONARY SYSTEM

Embryology

During the fourth week of gestation, an outpouching develops from the ventral surface of the primitive foregut.

A groove then separates this outpouching from the foregut (Fig. 2.14) (45). This groove (the laryngotracheal groove) develops from the formation of a thickened epithelial ridge that encroaches on the lumen of the foregut. As the groove develops, the outpouching also grows caudad and will eventually become the neotrachea. During this stage, cells of primitive mesenchyma from the mediastinal mesentery start to proliferate. These cells will eventually grow into the cartilage, muscle, and connective tissue of the lungs. During the cranial and caudal growth of the laryngotracheal groove, the epithelial ridges continue to grow, thereby separating the respiratory and alimentary tracts. Failure of complete separation can result in numerous congenital anomalies, including tracheoesophageal fistula, which may have dire consequences after birth (46–48).

As the neotrachea grows caudally, it bifurcates to form the right and left main-stem bronchus and two discrete lung buds. Initially, the level of the bifurcation is high in the cervical region, but by the sixth week it is descended to the level of the first thoracic vertebra, and at birth, it has reached T-4 or T-5. The primitive lung begins its true growth at approximately the 4th week of gestation and continues its critical glandular development until the 16th week. During this period, the lung bud is extremely susceptible to environmental influences, and any disruptions

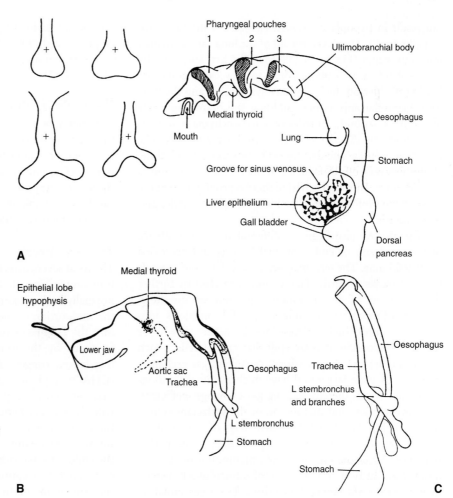

FIGURE 2.14 Development of trachea and bronchi. **A:** Four anterior views and lateral view of lung buds at the end of the fifth week (Horizon SIII). **B:** Lateral view at the middle of the sixth week (Horizon XV). **C:** Lateral view near the end of the sixth week (Horizon XVI). (From Streeter GL. Development horizons in human embryos. *Contrib Embryol* 1948;32: 133–203, with permission of the Carnegie Institution of Washington.)

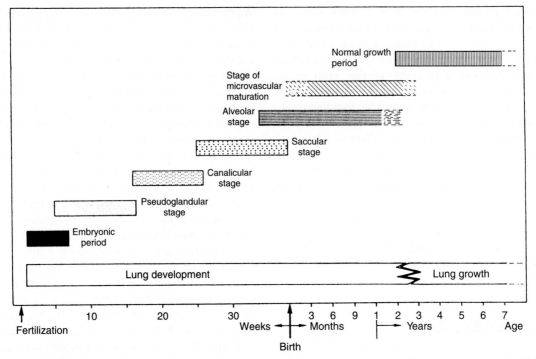

FIGURE 2.15   Diagram of the stages of fetal and postnatal lung development and growth. (From Burri PH. Fetal and postnatal development of the lung. *Ann Rev Physiol* 1984;46:617–628, with permission. Copyright 1984 by Annual Reviews Inc.)

can result in hypoplasia or even agenesis of the lung (see "Diaphragm"). The development of the lung can be divided into four stages (Fig. 2.15) (49–54). The first stage, or the pseudoglandular stage, lasts from 5 to 17 weeks of gestation. During this period the major airways develop and the lung has a glandular appearance. Budding and branching occur only if the surrounding mediastinal mesenchyma is present, suggesting that this tissue is the stimulus for growth. The next stage is the canalicular stage (17–26 weeks). By this time, all the airways from the trachea to the terminal bronchioles are laid down. During this period there is proliferation of the mesenchyma into cartilage, connective tissue, muscle, and blood vessels.

The airways also begin to differentiate, with evidence of increased size of endobronchial lumens and decreased epithelial lining. The terminal sac, or saccular stage, extends from 24 weeks to birth. This period is marked by further differentiation of the respiratory portion of the lung, with transformation of some terminal bronchioles into respiratory bronchioles. These are immature alveoli or sacculi and contain alveolar epithelial type II cells, which secrete surfactant. The sacculi are capable of gas exchange; however, they are larger and have thicker epithelial linings than true alveoli, thereby making gas exchange inefficient. The development and maturation of the surfactant system occurs during this stage. The fourth stage of growth starts just before term and continues postnatally. This period is marked by formation of alveoli, maturation of airways, and the production and secretion of numerous substances, including the surfactant within the lung. The larger immature

sacculi are divided by septa into alveolar sacs and ducts. Approximately 90% of alveoli form after birth. It is generally accepted that alveolar development continues until 8 years of age (51,53).

Pulmonary Anomalies

Anomalies of the respiratory tract are closely related to the stage of development when the abnormality occurs. However, no matter how severe the anomaly, it will usually not interfere with intrauterine life even if the defect is lethal in the immediate postnatal period. Tracheobronchial anomalies can be of variable severity and can run the spectrum from tracheal stenosis to tracheal and/or lung agenesis.

Tracheal Atresia

The most severe defect, tracheal atresia, is extremely rare and is incompatible with life. The tracheal primordium develops normally both proximally (larynx) and distally (lungs), but the midportion of the foregut fails to divide, and develops into the esophagus only. The origin of this defect is likely to occur by the fourth week of gestation. Fetuses with this lesion, congenital high airway obstruction syndrome (CHAOS) typically die at birth. Increasing numbers of these cases are now recognized prenatally. The fetuses present with very large, hyperinflated lungs due to retained lung fluid. In selected cases, these children can undergo *ex utero* intrapartum treatment (EXIT procedure). In this process, the child is partially delivered from the womb by a modified cesarean section approach. While the child is still attached to the mother and perfused through the placenta, access to the fetal airway is achieved and a tracheostomy performed before separating the infant from the placenta. This procedure requires a multidisciplinary approach and needs to be planned well ahead of the delivery. The outcome in these children is ultimately dependent on their lungs and other comorbidities.

Tracheal stenosis is a narrowing of the trachea. It can present with stridor in the newborn period. As with tracheal atresia, tracheal reconstruction is required.

Bilateral Agenesis of the Lungs

Bilateral agenesis is a rare disorder that is incompatible with life. It results from a failure of the progression of development of the distal or caudal tracheolaryngeal groove. This results in an absence of lung bud development and eventual pulmonary agenesis. In general, these defects are secondary to an abnormal division of the foregut endoderm and variable growth of the lung buds.

Unilateral Agenesis of the Lung

Unilateral agenesis is likely to be secondary to a failure to maintain normal development rather than a simple arrest of normal development. It seems likely that some environmental force acts to inhibit or slow normal growth on one side. A large number (>50%) of patients with unilateral agenesis also have associated anomalies, including esophageal atresia, tracheoesophageal fistula, spina bifida, fused ribs, laryngeal and palate malformations, imperforate anus, and cardiac defects (47,48,52). There is no clear underlying or common factor that has been discovered to date.

Pulmonary Hypoplasia

Pulmonary hypoplasia is an example of one model of environmental forces causing abnormal development, for example, diaphragmatic hernia. Factors that impinge on lung growth and development may result in pulmonary hypoplasia. These include space-occupying lesions (congenital lung and mediastinal masses) and herniated abdominal viscera. In addition, a normal amniotic fluid volume is important for lung development. Therefore, conditions associated with severe oligohydramnios or anhydramnios (e.g. renal agenesis) may also be associated with pulmonary hypoplasia.

In addition to various degrees of hypoplasia and agenesis, there are a number of other congenital pulmonary defects that may develop as a result of abnormal foregut differentiation (55–57).

Bronchogenic Cysts

Bronchogenic cysts, also called lung buds, are buds of developing embryonic lung that become separated from the developing tracheobronchial tree before the bronchi are formed. Because they arise from ectopic foregut, they may be lined with squamous epithelium. Although many of these cysts have ciliated columnar epithelium, they rarely have any connection to the normal bronchial lumens and may be located anywhere along the trachea or bronchi, either extraparenchymal or intraparenchymal, but most are in the posterior mediastinum at the level of the carina. Clinically, they present as space-occupying lesions, which may cause obstruction or become infected. During infancy they may partially obstruct one bronchus, thereby causing air trapping, and they may be confused clinically with congenital lobar emphysema or an intrabronchial foreign body. In many ways, they are the respiratory equivalent of foregut duplications. Treatment consists of simple excision.

Congenital Pulmonary Cysts

Congenital pulmonary cysts, like bronchogenic cysts, are a part of the developing lung bud that becomes entrapped. These cysts, however, communicate with the bronchi and may present as a thin-walled, large pneumatocele. Infants born with large lung cysts may develop acute respiratory distress and tension pneumothoraces, which may require emergency thoracotomy.

Pulmonary Sequestrations

Another type of anomaly in the spectrum of anomalous lung bud development is the pulmonary sequestrations (57,58). In this case, the isolated lung-bud segment returns or develops a systemic vascular circuit. It is not clear whether this happens because the initial separation of the sequestered segment occurs before the division of the pulmonary and aortic circulation or if persistence of the early embryonic splanchnic systems results in traction on a portion of the lung bud, causing this tissue to break away. In either case, the result is the development of accessory lung tissue that has no connection to the normal tracheobronchial tree and receives its blood supply directly from the systemic circulation (aorta). There are two types of sequestration: (i) intralobar, in which the venous drainage is into the pulmonary vein, and (ii) extralobar, which drains into the azygous system. It is likely that the more ectopic extralobar sequestration is a result of an isolation of the lung-bud segment at an earlier stage of development.

Adenomatoid Malformations

Adenomatoid malformation appears to be the result of an arrest in bronchial development while there is a persistence and, perhaps, overgrowth of mesenchymal elements. Histologically, this defect is characterized by the absence of cartilage in the bronchi and proliferation of terminal bronchioles, which gives the lung a cystic and glandular appearance. These lesions have been classified into three types on the basis of histologic and clinical presentation (1,56). Type I lesions are composed of a large single cyst or multiple cysts in which mucus-secreting cells and cartilage are rarely seen. Relatively normal alveoli are usually adjacent to these cysts. This type of lesion often causes marked mediastinal shift. Type II lesions are composed of multiple small cysts (<1 cm), again with a paucity of mucous cells or cartilage. Type III lesions are bulky noncystic lesions that often occupy the entire lobe. Bronchial-like structures are separated by masses of cuboidal epithelium–lined, alveolus-like structures. The most commonly affected portion of the lung is the left lower lobe, but multiple lobar involvement is frequent and can often be bilateral. Treatment consists of total excision, but the prognosis may be poor if there is multilobar involvement or there are type II and III lesions.

Increasing numbers of these fetal lung lesions are now being detected by prenatal ultrasound screening. Some of these lesions may grow relatively faster than the fetus, resulting in significant mediastinal shift, cardiac compression, and *in utero* heart failure (nonimmune hydrops fetalis). Without intervention, most of these fetuses will undergo *in utero* demise. Those with very large cystic lesions can be rescued by draining these cysts with a thoracoamniotic shunt draining the lung lesion into the amniotic fluid. For fetuses with lung masses without large dominant cysts, *in utero* resection of these masses may be possible in specialized centers. (Fig. 2.16) There is anecdotal evidence that regression in the size of some of these lesions may be induced with maternal glucocorticoid therapy. Glucocorticoids aid in lung maturation and are thought to decrease the lung fluid production by these lesions that results in their rapid growth.

Congenital Lobar Emphysema

Congenital lobar emphysema is usually limited to the upper lobes or right middle lobe and is characterized by severe air trapping and overdistention of the lung parenchyma. The dilated lobe causes compression of the adjacent lung parenchyma and can cause a shift of the mediastinum to the unaffected side. The etiology of this lesion may be manifold, but the common factor seems to be some pathologic entity that causes partial obstruction of the bronchi, resulting in a

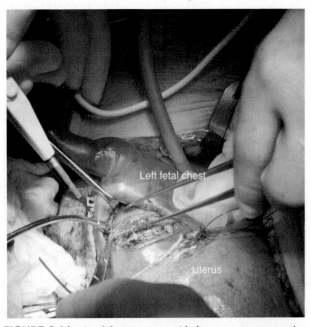

FIGURE 2.16 Fetal thoracotomy: with the uterus open, a portion of the left arm of the fetus is extruded while a thoracotomy is performed on the midgestation fetus to resect a large fetal lung lesion causing hydrops.

one-way, or ball valve, effect. This causes overexpansion of the lung with destruction of the normal alveolar architecture. Causes may include bronchial kinking, bronchomalacia, mucous plugging, external compression by aberrant vessels or lymph nodes, or intrinsic bronchial obstruction, that is, stenosis. In most cases no specific etiology can be discovered. Because the degree of lung destruction is irreversible, treatment consists of excision of the affected lobe.

DIAPHRAGM

The diaphragm evolves from four structures: the septum transversum, the pleuroperitoneal membranes, the esophagus and its mesentery, and ingrowth of muscular components from the lateral and dorsal body wall. The septum transversum first appears at the end of the third week as a thick plate of mesodermal tissue between the pericardium and the stalk of the yolk sac. The septum transversum becomes the central tendon of the diaphragm. The pleuroperitoneal folds develop as crescent-shaped folds along the caudal border of the pleural cavity. These folds form membranes that grow mediad to meet the esophageal mesentery in the midline, and dorsad and ventrad to fuse with the septum transversum to form the primitive diaphragm; complete partition of the thoracic and peritoneal cavities occurs by the seventh week (59). There is then an ingrowth of cells from the lateral body wall into the pleuroperitoneal membrane to form the muscular portion of the diaphragm, so that the membranous portion of the diaphragm in the newborn is very small. The crura of the diaphragm develop from the dorsal mesentery of the esophagus.

During the fourth week, the septum transversum begins to develop at the level of the third, fourth, and fifth cervical somites. Ventral folding and rapid growth of the dorsal and cephalic portions of the embryo result in an apparent caudal descent of the diaphragm. Whereas the dorsal part of the diaphragm lies at the level of the first lumbar vertebra, the motor innervation is from the ventral rami of C-3, C-4, and C-5, which lengthen and fuse into the phrenic nerve. Some of the sensory fibers come from the lower intercostal nerves (1). This explains diaphragmatic irritation being manifest as referred pain to the shoulder.

If the pleuroperitoneal membranes fail to develop by the eighth week, a posterior-lateral defect, Bochdalek hernia, occurs that allows the abdominal viscera to herniate into the chest (Fig. 2.17). This is particularly important because the midgut returns to the abdomen from the umbilical stalk during the eighth to tenth week of gestation. This is an early stage in the lung bud development, and the presence of the space-occupying abdominal viscera in the chest prevents normal lung development, causing the lung to become hypoplastic (60–62). Although the lung on the involved side is most severely affected, the contralateral lung may also be hypoplastic to varying degrees. In up to 30% of affected newborns, the lungs are so hypoplastic that survival is not possible. The right diaphragm seems to be protected

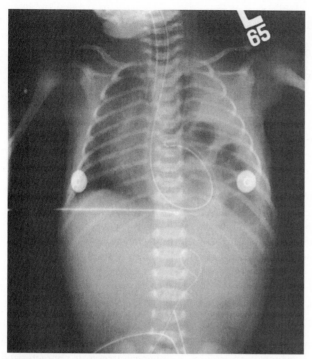

FIGURE 2.17 Roentgenogram of an infant with a left Bochdalek diaphragmatic hernia. The heart is shifted to the right, the position of the nasogastric tube indicates the stomach is in the left side of the chest, and the intestinal gas pattern is entirely within the chest.

during final development by the liver, and 90% of these hernias occur on the left.

Abnormal development of the diaphragm may result in hernias at various sites (Fig. 2.18) (1). Hernias may also occur directly behind the sternum through Morgagni foramen; these account for 2% to 6% of congenital diaphragmatic hernias. Morgagni hernias result from failure of the septum transversum to join the sternum. Most of these hernias are first recognized in middle-aged individuals, but they may also be symptomatic in the newborn (63). Depending on the size and amount of abdominal viscera herniated into the

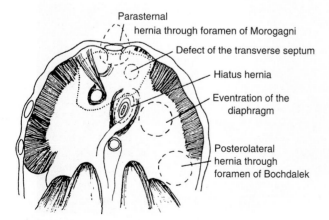

FIGURE 2.18 Sites of diaphragmatic anomalies. (From Gray SW, Skandalakis JE. *Embryology for surgeons.* Philadelphia: WB Saunders, 1972, with permission.)

chest, they can present with respiratory compromise and a clinical picture similar to that of a Bochdalek hernia (64). They may also be one component of a group of midline anomalies known as *pentalogy of Cantrell.*

Other uncommon anomalies of the diaphragm include eventration, congenital hiatal hernia, and phrenic nerve paralysis. Eventration may be difficult to differentiate from phrenic nerve paralysis and a small posterior-lateral hernia with a sac (65). In fact, many eventrations may be the result of phrenic nerve injury (66,67). Phrenic nerve injuries that occur during birth trauma are often associated with brachial plexus injuries or Erb palsy. The paralyzed hemidiaphragm typically rises to the fourth or fifth interspace, is thin and fibrotic, and moves paradoxically with respirations on fluoroscopic or ultrasound examination. Because newborn infants rely primarily on their diaphragms for ventilation, many of these infants are ventilator dependent. Many phrenic stretch injuries will recover if given time. Eventration of the diaphragm has also been associated with muscular dystrophy. Hiatal hernias, like Morgagni hernias, are usually seen later in life and are associated with obesity. When seen during infancy, they may be associated with a congenitally short esophagus.

GASTROINTESTINAL SYSTEM

Foregut Formation

The development of the foregut into the neotrachea and esophagus begins at approximately the third week of gestation. This differentiation involves three major processes (46,48,55). The first is the formation of two separate organ-forming fields from the primitive mesoderm. This causes differentiation of the ventral endoderm into the tracheal mucosa and differentiation of the dorsal endoderm into esophageal mucosa. Second, lateral ridges of proliferative ectoderm grow into the lumen of the foregut to divide into separate esophageal and tracheal tubes. The third major step is elongation of both the primitive tubes. This division becomes complete by approximately the fifth week, and the submucosa and circular muscle layer are apparent by the end of the sixth week. The outer longitudinal muscle layer is well formed by the ninth week. At no time during development does the esophagus become completely obliterated by the neoepithelium, so failure of recanalization is not a cause of esophageal atresia, as is the case with duodenal atresia. Most defects of the esophagus are a result of abnormal or incomplete separation of the trachea from the esophagus during the fourth and fifth weeks of gestation (1). The extent of malformation ranges from failure of separation of the trachea and esophagus (a persistent foregut) with a common lumen to a fistula or cleft between the trachea and esophagus. An example of the latter defect includes incomplete cranial growth of the septum. This will result in a laryngeal cleft or, in more severe cases, a laryngotracheoesophageal fistula. Local failure of septum formation will result in a simple tracheoesophageal fistula. In approximately 90% of these

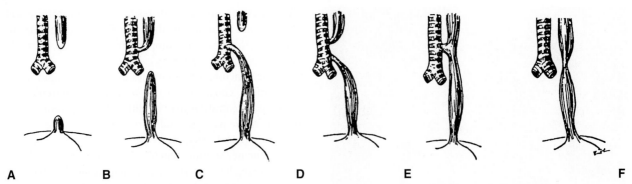

A   B   C   D   E   F

FIGURE 2.19   Types of congenital abnormalities of the esophagus. **A:** Esophageal atresia. There is no esophageal communication with the trachea; under such circumstances the lower esophageal end is apt to be quite short. **B:** Esophageal atresia. The upper segment communicates with the trachea. **C:** Esophageal atresia. The lower segment communicates with the back of the trachea; more than 90% of all esophageal malformations fall into this group. **D:** Esophageal atresia. Both segments communicate with the trachea. **E:** Esophagus has no disruption of its continuity but has a tracheoesophageal fistula. **F:** Esophageal stenosis. (From Gross RE. *The surgery of infancy and childhood*. Philadelphia: WB Saunders, 1953, with permission.)

cases, this is associated with the section of adjacent esophagus coming under the influence of the tracheal mesoderm, causing a local atresia of the esophagus. Any number of variations is possible based on relatively small alterations in the growth process. Figure 2.19 illustrates the classification of esophageal atresia and tracheoesophageal fistula proposed by Gross (67). Type C is the most common and accounts for

approximately 87% of these anomalies (Fig. 2.20) (68). Type A, which is an isolated esophageal atresia, is characterized by a gasless abdomen and esophageal atresia. Type A occurs in approximately 8% of infants in whom the anomaly is diagnosed at birth. Infants with type E anomalies usually present at an older age with recurrent respiratory tract infections or coughing when swallowing liquids. Types B and

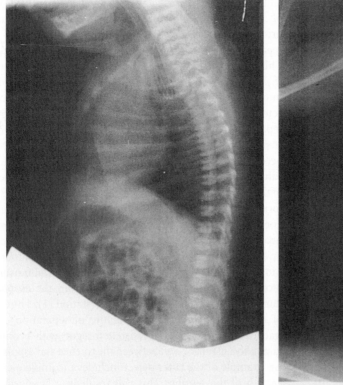

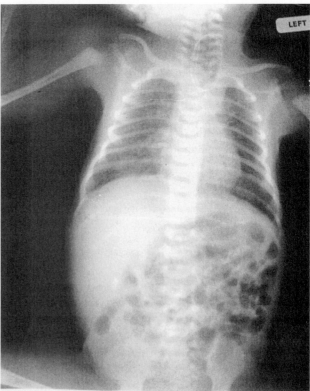

FIGURE 2.20   Lateral and PA roentgenograms of a newborn with an esophageal atresia and distal tracheoesophageal fistula (Type C). The catheter is curled in the blind upper esophageal pouch. Air has entered the intestine through the fistula.

D are uncommon. Anomalies of the trachea and esophagus have a high frequency of association with other defects (~50%) (69). One constellation of defects has been identified as the VATER or VACTERL syndrome. This classifies the association of tracheoesophageal anomalies with vertebral, cardiac, renal, radial bone, anal, and limb defects (70,71). All patients with tracheoesophageal fistula should be examined closely for other anomalies, and, in addition, a thorough family history should be obtained (72).

Stomach

The stomach begins to develop during the fifth week as a fusiform dilation of the lower end of the foregut. The dorsal portion grows faster than the ventral portion and forms the greater curvature. As the stomach grows, it undergoes a 90-degree clockwise rotation on its longitudinal axis so that the posterior wall, the greater curvature, becomes the left wall. The left wall and left vagus nerve are carried anteriorly, whereas the right wall and right vagus nerve move posteriorly. The dorsal mesentery is also carried to the left, forming a cavity to the right of the dorsal mesentery and dorsal to the stomach. This cavity is called the *omental bursa* or *lessor sac of the peritoneum*, and it communicates with the peritoneal cavity through the epiploic foramen or foramen of Winslow. Except for congenital pyloric stenosis and heterotrophic pancreatic mucosa, congenital anomalies of the stomach are rare.

Duodenum

The duodenum is formed by the distal foregut and proximal midgut, which are considered to meet just distal to the biliary ampullae. The duodenum is supplied by branches of the celiac artery, which supplies the foregut, and by branches of the superior mesenteric artery, which supplies the midgut. The proximal duodenum is pulled to the right by the bending of the stomach to form a C-shaped loop. The clockwise rotation and bending of the duodenum also draws the common duct behind the duodenum so that the biliary ampulla enters the posterior wall of the duodenum.

During the fifth and sixth weeks, the lumen of the duodenum becomes temporarily obliterated by proliferating epithelial cells from the gut lining. By the eighth week, the lumen is reestablished by a process of recanalization. Atresia and stenosis of the duodenum are thought to be the result of a failure of the recanalization process (73). Atresia or stenosis occurs most commonly at or just distal to the papilla of Vater, so that emesis is nearly always bilious (Fig. 2.21A–C) (74). The most common type of duodenal atresia is that caused by a diaphragm or web formed of mucosa and submucosa (Fig. 2.21 D). The membrane may become stretched by the peristaltic action on the swallowed amniotic fluid, forming a windsock anomaly (Fig. 2.21 E) (75). The ampulla of Vater is frequently located on or adjacent to the web, and great care must be taken when dissecting in this area.

Duodenal atresia is the most frequent location of intestinal atresia and is one of the more common major congenital anomalies requiring surgical correction to allow extrauterine

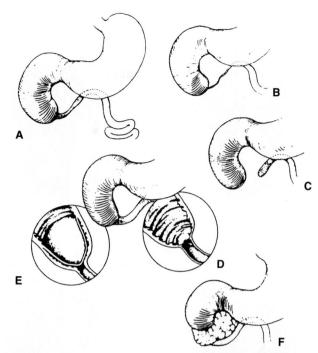

FIGURE 2.21 Various types of anomalies causing duodenal obstruction. **A:** Type 1 atresia with intact membrane producing marked discrepancy in size between proximal and distal segments. **B:** Blind ends of duodenum connected by a fibrous cord. **C:** Blind ends of duodenum are separated, and the mesentery is absent at the separation. **D:** Intraluminal membrane with a perforation. **E:** Windsock anomaly; note that an incision in the distal portion of the dilated segment would still be beyond the obstruction. **F:** Annular pancreas. (From Welch KJ, Randolph JG, Ravitch MM, et al. Duodenal atresia, stenosis and annular pancreas. In: Welch KJ, Randolph JG, Ravitch MM, et al. eds. *Pediatric surgery*, 4th ed. Chicago: Year Book Medical Publishers, 1986, with permission.)

survival (76). Associated anomalies are common and approximately 30% are associated with Down syndrome (74,76). Annular pancreas and malrotation may also present as duodenal obstruction (Fig. 2.21 F).

Liver and Pancreas

The liver primordium is first seen in the fourth week of development, but it is not identified as a separate organ until it grows from the septum transversum when the embryo is 6 to 8 mm in length. The bare area of the liver is the remaining evidence of the liver's intimate association with the septum transversum. The liver parenchyma arises from the hepatic bud of the distal foregut. This diverticulum grows into the transverse septum. The fetal liver is primarily an organ of hematopoiesis. At 9 weeks of gestation, the liver represents 10% of the body weight of the fetus. By birth, when it is no longer functioning as a hematopoietic organ, it represents approximately 5% of body weight. The most common anomaly of liver formation is the presence of an abnormal lobe, called *Riedel lobe*. This is an elongated, tonguelike lobe that extends from the right lobe. The lobe is functional and

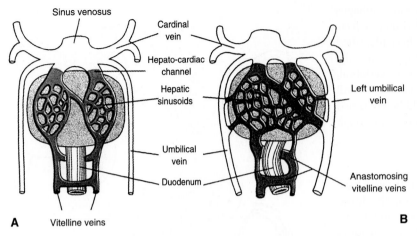

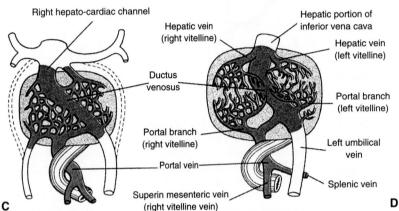

FIGURE 2.22 Schemes showing the development of the umbilical and vitelline veins. **A:** At the end of the fourth week; **B:** in the fifth week; **C:** in the sixth week; **D:** in the third month. Note the formation of the ductus venosus between the left umbilical vein and the inferior vena cava. (From Sadler TW. *Langman's medical embryology*, 8th ed. Baltimore: Williams & Wilkins, 2000, with permission.)

is only important in that it may be misdiagnosed as an abdominal mass if not recognized.

Conceptually, the most difficult, but also the most important for the surgeon, is the development of the blood vessels of the liver (Fig. 2.22) (77). The vitelline and umbilical veins start as paired structures, which are not associated with the liver parenchyma in the fourth week of gestation. The liver parenchyma envelops the vitelline veins by the end of the fifth week. At the same time, the extrahepatic portion of the vitelline veins undergoes a spontaneous anastomosis. The superior, or dorsal anastomosis, becomes the extrahepatic portal vein. The intrahepatic portion of the left umbilical vein becomes the ductus venosus, which shunts the placental blood through the liver to the fetal heart. The right umbilical vein regresses. In the newborn infant, the ductus venosus may remain patent for several days. This allows for passage of a catheter into the umbilical vein, through the ductus venosus and into a central venous position to sample blood or measure pressures in the newborn. In the adult, the umbilical vein remnant can be seen as a white, cordlike structure in the free edge of the falciform ligament, which extends to the umbilicus in the preperitoneal space. In patients with portal hypertension, the umbilical vein may recanalize and provide a spontaneous portosystemic shunt (caput medusae).

The pancreas is first identifiable as two pancreatic diverticular buds from the ventral and dorsal side of the foregut in the sixth week of gestation. The dorsal diverticulum

grows to form most of the body of the pancreas. As the duodenum elongates, the ventral diverticulum rotates inferiorly and mediad. This accomplishes two things: the common bile duct is brought into position to join the pancreatic duct at the sphincter of Oddi and the ventral diverticulum of the pancreas takes up a position inferior to the dorsal anlage, where it becomes the uncinate process (Figs. 2.23 and 2.24) (16). Each diverticular bud contains a pancreatic duct, but the proximal portion of the dorsal duct (duct of Santorini) regresses in 30% of individuals after it anastomoses with the ventral duct (duct of Wirsung).

There are two important anomalies of pancreatic development: anomalous pancreatic ducts and annular pancreas. Anomalous pancreatic ducts may occur if anastomosis between the two ducts fails (pancreatic divisum) or if both ducts enter the duodenum independently. There is some evidence that pancreas divisum may lead to pancreatitis in some patients. Annular pancreas occurs when the ventral anlage of the pancreas fails to rotate. In this condition, it remains anterior to the duodenum. Subsequent joining of the dorsal and ventral anlagen leads to a ring of pancreatic tissue around the second portion of the duodenum (78). This may be an incidental finding in a totally asymptomatic patient or may cause duodenal obstruction in the newborn. Heterotopic pancreatic tissue has been described throughout the gastrointestinal tract, although it is most often found in the duodenum or stomach. This too may be found incidentally

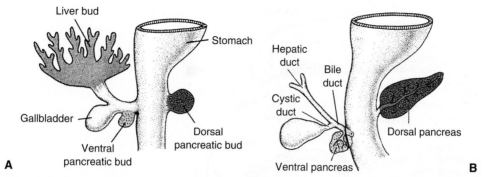

FIGURE 2.23 Successive stages in the development of the pancreas. **A:** At 30 days (~5 mm). **B:** At 35 days (~7 mm). The ventral pancreatic bud is initially located close to the hepatic diverticulum but later migrates posteriorly around the duodenum in the direction of the dorsal pancreatic bud. (From Sadler TW. *Langman's medical embryology*, 8th ed. Philadelphia: Lippincott Williams & Wilkins, 2000, with permission.)

at a laparotomy, when it may be confused with a neoplastic process. Ectopic pancreatic tissue may also act as a lead point for a small bowel intussusception.

Midgut

Embryologists consider the midgut to be that portion of the gut between the cephalic and caudal folds. On the other hand, the surgeon considers the midgut as the portion of the intestine that is supplied by the superior mesenteric artery; that is, beginning immediately distal to the entrance of the bile duct into the duodenum and terminating at the junction of the proximal two thirds of the transverse colon with the distal one third.

The primitive gut results from the cephalocaudal and lateral folding of the embryo to incorporate a portion of the endodermal-lined yolk sac (Fig. 2.25) (16). The middle part, or midgut, remains connected to the yolk sac by the vitelline duct. Whereas the epithelial lining of the digestive tract and the liver and the pancreas are derived from the endoderm, the muscular components of the gut form from the splanchnic mesoderm.

The midgut elongates rapidly, forming an intestinal loop that is connected through the vitelline duct at its apex with the

yolk sac. Failure of the vitelline duct to obliterate completely results in various anomalies, including Meckel diverticulum, vitelline cysts, and patent omphalomesenteric sinus or an umbilicoileal fistula (1,79–81). Although approximately 2% of the population has a Meckel diverticulum, only 4% of this group will produce symptoms (80,82). Meckel diverticulum typically presents with symptoms during early childhood (83). During the sixth week as the gut rapidly elongates, it enters the extraembryonic coelom in the umbilical cord. This process is known as *physiologic umbilical herniation*. The herniated intestine returns to the abdominal cavity before the 12th week of development.

The midgut normally undergoes a 270-degree rotation between the 6th and 12th week, when it has fully returned to the abdominal cavity (Fig. 2.26) (84). The point of reference of the rotation is the superior mesenteric artery (Fig. 2.27) (75). This rotation can be divided into two portions: the proximal (or duodenal) and the distal (or colonic) segments. The duodenum starts in the right side and rotates counterclockwise 270 degrees below the superior mesenteric artery to become fixed retroperitoneally in the left upper quadrant at the ligament of Treitz. The colon is located to the left and rotates counterclockwise 270 degrees over the

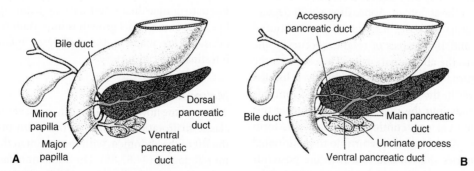

FIGURE 2.24 **A:** The pancreas during the sixth week of development. The ventral pancreatic bud is in close contact with the dorsal pancreatic bud. **B:** Drawing showing the fusion of the pancreatic ducts. The main pancreatic duct enters the duodenum in combination with the bile duct at the major papilla. The accessory pancreatic duct enters the duodenum at the minor papilla. (From Sadler TW. *Langman's medical embryology*, 8th ed. Philadelphia: Lippincott Williams & Wilkins, 2000, with permission.)

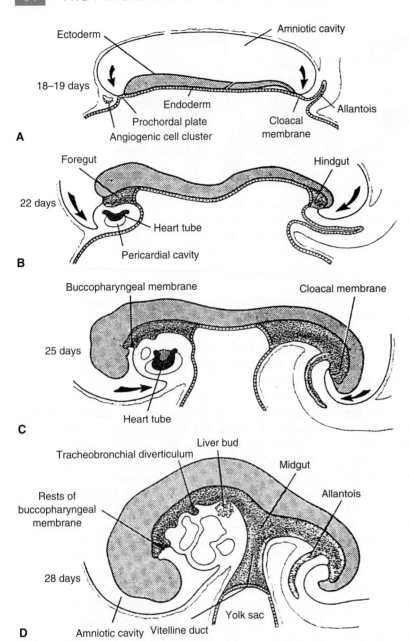

FIGURE 2.25 Schematic drawings of sagittal sections through embryos at various stages of development to demonstrate the effect of the cephalocaudal and lateral flexion on the position of the endoderm lined cavity. Note the formation of the foregut, midgut, and hindgut. **A:** Presomite embryo; **B:** 7-somite embryo; **C:** 14-somite embryo; **D:** at the end of the first month. (From Sadler TW. *Langman's medical embryology*, 8th ed. Philadelphia: Lippincott Williams & Wilkins, 2000, with permission.)

superior mesenteric artery and duodenum to become fixed on the right side of the abdomen. Approximately 90 degrees of this rotation occurs while the intestine is herniated out of the peritoneum, and 180 degrees of rotation occurs as the intestine returns to the abdominal cavity. The cecum is the last portion to return to the abdomen and, initially, is located just below the liver in the right upper quadrant. From this location, it descends into the right iliac fossa. During this time the small intestinal loops continue to elongate and form a number of loops. As the intestine returns to the abdominal cavity the mesenteries shorten and fuse with the posterior parietal peritoneum, resulting in fixing the position of the intestinal loops.

Intestinal length nearly doubles during the last trimester, from approximately 142 cm at 19 to 27 weeks of gestation to 304 cm at term (Fig. 2.28) (85). Patients with short gut syndrome who have undergone repeat surgery have been found to double their intestinal length during the first year of life (86). This normal growth is important to consider when decisions are made as to whether an infant with massive intestinal loss can survive.

Malrotation

Although the normal rotation can arrest at various stages, the classic malrotation consists of the colon malpositioned on the left of the abdomen, with the cecum in the right upper or mid-abdomen (84,87,88). The duodenum fails to undergo its normal counterclockwise rotation posterior to the superior mesenteric artery but rather descends retroperitoneally to the right of the vena cava. Peritoneal bands, known as *Ladd bands*, extend from the cecum and proximal colon across the duodenum to attach to the retroperitoneum on the

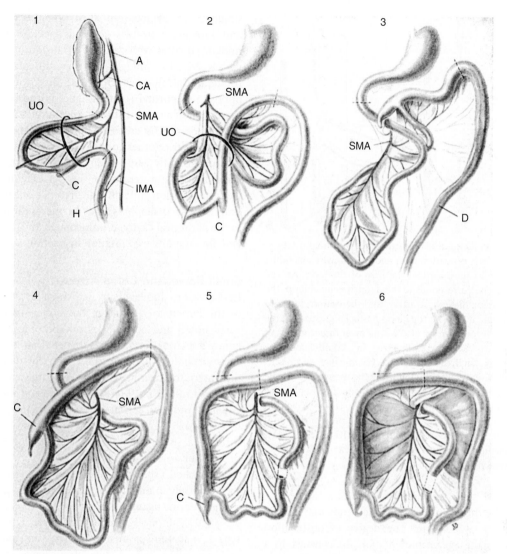

FIGURE 2.26 Schematic drawing of normal development, rotation, and attachment of the midgut. The midgut in each sketch is that part included between the dotted lines and represents that portion of the alimentary tract from duodenum to midtransverse colon that is supplied by the superior mesenteric artery. 1: Age: fifth week of fetal life, lateral view. The foregut, midgut, and hindgut with their respective blood supplies are indicated. Most of the midgut is extruded into the base of the umbilical cord where it normally resides from approximately the 5th to the 10th week. 2: Age: tenth week of fetal life. The intestine is elongating and the hindgut is displaced to the left side of the abdomen. The developing, intra-abdominal intestines come to lie behind the superior mesenteric artery. A portion of the midgut still protrudes through the umbilical orifice into the base of the cord. 3: Age: eleventh week of fetal life. The entire alimentary tract is withdrawn into the abdomen. The cecum lies in the epigastrium, beneath the stomach. 4: Age: late in the 11th week of fetal life. The colon is rotating; the cecum lies in the right upper quadrant of the abdomen. 5: rotation of the colon is complete, and the cecum lies in final position. There is a common mesentery; the mesocolon of the ascending colon is continuous with the mesentery of the ileum. There is no posterior attachment of this common mesentery except at the origin of the superior mesenteric artery. 6: Final stage in attachment of the mesenteries. The ascending and the descending mesocolons become fused to the posterior abdominal wall; thereby the mesentery of the jejunum and ileum gain a posterior attachment from the origin of the superior mesenteric artery obliquely downward to the cecum. *A*, aorta; *C*, cecum; *CA*, celiac axis; *D*, descending colon; *H*, hindgut; *IMA*, inferior mesenteric artery; *SMA*, superior mesenteric artery; *UO*, umbilical orifice. (From Welch KJ, Randolph JG, Ravitch MM, et al. Classification of the abnormalities of intestinal rotation. In: Welch KJ, Randolph JG, Ravitch MM, et al. eds. *Pediatric surgery*, 4th ed. Chicago: Year Book Medical Publishers, 1986:838–848, with permission.)

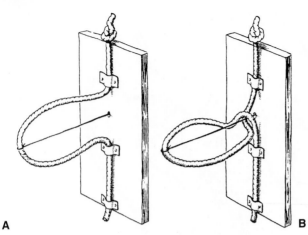

A   **B**

FIGURE 2.27 Mechanical demonstration of intestinal rotation. A rope is attached to a board at both ends with a wire extending at right angles from the board to the base of the loop. **A:** The top limb of the rope corresponds to the duodenojejunal loop; the wire, to the superior mesenteric artery; and the bottom limb, to the cecocolic segment. **B:** The rope loop has been grasped by the hand and rotated through an arc of 270 degrees, or three fourths, of a complete turn around the wire (the axis), in a counterclockwise direction. Therefore, in **B**, the top limb has become the bottom one, and the bottom limb the top. By following the movements of the two limbs around the wire close to the board, one can visualize the process of rotation of the intestine in the embryo. (From Welch KJ, Randolph JG, Ravitch MM, et al. Classification of the abnormalities of intestinal rotation. In: Welch KJ, Randolph JG, Ravitch MM, et al. eds. *Pediatric surgery*, 4th ed. Chicago: Year Book Medical Publishers, 1986:838–848, with permission.)

right side of the duodenum (89). These bands may entrap and obstruct the duodenum. The degree of obstruction is variable as is the age of presentation. In contrast to a duodenal atresia, which presents with a double bubble and no gas beyond the duodenum, an infant with a malrotation typically presents with a double bubble and small amounts of gas scattered beyond the duodenum. The amount of duodenal distention is also less than that seen with duodenal atresia. Although most cases present with signs of obstruction as newborns, 28% present after the neonatal period (90). In older children and adults, malrotation may present in one of three ways: (i) acute intestinal obstruction usually results from obstruction of the duodenum by peritoneal band; (ii) abdominal pain with or without vomiting occurs. The pain typically follows meals and is ascribed to peristaltic rushes in a dilated partially obstructed duodenum. Patients may get relief from the pain by vomiting the bile-stained meal; (iii) chronic diarrhea and malabsorption often with protein-losing enteropathy are present. These symptoms are usually associated with twisting and obstruction of the mesentery, which results in chronic lymphatic obstruction and edema of the bowel wall. This is associated with malabsorption and loss of protein into the intestinal lumen (91).

The entire mesentery of the malrotated midgut is very long and fixed to the retroperitoneum by a small pedicle containing the superior mesenteric artery and vein. This single point of fixation allows the entire small bowel and mesentery to twist on this pedicle, resulting in a midgut volvulus with vascular occlusion of the mesenteric vessels (92). In a midgut volvulus, the gut and mesentery rotate uniformly in a clockwise direction, which is the opposite of normal rotation. The diagnosis and operative correction of a midgut volvulus is a surgical emergency.

Malrotation is associated to a varying degree with a large number of other congenital anomalies (93). However, it is consistently associated with conditions in which the midgut does not return to the peritoneum by the 12th week of gestation and with the presence of gastroschisis and omphalocele. In diaphragmatic hernia, as the midgut returns to the peritoneal cavity, it immediately moves into the chest and does not undergo rotation or fixation.

Small Bowel and Colon Atresia

In contrast to duodenal atresia, which results from a failure of the lumen to recanalize, the lumen of the remaining small bowel and colon does not become obliterated and hence does not recannulate. Instead, atresia of the small intestine and colon occur as the result of a late intrauterine mesenteric occlusion, which results in varying lengths of intestinal infarction. Mesenteric occlusion may result from volvulus, intussusception, internal hernia, complications of meconium ileus, and herniation of the bowel and mesentery through a small abdominal wall defect such as a hernia or umbilical ring defect (94). Louw and Barnard (93) demonstrated a spectrum of intestinal atresia, similar to that seen clinically in infants, that could be produced in puppies by intrauterine ligation of the mesenteric vessels. Louw (75) classified jejunoileal atresia into three types (Fig. 2.29): type 1, a septum or membrane with an intact bowel wall and mesentery; type 2, two atretic ends connected by a fibrous cord and an intact mesentery; and type 3, two atretic ends with no connection and a gap in the mesentery (75). Other authors have added type 3b and type 4 (75,95). Type 3b is characterized by the loss of the majority of the midgut supplied by the superior mesenteric artery (96–98). A short segment of jejunum remains, which is supplied by collaterals from the celiac artery, and a segment of ileum remains, which is supplied by the ileocolic and right colic arteries through anastomotic arcades from the inferior mesenteric artery. The terminal ileum is wrapped in a spiral fashion about the ileocolic vessel. This unusual appearance gives the anomaly the name "apple-peel" or "Christmas-tree" deformity. Type 4 consists of multiple atresias that have the appearance of a "string of sausages" (99,100). Types 3b and 4 both have a familial pattern (101–103). Unlike duodenal atresia, which, most often, is type 1, jejunoileal atresias are most often types 2 and 3. In contrast to duodenal atresia, jejunoileal atresias are thought to occur later in fetal development as an intrauterine accident and are not commonly associated with extraperitoneal anomalies. Jejunoileal atresias are multiple in approximately 10% of cases (104).

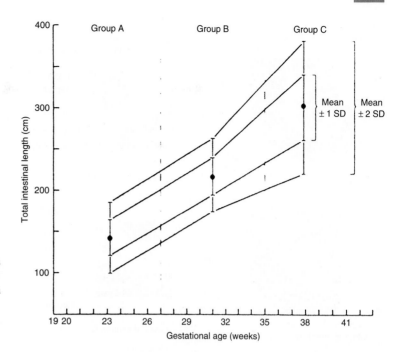

FIGURE 2.28 Mean total intestinal length 1 and 2 standard deviations, calculated by gestational ages from 19 to 27 weeks (Group A), 27 to 35 weeks (Group B), and older than 35 weeks (Group C). (From Touloukian RJ, Walker-Smith GJ. Normal intestinal length in preterm infants. *J Pediatr Surg* 1983;18:720–723, with permission.)

Hindgut

During the third week, because of cephalocaudal and lateral folding of the embryo, a portion of the endoderm-lined yolk sac becomes incorporated into the body of the embryo as the early gut. The tail region of this newly formed canal is the

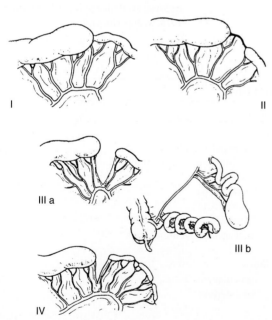

FIGURE 2.29 Classification of intestinal atresia. Type I, mucosal (membranous) atresia with intact bowel wall and mesentery. Type II, blind ends are separated by a fibrous cord. Type IIIa, blind ends are separated by a V-shaped mesenteric defect (gap). Type IIIb, apple-peel atresia. Type IV, multiple atresias (string of sausages). (From Grosfeld JL. Jejunoileal atresia and stenosis. In: Welch KJ, Randolph JG, Ravitch MM, et al. eds. *Pediatric surgery*, 4th ed. Chicago: Year Book Medical Publishers, 1986:838–848, with permission.)

hindgut. In addition, during this time, the hindgut terminates at the cloacal membrane (Fig. 2.30) (13). The caudalmost portion of the hindgut dilates to become the cloaca, which is then divided by a transverse ridge (the urorectal septum) into the urogenital sinus anteriorly and the anorectal canal posteriorly. This occurs by two processes; the first is a downgrowth of Torneaux septum, which stops its cranial to caudal growth at the level of the verumontanum or Müller tubercle. Below this point, the urorectal septum consists of an ingrowth from the lateral walls that fuse in the midline (Rathke fold). The point at which the Torneaux septum joins the Rathke fold is the site at which rectourethral fistulas occur most often in the male fetus (105). The urorectal septum completely separates the primitive rectum and urogenital sinus by the seventh week. Developmental failure of the urorectal septum results in the various fistulae between the rectum and the genitourinary tracts. At this time, the urorectal septum divides the cloacal membrane into an anal membrane and an anterior urogenital membrane. During the ninth week, the anal membrane ruptures at the anal pit to form an opening on to the perineum. Failure of the anal membrane to rupture results in an imperforate anus without a rectogenitourinary fistula. Whereas the proximal portion of the rectum is of endodermal origin and supplied by the inferior mesenteric artery, the distal third forms from ingrowth of ectodermal tissue of the anal pit and is supplied by branches of the internal iliac artery. The columnar endothelium of endodermal origin meets the squamous epithelium of ectodermal origin at the pectinate line.

Anomalies of the hindgut vary from anal stenosis to cloacal anomalies and are frequently associated with urogenital anomalies (Table 2.2) (106). Imperforate anus is a term used to describe a large number of hindgut anomalies characterized by an abnormally located and/or nonpatent anus (Fig. 2.31) (106).

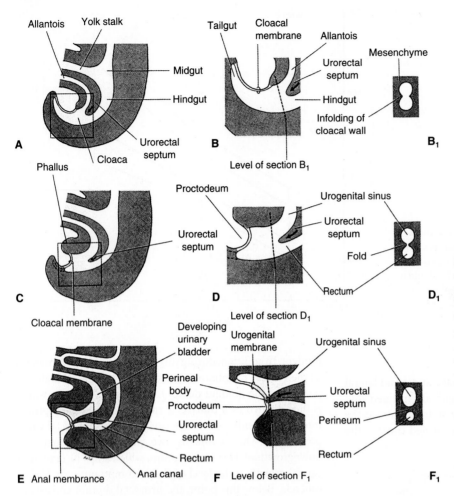

FIGURE 2.30 Drawings illustrating successive stages in the partitioning of the cloaca into the rectum and urogenital sinus by the urorectal septum. **A, C,** and **E** are views from the left side at 4, 6, and 7 weeks, respectively. **B, D,** and **F,** are enlargements of the cloacal region. **B1, D1,** and **F1** are transverse sections through the cloaca at the levels shown in **B, D,** and **F,** respectively. Note that the tailgut (shown in **B**) degenerates and disappears (shown in **C**), as the rectum forms from the dorsal part of the cloaca. (From Moore KL. *The developing human; clinically oriented embryology.* Philadelphia: WB Saunders, 1973, with permission.)

TABLE 2.2

Anatomic Classification of Anorectal Malformations

Female	*Male*
High	High
Anorectal agenesis	Anorectal agenesis
With rectovaginal fistula	With rectoprostatic urethral fistula[a]
Without fistula	Without fistula
Rectal atresia	Rectal atresia
Intermediate	Intermediate
Rectovestibular fistula	Rectobulbar urethral fistula
Rectovaginal fistula	Anal agenesis without fistula
Anal agenesis without fistula	
Low	Low
Anovestibular fistula[a]	Anocutaneous fistula[a]
Anocutaneous fistula[a,b]	Anal stenosis[a,c]
Anal stenosis[c]	
Cloacal malformations[d]	
Rare malformations	Rare malformations

[a]Relatively common lesion.
[b]Includes fistulae occurring at the posterior junction of the labia minora, often fourchette fistulae or vulvar fistulae.
[c]Previously called covered anus.
[d]Previously called rectocloacal fistulae. Entry of the rectal fistula into the cloaca may be high or intermediate, depending on the length of the cloacal canal.
From Welch KJ, Randolph JG, Ravitch MM, et al. eds. *Pediatric surgery,* 4th ed. Chicago: Year Book Medical Publishers, 1986, with permission.

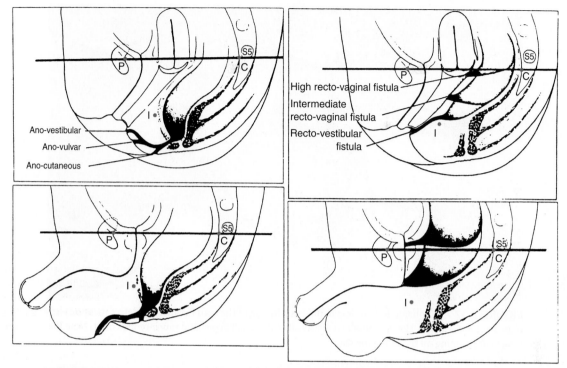

FIGURE 2.31 Imperforate anus and kinds of fistulae. **A:** Low-imperforate anus anomalies in women almost always have an external fistulous tract. The tract is named for the point at which it exits: cutaneous (perineal), vulvar (labia majora), or vestibular (just distal to the hymen). A hemostat placed inside all these fistulous tracts will pass posteriorly before turning cephalad to enter the rectum. **B:** Low-imperforate anus anomalies in the men usually have an external fistulous tract. The tracts are all anocutaneous, but they vary in how far removed the exit site is from the true anus. When the fistula extends up to and along the scrotal raphe, meconium can often be seen through the thin overlying skin. **C:** Intermediate and high-imperforate anus lesions in women are usually associated with a fistula to the posterior vagina. The passage of stool from above the hymen confirms the presence of an intermediate or high lesion. Patients with a vestibular fistula should be carefully evaluated because the underlying rectal pouch may be intermediate and not low. **D:** Intermediate and high-imperforate anus in men is usually associated with a fistula to the urinary tract. Most of these fistulae involve the prostatic urethra; the rectal pouch is therefore high. A few involve the bulbous urethra. Fistulae at this level are usually larger and enter the urethra more obliquely. P, pubis; C, coccyx; S5, 5th sacral vertebra. (From Templeton JM, O'Neill JA. Anorectal malformations. In: Welch KJ, Randolph JG, Ravitch MM, et al. eds. *Pediatric surgery*, 4th ed. Chicago: Year Book Medical Publishers, 1986:1022–1034, with permission.)

ABDOMINAL WALL

Omphalocele

The three embryonic folds that are important in the formation of the developing intestinal tract are also important in the formation of the anterior abdominal wall. Each of these folds is composed of somatic and splanchnic layers (107,108). The somatic layer of the cephalic fold forms the thoracic and epigastric wall and the septum transversum. Developmental failure of this layer results in an epigastric abdominal wall defect referred to as an *epigastric omphalocele*. This is often associated with features of pentalogy of Cantrell, including lower thoracic-wall malformations, anterior diaphragmatic defects (Morgagni hernia), and cardiac anomalies (109). Developmental failure

of the somatic layer of the caudal fold leads to a lower abdominal wall defect, which is referred to as a *hypogastric omphalocele*. This is usually associated with bladder exstrophy. If the splanchnic layer of the caudal fold is involved, the hindgut will be malformed most commonly as an imperforate anus with an intestinal fistula to the open bladder. Failure of the somatic layer of the lateral folds to develop completely and fuse at the umbilical ring causes the umbilical ring to remain open. This allows the extraembryonic coelom to communicate with the intraembryonic coelom and allows herniation of the midgut and, at times the liver, into the extraembryonic coelom (Fig. 2.32). An anomaly in which the umbilical ring is greater than 4 cm is referred to as an *omphalocele*; one smaller than 4 cm and containing only small bowel is referred to as a *hernia of the cord* (110). The herniated viscera are contained

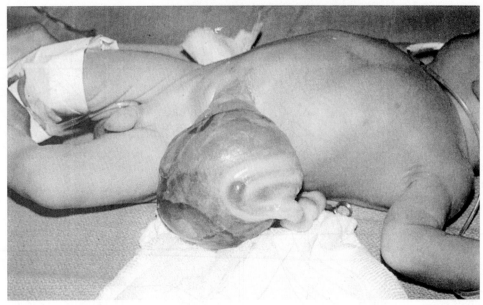

FIGURE 2.32 Omphalocele. This is classified as a hernia of the cord because the defect measures less than 4 cm in diameter. The sac contained nearly all of the small bowel and much of the colon. Note the intact cord coming off the top of the sac.

in a sac consisting of the avascular amniotic membrane that is an extension of the peritoneum.

As described in the section on the midgut, the midgut normally migrates into the cord or extraembryonic coelom during the 5th week and returns to the abdominal cavity by the 11th week. The finding of the gut in the cord after the 12th week by ultrasound is diagnostic of an omphalocele. Between 33% and 50% of infants with omphaloceles have other major anomalies, including cardiac and chromosomal anomalies, and should be evaluated for these. Beckwith-Wiedemann syndrome (omphalocele-macroglossia-gigantism and hypoglycemia) has a high association with hypoglycemia and should be considered in each infant who presents with an omphalocele. With improvements in neonatal care, survival of these infants is now limited only by the associated anomalies. Infants with isolated omphaloceles are expected to survive and develop normally. In infants with a giant omphalocele, in which most of the liver is extracorporeal in the omphalocele sac, the contribution of the liver to chest wall growth is limited. These infants have a narrow chest cavity with associated pulmonary hypoplasia. The severity of the pulmonary hypoplasia significantly impairs any attempt at reduction and closure of the omphalocele. These infants benefit from delayed closure where the amnion omphalocele covering is escharified with topical agents (silver- or iodine-based antibiotic creams) and epithelializes. The omphalocele is then wrapped and gradually reduced over many months as the child grows and the abdominal cavity increases in size.

Gastroschisis

Gastroschisis is a full-thickness defect in the anterior abdominal wall through which the stomach and the midgut herniate (Fig. 2.33). The following characteristics differentiate gastroschisis from omphalocele (111): (i) the abdominal wall defect is nearly always (97%) to the right of an intact umbilical cord; (ii) there is no sac; (iii) the liver and spleen rarely, if ever, herniate through the defect; (iv) the mesentery of the herniated bowel may be obstructed as it passes through the umbilical ring resulting in intrauterine infarction and small bowel atresia in 15% of the cases; and (v) other major congenital malformations are infrequent. Unlike patients with omphaloceles, those with gastroschisis rarely have associated anomalies outside the gastrointestinal tract (112). On the other hand, although malformations of the small bowel are rare in patients with omphalocele, approximately one in five patients with gastroschisis have an associated small bowel atresia (113,114). The jejunoileal atresia is thought to result from mesenteric vascular compromise that occurs as the intestine and mesentery herniate through the small umbilical ring (76,114).

Shaw (114) postulated that gastroschisis is a hernia of the umbilical cord in which rupture or tear of the membrane occurred before closure of the umbilical ring and fixation of the bowel in the peritoneal cavity. The rupture of the umbilical membrane occurs during a normal embryologic phase rather than as the result of a chromosomal or teratologic insult. This would explain the low incidence of associated anomalies. The occurrence to the right of the cord has been postulated to be the result of a weak area of the cord where the right umbilical vein disappears by the seventh week of development. The left vein remains on the left side of the cord and adds support to the left side of the sac in hernias of the cord. Glick et al. (115) have demonstrated the transformation of an antenatally ruptured hernia of the cord into a typical gastroschisis using serial antenatal ultrasound.

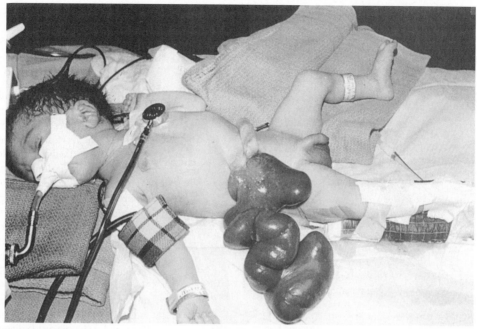

FIGURE 2.33 Gastroschisis. The intestine prolapses through a defect in the abdominal wall to the right of the umbilical cord. The intestine is edematous and appears short. As the inflammation resolves, the intestinal length will be normal.

The amniotic fluid is irritating to the exposed viscera and results in varying amounts of serosal edema and thickening (116,117). The bowel may be matted together, appear short, and exhibit poor peristalsis. It was formerly thought that the degree of serosal reaction corresponded to the length of time the bowel was exposed to the amniotic fluid. However, recent clinical studies with serial antenatal ultrasound examinations have shown poor correlation between the duration of exposure of bowel to amniotic fluid and the extent of serosal change (118). These serosal changes are reversible, once the intestine is returned to the peritoneal cavity and the defect closed shortly after birth (113).

Survival of patients with gastroschisis is approximately 95%. After a period of adaptation—which may last several weeks to allow the intestine to develop normal peristalsis—intestinal function is typically normal. Because there are rarely anomalies of other organ systems, patients with gastroschisis can be expected to grow and develop normally. Those with intestinal atresias may be saddled with the morbidity associated with short bowel syndrome.

UROGENITAL

Both the urinary and genital systems arise from the intermediate mesoderm and the mesodermal ridge from the level of the seventh somite caudad. The process of differentiation begins during the fourth and fifth weeks. The cephalad portions sequentially form the pronephros, then the mesonephros, and finally the metanephros or permanent kidney (Fig. 2.34) (16). The pronephros and mesonephros have degenerated and disappeared by the end of the first

and second months, respectively. The permanent kidney develops from the more caudad mesoderm known as the *metanephric mesoderm*. The collecting ducts form from the ureteric bud, an outgrowth of the mesonephric duct near the cloaca. The ureteric bud forms the major and minor calyces as well as the collecting tubules. The renal tubules continue to form until the end of the fifth month. From the ureteric bud develops the ureter, renal pelvis, calyces, and collecting tubules (Fig. 2.35) (16).

The excretory units develop from a metanephric tissue cap or blastema that forms at the distal end of each collecting tubule. This is known as *nephrogenesis*. Cells from the metanephric cap form small renal vesicles that form tubules, which, along with glomeruli and tufts of capillaries, make up the nephrons, or excretory units. The proximal end of the nephron forms the Bowman capsule. As the tubule lengthens, it forms the proximal convoluted tubule, the loop of Henle, and the distal convoluted tubule, before draining into the collecting tubule. Although development of the collecting system is nearly complete by the 20th week of gestation, nephrogenesis occurs primarily between the 20th and 30th week (Fig. 2.36) (119). Cystic dysplasia appears to be a developmental consequence of obstruction during the development of the excretory units (119).

Initial renal morphogenesis occurs in the area of upper sacral segments, but the kidney undergoes growth in a cranial direction, which is completely in the adult position by the ninth week. As the kidney ascends, it rotates 90 degrees so that the renal pelvis and ureter moves from the ventral to a medial position. If one kidney fails to ascend, it remains in the pelvis close to the iliac artery and is known as a *pelvic kidney*. The kidneys may be pushed together so that the lower

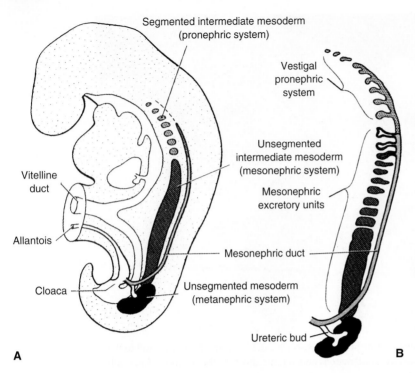

Segmented intermediate mesoderm
(pronephric system)

Vestigal
pronephric
system

Unsegmented
intermediate mesoderm
(mesonephric system)

Mesonephric
excretory units

Vitelline
duct

Allantois

Mesonephric duct

Cloaca

Unsegmented mesoderm
(metanephric system)

Ureteric bud

A

B

FIGURE 2.34 **A:** Schematic diagram showing the relation of the intermediate mesoderm of the pronephric, mesonephric, and metanephric systems. In the cervical and upper thoracic regions, the intermediate mesoderm is segmented; in the lower thoracic, lumbar, and sacral regions it forms a solid, unsegmented mass of tissue, the nephrogenic cord. Note the longitudinal collecting duct, initially formed by the pronephros, but later taken over the mesonephros. **B:** Schematic representation of the excretory tubules of the pronephric and mesonephric systems in a 5-week-old embryo. Note the remnant of the pronephric excretory tubules and longitudinal collecting duct. (From Sadler TW. *Langman's medical embryology*, 8th ed. Philadelphia: Lippincott Williams & Wilkins, 2000, with permission.)

poles fuse, resulting in the formation of a horseshoe kidney. The ascent of a horseshoe kidney is prevented by the root of the inferior mesenteric artery.

During the first year of life, renal function is immature. The glomerular filtration rate is low and the infant's ability to concentrate urine is decreased, which reflects immature tubular function (Table 2.3) (119). During this time, under

normal circumstances, the infant takes in only human milk, which provides a small excretory load. This decreased renal function requires a lower rate of energy expenditure at a time when calories are needed for rapid growth (119). However, the system may not adequately handle the increased excretory load associated with operative or other stress. This low urinary concentrating capacity also makes the infant more

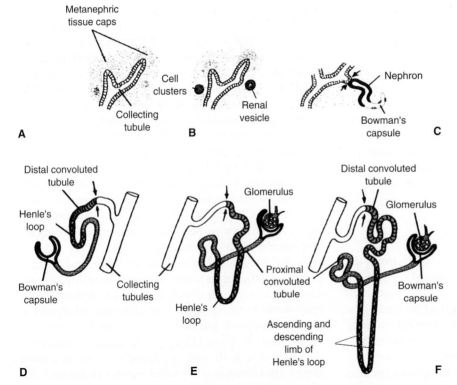

Metanephric
tissue caps

Cell
clusters

Collecting
tubule

A

Renal
vesicle

B

Nephron

Bowman's
capsule

C

Distal convoluted
tubule

Henle's
loop

Bowman's
capsule

Collecting
tubules

Henle's
loop

D

Glomerulus

Proximal
convoluted
tubule

Ascending and
descending
limb of
Henle's loop

E

Distal convoluted
tubule

Glomerulus

Bowman's
capsule

F

FIGURE 2.35 Schematic representation of the development of a metanephric excretory unit. Arrows indicate the place where the excretory unit establishes an open communication with the collecting system, thereby allowing for the flow of urine from the glomerulus into the collecting ducts. (From Sadler TW. *Langman's medical embryology*, 8th ed. Philadelphia: Lippincott Williams & Wilkins, 2000, with permission.)

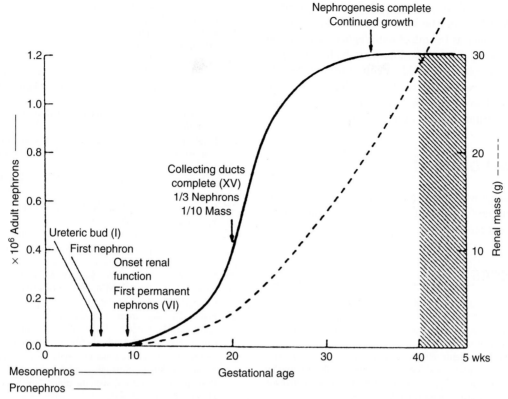

FIGURE 2.36 Fetal renal development is presented schematically. The branching of the collecting system (15 generations) is complete by 20 weeks, but the majority of nephrons and most of the functional mass form in the cortex after 20 weeks. Obstruction interferes with nephrogenesis; relief of obstruction may allow further development. (From Harrison MR, Golbus MS, Filly RA, et al. Management of the fetus with congenital hydronephrosis. *J Pediatr Surg* 1982;17:728–741, with permission.)

TABLE 2.3

Normal Values of Renal Function

	Age of Infant				
	Premature Infant		Term Infant		
	First 3 d	First 3 d	2 Wk	8 Wk	1 Yr
Daily excretion of urine mL/kg/24 h	15–75	20–75	25–120	80–130	40–100
Percentage fluid intake	40–80		50–70	45–65	40–60
Voiding size mL/kg per voiding	4–6	4–6	4–7	4–6	3–6
Maximal urine osmolality mOsmol/kg H$_2$O	400–500	600–800	800–900	1,000–1,200	1,200–1,400
Glomerular filtration rate mL/min per 1.73 m^2	10–15	15–20	35–45	75–80	90–110

From Holliday MA, Vernier RL, Barratt TM, et al. *Pediatric nephrology.* Baltimore: Williams & Wilkins, 1987, with permission.

sensitive to extrarenal water losses and the development of hypertonic dehydration. The newborn is able to dilute the urine so that as much as 165 mL of water/kg/day can be given without developing fluid retention. This high volume of water may be necessary to provide adequate urinary volume for the infant to excrete the solid load, which may result from tissue breakdown following stress or increased calories to satisfy the nutritional needs of the infant.

ACKNOWLEDGMENT

We wish to acknowledge the authors of the earlier editions whose contributions formed the basis for this edition. Also, the editorial assistance of Megan Fitch is appreciated.

REFERENCES

1. Gray SW, Skandalakis JE. *Embryology for surgeons.* Philadelphia: WB Saunders, 1972.
2. Fraser FC. Causes of congenital malformations in human beings. *J Chronic Dis* 1959;10:97–110.
3. Witschi E. Teratogenic effects from overripeness of the egg. In: Fraser FC, McKusick VA, Robinson R, eds. *Congenital malformations, proceedings of the third international conference.* Amsterdam: Excerpta Medica, 1969:157–169.
4. Hertig AT. Traumatic abortion and prenatal death of the embryo. In: Holt LE, Ingalls TH, Hellman LB, eds. *Prematurity, congenital malformation and birth injury.* New York: Association for the Aid of Crippled Children, 1953:174–176.
5. Erhardt CL. Pregnancy losses in New York city. *Am J Public Health* 1963;53:1337–1352.
6. Stickle G. Defective development and reproductive wastage in the United States. *Am J Obstet Gynecol* 1968;100:442–447.
7. Stevenson SS, Worcester J, Rice RG. 677 congenitally malformed infants and associated gestational characteristics. I. General considerations. *Pediatrics* 1950;6:37–50.
8. Smith DW. *Recognizable patterns of human malformation, genetic, embryologic, and clinical aspects,* 2nd ed. Philadelphia: WB Saunders, 1982.
9. Nadler HL, Sacks AJ, Evans MI. Genetics in surgery and prenatal diagnosis. In: Raffensperger JG, ed. *Swenson's pediatric surgery.* Chicago: Appleton, Century, Crofts, 1980.
10. Baraitser M, Winter R. *A colour atlas of clinical genetics.* London: Wolf Medical, 1984.
11. *Human Genome Project Information—SNP Fact Sheet.* Available at: http://www.ornl.gov/sci/techresources/Human_Genome/faq/snps.shtml. Accessed December 29, 2006.
12. Sachidanandam R, Weissman D, Schmidt SC, et al. International SNP Map Working Group. A map of human genome sequence variation containing 1.42 million single nucleotide polymorphisms. *Nature* 2001;409(6822):928–933.
13. Moore KL. *The developing human; clinically oriented embryology.* Philadelphia: WB Saunders, 1973.
14. Streeter GL. Developmental horizons in human embryos: age group XI, 13–20 somites, and age group XII, 21–29 somites. *Contrib Embryol* 1942;30:211.
15. Streeter GL. Developmental horizons in human embryos: age group XIII, embryos 4 or 5 mm long, and age group XIV, indentation of lens vesicle. *Contrib Embryol* 1945;31:26.
16. Sadler TW. *Langman's medical embryology,* 8th ed. Baltimore: Williams & Wilkins, 1996.
17. Seeds JW. Impaired fetal growth: definition and clinical diagnosis. *Obstet Gynecol* 1984;64:303–310.
18. Jones M, Battaglia F. Intrauterine growth retardation. *Am J Obstet Gynecol* 1977;127:540–549.
19. Kennedy WP. Epidemiologic aspects of the problem of congenital malformations. In: Bergsma D, ed. *Birth defects original article series.* New York: Alan R. Liss, 1967:1.
20. McIntosh R, Merritt KK, Richards MR, et al. Incidence of congenital malformations; a study of 5964 pregnancies. *Pediatrics* 1954;14:505–522.
21. Warkany J, Kalter H. Congenital malformations. *N Engl J Med* 1961;265:993.
22. Kalter H, Warkany J. Experimental production of congenital malformations in mammals by metabolic procedure. *Physiol Rev* 1959;39:69.
23. Wilson JG. *Environment and birth defects.* New York: Academic Press, 1973.
24. Wilson JG, Fraser FC. *Handbook of teratology,* Vols. 1–3. New York: Plenum Publishing, 1977.
25. Simmons RL, Sutherland DER, Lower RR, et al. Transplantation. In: Schwartz SI, ed. *Principles of surgery,* 5th ed. New York: McGraw-Hill, 1989:387–458.
26. Kosloske A, Stone HA. Surgical infections. In: Welch KJ, Randolph JG, Ravitch MM, et al. eds. *Pediatric surgery,* 4th ed. Chicago: Year Book Medical Publishers, 1986:78–88.
27. Rosen FS. The immunocompromised child. In: Welch KJ, Randolph JG, Ravitch MM, et al. eds. *Pediatric surgery,* 4th ed. Chicago: Year Book Medical Publishers, 1986:89–95.
28. Hoffman JIE. The circulatory system. In: Rudolph AM, ed. *Pediatrics,* 18th ed. Norwalk: Appleton & Lange, 1987:1219–1358.
29. Rudolph AM. Fetal and neonatal pulmonary circulation. *Ann Rev Physiol* 1979;41:383–395.
30. Anderson KD. Congenital diaphragmatic hernia. In: Welch KJ, Randolph JG, Ravitch MM, et al. eds. *Pediatric surgery,* 4th ed. Chicago: Year Book Medical Publishers, 1986:589–618.
31. Holder TM, Ashcraft KW. Cardiac disease. In: Welch KJ, Randolph JG, Ravitch MM, et al. eds. *Pediatric surgery,* 4th ed. Chicago: Year Book Medical Publishers, 1986:1385–1397.
32. Congdon ED. Transformation of the aortic-arch system during the development of the human embryo. *Contrib Embryol* 1922;14:47–110.
33. Kramer TC. The partitioning of the truncus and conus and the formation of the membranous portion of the interventricular septum in the human heart. *Am J Anat* 1942;71:343–370.
34. Waldhausen JA, Pae WE. Thoracic great vessels. In: Welch KJ, Randolph JG, Ravitch MM, et al. eds. *Pediatric surgery,* 4th ed. Chicago: Year Book Medical Publishers, 1986:1399–1419.
35. Krummel TM, Greenfield LJ, Kirkpatrick BV, et al. Alveolar-arterial oxygen gradients vs neonatal pulmonary insufficiency index for prediction of mortality in ECMO candidates. *J Pediatr Surg* 1984;19:380–384.
36. Fox WW, Duara S. Persistent pulmonary hypertension in the neonate: diagnosis and management. *J Pediatrics* 1983;103:505.
37. Colvin E. Cardiac embryology. In: Garson T, Bricker JT, McNamara DG, eds. *The science and practice of pediatric cardiology.* Philadelphia: Lea & Febiger, 1990:71–108.
38. Van Mierop LHS, Kutsche LM. Anatomy and embryology of the right ventricle. In: Hurst JW, ed. *The heart,* Vol. 1. 6th ed. Chicago: McGraw-Hill, 1986:3–16.
39. Pokorny WJ, Adams JM, McGill CW, et al. Ligation of patent ductus arteriosus in the neonatal intensive care unit. *Mod Probl Paediatr* 1985;23:133–142.
40. *Pediatrics.* Report of the task force on blood pressure control in children. 1977;59(suppl):799.
41. de Sweit M, Fayers P, Shinebourne EA. Systolic blood pressure in a population of infants in the first year of life: the Brompton study. *Pediatrics* 1980;65:1028–1035.
42. Hennekens CH, Jesse JM, Klein BE, et al. Aggregation of blood pressure in infants and their siblings. *Am J Epidemiol* 1976;103:457.

43. Greenwood RD, Rosenthal A. Cardiovascular malformations associated with tracheoesophageal fistula and esophageal atresia. *Pediatrics* 1976;57:87–91.

44. Streeter GL. Development horizons in human embryos. *Contrib Embryol* 1948;32:133–203.

45. Smith EI. The early development of the trachea and esophagus in relation to atresia of the esophagus and tracheoesophageal fistula. *Embryology* 1957;36:41.

46. DeLorimier AA. Congenital malformations and neonatal problems of the respiratory tract. In: Welch KJ, Randolph JG, Ravitch MM, et al. eds. *Pediatric surgery*, 4th ed. Chicago: Year Book Medical Publishers, 1986:631–644.

47. Randolph JG. Esophageal atresia and congenital stenosis. In: Welch KJ, Randolph JG, Ravitch MM, et al. eds. *Pediatric surgery*, 4th ed. Chicago: Year Book Medical Publishers, 1986:682–694.

48. Zeltner TB, Burri PH. The postnatal development and growth of the human lung. II. Morphology. *Respir Physiol* 1987;67:269–282.

49. Tooley WH. The respiratory system. In: Rudolph AM, ed. *Pediatrics*, 18th ed. Norwalk: Appleton & Lange, 1987:1359–1446.

50. Inselman LS, Mellins RB. Growth and development of the lung. *J Pediatr* 1981;98:1–15.

51. O'Brodovich HM, Huddad GG. The functional basis of respiratory pathology. In: Chernick V, Kendig EL, eds. *Kendig's disorders of the respiratory tract in children*, 5th ed. Philadelphia: WB Saunders, 1990.

52. Bucher U, Reid L. Development of the intrasegmental bronchial tree: the pattern of branching and development of cartilage of various stages of intrauterine life. *Thorax* 1961;16:207–218.

53. Burri PH. Fetal and postnatal development of the lung. *Ann Rev Physiol* 1984;46:617–628.

54. Heithoff KN, Sane SM, Williams HG, et al. Bronchopulmonary foregut malformations. *Am J Radiol* 1976;126:46–55.

55. Stocker JT, Madewell JE, Drake RM. Congenital cystic adenomatoid malformation of the lung. *Hum Pathol* 1977;8:155–171.

56. Side RM, Clouse M, Ellis FH. The spectrum of pulmonary sequestration. *Ann Thorac Surg* 1974;18:644–658.

57. Fowler CL, Pokorny WJ, Wagner ML, et al. Review of bronchopulmonary foregut malformations. *J Pediatr Surg* 1988;23:793–797.

58. Wells LJ. Development of the human diaphragm and pleural sacs. *Contrib Embryol* 1954;35:107.

59. DeLorimier AA, Tierney DF, Parker HR. Hypoplastic lungs in fetal lambs with surgically produced congenital diaphragmatic hernia. *Surgery* 1967;62:12.

60. Ohi R, Suzuki H, Kato T, et al. Development of the lung in fetal rabbits with experimental diaphragmatic hernia. *J Pediatr Surg* 1976;11:955.

61. Starrett RW, deLorimier AA. Congenital diaphragmatic hernia in lambs: hemodynamic and ventilatory changes with breathing. *J Pediatr Surg* 1975;10:575.

62. Comer TP, Clagett OT. Surgical treatment of hernia of the foramen of Morgagni. *Thorac Cardiovasc Surg* 1966;62:461–468.

63. Pokorny WJ, McGill CW, Harberg FJ. Morgagni hernias during infancy: presentation and associated anomalies. *J Pediatr Surg* 1984;19:394–397.

64. Berdon WE, Baker DH, Amoury RA. The role of pulmonary hyperplasia in the prognosis of infants with diaphragmatic hernia and eventration. *Am J Roentgenol* 1968;103:413.

65. Haller JA, Rickard LR, Tepas JJ, et al. Management of diaphragmatic paralysis in infants with special emphasis on selection of patients for operative plication. *J Pediatr Surg* 1979;14:779.

66. McNamara JJ, Paulson DJ, Urschel HC, et al. Eventration of the diaphragm. *Surgery* 1968;64:1013.

67. Gross RE. *The surgery of infancy and childhood*. Philadelphia: WB Saunders, 1953.

68. Waterson DJ, Bonham Carter RE, Aberdeen E. Oesophageal atresia, tracheoesophageal fistula—a study of survival in 218 infants. *Lancet* 1962;1:819.

69. Barry JE, Auldist AW. The VATER association: one end of a spectrum of anomalies. *Am J Dis Child* 1984;128:769.

70. Quan L, Smith DW. The VATER association. *J Pediatr* 1973;82:104–107.

71. Andrassy RJ, Mahour H. Gastrointestinal anomalies associated with esophageal atresia or tracheoesophageal fistula. *Arch Surg* 1979;114:1125–1128.

72. Tandler J. Zur entwicklungsgeschichte des menschlichen duodenums. *Morphol Jahrbuch* 1902;29:187.

73. Harberg FJ, Pokorny WJ, Hahn H. Congenital duodenal obstruction: a review of 65 cases. *Am J Surg* 1979;138:825–828.

74. Grosfeld JL. Jejunoileal atresia and stenosis. In: Welch KJ, Randolph JG, Ravitch MM, et al. eds. *Pediatric surgery*, 4th ed. Chicago: Year Book Medical Publishers, 1986:838–848.

75. Louw JH. Resection and end-to-end anastomosis in the management of atresia and stenosis of the small bowel. *Surgery* 1967;62:940.

76. DeLorimier AA, Fonkalsrud EW, Hays DM. Congenital atresia and stenosis of the jejunum and ileum. *Surgery* 1969;65:819.

77. Lecco TM. Zur morphologie des pankreas annulare. *Sitzungsb Akad Wissensch Cl* 1910;119:391.

78. Sibley WL. Meckel's diverticulum: dyspepsia Meckeli from heterotopic gastric mucosa. *Arch Surg* 1944;49:156–166.

79. Soltero MJ, Bill AH. The natural history of Meckel's diverticulum. *Ann Surg* 1937;105:44–55.

80. Soderland S. Meckel's diverticulum, a clinical and histologic study. *Acta Chir Scand Suppl* 1959;248:13–233.

81. Benson CD. Surgical implications of Meckel's diverticulum. In: Ravitch MM, Welch KJ, Benson DC, et al. eds. *Pediatric surgery*, 3rd ed. Chicago: Year Book Medical Publishers, 1979:955–960.

82. Amoury RA. Meckels diverticulum. In: Welch KJ, Randolph JG, Ravitch MM, et al. eds. *Pediatric surgery*, 4th ed. Chicago: Year Book Medical Publishers, 1986:859–867.

83. Snyder WH, Chaffin L. Embryology and pathology of the intestinal tract: presentation of 48 cases of malrotation. *Ann Surg* 1954;140:368–380.

84. Touloukian RJ, Walker-Smith GJ. Normal intestinal length in preterm infants. *J Pediatr Surg* 1983;18:720–723.

85. Pokorny WJ, Fowler CL. Isoperistaltic intestinal lengthening for short bowel syndrome. *Surg Gynecol Obstet* 1991;172:39–43.

86. Mall FP. Development of the human intestine and its position in the adult. *Int Abstr Surg* 1956;103:417–438.

87. Holder TM, Cloud DT, Lewis JE, et al. Esophageal atresia and tracheoesophageal fistula. A survey of its members by the Surgical Section of the American Academy of Pediatrics. *Pediatrics* 1961;34:542.

88. Ladd WE. Surgical diseases of the alimentary tract in infants. *N Engl J Med* 1936;215:705.

89. Brandt ML, Pokorny WJ, McGill CW, et al. Late presentations of midgut malrotation in children. *Am J Surg* 1985;150:767–771.

90. Stewart DR, Colodny AL, Daggett WC. Malrotation of the bowel in infants and children: a 15 year review. *Surgery* 1976;79:716–720.

91. Dott NM. Anomalies of intestinal rotation: their embryology and surgical aspects, with report of 5 cases. *Br J Surg* 1923;11:251–286.

92. Filston HC, Kirks DR. Malrotation—the ubiquitous anomaly. *J Pediatr Surg* 1981;16:614–620.

93. Louw JH, Barnard CN. Congenital intestinal atresia: observations on its origin. *Lancet* 1955;2:1065.

94. Langman J. *Medical embryology*, 3rd ed. Baltimore: Williams & Wilkins, 1975:245.

95. Weitzman JJ, Vanderhoof RS. Jejunal atresia with agenesis of the dorsal mesentery with "Christmas tree" deformity of the small intestine. *Am J Surg* 1966;111:443.

96. Zerella JT, Martin LW. Jejunal atresia with absent mesentery and a helical ileum. *Surgery* 1976;80:550.

97. Zwiren GT, Andrews HG, Ahmann P. Jejunal atresia with agenesis of the dorsal mesentery ("apple-peel small bowel"). *J Pediatr Surg* 1972;7:414.

98. Hays DM. Intestinal atresia and stenosis. *Curr Probl Surg* 1969;1:3–48.

99. Rittenhouse EA, Beckwith JB, Chappell JS, et al. Multiple septa of the small bowel: description of an unusual case with review of the literature and consideration of etiology. *Surgery* 1972; 71:371.

100. Guttman FN, Braun P, Garance PH, et al. Multiple atresias and a new syndrome of hereditary multiple atresias involving the gastrointestinal tract from stomach to rectum. *J Pediatr Surg* 1974;8:633.

101. Blyth H, Dickson JAS. Apple peel syndrome (congenital intestinal atresia): a family study of 7 index patients. *J Med Genet* 1969;6:275.

102. Seashore J, Collins F, Markwitz R, et al. Familial apple peel jejunal atresia: surgical, genetic and radiologic aspects. *Pediatrics* 1987;80:540.

103. Grosfeld JL. Alimentary tract obstruction in the newborn. *Curr Probl Pediatr* 1975;5:3–47.

104. Stephens FD, Smith ED. *Anorectal malformations in children*. Chicago: Year Book Medical Publishers, 1971.

105. Templeton JM, O'Neill JA. Anorectal malformations. In: Welch KJ, Randolph JG, Ravitch MM, et al. eds. *Pediatric surgery*, 4th ed. Chicago: Year Book Medical Publishers, 1986:1022–1034.

106. Duhamel B. Embryology of exomphalos and allied malformations. *Arch Dis Child* 1963;38:142–147.

107. Hutchin P. Somatic anomalies of the umbilicus and anterior abdominal wall. *Surg Gynecol Obstet* 1965;170:1075.

108. Cantrell JR, Haller JA, Ravitch MM. A syndrome of congenital defects involving the abdominal wall, sternum, diaphragm, pericardium and heart. *Surg Gynecol Obstet* 1958;107:602.

109. Benson CD, Penherthy GC, Hill EJ. Hernia into the umbilical cord and omphalocele (amniocele) in the newborn. *Arch Surg* 1949;58:833.

110. Schwaitzberg SD, Pokorny WJ, McGill CW, et al. Gastroschisis and omphalocele. *Am J Surg* 1982;144:650–654.

111. Pokorny WJ, Harberg FJ, McGill CW. Gastroschisis complicated by intestinal atresia. *J Pediatr Surg* 1981;16:261–263.

112. Schuster SR. Omphalocele and gastroschisis. In: Welch KJ, Randolph JG, Ravitch MM, et al. eds. *Pediatric surgery*, 4th ed. Chicago: Year Book Medical Publishers, 1986:740–763.

113. Moore TC. Gastroschisis and omphalocele: clinical difference. *Surgery* 1977;82:561.

114. Shaw A. The myth of gastroschisis. *J Pediatr Surg* 1975;10:235–244.

115. Glick LG, Harrison MR, Azick NS, et al. The missing link in the pathogenesis of gastroschisis. *J Pediatr Surg* 1985;20:406–409.

116. Moore TC. Gastroschisis with antenatal evisceration of intestines and urinary bladder. *Ann Surg* 1963;158:263.

117. Bond SJ, Harrison MR, Filly RA, et al. Severity of intestinal damage in gastroschisis: correlation with prenatal sonographic findings. *J Pediatr Surg* 1988;23:520–525.

118. Harrison MR, Golbus MS, Filly RA, et al. Management of the fetus with congenital hydronephrosis. *J Pediatr Surg* 1982;17:728–7741.

119. Holliday MA, Barratt TM, Vernier RL, eds. *Pediatric nephrology*. Baltimore: Williams & Wilkins, 1987.

CHAPTER 3

Fluids and Electrolytes

Andrew Z. Fenves, Archana Rao, and Michael Emmett

Fluid and electrolyte management in the surgical patient has become increasingly important over the last several decades. The advance of medical science and improved surgical techniques have allowed us to operate on higher risk patients; close attention to fluid balance constitutes a critical aspect of the care of these patients. This chapter focuses on the changes in fluid homeostasis and electrolyte balance that occur in the peri- and postoperative period. We will also review treatment options.

NORMAL FLUID SPACES AND DYNAMICS

In critically ill patients, the alteration in fluid balance is a dynamic process characterized by major hemodynamic changes and fluid shifts between body compartments. The extent of these changes is a function of the severity of the underlying disease process. Close monitoring of these fluid shifts helps the clinician to gauge the clinical course of the patient. Knowledge of the normal fluid distribution of the body is necessary to understand these changes.

In a normal human, approximately 60% of the total body weight is water (e.g., 42 L in a 70-kg man and slightly less in women). Approximately, two thirds of this fluid resides inside cells and is called *intracellular fluid* (ICF). The remaining one third of the water, the extracellular fluid (ECF), is outside the cells. The ECF is further separated into two compartments; the vascular compartment (plasma fluid) constitutes approximately one third of the ECF, and the fluid present between cells (interstitial fluid) constitutes approximately two thirds of the ECF. Within the vascular compartment (e.g., 4.6 L in the 70-kg man), approximately 85% of the fluid resides in the venous side of the circulation and 15% in the arterial side.

A number of forces govern the movement of fluid between, and the relative volumes of, the interstitial space and the vascular compartment. In the capillaries, a balance of forces exists between hydrostatic and oncotic pressure.

This concept is expressed mathematically by the Starling equation:

$$Qf = Kf \times (Pv - Pt) - \delta \times (COP - TOP)$$

where Qf is fluid flux, Kf is capillary filtration coefficient, Pv is vascular hydrostatic pressure, Pt is interstitial hydrostatic pressure, δ is a reflection coefficient (which defines the effectiveness of the membrane in preventing solute flow), COP is colloid osmotic pressure, and TOP is tissue osmotic pressure (1). Fluid leaves the capillary at the arterial end because hydrostatic pressure exceeds oncotic pressure. As blood continues to flow down the capillary, hydrostatic pressure falls and oncotic pressure increases as a result of increasing protein concentration. When the oncotic pressure exceeds the hydrostatic pressure—in the venous end of the capillary—fluid returns from the interstitium to the capillary. Some of the fluid that is not returned to the venous end of the capillaries by virtue of the Starling forces is eventually returned to the vascular compartment by lymphatic drainage. Under some circumstances, lymphatic flow can be massive. For example, in cirrhotic patients, hepatic fibrosis leads to high capillary hydrostatic pressures, which, in conjunction with low capillary oncotic pressures due to hypoalbuminemia, cause a 20-fold increase in daily lymphatic flow (from 1 to 20 L/d) (2). Serum albumin is the major determinant of capillary COP, and hypoalbuminemia can lead to excess transudation of fluid from the vascular to the interstitial compartment. As discussed later, this is one of the more important factors contributing to the development of interstitial edema and expansion of ECF volume in the surgical patient.

POSTOPERATIVE CHANGES IN BODY FLUID COMPARTMENTS

A number of perioperative events contribute to ECF volume expansion. These nonspecific events also occur with many other pathologic conditions such as sepsis, extensive burns, multiple trauma, pancreatitis, bone marrow transplants and so on. A major stimulus to ECF expansion is a reduced intravascular volume. First, hemorrhage may directly reduce blood volume. Second, a generalized increase in capillary permeability occurs in many patients, especially after major abdominal and chest surgery. This results from a loss of endothelial integrity and the opening of intercellular clefts. The mediators that cause increased capillary permeability are probably identical to those responsible for some elements of the inflammatory response. These include, but may not be limited to, cytokines (interleukin 1, interleukin 6, tumor necrosis factor), integrins, thrombin, bradykinin, and platelet-activating factor (1). As a result of increased capillary permeability, protein-rich fluid escapes from the vascular compartment and expands the interstitial fluid. Third, negative interstitial fluid hydrostatic pressure may develop and *increase* the intravascular to interstitial pressure gradient generating interstitial edema (3).

The above alterations lead to reduced cardiac output and decreased effective blood volume. The sensors for effective blood volume are in the intra-arterial side of the intravascular compartment. In response to these signals, volume is regulated by modulation of renal sodium and water reabsorption. A decrease in cardiac output, increase in peripheral arterial vasodilation, or any combination thereof leads to arterial underfilling, and thereby initiates and sustains a sodium- and water-retaining state (4).

Failure to maintain adequate intravascular volume leads to systemic hypoperfusion, decreased oxygen delivery, lactic acidosis, and ultimately tissue death. Therefore, it is imperative to replace intravascular volume with appropriate amounts of colloid and crystalloid. The aim is to maintain a systolic blood pressure above 100 mm Hg, and a urinary output of approximately 30–50 mL/h. However, in some patients, aggressive volume expansion markedly increases ECF volume, while producing only a limited increase in the intravascular volume. Under these circumstances, avid renal sodium and water retention persists because the effective blood volume remains low. Indeed, increases in body weight of 10% to 30% are common after major surgery, trauma, or sepsis. Bock et al. found a 55% expansion of the interstitial compartment following the resuscitation of severely traumatized patients with isotonic salt solution (5). Generalized pitting edema indicates an excess of ECF, but the intravascular volume may be decreased, normal, or increased. Intravascular volume status should be estimated whether generalized edema is present or not.

No known direct treatment can reverse the increased capillary permeability that develops in such patients. As patients recuperate from their underlying illness, the "capillary leak" resolves. Although substances that counteract the proinflammatory mediators could theoretically attenuate this pathologic state, none have proved to be effective. As long as clinical parameters suggest low effective intravascular volume, the best approach is the judicious administration of balanced electrolyte solutions and colloid to expand this compartment. Acceptable cardiac output and tissue

perfusion remain the paramount concerns, even at the price of a marked increase in ECF and total body weight. In the severely anemic or bleeding patient, blood transfusions are used to expand intravascular volume and improve tissue oxygen delivery. To optimize intravascular volume replacement, pulmonary arterial pressure monitoring can be accomplished through a Swan-Ganz catheter, which measures pulmonary capillary wedge pressure and cardiac output. A pulmonary capillary wedge pressure of 16 to 18 mm Hg and a stable blood pressure is consistent with optimal fluid resuscitation in the patient with normal cardiac function. When the pulmonary capillary wedge pressure rises above 18 mm Hg, the rate of fluid infusion should be decreased to reduce the risk of pulmonary edema.

Adult respiratory distress syndrome (ARDS) may develop as a consequence of major surgical procedures, sepsis, burns, or multiple trauma. ARDS is a state of noncardiogenic pulmonary edema stemming from pulmonary capillary endothelial damage and functional disruption of the capillary–alveolar epithelial permeability barrier (6). Endothelial injury favors the exudation of the protein-rich fluid into the interstitial spaces of the lungs and fluid accumulated in the alveoli. Patients with ARDS may require lower pulmonary capillary wedge pressures, in the range of 10 to 12 mm Hg, to reduce pulmonary congestion and facilitate hemoglobin oxygenation.

Another indirect measure of intravascular volume status is the fractional excretion of sodium calculated from measurements of sodium and creatinine in urine and blood.

$$\frac{U_{Na} \times P_{cr}}{U_{cr} \times P_{Na}} \times 100 = FeNa$$

where U_{Na} = urinary sodium; U_{cr} = urinary creatinine; P_{cr} = plasma creatinine; P_{Na} = plasma sodium.

When patients develop oliguria, usually defined as a urine output of less than 600 mL of urine per 24 hours, distinguishing between intrinsic acute renal failure and intravascular volume depletion or prerenal renal dysfunction is critical. A fractional excretion of sodium lower than 1% in this setting suggests intravascular (absolute or relative, i.e., effective) volume contraction and renal hypoperfusion. As long as renal function is normal, the kidneys will retain salt and water until intravascular volume is optimized.

Resuscitation fluids can be divided into two groups: colloid and crystalloid. Colloid refers to albumin or protein solutions (i.e., plasmanate) or synthetic hydroxy ethyl starch (hetastarch). Crystalloid refers to salt solutions such as normal saline or Ringers lactate solution. A larger volume of crystalloid than colloid is required to produce an equal expansion of the ECF. Albumin solutions are much more expensive, and usually offer little advantage over synthetic colloid solutions.

A recent multicenter trial comparing the use of albumin versus saline found no difference in overall mortality between the patients treated with either crystalloid or colloid (7). In the subset of trauma patients, however, they found a trend toward better outcomes with crystalloid (i.e., saline). Among the crystalloid solutions, one could use normal saline or

TABLE 3.1

Composition and Osmolality of Intravenous Solutions

	Na (mEq/L)	Cl (mEq/L)	Glucose (gm/L)	Osmolality (mOsm/kg)
Ringers lactate[a]	130	109	—	272
0.9% NaCl (normal saline)	154	154	—	308
0.45% NaCl (1/2 normal saline)	77	77	—	154
5% D/W	—	—	50	252
10% D/W	—	—	100	505
50% D/W	—	—	500	2520
3% NaCl (hypertonic saline)	513	513	—	1026

[a]Also contains K^+ (4 mEq/L), Ca^{2+} (3 mEq/L), and lactate (28 mEq/L).
D/W, dextrose in water.

Ringers lactate. Table 3.1 depicts the electrolyte composition and osmolality of various intravenous solutions.

Although it is tempting to use diuretics during the early phase of resuscitation of oliguric critically ill patients, oliguria in this early phase may be appropriate and may simply reflect decreased intravascular volume and cardiac output. In that case, diuretics are contraindicated because they could further reduce circulatory volume, peripheral perfusion, and thereby contribute to the development of lactic acidosis and acute renal failure.

Diuretics are appropriate when cardiogenic pulmonary edema develops following aggressive fluid resuscitation or when progressive ARDS occurs. Also, during the recovery phase, a large amount of interstitial fluid may reenter the intravascular compartment leading to pulmonary edema. Diuretics may then be required. Generally, loop diuretics are selected because they are most potent. Loop diuretics have several important beneficial effects: (i) they inhibit active sodium absorption in the thick ascending limb of Henle; (ii) they increase blood flow to the kidney by stimulating vasodilatory prostaglandins; and (iii) they increase venous capacitance, which can quickly relieve pulmonary edema, even before diuresis and natriuresis have occurred. Loop diuretics, such as furosemide or bumetanide, are extensively protein bound and must reach their intratubular site of action through active proximal tubular secretion. Usually, they are administered as intermittent intravenous boluses every 4 to 12 hours. When patients are found to be resistant to bolus doses of loop diuretics, continuous intravenous infusion may be used; for example, bumetanide may be infused at a dose of 0.5 to 1.0 mg/h. This method of administration can produce as much as a 30% increase in urine volume compared with conventional intermittent intravenous doses. A schematic representation of the human nephron is depicted in Figure 3.1 showing the primary site of action of various diuretics.

The role of low-dose intravenous dopamine in postoperative fluid management remains controversial. Some advocate the continuous infusion of dopamine at a dose of 1 to 2 μg/kg/min to cause an increase in the cortical perfusion of the kidney and thereby an increased urinary output (i.e., "renal dose dopamine"). This effect occurs by both increased cardiac output and renal vasodilation. It also directly inhibits renal tubular sodium reabsorption. The major potential side effect of dopamine is tachycardia, and occasionally tachyarrhythmias, myocardial ischemia, and even intestinal ischemia may occur. It may be used when diuresis is needed and diuretics alone are not producing an adequate effect.

There is also a strong tendency by some clinicians to use low-dose dopamine therapy to try to prevent postoperative acute renal failure. However, there is a growing body of evidence that this therapy does not confer clinically significant protection from renal dysfunction in critically ill patients (8,9). Furthermore, at higher doses (between 2 and 5 μg/kg/min) dopamine binds to β-adrenergic and α-receptors so that urine output may decrease as a result of "pressor-like" effects.

Hemodialysis or peritoneal dialysis should be considered if pulmonary edema exists and the maneuvers described in the preceding text are ineffective. Peritoneal dialysis removes volume much slower than hemodialysis, and the initial instillation of fluid into the abdomen may compromise respiratory status as the diaphragm is forced upward. In addition, peritoneal dialysis may not be feasible after major abdominal procedures. Hemodialysis, on the other hand, may be less well tolerated hemodynamically and can produce hypotension and cardiac arrhythmias.

Recently, continuous forms of renal replacement therapy have been advocated by several investigators. These include several different modalities such as continuous arteriovenous hemodialysis (CAVHD) and continuous venovenous hemodialysis (CVVHD). The presumed benefits of continuous renal replacement therapy (CRRT) include improved solute removal, improved fluid management, and less hemodynamic instability (10). There is increasing evidence that in selected patients with severe acute renal failure in the postoperative setting CRRT may lead to improved survival.

In summary, appropriate peri- and postoperative fluid management is critically important. Effective arterial blood volume must be optimized, even at the price of an

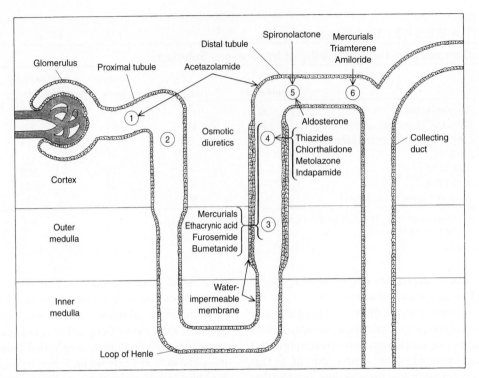

FIGURE 3.1 Diuretics primarily inhibit tubular reabsorption of sodium to increase excretion. However, other tubular functions are also affected at the discrete sites along the nephron where diuretics act. Therefore, the proximal tubule is sensitive to diuretics inhibiting carbonic anhydrase and hydrogen ion section *1*. Proximal-acting diuretics increase delivery of sodium and water to the ascending limb of Henle and more distal nephron and ultimately increase free water reabsorption or production, depending on antidiuretic hormone (ADH) activity or its absence. An osmotic diuretic (e.g., mannitol) acting in the proximal tubule *2* would also enhance free water reabsorption or production. If a diuretic works in the medullary diluting segment of the ascending limb *3*, it inhibits sodium chloride reabsorption at a site where major free water generation would also be inhibited. At the same time, such an agent impedes delivery of osmotically active material into the medullary interstitium, impairing its ability to reabsorb free water. A diuretic acting solely in the cortical diluting segment *4* affects free water production but not reabsorption. Diuretics that enhance sodium passage proximal to the distal nephron will enhance potassium secretion, thereby increasing potassium loss. Diuretics acting in the distal tubule conserve potassium either by inhibiting the action of the aldosterone *5* or independently of aldosterone *6*. (From Thier SO. Diuretic mechanism as a guide to therapy. *Hosp Pract* 1987;7:69, with permission.)

expanded ECF volume and increased total body weight. Close monitoring of the intravascular compartment permits the physician to adjust to the various stages of recovery and the dynamic fluid shifts between compartments.

ELECTROLYTE DISTURBANCES

Electrolyte disturbances occur commonly in the postoperative patient and may produce significant morbidity and mortality. This section focuses on hypo- and hypernatremia, hypo- and hyperkalemia, hypomagnesemia, and hypocalcemia. Metabolic alkalosis will also be discussed.

Hyponatremia

Hyponatremia is one of the most frequent electrolyte abnormalities that occur in hospitalized patients. Hyponatremia is usually equated with hypo-osmolality with two exceptions.

Pseudohyponatremia results when some unusual biochemical abnormality interferes with correct measurement of the sodium concentration. For example, marked hyperlipidemia or hyperproteinemia displaces water and generates measured hyponatremia with flame photometry. Introduction of newer instruments using direct ion-selective electrodes has eliminated many of these problems. Hyponatremia can also be produced by very high concentrations of glucose, mannitol, glycine, or the presence of other impermeant solutes, which can shift water from the intracellular to the extracellular space and thereby dilute other ECF solutes.

If these problems are excluded, hyponatremia usually indicates hypo-osmolality. Plasma osmolality can be measured directly by an osmometer or estimated using the following equation:

$$P_{osm} = 2 \times Na(mEq/L) + \frac{glucose(mg\%)}{18} + \frac{BUN(mg\%)}{2.8}$$

Where BUN stands for blood urea nitrogen. Usually, simply doubling the serum sodium concentration gives a good approximation of the plasma osmolality.

Hypo-osmolality indicates excess water relative to solute in the ECF. Water moves freely across most cell membranes so the ICF and ECF will have the same osmolality. Therefore, hypo-osmolality in the plasma equals hypo-osmolality in the ICF. In general, intracellular hypo-osmolality is caused by increased intracellular water, i.e., cell swelling, rather than reduced intracellular solute.

Hyponatremia develops in 4% to 5% of all postoperative patients (conversely, approximately 25% of all episodes of hospital-acquired hyponatremia affect postoperative patients) (11). In most cases, the serum sodium concentration falls between 125 and 140 mEq/L, and these patients are generally asymptomatic. When the serum sodium falls below 125 mEq/L, clinical signs and symptoms may occur. These include headache, nausea, lethargy, hallucinations, seizures, hypothermia, bradycardia, hypoventilation, and occasionally coma.

One of the most important factors contributing to the development of hyponatremia in the perioperative period is persistent secretion of antidiuretic hormone (ADH). Usually, the osmolality of the ECF is the major factor controlling ADH secretion. Hyperosmolality stimulates ADH, whereas hypo-osmolality is a potent inhibitor. However, some nonosmotic stimuli can override the inhibition produced by hypo-osmolality. Potent nonosmotic stimuli to ADH include intravascular volume depletion, nausea, anxiety, pain, and potent narcotics. All these factors contribute to postoperative "inappropriate" (for osmolality) ADH secretion. Postoperative ADH levels are 5- to 50-fold higher than preoperative values (12). ADH levels generally decline to control values by the third to fifth postoperative day. A second important factor contributing to postoperative hyponatremia is decreased renal function. Postoperative hypotension decreases the glomerular filtration rate (GFR), which in turn reduces fluid delivery to the distal nephron. This limits the renal capacity to excrete free water and sets the stage for hyponatremia. The functional processes for regulation of salt and water transport are illustrated schematically in Figure 3.2.

A third factor contributing to postoperative hyponatremia is the administration of excessive free water in the form of hypotonic intravenous fluids. The perioperative patient with elevated ADH levels and decreased renal perfusion is likely to retain hypotonic intravenous fluids and thereby develop hyponatremia. Women in their reproductive years seem to be unusually susceptible to the neurologic complications of hyponatremia. As little as 3 L of intravenous water over 36 hours can lead to devastating symptoms of hyponatremia, severe neurologic morbidity, and death (13,14). Although the exact mechanism responsible for this unusual syndrome has not been fully elucidated, the administration of hypotonic fluid perioperatively has clearly played a major role. In high-risk patients, only isotonic fluids should be used, and the serum sodium should be evaluated frequently.

Another important, often overlooked hyponatremic syndrome occurs in patients undergoing a transurethral prostate resection (15). During this procedure, the prostatic bed is irrigated with large volumes of hypotonic glycine–containing solutions. Absorption of this fluid into the intravascular space can generate hyponatremia, whereas the plasma osmolality may only be reduced slightly (as a result of the glycine). When the syndrome is severe, these men become hypertensive, confused, dyspneic, and nauseated. Hypotension, seizures, coma, and even death can follow. The altered mental and hemodynamic status may be caused by hyponatremia, ammonia generated from the glycine, or a direct toxic effect of the glycine itself (15). The full-blown syndrome occurs in 1% to 7% of patients undergoing a transurethral resection of the prostate.

Diuretic administration is the most common cause of hypovolemic hyponatremia in hospitalized patients. Thiazide diuretics are more likely than loop diuretics to cause hyponatremia because of their site of action in the distal convoluted tubule where urinary diluting capacity is blunted. Although hyponatremia secondary to thiazide diuretics is usually mild and asymptomatic, on occasion it can be acute, develop over 48 hours, and be severe. Furthermore, many diuretics will also produce significant urinary potassium and magnesium losses, further complicating the postoperative care of patients. It is often best to limit diuretic use in the postoperative patient and allow spontaneous diuresis to occur as interstitial fluid floods the intravascular compartment.

The treatment of hyponatremia in the postoperative patient is guided by identifying the cause of the hypo-osmolality. Administration of excess free water should be discontinued. If diuretics have generated volume depletion, infusion of normal saline to expand the ECF will cause a brisk water diuresis and correction of the hyponatremia. In severely hyponatremic patients who are symptomatic, especially when the hyponatremia develops acutely, hypertonic saline may be used.

Recent advances in the treatment of hyponatremia due to syndrome of inappropriate secretion of antidiuretic hormone (SIADH) include the use of vasopressin receptor antagonists (16). This class of drugs can be used to treat patients especially those with chronic hyponatremia related to ADH secretion. The therapeutic goal in these patients with profound hyponatremia is not to restore the sodium concentration to normal; rather, it is to aim for a sodium concentration of approximately 120 mEq/L and improvement of the neurologic symptoms. The serum sodium level should be monitored closely during the correction phase.

Hypernatremia

Hypernatremia occurs much less commonly than hyponatremia in the perioperative patient. A high serum sodium concentration is always associated with a high serum osmolality and hypertonicity, and water is needed to restore isotonicity. Hypernatremia is normally a potent stimulus to thirst. Therefore, for a patient to develop hypernatremia, some impairment of water intake must exist, such as an

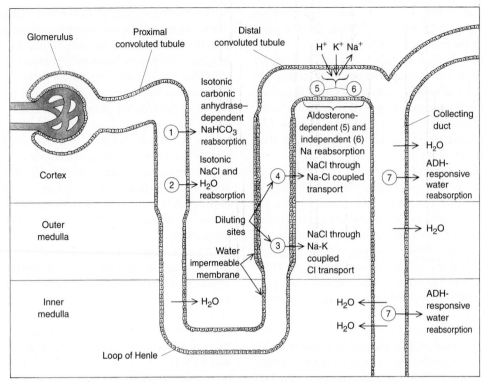

FIGURE 3.2 Functional processes for regulation of salt and water transport are illustrated schematically. Fluid formed by glomerular filtration of plasma is modified by transtubular reabsorption of sodium in the proximal tubule. Solute reabsorption in the proximal tubule is isotonic, being accompanied by reabsorption of water. In the first portion, the principal anion accompanying sodium reabsorption is bicarbonate *1*; farther along, sodium is reabsorbed mainly with chloride *2*. Differing permeability properties in the loop of Henle provide for water reabsorption in the descending thin limb and some sodium chloride reabsorption in the ascending thin portion. The thick ascending limb, impermeable to water, is a major site for reabsorption of sodium chloride *3, 4*. Two mechanisms are operative in the ascending limb: the first is a sodium–potassium transport coupled to chloride transport; the second is a coupled sodium–chloride transport in the cortical diluting segment. Sodium reabsorption in the distal tubule is related to potassium and hydrogen ion secretion *5, 6*. Last, in the presence of antidiuretic hormone, the cortical and medullary collecting ducts become permeable to water; this produces further water reabsorption and concentrates the urine *7*. (From Thier SO. Diuretic mechanism as a guide to therapy. *Hosp Pract* 1987;7:69, with permission.)

inappropriate lack of thirst or no access to water. Excessive water loss or salt intake may contribute as well. The ECF volume status of hypernatremic patients is high when they have excess total body solute; normal when total body solutes are normal but water is inadequate, or low when total body solutes are low and water is reduced even more. For example, excessive sweating and large evaporative losses from the skin and lungs, especially with fever or high environmental temperatures, may cause a disproportionate loss of water compared with the loss of salt from the body. This can generate severe hypernatremia. In such instances, both solute and water are depleted, but water loss exceeds solute loss. Initial therapy with isotonic saline is usually indicated to restore normal intravascular volume before addressing the free water deficit.

Similarly, when diarrhea is induced by osmotic cathartics such as lactulose, sorbitol, or by carbohydrate malabsorption, large quantities of hypotonic fluid will be lost in the stool and can cause severe hypernatremia. However, this occurs only when patients have no access to water or lack appropriate thirst mechanisms.

An often overlooked and relatively common cause of an elevated serum sodium is osmotic diuresis, such as that produced by prolonged glycosuria. The glucose acts as an osmotic agent and generates large losses of electrolyte-free water into the urine. Osmotic diuresis can also occur in catabolic postoperative patients who develop severe prerenal azotemia. Later, as renal function improves and urea is excreted, it generates an osmotic diuresis leading to hypernatremia.

Whenever hypernatremia develops, a relative free water deficit exists and must be replaced. The water deficit can be approximated using the formula:

$$\text{water deficit} = \text{total body water}$$
$$\times (1 - 140 \div \text{serum sodium})$$

Usually, the rate of correction of hypernatremia should not exceed 12 mEq/L/d (17). The aim should be to correct approximately half the deficit over the first 24 hours. Too rapid a correction of hypernatremia may lead to cerebral edema and seizures.

Hypokalemia

Hypokalemia is an important and common electrolyte abnormality in the surgical patient. It is defined as a plasma potassium concentration below 3.5 mEq/L. Most of thepotassium stores of the body are intracellular, and the degree of hypokalemia correlates poorly with total body potassium deficit.

Hypokalemia can have profound physiologic consequences. Of greatest clinical concern are cardiac arrhythmias and exacerbation of digitalis toxicity. Muscle weakness, cramps, myalgias, paralysis, and when severe, rhabdomyolysis can result. Hypokalemia also enhances renal acid excretion, which can generate and maintain metabolic alkalosis.

Potassium may be lost through the gastrointestinal (GI) tract, primarily in patients with diarrhea, and through the kidneys. The most important cause of renal potassium loss is diuretics. Metabolic alkalosis also contributes to renal potassium wasting. Whenever large quantities of $NaHCO_3$ transit the distal parts of the nephron, potassium secretion is stimulated. High levels of aldosterone, whether due to volume depletion or autonomous secretion, also stimulate potassium secretion. When hypokalemia develops in patients with vomiting or nasogastric suction, it is primarily caused by renal potassium losses, and not the small amount of potassium lost in the vomitus. The high aldosterone levels and metabolic alkalosis associated with the gastric losses combine to stimulate renal potassium excretion. The electrolyte content of sweat and GI secretions is shown in Table 3.2.

The treatment of hypokalemia should be guided by the severity of the disorder and by the presence of complications such as cardiac arrhythmias or musculoskeletal symptoms. If no medical indication exists to rapidly correct the potassium deficit, oral or slow intravenous replacement (i.e., 40 mEq/L over 8 to 12 hours) is adequate. When rapid replacement becomes necessary and the hypokalemia is severe, a central venous access should be used to correct the deficit. This avoids discomfort, venous irritation or sclerosis, and potential severe tissue damage if the fluid extravasates (10 to 20 mEq KCl can be dissolved in 50 to 100 cc of fluid). The rate of intravenous potassium repletion should not exceed 20 mEq/h.

Hyperkalemia

Hyperkalemia is defined as a plasma potassium concentration above 5.4 mEq/L, and it is considered severe if the concentration exceeds 7.0 mEq/L. Hyperkalemia developing in the perioperative patient may be the result of excessive intake, decreased excretion, redistribution of potassium from the ICF to the ECF compartment, or any combination of these derangements. Excessive intake is usually the result of overzealous intravenous potassium

administration. Sometimes, excessive oral intake occurs when potassium-containing salt substitutes are used. Decreased excretion is usually caused by acute, chronic, or acute superimposed on chronic renal failure. Addison disease, mineralocorticoid deficiency, potassium-sparing diuretics, angiotensin-converting enzyme inhibitors, nonsteroidal anti-inflammatory drugs, and cyclosporine are other conditions and drugs that reduce renal potassium excretion.

Several circumstances may cause a shift of potassium out of cells into the ECF compartment. The cells may be damaged or destroyed with hemolysis or rhabdomyolysis, for example. Hyperosmolality (i.e., hyperglycemia) will also produce a shift of potassium into the ECF. Certain drugs, such as β-adrenergic antagonists, digitalis, or succinylcholine, can also produce such potassium shifts. The most important clinical consequences of hyperkalemia are cardiac in nature. Typical electrocardiographic changes include peaked T waves, prolonged PR interval, widening of the QRS complex, and eventually loss of P waves. Wide complex ventricular tachycardia, ventricular fibrillation, and asystole may result. Severe hyperkalemia can also produce profound neuromuscular dysfunction, including flaccid paralysis and respiratory failure.

Severe hyperkalemia is a medical emergency because of potential life-threatening cardiac arrhythmias. Sodium bicarbonate is often given intravenously to promote cellular entry of potassium, but it is not an effective therapy except in cases of inorganic acid metabolic acidosis. Potassium can also be shifted into cells by the administration of glucose and insulin. Inhaled β-adrenergic agents such as albuterol may also be useful in shifting potassium back into cells. When severe hyperkalemia results in dangerous cardiac arrhythmias, calcium salts (chloride or gluconate) may be injected intravenously. This will quickly suppress cardiac excitability by altering the cell membrane threshold potential. However, it is often necessary not only to shift potassium into cells, but also to remove it from the body. If kidney function is adequate, this can be accomplished by inducing a brisk diuresis with diuretics. In addition, the cation exchange resin, sodium polystyrene, can be given by mouth or enema to bind potassium in the GI tract and remove it through the stool. When a large load of plasma potassium needs to be removed, hemodialysis may be necessary.

Hypomagnesemia

Hypomagnesemia is a less common and frequently overlooked electrolyte abnormality. It should be suspected in patients on an insufficient diet, especially alcoholics, or in patients chronically using diuretics. Both alcohol and most diuretics increase renal magnesium excretion. Hypomagnesemia is clinically important not just because it has direct effects, but also because it can produce hypocalcemia and contribute to the persistence of hypokalemia. Magnesium deficiency will cause renal potassium wasting. When hypokalemia and hypomagnesemia coexist, magnesium should be aggressively replaced to restore potassium balance. The

TABLE 3.2

Electrolyte Content of Sweat and Gastrointestinal Secretions

Sweat or Gastrointestinal Secretion	Electrolyte Concentration (mEq/L)					Replacement Amount for Each Liter Lost			
	Na+	K+	H+	Cl⁻	HCO₃⁻	Isotonic Saline (mL)	5% D/W (mL)	KCl (mEq)	NaHCO³ (mEq)
Sweat	30–50	5		45–55		300	700	5	
Gastric secretions	40–65	10	90	100–140		300	700	20	
Pancreatic fistula	133–155	5		55–75	70–90	250	750	5	90
Biliary fistula	135–155	5		80–110	35–50	750	250	5	
Ileostomy fluid	120–130	10		50–60	50–70	300	700	10	67.6
Diarrhea fluid	25–50	35–60		20–40	30–45		1,000	35	45

same is true for hypocalcemia. The level of plasma magnesium is a poor indicator of the degree of total body magnesium stores. Magnesium should be replaced until the plasma level returns to the upper normal range. Magnesium can be replaced either intravenously or, in less acute circumstances, through oral supplements. Gastrointestinal absorption of this cation, which occurs with greatest facility in the duodenum, is variable. In addition, all magnesium salts have a laxative effect when taken by mouth.

Hypocalcemia

Most of the body's calcium is contained within the bone matrix; approximately 0.1% of body calcium is in the ECF. Normally, the serum calcium concentration is maintained at a level between 9.0 and 10.4 mg/dL or 2.25 and 2.6 mmol/L. Calcium in the serum is found in three forms: approximately 40% is protein bound, 10% is complexed to phosphate and other anions, and 50% exists in the ionized form. Normally, the concentration of ionized calcium is remarkably constant despite marked variations in the level of total calcium concentration. A fall in serum albumin of 1 g/dL usually is associated with a 0.8 mg/dL fall in total calcium concentration, yet the ionized calcium may remain normal. Alterations in systemic pH will affect albumin binding of calcium. Metabolic acidosis decreases protein binding and increases the ionized calcium concentration, whereas metabolic alkalosis has the opposite effect. Direct measurement of the ionized calcium can be done with special electrodes and is often helpful.

Of clinical importance, hypocalcemia may be defined as a reduction in the ionized component of serum calcium. Patients with hypoalbuminemia and a low total serum calcium concentration may or may not have a reduction in ionized calcium. Consequently, the clinical presentation of the patient with hypocalcemia is crucial when deciding whether therapy is indicated.

The principal clinical manifestations of hypocalcemia are neurologic and include, in order of increasing severity: perioral paresthesias, carpal pedal spasm, tetany, and generalized seizures. Chvostek sign (twitching of the corner of the mouth produced by tapping over the facial nerve) and Trousseau sign (spasm of the fingers produced by inflating a blood pressure cuff above systolic) are also manifestations of neuromuscular irritability. Electrocardiographic changes include prolonged corrected QT and ST intervals and peaked T waves. Rarely, heart block may develop.

Perioperative hypocalcemia may be the result of hypomagnesemia, acute renal failure, septic shock, rhabdomyolysis, or acute pancreatitis. Hypocalcemia associated with acute renal failure is usually not severe and rarely requires specific therapy. When rhabdomyolysis occurs, it produces extensive skeletal muscle necrosis and results in calcium deposition in the injured tissue and subsequent hypocalcemia. Similarly, when acute pancreatitis results in the local release of pancreatic enzymes, retroperitoneal and omental fat digestion releases fatty acids that bind calcium. Though severe hypocalcemia may develop, only clinically symptomatic hypocalcemia should be treated with calcium supplementation. Aggressive calcium infusion will often cause a period of hypercalcemia in patients who recover from the acute insult and in whom deposited calcium is released.

Metabolic Alkalosis

Metabolic alkalosis in the postoperative patient is associated with increased morbidity and mortality (18). The pathogenesis of this acid–base disorder may be divided into two distinct phases: the generation of excessive bicarbonate, and the maintenance of the metabolic alkalosis (19). The generation of excess bicarbonate results either from renal or extrarenal acid loss or the addition of base to the ECF. In the perioperative patient, metabolic alkalosis is most often due to vomiting or gastric drainage. When hydrochloric acid is secreted by the gastric mucosa, an equal amount of bicarbonate is added to the ECF compartment. Normally, the HCl is neutralized by bicarbonate in the duodenum and small bowel, resulting in no net acid–base imbalance. However, if the HCl is removed through vomiting or nasogastric suction, then net bicarbonate addition to the ECF results. Diuretics also contribute to the metabolic alkalosis in many patients. Bicarbonate may be infused through intravenous solutions, total parenteral nutrition (TPN), or blood products that contain sodium citrate, a bicarbonate precursor.

The kidneys have an enormous capacity to rapidly excrete large quantities of bicarbonate. Consequently, for metabolic alkalosis to persist, impaired renal corrective mechanisms, or strong signals to the kidney to retain bicarbonate, must exist. If renal function is impaired markedly, the kidney cannot excrete the generated bicarbonate load. If renal function is preserved, then three major stimuli act to enhance bicarbonate reabsorption: (i) effective arterial volume depletion, (ii) mineralocorticoid excess, and (iii) hypokalemia. Decreased effective arterial volume increases proximal tubular bicarbonate reabsorption. Hypokalemia also increases proximal reabsorption of bicarbonate and stimulates distal acid excretion. Mineralocorticoid increases distal acid excretion and also contributes to the development of hypokalemia.

The therapy of metabolic alkalosis requires reversal of those factors generating bicarbonate (i.e., stopping diuretics, decreasing gastric acid secretions), and also reversing those factors which act to maintain the alkalosis. To the extent possible, renal function should be normalized, effective intra-arterial volume should be restored, and hypokalemia should be corrected. Therefore, if renal function is reasonable, the simple infusion of isotonic saline will quickly produce bicarbonaturia and correct the metabolic alkalosis.

Metabolic Acidosis

Metabolic acidosis is characterized by a fall in the serum bicarbonate concentration, which, if unopposed, reduces the arterial pH (or a rise in the hydrogen ion concentration). This acid–base disorder can develop in several ways: (i) bicarbonate may be lost from the body through the GI tract or the kidney, (ii) the kidney may fail to regenerate bicarbonate due to inadequate acid excretion, or (iii) bicarbonate may be consumed in the titration of excessive endogenously produced acid (e.g., lactic acidosis/ketoacidosis), or by the ingestion of exogenous acid producing compounds, such as methanol or ethylene glycol.

The kidney plays a pivotal role in maintaining acid–base balance in the human body. The metabolism of an average Western protein-containing diet will generate approximately 1 mEq/kg body weight of acid. This daily acid is titrated in the ECF, primarily by the bicarbonate anion. The role of the kidney is twofold: (i) it must reclaim all of the bicarbonate that is filtered and (ii) it must excrete the acid anion produced and regenerate the bicarbonate that was consumed by the titration outlined in the preceding text.

Bicarbonate is regenerated by tubular pumping of hydrogen ions, which are buffered as titratable acid (mainly phosphate), and by ammonia. When the kidney is unable to excrete an adequate quantity of acid (such as NH_4), a variety of distal renal tubular acidoses may result. When the ability of the kidney to reabsorb all of the filtered bicarbonate is impaired, then bicarbonate wastage results in proximal renal tubular acidosis.

Patients with chronic renal insufficiency (a decreased GFR) generally have reduced acid excretory capacity. Chronic metabolic acidosis must be recognized in such patients preoperatively because worsening renal function and more severe metabolic acidosis may ensue in the postoperative period. The development of postoperative severe metabolic acidosis can adversely affect cardiac function, vascular resistance, and the response to catecholamines. Metabolic acidosis must be addressed appropriately and treated according to the clinical circumstances.

ACKNOWLEDGMENT

The authors wish to express their appreciation to Ann Drew for her assistance in preparation of this manuscript.

REFERENCES

1. Weissman C. Ensuring perioperative fluid homeostasis in critically ill patients. *J Crit Illn* 1994;9:1077–1093.
2. Schrier RW. The edematous patient: cardiac failure, cirrhosis and nephrotic syndrome. In: Schrier RW, ed. *Manual of nephrology*, 4th ed. Boston: Little, Brown and Company, 1995:1–19.
3. Lund T, Wiig H, Reed RK. Acute postburn edema: role of strongly negative interstitial fluid pressure. *Am J Physiol* 1988;255:H1069–H1074.
4. Schrier RW. A unifying hypothesis of body fluid volume regulation. *J R Coll Physicians Lond* 1992;26:297.
5. Bock JC, Barker BC, Clinton AG, et al. Post-traumatic changes in, and effect of colloid osmotic pressure on the distribution of body water. *Ann Surg* 1989;210:395–405.
6. Raffin TA. ARDS: mechanisms and management. *Hosp Pract (Off Ed)* 1987;15:65–80.
7. Finfer S, Bellomo R, Boyce N, et al. SAFE Study Investigators. A Comparison of albumin and saline for fluid resuscitation in the intensive care unit [Clinical Trial] *N Engl J Med* 2004;350(22):2247–2256.
8. Denton MD, Chertow GM, Brady HR. "Renal-dose" dopamine for the treatment of acute renal failure: scientific rationale, experimental studies and clinical trials. *Kidney Int* 1996;50:4–14.
9. The Australian and New Zealand Intensive Care Society (ANZICS) Clinical Trial Group. Low-dose dopamine in patients with early renal dysfunction: a placebo-controlled randomized trial. *Lancet* 2000;356:2139–2143.
10. Yagi N, Paganini EP. Acute dialysis and continuous renal replacement: the emergence of a new technology involving the nephrologist in the intensive care setting. *Semin Nephrol* 1997;17:306–320.
11. Chung HM, Kluge R, Schrier RW, et al. Postoperative hyponatremia: a prospective study. *Arch Intern Med* 1986;146:333–336.
12. Carlos AJ, Arieff AI. Symptomatic hyponatremia: making the diagnosis rapidly. *J Crit Illn* 1990;5:846–856.
13. Arieff AI. Hyponatremia, convulsions, respiratory arrest, and permanent brain damage after elective surgery in healthy women. *N Engl J Med* 1986;314:1529–1535.
14. Fraser CL, Arieff AI. Fatal central diabetes mellitus and insipidus resulting from untreated hyponatremia: a new syndrome. *Ann Intern Med* 1990;112:113–119.
15. Agarwal R, Emmett M. The post-transurethral resection of prostate syndrome: therapeutic proposals. *Am J Kidney Dis* 1994;24:108–111.
16. Soupart A, Gross P, Legros J-J, et al. Successful long-term treatment of hyponatremia in syndrome of inappropriate antidiuretic

hormone with satavaptan (SR121462B), an orally active nonpeptide3 vasopressin V2-receptor antagonist. *Clin J Am Soc Nephrol* 2006;1(6):1154–1160.

17. Sterus R. Hypernatremia. In: Greenberg A, ed. *Primer on kidney diseases*. New York: Academic Press, 1994:370–371.

18. Jones ER. Metabolic alkalosis. In: Greenberg A, ed. *Primer on kidney diseases*. New York: Academic Press, 1994:382–387.

19. Emmett M, Seldin DW. Metabolic acidosis and metabolic alkalosis. In: Seldin DW, Giebish G, eds. *The kidney: physiology and pathophysiology*. New York: Raven Press, 1985:1567–1639.

CHAPTER 4

Shock and Hypoperfusion States

Herbert A. Phelan, Alexander L. Eastman, Amin Frotan, and Richard P. Gonzalez

The clinical picture of a patient in shock is compelling, and it tends to leave a lasting impression on young surgeons-in-training. The gravity of the situation, the clinical skills required for effective delivery of care, and knowledge of the consequences of failure combine to make surgical critical care simultaneously exciting and daunting. The sheer *sickness* of these patients is as impressive now as ever, and was what led to attempts to characterize the shock state as long ago as 1575 when Ambroise Pare wrote the first classical description of the manifestations of traumatic shock (1). The first use of the word "shock" was credited to the French surgeon, H. LeDran in 1743 (2), and soon thereafter as the term *shock* began to evolve its definition became more varied. In 1815, G. J. Guthrie cautioned surgeons to delay surgeries "until the alarm and shock have subsided (3)," and it was discovered that situations other than the hemorrhage of trauma could be associated with shock. According to Wiggers (4), O'Shaughnessey described the presence of circulatory collapse in patients suffering from cholera in 1831, and in 1876 Blum (5) described shock in association with burns and strangulated hernias.

As the 19th century came to a close, most investigators continued to focus on circulatory failure as the most important feature of shock. Crile (6,7) was one of the first investigators who could consistently reproduce the shock state in various experimental models.

During World War I, American, British, and French physicians observed and carried out numerous studies and experiments on victims of traumatic shock. Shortly thereafter, Macleod (8) demonstrated that following a reduction in oxygen to tissues, a liberation of metabolic acids occurred. This led him to discover the presence of lactic acid in the advanced hypovolemic state.

Before World War II, the definitions of shock began to become more precise. In 1940, Freeman defined shock as, "The clinical condition characterized by progressive loss of the circulating blood volume, which brought about the tissue anoxia which results from inadequate circulation" (9).

In the aftermath of World War II, further hemodynamic data on shock was obtained through the application of cardiac catheterization. Because most of the human data were the result of battle injuries, almost all of the observations were on patients who were hypovolemic secondary to blood loss. Research continued aggressively as the United States entered the Korean War and emphasis was placed on the renal failure resulting from severe shock. The era of the Vietnam War subsequently saw research interests change toward crystalloid resuscitation and the development of pulmonary failure.

The 1970s saw the creation of dedicated intensive care units (ICUs) as well as the development of the Swan-Ganz catheter which allowed the relations of preload, afterload, and myocardial contractility to the shock state to be elucidated. The pathophysiology of the septic state and the respiratory distress syndrome began to be understood. Now the discovery of the cytokine milieu holds the promise of immunomodulatory therapies for multiple organ failure (MOF).

WHAT IS SHOCK?

Very few things about the pathophysiology of shock are simple, but one relatively straightforward aspect of the syndrome is that while any number of etiologies are capable of severely disrupting normal physiology, the final sequelae of their damage tends to be similar regardless of the cause (Fig. 4.1). Indeed, the commonality of this final pathway is what led R. Adams Cowley to define shock as "a momentary pause in the act of dying."

The metabolic consequence of this multitude of etiologies is cellular hypoperfusion with an attendant tissue hypoxia. At its simplest and clearest level, this is probably the single best definition of what constitutes shock: cells not getting enough oxygen, generally from a lack of perfusion. Consequently, this discussion will cover both the numerous causes of the shock state as well as their final pathway. Let us begin with the easier of the two by examining how oxygen is delivered and handled.

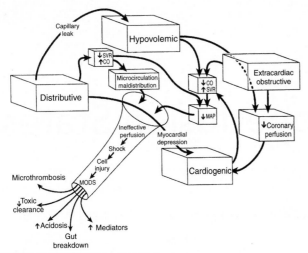

FIGURE 4.1 The various causes of shock and their final common pathway. Despite a spectrum of etiologies, the fundamental pathophysiology of shock (i.e., cellular hypoperfusion) is the same regardless of the source. CO, cardiac output; SVR, systemic vascular resistance; MAP, mean arterial pressure; MODS, multiorgan dysfunction syndrome. (From Civetta JM, Taylor RW, Kirby RR, eds. *Critical Care*, 3rd ed. Philadelphia: Lipincott-Raven Publishers, 1997:362, with permission.)

OXYGEN AVAILABILITY AND UTILIZATION

Now that we have a simpler definition of shock, namely the inadequate delivery of oxygen (Do_2) substrate to cells, we can examine the determinants of oxygen availability to the microenvironment. In approaching this discussion with students and residents, we have found it helpful to construct an analogy for oxygen delivery using the idea of a railroad in which boxcars represent hemoglobin molecules carrying varying "loads" of oxygen molecules down the rail line of the microcirculation. Using this construct, the idea makes intuitive sense that to deliver more oxygen one must either increase the number of boxcars (increase the hemoglobin level through transfusions), increase the number of oxygen molecules carried by a given boxcar (augment the hemoglobin saturation), or accelerate the speed at which the boxcars go by [increasing cardiac output (CO)]. Although a simple analogy, it is also effective and one to which we will return as the discussion proceeds.

Aerobic and Anaerobic Metabolism

The basic requirement for oxygen is the rate at which it is metabolized to water in cellular mitochondria. When the circulatory supply meets the mitochondrial demand, aerobic metabolism occurs and glucose is completely oxidized. Under normal circumstances, only 20% to 25% of oxygen available in capillary blood is utilized by the tissues to support aerobic metabolism. When the Do_2 by the microcirculation is impaired, tissues are capable of increasing this percentage to as high as 50% to 60% in order to maintain aerobic metabolism (10). When oxygen delivery is decreased below a

critical threshold, however, a portion of glucose utilization is converted to anaerobic metabolism (Fig. 4.2). Not only does the energy yield drop precipitously, [2 adenosine 5-triphosphate (ATP) versus 36 ATP/mol glucose], but breakdown products of the anaerobic pathway accumulate (lactate, pyruvate, and hydrogen ions). The lactate produced is not removed from the microenvironment as easily as carbon dioxide, and a significant metabolic (lactic) acidosis ensues. This acidosis impairs the ability of first cells, and then whole organs, to function effectively. Consequently, with the impairment of organ function, cellular perfusion can be further reduced. Unless this cycle is halted, the damage continues to accrue until cell function is irreversibly damaged. Therefore, it is easy to see how shock can become a self-perpetuating condition.

Determinants of Oxygen Content

At its simplest level, the amount of oxygen that will be available for cellular utilization can be understood as the amount of oxygen that a given volume of blood carries multiplied by the speed at which it is carried to the cellular environment. The first point is formally described by the equation for the content of oxygen in arterial blood (Cao_2):

$$Cao_2 = (1.34 \times Hgb \times Sao_2) + (0.003 \times Pao_2)$$

In this equation, Hgb is the hemoglobin concentration, Sao_2 the arterial oxygen saturation, and Pao_2 is the partial pressure of oxygen dissolved in plasma. The constant 1.34 signifies the amount of oxygen in milliliters that each gram of hemoglobin can carry when fully saturated. A cursory inspection of this equation shows that to increase the amount of oxygen that a particular amount of blood carries, one can attempt to increase the hemoglobin mass (again, the number of boxcars), the saturation of the existing hemoglobin mass (the number of oxygen molecules on each boxcar), or the amount of oxygen dissolved in the plasma and not bound by hemoglobin. A closer look at these variables, however, shows the minimal contribution of dissolved oxygen to the total oxygen carried. After multiplying the amount of dissolved oxygen by its solubility coefficient (0.003), the amount of oxygen available for extraction is minor.

Determinants of Oxygen Delivery

Now that the concept of oxygen content is hopefully clear, it should be only a short leap to an understanding of oxygen delivery. If a given unit of blood contains a given amount of oxygen, the only other variable left to account for is that of the rate at which the oxygen content is delivered to the periphery (i.e., the speed at which the boxcars move). On a practical level, this is represented by the CO. Therefore, the equation describing the Do_2 is:

$$Do_2 = CO \times Cao_2$$

or

$$Do_2 = CO \times [(1.34 \times Hgb \times Sao_2) + (0.003 \times Pao_2)]$$

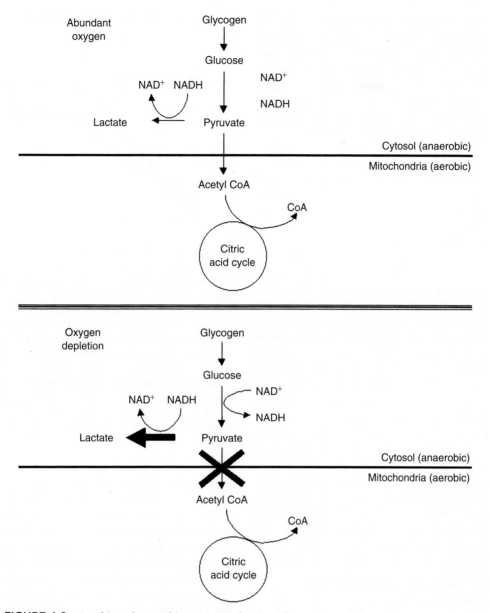

FIGURE 4.2 Aerobic and anaerobic energy production. The upper panel shows glycolysis occurring under circumstances of adequate oxygen delivery to the cell. Pyruvate can be transported across the mitochondrial membrane, converted to Acetyl-coenzyme A, and participate in the energy-efficient citric acid cycle. The bottom panel shows the metabolic block that occurs when the delivery of oxygen is insufficient to maintain aerobic metabolism. Anaerobic metabolism is confined to the cytosol. The excess pyruvate and the need to regenerate the oxidized form of nicotinamide adenine dinucleotide (NAD^+) drive the reaction to produce lactate.

The definition of CO makes intuitive sense: the number of heart beats per minute multiplied by the amount of blood per beat. To keep a stable CO, decreases in one of these variables necessitate an increase in the other. Tachycardia is one of the earliest and most effective mechanisms of the body for offsetting decreases in CO. The ability of an increased heart rate to augment CO generally begins to drop off at rates greater that 150 beats/min. At these rates, there is not enough time during diastole for the heart to fill. Conversely, bradycardia can also impair CO for obvious reasons. The stroke volume is the result of a complex interplay between the head of pressure driving blood into the ventricle, the distensibility and activity of the ventricle, and the pressure head against which the ventricle is working. These are known more formally as preload, contractility, and afterload, and will be discussed shortly.

Determinants of Oxygen Uptake

The discussion to this point has focused on the factors that affect the DO_2 to the cellular microenvironment. We turn our attention now to the relation governing the ability of tissues to utilize the oxygen with which they have been presented.

Technologic constraints limit our ability to directly measure the efficiency with which this process takes place. We can, however, measure the oxygen content of blood as it enters the cellular environment on the arterial side as well as when it exits the environment on the venous side. From the difference between these two values, we may make some inferences as to the magnitude of the oxygen consumption ($\dot{V}_{O_2}$). Mathematically, this relation is expressed as:

$$\dot{V}_{O_2} = CO \times (Ca_{O_2} - Cv_{O_2})$$

This equation states that the O_2 consumption is equal to the CO multiplied by the difference of the Ca_{O_2} and the oxygen content of venous blood (Cv_{O_2}). After isolating terms and converting units, the result is intuitively obvious to even the most casual of observers and can be rewritten as:

$$\dot{V}_{O_2} = CO \times 13.4 \times Hgb \times (Sa_{O_2} - Sv_{O_2})$$

The Sa_{O_2} is easily measured by using standard transcutaneous sensors or arterial blood gas determination. This value reflects the saturation of hemoglobin in the arterial system before passing through the capillary bed where oxygen extraction occurs. A normal value is approximately 95% to 100% on room air. The mixed venous oxygen saturation (Sv_{O_2}) is a measure of the saturation of hemoglobin with oxygen *after* exiting the capillary bed. Its normal value is in the range of 70%. This generally requires the use of a pulmonary artery catheter with a special transducer at its tip. Only 20% to 30% of delivered O_2 is utilized under normal conditions, which would seem to imply that a considerable pool of oxygen is available as a reserve in times of inadequate oxygen supply. This is indeed the case. As previously cited, the cellular microenvironment is capable of drawing off 50% to 60% of the oxygen present in the capillary blood flow during times of decreased supply or increased demand. This relation is formally described by the oxygen extraction ratio (O_2ER):

$$O_2ER = \text{Oxygen consumed/oxygen delivered}$$
$$O_2ER = \dot{V}_{O_2}/D_{O_2}$$

This compensatory mechanism of extracting larger and larger percentages of hemoglobin-bound oxygen is an attempt to maintain aerobic metabolism in the cellular milieu. Once the point of maximal extraction is reached, however, further decreases in the D_{O_2} result in cellular hypoxia. This is illustrated graphically in Figure 4.3 (11).

The flat horizontal part of the curve depicts aerobic metabolism in which supply exceeds demand. When D_{O_2} decreases to some critical value, the $\dot{V}_{O_2}$ curve becomes linear. This point is known as the point of critical oxygen delivery and the down-sloping portion of the curve is known as the region of *supply dependency*, which indicates progressive reliance on anaerobic metabolism. The breakpoint between the linear and the flat portion of the curve is the point of maximal O_2ER.

Oxyhemoglobin Dissociation

Note that we have largely ignored the role of Pa_{O_2} when concerning ourselves with the oxygen content of blood

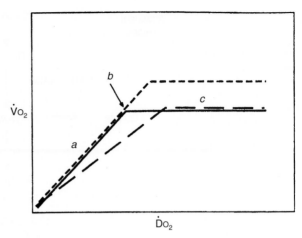

FIGURE 4.3   The relation between oxygen consumption ($\dot{V}_{O_2}$) and delivery of oxygen (D_{O_2}). During cellular hypoperfusion, oxygen utilization by tissues is limited by delivery (*a*). This sloped portion of the curve is known as the region of "supply dependency" and is marked by anaerobic metabolism and elevated oxygen extraction ratios. Augmenting D_{O_2} will increase cellular uptake until a point at which enough oxygen is present to support aerobic metabolism (*b*). Further increases in D_{O_2} do not yield increases in $\dot{V}_{O_2}$ (*c*). Patients with sepsis or systemic inflammation can have an elevated saturation $\dot{V}_{O_2}$ plateau (*dotted line*). The slope of the supply-dependency portion of the curve is a graphic illustration of a patient's ability to extract oxygen from the periphery. Impaired extraction would depress the slope (*dashed line*). (From *J Surg Res* 2000; 92:120–141, with permission.)

because of its small overall contribution to the total oxygen load. It does play a part, however, through its contribution to determining the saturation of hemoglobin with oxygen. If the relation between the Sa_{O_2} and the Pa_{O_2} are plotted against one another, an "S"-shaped curve results (Fig. 4.4). This curve describes the affinity that hemoglobin has for oxygen at various partial pressures of oxygen. At high Pa_{O_2}, the hemoglobin molecule is nearly completely bound and has a high affinity for oxygen molecules (thereby explaining the flat portion of the curve at these values). As the ambient Pa_{O_2} in the hemoglobin molecule's microenvironment falls, the hemoglobin molecule's affinity for oxygen lessens and it readily unloads its oxygen cargo.

Further, the affinity of the hemoglobin molecule for oxygen can be changed by various physiologic conditions. In practice, this means that the curve can shift left or right depending on whether the new condition makes the hemoglobin molecule want to bind more tightly to oxygen, or to have a relatively weaker bond. Factors that shift the curve to the left are ones which cause an increased affinity such as a decrease in temperature, an increase in pH, a decrease in Pa_{CO_2}, or low levels of 2,3-diphosphoglycerate [(2,3-DPG), which is an organophosphate created in red blood cells (RBCs) during glycolysis which binds to hemoglobin and decreases its affinity for oxygen]. Conversely, a right shift of the curve causes a lower affinity of hemoglobin for oxygen and is caused by an increase in temperature, lowering of pH, an increase in Pa_{CO_2}, or high levels of 2,3-DPG. The

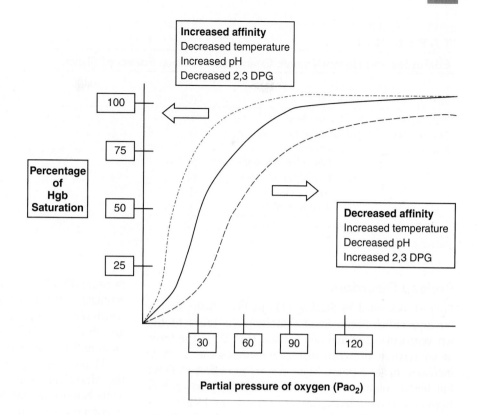

FIGURE 4.4 The oxyhemoglobin dissociation curve.

production of 2,3-DPG is probably an adaptive mechanism because its production increases during times of diminished peripheral tissue O_2 availability.

Rather than trying to memorize all of these factoids, we find it is easier to think about the oxyhemoglobin dissociation curve conceptually. If you can just remember that the curve is sigmoid-shaped with saturations on the y-axis and Pa_{O_2} on the x-axis, the things that shift the curve can be figured out. Say you are trying to remember what direction the curve is shifted by physiologic stress such as acidosis and fever. Remember that the body deals with physiologic stressors by increasing D_{O_2}, and this is accomplished by unloading more oxygen from a given hemoglobin molecule. Looking at the normal curve, a Pa_{O_2} of 27 mm Hg corresponds with a saturation of 50%. Hypothetically, if the curve moved a little to the left we see that the new saturation of a hemoglobin molecule at that same Pa_{O_2} would actually be a little *increased* to a new value in the 60% saturation range (indicating a higher affinity of the hemoglobin molecule for oxygen, or less of a willingness to unload oxygen). Physiologically, this would make no sense. Why would hemoglobin want to hang on to oxygen more avidly in the starving environment of the tissues during stress? Now let us look at what would happen with a right shift of the curve during stress. Again, assuming a starting Pa_{O_2} of 27 mm Hg and a saturation of 50% (values that have a funny way of showing up on standardized tests, by the way), what would a right shift of the curve do to oxygen affinity? We see that at the same Pa_{O_2} we would now have a saturation in the 40% range, indicating an increased willingness of hemoglobin to unload oxygen. This makes more physiologic sense, and

indeed is the correct answer. Again, as long as you can remember that Pa_{O_2} is on the x-axis, saturation is on the y-axis, and that the curve is S-shaped, most of the rest can be reasoned through. As for the effect of 2,3-DPG: well, just memorize it.

CATEGORIZATION

As mentioned earlier, definitions of shock have evolved from the classic descriptions of simple hypotension to a more sophisticated view that centers on inadequate perfusion. The complex interplay between the head of pressure driving blood into the ventricle, the distensibility and activity of the ventricle, and the pressure head against which the ventricle is working normally meet the demands of the body with a great deal of reserve. Clinically, these determinants are known more formally as preload, contractility, and afterload (Table 4.1). Although numerous conditions can cause a breakdown of normal circulation and perfusion, we tend to group these etiologies of the shock state by the aspect of cardiovascular physiology primarily affected. One of the authors, despite being board-certified in surgical critical care, still begins every resuscitation of a critically ill patient by asking himself, "Is this a preload problem, a pump problem, or an afterload problem?" Although the overlap that can exist between the groups should be recognized, this overly simple question not only serves as a good segue into a discussion of the pathophysiology and treatment of different types of shock, but as a useful real-life starting point in the beginning of a resuscitation as well.

TABLE 4.1

Etiologies and Hemodynamic Changes in Various Forms of Shock

Etiology of Shock	Example	CVP	Cardiac Output	Systemic Vascular Resistance	Venous O_2 Saturation
Preload	Hypovolemic	↓	↓	↑	↓
Contractility	Cardiogenic	↑	↓	↑	↓
Afterload	Distributive				
	Hyperdynamic septic	↑↓	↑	↓	↑
	Hypodynamic septic	↑↓	↓	↑	↑↓
	Neurogenic	↓	↓	↓	↓
	Anaphylactic	↓	↓	↓	↓

CVP, central venous pressure.

Preload Disorders

Preload, described by Starling (12) in 1915, is the stretch on myocardial fibers. In clinical terms, it refers to the left ventricular end-diastolic volume (LVEDV). The force of contraction of ventricular fibers increases as LVEDV increases, up to a point. Many factors can affect LVEDV, but blood volume and distribution are the most critical. Beyond a certain level, further increases in LVEDV no longer increase CO. This is demonstrated by the Frank Starling Curve and occurs on the flat, upper part of the curve (Fig. 4.5). At this part of the curve, cardiac failure, and pulmonary edema occur. The most common clinical tool for estimating LVEDV is a pulmonary artery catheter passed through the right heart as described by Swan (13). Once the balloon at the end of the catheter is inflated and "wedged" in the pulmonary artery, it obscures any pressure influence of the right ventricle. There are no valves within the pulmonary circulation leaving a direct column of blood from the end of the catheter in the pulmonary artery, through the lung capillary bed, to the pulmonary vein, and finally to the left atrium. Pulmonary capillary wedge

pressure (PCWP) estimates left atrial pressure, which in turn estimates left ventricular end-diastolic pressure (LVEDP), which serves as a proxy for LVEDV (preload). Many factors and disease processes affect these measurements and can confound attempts to measure preload.

Hypovolemic shock results from any insult that reduces the intravascular volume and, therefore, preload. Classically, acute hemorrhage has been the model used to describe this phenomenon, but any other number of insults can account for a similar physiologic state. Diarrhea and vomiting, high urinary outputs from hyperosmolar states, and capillary leakage into the third space are just a few examples of other etiologies which can result in this type of shock syndrome. Taken together, it is easy to see why hypovolemia is the most common category of shock dealt with by surgeons.

Clinical Signs

The degree to which the signs and symptoms of shock are manifested is dependent on the rate and volume of fluid loss as well as the ability of the individual to compensate. These responses describe a spectrum of physiologic changes ranging from the very minor to impending circulatory collapse. These compensatory mechanisms are most evident by looking at the example of acute blood loss. Hemorrhagic shock is categorized by the amount of volume lost, and each class has a predictable set of physiologic signs (14).

Class I: Loss of 15% or Less of Blood Volume

Urine output and blood pressure are maintained and tachycardia is either absent or minimal. This is akin to the changes seen after blood donation, and blood volume replacement is unnecessary.

Class II: Loss of 15% to 30% of Blood Volume

This corresponds to a blood loss of approximately 800 to 1,500 mL in a 70-kg male. These patients will usually manifest the earliest signs of compensation for blood loss. Although urine output and blood pressure are still largely maintained, a resting tachycardia and orthostatic blood pressure changes may be seen. Further, a decrease in pulse pressure may be noted secondary to a catecholamine-induced rise in the

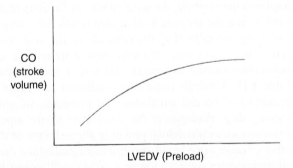

FIGURE 4.5 The Frank-Starling Curve. This curve shows the relation between left-ventricular end-diastolic volume (LVEDV) and cardiac output (CO). Increasing the LVEDV yields increasing stroke volumes to a point. After that, the myocardial fibers are stretched to the point that their contractions become less efficient and CO plateaus then fall. (From O'Leary, JP, ed. *The physiologic basis of surgery*, 2nd ed. Baltimore: Williams and Wilkins, 1996:85, with permission.)

peripheral resistance and, thus, the diastolic pressure. The shunting of blood away from organs designed to tolerate some ischemia may first be detected. This is often most noticeable in the skin, as blood shunted away from the integument by peripheral vasoconstriction can result in cool, clammy extremities. This stage requires some volume replacement.

Class III: Loss of 30% to 40% of Total Blood Volume

This stage corresponds to a blood loss of approximately 2,000 mL. Compensatory mechanisms for blood loss begin to fail at this point as blood pressure begins to drop.

The shunting of blood past the skin increases, and vasoconstriction begins to affect blood flow to the kidneys resulting in a pronounced drop off in urine output. These patients can often begin to act anxious and combative, and they will usually require transfusion of RBC for an adequate resuscitation.

Class IV: Loss of More Than 40% of Total Blood Volume

At this point, blood flow to the brain is insufficient for higher function and the patient will frequently become obtunded. Adrenergic discharge is maximal, yet hypotension and profound oliguria are seen. The patient is in imminent danger of circulatory collapse, and immediate resuscitative measures and hemostatic maneuvers are required to prevent organ damage or death.

Compensatory Mechanisms

As previously mentioned, the central perturbation in hypovolemic shock is a reduction in intravascular volume. Most of the physiologic sequelae seen in the syndrome are mechanisms designed to compensate for this insult. The immediate consequence of decreased blood volume is a reduction in venous return to the heart (preload) with a commensurate drop in ventricular filling pressures, stroke volume, and CO. Referring back to the equation for the arterial oxygen content of blood, we see that the D_{O_2} is inhibited in hypovolemia by a drop in CO, and in the case of hemorrhage by a drop in hemoglobin as well. As perfusion at the cellular level is decreased, the body's attempt to offset these losses begins.

The earliest compensatory mechanism elicited by a drop in blood pressure is an increase in sympathetic activity. This is mediated largely by the action of baroreceptors located in the aortic arch, atria, and carotid bodies. When stimulated, these receptors positively regulate parasympathetic discharge. A decrease in systolic blood pressure effectively inhibits them, and the result is an increase in sympathetic drive. Norepinephrine and epinephrine are released and act on adrenergic receptors in the myocardium and vascular smooth muscle. Consequently, heart rate and contractility are increased (thereby augmenting CO), and peripheral vascular resistance is elevated in an attempt to increase perfusion pressure. A key aspect of this mechanism is its selectivity. Organ systems taking the brunt of this shunting phenomenon are those that are the least oxygen-dependent, because blood flow to the skin, skeletal muscle, and splanchnic circulation is reduced first while that of the kidneys is initially spared. If the hypotensive state persists, however, the kidneys will also eventually feel the effects of vasoconstriction. The result is the body's attempt to preserve blood flow to the heart and brain.

As the kidney begins to feel the effects of vasoconstriction, another aspect of the body's compensatory mechanisms comes into play as hormonal mediators of volume control are released. When renal perfusion pressures begin to fall, the juxtaglomerular cells of the afferent arterioles release renin into the systemic circulation. This enzyme cleaves angiotensin I from angiotensinogen. Angiotensin I is further cleaved to angiotensin II, the active form of the hormone. Angiotensin II stimulates increased sympathetic drive at the level of the nerve terminal through the release of hormones from the adrenal medulla and through a centrally acting increase in sympathetic tone. It also causes increased sodium reabsorption through a direct action on renal tubules, and stimulates the release of aldosterone in order to further augment sodium reabsorption. Concurrently, baroreceptors found in the atria and the juxtaglomerular apparatus of the kidney send afferent signals to the supraoptic and paraventricular nuclei in the brain. Decreased stimulation of these volume receptors results in the release of antidiuretic hormone (ADH) from the posterior pituitary. ADH causes retention of free water at the level of the kidney, and has powerful vasoconstrictive properties of its own. Taken together, these effects serve to increase vascular tone while simultaneously expanding the intravascular volume.

As the shock state progresses, the body's attempts to counteract volume loss continue as there is a shift of fluid from the extracellular compartment into the intravascular space. This fluid shift helps to restore blood volume, and in the setting of hemorrhagic shock, the hematocrit will fall as this fluid shift into the intravascular space dilutes out the remaining red cells. A word of caution is warranted here about interpreting spun hematocrits in the setting of sudden, massive hemorrhage. The blood lost in an episode of hemorrhage such as this contains roughly the same proportions of red cells and plasma as that of whole blood. Consequently, the rapidity with which a spun hematocrit can be performed in the resuscitation room can conspire with a lack of time for the body to mobilize third spaced fluids to yield an artificially high hematocrit for several minutes after a hemorrhagic episode. The importance of correlating the patient's clinical appearance with the spun hematocrit while maintaining a high index of suspicion cannot be overemphasized.

The mechanism for this shift of extravascular fluid into the intravascular space is based on a reduction of hydrostatic pressure in the capillary beds (Fig. 4.6). This pressure decrease is a consequence of the arteriolar vasoconstriction of the precapillary sphincters, which is greater than the vasoconstriction of postcapillary sphincters in the venule. Therefore, the fall in the capillary hydrostatic pressure results

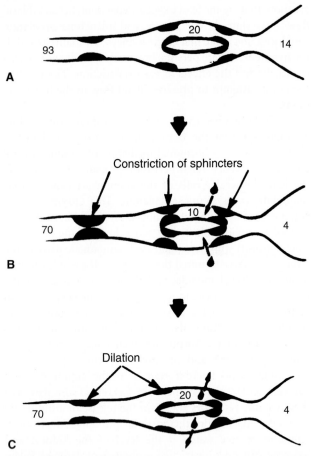

FIGURE 4.6 Mechanisms of compensation for and irreversibility of hypovolemic shock. **A:** In a normal arteriole the mean arterial, capillary, and venular pressures are 93, 20, and 14 mm Hg, respectively. **B:** With hypoperfusion, the precapillary sphincters constrict more than the postcapillary sphincters. This reduction of intracapillary pressure results in inflow of interstitial fluid to the vascular space. **C:** In late shock, the precapillary sphincters dilate while the postcapillary sphincters stay constricted, thereby elevating the intracapillary pressure and driving fluid back into the interstitium. (From Sabiston DC. *Textbook of surgery*, 13th ed. Philadephia: WB Saunders, 1986:42, with permission.)

from a combination of the precapillary vasoconstriction plus the already present systemic arterial hypotension and a decreased resistance to outflow on the venule end. The low hydrostatic pressure that results allows redistribution of water and electrolytes from the extracellular space into the vascular space.

These compensatory mechanisms have finite capacities. One of the first signs that they are being overwhelmed is when the interstitial oncotic pressure becomes greater than the plasma oncotic pressure. This reversal occurs in moderate-to-severe shock because the capillary permeability becomes altered, with proteins extravasating out of the plasma and into the interstitial space. A decrease in coronary perfusion pressure occurs, resulting in myocardial ischemia. If the acidosis in the cellular milieu becomes profound enough, it can override the stimuli of the sympathetic

discharge and promote arteriolar vasodilation and relaxation of the precapillary sphincters. These effects favor shifting of fluid back into the interstitium, and the acidosis further exacerbates the negative cardiac inotropic effect. If allowed to progress in this direction, the acidosis will worsen to the point that the shock state becomes irreversible and death results.

Treatment

The ultimate goal of treatment of hypovolemic shock is the restoration of perfusion at the cellular level sufficient to result in aerobic respiration. This requires identification of the etiology of volume loss as well as managing its replacement. The debate between the use of crystalloid or colloid solutions for resuscitation from shock has gone on for decades. Recently, the Saline versus Albumin Fluid Evaluation (SAFE) group conducted a multicenter, double-blinded trial of almost 7,000 patients randomized to resuscitation with 4% albumin or normal saline (NS). No differences in outcome were noted (15). Other meta-analyses have shown similar results (16) and given that colloids are considerably more expensive, the current consensus is that a balanced salt solution should be used for the acute resuscitation of the patient in shock. If the source of hypovolemia is thought to be hemorrhage, blood and blood products should be used as well.

When considering the adequacy of resuscitation efforts, the clinical endpoints that are frequently used are normalization of blood pressure and heart rate, and restoration of adequate urine output (0.5 mL/kg of body weight per hour). Although seeing the unstable patient respond to resuscitation efforts with a normalization of systolic blood pressure, heart rate, and urine output is encouraging, any reassurance should be tempered by the knowledge that up to 80% of critically ill trauma patients with normal vital signs and an adequate urine output have evidence of tissue hypoperfusion (17).

More sensitive measures of the adequacy of cellular oxygenation are the base deficit and serum lactate. The base deficit is a measure of the number of millimoles of base required to correct the pH of a liter of whole blood to 7.40, and its normal value is −3 to +3. This determination is readily available as it can be measured on a blood gas analysis, and it has been shown to correlate with severity of shock (18–20). Rutherford showed that a base deficit of 8 carried a 25% mortality for patients older than 55 with no head injury or younger than 55 with a head injury (Fig. 4.7) (21). Should it remain elevated during attempted resuscitation, it should be taken as a sign that adequate cellular oxygenation may not yet have been achieved. Its largest drawback lies in the fact that it can be elevated in other situations other than under-resuscitation, particularly renal dysfunction and hyperchloremia. The latter is especially prevalent in patients who have gotten large amounts of NS with a consequent hyperchloremic nongap acidosis. Nevertheless, the base deficit is a useful guide to the adequacy of resuscitation efforts in the early stages.

Lactate is a byproduct of anaerobic metabolism and a fairly specific marker for tissue dysoxia. Although its

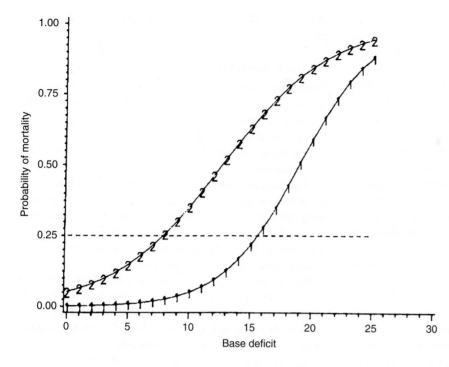

FIGURE 4.7 Relation of increasing base deficit and mortality. Mortality curves for (*1*) age less than 55 years and no head injury; and (*2*) age younger than 55 years and a head injury or age 55 or older and no head injury. Note that a 25% mortality is seen for (i) base deficit of approximately 15 in ages younger than 55 with no head injury, (ii) base deficit of approximately 8 in ages younger than 55 *with* a head injury, or (iii) base deficit of approximately 8 in those older than 55 *without* a head injury. (From *J Trauma* 1992; 33:417–423, with permission.)

clearance is a matter of some controversy, most believe that it has a half-life of approximately 3 hours. It has been shown to be a predictor of mortality and serial measurements of the serum lactate serve as a useful guide for the adequacy of resuscitation efforts (22–26). Its largest drawbacks consist of the fact that the value takes longer to obtain than a blood gas, and it must be drawn from an arterial or central venous source (to avoid sampling of a region rather than the whole body). It is worth remembering that lactate is partially cleared through the liver, making it of much less utility in patients with liver failure and/or cirrhosis as their levels can be elevated even in the face of adequate resuscitation.

Another method that some have advocated for identification of oxygen deficits is the use of gastric tonometry. This technique measures the adequacy of blood flow to the gastrointestinal tract through placement of a carbon dioxide (CO_2)-permeable balloon filled with saline in the stomach of a patient after gastric acid suppression. The balloon is left in contact with the mucosa of the stomach for 30 minutes, allowing the CO_2 of the gastric mucosa to pass into the balloon and equilibrate. The saline and gas are withdrawn from the balloon and the partial pressure of CO_2 measured. This value, in conjunction with the arterial bicarbonate (HCO_3), is used through the Henderson-Hasselbach equation to calculate the pH of the gastric mucosa, and, by inference, the adequacy of blood flow to the splanchnic circulation (27–29). The logistical difficulties involved with this method, in conjunction with data suggesting that it is not able to distinguish survivors from nonsurvivors during resuscitation (30), has limited its popularity.

If the total picture of vital signs, urine output, and base deficit/lactate clearance do not follow a predictable trajectory toward normalization fairly quickly, the general consensus of the critical care community is that more

aggressive monitoring methods are indicated. Specifically, this means placement of a pulmonary artery catheter. Although controversial, these catheters allow calculation of the Do_2. Remember that the main variables that go into Do_2 are the hemoglobin concentration, the Sao_2, and the CO. The pulmonary artery catheter not only allows measurement of the CO, but it also provides essential information about preload. After placing the catheter, a Starling curve should be constructed to find the optimal PCWP beyond which CO is not augmented. If maintenance of this filling pressure still does not yield a satisfactory Do_2 to avoid anaerobic metabolism, inotropic agents should be considered.

When the Do_2 is normalized for body surface area, the resulting value is termed the *delivery of oxygen index* (Do_2I). Since the early 1980s, intensivists have debated the role of increasing Do_2I in an attempt to counter poor oxygen delivery to end organs in the shock state in the hope of improving outcomes. This resuscitation model of pulmonary artery catheter placement and using a given Do_2I value as an endpoint for resuscitation has been termed *goal-directed* resuscitation. Led by the thought that if some is good a lot might be better, others have advocated not only normalizing the Do_2, but driving it to supranormal numbers using liberal transfusions and pressors. This latter resuscitation strategy for patients in shock showed promise in a few initial studies. Multiple authors have shown trends toward improvements in survival when early (i.e., <12 hours after surgery or trauma) goal-directed therapy is instituted (31–34). However, a large meta-analysis on the subject found that despite achieving supranormal Do_2I levels, there was no significant reduction in mortality in this cohort of critically ill patients (35).

Moore et al. from UT-Houston and the Hermann Memorial Hospital Trauma Center have done a significant amount of work in trying to answer the question of whether or not supranormal Do_2I levels are of value in the resuscitation of patients in shock. They have eloquently described their protocol for shock resuscitation using goal-directed endpoints. In the time since its inception, they have computerized their protocol to provide the clinician real-time, data-driven decision support at the bedside. Additionally, in response to an article by Shoemaker himself that called into question his previous claim of benefit to the use of supranormal delivery levels (36), they have reduced their resuscitation endpoint from a Do_2I of 600 mL/min/m^2 to 500 mL/min/m^2 (37) after finding that shock resuscitation response was indistinguishable between the two groups, and that the group with the normal Do_2I endpoint was adequately resuscitated despite receiving less lactated Ringers solution and a trend toward less blood transfusion. Despite being a relatively small study, there seemed to be no significant benefit to a supranormal oxygen delivery goal.

The use of supranormal Do_2I was dealt what many have felt to be its final blow with the publication of two prospective trials that showed no survival benefit from the technique in the resuscitation of patients in septic shock (38,39). These two studies provided what is considered the most definitive answer to date, that while goal-directed therapy probably has a role in the resuscitation of patients in shock, the goal likely should be a more normal level of Do_2I (approximately 500 mL/min/m^2).

Historically, a hemoglobin level of 10 g/dL or a hematocrit of 30% were the generally accepted minimum levels consistent with patient safety, particularly in the surgical setting. First proposed in 1942, the "10/30" rule was a dogmatic rather than evidence-based recommendation as a trigger for the transfusion of red cells (40). In 1972, almost 90% of anesthesiology departments required preoperative hemoglobin of 10 g/dL, and even into the mid-1980s, this remained true for two thirds of anesthesiologists surveyed (41). The gradual recognition of the significant infectious and immunomodulatory side effects of blood transfusion led to more rigorous study of this practice. The Transfusion in Critical Care (TRICC) trial was a prospective randomized investigation comparing the effects of liberal and restrictive transfusion regimens in resuscitated, critically ill patients (42). The study utilized a protocol of transfusing patients to keep their hemoglobin levels at 10 g/dL or greater versus holding transfusions until the hemoglobin level reached 7 g/dL. The TRICC trial showed that when examining short-term mortality, an allogeneic RBC transfusion threshold as low as 7 g/dL was at least as safe as, and possibly superior to, a transfusion trigger of 10 g/dL. The one exception to this finding was in patients undergoing acute coronary syndromes (ACSs) who did benefit from having a hemoglobin level kept at 10 g/dL or greater. Again, the point should be emphasized that these were hemodynamically stable, well-resuscitated patients. Disappointingly, despite the strength of this class I data research has shown that these results have been slow to be incorporated into the practice patterns of many physicians (43).

Pump Disorders

Contractility refers to the force of contraction of the myocardial musculature independent of preload and afterload. This so-called inotropic state describes the ability of the heart to squeeze at a constant preload and afterload. The most important factor governing contractility is perfusion of the myocardium.

Cardiogenic shock can be thought of as failure of the heart to function effectively enough as a pump to provide adequate blood flow. This can be the result of intrinsic myocardial dysfunction or caused by extrinsic factors that limit the ability of the heart to function normally. When hemodynamic parameters are measured, a more precise definition would include a low systolic blood pressure (<90 mm Hg or 30 mm Hg below basal levels for 30 minutes), an elevated arteriovenous oxygen difference (>5.5 mL/dL), a depressed cardiac index (<2.2 L/min/m^2), and an adequate or elevated wedge pressure (>15 mm Hg).

Before diagnosing cardiogenic shock, it is critical to correct or exclude nonmyocardial factors that contribute to hypoperfusion, with the most common being hypovolemia. Once satisfied that the etiology likely stems from cardiac dysfunction, the next step in the process is to decide if the problem lies at the level of the heart muscle or in thoracic problems that affect normal cardiac performance.

Several causes of primary myocardial dysfunction are seen frequently in patients with cardiogenic shock. The most common of these is myocardial infarction with loss of at least 40% of functioning left ventricular myocardium. The primary insult is that of weakened myocardial contraction strength, with a commensurate drop in stroke volume and CO. Consequently, end diastolic volume (preload) increases causing an increased wedge pressure. The increased pressure head is transmitted to the lungs, and pulmonary edema with hypoxia can result. The hypoperfusion is therefore aggravated by both a decreased content and delivery of oxygenated blood. Although the phenomenon of right ventricle infarction predisposing to a shock state caused by bundle branch blocks and arrhythmias has long been recognized, the ability of isolated right ventricular infarction to cause cardiogenic shock is a matter of controversy.

As previously mentioned, arrhythmias can also produce a state of hypoperfusion. Tachycardia is a useful compensatory mechanism for hypoxia, but at heart rates above 150 beats/min, the time allowed for diastolic filling can become so short that an insufficient volume enters the ventricle to maintain an adequate CO. Further, the coronary arteries are perfused during diastole. A decrease in diastolic perfusion time decreases coronary filling and can render the myocardium ischemic, further exacerbating the problem. Bradycardia can be equally harmful. When one considers that the determinants of CO are stroke volume multiplied by heart rate, it is apparent that a decrease in the pulse rate with maintenance of stroke volume will adversely impact the amount of blood delivered to the periphery.

Although myocardial infarction causes a loss of muscle mass, it also poses a serious hazard in that it predisposes to the development of mechanical defects. In this situation, ischemic or necrotic myocardium not only loses its ability to contract effectively, but it also ceases to support the structures vital to the pumping mechanism. Damage to myocardium acting as the foundation for the papillary muscles and chordae tendineae can result in their rupture with consequent insufficiency of the mitral valve. Infarction of the septal perforating branches of the left anterior descending artery can cause necrosis of this muscle and a ventricular septal defect. This finding usually presents with the abrupt onset of heart failure and a new murmur 3 to 5 days after a myocardial infarction. Large transmural infarcts involving the left ventricle predispose to free-wall rupture after 5 to 7 days. This usually presents with sudden death. A more common complication is left ventricular aneurysm formation, which has been estimated to occur in 15% of infarction survivors, and can result in loss of cardiac function (44). Cardiogenic shock resulting from any of these peri-infarct mechanical perturbations is associated with a very high mortality.

The extrinsic causes of cardiogenic shock have an end result of decreased CO similar to that of intrinsic disease. However, in these circumstances, normal myocardium is laboring under the influence of an external insult until the very end stages. Venous inflow can be blocked by mechanical kinking with tension pneumothorax, or by luminal obstruction with caval obstruction or pulmonary embolism. The syndrome can also be seen in pericardial tamponade, which progressively decreases diastolic filling volumes of the left ventricle.

No matter what the etiology of the pump's failure, the body's compensatory mechanisms are largely the same. As stroke volume falls, hypotension results. Reflex responses, namely the baroreceptor mechanism and sympathetic output, serve to increase peripheral vascular resistance. The extent and location of the cumulative myocardial damage will determine whether these compensatory mechanisms are able to achieve hemodynamic stability. In the favorable situation, the uninvolved myocardium is able to compensate, peripheral perfusion is maintained, and the patient usually has an uncomplicated convalescence. When compensatory mechanisms cannot offset the degree of myocardial damage, CO continues to fall and shock ultimately ensues. Adequate intravascular volume must be established to differentiate between these two scenarios.

Cardiogenic shock can present in a manner similar to that of hypovolemic shock in that both sets of patients will experience increased peripheral vasoconstriction, with pale, cool extremities and decreased urine output. Those with a cardiac etiology who are still lucid will often give a characteristic history of chest pressure or pain and shortness of breath. Frequently, a long history of cardiac problems will be found on questioning. On physical examination, these patients will often have crackles suggestive of pulmonary edema, and murmurs or gallops indicative of heart failure. Jugular venous distention, hepatomegaly, and peripheral edema are sometimes found. These findings point away from hypovolemia as an etiology for the shock state and should prompt an appropriate cardiac workup.

Once comfortable with the diagnosis of intrinsic cardiac dysfunction, therapy should be delivered in a systematic manner. The first priority in the stabilization of a patient in cardiogenic shock is the airway, breathing, and circulation (ABC) of any resuscitation. Once maintenance of an airway and oxygenation are secured, attention should be turned to the patient's hemodynamics. Low ventricular fillings pressures should be augmented with volume until PCWPs are at least 15 mm Hg. If the CO remains low despite this intervention, one can be reasonably confident in the diagnosis of cardiogenic shock. In this instance, hypotension in the face of euvolemia warrants pharmacologic support with a vasopressor dictated by the patient's systemic vascular resistance (SVR).

Hypotension with an elevated SVR is best treated initially with an agent that increases contractility while simultaneously gently dilating the periphery. This not only increases CO, but also decreases the pressure head against which the left ventricle must work. Dobutamine, a synthetic agent that acts primarily on β-1 receptors in the myocardium, is an ideal drug for this effect. An alternative agent is amrinone. This phosphodiesterase inhibitor works by inhibiting the degradation of cyclic adenosine monophosphate (cAMP) in myocardial cells, and has an action profile similar to that of dobutamine. If the inotropic agent alone is not enough to decrease the SVR, an afterload reducing agent such as nitroprusside may be added. A word of caution should be given regarding attempts at afterload reduction alone in the face of hypotension and an elevated SVR. This should only be undertaken with extreme caution, as the increased peripheral resistance may be the principal mechanism preventing the patient's pressure from dropping further.

Should invasive monitoring reveal a low or normal SVR in the face of hypotension, an agent which will "tighten up" the periphery is indicated. In this regard, dopamine has a dose-dependent action profile. At low doses, dopamine causes dilation of renal blood vessels and increased renal blood flow. At slightly higher does (i.e., 5–10 μg/kg/min), it results in stimulation of β-1 receptors at the level of the myocardium, and has a largely inotropic function. At doses higher than 10 μg/kg/min, it begins to stimulate α receptors in the periphery, with a consequent increase in SVR. Another drug that potently stimulates both α and β receptors is epinephrine.

Failure to respond to pharmacologic support warrants consideration of mechanical support of the heart. Initially, intra-aortic balloon pump (IABP) counter pulsation is usually employed. The IABP is positioned in the descending aorta where it is linked to the electrocardiography (EKG) to inflate 40 ms before the T wave and to deflate with the P wave. This results in inflation during diastole and deflation during systole. The physiologic effect is to increase coronary perfusion pressure during diastole and decrease afterload during systole. The net effect is an increase in myocardial oxygen supply and a decrease in demand, thereby improving ischemia. The IABP is most useful if myocardial dysfunctional is expected to be transient. Generally, patients are weaned from it over a few days by decreasing its rate of inflation from every beat to every other beat. This is gradually decreased to inflating with every third beat of the heart followed by discontinuation.

The management of cardiogenic shock complicating ACS has been made difficult by the fact that a majority of trials for various ACS interventions such as medical management alone, percutaneous angioplasty, and emergency coronary artery revascularization have excluded patients with cardiogenic shock because of the extremely high mortality rate when the two conditions are superimposed. Early exceptions were the Global use of Strategies to Open Occluded Coronary Arteries (GUSTO) trials conducted from 1990 to 1993 (GUSTO I) (45) and 1995 to 1997 (GUSTO III) (46). Among other findings, they noted that mortality for ACS complicated by cardiogenic shock was lower at centers in the Unites States as opposed to Europe, and that invasive revascularization techniques were also performed more commonly in the United States as well. With the very large caveat that these findings were in patients who had been selected rather than randomized, these studies were the first evidence that invasive revascularization may carry a benefit over thrombolytics and medical management in these patients. The Should We Emergently Revascularize Occluded Coronaries for Cardiogenic Shock (SHOCK) trial was a large, randomized prospective trial conducted from 1993 to 1998 which examined the effects of emergency angioplasty or bypass grafting versus medical management consisting of treatment with a balloon pump and thrombolytics if indicated. No significant difference was seen in 30-day mortality rates between the arms. However, in the revascularization group, the subgroup analysis showed that patients younger than 75 clearly benefited from a revascularization procedure. In addition, there was an overall benefit with revascularization when considering 6-month mortality (47). Subsequent studies of these patients have shown that the overall survival advantage of the emergency revascularization group persisted at 1 year (48) and 6 years of follow-up (49).

Afterload Disorders

Afterload is the resistance against which the heart muscle contracts. It is physiologically equivalent to ventricular wall tension during systole. Clinically, the SVR is the entity that estimates afterload. It can be calculated using Ohms law, which is:

$$V = IR$$

and therefore

$$R = V/I$$

Where V is the pressure difference across the capillary bed (R). Physiologically, this is equivalent to the mean arterial pressure (MAP) minus the central venous pressure (CVP). In this equation, I is the flow or CO. Eighty is a conversion factor, resulting in:

$$SVR = \frac{MAP - CVP}{CO} \times 80$$

The normal value is 900 to 1,400 dynes/s/cm^5.

Disturbances of afterload are frequently referred to as distributive shock, and they arise when the SVR drops to the point that, regardless of CO, the periphery is underperfused. Distributive shock can arise from any process that interferes with the control of vasomotor tone by the nervous system, or that causes the release of immunologic mediators that dilate the periphery. On the basis of etiology, it can be further broken down into neurogenic shock, septic shock, and anaphylactic shock.

Neurogenic shock is a hypotensive state that results from trauma to the thoracic or cervical regions of the spinal cord sufficient to interrupt the sympathetic outflow tracts responsible for vascular tone. This loss of vasoconstriction results in blood pooling in the now-maximally dilated periphery and a consequent decrease in venous return to the heart and ventricular filling pressures. Although cord injury is the classic model for this category of shock, the same clinical picture can be seen with spinal anesthesia or any event that causes massive vagal stimulation (i.e., acute gastric dilatation, a grief reaction, the sight of blood). The patient in neurogenic shock will manifest all of the signs and symptoms of hypotension without vasoconstrictive compensation. Peripheral pulses will be weak, urine output is usually adequate, capillary refill is brisk, and the extremities are warm and dry. Further, the pulse rate will be low secondary to the unopposed vagal stimulation of the heart. Finally, when spinal cord injury is the etiology, the patient in neurogenic shock will usually manifest motor and sensory deficits as well as decreased sphincter tone. A note of caution in evaluating patients presumed to have neurogenic shock after spinal trauma is in order. The energy required to cause damage to the spinal cord puts the patient at significant risk for concomitant intra-abdominal or skeletal injuries. Concurrent hemorrhagic shock must be considered and ruled out in these patients lest an occult injury be missed.

Septic shock results from the response of the body to an overwhelming infection. In the course of infection, bacterial wall components are released. One such component is endotoxin, a lipopolysaccharide found in the cell wall of gram-negative bacteria. It is the body's response to endotoxemia which is one of the most common causes of septic shock in that inflammatory mediators become activated and result in characteristic hemodynamic derangements including profound vasodilation.

The changes that occur with septic shock constitute a spectrum of disease. These changes are classically described as "hyperdynamic" in the early stages of the shock process, and "hypodynamic" in the later, decompensated stages. The hyperdynamic stage is marked by a low SVR with an increased CO and warm extremities. Increased venous pooling and capillary permeability lead to an effective decrease in circulating volume and tissue perfusion. Further, while the peripheral system as a whole has decreased resistance, the splanchnic system is markedly vasoconstricted. As the disease process worsens, the endotoxin-induced metabolic derangements begin to exert a myocardial-depressive effect, and the patient decompensates into the hypodynamic stage of the disease. CO drops, the extremities become cool and pale, and oliguria develops.

A hallmark of septic shock is an endotoxin-induced metabolic derangement that results in inefficient extraction and/or utilization of oxygen from the microcirculation. This occurs to such a degree that it is not uncommon to see normal or even increased mixed Svo_2 in profoundly acidotic patients. The mechanism behind this finding is still under investigation.

Anaphylactic shock is a consequence of a hypersensitivity reaction caused when immunoglobulin E (IgE) on the surface of mast cells and basophils binds a particular antigen. This binding causes the mast cells and basophils to degranulate and release a host of immunologic mediators. When released in large enough quantity, these mediators cause capillary leakage and a drop in peripheral resistance similar to that seen with septic shock.

Treatment

Treatment of distributive shock depends on its etiology. In neurogenic shock, initial therapy consists of simply "filling the tank" after ensuring that a concurrent source of hemorrhagic shock does not exist. Because the circulatory capacity is suddenly much larger than the normal blood volume, fluid expansion of this compartment is often adequate treatment and many patients in neurogenic shock will respond to a standard 2 L bolus of crystalloid solution with stabilization of the systolic blood pressure. Should fluid resuscitation in a patient with a high cord injury not stabilize the blood pressure, a vasopressor which augments *a*-adrenergic discharge should be utilized. Once hemodynamic stability is achieved, most patients will not need ongoing support as their spinal cords eventually begin to function independently and restore sympathetic discharge enough to avoid pacemaker placement and pharmacologic blood pressure support.

The treatment of septic shock is much more complex as the metabolic derangements are more severe than in the other types of distributive shock, and multiple priorities must be addressed simultaneously. The complexity of the subject led 11 leading international critical care and infection societies to create the Surviving Sepsis Campaign in 2003. This effort was designed to promulgate a set of evidence-based guidelines for the management of severe sepsis and septic shock in order to improve outcomes (50), and should be required reading for any physician caring for these patients. Although the treatment of septic shock could merit its own chapter, some of the more salient topics will be discussed here.

In 2001, an important study was published emphasizing that the timeliness of an intervention for sepsis is as important as the intervention itself. Rivers et al. randomized septic patients presenting to the emergency room into arms that received early central venous saturation monitoring with crystalloid infusion, blood transfusion, and pressor utilization as needed to achieve predetermined resuscitation endpoints, or to standard therapy which included delaying invasive monitoring until the patient arrived in the ICU. They found a significantly lower mortality rate in those patients who had early interventions (51). This study emphasizes the importance of acting quickly and aggressively in this patient population.

Early volume challenge with boluses should be used to augment filling pressures. If blood pressure fails to quickly normalize and evidence of ongoing tissue dysoxia persists, invasive monitoring with an α-agonist is warranted. The finding that septic patients requiring increasing dosages of vasopressors have lower-than-expected endogenous vasopressin levels has led to a hypothesis that these patients suffer from a "relative vasopressin deficiency," and should be supplemented with low doses of vasopressin infusions (i.e., 0.01–0.04 U/min). This subject is a focus of ongoing trials.

It is the position of the Surviving Sepsis Campaign that appropriate broad spectrum antibiotics likely to cover the suspected pathogen should be initiated within the first hour of sepsis is recognized and cultures are drawn (50). Source control is paramount as the etiology of sepsis should be aggressively sought. If the source is surgically amenable, it should be dealt with expeditiously: abscesses should be drained, necrotic skin debrided, and infected devices removed.

Hyperglycemia is common in critically ill patients, even in patients without a pre-existing diagnosis of diabetes. Elevated blood glucose has an effect of "coating" phagocytes, impairing their ability to function in a manner that is proportional to the level of hyperglycemia. This practical immunosuppression led Van den Berghe et al. to randomize critically ill patients to tight blood sugar control of 80 to 110 mg/dL versus standard therapy (52). The patients with tight control of their blood sugars had a significantly higher survival rate, and this effect was most pronounced in their septic patients. Consequently, it is the consensus of the ICU community that all septic patients should have their blood glucose maintained between these parameters with insulin drips.

Many studies have shown that protein C is depleted in both adult and pediatric patients with sepsis and that there is an inverse correlation between the level of protein C and mortality and morbidity in these patients (53–57). Mesters et al. (58) reported that a decrease in plasma protein C levels preceded the onset of the clinical symptoms of severe sepsis and septic shock by a median of 12 hours, indicating that depletion of protein C occurs early in the disease course. This early decrease in protein C levels in the pathogenesis of sepsis is further supported by the prevalence (90%) of acquired protein C deficiency in patients with severe sepsis (59). This depletion is probably caused by a combination of degradation of protein C by neutrophil elastase (60) which is released during sepsis, depletion of the plasma pool of protein C during the continuous and rapid conversion of protein C to activated protein C that occurs in sepsis, and inadequate biosynthesis of protein C to replenish the circulating pool (61).

Recombinant Protein C is an inhibitor of factor Va, VIIIA, and plasminogen activator inhibitor-1, thereby regulating the clotting cascade. Other proposed effects include blocking of leukocyte adhesion, and limitation of thrombin-induced inflammation. This results in the activated form of protein C having anticoagulant, fibrinolytic, and anti-inflammatory properties. At suprapharmacologic concentrations, protein C inhibits neutrophil-endothelial adhesion by acting as an alternative ligand for E-selectin. In sepsis, this results in a clinical effect of improved microcirculation, Do_2, and limitation of endothelial inflammation and vascular permeability.

The administration of activated protein C to patients with severe sepsis was associated with a significant reduction in mortality in the Recombinant Human-Activated Protein C Worldwide Evaluation in Severe Sepsis (PROWESS) trial where the absolute survival benefit was 6% overall and 13% in the high-risk population (62). Interestingly, in *post hoc* subgroup analysis there was a large, highly significant survival benefit with therapy in subjects with more severe degrees of illness, but no evidence of benefit in subjects who were not as sick. Recombinant activated protein C was subsequently approved by the U.S. Food and Drug Administration (FDA) for the treatment of severe sepsis associated with organ dysfunction in adults at high risk of death.

A major risk associated with activated protein C is hemorrhage, and this limits its use in many surgical patients. Caution is advised in the use of activated protein C in patients with an international normalized ratio (INR) greater than 3.0 or a platelet count of less than 30,000 per cubic millimeter. Currently, activated protein C is approved only for use in patients with sepsis who have the most severe organ compromise and the highest likelihood of death based on the Acute Physiology and Chronic Health Evaluation (APACHE) scoring system.

Given the inflammatory and immunologic dyscrasias that are seen in the severely septic state, it should not be surprising that the role of adjunctive steroid use in the treatment of the condition was an area of intense interest for many years. Unfortunately, several randomized, multicenter trials in the 1980s yielded results which demonstrated that there was no role for high-dose corticosteroid therapy in the treatment of severe sepsis (63–65). The subject of corticosteroids in the treatment of sepsis was largely considered settled in the critical care community for a matter of years.

In the early 1990s, however, interest in corticosteroids as a therapy in septic shock was renewed, this time using more physiologic doses for longer durations of time. It came to be appreciated that there was a subclass of septic patient who had a "relative" adrenal insufficiency. These patients have elevated serum cortisol levels as would be expected in such a stress state. If, however, they were administered a dose of an adrenal gland stimulant (such as adrenocorticotropic hormone), the serum cortisol levels would not increase as would be expected, therefore signifying that the adrenal glands were working maximally and not capable of further augmentation of output. If this level of cortisol output was not sufficient to meet the body's requirements, they were considered to be relatively adrenal insufficient (66). Annane et al. tested this notion in patients with vasopressor-dependent sepsis who did not increase their serum cortisol levels by greater than 9 μg/dL in response to an adrenocorticotropin hormone stimulation test. In this multicenter, randomized, blinded study they found a significant survival benefit in patients treated with the low-dose steroid replacement regimen (67). It is now the consensus of the critical care community that septic patients who require vasopressors to support their blood pressure should be treated for 7 days with 300 mg/d of hydrocortisone divided among 3 or 4 doses. The issue of whether or not they should undergo adrenal gland stimulation before treatment is controversial.

Anaphylactic shock requires early attention to the patient's airway. Edema of the soft tissues of the neck can cause aerodigestive compromise, and early intubation for true anaphylaxis should be strongly considered. In addition to the usual volume infusion, treatment with antihistamines is standard. In instances of shock, the use of epinephrine is also desirable because of its dual role as a sympathetic agonist and its ability to block the release of inflammatory mediators by mast cells and basophils (68).

THE LETHAL TRIAD

An appreciation for the consequences of the hemorrhagic shock state has led to a revision of trauma surgery principles over the last two decades. This was spawned by the observation that surgeries with good technical results were resulting in bad patient outcomes secondary to irreversible metabolic distress. This combination of acidosis, coagulopathy, and hypothermia has come to be known as the *lethal triad*, as each contributes to the other in a cycle that frequently proved fatal. The recognition that this phenomenon was time dependent prompted surgeons to begin truncating initial procedures on severely injured patients after achieving hemostasis and controlling spill from the alimentary tract. These temporized patients would undergo aggressive correction of their acidosis, coagulopathy, and hypothermia in the ICU with plans for a return trip to the operating room for definitive management of their injuries if they survived their resuscitation. This technique of quickly and solely controlling hemorrhage and contamination in order to expedite reestablishing a survivable physiology has come to be known as *damage control* surgery, and its use has resulted in improved mortality rates (69–76). Although its application in abdominal trauma is now routine, the concept has also begun to be utilized in thoracic trauma, albeit with some modifications. The principle of expediting the operative management of unstable patients still holds in thoracic damage control. In addition to abdominal damage control's emphasis on temporizing injuries, however, thoracic damage control also entails performing definitive techniques which are rapid and relatively simple. The utilization of damage control thoracotomy has led to better-than-expected survival rates for these badly injured patients (77).

Coagulopathy

The coagulopathy seen in damage control patients is multifactorial. It is consumptive, dilutional, and functional as the kinetics of the clotting enzyme cascades are trying to work outside their optimal pH and temperature ranges. Similarly, correction of coagulopathy must be simultaneously directed at replacement of clotting factors as well as reestablishment of a favorable physiologic environment. One thing to keep in mind when testing a patient's coagulation profile is that most labs normally warm the sample sent to them to 37°C in order to run the test. Consequently, this value may underestimate the true level of coagulopathy in the hypothermic patient. Hypothermia also confounds the process of testing for coagulopathy by inhibiting thromboxane B_2 production (78). This results in abnormal platelet function, even in the presence of adequate platelet levels.

Standard therapy for clotting factor replacement has been liberal transfusion with fresh frozen plasma and platelet concentrates. Additionally, the importance of cryoprecipitate transfusion, as it is rich in fibrinogen, and calcium administration for its role in the coagulation cascade, cannot be overemphasized. The citrate in banked blood binds calcium thereby lowering the serum levels, and in the setting of massive transfusion its empiric administration is advisable. In recent years, there has been increasing interest in the use of recombinant activated factor VII (rfVII) as an adjunct in the resuscitation process. Originally approved as a treatment for hemophiliacs who had become sensitized to donor pools of Factor VIII and IX in 1998, it has been utilized off-label for the management of nonsurgical bleeding in trauma patients in a number of case reports and small series (79–82). Interestingly, although acidosis appears to diminish the hemostatic efficacy of the drug, hypothermia does not (83). Although early anecdotal evidence generally showed a strongly positive effect on hemostasis, research efforts have been hindered by institutional variations in dosing and timing regimens, its frequent use as a treatment of last resort (and consequent difficulty with cohort matching), and the cost of the drug ($3,000–$8,000 per 50–100 μg/kg dose) (84). Further, those studies which did retrospectively utilize controls did not show a survival benefit to rfVII utilization (85,86). Boffard et al. (87) recently reported the results of parallel randomized, double-blinded placebo controlled trials of rfVII in more than 300 blunt and penetrating injuries. In both trials, patients receiving their sixth unit of packed red cell transfusion in 4 hours were randomized to receive 200 μg/kg of rfVII followed by 100 μg/kg at 1 and 3 hours after the first dose, or placebo. Neither arm showed a mortality benefit, while patients suffering from a blunt mechanism had a significantly lower transfusion requirement and lower incidence of massive transfusion. In an effort to define those patients in whom rfVII use was futile, Stein et al. (84) identified a prothrombin time of 17.6 seconds and a Revised Trauma Score of 4.09 as independent predictors of a lack of rfVII effect. Further investigations into the role of rfVII in resuscitation continue. Only bench work and anecdotal evidence exist for the use of the antifibrinolytic aprotinin in treating coagulopathy (88,89) and its use in trauma resuscitations cannot be recommended at this time.

Hypothermia

The lethality of hypothermia in the setting of trauma is well documented as previous work has shown a 100% mortality when core temperatures are allowed to drop below 32°C (Table 4.2) (90). All fluids should be transfused through warmers, and ventilator gases should be warmed and humidified. Warm air blankets as well as warmed sheets should be used, and care should be taken to bundle them around the patient's head as this is a significant source of heat loss. Gentilello (91) et al. described the use of continuous arteriovenous rewarming as a method of rapidly correcting a cold core body temperature. In this technique, percutaneously placed arterial and venous femoral catheters are connected to the inflow and outflow ports of a fluid warmer in order to use the patient's own arterial pressure to drive blood flow through the circuit and warm it extracorporeally. Its major limitation lies in the requirement of an adequate MAP to drive flow. When utilized, however, it has resulted in significantly faster rewarming times (39 minutes to correction of hypothermia versus 3.2 hours in a control arm) and better outcomes (92). Other technologies utilizing venovenous rewarming and a pump have shown promise in the preclinical setting, but have yet to make the leap to the bedside (93).

Acidosis

As has been previously discussed, hypoperfusion at the level of the cell is the etiology of the metabolic acidosis manifested by patients in hemorrhagic shock, and its correction centers around optimizing volume status and shifting cellular metabolism from anaerobic to aerobic. Again, the main determinants of oxygen delivery are cardiac index, hemoglobin concentration, and oxygen saturation of hemoglobin. Treatment should center on assuring the adequacy of each of these variables without overzealously "flooding" the patient. Excessive and unnecessary fluid administration can exacerbate lung injuries and cause visceral edema. It is incumbent on the surgeon to be alert for signs that this edema and its obligatory increase in intra-abdominal pressure have progressed to the development of an abdominal

TABLE 4.2

Analysis of Injury Severity Score (ISS), Lowest Core Temperature, and Mortality

| | | | 34°C | | 33°C | | 32°C | |
| | | | *Colder* | *Warmer* | *Colder* | *Warmer* | *Colder* | *Warmer* |
	n	*Percentage of Mortality*	*Percentage of Mortality*	*Percentage of Mortality*	*Percentage of Mortality*	*Percentage of Mortality*	*Percentage of Mortality*	*Percentage of Mortality*
Total	71	21	40	7	69	7	100	10
ISS 25–29	35	11	33	0	50	4	100	3
ISS 30-29	17	0	0	0	0	0	—	0
ISS 40–49	9	44	33	67	67	33	100	38
ISS >50	10	70	66	100	100	25	100	40

Relation between hypothermia and mortality. Note that at core temperatures below 32°C, mortality was 100%. (Adapted from Jurkovich GJ, Greiser WB, Luterman A, et al. Hypothermia in trauma victims: an ominous predictor of survival. *J Trauma* 1987; 27:1019–1024.)

compartment syndrome, which can require a decompressive laparotomy even in the absence of abdominal injuries.

The Abdominal Compartment Syndrome

Hopefully as hypothermia and coagulopathy are addressed and oxygen delivery is optimized with volume loading and packed red cell transfusion, the resuscitation will proceed smoothly with a rapid move toward reestablishing a survivable physiology. If it does not, a decision must be made as to whether surgical bleeding still exists and a return trip to the operating room is required. One of the most difficult scenarios with which a surgeon contends is deciding whether ongoing postoperative bleeding is due to coagulopathy or a missed source requiring surgical intervention, because judging incorrectly is usually a fatal error. Just as a missed source of surgical bleeding dooms the patient, so too can the effects of an open body cavity and general anesthesia on an unstable patient being returned to the operating room for the bleeding that accompanies being cold and coagulopathic. A threshold of 6 units of packed red cell transfusion in 6 hours without a change in hematocrit has been put forth by some authors as a trigger for returning to the operating room (94). Reoperation may also be required if resuscitation efforts result in visceral edema profound enough to impair diaphragmatic excursion. This "abdominal compartment syndrome" manifests as increased peak inspiratory pressures on the ventilator, hypercarbia, and oliguria. If the diagnosis is in doubt, bladder pressure should be checked as the bladder acts as a passive conduit for intraperitoneal pressure. This is performed by instilling 100 mL of saline into the bladder followed by clamping of the Foley tube, leveling of the pressure-sensing diaphragm on the Foley with the pubic symphysis, and sticking the diaphragm with a zeroed needle hooked up to a pressure transducer. A value of 30 mm Hg is indicative of a degree of pressure which should be addressed. Having said that, we prefer to diagnose the syndrome clinically. The treatment is to reopen the laparotomy, or perform one if the abdominal compartment syndrome is secondary to a massive volume resuscitation for

other reasons such as pancreatitis or a burn. The bowel is subsequently eviscerated. Once the compartment syndrome has been alleviated, a vacuum-based dressing can be placed over the bowel if ongoing bleeding is not a concern, while a sterile cassette drape or 3 L IV bag can be opened up and sutured to the skin edges if bleeding is an issue and a vacuum application is contraindicated.

THE INFLAMMATORY RESPONSE AND ORGAN FAILURE SYNDROMES

Commensurate with improvements in prehospital care, the development of organized trauma systems, increased understanding of the pathophysiology of shock, and improvements in critical care technology, intensivists began to see an increase in the severity of injury from which patients could be salvaged. As these massively injured patients began to survive their resuscitations and went on to have prolonged ICU stays, anecdotal reports began to appear in the literature of a syndrome that often culminated in death from progressive, irreversible organ damage. The pattern of this clinical course led Eiseman to coin the phrase "multiorgan failure (MOF)" in 1977 (95). As experience with the entity of MOF became more common, it became clear that death from traumatic injury was following a trimodal distribution. Death in the first subset occurs at the scene of injury, whereas the second peak occurs within 6 hours of injury and usually results from unsuccessful resuscitation. The third occurs within 30 days from MOF (96). The only interventions applicable to the first population are prevention measures, and advances in prehospital care have been used successfully to counter the second. The last group has been considerably more challenging as it has required elucidation of the body's natural response to stress and injury as well as the pathologic response seen in these badly injured patients before being able to create therapeutic strategies aimed at its modulation.

It is now widely accepted that the basic physiologic insult in this last group of patients appears to be an exaggeration

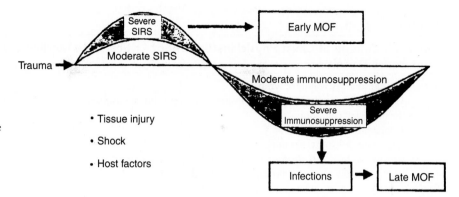

FIGURE 4.8 The proposed relation underlying the immunologic pathophysiology of multiple organ failure (MOF). SIRS, systemic inflammatory response syndrome. (From *American Journal of Surgery* 1999;178:449–453 with permission.)

of the body's normal homeostatic response to an injury or infection. Here, these critically ill patients experience the development of a body-wide inflammatory state known as the systemic inflammatory response syndrome (SIRS). SIRS is a sterile phenomenon with an immunologic profile dominated in the early hours by proinflammatory cytokines. With time, counter-regulatory mechanisms result in an inhibition of the inflammatory response and a mild immunosuppression. This is probably an adaptive response. If the process overcompensates, however, a severe immunosuppressive state can result leaving the patient at risk for infection (i.e., sepsis) (Fig. 4.8) (97,98). The confusion and inconsistency of the terms SIRS, sepsis, septic shock, and MOF led the American College of Chest Physicians and Society of Critical Care Medicine to propose diagnostic criteria to accompany each of these terms (Table 4.3) (99). Interestingly, a revisitation of these definitions at a consensus conference in 2001 showed them to be suprisingly durable, and no major changes were made beyond expanding the list of signs and symptoms of sepsis (100). A glance at the criteria shows the ubiquity of these syndromes in the average ICU population.

Let us begin by examining the mechanisms behind the proinflammatory state during shock. The initial physiologic changes that occur with hemorrhage are the result of complex interactions between humoral and cellular systems. The earliest of the humoral systems to be involved is the complement cascade. With hemorrhage, complement is activated with release of the biologically active anaphylotoxins C3a and C5a. These substances cause granulocyte activation and aggregation, increased vascular permeability, smooth muscle contraction, and release of histamine and arachidonic acid metabolites. They have also been shown to induce the release of the proinflammatory cytokines tumor necrosis factor (TNF) and interleukin 1 (IL-1) (101). These cytokines are macrophage-derived proteins, and are the key mediators of the inflammatory response. The infusion of low doses of TNF-α and IL-1β can precipitate many of the signs of sepsis including fever, hypotension [by stimulating inducible nitric oxide (NO) synthase], fatigue, and anorexia. TNF-α promotes adhesion of white blood cells to the endothelium, induces neutrophil activation, and mediates the production and release of numerous other proinflammatory cytokines. IL-1β shares many of these properties. Blockade of TNF-α

and IL-1β stunts the inflammatory response in an additive manner. Other proinflammatory mediators are IL-6 and IL-8. IL-6 is key to the induction of T and B cells and the acute phase response. IL-8 helps to recruit and activate inflammatory cells at the site of injury (102).

The cells that represent the first line of defense against tissue damage or pathogenic invaders are the polymorphonuclear cells (PMNs). When injury or infection occurs, PMNs follow a chemotactic gradient to the site of injury, where they are activated and release their metabolic products. These substances, such as proteolytic enzymes and reactive oxygen species, help to destroy and remove damaged tissue. Further, PMNs also release vasoactive substances such as leukotrienes, eicosanoids, and platelet activating factor (PAF). Some of these substances cause the local endothelium to elaborate adhesion molecules known as selectins (E-selectin and P-selectin),intracellular adhesion molecules (ICAMs), and vascular cell adhesion molecules (VCAMs). PMNs in the vessel lumen express their own adhesion molecules known as L-selectins and the CD11/CD18 receptor complex. These allow the PMNs to bind to the endothelial adhesion molecules (103,104). Once bound, this second wave of PMNs migrates through the endothelium to the site of injury where they too release their own proinflammatory granules. When locally limited to the site of an insult, this is a vital function. In SIRS, however, there is the unregulated elaboration of these toxic metabolites, which are largely responsible for the damage caused by this condition.

As previously mentioned, the proinflammatory stimuli dominate the early phases of injury. It is thought that an anti-inflammatory response begins to eventually manifest and attempts to bring the organism back to a state of homeostasis. The chief mediators of this response are IL-4 and IL-10. Both of these cytokines act to inhibit TNF-α, IL-1, IL-6, and IL-8. These brakes on the inflammatory cascade may limit TNF-α–induced cellular damage.

As this overview of the cytokine milieu was elucidated, efforts began to center on piecing together how they resulted in the clinical entity of MOF. Some advocated what has come to be referred to as the *two-hit* hypothesis as a possible etiology for the development of MOF (Fig. 4.9) (105). In this paradigm, the individual mounts an immunologically

TABLE 4.3

American College of Chest Physicians/Society of Critical Care Medicine (ACCP/SCCM) Consensus Conference Definitions

Systemic inflammatory response syndrome

The systemic inflammatory response to a variety of severe clinical insults; the response is manifested by two or more of the following conditions

Temperature, $>38°C$ or $<36°C$

Heart rate, >90 beats per minute

Respiratory rate >20 breaths per minute or $Pa_{CO_2} <32$ mm Hg

WBC $>12,000/$ mm^3, $4,000/$mm^3, or $>10\%$ bandemia

Sepsis

The systemic responses to infection; this systemic response is manifested by two or more of the following conditions as a result of infection

Temperature $>38°C$ or $<36°C$

Heart rate >90 beats per minute

Respiratory rate >20 breaths per minute or $Pa_{CO_2} <32$ mm Hg

WBC $>12,000/$ mm^3, $<4,000/$mm^3, or $>10\%$ bandemia

Severe sepsis

Sepsis associated with organ dysfunction, hypoperfusion, or hypotension

Hypoperfusion and perfusion abnormalities may include, but are not limited to lactic acidosis, oliguria, or an acute alteration in mental status

Septic shock

A subset of severe sepsis; sepsis with hypotension despite adequate fluid resuscitation along with the presence of perfusion abnormalities that may include, but are not limited to, lactic acidosis, oliguria, or an acute alteration in mental status; patients who are on inotropic or vasopressor support may not be hypotensive at the time that perfusion abnormalities are measured.

Multiple organ dysfunction syndrome

Presence of altered organ function in an acutely ill patient such that homeostasis cannot be maintained without intervention.

From Members of the American College of Chest Physicians/Society of Critical Care Medicine Consensus Conference Committee. American College of Chest Physicians/Society of Critical Care Medicine Consensus Conference: definitions for sepsis and organ failure and guidelines for the use of innovative therapies in sepsis. (*Crit Care Med* 1992;20:864–874, with permission.)

appropriate response to an insult. The recovery from this episode, however, leaves the host with a "primed" immune system. With the onset of a second challenge, the organism manifests an exaggerated immune response that culminates in SIRS and possible MOF (105).

Other investigators centered their interest on the possible role of the alimentary tract. It has long been known that one of the compensatory mechanisms of shock is to produce splanchnic vasoconstriction in an attempt to shunt blood to more vital structures. As a result of this process, the gastrointestinal tract may become ischemic, followed by reperfusion, which has been shown to produce cell injury. The gut was first implicated as a potential player in the development of MOF as a way to account for the fact that no identifiable source of infection could be found in up to 30% of patients with bacteremia who later died of MOF (106). Most investigators have ascribed this to the breakdown of gut mucosal integrity, the result of an ischemic insult. This was supported by evidence that intestinal mucosa becomes permeable in the septic state (107). Whether this feature promotes the inflammatory response by the translocation of bacteria across the gut wall or from the release of cytokines from intestinal lymphoid tissue is still debated. The working

model for the role of the gut in the development of MOF has centered upon early mediator release exacerbating the SIRS response, whereas late bacterial translocation contributes to infection during the relative immunosuppression seen later in the disease course (97).

The last decade has brought an appreciation for the role of blood transfusions in the development of MOF. The immunomodulatory effects of red cell transfusions have been known since early studies which showed lower rejection rates for transfused kidney transplant patients as well as higher recurrence rates for patients with colorectal malignancies who received transfusions at the time of surgery (108–115). These intriguing findings led to the discovery that red cell transfusion is an *independent* risk factor for MOF in trauma patients (116), with a threshold of 6 units of red cell transfusion within the first 12 hours postinjury serving as an early independent predictor for the subsequent development of multiorgan failure (117). Interestingly, evidence began to accumulate that one of the explanations for the immunomodulatory effects of blood transfusion seemed to lie in the length of time that a unit of blood sat in the blood bank before transfusion. Purdy showed that transfusion of older

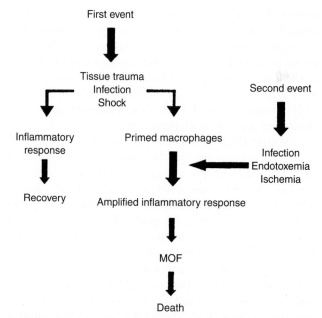

First event

Tissue trauma
Infection
Shock

Second event

Inflammatory
response

Primed macrophages

Infection
Endotoxemia
Ischemia

Recovery

Amplified inflammatory response

MOF

Death

FIGURE 4.9 The "two-hit" hypothesis of multiple organ failure (MOF). This idea holds that an initial insult leaves the immune system primed. A second physiologic hit is met with an overly aggressive immune response that can lead to multiple organ failure. (From *Surg Clin N Am* 1999;79:1471–1488, with permission.)

As evidence accumulated linking the age of transfused blood with the immunologic sequelae commonly seen in critically ill trauma patients, attention has turned to elucidating the etiology of these effects. One hypothesis for the mechanism of transfusion-related effects on immunity centers on the role of leukocytes in the donor units. Data was published showing that these "passenger" leukocytes secrete cytokines in a time-dependent manner after donor unit storage (121,122). Others showed that lipid mediators capable of priming neutrophils accumulate in donor unit plasma, postulating that this may be a function of leukocyte activity on red cell membranes (123–127).

Subsequently, interest arose in removing these white cells before storage with the thought that this would presumably abrogate any immunomodulatory effect resulting from passenger leukocyte storage and transfusion. This process of "prestorage leukoreduction" removes 99.9% of donor white blood cells, and has been implemented by many centers in the United States and all of Canada.

The largest clinical trial demonstrating a positive effect of leukoreduction on outcomes was a retrospective before-and-after cohort study performed in Canada after its nation-wide institution of the practice. This study examined 14,786 postoperative patients, and found a significant decrease in mortality rates from 7.03% in those patients transfused before universal leukoreduction to 6.19% after its institution (128). Interestingly, this improvement in mortality rates occurred without a commensurate decrease in serious nosocomial infections. Others have described leukoreduced blood product utilization as being associated with lower rates of rejection in liver transplantation (129), decreased sepsis from indwelling venous access (130), and decreased low cardiac output syndrome (LOS) in open-heart surgery (131). One of the authors has also shown that, while leukoreduction of transfused blood does not impact mortality in trauma patients, it does result in a lower rate of infectious complications which is dose

blood to ICU patients with severe sepsis was associated with increased mortality (118), and Offner found higher infection rates in trauma patients transfused with blood banked for longer than 14 and 21 days (119). Zallen et al. also identified the age of blood transfused in the first 12 hours postinjury as an independent risk factor for multiorgan failure, finding that these patients received both blood banked for longer on average as well as a greater number of units banked for longer than 14 and 21 days (Fig. 4.10) (120).

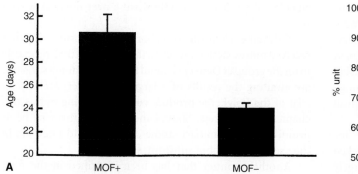

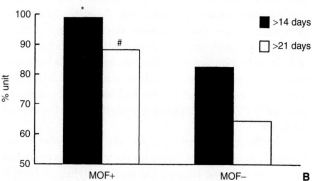

FIGURE 4.10 **A:** the age of transfused blood was analyzed in patients who developed multiple organ failure (MOF+) and was compared with patients who did not develop MOF (MOF−). The age of blood was significantly older in the MOF+ group (*p* <0.05 compared with MOF). **B:** the percentage of transfused blood units banked for longer than 14 and 21 days were analyzed in the MOF+ and MOF− groups. The MOF+ group received significantly more units of blood banked for longer than 14 and 21 days.**p* <0.05 compared with MOF−, >14 days. #*p* <0.05 compared with MOF−, >21 days. (From *Am J Surg* 1999;178:570–572, with permission.)

dependent (132,133). The literature is not unanimous as a myriad of smaller trials exist which do not show an effect on various clinical outcomes after initiation of institutional leukoreduction (134–138).

The logical first step in the treatment of a condition largely mediated by cytokines would seem to lie in the blockade of the actions of these cytokines. Early promising bench results have not been duplicated in humans. The North American Sepsis Trail (NORASEPT) (139) and the International Sepsis Trial (INTERSEPT) (140) were prospective, randomized, multicentered, double-blinded trails that examined the 28-day mortality of critically ill patients who received anti-TNF antibody. Neither showed a statistically significant improvement in the treated group. The list of other failed randomized controlled trials which followed promising bench results is depressing: anti-IL-1 receptor (141), antiendotoxin antibodies (142), bradykinin antagonists (143), PAF receptor antagonists (144), immunoglobulin administration (145), and NO synthase inhibition (146). It is becoming increasingly likely that efforts to attack the "upstream" immunomodulatory etiologies of MOF will require multiagent treatment. This paradigm has proved effective in the treatments of cancer, human immunodeficiency virus (HIV), and transplantation. It remains to be seen whether the pathology of SIRS/MOF will be similarly responsive.

FUTURE DIRECTIONS

Several areas hold promise for future targets of intervention in the immunologic cascade that results from severe infection or injury. Not surprisingly, many of them deal with blood products and transfusions.

If prospective, randomized trials continue to show that leukoreduction is beneficial and that the age of transfused blood is an independent risk factor for MOF, a possible area for impacting the cascade lies in changing blood banking practices so that only relatively fresh blood would be made available for massive resuscitations. To date, limitations in resources have made studying this question practical. Additionally, given that the data on the beneficial effects of leukoreduction are not universal, interest has arisen in poststorage washing of red cells as a means of decreasing their immunogenicity. Bench research in this area has shown promise (147,148), but it has not made its way to the clinical arena yet.

Despite intense research, an effective substitute for human hemoglobin, and hence for the transfusion of packed RBC in the anemic patient, has remained elusive. Largely driven by caregivers in environments where packed red cell transfusion is not readily available or feasible, new research has focused on the development of a compound capable of carrying oxygen without the immunologic sequelae of red cell transfusion.

These hemoglobin-based oxygen carrier (HBOCs) appeared promising in the early 1980s, but problems quickly came to light which precluded their widespread use. These initial hemoglobin substitutes were tetrameric, cross-linked structures. Their combination of decreased colloid-based osmotic pressure as well as a relatively short retention time in the intravascular space reduced the effectiveness of these early solutions as resuscitation adjuncts. Additionally, these early products induced a clinically significant amount of vasoconstriction upon administration.

EmAssist (Baxter Healthcare, Boulder, CO) was the only one of these early products to come to Phase III clinical trial. The results of this major, multicenter US trial nearly heralded the end of the HBOC era. The primary endpoint of the study, 28-day mortality, was 46% in the HBOC group and 17% in the control/NS group. This near tripling of mortality was a major concern even to those advocating the use of hemoglobin substitute solutions (149).

Two products were developed to address these early shortcomings. Both are polymerized (rather than tetramerized) hemoglobin products. It is believed that this polymerization represents an advance through two predominant mechanisms. First, due to a much higher molecular weight (>130 kDa versus 65 kDa) the polymerized HBOCs tend to stay intravascular longer without significant endothelial extravasation. Second, some have proposed that by avoiding contact with extravascular NO, the NO remains unbound and attenuates the vasoconstriction seen with previous products. Despite these improvements, concerns regarding HBOC-induced vasoconstriction remain.

Hemopure (Biopure Corp., Cambridge MA), made from bovine hemoglobin, was the first of the polymerized HBOCs to show clinical efficacy at reducing dependence on allogeneic packed red blood cell transfusion. Initial benefits were described in aortic repair (150) and hepatic resection (151). A relatively large, randomized trial in elective cardiac surgery (152) remains the most convincing evidence to date for its use. A large, U.S. Navy-sponsored trial of Hemopure in the prehospital management of hemorrhagic shock has been designed and funded, but currently awaits FDA approval to proceed. It is hoped that this large, multicenter trial will help elucidate the role for this HBOCs use over the next several years.

Polyheme (Northfield Laboratory, Evanston, IL) has received more extensive study in the trauma setting, primarily from the group at Denver General Hospital. Trauma surgeons are awaiting the results of a large multicenter, prehospital trial of the Polyheme product currently closing out as this chapter goes to press. Should the results of this trial be as promising as preliminary studies, it may herald a new era in the use of hemoglobin substitutes.

Another frontier that has been identified in the fight against immunomodulation is that of the time frame in which trauma patients are evaluated and treated. Given Rivers' impressive results on the importance of early goal directed therapy, it would seem intuitive that this would apply to the resuscitation of trauma patients as well. Unfortunately, the early hours of a trauma patient's course are frequently marked by interhospital transfers, hours in the angiography suite, or waiting for an ICU bed to open up. The challenge will be to find a bedside method of assessing global oxygen delivery and consumption which is easy, simple, portable, and reliable so that the process of goal-directed therapy can be begun as early as the time of transport and can continue until the patient arrives at an ICU where they can receive a pulmonary artery catheter.

Finally, the undertaking which is broadest in scope is that of the Inflammation and Host Response to Injury Program sponsored by the National Institute of General Medical Sciences (NIGMS), a division of the National Institutes of Health. Frustration over the fact that two different patients with identical demographics and severity of injury can receive identical care yet have radically different outcomes led to the creation of this interdisciplinary effort to tease apart the molecular basis of the host immunologic response to injury. Referred to as the *glue grant* since the NIGMS funding acts as the glue to bring together established investigators and centers of excellence across multiple fields, one of its goals is the identification of the genotype and phenotype associated with a predilection for an exaggerated inflammatory response. Once these are identified, it is hoped that this would serve as a basis for molecular therapies to blunt the syndrome. This exciting project is ongoing.

CONCLUSION

The pathophysiology of shock can be brought on by any number of etiologies. The central pathway of these numerous insults, however, is the inadequate availability of oxygen for use at the level of the cell. The hemodynamic disturbances that characterize this state are best thought of as disorders of preload, contractility, or afterload. As our understanding of the shock process has grown (and our treatments have become more specialized), there has been a commensurate drop in the early mortality associated with the shock syndrome. Late deaths have not been similarly impacted despite intensive investigations into the immunologic cascades that balance the pro- and anti-inflammatory states. These cytokine systems remain an area of active investigation and with a better understanding of the process, the hope for control of the systemic inflammatory response and multiorgan failure syndrome.

ACKNOWLEDGMENTS

We wish to acknowledge the contribution of Daniel Jurusz and Jared Gilmore for those portions of the previous chapter in the second edition of *The Physiologic Basis of Surgery* that we maintained in the current work.

We would also like to acknowledge the assistance of Shaunda Fakaha and Robert Earl Keen for their assistance and support in the preparation of this manuscript.

REFERENCES

1. Pare A. *Les Oeuvres d' Ambroise Pare.*Paris: Dupuye, 1582.
2. LeDran HF. *A treatise or reflection drawn from practice on gunshot wounds.* London: Longman, 1815.
3. Guthrie GJ. *On gunshot sounds of the extremities.* Longman, 1815.
4. Wiggers CJ. *Physiology of shock.* New York: The Commonwealth Fund, 1950:1–25.
5. Blum A. Du choc traumatique. *Arch gen de med* 1876;1:5.
6. Crile GW. *An experimental research into surgical shock.* Philadelphia: J.B. Lippincott, 1899.
7. Crile GW, Lower WE. *Surgical shock and the shockless operation through anoci-association.* Philadelphia: WB Saunders, 1920:17–24.
8. MacCleod JJ. The concentration of lactic acid in the blood on anoxemia and shock. *Am J Physiology* 1991;55:184.
9. Freeman NE. Cortin and traumatic shock. *Science* 1933;77:211–212.
10. Leach RM, Treacher DF. The relationship between oxygen delivery and consumption. *Dis Mon* 1994;39:301–368.
11. Blinman T, Maggard M. Research review-rational manipulation of oxygen delivery. *J Surg Res* 2000;92:120–141.
12. Starling EH. *The Linacre lecture on the law of the heart.* London: Longmans, Green, 1918.
13. Swan HJC, Ganz W, Forrester J, et al. Cardiac catheterization with a flow directed balloon-tipped catheter. *N Engl J Med* 1970;283:447–451.
14. ACS Committee on Trauma. Shock. In: *Advanced trauma life support course,* 6th ed. USA: First Impression, 1997.
15. The SAFE Study Investigators. A comparison of albumin and saline for fluid resuscitation in the intensive care unit. *N Engl J Med* 2004;350:2247–2256.
16. Choi PTL, Gordon Y, Quinonez LG, et al. Crystalloids vs. colloids in fluid resuscitation: a systematic review. *Crit Care Med* 1999;27(1):200–210.
17. Scalea TM, Maltz S, Yelon J, et al. Resuscitation of multiple trauma and head injury: role of crystalloid fluids and inotropes. *Crit Care Med* 1994;22:1610–1615.
18. Bannon MP, O'Neill CM, Martin M, et al. Central venous oxygen saturation, arterial base deficit, and lactate concentration in trauma patients. *Amer Surg* 1995;61:738–745.
19. Davis JW, Kaups KL, Parks SN. Base deficit is superior to pH in evaluating clearance of acidosis after traumatic shock. *J Trauma* 1998;44:114–118.
20. Davis JW, Shackford SR, Holbrook TL. Base deficit as a sensitive indicator of compensated shock and tissue oxygen utilization. *Surg Gynecol Obstet* 1991;173:473–478.
21. Rutherford EJ, Morris JA Jr, Reed GW, et al. Base deficit stratifies mortality and determines therapy. *J Trauma* 1992;33:417–423.
22. McNelis J, Marini CP, Jurkiewicz A, et al. Prolonged lactate clearance is associated with increased mortality in the surgical intensive care unit. *Am J Surg* 2001;182:481–485.
23. Abramson D, Scalea TM, Hitchcock R, et al. Lactate clearance and survival following injury. *J Trauma* 1993;35:584–588.
24. Manikis P, Jankowski S, Zhang H, et al. Correlation of serial blood lactate levels to organ failure and mortality after trauma. *Am J Emerg Med* 1995;13:619–622.
25. Jeng JC, Jablonski K, Bridgeman A, et al. Serum lactate, not base deficit, rapidly predicts survival after major burns. *Burns* 2002;28:161–166.
26. Husain FA, Martin MJ, Mullenix PS, et al. Serum lactate and base deficit as predictors of mortality and morbidity. *Am J Surg* 2003;185:485–491.
27. Creteur J, De Backer D, Vincent JL. Does gastric tonometry monitor splanchnic perfusion? *Crit Care Med* 1999;27:2480–2484.

28. Morgan TJ, Venkatesh B, Endre ZH. Accuracy of intramucosal pH calculated from arterial bicarbonate and the Henderson-Hasselbach equation: assessment using stimulated ischemia. *Crit Care Med* 1999;27:2495–2499.

29. Robbins MR, Smith RS, Helmer SD. Serial pH measurement as a predictor of mortality, organ failure, and hospital stay in surgical patients. *Amer Surg* 1999;65:715–719.

30. Joynt GM, Lipman J, Gomersall CD, et al. Gastric intramucosal pH and blood lactate in severe sepsis. *Anaesthesia* 1997;52:726–732.

31. Shoemaker WC, Appel PL, Kram HB, et al. Prospective trial of supranormal values of survivors as therapeutic goals in high-risk surgical patients. *Chest* 1988;94:1176–1186.

32. Shoemaker WC, Appel PL, Kram HB. Hemodynamic and oxygen transport responses in survivors and nonsurvivors of high-risk surgery. *Crit Care Med* 1993;21:977–990.

33. Boyd O, Grounds M, Bennett D. Preoperative increase of oxygen delivery reduces mortality in high-risk surgical patients. *JAMA* 1993;270:2699.

34. Yu M, Levy MM, Smith P, et al. Effect of maximizing oxygen delivery on mortality and mortality rates in critically ill patients: A prospective randomized controlled study. *Crit Care Med* 1993;21:830–838.

35. Heyland DK, Cook DJ, King D, et al. Maximizing oxygen delivery in critically ill patients: A methodological appraisal of the evidence. *Crit Care Med* 1996;24:517–524.

36. Velmahos GC, Demetriades D, Shoemaker WC. Endpoints of resuscitation of critically injured patients: normal or supranormal? A prospective randomized trial. *Ann Surg* 2000;232:409–414.

37. McKinley BA, Kozar RA, Cocanour CS, et al. Normal versus supranormal oxygen delivery goals in shock resuscitation: the response is the same. *J Trauma* 2002;53:825–832.

38. Gattinoni L, Brazzi L, Pelosi P, et al. A trial of goal-oriented hemodynamic therapy in critically ill patients. *N Engl J Med* 1995;333:1025–1032.

39. Hayes MA, Timmins AC, Yau EHS, et al. Elevation of systemic oxygen delivery in the treatment of critically ill patients. *N Engl J Med* 1994;330:1717–1722.

40. Adam RC, Lundy JS. Anesthesia in cases of poor risk. Some suggestions for decreasing the risk. *Surg Gynecol Obstet* 1942;74:1011–1101.

41. Stehling LC, Ellison N, Faust RJ, et al. A survey of transfusion practices among anesthesiologists. *Vox Sang* 1987;52:60–62.

42. Hebert PC, Wells G, Blajchman MA, et al. A multicenter, randomized, controlled clinical trial of transfusion requirements in critical care. Transfusion Requirements in Critical Care Investigators. Canadian Critical Care Trials Group. *N Engl J Med* 1999;340:409–417.

43. Corein HL, Gettinger A, Pearl RG, et al. The CRIT study: Anema and blood transfusion in the critically ill- current clinical practice in the United States. *Crit Care Med* 2004;2:39–52.

44. Visser CA, Kan G, David CK, et al. Echocardiographic cineangiographic correlation in detecting left ventricular aneurysm. *Am J Cardiology* 1982;50:337.

45. Holmes DR, Bates ER, Kleinman NS, et al. Contemporary reperfusion therapy for cardiogenic shock: the GUSTO-I trial experience. The GUSTO-I Investigators. Global Utilization of Streptokinase and Tissue Plasminogen Activator for Occluded Coronary Arteries. *J Am Coll Cardiology* 1995;26:668–674.

46. The Global Use of Strategies to Open Occluded Coronary Arteries (GUSTO III) Investigators. A comparison of reteplase with alteplase for acute myocardial infarction. *N Eng J Med* 1997;337:1118–1123.

47. Hochman JS, Sleeper LA, Webb JG, et al. Early revascularization in acute myocardial infarction complicated by cardiogenic shock. SHOCK Investigators-Should We Emergently Revascularize Occluded Coronaries for Cardiogenic Shock. *N Engl J Med* 1999;341:625–634.

48. Hochman JS, Sleeper LA, White HD, et al. One year survival following early revascularization for cardiogenic shock. *JAMA* 2001;285:190–192.

49. Hochman JS, Sleeper LA, Webb JG, et al. Early revascularization and long-term survival in cardiogenic shock complicating acute myocardial infarction. *JAMA* 2006;295:2511–2515.

50. Dellinger RP, Carlet JM, Masur H. Surviving sepsis campaign guidelines for management of severe sepsis and septic shock. *Crit Care Med* 2004;32:858–873.

51. Rivers E, Nguyen B, Havstad S, et al.. Early goal directed therapy in the treatment of severe sepsis and septic shock. *N Eng J Med* 2001;345:1368–1377.

52. Van den Berghe G, Wouters P, Weekers F, et al. Intensive insulin therapy in the critically ill. *N Eng J Med* 2001;345:1359–1367.

53. Boldt J, Papsdorf M, Rothe A, et al. Changes of the hemostatic network in critically ill patients: Is there a difference between sepsis, trauma, and neurosurgery patients? *Crit Care Med* 2000;28:445–450.

54. Fisher CJ, Yan SB. Protein C levels as a prognostic indicator of outcome in sepsis and related diseases. *Crit Care Med* 2000;28 (Suppl):S49–S56.

55. Fourrier F, Chopin C, Goudemand J, et al. Septic shock, multiple organ failure and disseminated intravascular coagulation: Compared patterns of antithrombin III, protein C, and protein S deficiencies. *Chest* 1992;101:816–823.

56. Lorente JA, Garcia-Frade LJ, Landin L, et al. Time course of hemostatic abnormalities in sepsis and its relation to outcome. *Chest* 1993;103:1536–1542.

57. Powars D, Larsen R, Johnson J, et al. Epidemic meningococcemia and purpura fulminans with induced protein C deficiency. *Clin Infect Dis* 1993;17:254–261.

58. Mesters RM, Helterbrand J, Utterback BG, et al. Prognostic value of protein C levels in neutropenic patients at high risk of severe septic complications. *Crit Care Med* 2000;28:2209–2216.

59. Yan SB, Helterbrand JD, Hartman DL, et al. Low levels of protein C are associated with poor outcome in severe sepsis. *Chest* 2001;120:915–922.

60. Philapitsch A, Schwarz HP. The effect of leukocyte elastase on protein C and activated protein C. *Thromb Haemost* 1993;69:726.

61. Dhainaut JF, Marin N, Mignon A, et al. Hepatic response to sepsis: interaction between coagulation and inflammatory processes. *Crit Care Med* 2001;29:S42–S47.

62. Bernard GR, Vincent JL, Laterre PF, et al. Efficacy and safety of recombinant human activated protein C for severe sepsis. *N Eng J Med* 2001;344:699–709.

63. Bone RC, Fisher CJ Jr, Clemmer TP, et al. A controlled clinical trial of high-dose methylprednisolone in the treatment of severe sepsis and septic shock. *N Engl J Med* 1987;317:653–658.

64. Bone RC, Fisher CJ Jr, Clemmer TP, et al. Early methylprednisolone treatment for septic syndrome and the adult respiratory distress syndrome. *Chest* 1987;92:1032–1036.

65. Veterans Administration Systemic Sepsis Cooperative Study Group. Effect of high-dose glucocorticoid therapy on mortality in patients with clinical signs of systemic sepsis: the Veterans Administration Systemic Sepsis Cooperative Study Group. *N Engl J Med* 1987;317:659–665.

66. Annane D, Sebille V, Troche G, et al. A 3-level prognostic classification in septic shock based on cortisol levels and cortisol response to corticotropin. *JAMA* 2000;283:1038–1045.

67. Annane D, Sebille V, Charpentier C, et al. Effect of treatment with low doses of hydrocortisone and fludrocortisone on mortality in patients with septic shock. *JAMA* 2002;288:862–871.

68. Chiolero R, Flatt JP, Revelly JP, et al. Effects of catecholamines on oxygen consumption and oxygen delivery in critically ill patients. *Chest* 1991;100:1676–1684.

69. Stone HH, Strom PR, Mullins RJ. Management of the major coagulopathy with onset during laparotomy. *Ann Surg* 1983;197:532–535.

70. Feliciano DV, Burch JM, Spjut-Patrinely V, et al. Abdominal gunshot wounds: an urban trauma center's experience with 300 consecutive patients. *Ann Surg* 1988;208:362–370.

71. Sharp KW, Locicero RJ. Abdominal packing for surgically uncontrollable hemorrhage. *Ann Surg* 1992;215:467–474.

72. Rotondo MF, Schwab CW, McGonigal MD, et al. "Damage Control": an approach for improved survival in exsanguinating penetrating abdominal injury. *J Trauma* 1993;35:375–383.

73. Carillo C, Fogler RJ, Shaftan GW. Delayed gastrointestinal reconstruction following massive abdominal trauma. *J Trauma* 1993;34:233–235.

74. Hirshberg A, Wall MJ, Mattox KL Jr. Planned reoperation for trauma: a two year experience with 124 consecutive patients. *J Trauma* 1994;37:365–369.

75. Johnson JW, Gracias VH, Schwab W, et al. Evolution in damage control for exsanguinating penetrating abdominal injury. *J Trauma* 2001;51:261–271.

76. Nicholas JM, Rix EP, Easley KA, et al. Changing patterns in the management of penetrating abdominal trauma: the more things change, the more they stay the same. *J Trauma* 2003;55:1095–1110.

77. Vargo DJ, Battistella FD. Abbreviated thoracotomy and temporary chest closure—an application of damage control after thoracic trauma. *Arch Surg* 2001;136:21–24.

78. Valeri CR, Feingold H, Cassidy R, et al. Hypothermia-induced reversible platelet dysfunction. *Ann Surg* 1997;205:175–181.

79. Martinowitz U, Kenet G, Segal E, et al. Recombinant activated factor VII for adjunctive hemorrhage control in trauma. *J Trauma* 2001;51:431–439.

80. O'Neill PA, Bluth M, Gloster ES, et al. Successful use of recombinant activated factor VII for trauma-associated hemorrhage in a patient without preexisting coagulopathy. *J Trauma* 2002;52:400–405.

81. Christians K, Brasel K, Garlitz J, et al. The use of recombinant activated factor VII in trauma-associated hemorrhage with crush injury. *J Trauma* 2005;59:742–746.

82. Benharash P, Bongard F, Putnam B. Use of recombinant factor VIIa for adjunctive hemorrhage control in trauma and surgical patients. *Amer Surg* 2005;71:776–780.

83. Martinowitz U, Michaelson M. Guidelines for the use of recombinant activated factor VII in uncontrolled bleeding: a report by the Israeli Multidisciplinary rFVIIa Task Force. *J Thromb Haemost* 2005;3:640–648.

84. Stein DM, Dutton RP, O'Connor J, et al. Determinants of futility of administration of recombinant factor VIIa in trauma. *J Trauma* 2005;59:609–615.

85. Dutton RP, McCunn M, Hyder M, et al. Factor VIIa for correction of traumatic coagulopathy. *J Trauma* 2004;57:709–719.

86. Harrison TD, Laskosky J, Jazaeri O, et al. "Low-dose" recombinant activated factor VIIa results in less blood and blood product use in traumatic hemorrhage. *J Trauma* 2005;59:150–154.

87. Boffard KD, Riou B, Warren B, et al. Recombinant factor VIIa as adjunctive therapy for bleeding control in severely injured trauma patients: two parallel randomized, placebo-controlled, double-blind clinical trials. *J Trauma* 2005;59:8–18.

88. Valentine S, Williamson P, Sutton D. Reduction of acute haemorrhage with aprotinin. *Anaesthesia* 1993;48:405–406.

89. Paran H, Gutman M, Mayo A. The effect of aprotinin in a model of uncontrolled hemorrhagic shock. *Am J Surg* 2005;190:463–466.

90. Jurkovich GJ, Greiser WB, Luterman A, et al. Hypothermia in trauma victims: an ominous predictor of survival. *J Trauma* 1987;27:1019–1024.

91. Gentilello LM, Rifley WJ. Continuous arteriovenous rewarming: report of a new technique for treating hypothermia. *J Trauma* 1991;31:1151–1154.

92. Gentilello LM, Cobean RA, Offner PJ, et al. Continuous arteriovenous rewarming: rapid reversal of hypothermia in critically ill patients. *J Trauma* 1992;32:316–327.

93. Janczyk RJ, Park DY, Howells GA, et al. High-flow venovenous rewarming for the correction of hypothermia in a canine model of hypovolemic shock. *J Trauma* 2002;53:639–645.

94. Martin RR, Byrne M. Postoperative care and complications of damage control surgery. *Surg Clin Nor Amer* 1997;77:930–942.

95. Eiseman B, Beart R, Norton L. Multiple organ failure. *Surg Gynecol Obstet* 1977;144:323–326.

96. Committee on Trauma Research, National Research Council, and the Institute of Medicine. *Injury in America, a continuing public health problem*. Washington, DC: National Academy Press, 1985:65–80.

97. Moore FA. The role of the gastrointestinal tract in postinjury multiple organ failure. *Am J Surg* 1999;178:449–453.

98. Bone RC, Grodzin CJ, Balk RA. Sepsis: a new hypothesis for pathogenics of the disease process. *Chess* 1997;112:235–243.

99. Members of the American College of Chest Physicians/Society of Critical Care Medicine Consensus Conference Committee. American College of Chest Physicians/Society of Critical Care Medicine Consensus Conference: definitions for sepsis and oran failure and guidelines for the use of innovative therapies in sepsis. *Crit Care Med* 1992;20:864–874.

100. Levy MM, Fink MP, Marshall JC, et al. 2001 SCCM/ESICM/ACCP/ATS/SIS International Sepsis Definitions Conference. *Crit Care Med* 2003;31:1250–1256.

101. Cavaillon JM, Fitting C, Haeffner-Cavaillon N. Recombinant C5a enhances interleukin 1 and tumor necrosis factor release by lipopolysaccharide-stimulated monocytes and macrophages. *Eur J Immunol* 1990;20:253–257.

102. Kim PK, Deutschman CS. Inflammatory responses and mediators. *Surg Clin N Am* 2000;80:885–894.

103. Barnett CC, Moore EE, Moore FA, et al. Intercellular adhesion molecule-1 promotes neutrophil-mediated cytotoxicity. *Surgery* 1995;118:171–175.

104. Springer T. Traffic signals on endothelium for lymphocyte recirculation and leukocyte emigration. *Ann Rev Physiol* 1995;57:827–872.

105. Deitch EA, Goodman ER. Prevention of multiple organ failure. *Surg Clin N Am* 1999;79:1471–1488.

106. Goris RJ, Beokorst PA, Nuytinck KS. Multiple organ failure: generalized autodestructive inflammation. *Arch Surg* 1985;120:1109–1115.

107. Ziegler TR, Smith RJ, O'Dwyer ST, et al. Increased intestinal permeability associated with infection in burn patients. *Arch Surg* 1988;123:1313–1319.

108. Opelz G, Sengar DP, Mickey MR, et al. Effect of blood transfusions on subsequent kidney transplants. *Transplantation Proceedings* 1973;5:253–259.

109. Opelz G, Teraski PI. Improvement of kidney-graft survival with increased numbers of blood transfusions. *N Eng J Med* 1978;299:799–803.

110. Foster RS Jr, Costanza MC, Foster JC, et al.. Adverse relationship between blood transfusions and survival after colectomy for colon cancer. *Cancer* 1985;55:1195–1201.

111. Creasy TS, Veitch PS, Bell PR. A relationship between perioperative blood transfusion and recurrence of carcinoma of the sigmoid colon following potentially curative surgery. *Ann of Royal Coll Surg of England* 1987;69:100–103.

112. Blumberg N, Heal J, Chuang C, et al. Further evidence supporting a cause and effect relationship between blood transfusion and earlier cancer recurrence. *Ann Surg* 1988;207:410–415.

113. Chung M, Steinmetz OK, Gordon PH. Perioperative blood transfusion and outcome after resection for colorectal carcinoma. *BJS* 1993;80:427–432.

114. Edna TH, Bjerkeset T. Association between transfusion of stored blood and infective bacterial complications after resection for colorectal cancer. *European J Surg* 1998;164:449–456.

115. Chiarugi M, Buccianti P, Disarli M, et al. Effect of blood transfusions on disease-free interval after rectal cancer surgery. *Hepato-Gastroenterology* 2000;47:1002–1005.

116. Moore FA, Moore EE, Sauaia A. Blood transfusion. An independent risk factor for postinjury multiple organ failure. *Arch Surg* 1997;132:620–625.

117. Sauaia A, Moore FA, Moore EE, et al. Early predictors of postinjury multiple organ failure. *Arch Surg* 1994;129:39–45.

118. Purdy FR, Tweeddale MG, Merrick PM. Association of mortality with age of blood transfused in septic ICU patients. *Can J Anaesth* 1997;44:1256–1261.

119. Offner PJ, Moore EE, Biffl WL, et al. Increased rate of infection associated with transfusion of old blood after severe injury. *Arch Surg* 2002;137:711–717.

120. Zallen G, Offner PJ, Moore EE, et al. Age of transfused blood is an independent risk factor for postinjury multiple organ failure. *Am J Surg* 1999;178:570–572.

121. Nielsen HJ, Reimert CM, Pedersen AN, et al. Time-dependent, spontaneous release of white cell- and platelet-derived bioactive substances from stored human blood. *Transfusion* 1996;36:960–965.

122. Kristiansson M, Soop M, Saraste L, et al. Cytokines in stored red blood cell concentrates: promoters of systemic inflammation and simulators of acute transfusion reactions. *Acta Anaesthesiologica Scandinavica* 1996;40:496–501.

123. Silliman CC, Clay KL, Thurman GW, et al. Partial characterization of lipids that develop during the routine storage of blood and prime the neutrophil NADPH oxidase. *J Lab Clin Med* 1994;124:684–694.

124. Silliman CC, Dickey WO, Paterson AJ, et al. Analysis of the priming activity of lipids generated during routine storage of platelet concentrates. *Transfusion* 1996;36:133–139.

125. Silliman CC, Boshkov LK, Mehdizadehkashi Z, et al. Transfusion-related acute lung injury: epidemiology and a prospective analysis of etiologic factors. *Blood* 2003;101:454–462.

126. Silliman CC, Paterson AJ, Dickey WO, et al. The association of biologically active lipids with the development of transfusion-related acute lung injury: a retrospective study. *Transfusion* 1997;37:719–726.

127. Silliman CC, Voelkel NF, Allard JD, et al. Plasma and lipids from stored packed red blood cells cause acute lung injury in an animal model. *J Clin Inv* 1998;101:1458–1467.

128. Hebert PC, Fergusson D, Blajchman MA, et al. Clinical outcomes following institution of the Canadian universal leukoreduction program for red blood cell transfusions. *JAMA* 2003;289:1941–1949.

129. Tzimas GN, Deschenes M, Barkun JS, et al. Leukoreduction and acute rejection in liver transplantation: an interim analysis. *Transplantation Proceedings* 2004;36:1760–1762.

130. Blumberg N, Fine L, Gettings KF, et al. Decreased sepsis related to indwelling venous access devices coincident with implementation of universal leukoreduction of blood transfusions. *Transfusion* 2005;45:1632–1639.

131. Fung MK, Rao N, Rice J, et al. Leukoreduction in the setting of open heart surgery: a prospective cohort-controlled study. *Transfusion* 2004;44:30–35.

132. Phelan HA, Sperry J, Friese R. Leukoreduction of packed red cells prior to transfusion does not affect survival in transfused trauma patients. *J Surg Res.* 2007;138(1):32–36. (In press)

133. Friese R, Sperry J, Phelan HA, et al. The use of leukoreduced red cell products is associated with fewer infectious complications in trauma patients. Unpublished data in review.

134. Baron JF, Gourdin M, Bertrand M, et al. The effect of universal leukodepletion of packed red blood cells on postoperative infections in high-risk patients undergoing abdominal aortic surgery. *Anesthesia and Analgesia* 2002;94:529–537.

135. Llewelyn CA, Taylor RS, Todd AA, et al. The effect of universal leukoreduction on postoperative infections and length of hospital stay in elective orthopedic and cardiac surgery. *Transfusion* 2004;44:489–500.

136. Titlestad IL, Ebbesen LS, Ainsworth AP, et al. Leukocyte-depletion of blood components does not significantly reduce the risk of infectious complications. Results of a double-blinded, randomized study. *Int J Colorectal Dis* 2001;16:147–153.

137. Wallis JP, Chapman CE, Orr KE, et al. Effect of WBC reduction of transfused RBCs on postoperative infection rates in cardiac surgery. *Transfusion* 2002;42:1127–1134.

138. Dzik WH, Anderson JK, O'Neill EM, et al. A prospective, randomized clinical trial of universal WBC reduction. *Transfusion* 2002;42:1114–1122.

139. Abraham EA, Wunderink R, Silverman H, et al. Efficacy and safety of monoclonal antibody to human tumor necrosis factor-alpha (in patients with sepsis syndrome): a randomized, controlled, pha (in patients with sepsis syndrome): a randomized, controlled, double-blind multicenter trail. *JAMA* 1995;273:934–941.

140. Cohen J, Carlet J. INTERSEPT: an international, multicenter, placebo-controlled trial of monoclonal antibody to human tumor necrosis factor-alpha in patients with sepsis. *Crit Care Med* 1996;24:1431–1439.

141. Fisher CJ, Dhainaut JF, Opal SM, et al. Recombinant human interleukin-1 receptor antagonist in the treatment of patients with sepsis syndrome: results from a randomized, double-blind, placebo-controlled trail. *JAMA* 1991;266:1097–1102.

142. Bone RC, Balk RA, Fein AM, et al. A second large controlled clinical study of E5, a monoclonal antibody to endotoxin: results of a prospective multicenter, randomized, controlled trail. *Crit Care Med* 1995;23:994–1006.

143. Fein AM, Bernard GR, Criner GJ, et al. Treatment of severe systemic inflammatory response syndrome and sepsis with a novel bradykinin antagonist, deltibant (CP-0127). Results of a randomized, double-blind, placebo-controlled trial. CP-0127 SIRS and Sepsis Study Group. *JAMA* 1997;277:482–487.

144. Dhainaut JF, Tenaillon AL, Tulzo Y, et al. Platelet-activating factor receptor antagonist BN 52021 in the treatment of severe sepsis: a randomized, double-blind, placebo-controlled, multicenter clinical trial. BN 52021 Sepsis Study Group. *Crit Care Med* 1994;22:1720–1728.

145. Schedel I, Dreikhausen U, Nentwig B, et al. Treatment of gram-negative septic shock with an immunoglobulin preparation: a prospective, randomized clinical trial. *Crit Care Med.* 1991;19:1104–1113.

146. Lopez A, Lorente JA, Steingrub J, et al. Multiple-center, randomized, placebo-controlled, double-blind study of the nitric oxide synthase inhibitor 546C88: effect on survival in patients with septic shock. *Crit Care Med* 2004;32:21–30.

147. Biffl WL, Moore EE, Offner PJ, et al. Plasma from aged stored red blood cells delays neutrophil apoptosis and primes for cytotoxicity: abrogation by poststorage washing but not prestorage leukoreduction. *J Trauma* 2001;50:426–431.

148. Rao RS, Howard CA, Teague TK. Pulmonary endothelial permeability is increased by fluid from packed red blood cell units but not by fluid from clinically available washed units. *J Trauma* 2006;60:851–858.

149. Sloan EP, Koenigsberg M, Gens D, et al. Dispirin cross-linked hemoglobin (DCLHb) in the treatment of severe traumatic hemorrhagic shock: a randomized controlled efficacy trial. *JAMA* 1999;282:1857–1864.

150. LaMuraglia GM, O'Hara PJ, Baker WH, et al. The reduction of the allogenic transfusion requirement in aortic surgery with hemoglobin-based solution. *J Vasc Surgery* 1998;31:229–308.

151. Standl T, Burmeister MA, Horn EP, et al. Bovine hemoglobin-based oxygen carrier for patients undergoing haemodilution before liver resection. *Br J Anaesth* 1998;80:189–194.

152. Levy JH, Goodnough LT, Greilich P, et al. Polymerized bovine hemoglobin solution as a replacement for allogenic red blood cell transfusion after cardiac surgery: results of a randomized, double-blind trial. *J Thorac Cardiovasc Surg* 2002;124:35–42.

CHAPTER 5

Nutrition and Metabolism

Robert G. Martindale and Minhao Zhou

OVERVIEW OF METABOLISM

The significance of nutrition in the surgical setting cannot be overstated. This significance is particularly noted in the realm of surgical intensive care. Over the past three decades, physicians have begun to understand the molecular and biologic effects of nutrients in maintaining homeostasis in the perioperative setting. Since the turn of the century, investigators have alluded to the importance of nutrition in optimizing surgical outcomes (1), but only recently have these assumptions been verified with well-designed clinical studies (2–4). Traditionally, nutritional support in the surgical population has had three main objectives: attempt to preserve lean body mass, maintenance of immune function, and averting metabolic complications. Recently these goals have become more focused toward attenuation of the metabolic response to surgical stress, prevention of oxidative cellular injury, and favorable modulation of the immune response. Nutrient modulation of the immune response includes aggressive enteral nutrition, appropriate macro- and micronutrient delivery, and meticulous glycemic control. Nutrient delivery in the clinical setting can be a technically involved modality that can potentially yield significant benefits but can result in significant morbidity and possible mortality when approached improperly or with inadequate knowledge (5). Outcomes from large randomized clinical studies over the last 20 years highlight the potential benefits and risks involved (5,6).

In terms of nutritional support in the surgical patient, it is generally accepted that: (i) enteral feeding when done appropriately is vastly superior to parenteral; (ii) earlier feeding is better than later; (iii) the quality of nutrition appears to be more important than the quantity; (iv) select populations show additional benefits from specific nutrient supplementation (4). These new concepts in nutritional support of the surgical patient require a shift in the mindset from nutritional support to one of nutritional therapy. When nutrition is considered a therapy, one must then assume that the nutrient delivered must reach a therapeutic level.

Consideration must also be made for appropriate timing, dosing, and the metabolic state of the host.

The nutritional implications in surgical diseases are numerous and include anorexia, sodium and fluid retention, accelerated gluconeogenesis, hyperglycemia, insulin resistance, and lipid intolerance (7,8). During the metabolic response to stress, starvation, and sepsis, neuroendocrine reflexes result in very complex and integrated attempts to mobilize sufficient nutrient substrates to maintain energy requirements for essential bodily function. These metabolic alterations following either hypermetabolic stress or starvation, involve the significant redistribution of all three nutrient substrates, carbohydrate, protein, and lipid. In reviewing body nutrient metabolism, one must consider body energy stores and fuels immediately available (Table 5.1). Cahill, in a classic group of studies, showed that fuels immediately available in the serum include only approximately 113 cal (9). The estimated stored fuels in a 70-kg male include triglycerides 140,000 cal in adipose, muscle 2,000 cal as glycogen, and liver 300 cal as glycogen. (9). Muscle contains approximately 24,000 cal as protein, 2,000 cal as glycogen, and 3,000 cal as triglyceride. Liver contains approximately 300 cal of glucose in the form of glycogen and 500 cal as triglyceride. During unstressed starvation, the body mainly relies on mobilization of endogenous adipose stores (10). Glycogen storage is limited and is usually metabolized within 24 hours in the

TABLE 5.1

Body Energy Stores

Tissue	Fuel	Energy (kcal)
Adipose	Triacylglycerol	140,000
Muscle	Protein	24,000
	Glycogen	2,000
	Triacylglycerol	3,000
Liver	Glycogen	300
	Triacylglycerol	500

unfed, unstressed state. It is important to realize that there is no protein storage available *per se* and any protein utilized for gluconeogenesis and acute-phase protein synthesis should be considered as loss of functional protein. During the first 24 to 48 hours of unstressed starvation, the basic energy need will be supplied from glycogen and proteins, with minimal contribution from fat stores. Starvation will initially result in increased production of urinary urea nitrogen that reflects the mobilization of endogenous protein to meet energy and vital protein synthetic needs. Following the initial 48 to 72 hours of unstressed starvation, there is a relative increased utilization of adipose stores, and most tissues, with the exception of red cells, white cells, and the renal medulla, begin to oxidize lipid stores as their primary oxidative fuel source. The brain has an obligate glucose requirement; however, over 3 to 5 days the brain will transition to mainly utilizing fatty acids for energy (7). During unstressed starvation, there is a general decrease in energy expenditure and a change in the insulin–glucagon ratio favoring mobilization of stored fuels and minimizing the loss of lean body mass (7).

Hypermetabolism associated with major catabolic illness, surgery, or trauma results in a significant change in nutrient homeostasis from the unstressed starvation described earlier. The hormonal response to the metabolic insult results in increased adrenocorticotropic harmone (ACTH), epinephrine, glucagon, and cortisol production (8). Secondarily, we see major alteration in carbohydrate, fat, and protein metabolism. Glycogen stores are exhausted within 4 to 6 hours. In contrast to unstressed starvation during hypermetabolism, gluconeogenesis continues at an accelerated rate (7). Gluconeogenesis from protein provides the main carbohydrate source for the tissues that require glucose. Muscle protein, in addition to providing a source for gluconeogenesis, serves as a substrate for acute-phase protein synthesis by providing necessary amino acids. As a result of the catabolic insult, the liver reprioritizes its protein synthesis from the production of visceral proteins to acute-phase proteins induced by the catabolic insult (9). Increased levels of glutamine and alanine are released from the muscle delivering glutamine to the gastrointestinal (GI) tract and alanine to the liver for gluconeogenesis. Hyperglycemia is a common occurrence during hypermetabolic stress and results from the accelerated gluconeogenesis and relative insulin resistance (11).

Carbohydrate

Dietary carbohydrates consist of significant amounts of monosaccharides and disaccharides, in addition to large molecular weight polysaccharides such as starch and glycogen. Carbohydrates are absorbed by the enterocytes exclusively as monosaccharides. Therefore, the polysaccharides and disaccharides in the diet have to undergo complete digestion in the intestinal lumen before absorption can occur.

Starch and glycogen are substrates for the endosaccharidase α-amylase, which is secreted from the pancreas in response to a large intake of starch. Amylase is also present in saliva although in less significant amounts. The products of amylase digestion are the disaccharide maltose, the

trisaccharide maltotriose, and the so-called limit dextrins. The di- and oligosaccharides arising from α-amylase digestion are further broken down to monosaccharides by surface saccharidases, found on the enterocyte. Oligosaccharides, including disaccharides and trisaccharides, which cannot be broken down by α-amylase or intestinal saccharidases, cannot be absorbed and are fermented by bacteria in the large intestinal tract, providing end products of short-chain fatty acids (SCFAs) which are the primary fuel of the colonocyte (12–14).

Absorption of the major monosaccharides arising from the digestion of disaccharides and polysaccharides, D-glucose, D-galactose and D-fructose occurs through carrier-mediated mechanisms. At least four glucose transporters have been identified in the mammalian enterocyte and others are under investigation (14). Glucose transporter-1 (GLT1) is very well characterized and serves in the Na^+-dependent glucose and galactose uptake at the luminal membrane of the intestinal epithelial cell. A different, Na^+-independent D-fructose transporter has also been identified in the enterocyte. Altogether, seven members of the glucose transporter family have been identified, but not all are fully characterized.

Carbohydrates serve as the main energy source for cellular metabolism when energy is rapidly required following stress. Each gram of carbohydrate yields approximately 4 kcal/g. Carbohydrates, in addition to their use as an energy source, are important in membranes as glycoproteins and glycolipids, as well as in the carbon backbone of lipid and nonessential amino acids (NEAAs) (14). As mentioned previously, many tissues including the brain, red cells, white cells, and wounds are to a large extent glucose-dependent tissues. Several sugars are required for homeostasis and metabolism of which glucose, galactose, and fructose serve as the main six carbon sugars. Carbohydrate is stored as glycogen that is contained in the liver, skeletal muscle, and cardiac muscle. Muscle glycogen is used primarily by the muscle itself and is not available as a glucose source to other tissues. Muscle does not contain the enzyme glucose 6-phosphatase, which is responsible for the terminal step of glycogenolysis and would allow net release of glucose from the muscle into the circulation. Liver glycogen serves as the only source of free glucose available systemically from carbohydrate stores. It has been estimated that hepatic glycogen reserve in a 70-kg man is approximately 75 g and muscle glycogen reserve is approximately 105 g (9,10). Glucose, serving as the main energy source in metabolic stress, yields 38 high-energy phosphate bonds [adenosine triphosphate (ATP)] per glucose molecule when completely metabolized to carbon dioxide (CO_2) and water. In cells unable to utilize the Krebs cycle, glycolysis yields two high-energy phosphate bonds in the glucose to lactate conversion (Fig. 5.1).

Protein

Protein intake differs significantly from carbohydrate intake in that the amount of free amino acids and small peptides are minimal in the normal diet, and are obtained principally

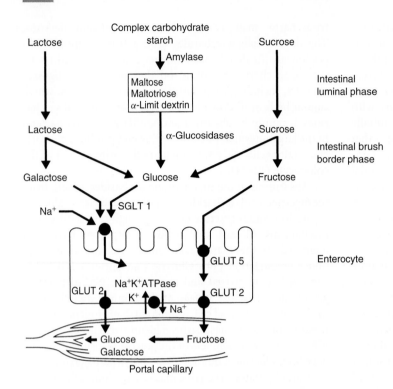

FIGURE 5.1 Luminal digestion of carbohydrate substrates and absorption of digestion products in the gastrointestinal tract. SGLT-1, glucose transporter 1; GLUT-2, glucose transporter 2; GLUT-5, glucose transporter 5.

in the form of protein. In contrast to carbohydrate digestion in the intestinal lumen, protein digestion is incomplete and leads to a mixture of free amino acids and oligopeptides, in which the peptide fraction predominates (Fig. 5.1). The major end products of protein digestion are absorbed by the luminal epithelial cell as small peptides which are subsequently digested to free amino acids inside the cell (15). Digestion of protein occurs in two phases defined by the site of digestion along the GI tract: a gastric phase and an intestinal phase. For convenience, the intestinal phase can be subdivided into the luminal phase, brush border phase, and intracellular phase, again defined by the exact location of digestion in the intestine. The overall scheme of protein digestion in the GI tract is given in Figure 5.2 (16).

In addition to protein in the diet, substantial amounts of endogenous proteins enter the GI tract and are digested and assimilated just as dietary proteins. These endogenous proteins arise partly from the saliva and the gastric, biliary, pancreatic, and intestinal secretions and partly from desquamated epithelial cells of the GI tract (16). The endogenous secretions account for approximately 20 to 30 g of proteins per day, and desquamated cells account for an additional 30 g/d.

Proteins and amino acids are essential components of all living cells and are involved in virtually all bodily functions. These molecules serve as enzymes, hormones, neurotransmitters, immunoglobulins, and transport proteins. Proteins and amino acids also serve as components of essential cell function including receptor binding, transport systems, and contractile elements. Total body protein is only 15% to 18% of body weight in a healthy man (7). It is important to remember that protein is not stored and that all protein in the body should be considered functional.

As a result of its widespread metabolic and cellular requirements to maintain normal bodily function, there is an obligate protein turnover rate. During homeostasis, approximately 2.5% of total body protein is broken down and resynthesized every 24 hours (7). More than half of this turnover is accounted for by the daily digestive process, hemoglobin turnover, muscle protein synthesis, and maintenance of normal immune function. This turnover does change slightly with age. The neonate has significantly increased daily protein turnover associated with growth and development, whereas the elderly undergo significantly diminished daily protein turnover (17). Protein utilized for energy, yields approximately 3.5 cal/g. In the clinical setting, adult protein requirements range from 1.0 to 2 g/kg/d depending on the degree of metabolic stress. Most postoperative surgical patients do well with 1.5 to 1.75 g/kg/d. Adjustments may be necessary according to hepatic and renal function.

Lipids

Where carbohydrate and protein are fairly soluble in aqueous solution, lipids are characterized by poor solubility in aqueous solution and good solubility in organic solvents. Because the lipid substrates are not accessible to the digestive enzymes in the aqueous phase, lipid digestion presents some unique problems in many surgical settings. To overcome these problems, unique conditions involving changes in the physical and chemical properties have evolved for the digestion and absorption of lipids in the GI tract (18) (Fig. 5.3). The nonpolar and hydrophobic properties of lipids confer features suitable for specific roles in biologic systems. Lipid compounds play a key role in four major functions and numerous minor functions.

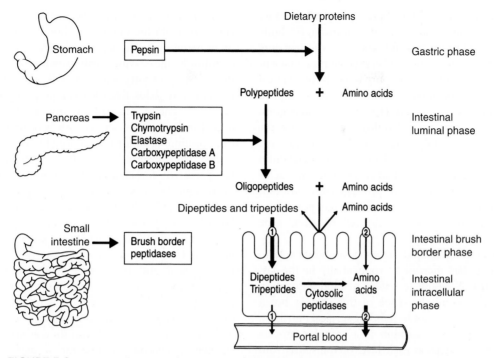

FIGURE 5.2 Luminal digestion of protein and absorption of protein digestion products in the gastrointestinal tract. Transport system for dipeptides and tripeptides (*1*); transport system for free amino acids (*2*).

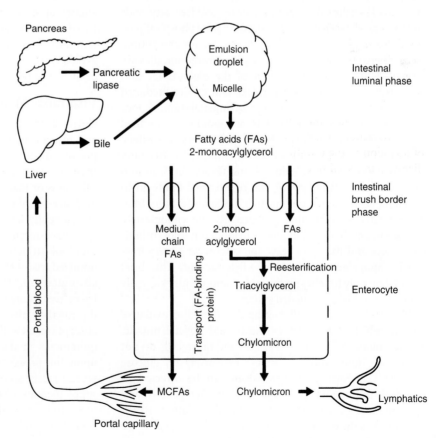

FIGURE 5.3 Luminal digestion of lipid substrates and absorption of fatty acids in the gastrointestinal tract. MCFAs, medium-chain fatty acids.

The major roles for dietary lipids include a primary energy source, cell membrane structure, lubricant for body surfaces, joints, and mucous membranes, and cell signaling components (19,20). As mentioned earlier, adipose tissue in the average 70-kg man contains approximately 140,000 cal and serves as a major metabolic storage site. Complete oxidation of lipid to CO_2 and H_2O yields 9 kcal/g. In addition to energy storage and utilization, lipids are the main component in cellular and subcellular membranes. Lipids also serve as the precursors for prostaglandin synthesis. Linoleic and linolenic acid are essential fatty acids (EFAs) that serve as precursors for prostaglandin synthesis. Prostaglandins then become key regulatory components in metabolism, and are involved in the cell signaling, gene expression, and inflammation.

The understanding of lipid metabolism and its role in surgical nutrition has increased exponentially in the last two decades (18). A complete review of lipid absorption and digestion is beyond the scope of this chapter but a brief review is essential for understanding surgical nutrition. Luminal digestion and absorption is a complex process involving numerous steps at each level of transport from lumen, to enterocyte, to lymphatics, and to blood. Lipid digestion begins in the gastric lumen with gastric lipase. The lipid emulsion then enters the small intestine as small 0.5 mm droplets. Here it is mixed with bile and pancreatic enzymes, mainly lipase and colipase, forming micelles. Pancreatic lipase works at the oil/water interface to yield free fatty acids and monoacylglycerol. Phospholipids require phospholipase and cholesterol requires cholesterol esterase for absorption. Once cleaved by the respective enzymes, mixed micelles are formed which allow permeation of the digested fat into the enterocytes. Both passive uptake and carrier-mediated transport have been supported in experimental studies. Once taken up by the enterocyte, fats are rapidly re-esterified into triacylglycerol, phospholipids, and cholesterol esters. This rapid re-esterification allows the intracellular free fatty acid concentration to remain low and favors diffusion into the cell. Once in the cytosol, the re-esterified lipids go to the endoplasmic reticulum through mechanisms thought to involve fatty acid binding proteins. At the endoplasmic reticulum, apolipoprotein and chylomicron biosynthesis takes place and the lipids leave the enterocyte as very low-density lipoproteins (VLDL) or chylomicrons. This brief description only touches on the high points of this extremely complex and highly regulated system.

Tissues capable of utilizing lipids as a major oxidative fuel include the liver, kidney, heart, and skeletal muscle. The red blood cell, white blood cell, and nerve cells do not metabolize lipids and rely almost exclusively on glucose for fuel (7). Fatty acid metabolism can be directed in one of three potential pathways: lipolysis, ketogenesis, and lipogenesis (18). The first pathway is β-oxidation, which takes place in the outer mitochondrial membrane to produce fatty acyl-coenzyme A (CoA). Fatty acyl-CoA is subsequently shuttled to the inner mitochondrial membrane where it is metabolized to carbon dioxide, water, and ATP. Carnitine, a nonprotein amino acid, serves as the carrier for the fatty acyl-CoA from the outer mitochondrial membrane to the inner membrane. The acyl-CoA is linked for transport with carnitine by the enzyme carnitine palmitoyltransferase. Only the first step of fatty acid metabolism is energy requiring. β-Oxidation yields five high-energy phosphate bonds per acyl-CoA. The second pathway involves ketogenesis in the liver. Ketone synthesis starts with two molecules of acetyl-CoA combining to form acetoacetyl-CoA. The acetoacetyl-CoA is then converted to 3-hydroxy, 3-methylglutaryl-CoA, the precursor for cholesterol synthesis and ketone body formation. Three ketone bodies are produced including acetoacetate, β-hydroxy butyrate, and acetone. These ketone bodies are released by the liver and can be utilized by a variety of peripheral tissues such as cardiac and skeletal muscle. The third pathway for acetyl-CoA metabolism is fatty acid and triglyceride synthesis. Lipogenesis (as opposed to β-oxidation) requires malonyl-CoA that is produced directly from acetyl-CoA by the enzyme acetyl-CoA carboxylase. When mitochondrial concentrations of malonyl-CoA are elevated, carnitine acyltransferase I, (the enzyme responsible for transport of acyl groups into the mitochondria) is secondarily inhibited. In contrast, when intracellular concentrations of fatty acids are elevated, acetyl-CoA carboxylase, the rate-limiting step in malonyl-CoA synthesis, is inhibited. This serves as an efficient regulator promoting malonyl-CoA and thereby lipogenesis when energy supply is abundant. When energy supplies are limited, β-oxidation of fatty acids predominates. This is a classic example of reciprocal utilization in a biologic system. This avoids synthesis and degradation of the same molecule from occurring at the same time.

Vitamins, Minerals, and Trace Elements

Currently there are no specific guidelines regarding vitamins and mineral requirements in the surgical population. It is presumed and supported by animal data and limited human trials that the antioxidant needs are increased during surgical illness or major metabolic insults (21,22). However, the evidence-based reports to support routine supplementation are currently lacking. The antioxidant vitamins and minerals have recently received much attention, and although they look attractive in theory, require large multicenter randomized trials before large quantity supplementation can be advocated (23,24). Factors causing variations in micronutrient requirement levels include the interactions between the micronutrient excretion, utilization, distribution, and absorption, as well as storage levels (25). Micronutrient requirements in the acute setting will be largely dependent upon the preexisting nutritional status. There have been several recent studies using single nutrient supplements or supplementation with "antioxidant cocktails"(26). Many of these studies have shown significant benefits in outcome. Despite these studies, there is currently inadequate clinical data to support routine supplementation. The patient populations that will be of highest risk for antioxidant and micronutrient deficiency are those patients on ventilators with high levels of fraction of inspired oxygen (FiO_2) and those who have sustained ischemic reperfusion injuries. Other surgical illnesses that may predispose the patient to vitamin deficiency include long term total parenteral nutrition (TPN) with inadequate supplementation, malnutrition before surgical intervention, preexisting diseases with increased loss or increased demand in vitamin and micronutrients. Patients with high-output fistulas or proximal ostomies are excellent examples of patients at risk from excessive loss of micronutrients, such as trace minerals zinc and copper. Supplementation in these high-risk patient populations should be strongly considered (27).

Each micronutrient has both a beneficial and potential detrimental effect, with only a relatively narrow range of optimal supplementation yielding maximal clinical outcome (26,28,29). The interactions between micronutrients, medications, and disease process will have an impact on the supplementation of nutrients. It must be kept in mind that absolute micronutrient deficiency is extremely rare in the routine surgical patient, with the exception of those patients with inborn errors in metabolism and exceedingly high losses as mentioned earlier. Although it is intriguing to review the theoretic and nutrient supplementation studies, it is very difficult to extrapolate these studies to the general population of surgical patients. Numerous questions still remain on the quantity of micronutrient to be supplemented, the timing of this supplementation, as well as the background substrate which will provide optimal supplementation. Until these questions are answered, the risk-versus-benefit ratio of large doses of supplements is not supported for the routine surgical patient. Data does clearly support that it is essential that patients receive at least the recommended dietary allowance for micronutrients except when contraindicated for specific disease states (22) (Table 5.2).

Specific Antioxidants

Oxidative stress is induced by surgery and critical illness where balance is tilted toward the production of reactive oxygen species (ROS). Oxygen-free radicals and other ROS are capable of attacking nucleic acids, proteins, polysaccharides, and polyunsaturated fatty acids resulting in cellular damage and tissue dysfunction (21,22). Activation of nuclear factor κB (NF-κB) by ROS leads to expression of gene products critical in the initiation and perpetuation of the systemic inflammatory response (24). Nonenzymatic antioxidants include vitamin E, vitamin C, β-carotene, and heme-binding proteins. Enzymatic scavenger systems include superoxide dismutase, catalase, and glutathione peroxidase with their associated cofactors selenium, zinc, manganese, and iron. There have been multiple clinical studies, including two recent meta-analyses (24,30) evaluating the possible benefits of antioxidant supplementation during critical illness. Major drawbacks with most of these studies are the relative small sample size, differences in the antioxidant combinations used, monotherapy versus combination therapy, dosages used, route of administration (parenteral versus enteral), and timing of supplementation. Taking these limitations into account, most of these studies show a benefit in select

TABLE 5.2

American Medical Association Recommendations for Daily Parenteral Vitamin and Mineral Intake

Intake	Amount
Vitamin	
Vitam A	3,300 IU
Vitamin D	200 IU
Vitamin E	10 IU
Vitamin C (ascorbic acid)	100 mg
Folacin	400 μg
Niacin	40 mg
Riboflavin	3.6 mg
Thiamine	3 mg
Vitamin B_6 (pyridoxine)	4 mg
Vitamin B_{12} (cyanocobalamin)	5 μg
Pantothenic acid	15 mg
Biotin	60 μg
Mineral	
Zinc	2.5–4 mg[a]
Copper	0.5–1.5 mg
Manganese	150–180 μg
Chromium	10–15 μg
Selenium[b]	40–80 μg

[a]Additional amounts; 2.0 mg/d in acute catabolism; 12.2 mg/L of small bowel fluid losses; 17.1 mg/kg of stool or ileostomy output.
[b]Suggested intake.
Adapted from Multivitamin preparations for parenteral use. A statement by the Nutrition Advisory Group. *J Parenter Enteral Nutr* 1979;3:258, 263, with permission.

populations with antioxidant supplementation as evidenced by decrease in mortality, decrease in duration of mechanical ventilation, and decrease in intensive care unit (ICU) days (24,30). One key variable in antioxidant supplementation is timing of intervention. Antioxidants lack therapeutic effect once tissue damage is irreversible. Ideal therapy must be started early after admission to the surgical ICU (30). Future large multicenter trials will be needed to clarify the antioxidants to use, their dosage, route of administration, and timing.

NUTRITION ASSESSMENT

The purpose of performing a nutritional assessment is to evaluate the current nutritional status as well as identify those patients at risk for developing malnutrition. Over the last several decades many nutritional assessment tools have been developed. However, there is no single method that can be considered perfect as an indicator of nutritional assessment (31,32). In the clinical setting, the nutrition assessment tool needs to be practical, user friendly, cost effective, and be able to produce accurate and reproducible measurements. Nutrition assessment involves both clinical and biochemical assessments (33).

Clinical Assessment

The history and physical examination are part of a comprehensive approach to the assessment of nutritional status along with anthropometric measurements. The physical examination remains the primary nutritional assessment tool, relying on subjective and descriptive information. The main objective is to establish signs and symptoms of nutrient deficiencies or toxicities, and tolerance of current nutrient provision. A thorough history includes demographic information, chief complaint, present and past illnesses, current health, family history, dietary history, socioeconomic status, personal stress, coping mechanisms and review of systems focusing on nutrient deficiencies (34). There are more than a 100 different physical signs and symptoms of nutritional deficiencies or excesses (Table 5.3). A nutrition health history can provide approximately 80% of information on nutritional status; it should include any changes in the patient's current intake, types of foods consumed, duration of change, and reasons for altered intake. The patient's medications should also be examined for potential drug–nutrient interactions, nutritionally related side effects, and increased nutrient requirements (Table 5.4).

The results of the physical examination should be viewed in relation to nutritional status. Vital signs can afford insight into the functional capacity of specific organs (e.g., heart and lung). Micronutrient deficiencies or interferences to optimal nutrient intake can be discovered by examining the hair, nails, skin, and oral cavity (e.g., dentition, ulcers, gums). The abdomen should be examined for enlargement or wasting. The thyroid should also be evaluated for enlargement. The extremities should be examined for skeletal deformities, tenderness, or edema. A detailed neurologic examination is needed to evaluate orientation, memory, cranial nerves, motor performance, reflexes, and sensation—all of which can indicate nutritional deficiency (35).

Anthropometric and Body Composition Assessment

An accurate height and body weight measurement should be obtained on all patients. The history should reveal the patient's usual weight and comparison should be made to actual weight with reference to the period of time elapsed. The key is to estimate weight loss properly and assess its impact on physiologic function. Any unintentional weight loss, whether in obese or normal weight individuals, greater than 5% over the preceding month or greater than 10% over the last 6 months is important and suggestive of nutritional risk (31,34) and increased morbidity and mortality (36). The overall impact of the weight loss on physiologic function is assessed from the history and by examination. Organomegaly, ascites, or massive tumor growth may mask progressive loss of lean body weight, whereas rapid weight gain usually reflects fluid retention, ascites, or adipose weight gain (31). Weight should preferably be measured weekly noting that acute weight changes are most likely due to fluid shifts; a standardized weight measuring protocol should be followed. Body mass indices (BMI) such as the Quetelet index [weight (kg)/height (m^2)] have been developed to provide a fairly accurate measurement of body mass. An excessive disease risk and death rate is noted at both ends of the index; survival in a patient with a BMI less than 14 is unusual (Table 5.5).

Numerous methods have been developed to assess body composition. Few of these are relatively cost effective, noninvasive, reproducible and convenient to the surgical patient.(31). The measurement that is probably the most inaccurate, yet most frequently used, is skin-fold thickness assessment. Skin-fold thickness measurement of various points on the body [triceps, biceps, subscapular, suprailiac (women), and abdomen (men)] is used as an indirect measurement of subcutaneous fat. Drawbacks in using these measurements in the clinical setting include the following: fluid shifts and changes in hydration status affect measurements, the available standards do not reflect variations in bone size and skin compressibility, and the technique is affected by interobserver variability. This measurement is useful to study populations but is essentially useless in the acute clinical setting on a single patient (37).

Creatinine height index (CHI) is a method used to assess skeletal muscle mass. It assumes that creatinine excretion correlates with lean body mass and body weight. It is estimated that 18 to 20 kg of muscle is needed to produce 1 g of creatinine. Dietary protein sources may contribute up to 20% of the excreted creatinine (36). CHI is calculated by comparing the actual measured creatinine excretion value with an expected value from a normal individual of the same height and gender. Several factors affect the reliability of CHI: decline in lean body mass with malnutrition; advanced age results in decreased creatinine excretion; renal impairment reduces the amount of creatinine filtered through the kidney and urine output is also diminished; rhabdomyolysis, bed rest, and catabolic states increase short-term creatinine excretion; and incomplete 24-hour urine collection will invalidate creatinine excretion results (37).

Bioelectric impedance (BIA) measures fat-free mass by determining differences in electrical conductivity between fat and lean body mass. Lean tissue has a far greater conductivity as a result of its electrolyte content. An imperceptibly small electrical current passes through electrodes attached to the extremities of the patient to obtain electrical and resistance measurements (37). This technique is safe, noninvasive, inexpensive, and requires little patient cooperation. Factors that affect reliable BIA measurements include fever, electrolyte imbalance, obesity, hydration issues, and lack of standards that consider variations in individual body size. BIA is of little use in the critically ill or acute surgical populations. BIA use is not recommended in individual patients, but rather for population studies (37,38). Other techniques for measuring body composition include dual-energy x-ray absorptiometry, computed tomography, ultrasonography, magnetic resonance imaging, total body potassium counting, neutron activation analysis, and isotope dilution techniques. These techniques are not readily available for clinical use and

TABLE 5.3

Nutrient Deficiencies Revealed by Physical Examination

Deficient Nutrient	Findings
General	
Protein, calories	Loss of weight, muscle mass, or fat stores; growth retardation; infection; poor wound healing
Protein, thiamine	Edema (ankles and feet; rule out sodium and water retention, pregnancy, protein-losing enteropathy)
Obesity	Excessive fat stores
Vitamin A	Poor growth
Iron	Anemia, fatigue
Skin	
Protein, vitamin C, zinc	Poor wound healing, pressure ulcers
Fat, vitamin A	Xerosis (rule out environmental cause, lack of hygiene, aging, uremia, hypothyroidism), follicular hyperkeratosis, mosaic dermatitis (plaques of skin in center, peeling at periphery on shins)
Vitamin C	Slow wound healing
Niacin	Red, swollen skin lesions
Zinc	Delayed wound healing, acneiform rash, skin lesions, hair loss
Vitamin K or C	Excessive bleeding, petechiae, ecchymoses; small red, purple, or black hemorrhagic spots
Dehydration (fluid)	Poor skin turgor
Nails	
Iron	Koilonychia (rule out cardiopulmonary disease)
Protein deficiency	Dull, lusterless with transverse ridging across nail plate
Vitamin A, C	Pale, poor blanching, irregular, mottled
Protein, calories	Bruising, bleeding
Vitamin C	Splinter hemorrhages
Hair	
Protein	Hair lacks shine, luster (cause may be environmental or chemical)
Protein, copper	Dyspigmentation (lightening of normal hair color, consider if hair is bleached or dyed)
Copper	Corkscrew hair (Menkes syndrome)
Face	
Protein	Diffuse pigmentation, swelling
Calcium	Facial paresthesias
Eyes	
Iron, folate, or vitamin B_{12}	Pale conjunctivae (anemia)
Vitamin A	Bitot spots (more common in children), conjunctival xerosis (rule out chemical or environmental irritation), corneal xerosis, keratomalacia
Pyridoxine, niacin, riboflavin	Angular palpebritis
Hyperlipidemia	Corneal arcus, xanthelasma
Nose	
Riboflavin, niacin, pyridoxine	Seborrhea on nasolabial area, nose bridge, eyebrows, and back of ears (rule out poor hygiene)
Lips and mouth	
Niacin, riboflavin	Cheilosis, angular scars
Riboflavin, pyridoxine, niacin, iron	Angular stomatitis
Tongue	
Niacin, riboflavin, folic acid, iron	Atrophic filiform papillae
Vitamin B_{12}	Glossitis
Zinc	Taste atrophy
Riboflavin	Magenta tongue
Teeth	
Excess sugar, vitamin C	Edentia, caries
Fluorosis	Mottled
Gums	
Vitamin C	Spongy, bleeding, receding

(Continued)

TABLE 5.3

(Continued)

Deficient Nutrient	Findings
Neck	
Iodine	Enlarged thyroid gland
Protein, bulimia	Enlarged parotid glands (bilateral)
Excess fluid	Venous distention, pulsations
Thorax	
Protein, calories	Decreased muscle mass and strength, shortness of breath, fatigue, decreased pulmonary function
Cardiac system	
Thiamine	Heart failure
Gastrointestinal system	
Protein, calories, zinc, vitamin C	Poor wound healing
Protein	Hepatomegaly
Urinary tract	
Dehydration	Dark, concentrated urine
Overhydration	Light colored, dilute urine
Musculoskeletal system	
Vitamin D, calcium	Rickets, osteomalacia
Vitamin D	Persistently open anterior fontanel (after age 18 months), craniotabes (softening of skull across back and sides before age 1 year); epiphyseal enlargement (painless) at wrist, knees, and ankles; pigeon chest and Harrison sulcus (horizontal depression on lower chest border)
Protein	Emaciation, muscle wasting, swelling, pain, pale hair patches
Vitamin C	Swollen, painful joints
Thiamine	Pain in thighs, calves
Nervous system	
Protein	Psychomotor changes (listless, apathetic), mental confusion
Thiamine, vitamin B_6	Weakness, confusion, depressed reflexes, paresthesias, sensory loss, calf tenderness
Niacin, vitamin B_{12}	Dementia
Calcium, magnesium	Tetany

none of these body composition measurements have been shown to consistently predict clinical outcome (3).

Subjective global assessment (SGA) assesses nutritional status and malnutrition based on historic factors (weight change, dietary intake change, GI symptoms that have persisted for greater than 2 weeks, functional capacity, underlying disease, and effect on metabolic stress), and physical findings (loss of subcutaneous fat, muscle wasting, ankle edema, sacral edema, and ascites). Patients are rated as being well nourished, moderately or severely malnourished (31). SGA is considered a relatively reliable indicator for nutritional compromise, but may not be sensitive enough to reflect a patient's early response to nutrition support, thereby limiting its use in surgery and critical care. SGA has proved very useful in the preoperative setting to estimate surgical risk and outcome.

Biochemical Assessment

The selection and frequency of biochemical parameters to aid in nutrition assessment should be based on findings from the patient history and physical examination and clinical relevance.

Immune Competence

Immune competence is measured by delayed cutaneous hypersensitivity (DCH) and total lymphocyte count (TLC), which is reduced in malnutrition. The following factors nonspecifically alter DCH in the absence of malnutrition: infection, uremia, cirrhosis, hepatitis, trauma, burns, hemorrhage, steroids, immunosuppressants, cimetidine, coumadin, general anesthesia, and surgery (39). Non-nutritional factors that affect TLC include hypoalbuminemia, metabolic stress, infection, cancer, and chronic diseases. Therefore, critically ill patients have multiple factors that can alter DCH and TLC, making them valueless in assessing nutritional risk and status.

Nitrogen Balance Studies

Nitrogen balance studies are commonly used in the acute care setting to determine protein turnover and whether the patient is in a state of anabolism or catabolism. Nitrogen is released as the result of catabolism of amino acids in proteins and is excreted in the urine in the form of urea. Nitrogen balance is calculated by subtracting the excreted nitrogen [24-hour urine urea nitrogen (UUN) collection

TABLE 5.4

Drug-Induced Nutritional and Metabolic Alterations

Altered taste

Chemotherapeutic agents (carboplatin, cisplatin, etoposide, interferon-α, teniposide)

Metallic taste: captopril, metronidazole (Flagyl)

Sulfonylureas

Disulfiram

Appetite changes

Increased

Steroids, megestrol, androgens, benzodiazepines, antihistamines, insulin, phenothiazines, sulfonylureas

Decreased

Antibiotics, antineoplastics, anticonvulsants, levodopa, thiazides, fluoxetine, amphetamines, diet products

Dry mouth

Radiation therapy, diuretics, antihistamines, tricyclic antide-pressants, atropine-like drugs

Nausea/emesis

Antibiotics, thiazides, chemotherapeutic agents

Diarrhea

Antibiotics, magnesium-containing medications, hyperosmolar medications, sorbitol-containing medications, prokinetic agents, cathartics, cholinergics, lactulose, neomycin

Constipation

Barbiturates, vecuronium bromide, opiates (morphine, codeine)

Hyperglycemia

Steroids, theophylline, chemotherapeutic agents (asparaginase, interferon, methotrexate)

Hypoglycemia

Pentamidine, insulin, oral hypoglycemia agents

Altered fat metabolism/absorption

Cyclosporine, androgens, estrogen, progestin, cholestyramine, aluminum-containing antacids

Sodium alterations

Loss: laxatives, diuretics, probenecid

Excess: penicillin G sodium, increased amounts of normal saline

Potassium alterations

Loss: diuretics, laxatives, probenecid, amphotericin B

Excess: spironolactone, penicillin G potassium

Phosphorus loss

Binders (sucralfate, aluminum, calcium, magnesium), corticosteroids, furosemide, thiazides

Magnesium loss

Diuretics, amphotericin B, ciprofloxacin, cyclosporine, probenecid, carbenicillin, pentamidine, cisplatin

Calcium loss

Furosemide, triamterene, probenecid, corticosteroids, cisplatin, amphotericin B, calcitonin, phenytoin, pentamidine, mithramycin

TABLE 5.5

Body-Mass Index (BMI) Categories and Interpretation

BMI Category	BMI	Disease Risk
<20, underweight	<20	Very high
20–25, normal	20–25	Very low
25–30, overweight	25–30	Low
>30, obese	30–35	Moderate
	35–40	High
	>40	Very high

BMI = weight (kg)/height (m²).

A positive nitrogen balance in the range of 2 to 4 g of nitrogen per day, indicating an anabolic state, is desired, but often difficult to achieve. Measurement of nitrogen balance does not indicate gains or losses of individual organs, because nitrogen balance is the sum total of body gains and losses. Validity of nitrogen balance is affected by severe nitrogen retention disorders (e.g., creatinine clearance <50 mL/min or severe hepatic failure), massive diuresis, accuracy of the 24-hour urine collection, abnormal nitrogen losses through diarrhea or large draining wounds, skin exfoliation as in burns, and completeness of protein or amino acid intake data (31,37).

Serum Proteins

Because of the numerous flaws and labor-intensive expense associated with nitrogen balance studies, monitoring of serum protein levels is often used as a surrogate to nitrogen to help assess a patient's nutritional status. Serum albumin, transferrin, thyroxine-binding prealbumin, and retinol-binding protein are most commonly used in the clinical setting (Table 5.6). All of these proteins have transport functions separate from their use in nutrition assessment. The use of serum proteins for nutrition assessment assumes incorrectly that decreased levels are solely caused by malnutrition.

When evaluating serum-protein concentration, determinants such as synthesis, degradation, and distribution, all must be considered to produce a valid interpretation. The visceral proteins mentioned earlier are produced by the liver; therefore several factors can affect their synthesis including hepatic synthetic function, metabolic state, and amino acid availability.

The use of these transport proteins in the critically ill surgical population to assess nutrition status should be undertaken with caution. Following a metabolic insult, inflammatory cytokines tumor necrosis factor (TNF) and interleukin 1 (IL-1) are released in response to the injury. With resultant proinflammatory cytokine release, hepatic reprioritization occurs leading to upregulation and increased synthetic rates of acute phase reactants such as C-reactive protein, fibrinogen, ceruloplasmin, and α_1-antitrypsin and downregulation with decreased synthetic rates of transport proteins (40–44). This, along with volume shifts associated with the inflammatory process, commonly results in a

plus insensible losses] from the nitrogen intake provided in the nutrition support regimen:

Nitrogen balance g/d =

(protein or amino acid intake/6.25) − (UUN + 4)

TABLE 5.6

Serum Transport Protein Features in Nutrition Assessment

Serum Protein	Normal Value	Half-Life	Function	Clinical Significance and Other Comments
Albumin	3.5–5.0 g/dL <2.1, severe depletion; 2.1–2.8, moderate depletion; 2.8–3.5, mild depletion	21 d	Maintains plasma oncotic pressure, carrier for amino acids, zinc, magnesium, calcium, free fatty acids, drugs	Routinely available Useful in long-term nutritional assessment Limited value in short-term nutrition indicator because of long half-life and other variables (albumin infusion, hydration status) Reliable prognostic indicator of morbidity and mortality Synthesized in liver (low levels with hepatic disease) >60% total body albumin found extravascular
Transferrin	200–400 mg/dL <100, severe depletion; 100–150, moderate depletion; 150–200, severe depletion	8–10 d	Binds iron in plasma and transports to bone	Strongly influenced by iron status Synthesized in liver and found primarily extravascular Increased levels with pregnancy estrogen and iron therapy, acute hepatitis, iron-deficiency anemia, chronic blood loss, and dehydration Decreased levels with hepatic disease, protein-losing states (nephrotic syndrome), hemolytic anemia, metabolic stress
Prealbumin	10–40 mg/dL <5, severe depletion; 5–10, moderate depletion; 10–15, mild depletion	2–3 d	Binds thyroxin, carrier, or RBP	Useful as short-term nutritional index Better index of visceral protein, especially in acute states of protein-calorie malnutrition Synthesized in the liver Increased levels with renal dysfunction Decreased levels with acute catabolic states, postsurgery, hyperthyroidism, liver disease, protein-calorie malnutrition
Retinol-binding protein (RBP)	2.7–7.6 mg/dL	12 h	Transports vitamin A in plasma, binds to prealbumin	Reflects acute changes in protein malnutrition and changes in dietary intake Limited use in renal failure because it is metabolized by the proximal tubular cells Increased levels in chronic renal failure and in patients on oral contraceptives Decreased levels with vitamin A deficiency, protein-calorie malnutrition, acute catabolic states, postsurgery, hyperthyroidism, liver disease

rapid decrease in serum protein levels. This so-called reprioritization of protein synthesis by the hepatocyte returns to normal within several days of surgery or stress, unless continued hypermetabolic complications, such as sepsis, ensue (45). These changes have been described in many clinical situations such as severe multiple trauma, postoperative course, sepsis, and burn injury (43). Therefore, it is common to find subnormal transport protein levels within the first several days of trauma or major surgery.

These initially low levels are more reflective of illness severity and intravascular to extravascular volume shifts rather than nutritional status. In addition, due to the long half-life of serum albumin ($t^{1/2} \sim 20$ days) and its depletion with large fluid volumes, it is of little-to-no value to rely on albumin levels as a nutritional marker in the acute postoperative or post trauma period, or during critical illness. Despite the problems associated with using albumin in the postoperative and critical care settings, albumin remains an excellent and inexpensive marker for preoperative assessment of nutritional status. Kudsk et al. have recently shown a direct linear correlation between albumin levels and risk of major complication in various GI surgery procedures (46).

Critically ill surgical patients are at high risk for developing nutritional deficiencies. Decreased levels of some of the shorter half-life transport protein levels may assist in rapid identification of the potential nutritional risk and otherwise unidentified inflammatory process (38,40). Prealbumin with a $t^{1/2}$ of 48 hours is currently the visceral protein most commonly used as a monitor of nutritional status in the surgical ICU setting. Several centers have started using ratios of visceral protein such as prealbumin and acute phase proteins such as C-reactive protein as early indicators of increased inflammatory focus, that is, sepsis, abscess or pneumonia, and synthetic potential of visceral proteins (47).

Other Biochemical Parameters

Various other laboratory tests exist that reflect a change in nutritional status, tolerance, or response to nutritional therapy. Electrolyte and micronutrients should be evaluated when deficiencies or toxicities are suspected. Liver, renal, and respiratory function strongly affects a patient's dietary prescription and should be included in the nutrition assessment and monitoring process. Iron levels, iron transport proteins, hemoglobin, and hematocrit with indices may determine an anemia of nutritional origin. It should be noted that serum magnesium and calcium levels must be corrected for albumin levels.

ENERGY REQUIREMENTS

In the acute setting, especially the surgical critically ill and recent major surgical patients, the goal of nutritional support is maintenance, not repletion, and should serve as an adjunct to other critical therapies. Numerous hormonal and inflammatory factors are present that limit the effectiveness of exogenously administered nutritional substrates. Routine nutrition support alone should not be expected to convert a catabolic septic patient into an anabolic state. Many undesirable metabolic complications occur when attempting to push excessive calories in the catabolic patient. These complications include hypercapnia, hyperglycemia, hypertriglyceridemia, hepatic steatosis, and azotemia (4,48–50). Once the hypermetabolic process is corrected then anabolism is favored and repletion can occur.

There are multiple methods for determining energy requirements. Indirect calorimetry involves the actual measurement of energy expenditure and remains the "gold standard" (51). However, there are many downsides to this method including expense, requirement of trained personnel, and inaccurate readings in patients with F_{IO}^2 greater than or equal to 50%, malfunctioning chest tubes, endotracheal tubes, or bronchopleurofistulas. These problems have limited the routine clinical application of indirect calorimetry. Most

institutions rely heavily upon predictive equations. Predicting energy needs can be difficult because of uncertainties in estimating energy expenditure (Table 5.7). Predictive equations commonly overestimate energy needs for those mechanically ventilated and sedated patients. For example, neuromuscular paralysis decreases energy requirements by as much as 30% (52). Calculated results are only as accurate as the variables used in the equation. Obesity and resuscitative water weight complicate the use of these equations and lead to a tendency for overfeeding (53). It is unclear as to whether ideal body weight (IBW) or total body weight should be used in predictive energy equations. It has been reported that obese patients should receive 20 to 30 kcal/kg IBW per day (54). Other methods in obese patients use adjusted body weight, particularly in those greater than 130% IBW (53). Predictive equations have been developed to account for obesity, using actual body weight, as well as trauma, burns, and ventilatory status (55). Patino et al. reported a hypocaloric nutrition regimen with adequate protein provided during the first days of the flow phase of the adaptive response to injury, sepsis, and critical illness (56). The regimen consists of a daily supply of 100 to 200 g of glucose and 1.5 to 2.0 g of protein per kg IBW. Irrespective of the method of estimating or calculating energy requirements, energy requirements for surgery patients range from 20 to 35 kcal/kg usual body weight per day (57).

TABLE 5.7

Influences on Resting Energy Expenditure

Clinical Condition	Percentage of REE
Elective uncomplicated surgery	Normal
Major abdominal, thoracic, and vascular surgery	
ICU and mechanical ventilation	105–109 ± 20–28
Cardiac surgery	
ICU and mechanical ventilation	119 ± 21
Multiple injury	
ICU and mechanical ventilation	138 ± 23
Spontaneous ventilation	119 ± 7
Head and multiple injury	150 ± 23
ICU and mechanical ventilation	
Head injury	
ICU and spontaneous ventilation	126 ± 14
ICU and mechanical ventilation	104 ± 5
Infection	
Sepsis and spontaneous ventilation	121 ± 27
ICU, septic shock, and mechanical ventilation	135 ± 28
Sepsis and mechanical ventilation	155 ± 14
Septic shock and mechanical ventilation	102 ± 14
Multiple injury, sepsis, mechanical ventilation, and TPN	191 ± 38

Data are percentages of reference value (± SD). REE, resting energy expenditure; ICU, intensive care unit; TPN, total parenteral nutrition.

Permissive Underfeeding

The caloric requirement for the perioperative and ICU patient is evolving. The concept of permissive underfeeding of these patients during the early phases of the catabolic stress is gaining support in a series of animal and human studies. A teleologic argument states that a relative "anorexia of illness" develops with significant injury or stress to the host and that supplying excessive nutrients during this period induces a proinflammatory state which then exacerbates the condition (4,58–60). Several retrospective studies and a few prospective studies have evaluated caloric delivery and outcome. Krishnan et al. (61) reported in a prospective cohort study that underfed patients compared with patients fed near goal in a medical ICU resulted in a small improvement in survival. In a study evaluating TPN and caloric delivery, McCowan et al. (62) demonstrated an interesting but not statistically significant trend in decreasing infectious complications; however, nitrogen balance was statistically more negative in the hypocaloric group. Several studies in critically ill obese patients use a hypocaloric high-protein regimen with excellent metabolic results (51,63,64). Although the optimal caloric load for the hypermetabolic surgical patient remains in transition, the caloric delivery currently considered safe for the perioperative period is in the range of 20 to 30 kcal/kg/d (excluding the morbidly obese).

Preoperative Carbohydrate Loading

One of the dogmas of surgical practice is making patients NPO after midnight of the day before any planned surgical procedure. This practice, however, has recently been called into question especially with regard to preoperative intake of liquids. The most recent Cochrane review by Brady et al. reviewed 38 randomized controlled trials on preoperative fasting practices and concluded that there was no evidence to suggest overnight fasting for fluids results in a decrease in perioperative aspiration risk or related morbidity (65). Moreover, the practice guidelines for preoperative fasting by the American Society of Anesthesiologist Task Force in 1999, recommends fasting time before anesthesia for clear fluids to be 2 hours and 6 hours for solids for otherwise healthy patients (66). There is emerging evidence suggesting that preoperative overnight fasting, which is the current standard of care, is not only unnecessary, but may be harmful. Surgical stress causes increases in postoperative insulin resistance, increases in immunosuppression, decreases in lean body mass, and increases in perioperative patient discomfort (67,68). Preoperative "carbohydrate loading" has been shown to attenuate these adverse effects by decreasing postoperative insulin resistance, decreasing surgery-induced immunosuppression, decreasing lean body mass loss, and decreasing perioperative patient discomfort (69–74). Preoperative "carbohydrate loading" involves giving a carbohydrate-rich drink the night before and 3 hours before the scheduled procedure. A commercially available product is Nutricia preOp (12.6% carbohydrates, 50 kcal/100 mL, 240 mOsm, pH 4.9, Nutricia, Wiltshire, UK).

ENTERAL FEEDING

Historically, enteral feeding has been attempted since ancient Egypt and Greece. When the patient was unable to take adequate oral calories, nutrient enemas using various combinations of wine, milk, broth, grains, and raw eggs were used with limited success (75). Colonic delivery of nutrients was continued until the early 1900s despite lack of any outcome data to support the procedure. Of historical interest, following an attempted assassination, President James Garfield was given nutrient enemas every 4 hours for 79 days before he succumbed to his injuries (75)!

The first reports of enteral feeding through "feeding tubes" into the esophagus were in 1598 using a tube made of eel skin. In 1790, John Hunter initiated the modern era of GI access with his reports of gastric feeding (75). Tubes remained very primitive and extremely uncomfortable until rubber manufacturing allowed an array of tubes similar to the current selection. From gastric feeding, nasojejunal tubes evolved and the implementation of orojejunal tube feeding in surgical patients was described by Ravdin and Stengal in 1939 (75).

Before the 1950s, enteral nutrients used in the feeding tubes were mainly milk-based with various additions for specific diseases. Chemically defined diets were developed as part of a National Aeronautics and Space Administration (NASA) study investigating possibilities in minimizing fecal output during space travel (75). In the late 1960s, chemically defined diets were first reported used in critically ill surgical patients and considered as a "medical colostomy." Enteral formulations have evolved into an entire industry and now exist for nearly every metabolic disease state.

Rationale and Benefits

Enteral nutrition is now considered the preferred route of nutrient delivery. The enteral route should always be the primary approach unless safe enteral access is unattainable or unsuccessful in delivery of adequate macro and micronutrients. Extensive review of the myriad benefits of enteral nutrition is beyond the scope of this chapter and is only briefly addressed. Available reviews provide more extensive background in these areas (76,77).

These benefits include maintenance of the gut-associated lymphoid tissue (GALT) (77), enhancing mucosal blood flow (78), and maintenance of mucosal barrier (76). When compared with parenteral nutrition, enteral nutrient delivery attenuates the metabolic response to stress (77) yields better glycemic control, accelerates the return to positive nitrogen balance, and reduces clinical infections in the abdominal cavity and respiratory tract (77,79).

Indications and Contraindications

Enteral nutrition through feeding tubes is indicated when patients are unable to maintain adequate volitional oral intake and a functional GI tract is available and accessible. Absolute and relative contraindications are few and found in Table 5.8. Patient intolerance to enteral feeding is often not

TABLE 5.8

Enteral Feeding Contraindications

- Bowel obstruction
- Persistent intolerance (e.g., emesis, diarrhea)
- Hemodynamic instability
- Major upper gastrointestinal bleeding
- Unable to safely access

Relative contraindications

- Significance bowel-wall edema
- Persistent ileus
- High-output fistula (>800 mL/d)

TABLE 5.10

Methods of Gastrointestinal Access

Nasoenteric feeding tubes	Percutaneous feeding tubes
Spontaneous passage	Percutaneous endoscopic
Bedside, prokinetic agent	gastric (PEG)
Active passage	Gastric/jejunal (PEG/J)
Bedside-assisted	Direct jejunal (DPEJ)
Endoscopic	Laparoscopic
Fluoroscopic	Gastrostomy
Operative	Jejunostomy
	Surgical
	Gastrostomy
	Jejunostomy

PEG, percutaneous endoscopic gastrostomy; PEG/J, percutaneous gastr/jejunostomy; DPEJ, direct percutaneous endoscopic jejunostomy.

easy to predict. If patients fail repeated attempts at enteral feeding, parenteral nutrition should be instituted to provide supplemental or total calorie requirement as indicated.

Enteral Access

Route of administration and method of access is usually determined by the expected duration of exogenous nutrition support, risk of aspiration (Table 5.9), and local technical expertise (80). Nasoenteric or oroenteric feeding tubes are generally used when therapy is anticipated to be of short duration (i.e., 3 weeks) or for interim access before the placement of a long-term device. Long-term access requires a percutaneous or surgically placed feeding tube (81). For various methods of access, see Table 5.10.

Enteral Formulations

The continued success of enteral feeding over the last 30 years has resulted in an explosion in the number of enteral nutrition products available. These enteral products are classified as medical foods and do not currently require U.S. Food and Drug Administration (FDA) approval for their proposed clinical uses. Table 5.11 provides an overview of various categories of supplements specifying the types of macronutrients and physical properties. The appropriate selection and administration of enteral formula requires a thorough knowledge of physiology and pathophysiology of digestion and absorption. The physical form and quantity

TABLE 5.9

Risk Factors for Aspiration

Altered mental status with inability to protect airway
Swallowing dysfunction
Central nervous system insult (cerebrovascular accident)
Local injury (vagal disruption, trauma)
History of aspiration
Severe gastroesophageal reflux
Gastric outlet obstruction
Gastroparesis
Patient position restrictions (supine vs. semirecumbent)

of each nutrient may determine the extent of absorption of and tolerance to the formula (e.g., long-chain versus medium-chain triglyceride).

Macronutrients
Carbohydrate
The molecular form of carbohydrate in enteral formula ranges from simple sugar to starch. The molecular form contributes to the characteristics of osmolality, sweetness, and digestibility. In general, the larger molecular weight carbohydrate molecules (e.g., starch) exert less osmotic pressure, are less sweet, and require more digestion before absorption. The simple sugars found in formulas are maltodextrin, sucrose, and corn syrup solids. In most surgical settings, optimal carbohydrate delivery should be at a level to allow maximal protein sparing while minimizing hyperglycemia (82). This optimal level for the postoperative or hypermetabolic patient is 4 to 6 mg/kg/min (82).

Fiber
Fiber has been reported to be beneficial in the control of a myriad of GI disorders, as well as treatment of hyperlipidemia, and control of blood glucose (83). Fiber-containing formulas usually contain between 5 g and 14 g of total dietary fiber per liter. The form of fiber used is primarily insoluble fiber (e.g., soy fiber), but the more recently developed formulas also contain additional soluble fiber in the form of guars, gums, and pectins. The insoluble fiber is beneficial with regard to colonic function and bowel regulation. The soluble fibers are reported to slow gastric emptying and attenuate the rise in postprandial blood glucose levels. Soluble fibers also bind bile acids and dietary cholesterol, thereby lowering serum cholesterol levels. In addition to the physical properties discussed earlier, soluble fibers serve as substrates for bacterial fermentation in the colon. This fermentation yields SCFAs, carbon dioxide, methane, hydrogen, and water. SCFAs are now known to be the primary fuel for the colonocyte and recent data also support the concept that SCFAs have numerous benefits

TABLE 5.11

Overview of Select Enteral Formulas

Formula Category	Protein Sources	Calories from Protein (%)	Carbohydrate Sources	Calories from Carbohydrate (%)	Fat Sources
Oral supplements	Sodium and calcium caseinates, soy protein isolate	14–24	Corn syrup, sugar, sucrose, maltodextrin	47–64	Corn oil, canola oil, soy oil, sunflower oil, safflower oil
Standard tube feedings	Sodium and calcium caseinates, soy protein isolates	13–18	Corn syrup, maltodextrin	45–57	Soy oil, corn oil, canola oil, MCT, safflower oil
Standard tube feedings with fiber	Sodium and calcium caseinates, soy protein isolate	14–18	Corn syrup, maltodextrin, corn syrup solids, soy fiber, guar gum, oat fiber FOS	44–57	Canola oil, soybean oil, corn oil, MCT
High-protein tube feedings	Sodium and calcium caseinates	22–25	Hydrolyzed cornstarch, maltodextrin, sucrose, fructose, oat fiber, soy fiber	38–52	Canola oil, MCT, soybean oil, safflower oil
Elemental and semielemental	Free amino acids, soy hydrolysates, hydrolyzed whey, hydrolyzed casein, hydrolyzed soy	12–25	Hydrolyzed cornstarch, maltodextrin, sucrose, modified cornstarch	36–82	Soybean oil, safflower oil, canola oil, MCT, sunflower oil
Pulmonary	Sodium and calcium caseinates	17–20	Hydrolyzed cornstarch, corn syrup, sucrose, maltodextrin, sugar	27–40	Canola oil, soybean oil, MCT, corn oil, safflower oil, sardine oil, borage oil
Renal	Sodium and calcium caseinates, whey, L-amino acids	7–15	Corn syrup, sucrose, fructose, maltodextrin, sugar	40–58	Corn oil, safflower oil, canola oil, MCT
Diabetic	Sodium and calcium caseinates, beef, milk protein, soy protein isolate	16–24	Maltodextrin, hydrolyzed cornstarch, fructose, sucrose, guar gum, vegetables, fruits, soy fiber	34–40	Sunflower oil, soybean oil, canola oil, MCT, safflower oil
Immune modulated	Sodium and calcium caseinates, L-arginine, L-glutamine, BCAA	22–32	Hydrolyzed cornstarch, maltodextrin, soy fiber	38–53	Canola oil, structured lipids; sunflower oil and menhaden fish oil, MCT
Hepatic	L-amino acids, whey	11–15	Sucrose, maltodextrin, modified cornstarch	57–77	Soybean oil, MCT, canola oil, corn oil, lecithin

MCT, medium-chain triacylglycerol; FOS, fructooligosaccharide; BCAA, branched-chain amino acid.

systemically (13). It has been estimated that up to 400 cal/d can be absorbed from the colon in the form of SCFAs when patients are given a diet high in soluble fibers. It is believed that SCFAs are required to maintain optimal colonocyte function and colonic luminal pH (84). In patients requiring long-term tube feeding, a fiber-containing formula may help to regulate GI motility.

Fructooligosaccharides

Fructooligosaccharides (FOS) are indigestible sugars that occur naturally in food (e.g., onions, blueberries). These sugars consist of a sucrose molecule linked to one, two, or three additional fructose units. These oligosaccharides appear to remain intact in the stomach and small intestine and pass into the colon unaltered, where they are fermented

Calories from Fat (%)	Caloric Density (Calories/mL)	NPC:g N	mL for 100% RDI	Percentage of Free Water	Water (mOsmol/kg)	Product Names (Select Number)
21–39	1.0–2.0	78–154:1	946–2,000	73–85	480–870	Ensure, Ensure Plus, Sustacal, Sustacal with Fiber, Resource Plus, NuBasics, Sustacal Plus, Boost
29–39	1.0–1.5	116–167:1	830–1,890	77–85	270–500	Isocal, IsoSource HN, Nutren 1.0, Nutren 1.5, Osmolite, Osmolite HN, Comply
29–37	1.0–1.2	110–149:1	933–1,500	78–85	300–500	Fibersource, Jevity, Jevity Plus, ProBalance, Ultracal, Nutren 1.0 with Fiber
23–40	1.0–1.5	75–91:1	1,000–2,000	78–85	300–490	IsoSource VHN, Replete with Fiber, Promote, Protain XL, TraumaCal
3–39	1.0–1.5	67–175:1	1,150–2,000	76–86	270–650	Vivonex Plus, Crucial, Peptamen, Perative, Reablin, AlitraQ, Sandosource Peptide, Subdue, Optimental
40–55	1.5	102–125:1	933–1,420	76–79	330–650	Nutrivent, Pulmocare, Respalor, Novasource Pulmonary, Oxepa
35–45	2.0	140–340:1	947–1,000	70–71	570–700	Nepro, Magnacal Renal, Novasource Renal, RenalCal
40–49	1.0–1.06	79–125:1	1,000–1,890 or N/A	85	355–450	Glucerna, Glytrol, Choice Dm, DiabetiSource, Resource Diabetic
20–40	1.0–1.5	52–71:1	1,250–2,000	78–86	375–550	Impact, Impact 1.5 ImmunAid, Crucial, Intensical, Optimental
12–28	1.2–1.5	148–209:1	N/A–1,000	76–82	560–690	NutriHep, Hepatic Aid II

by colonic microorganisms (e.g., bifidobacteria) to lactate and SCFAs (84). These fermentation products produce a colonic mucosal microenvironment favoring proliferation of bifidobacteria species. The presence of FOS and the consequent production of the fermented byproducts, acetate, and lactate, produce an environment undesirable for several of pathogenic bacteria such as *Clostridium difficile* by lowering the colonic pH. Several enteral formulations now contain

FOS but proposed benefits remain to be elucidated in large clinical studies (13).

Lipid

The major sources of fat in standard lactose-free formulas are corn, soy, safflower, and canola oils. Variable amounts of lecithin, and medium-chain triacylglycerol (MCT) are also available in some formulas. In addition to their significance as a concentrated caloric source (9 cal/g) fat is required as the EFAs linoleic and linolenic acid and serves as a carrier for the fat-soluble vitamins. Fat also enhances the flavor and palatability of enteral formulas without increasing the osmality significantly. Dietary long-chain triacylglycerol (LCT) is the main source of EFAs, linoleic and linolenic acid. The estimated daily requirement for EFAs is only 3% to 4% of total calories. Recently LCTs, especially in the parenteral form, have come under increased scrutiny secondary to their poor utilization in hypermetabolism, and immunosuppressive influence when given in large quantities (85). Most enteral formulas now contain a mixture of MCT and LCT.

Medium-chain triglycerides are 6 to 12 carbons long and are prepared from tropical oils. MCT has the benefit of being more rapidly hydrolyzed and has greater water solubility than LCT. These smaller carbon chains require little or no pancreatic lipase or bile salts for absorption, and can be transported directly into the portal vein. This yields two separate mechanisms of absorption for MCT through the portal vein and through the lymphatic system (86). In addition to the benefit in absorption, MCTs are also able to cross from the outer mitochondrial membrane to inner membrane for β-oxidation without an acyl-carnitine carrier, thereby enhancing utilization in hypermetabolic patients (87). They are generally well tolerated by the enteral route but can occasionally result in some GI symptoms such as nausea, vomiting, and diarrhea. As MCTs are ketogenic, they should not be used in patients who are prone to high ketone levels.

Recent animal and clinical research has led to the incorporation of omega (Ω)-3 fatty acids into several enteral formulas. Ω-3 Fatty acids found in fish [eicosapentanoid acid (EPA) and docohexanoic acid (DHA)] have multiple beneficial effects in the perioperative period, including modulation of leukocyte function and regulation of cytokine release through nuclear signaling and gene expression (88). In addition Ω-3 fatty acids are metabolized to a new group of prostaglandin derivatives called *resolvins* and *neuroprotectins*, which play a role in accelerating the resolution of the proinflammatory state (89). In contrast to Ω-3 fatty acids, Ω-6 fatty acids are associated with higher inflammatory response and are precursors to leukotrienes, thromboxane, and prostaglandins that are vasoconstrictive, and induce platelet aggregation (90,91). In a recent study involving 661 surgical and ICU patients, the administration of Ω-3 fatty acids intravenously demonstrated a statistically significant decrease in mortality, antibiotic use, and length of hospital stay (92). Numerous reports using various *in vivo* and *in vitro* models suggest that the slight structural difference between Ω-3 and Ω-6 fatty acids supports the anti-inflammatory, antithrombotic, antiarrhythmic, hypolipidemic, and antiatherosclerotic effects of the Ω-3 compounds (19,93).

Structured lipids are a synthetic mixture of LCTs and MCTs incorporated onto the same glycerol backbone. Structured lipids offer several theoretic advantages over LCT or MCT. Structured lipids are reported to decrease infection

and improve survival by producing fewer proinflammatory and immunosuppressive eicosanoids as compared with conventional triacylglycerols. Enteral formulas, particularly the immune-modulated category, are beginning to include structured lipids as a source of fat.

Protein

The protein component of enteral formulas can be in the form of intact protein (e.g., lactalbumin, casein, caseinates), partially hydrolyzed protein (e.g., oligopeptides, dipeptides, or tripeptides) or crystalline L-amino acids. Intact protein and protein hydrolysates (>4 amino acid residues) require further digestion by pancreatic and/or brush border proteases into peptides (dipeptides or tripeptides) and free amino acids, which are then rapidly and efficiently absorbed by the enterocyte primarily in the proximal small bowel (16). Most protein digestion products are absorbed through the peptide transporter 1 (PEPT1) as dipeptides or tripeptides (15). Once in the enterocyte, they are subsequently digested to free amino acids. The single amino acid carriers, of which several have been characterized, play a less significant role in protein absorption. Intact proteins do not add appreciably to the osmolality of the formula, unlike hydrolyzed or crystalline amino acids. The higher the percentage of hydrolyzed protein or free amino acids, the greater the solution osmolality will be. An understanding of the various protein sources is crucial when deciding on the optimal protein substrate for patients with defects in either protein digestion (e.g., pancreatic insufficiency) or absorption (e.g., short bowel syndrome).

Multiple surgical conditions alter protein metabolism and absorption (94–96). Provision of free amino acid solutions for patients with decreased absorptive surface area, ischemic injury to the mucosa, or malabsorption has been reported to be beneficial. At present in patients with intact mucosal brush border surface and adequate pancreatic exocrine function, no clear consistent clinical data support the use of solutions in which protein is in the form of free amino acids or hydrolysates. This may be due to the fact that the small bowel has a very adaptive and redundant absorptive surface. The normal human small intestine is 300 to 500 cm and most patients will survive without parenteral supplementation if approximately 100 cm remains functional (97). Although patients with maldigestion and/or malabsorption may benefit from a peptide or crystalline amino acid–based enteral formula, the higher cost of these formulas and lack of clinical supportive data discourage the routine use in patients with normal GI physiology.

Glutamine

Glutamine is the most abundant amino acid in the body and makes up greater than 50% of the free amino acid pool (98). It contains 5 carbons and 2 nitrogen moities, making it the major interorgan donor of nitrogen and carbon. In contrast to the demand for glutamine during normal homeostasis, the demand for glutamine during major catabolic insults is greater than supply, consequently making glutamine a conditionally essential amino acid (EAA) (99). Glutamine can be synthesized in most tissues of the body, but skeletal muscle, by virtue of which it mass produces the most endogenous glutamine. Glutamine is the primary fuel for many rapidly dividing tissues such as the small bowel and proliferating lymphocytes (100). Glutamine has numerous metabolic roles including maintenance of acid–base status, as a precursor of urinary ammonia, as the primary fuel source for enterocytes, as fuel source for lymphocytes and macrophages, and as a precursor for nucleotides, arginine, glutathione, and glucosamine (101). Glutamine is also a major contributor to gluconeogenesis and is the primary substrate for renal gluconeogenesis (101). Recent reports also show glutamine being important in decreasing peripheral insulin resistance in stressed models (101). During catabolic illness, glutamine uptake by the small intestine and immunologically active cells may exceed glutamine synthesis and release from skeletal muscle (98,102).

There is a rapidly growing volume of human data regarding the use of enteral glutamine supplementation (103). The majority, estimated at 70% to 80%, of enterally supplied glutamine is metabolized by the enterocyte with minimal glutamine reaching the systemic circulation. Clearly, the target for enterally supplied glutamine is the splanchnic bed and GALT. In animal models, supplemental glutamine has been shown to enhance intestinal adaptation after massive small bowel resection (97), to attenuate intestinal and pancreatic atrophy (103), and to prevent hepatic steatosis associated with parenteral and elemental enteral feeding (101). Glutamine appears to help maintain GI tract mucosal thickness, maintain deoxyribonucleic acid (DNA) and protein content, reduce bacteremia and mortality after chemotherapy, and reduce bacteremia and mortality following sepsis or endotoxemia (101).

In humans undergoing surgical stress, glutamine-supplemented parenteral nutrition appears to help maintain nitrogen balance and the intracellular glutamine pool in skeletal muscle (104). A recent trauma study reported a greater than 50% decrease in pneumonia compared to an isonitrogenous, isocaloric control population (105). In critically ill patients, glutamine supplementation may attenuate villous atrophy and the increased intestinal mucosal permeability associated with parenteral nutrition. Glutamine supplementation in a randomized blinded trial of 84 critically ill patients showed significant improvement in mortality (106). Parenteral nutrition supplemented with glutamine has also resulted in fewer infections, improved nitrogen balance, and significantly shorter mean hospital length of stay in bone marrow transplantation patients. Glutamine supplementation may also play a role in protecting the GI tract against chemotherapy-induced toxicity (107). Oral glutamine supplementation reduced the severity and decreased the duration of stomatitis that occurs during chemotherapy in bone marrow transplantation (108). Glutamine supplementation at 30 g/dL in esophageal cancer patients undergoing radiation had preserved lymphocyte response and decreased gut permeability (109).

One possible mechanism recently discovered that may explain the numerous benefits of glutamine supplementation is its enhancement of heat shock protein (HSP) expression (HSP-70, HSP-32, HSP-27) (110). HSPs are a family of highly conserved cytosolic chaperone proteins involved in cellular protection during times of stress. In animal models of sepsis, administration of glutamine as a single-dose 1 hour following the initiation of sepsis significantly enhanced lung and tissue expression of HSP-70 and HSP-25, decreasing mortality and preventing the development of adult respiratory distress syndrome (ARDS) (111). Treatment with quercetin (a chemical inhibitor of HSP-70) blocked all beneficial effects of glutamine administration. A recent clinical trial looked at glutamine administration through TPN compared to isonitrogenous control and examined HSP-70 expression after 7 days (112). The glutamine group demonstrated a 3.7-fold increase in serum HSP-70 expression that correlated with a decrease in ICU length stay (112).

Although a large volume of animal and human data supports the concept that glutamine is beneficial in a variety of experimental models, the benefit of routine enteral glutamine supplementation in critically ill human patients remains controversial. Well-designed clinical trials with clearly defined endpoints and adequate statistical power are needed to assess whether the beneficial effects demonstrated in GI physiology, immune function, and postoperative metabolism translate into a reduction in hospital stay and mortality rate. It is clear that glutamine is a major contributor to homeostasis in the surgical population. Adequate clinical studies are available to support the concept that glutamine is required for optimal gut growth, repair, and function, as well as decreasing gut origin sepsis, and enhancing nitrogen balance.

Arginine

Arginine, like glutamine, is classified as an NEAA in unstressed conditions because the body synthesizes adequate arginine for normal maintenance of tissue metabolism, growth, and repair (103). During major catabolic insults such as trauma or surgery, an increase in urinary nitrogen, excreted largely as urea, represents the end products of increased lean body tissue catabolism and reprioritized protein synthesis. As the activity of the urea cycle increases, so does the metabolic demand for arginine and like glutamine, arginine becomes conditionally essential.

Studies indicate that supplemental dietary arginine is beneficial for accelerated wound healing, enhanced immune response, and positive nitrogen balance (113). The exact mechanisms for these benefits are yet to be entirely understood but may in part be the result of arginine's role as a potent anabolic hormone secretogogue. Growth hormone, glucagon, prolactin, and insulin release are all increased with supplemental arginine. Arginine is also the substrate for nitric oxide synthase producing nitric oxide and citrulline. Nitric oxide is a ubiquitous molecule which plays important roles in the maintenance of vascular tone, coagulation cascade, immunity, and the GI tract function (114). Nitric oxide has been implicated as a participant in numerous disease states as diverse as sepsis, hypertension, and cirrhosis. In addition to nitric oxide synthesis, arginine is also the substrate for the enzyme arginase with end products urea and ornithine. Ornithine then serves as a precursor for polyamine synthesis that regulates lymphocyte mitogenesis following a stimulus. Polyamines play a pivotal role in cell division, and DNA synthesis (115).

In animal models, arginine supplementation has been associated with improved wound healing, with increased wound tensile strength, and collagen deposition. Using a wound healing model, Barbul et al. showed enhanced collagen deposition in human volunteers with supplemental arginine (113). Arginine-supplemented rats have been shown to have improved thymic function as assessed by thymic weight, the total number of thymic lymphocytes, and the mitogenic reactivity of thymic lymphocytes to phytohemagglutinin and concanavalin A (114). Animal studies using supplementation arginine have shown improved survival in burns, intraperitoneal bacterial challenge, cecal ligation, and puncture, and tumor implantation models (114). Although supplemental arginine has been shown to improve survival in various animal models and to improve a number of *in vitro* measures of immune function in both animal and human studies, most of these studies have used arginine in combination with other nutrients such as EPA, glutamine, and nucleic acids. The benefit of arginine supplementation alone needs further large-scale human studies to confirm its use as a single agent. Certainly, the early data suggests that arginine supports immune function, enhances nitrogen balance, and appears to have multiple beneficial effects in the surgical population (91).

As mentioned earlier, multiple human clinical trials have been conducted comparing the use of various enteral formulations that contain arginine as well as other supplemental nutrients (e.g., glutamine, Ω-3 fatty acids, nucleotides) to a standard nonsupplemented formula. Results of these trials have found the supplemented formula groups to have several improved outcomes such as decreased number and severity of septic complications, decreased antibiotic use, and decreased hospital and ICU stay (116,117).

Vitamins and Minerals

Virtually all nutritionally complete commercially available formulas now contain currently recommended quantities of vitamins and minerals when a sufficient volume of formula to meet energy and macronutrient needs is provided. Select disease-specific formulas are nutritionally incomplete in relation to vitamin and mineral content (e.g., hepatic formulas). Liquid vitamin and mineral supplements may be indicated for patients receiving nutritionally incomplete or diluted formulas for prolonged periods of time. In patients with fat malabsorption, supplementation of the fat-soluble vitamins A, D, E, and K may be indicated. For patients on Coumadin it is important to compensate dosing when patients receive enteral feeding as most commercial formulas contain vitamin K.

Physical Properties

Osmolality

Osmolality is a function of size and quantity of ionic and molecular particles (protein, carbohydrate, electrolytes, and minerals) within a given volume. The unit of measure for osmolality is mOsm/kg of water versus the unit of measure for osmolarity, which is mOsm/L. Osmolality is considered the preferred term to use in reference to enteral formulas.

In the clinical setting osmolality is important because of its role in maintaining the balance between intracellular and extracellular fluids. Several factors affect the osmolality of enteral formulas. The smaller the chain length of carbohydrates and proteins, the greater the osmolality will be. Hence, formulas containing increased amounts of simple sugars or free amino acids and/or dipeptides and tripeptides will have a greater osmolality as opposed to those containing starch and longer-chain intact proteins. Lipids contribute minimally to the osmolality of an enteral formula, with the exception of MCT owing to their water solubility. Because of dissociation properties and small size, minerals and electrolytes also increase the osmolality.

GI tolerance (e.g., gastric retention, abdominal distention, diarrhea, nausea, and vomiting) is influenced by the osmolality of enteral formulas. Generally, the greater the osmolality the greater the likelihood of GI intolerance. Administering hypertonic formulas at a slow continuous rate initially (10–20 cc/h), with a gradual titration to the final volume while monitoring for GI complications, can reduce the incidence of GI intolerance. What may be more important than the osmolality of the enteral formula is the osmotic contribution from liquid medications, either infused with the enteral formula, or "bolused" through the feeding tube. The average osmolality range of commercially prepared liquid medications is reported to be between 450 and 10,950 mOsm/kg. The osmolality of enteral formulas ranges from 270 to 700 mOsm/kg.

Calorie-Nutrient Density

The calorie density of enteral formulas generally ranges from 1.0 to 2.0 cal/mL. This is important as it not only determines how many calories, but also other macro- and micronutrients the patient receives. Obviously as a formula becomes more nutrient dense, it contains less free water.

Caloric density often affects the patient's tolerance for tube feeding. Delayed gastric emptying frequently occurs in patients who are given concentrated formulas, especially the high fat formulas. Lipids significantly slow gastric emptying. Because the patient's nutrient needs are met by a decreased volume of this class of formula, free water supplementation should be considered to ensure that fluid requirements are met, and to prevent dehydration, electrolyte imbalance, and constipation. Generally these products are best tolerated as voluntary oral supplements and not as tube feeding.

Nonprotein Calorie to Gram of Nitrogen Ratio

In general, the average healthy adult requires a nonprotein calorie to gram of nitrogen (NPC:g N) ratio of 150:1 to 250:1.

As described earlier, during a hypermetabolic stress, the body catabolizes lean body mass as a nitrogen and energy source. Commercial formulas have NPC:g N ratios of 80:1 to 200:1. For the postoperative catabolic conditions, 100:1 to 150:1 are recommended (8). This protein content of enteral formulas becomes extremely important in patients who require wound healing due to trauma, burns, metabolic stress, infection, and increased wound healing requirements.

Renal Solute Load

Renal solute load refers to the constituents in the formula that must be excreted by the kidneys. Major contributors to renal solute load in enteral formulas are protein, sodium, potassium, and chloride. There is an obligatory water loss for each unit of solute. Therefore, as a formula becomes more concentrated or its renal solute load increases, then the patient will require more free water. Pediatric and geriatric patients should be monitored closely for hydration status as well as those with diarrhea, emesis, fistulas, or fevers.

Disease-Specific Formulations

Most routine surgical patients that require enteral nutrition can be supported safely with a standard enteral formula. Various clinical conditions such as severe hypercatabolism, renal or hepatic failure, pulmonary insufficiency, or malnutrition alters nutrient metabolism, and may thereby warrant an enteral formulation tailored to the specific disease process. Determining the location of enteral nutrient delivery, timing, and mode of delivery, the patient's overall current clinical condition, as well as past medical history, is necessary for appropriate cost-effective formula selection.

Renal Formulas

The clinical status of patients with renal failure is variable; therefore, prescribed nutrient intake differs greatly among patients and should depend on individual nutritional status, catabolic rate, residual glomerular filtration rate, and intensity of dialysis or hemofiltration therapy. Currently formulas for renal insufficiency do not clearly distinguish the difference between patients with acute and chronic renal failure.

Renal enteral formulas were first developed as oral supplements; therefore, they tend to be hyperosmolar secondary to their large simple sugar content for flavor enhancement. This hypertonicity often causes GI intolerance. The simple sugar content can also be problematic, causing impaired glycemic control in those patients who are hypermetabolic, insulin resistant, or diabetic. The goal of feeding patients with renal failure is to provide optimal nutrients without further accumulation of nitrogenous compounds, volume, and electrolytes, mainly potassium and phosphate (118). Hence, renal formulas are all calorically rich, usually providing 2 cal/mL and containing low-to-moderate amounts of protein, electrolytes, and various minerals. EAA formulas were developed to decrease the need for dialysis. Recent guidelines recommend the use of EAAs and NEAAs for enhanced protein synthesis and correction of low plasma NEAA values (119). The development of fluid and electrolyte disorders or accumulation of metabolic waste products should not solely be minimized by nutrient restriction, but also by adjusting the intensity of dialysis treatment as tolerated (120). Many patients with stable levels of creatinine, blood urea nitrogen (BUN), and electrolytes with or without dialysis can be fed with standard complete enteral formulas.

Pulmonary Formulas

Respiratory insufficiency and ventilator dependence can have a major impact on the feeding of critically ill and surgical patients. Often these patients do not receive their required nutrient needs due to the increased work of breathing, carbon dioxide retention, and fluid and electrolyte restrictions (121). This reduced nutrient intake results in further catabolism of muscle (e.g., intercostals, diaphragm) and malnutrition that in turn leads to fatigue and further difficulty with liberation from the ventilator.

β-Oxidation of lipids produces less carbon dioxide per oxygen utilized than oxidation of either glucose or protein. The respiratory quotient (RQ) (CO_2 produced per O_2 utilized) is 1.0 for carbohydrate and 0.7 for fat. This lower RQ (CO_2 production) has been the basis for the development of relatively high fat (~45%–55% of calories) and high caloric density (1.5 cal/mL) enteral formulas. Originally the lipid component of these products consisted of 100% LCTs, which, when given in excess, can suppress the immune system as well as induce malabsorption. Pulmonary formulas now contain a variety of lipids including medium chain triacylglycerol, Ω-6 and Ω-3 fatty acids, and more recently, γ-linolenic acid (GLA).

Research has shown that animals fed with Ω-3 fatty acids produce reduced amounts of proinflammatory eicosanoids relative to those fed with Ω-6 fatty acids (121). In another study, animals fed diets enriched by GLA, as borage oil, were found to have higher levels of GLA and dihomogamma-linolenic acid (DGLA) with reduced levels of prostaglandin E2 (PGE2) and leukotrienes, suggesting that GLA modulates inflammatory status in a manner similar to that of Ω-3 fatty acids (122). In another animal study, the authors concluded that dietary fish (primarily eicosapentaenoic acid) and borage oil, as compared with corn oil may ameliorate endotoxin-induced acute lung injury (ALI) by suppressing the levels of proinflammatory eicosanoids in bronchoalveolar lavage fluid and reduce pulmonary neutrophil accumulation (123).

In human studies, Gadek et al. was able to show in 146 patients with ARDS, a decrease in ICU length of stay, and decreased ventilator days in patients who received formulas high in Ω-3 fatty acids and borage oil (124). However, Nelson et al. was unable to reproduce these results and found no significant changes in ARDS patients receiving a diet high in Ω-3 fatty acids in 98 patients. This may be attributed to the design of the study and is under debate (125).

One of the best-designed studies was published by Pacht et al. using Ω-3 fatty acids in 67 patients with ALI or ARDS (126). In this study, patients underwent bronchoalveolar lavage and the bronchial fluid was analyzed for inflammatory markers such as proinflammatory cytokines and white blood cell concentration. Those patients who received the diet enriched with Ω-3 fatty acids from fish oil, showed significantly decreased LTB$_4$, IL-8, and neutrophils (all proinflammatory indicators) as compared with those patients who did not receive the fish oil enriched diet (126). Mayer et al. published in a study of 63 patients who were septic, a diet high in Ω-3 fatty acids resulted in suppressed inflammatory cytokine profiles as compared with patients who received the control diet (127).

Heller et al. conducted one of the most recent published studies using an intravenous emulsion containing EPA and DHA. A total of 661 patients with a variety of critical care conditions were enrolled in a prospective, open-labeled trial, where investigators delivered different doses of IV fish oil (available in Europe) and measured the length of hospital stay and antibiotic days in association with dose amount. Researchers found that doses of 0.1 to 0.23 g/kg of fish oil delivered intravenously had a positive correlation with decreased hospital and ICU days, as well as less antibiotic days and decreased rates of multiple organ failure. Although this research is done with an IV lipid emulsion, the authors concluded the positive correlation with this dosing of fish oil can be a starting point for further research to come using both IV fish oil and enterally delivered fish oil (92).

Aside from the previously mentioned studies using specific lipid substrates in ARDS patients, early research evaluating the use of specific pulmonary enteral formulas of high total fat and low carbohydrate have not demonstrated a clear benefit. It appears that overfeeding, especially with carbohydrates, has a far greater influence on PCO_2 than attempting to manipulate the RQ between 0.7 and 1.0. Close attention should be given to the avoidance of overfeeding by providing energy intakes from 1.2 to 1.5 times the predicted resting energy expenditure or by measuring energy expenditure through indirect calorimetry.

There are potential detrimental effects in using a high-fat, low-carbohydrate enteral formula. It is well known that high fat diets can impair gastric emptying (128). Delayed gastric emptying can result in increased gastric residual volumes with subsequent increased risk of aspiration. During intense use of respiratory muscles following extubation and during weaning depleted muscle glycogen stores may limit muscle endurance and strength. Nutrition support for the pulmonary-compromised patient requires a balanced energy mix so that prompt replenishment of respiratory muscle glycogen can occur. Pulmonary formulas, with their low carbohydrate levels, reveal a potential disadvantage to fully support muscle glycogen during attempted ventilator weaning.

Literature and clinical practice clearly demonstrate that most patients who have limited pulmonary reserves can have their caloric requirement met with a standard enteral product (~30% calories as fat) (129).

Diabetic Formulas

Nutrition is an integral component in the management of diabetes mellitus (DM). Whether during critical illness or long-term support, it can be extremely challenging. Over the last several years, a number of enteral formulas have been developed for the purpose of obtaining better glycemic control for patients with DM. These formulations contain a relatively high-fat low-carbohydrate nutrient ratio, with actual ingredients varying among the manufacturers (Table 5.11). The carbohydrate sources include fructose and fiber to assist in glycemic management. Some fat sources have been modified to contain a higher ratio of monounsaturated fatty acids than saturated fatty acids to better meet the 1994 guidelines of the American Diabetes Association.

Few large outcome studies have been conducted to determine the benefit of providing these formulations in gaining optimal glycemic control (130,131). Overall, the recommendation is to begin by administering a standard, fiber-containing enteral formula with moderate carbohydrate and fat content. Blood glucose levels will vary based on the patient's preexisting diabetic history, metabolic stress level, and nutrient delivery method. Blood glucose levels should be monitored closely in an attempt to keep blood sugars less than 150 mg/dL with appropriate insulin management. Frequent monitoring should be done, especially with any interruptions or changes in delivery. If metabolically stable diabetic patients do not meet desired glycemic control with a standard formula, then a diabetic enteral formula may be beneficial.

Hepatic Disease Formulas

The specialized formulas for patients with cirrhosis and hepatic failure are designed to reestablish a normal serum amino acid profile. The liver is primarily responsible for metabolism of the aromatic amino acids (AAAs). Consequently, in hepatic failure, amino acid metabolism is altered, resulting in increased plasma AAAs (132). The branched-chain amino acids (BCAAs) are primarily utilized by muscle. Because most hepatic failure patients are relatively catabolic and show increased utilization of BCAA, a significant change in the BCAA to AAA ratio is noted (132). This change results in altered blood–brain barrier transport with production of false neurotransmitters. This, along with other metabolic abnormalities noted such as hyperammonaemia, results in hepatic encephalopathy (132). Specialized formulas for hepatic encephalopathy have been designed to reduce the availability of AAAs and attempt to reestablish more normal serum AA pattern (133,134). Therefore, these formulas contain low quantities of AAAs and methionine and high quantities of BCAAs.

In metabolically stressed, malnourished cirrhotic patents with encephalopathy, the effectiveness of the BCAA-enriched formulas may lie in correcting malnutrition by increasing nitrogen intake without aggravating the encephalopathy. However, the life-threatening derangements in liver failure, such as portal hypertension and esophageal varices, are unaffected by nutritional repletion. Therefore, these formulas should be provided only in malnourished patients with liver failure and concomitant encephalopathy who have failed to respond to conventional medical and nutritional therapy. Also noteworthy is the fact that due to the incidence of associated fluid and electrolyte abnormalities, these enteral formulas are calorically concentrated and contain minimal amounts of electrolytes, with some formulations failing to provide 100% of the recommended daily intake by the United States. Therefore, patients receiving these incomplete enteral formulations should be monitored closely to ensure that additional nutrient deficiencies do not occur.

Immune-Modulated Formulas

Over the last several decades, numerous animal models have shown that certain individual nutrients are able to enhance immune function. Several nutrients have been shown to be beneficial but most of the current literature involves the nutrients arginine, glutamine, Ω-3 fatty acids, and nucleotides (135). As a result of these promising animal and early clinical studies, several enteral formula manufacturers have developed "immune-modulated" enteral formulas to potentially improve clinical outcomes in high-risk surgical and/or critically ill patients. These products all vary in the quantity and quality of the "neutraceuticals" they contain. More than 34 human studies have been conducted to determine if surgical, medical, critically ill or other immune-compromised individuals experience positive outcomes as a result of receiving these formulations (116,117). Results of these studies vary; they have been extensively scrutinized for several variables including lack of feeding comparisons, lack of homogeneous study population comparisons, and the manner in which the data were analyzed. Despite the minor study design variations, most of these studies show clear benefit of reduced rates of infection, decreased antibiotic use, lowered incidence of intra-abdominal abscesses, and reduced ICU and hospital length of stay (135). The vast majority of the 34 currently published peer-reviewed studies report benefit in the surgical population with only a few reporting no significant change (60,136). In addition to the greater than 30 individual studies, 5 meta-analyses have now been completed all showing similar outcome benefit in the surgical population (116,117,137–139).

In summary, the literature suggests that these immune-modulated formulas may be beneficial in certain patient populations. These populations include those who will undergo or have undergone complicated GI surgery, especially if malnourished, sustained severe trauma, or had complicated ICU stays (135). The immune-modulated formulas were associated with decreased incidence of infections and hospital length of stay. These formulas have not shown to consistently reduce mortality in severely injured and immune-compromised patients. Continued research is necessary to determine the optimal timing of nutrient delivery and duration of therapy for which these formulas may be appropriate.

Probiotics and Prebiotics

The human GI tract harbors approximately 300 to 500 protective and pathogenic bacterial species that maintain a constant homeostasis in healthy individuals. Bacteria colonize the alimentary tract soon after birth and the composition of the intestinal microflora remains relatively constant thereafter. The foregut and small intestine harbors relatively small numbers of bacteria secondary to gastric acid and constant peristalsis. Concentrations of bacteria in the colon can reach 10^{12} CFU/mL, comprised mainly of anaerobes such as *Bacteroides, Bifidobacterium, Clostridium,* and *Lactobacillus,* with anaerobic bacteria outnumbering aerobic bacteria by a factor of 100:1 to 1000:1. The protective enteric bacterial floras provide four key functions: immunomodulation, colonization resistance, mucosal barrier support, and nutritional contributions (140). Nutritional contributions include salvage of unabsorbed dietary sugars by bacterial disaccharidases that are converted to SCFAs and used as an energy source by the colonic mucosa. Enteric bacteria also produce vitamins and nutrients such as folate and vitamin K. Colonization resistance is thought to be by competitive inhibition of exogenous and pathogenic bacterial species and enhancement of the mucosal barrier. Immunomodualtion is through the interactions with GALT, induction of immune tolerance, and secretion of immunoglobulin A. With antibiotic use and during periods of stress such as major surgery or sepsis, this luminal bacterial homeostasis becomes disrupted and favors growth of pathogenic bacteria.

Probiotics, defined as live organisms when ingested in adequate amounts, exert a health benefit on the host. The most widely available probiotics are *Lactobacillus* and *Bifidobacterium* species. Human trials with probiotic use after major surgery and critical illness have yielded conflicting results depending on the model used and species of bacteria being studied. Several randomized prospective trials in several surgical models have reported benefits in lowering infectious complications in surgical patients (141,142). It is difficult to make direct comparisons between these various clinical trials given the variations of probiotics used, dosing, and timing of therapy. The benefits of probiotics with regard to antibiotic-associated diarrhea such as *C. difficile* infection are better established. There are two meta-analyses of randomized, double blind, controlled trials that determined the odds ratio for development of antibiotic-associated diarrhea with protiotic supplementation is between 0.34 to 0.39 (143,144).

Prebiotics are defined as nondigestible foods that can be fermented by colonic bacteria to beneficially affect the host by selectively stimulating the growth and activity of protective bacterial species in the colon. The prototypic prebiotic are oligosaccharides found in human breast milk which facilitate the preferential growth of *Bifidobacteria* and *Lactobacilli* in the colon in exclusively breast-fed babies (145). Fruits and vegetables including wheat, garlic, onion, and bananas are rich in prebiotics consisting of inulin-type fructans, and fructooligosaccharides. These molecules are fermented in the colon by endogenous bacteria to lactic and short-chain carboxylic acids to act as energy and metabolic substrates. Currently, there is a lack of clinical studies evaluating prebiotics in the setting for surgical and critically ill patients.

Administration Methods

Administration methods for enteral tube feeding are limited to the type and site of enteral feeding access. The formula delivery method selected for the patient also depends on the patient's hemodynamic stability, gastric emptying rate, GI tolerance to tube feeding, type of formula selected, nutrient needs, patient mobility, and ease of administration. The main methods of tube feeding are by continuous, intermittent, or bolus delivery. Each institution should have an established protocol for the initiation and advancement of enteral feedings.

Bolus Feeding

Bolus feedings involve the delivery of larger amounts of formula over short periods of time, usually 5 minutes or less. The bolus method should only be used with gastric delivery. The stomach can act as a reservoir to handle relatively large volumes of formula (e.g., 400 mL) over a short time. Bolus feedings are usually administered through a gastrostomy tube, owing to the large lumen, but they can also be given through a small-bore nasogastric tube. Usually a syringe or bulb is used to push 200 to 500 mL of formula into the feeding tube several times a day. A patient should demonstrate adequate gastric emptying and the ability to protect their airway (i.e., an intact gag reflex) before initiating bolus feedings, especially in the critical care setting.

Bolus feedings are considered the most physiologic method of administration. They are also the easiest to administer because a pump is not required. Bolus feedings also allow for increased patient mobility because they are delivered intermittently and do not require continuous attachment to a pump. For these reasons, the bolus method of nutrient delivery is most desirable for stable patients who are going home or to an extended care facility.

Intermittent Feedings

This method of feeding involves the formula to be infused over a 20- to 30-minute period. A feeding container and gravity drip is usually used for this method. Intermittent feedings are less likely than bolus feeding to cause GI side effects since the formula is administered over a longer interval. Depending on the volume delivered, this method may be used for gastric as well as small bowel formula delivery.

Continuous Feedings

Continuous formula delivery is usually the best tolerated enteral delivery method, especially in the ICU or immediate perioperative period. Continuous feedings are delivered slowly over 12 to 24 hours, typically with an infusion pump. In order to avoid accidental bolus delivery, continuous pump infusion is preferred over gravity as a constant infusion rate can be programmed in a pump. Postpyloric feedings require continuous infusion. The small bowel acts as a poor reservoir for large volumes of fluid within a short time, and GI complications involving pain and diarrhea usually arise if feedings are delivered into the small bowel in bolus manner.

Initiation and progression of continuous feedings should be individualized and based on the patient's clinical condition and feeding tolerance. Typically, feedings may be initiated at 10 to 50 mL/h, with the lower range for the critically ill and early postoperative patient. Progression of tube feedings may range from 10 to 25 mL/h every 4 to 24 hours, depending on the patient's tolerance, until the desired goal rate is achieved. As a patient is beginning to transition to oral intake, the tube feedings may be cycled to allow for appetite stimulation, or to allow for bowel rest and time away from the pump. Once the patient is stable, the feedings may be administered at night and held during the day to allow for increased patient mobility and an opportunity to eat.

Enteral Feeding Complications

Although enteral nutrition is clearly the preferred route of nutrient provision in those individuals unable to consume adequate nutrients orally, it does not exist without complications. Compared with parenteral nutrition, enteral nutrition complications are fewer and usually less serious. Appropriate precautions and knowledgeable staff can prevent most complications. Appropriate patient assessment for needs and risks, proper feeding route, and formula selection, in addition to appropriate monitoring of the enteral nutrition feeding regimen can increase the success of enteral feeding. The most common complications can be categorized as mechanical, metabolic, or GI. Table 5.12 lists some of the common complications; their possible causes, and suggested corrective measures.

Summary—Enteral Nutrition

Enteral feeding is clearly the preferred method of providing nutrition in those patients with inadequate volitional intake. Enteral feeding has many advantages over parenteral nutrition, including preservation of the structure and function of the GI barrier and gut associated lymphoid tissue, more efficient nutrient utilization, better glycemic control, fewer infectious and metabolic complications, easier administration, and significantly lower cost (146). In order for enteral nutrition to be successful, an understanding of nutrient metabolism in various disease states is essential. In addition, assessment for the optimal access site, appropriate formula selection, nutrient requirements, monitoring, and trouble-shooting complications is required.

PARENTERAL NUTRITION

Parenteral nutrition can be considered one of the 20th century's major advances in management of medical and surgical patients. Its discovery and first implementation in the 1960s launched modern nutrition into the medical

TABLE 5.12

Common Nutrition-Related Complications Associated with Enteral Feeding (55,56)

Complication	Suggested Possible Causes	Corrective Measures
Mechanical		
Obstructed feeding tube	Formula viscosity excessive for feeding tube	Use less viscous formula or larger-bore tube
	Obstruction from crushed medications administered through tube	Flush tube before and after feeding
	Coagulation of formula protein in tube when in contact with acidic medium (medication flushing solution)	Give medications as elixir or ensure medications are crushed thoroughly
		Flush tube before and after delivering each medication
		Flush feeding tube with warm water only; Avoid flushing with sodas, coffee, juices, or any other acidic medium
Metabolic		
Hyperglycemia	Metabolic stress, sepsis, trauma	Treat origin of stress and provide insulin as needed
	Diabetes	Avoid excessive carbohydrate delivery
		Give appropriate insulin dose
Elevated or depressed serum electrolytes	Excessive or inadequate electrolytes in the formula	Change formula
	Refeeding syndrome	Monitor electrolytes closely (e.g., potassium, magnesium, phosphorus) and replace as indicated
Dehydration	Osmotic diarrhea caused by rapid infusion of hypertonic formula	Infuse formula slowly
	Excessive protein, electrolytes, or both	Change to isotonic formula or dilute with water
	Inadequate free-water provision	Reduce protein, electrolytes or increase fluid provision
		Ensure that patient receives adequate free water, especially if provided calorically dense formula
Overhydration	Excessive fluid intake	Assess fluid intake; monitor daily fluid intake and output
	Rapid refeeding in malnourished patient	Monitor serum electrolytes, body weight daily; weight change >0.2 kg/d reflects decrease or increase or extracellular fluid
	Increased extracellular mass catabolism causing loss of body cell mass with subsequent potassium loss	Use calorically dense formula to decrease free water if needed
	Cardiac, hepatic, or renal insufficiency	Diuretic therapy
Gradual weight loss	Inadequate calories	Ensure that patient is receiving prescribed amount of calories
		Ensure monitoring of patient over time, as nutrient requirements may change as a result of metabolic alterations
Excessive weight gain	Excess calories	Change formula or decrease volume per day
Visceral protein depletion	Inadequate protein or calories	Increase protein provision
EFA deficiency	Inadequate EFA intake	Include at least 4% of kcal needs as EFAs
	Prolonged use of low-fat formula	
Gastrointestinal		
Nausea and vomiting	Improper tube location	Reposition or replace feeding tube
	Excessive formula volume or rate infusion	Decrease rate of infusion or volume infused
	Very cold formula	Administer formula at room temperature
	High osmolality formula infused	Change to isotonic formula or dilute with water before infusing
	Smell of enteral formulas	Change to lower fat formula
		Add flavorings to formula; use polymeric as has less offensive odor

(Continued)

TABLE 5.12

(Continued)

Complication	Suggested Possible Causes	Corrective Measures
Diarrhea	Too rapid infusion Lactose intolerance Bolus feedings into small bowel High osmolality formula infused Hyperosmolar medication delivery Altered gastrointestinal anatomy or short gut	Decrease rate of infusion Use lactose-free formula Only provide continuous or slow-gravity feedings into small bowel Change to isotonic formula or dilute with water before infusing Change medications or dilute with water to make isotonic before delivery Change to hydrolyzed or free amino acid formula with MCT oil
Vomiting and diarrhea	Contamination	Check sanitation of formula and equipment, ensure proper handling techniques
Abdominal distention, bloating, cramping, gas	Rapid bolus or intermittent infusion of cold formula Rapid infusion through syringe Nutrient malabsorption Rapid administration of MCT	Administer formula at room temperature Infuse continuously at low rate and gradually increase to goal Use hydrolyzed formula, MCT-containing, lactose-free Administer MCT gradually as tolerated
Constipation	Lack of fiber Inadequate free water Fecal impaction, gastrointestinal obstruction Inadequate physical activity	Use high-fiber formula or add stool softener Increase free water intake Rectal examination, digital disimpaction Increase ambulation if able
Aspiration or gastric retention	Altered gastric motility, diabetic gastroparesis, altered gag reflex, altered mental status Head of bed <30 degrees Displaced feeding tube Ileus or hemodynamic instability Medications that may slow gastric motility (e.g., opiates, anticholinergics) Gastric or vagotomy surgery	Ensure postpyloric nutrient delivery with continuous infusion Add prokinetic agent if changed feeding position does not help Elevate head of bed to >30 degrees if possible Verify feeding tube placement and replace as needed If small bowel feedings not tolerated, then hold feedings and initiate TPN for prolonged intolerance Evaluate medications and change if feasible

EFA, essential fatty acid; MCT, medium-chain triacylglycerol; TPN, total parenteral nutrition.

forefront by providing a means for complete and safe feeding of patients with significant GI disease preventing adequate volitional intake. Experimentation with intravenous feeding can be traced as far back as the 1600s when sharpened quills were used to administer various mixtures of milk and wine into the veins of experimental animals (147). The 1800s brought the administration of saline, and by the 1930s, 5% dextrose and protein hydrolysates were being infused intravenously (148). Numerous limitations prevented safe infusions, including large volumes, venous endothelial injury, and occlusion from excessive osmolality (148). Solutions of greater than 800 mOsm are not tolerated through peripheral veins. These limitations led to experimentation with alternative fuel substrates, such as alcohol and fat, due to their increased caloric density of 7 and 9 cal/g, respectively. Intravenous fat delivery was an enticing alternative due to its high caloric load and low osmolality. Initially, provisions of intravenous fat was extracted from cottonseed oil in the 1950s (149). However, it was rapidly removed from clinical use, as it was associated with jaundice, fever, pulmonary compromise, and coagulopathy. Research continued in Europe to where emulsions made from soybean oil and safflower oil were successfully administered (129).

Technical advancement came in 1967 when cannulation of the subclavian vein was introduced to administer intravenous nutrients. Dudrick and Wilmore (150) first reported successful provision of centrally administered nutrition to an infant following bowel resection for intestinal atresia. The early clinical use of TPN was limited by high infection rates and access complications. By the 1970s refinements continued with the use of crystalline amino acids rather than protein hydrolysates of casein and fibrin. The 1970s also brought recommendations for standard amounts of vitamins and minerals, and the

TABLE 5.13

Development of Guidelines for Total Parenteral Nutrition

Organization	Year
American Society for Parenteral and Enteral Nutrition	1986, 1993, 2002
American College of Physicians	1987, 1989
American Gastroenterology Association	1989
U.S. Department of Health and Human Services	1990

reintroduction of safe intravenous lipid emulsions in the United States (147). During the 1980s, the focus turned to fine-tuning the parenteral solutions with the development of specialized amino acid solutions for specific disease states, approval of total nutrient admixtures (TNAs) by the FDA, and development of new access devices and delivery systems (147).

Rationale for Use of Parenteral Nutrition

Parenteral nutrition was first developed to provide nutrition to those unable to take adequate nutrition through the GI tract due to loss of absorptive surface and/or the inability to digest nutrients. This still remains the primary indication

for parenteral nutrition, a nonfunctioning GI tract and/or failure to tolerate enteral nutrition. There are several other indications for parenteral nutrition that need consideration such as being nutritionally at risk and the projected inability to consume anything by mouth for at least 7 to 14 days (119). Over the last two decades, several organizations have developed practice guidelines to identify the appropriate uses for parenteral nutrition (Table 5.13). Diagnoses that commonly need parenteral nutrition include short bowel syndrome, chronic malabsorption, bowel obstruction, intractable diarrhea or vomiting, prolonged ileus, and high output GI fistulas (119,149,151,152) (Table 5.14).

Comparison of Parenteral and Enteral Nutrition

Although parenteral nutrition can be lifesaving when used appropriately, it may also potentiate adverse clinical outcomes. The GI tract not only functions to digest and absorb nutrients, but it is also the body's largest immunologic organ. It serves as a protective barrier against intraluminal toxins and bacteria. Approximately 60% of the body's immunoglobulin producing cells line the GI tract with 80% of the body's manufactured immunoglobulin being secreted across the GI tract (76). During severe physiologic stress, relative or absolute gut ischemia can occur, leading to mucosal compromise and disruption of the gut's barrier function and ultimately passage of bacteria and toxins into the bloodstream or mesenteric lymphoid

TABLE 5.14

Indications for Total Parenteral Nutrition

Clinical Situation	Consensus
Short bowel syndrome	Inability to absorb adequate nutrients orally <60-cm small bowel may require indefinite use
Severe pancreatitis	Recommended if enteral nutrition causes abdominal pain, ascites, or elevated amylase/lipase Increased fistula output with enteral feedings Intravenous lipids are considered safe if serum triglyceride levels are <400 mg/dL
Enterocutaneous fistula	Fistula that exhibits increased output with enteral nutrition
Intractable diarrhea or vomiting	Recommended for losses >500–1,000 mL/d with inability to maintain adequate nutritional status
Bowel obstruction, ileus	With obstruction and malnutrition awaiting surgery >7 days Prolonged ileus >5–7 days with poor nutritional status
Perioperative support	Preoperative support is indicated for severely malnourished patients with expected postoperative NPO status >10 days For those with postoperative complications rendering NPO >10 days
Inflammatory bowel	If enteral nutrition not tolerated or if precluded by GI fistulas
Critical care	Unable to gain enteral access, instability, abdominal distention with prolonged reflux of enteral feedings, expected to remain NPO >7 days
Eating disorders	Severe malnutrition and inability to tolerate enteral feeding for psychological reasons
Pregnancy	Safe in pregnancy; hyperemesis gravidarum

GI, gastrointestinal; NPO, nothing by mouth.

system. In addition, common clinical practices such as broad-spectrum antibiotics, proton pump inhibitors, H2 blockers, and narcotic administration, as well as physiologic changes during acute stress, can lend to bacterial overgrowth in the proximal GI tract and impact the gut's protective barrier (153,154). Whether or not bacterial translocation occurring in animals and humans during acute stress is clinically significant remains hotly debated. Animal studies support the statement that enteral rather than parenteral nutrition maintains gut integrity, immune responsiveness and prevents bacterial translocation (76,154–157).

Parenteral nutrition is associated with several metabolic disadvantages when compared with enteral (158,159). The metabolic response to intravenous glucose differs from oral glucose (160). This is partially due to the fact that the insulin-independent hepatic uptake of glucose from the portal vein during first pass physiology is significant when glucose is provided orally resulting in less systemic hyperglycemia and hyperinsulinemia (160). A meta-analysis comparing enteral and parenteral nutrition also concluded that plasma glucose concentrations are lower during enteral than parenteral nutrition. Plasma glucose and insulin concentrations, glucose oxidation, CO_2 production and minute ventilation increase in a linear relation with calories administered in TPN (161). Prolonged infusion of high rates of glucose (>4 mg/kg/min) results in *de novo* lipogenesis in most critically ill patients. Furthermore, several well-designed studies now confirm that TPN is associated with increased septic morbidity (6,77,159,162) and increased cost (159) when compared with enteral nutrition in trauma and mixed-surgical populations.

Parenteral Carbohydrate

Carbohydrate remains the primary energy source in parenteral solutions. The amount of carbohydrate provided should be based on the patient's individual nutrient requirements and ability to oxidize glucose (163,164). Although the exact requirement is individually based, guidelines are available. It is estimated that 100 g of glucose is the minimum needed for tissues with obligate glucose requirement such as central nervous system (CNS), white blood cells, red blood cells, and renal medulla (82). The maximum rate of glucose oxidation in adults is 4 to 7 mg/kg/min, or approximately 350 to 450 g for a 70-kg person (164). The lower range is suggested for critically ill hypermetabolic patients secondary to endogenous glucose production that is not reversed by external carbohydrate supply (165). Excessive carbohydrate provision is associated with hyperglycemia, increased carbon dioxide production, and hepatic steatosis (166–168).

Currently in the United States, carbohydrate is provided as dextrose monohydrate in parenteral solutions. Each gram of hydrated dextrose provides 3.4 kcal/g. Commercial dextrose preparations are available in concentrations from 5% to 70% (Table 5.15). Dextrose solutions have an acidic pH (3.5–5.5) and are stable after autoclave sterilization. Additional carbohydrates have been tried in various experimental

TABLE 5.15

Intravenous Dextrose Solutions

Dextrose Concetration (%)	Carbohydrate (g/L)	Calories (kcal/L)	Osmolarity (mOsmol/L)
5	50	170	250
10	100	340	500
20	200	680	1,000
30	300	1,020	1,500
50	500	1,700	2,500
70	700	2,380	3,500

protocols with glycerol being the only other carbohydrate used clinically to any extent (169).

Glycerol is a 3 carbon glycolytic intermediate which has shown some success in parenteral systems. Glycerol yields 4.3 kcal/g when oxidized to carbon dioxide and water and does not require insulin for cellular uptake. When provided in low concentrations (3%) with amino acids, it has been found to be protein sparing (170). Because of these advantages, glycerol is used as an alternative source of calories in some parenteral formulations, primarily through the peripheral route.

Lipid

Since its introduction in Europe in the mid-1960s, intravenous fat emulsions have been extensively used as an alternative or complementary nutrient source in parenteral nutrition. Triacylglycerol emulsions became available in the United States in 1976. The current lipid emulsions available in the United States are long-chain triglycerides from soybean and safflower oil. Therefore, the lipid emulsions not only provide a concentrated caloric source but also provide EFAs. These products contain egg yolk phospholipid as an emulsifying agent and glycerol that make the products nearly isotonic. The glycerol raises the caloric concentration of the 10% emulsion to 1.1 kcal/mL and the 20% emulsion to 2.0 kcal/mL. The phospholipids may contribute to the phosphorus intake of patients who receive large amounts of lipids (>500 mL/d). Various combinations of long-chain triglycerides including olive oil, fish oil, and medium-chain triglyceride emulsions have been available and used safely throughout most of the world with the exception of the United States for several years. FDA regulations have prevented the use of these novel more physiologic lipid compounds in the United States.

Most patients tolerate daily infusion of lipids when provided as an intermittent or continuous infusion. Often lipids are combined with the other nutrient solution as part of a TNA (129). Continuous lipid delivery with a moderate dose is favored over intermittent infusion due to fewer fluctuations in serum triglyceride levels and improved fat oxidation (171). Extremely rarely, reactions to the lipid emulsions occur so patients should still be monitored for fever, chills, headache, and back pain during the first dose of intravenous lipid. Absolute contraindications to intravenous fat emulsions include pathologic hyperlipidemia, lipoid nephrosis, severe egg allergy, and lipid-induced acute pancreatitis with the etiology of the pancreatitis being hyperlipidemia (172). Intravenous lipids should be delivered cautiously to patients with severe liver disease, ARDS, or severe hypermetabolic stress. If serum triglyceride levels are greater than 500 mg/dL, then lipids should be held with only the minimal EFA requirements provided to avoid further metabolic complications.

EFA requirements are met by providing at least 4% of calories as EFAs. Delivering 10% to 15% of calories as a commercial lipid emulsion from safflower oil will prevent EFA deficiency. Because lipid emulsions vary in their composition of EFA, the minimum amount provided is based on the EFA content rather than a percentage of total calories. Recommendations for optimal intravenous lipid delivery have evolved over the last 25 years. It was once common practice to provide 40% to 50% of calories as lipid to take advantage of its concentrated energy source and decreased volume. However, more recent animal and clinical research have confirmed the concepts that parenteral long-chain triglycerides in excess volume impair neutrophil function, endotoxin clearance, and complement synthesis (129). As a result of these adverse effects, it is now recommended to limit lipid administration to 1 g/kg/d or 25% to 30% of total calories. In patients with severe infections or sepsis, intravenous lipids should be given at a minimum to meet the EFA needs (87).

Parenteral Protein

The primary function of protein in parenteral nutrition is to provide nitrogen in an attempt to minimize protein degradation to provide substrate for gluconeogenesis or provide amino acids for protein synthesis. The nitrogen source utilized in parenteral nutrition is in the form of crystalline amino acids. Parenteral amino acid products can be divided into standard and modified. Standard amino acid products are suitable for the vast majority of surgical patients. They contain a balanced or physiologic mixture of essential and NEAAs in which the ratios are based on Food and Agricultural Organisation of the United Nation (FAO)/World Health Organisation (WHO) recommendations for optimal proportions of EAAs. Standard formulations are available in a range of concentrations from 3% to 15%. Most institutions stock 10% and 15% concentrations because more dilute solutions can be made easily by adding sterile water with an automated compounder in the pharmacy.

The modified amino acid solutions are designed for patients with disease- or age-specific amino acid requirements. Formulations are commercially available for adults with hepatic failure, renal dysfunction, metabolic stress, and for neonates with special requirements for growth and development. These modified formulations are significantly more expensive than the standard formulations and rarely prove as cost effective in the adult; therefore, strict criteria should be established for their use.

Patients with hepatic failure develop multiple metabolic abnormalities to include electrolyte disturbances and alterations in amino acid metabolism. In end-stage or severe acute hepatic disease, hepatic encephalopathy commonly occurs. In addition to elevated ammonia levels observed during hepatic encephalopathy, a decrease in serum BCAAs and an elevation in AAAs and methionine levels are observed. Patients with hepatic disease without significant encephalopathy may be provided with moderate levels of standard amino acids while monitoring their mental status. When hepatic encephalopathy is severe (>Grade II), then a modified hepatic protein formulation may be beneficial in temporarily correcting the altered serum and CNS amino acid ratios. These formulations have high concentrations of BCAA (~45% of protein) and low concentrations of AAA and methionine. Improvements in hepatic encephalopathy and lower mortality have been found in some patients who received this formulation. The BCAA formulations should be adjunctive therapy to all other medical means to reduce nitrogenous metabolic products such as oral nonabsorbed antibiotics and Lactulose.

There are modified formulations still marketed for patients with renal failure, although the indications are exceedingly rare. These formulas contain mainly EAAs. These solutions were designed on the premise that only essential nitrogenous products should be given and all nonessental amino acids could be produced through transamination reactions. This hypothesis has been recently challenged, thereby questioning the usefulness of these formulas (163). Prospective, randomized, controlled studies have demonstrated that standard amino acids are as effective as modified amino acids in patients who have renal failure and who require parenteral nutrition (118). Therefore, patients with severe azotemia (BUN >100–150 mg %) with uremic complications may be given standard amino acids as part of parenteral nutrition in most clinical situations. In the critically ill or surgical patient the EAA solutions are not indicated because the proteins delivered by these solutions are inadequate to meet the needs of these patients.

A parenteral formulation with an enhanced BCAA formulation is marketed for patients with metabolic stress, such as that caused by major trauma, burns, and sepsis. Metabolic stress causes an efflux of amino acids from skeletal muscle and the gut to the liver for gluconeogenesis and support of acute phase protein synthesis. Metabolically stressed patients have also been shown to have increased serum levels of AAAs and decreased BCAA levels. Therefore, the rationale of using a high BCAA formula in these patients is to reestablish more normal serum amino acid levels to optimize protein synthesis and minimizes negative nitrogen balance. There have been multiple clinical studies evaluating the benefits of high BCAA formulations in metabolic stress (173–177). Some studies have shown positive benefits when using these formulations such as nitrogen retention, improved visceral protein levels, reversal of skin test anergy, but no major difference in morbidity or mortality. Other studies have failed to exhibit significant outcome advantages of BCAAs over standard amino acid formulas in metabolic stress. Therefore, since the cost-effectiveness of high BCAA solutions has not been clearly demonstrated, initiation of nutrition support with a standard amino acid solution is recommended in patients with significant metabolic stress.

Recently, novel intravenous amino acids such as glutamine or glutamine dipeptide, are undergoing large clinical trials in the United States. In the case of glutamine dipeptide, it is already in routine clinical use in Europe, Asia, and South America. Free glutamine is only temporarily stable in solution and requires specialty preparations in the pharmacy. This issue makes the commercial production and clinical use of free glutamine not feasible. Glutamine dipeptide currently available in Europe, Asia, and South America, shows promise as a means to supplement glutamine (106,107,178,179). The dipeptide is rapidly cleaved intracellularly, providing glutamine to tissues. Recent studies in surgical populations have shown benefits of glutamine dipeptide supplementation in parenteral nutrition in lowering infections and decreasing length of hospital stay (99,180).

Protein requirements are based on the patient's clinical condition. For normal healthy adults, the protein recommendation is 0.8 g/kg/d. In the critically ill/surgical population free of renal and/or hepatic disease, a range of 1.5 to 2.0 g/kg/d is appropriate, with higher levels showing no further improvement in nitrogen utilization. For patients with renal or hepatic disease, protein recommendations vary according to the disease stage and its intervention. For those with renal disease undergoing peritoneal dialysis, 1.2 to 1.5 g/kg/d of IBW is recommended for maintenance or repletion. For hemodialysis, 1.1 to 1.4 g/kg/dof IBW is recommended for maintenance or repletion. For those with uncomplicated hepatic dysfunction, 0.8 to 1.5 g/kg/d dry weight is suggested. For end-stage liver disease with encephalopathy, 0.5 to 0.7 g/kg/d is recommended. If a high BCAA formula is used, then 0.8 to 1.2 g/kg/d is suggested. In patients with major burns, high-output proximal fistulas, large open wounds, or open abdomens, protein levels can be increased to greater than 1.7 g/kg/d. Levels greater than 2.0 g/kg/d is rarely indicated and usually results in increased urea genesis and other metabolic complications.

Electrolytes

Electrolytes are added to parenteral solutions based on individual need. The amount added daily varies based on the patient's weight, disease state, renal and hepatic function, nutrition status, pharmacotherapy, acid–base status, and overall electrolyte balance. Extrarenal electrolyte losses may be a result of diarrhea, ostomy output, vomiting, fistulas, or nasogastric suctioning. As a patient becomes anabolic following resolution of the stress response, parenteral nutrient delivery is commonly associated with increased requirements for the major intracellular electrolytes (potassium, phosphorus, and

TABLE 5.16	
Parenteral Electrolyte Recommendations	
Sodium	60–150 mEq/d
Potassium	70–150 mEq/d
Phosphorus	20–30 mmol/d
Magnesium	15–20 mEq/d
Calcium	10–20 mmol
Chloride	Equal to Na^+ to prevent acid–base disturbances

magnesium) (181). During refeeding of undernourished patients, these electrolytes should be monitored frequently and replenished accordingly.

Electrolytes as macronutrients need careful monitoring. General recommendations for electrolyte provision are provided in Table 5.16. Electrolyte products are commercially available and the composition of the parenteral solution is dependent upon the compatibility of each electrolyte with the other components of the admixture and the order in which they are mixed. For calcium provision, calcium gluconate is the preferred form for parenteral formulations due to its stability in solution and decreased chance of dissociating and forming a precipitate with phosphorus. The decision to provide an electrolyte as a chloride or an acetate salt depends on the patient's acid–base status. Generally, acid–base balance is maintained with providing chloride and acetate in a 1:1 ratio. If a patient has altered acid–base status, then the chloride:acetate ratio can be adjusted to facilitate correction. Acetate and chloride are also present in the base amino acid solutions in various amounts and should be considered when attempting to calculate electrolyte balance.

Electrolytes increase the osmolarity of the parenteral solution; however, large amounts can be added to solutions with amino acids and dextrose without affecting the stability. When lipids are added to the parenteral solutions as TNA, caution is needed when adding electrolytes as there are limitations and hazards. An insoluble precipitate can form when there are excess cations in the parenteral solutions; as with calcium and phosphate, these precipitates may not be seen in TNAs. Crystal formation in the lungs with subsequent death has been reported in patients as a result of precipitate formation in TPN solutions. The solubility of calcium and phosphorus vary with the volume of the solution, its pH, the type of calcium preparation, the temperature at which the solutions are stored, and the order of admixture. Solutions can be prepared with a range of calcium and phosphorus contents as long as the product of calcium (in mEq) and phosphorus (in mmols) is less than 200.

Parenteral Vitamins and Trace Elements

Vitamins are typically added to every parenteral formulation in doses consistent with the American Medical Association

TABLE 5.17

Mechanical Complications of Parenteral Nutrition

Complication	Possible Cause	Symptom(s)	Treatment	Prevention
Pneumothorax	Catheter placement by inexperienced personnel	Tachycardia, dyspnea, persistent cough, diaphoresis	Large pneumothorax may require chest-tube placement	Experienced personnel to place catheter
Catheter embolization	Pulling catheter back through needle used for insertion	Cardiac arrhythmias	Surgical removal of catheter tip	Avoid withdrawing catheter through insertion needle
Air embolism	Air is inspired while line is interrupted and uncapped	Cyanosis, tachypnea, hypotension, churning heart murmur	Immediately place patient on left side and lower head of bed to keep air in apex of the right ventricle until it is reabsorbed	Experienced personnel to place catheter
Venous thrombosis	Mechanical trauma to vein, hypotension, hyperosmolar solution, hypercoagulopathy, sepsis	Swelling or pain in one or both arms or shoulders or neck	Anticoagulation therapy with urokinase or streptokinase; catheter removal	Silicone catheter, adding heparin to TPN, low-dose warfarin therapy
Cathether occlusion	Hypotension, failure to maintain line patency, formation of fibrin sheath outside the catheter, solution precipitates	Increasing need for greater pressure to maintain continuous infusion rate	Anticoagulation therapy with urokinase or streptokinase	Larger diameter catheter routine catheter flusing, monitor solution for a precipitate
Phlebitis	Peripheral administration of hypertonic solution	Redness, swelling, pain at peripheral site	Change peripheral line site, begin central TPN if necessary	Maintain osmolarity of peripheral solution <900 mOsmol/kg
Catheter-related sepsis	Inappropriate technique of line placement, poor catheter care, contaminated solution	Unexplained fever, chills, red and indurated area around catheter site	Remove catheter and replace at another site	Follow strict protocols for line placement and care

TPN, total parental nutrition.

Nutrition Advisory Group's recommendations (182). These guidelines are established for the 12 essential vitamins (Table 5.17). Most institutions use a commercially available multiple-entity product that contains all 12 essential vitamins for adults. The multivitamin preparations for adults do not contain vitamin K as it can adversely affect the anticoagulation effect of Coumadin. In adults, vitamin K may be administered by adding 1 to 2 mg/d to the parenteral solution or by giving 5 to 10 mg/wk intramuscularly or subcutaneously. Individual vitamin preparations are also available and are used to supplement the multivitamin doses when a deficiency state exists or with increased needs due to disease, medical condition, or excessive loss.

Trace minerals are essential to normal growth and metabolism. They function as metabolic cofactors essential for the optimal activity of numerous enzyme systems. Although the requirements are minute, deficiency states develop rapidly in clinical settings secondary to increased metabolic demands or excessive losses. Most clinicians supplement parenteral solutions with micronutrients daily; however there are clinical conditions necessitating trace mineral restriction and therefore adjustments in the daily intakes. This is especially important in cholestatic liver disease where copper and manganese are excreted in the bile.

The Nutrition Advisory Group of the American Medical Association has also published guidelines for four trace elements known to be essential in human nutrition (183). The suggested amounts of zinc, copper, manganese, and chromium for adults are listed in Table 5.18. Since the original recommendations, it has become more evident that

TABLE 5.18

Metabolic Complications of Parenteral Nutrition

Complication	Possible Cause	Treatment
Hypovolemia	Inadequate fluid provision, over diuresis	Increase fluid delivery
Hypervolemia	Excess fluid delivery, renal dysfunction, congestive heart failure, hepatic failure	Fluid restriction, diuretics, dialysis
Hypokalemia	Refeeding syndrome, inadequate potassium provision, increased losses	Increase intravenous or parenteral potassium
Hyperkalemia	Renal dysfunction, too much potassium provision, metabolic acidosis, potassium-sparing drugs	Decrease potassium intake, potassium binders, dialysis in extreme cases
Hyponatremia	Excessive fluid provision, nephritis, adrenal insufficiency, dilutional states	Restrict fluid intake, increase sodium intake as indicated clinically
Hypernatremia	Inadequate free-water provision, excessive sodium intake, excessive water losses	Decrease sodium intake, replete free-water deficit
Hypoglycemia	Abrupt discontinuation of parenteral nutrition, insulin overdose	Dextrose delivery
Hyperglycemia	Rapid infusion of large dextrose load, sepsis, pancreatitis, steroids, diabetes, elderly	Insulin, reduce dextrose delivery
Hypertriglyceridemia	Inability to clear lipid provision, sepsis, multisystem organ failure, medications altering fat absorption, history of hyperlipidemia	Decrease lipid volume provided, increase infusion time, hold lipids up to 14 d to normalize level
Hypocalcemia	Decrease vitamin D intake, hypoparathyroidism, citrate binding of calcium resulting from excessive blood transfusion, hypoalbuminemia	Calcium supplementation
Hypercalcemia	Renal failure, tumor lysis syndrome, bone cancer, excess vitamin D delivery, prolonged immobilization-stress hyperparathyroidism	Isotonic saline, inorganic phosphate supplementation, corticosteroids, mithramycin
Hypomagnesemia	Refeeding syndrome, alcoholism, diuretic use, increased losses, medications, diabetic ketoacidosis, chemotherapy	Magnesium supplementation
Hypermagnesemia	Excessive magnesium provision, renal insufficiency	Decrease magnesium provision
Hypophosphatemia	Refeeding syndrome, alcoholism, phosphate-binding antacids, dextrose infusion, overfeeding, secondary hyperparathyroidism, insulin therapy	Phosphate supplementation, discontinue phosphate-binding antacids, avoid overfeeding, initiate dextrose delivery cautiously
Hyperphosphatemia	Renal dysfunction, excessive provision	Decrease phosphate delivery, phosphate binders
Prerenal azotemia	Dehydration, excessive protein provision, inadequate nonprotein calorie provision with mobilization of own protein stores	Increase fluid intake, decrease protein delivery, increase nonprotein calories
Essential fatty acid deficiency	Inadequate polyunsaturated long-chain fatty acid provision	Lipid administration

selenium is essential and should be added on a daily basis with the other four trace elements (184). Most institutions use a commercially available multiple-entity product, but there are also single-entity mineral solutions available for use during times of increased requirements or when specific mineral are contraindicated. Zinc requirements are felt to be increased during metabolic and surgical stress due to increased urinary losses and with excessive GI losses common with diarrhea and increased ostomy output. Manganese

and copper are excreted through the biliary tract, whereas zinc, chromium, and selenium are eliminated through renal mechanisms. Therefore, copper and manganese should be restricted or withheld from the parenteral nutrition in patients with cholestatic liver disease but should be considered for supplement with complete external biliary diversion. Selenium depletion is commonly reported in patients receiving long-term nonsupplemented TPN, as well as with thermal injury, acquired immunodeficiency syndrome, liver failure, and long-term hypermetabolic states.

Other Additives

Many patients receiving TPN are also receiving multiple additional intravenous medications. Using TPN as a drug delivery vehicle is very tempting as it may allow for continuous medication infusion in addition to minimizing fluid volume by eliminating the need for a separate diluent for each medication administered. However, communication with the pharmacy is needed before adding medications to the TPN solution, as there is potential for serious adverse drug–drug and drug–nutrient interactions. Issues needing scrutiny include medication compatibility with macro- and micronutrients the effect of pH changes on TPN compatibility and drug effectiveness, whether the infusion schedule of the TPN is appropriate to achieve therapeutic levels of the drug, and the potential for drug–drug interactions. Medications that are most frequently added to TPN include albumin, aminophylline, cimetidine, famotidine, ranitidine, heparin, hydrochloric acid, and regular insulin.

Methods of Administration

Serious complications can occur with TPN if careful initiation and monitoring methods are not followed. TPN solutions may be infused continuously over a 24-hour period or in stable patients cycled over shorter time intervals. If a patient is critically ill or just initiating TPN, it is suggested to infuse the TPN over a 24-hour period until patient tolerance and stability are demonstrated. TPN in the surgical or hypermetabolic patient should not be initiated at goal caloric rates as many patients may not tolerate either the acute volume increase or caloric load. Proportional increases in carbohydrate-dependent electrolytes such as magnesium and phosphorus, and protein-dependent electrolytes such as potassium, and volume-dependent electrolytes such as sodium should be given as these macronutrients are increased.

For patients with DM, stress-induced hyperglycemia, systemic steroid administration, or risk for refeeding syndrome, dextrose should be limited initially to approximately 100 to 150 g/d. For other patients with normal glucose tolerance, dextrose may be initiated at 200 to 250 g/d. If after 24 hours glycemic control is acceptable, then the dextrose may be advanced to goal over the next 24 to 48 hours as tolerated. Capillary glucose measurements should be obtained at least three to four times daily until the values are normal for 2 consecutive days. Regular insulin may be administered according to a sliding scale. Most hospitals now have standard protocols for continuous intravenous insulin infusions for dealing with persistent hyperglycemia associated with TPN. Insulin may also be added to the TPN solution. However, the ordering team must be cognizant that exogenous stress during perioperative periods may only temporarily elevate glucose. If these hyperglycemic stresses resolve inadvertent hypoglycemia can result. For patients requiring insulin before TPN institution, approximately half of the established insulin requirement may be included as regular insulin in the initial bag of TPN formula. If blood glucose levels are less than 200 mg/dL, approximately two thirds of the previous day's subcutaneous insulin dose may be added to the TPN as regular insulin. Regardless of the method of insulin delivery, the goal is to consistently maintain blood glucose levels between 100 and 180 mg/dL.

Lipids may be infused on a daily basis and for up to 24 hours. Irrespective of the method of lipid delivery, either through TNA or as a separate infusion, maximal lipid infusion rates should not exceed 0.1 g/kg/h. The adverse effects of intravenous lipids, mainly the immunosuppressive effects, are noted when infusion rates exceed that stated earlier (185). It is suggested to maintain triglyceride levels to less than or equal to 400 mg/dL while lipids are being infused. If serum triglyceride levels exceed the recommended level, intravenous lipids should be held until levels normalize. For persistent or severe hypertriglyceridemia or for patients with egg allergy, safflower oil or any oil high in EFA can be administered through feeding tube or orally in attempts to alleviate the symptoms of EFA deficiency. Several commonly used intravenous medications are now available in lipid formulations, that is, propofol. The amount of lipid given as vehicles in drug delivery should be considered in the final TPN caloric calculation to avoid iatrogenic excessive long-chain triglyceride and caloric delivery.

Although parenteral nutrition is usually provided over a 24-hour continuous rate, it may also be delivered in a cyclic pattern. Cyclic TPN has been suggested for patients who are stable and receiving TPN for an extended duration. Cyclic TPN also allows for some liberation from the TPN pump system allowing for easier patient mobility. Also for those individuals with limited vascular access, cyclic infusion may be required in order to administer necessary medications or blood products. Conversion from 24-hour continuous infusion to cyclic infusion is usually accomplished over 2 to 3 days. The largest concern that is commonly overstated is with the initiation and discontinuation of the carbohydrate infusion and potential for hyperglycemia and rebound hypoglycemia. Another concern is with the increased volume delivery over a shorter time frame in patients with limited cardiac compensation mechanisms. Most stable patients can tolerate cyclic TPN over 8 to 16 hours.

Parenteral Nutrition Discontinuation

Eventually in all patients, the goal is to transition the patient from TPN to enteral nutrition, tube feeding or oral intake. Before discontinuing the TPN, assurance that the patient is consuming and absorbing adequate nutrients enterally is imperative. TPN should be sequentially decreased as the enteral intake and tolerance improves to avoid the complications of overfeeding. TPN may be discontinued once the patient is tolerating approximately 65% to 75% of goal calories. For patients who are eating, TPN may be reduced and stopped over a 12- to 24-hour period. If TPN is inadvertently discontinued abruptly in patients who are not eating, all insulin should be stopped and blood glucose levels should be monitored for 30 to 120 minutes after discontinuation of TPN. On the basis of the blood glucose levels, appropriate therapy for hypoglycemia should be implemented. Previously, most clinicians felt D_{10} should be immediately started if TPN is abruptly discontinued but most now feel that this is unnecessary and patient monitoring is adequate. Lastly, if the TPN was used as a vehicle for medication or electrolyte administration, an alternate plan should be made once it is discontinued.

Complication of Parenteral Nutrition

Complications of parenteral nutrition have been widely reported. However, TPN is safe with minimal complications when it is managed and monitored by a multidisciplinary team of trained professionals. The complications that may arise are diverse and for simplicity can be subdivided into mechanical, infectious, and metabolic complications (158, 166,185,186).

Potential mechanical complications of catheter insertion are almost unlimited but the majority (Table 5.17) includes pneumothorax, hydrothorax, and great vessel injury. Catheter malposition may result in venous thrombosis, causing head, neck, or arm swelling, or possibly a pulmonary embolus. Catheter-related infections are a significant morbidity and can result in mortality. A catheter infection rate greater than 3% is considered unacceptable, with most major centers now reporting less than 1%. Appropriate use of sterile technique is essential to maintain an acceptable catheter infection rate. Nursing protocols should be established for dressing changes and line manipulation. Dressings should be changed every 48 hours and should include local sterilizing ointment and an occlusive dressing.

With adequate monitoring of TPN, metabolic complications (Table 5.18) can be avoided. Despite being widely reported, these mainly iatrogenic complications still occur. Refeeding syndrome may be defined as a constellation of fluid, micronutrient, electrolyte, and vitamin imbalances that occur within the first few days of nutrient infusion in a chronically starved patient (181). Refeeding syndrome can include hemolytic anemia, respiratory distress, paresthesias, tetany, and cardiac arrhythmias. Typical laboratory findings include hypokalemia, hypophosphatemia, and hypomagnesemia. Reported risk factors for refeeding syndrome include alcoholism, anorexia nervosa, marasmus, rapid refeeding, and excessive dextrose infusion. To prevent the syndrome from occurring, it is recommended to (i) aggressively monitor and replete serum potassium, phosphorus, and magnesium concentrations before beginning full caloric TPN; (ii) limit initial carbohydrate infusion to 150 g/d, fluid to 800 mL/d, and sodium intake to no more than 20 mEq/d in at-risk patients; (iii) include adequate amounts of potassium, magnesium, phosphorus, and vitamins in the TPN solution; (iv) increase carbohydrate-dependent minerals in proportion to increases in carbohydrate when TPN is advanced.

Hyperglycemia (nonfasting blood glucose >200 mg/dL) is the most common metabolic complication of TPN (62). Risk factors include metabolic or surgical stress, medications,

obesity, diabetes, and excess dextrose administration. Careful glucose monitoring, especially in the first 72 hours of TPN administration, can help guide advancement of dextrose to goal. Administration of dextrose in amounts less than the maximum glucose oxidation rate (4–7 mg/kg/min) and initiating dextrose in reduced amounts (100–150 g/d) in at-risk patient may help minimize the occurrence of hyperglycemia.

Patients receiving TPN often experience fluid and electrolyte abnormalities and routine monitoring is recommended. The etiology of the abnormalities is related to several factors including the patient's preexisting and current medical condition and treatment, medications, or excessive or inadequate free water provision.

Summary—Parenteral Nutrition

Parenteral nutrition has seen major medical advancements over the last several decades. The recent trends in clinical studies showing the numerous benefits of enteral over parenteral nutrition have taken away much of the early luster of parenteral nutrition. There is no question that the now routine use of TPN has saved thousands of lives. The next several decades will most likely bring more advances in the technology and science of parenteral nutrition. Most TPN research is now focused on developing a more complete and balanced solution containing the amino acids such as glutamine that have previously been omitted secondary to solubility characteristics and safety issues. In addition to the amino acid changes, the development and availability of much more physiologic and safe lipid emulsions containing fish oil, olive oil, and medium chain triglycerides should be available soon in the United States. With careful selection, implementation, and monitoring, parenteral nutrition continues to be a lifesaving nutritional delivery system for those unfortunate patients with a temporary or permanently nonfunctioning alimentary system.

SUMMARY

An understanding of the basic scientific principles of nutrition is essential to surgical practice. Nutrition support has consistently proved its value as one of the most important clinical interventions available to minimize surgical morbidity and mortality. The advances in clinical nutrition over the last 30 years have incorporated physiology, biochemistry, immunology, and molecular biology to begin to unravel the complex, highly integrated attempt by the body to maintain sufficient nutrient substrates to withstand surgical or metabolic insult. Nutrition support for the surgical patient is no longer just the provision of calories for postoperative nitrogen sparing. Surgical nutrition should be considered a therapeutic tool just as any other surgical intervention or medical therapy. The surgeon should consider the use of specific substrates such as Ω-3 fatty acids or its derivatives, glutamine, and arginine in treatment of complex surgical and critical care conditions. The challenge for the future is for surgeons to adapt the scientific information currently available in regard to route, timing, and type of nutrition to surgical practice. Undoubtedly, attention to the patient's nutritional status will improve outcome, shorten hospital stay, and lower morbidity and mortality.

REFERENCES

1. Studley HO. Percentage of weight loss: a basic indicator of surgical risk in patients with chronic peptic ulcer 1936. *Nutr Hosp* 2001;16:141–143. Discussion 140–141.

2. Alexander JW, MacMillan BG, Stinnett JD, et al. Beneficial effects of aggressive protein feeding in severely burned children. *Ann Surg* 1980;192:505–517.

3. Klein S, Kinney J, Jeejeebhoy K, et al. Nutrition support in clinical practice: review of published data and recommendations for future research directions. National Institutes of Health, American Society for Parenteral and Enteral Nutrition, and American Society for Clinical Nutrition. *J Parenter Enteral Nutr* 1997;21:133–156.

4. Martindale RG, Maerz LL. Management of perioperative nutrition support. *Curr Opin Crit Care* 2006;12:290–294.

5. Moore EE, Jones TN. Benefits of immediate jejunostomy feeding after major abdominal trauma-a prospective, randomized study. *J Trauma* 1986;26:874–881.

6. Moore FA, Feliciano DV, Andrassy RJ, et al. Early enteral feeding, compared with parenteral, reduces postoperative septic complications. The results of a meta-analysis. *Ann Surg* 1992;216:172–183.

7. Amaral JF, Shearer JD, Mastrofrancesco B, et al. The temporal characteristics of the metabolic and endocrine response to injury. *J Trauma* 1988;28:1335–1352.

8. Townsend CM. Sabiston textbook of surgery. In: Tawa NE, Maykel JA, Fischer JE, ed. *Metabolism in surgical patients*, 17th ed. Philadalphia: WB Saunders, 2004;137–182.

9. Cahill GF Jr. Starvation in man. *N Engl J Med* 1970;282:668–675.

10. George FC. Fuel metabolism in starvation. *Annu Rev Nutr* 2006;26:1–22.

11. Cresci G. Nutrition support for the critically ill patient. In: Toulson MI, ed. *Metabolic response to stress*, 1st ed. Boca Raton: CRC Press, 2005;3–14.

12. Andoh A, Tsujikawa T, Fujiyama Y. Role of dietary fiber and short-chain fatty acids in the colon. *Curr Pharm Des* 2003;9:347–358.

13. Wong JM, de Souza R, Kendall CW, et al. Colonic health: fermentation and short chain fatty acids. *J Clin Gastroenterol* 2006;40:235–243.

14. Yamada T. Textbook of gastroenterology. In: Traber PG, ed. *Carbohydrate assimilation*, 4th ed. Philadelphia: Lippincott Williams & Wilkins, 2003;389–412.

15. Leibach FH, Ganapathy V. Peptide transporters in the intestine and the kidney. *Annu Rev Nutr* 1996;16:99–119.

16. Yamada T. Textbook of gastroenterology. In: Ganapathy V, Ganapathy ME, Leibach, FH, ed. *Protein digestion and assimilation*, 4th ed. Philadelphia: Lippincott Williams & Wilkins, 2003;438–448.

17. Morais JA, Chevalier S, Gougeon R. Protein turnover and requirements in the healthy and frail elderly. *J Nutr Health Aging* 2006;10:272–283.

18. Stipanuk MH. Biochemical and physiologic aspects of human nutrition. In: Goodridge AG, Sul HS, ed. *Lipid metabolism-synthesis and oxidation*, 1st ed. Philadelphia: WB Saunders, 2000;305–346.

19. Alexander JW. Immunonutrition: the role of omega-3 fatty acids. *Nutrition* 1998;14:627–633.

20. Stipanuk MH. Biochemical and physiologic aspects of human nutrition. In: Small DM, ed. *Structure and properties of lipids*, 1st ed. Philadelphia: WB Saunders, 2000;43–62.

21. Heyland DK, Dhaliwal R, Day AG, et al. Reducing deaths due to oxidative stress (The REDOXS Study): rationale and study design for a randomized trial of glutamine and antioxidant supplementation in critically-ill patients. *Proc Nutr Soc* 2006;65:250–263.

22. Heyland DK, Dhaliwal R, Suchner U, et al. Antioxidant nutrients: a systematic review of trace elements and vitamins in the critically ill patient. *Intensive Care Med* 2005;31:327–337.

23. Demling RH, DeBiasse MA. Micronutrients in critical illness. *Crit Care Clin* 1995;11:651–673.

24. Nathens AB, Neff MJ, Jurkovich GJ, et al. Randomized, prospective trial of antioxidant supplementation in critically ill surgical patients. *Ann Surg* 2002;236:814–822.

25. Said HMP, Kumar CP. Intestinal absorption of vitamins. *Curr Opin Gastroenterol* 1999;15:172.

26. Shenkin A. Micronutrients in adult nutritional support: requirements and benefits. *Curr Opin Clin Nutr Metab Care* 1998;1:15–19.

27. Okada A, Takagi Y, Nezu R, et al. Zinc in clinical surgery-a research review. *Jpn J Surg* 1990;20:635–644.

28. Berger MM, Cavadini C, Chiolero R, et al. Copper, selenium, and zinc status and balances after major trauma. *J Trauma* 1996;40:103–109.

29. Mertz W. Risk assessment of essential trace elements: new approaches to setting recommended dietary allowances and safety limits. *Nutr Rev* 1995;53:179–185.

30. Crimi E, Sica V, Williams-Ignarro S, et al. The role of oxidative stress in adult critical care. *Free Radic Biol Med* 2006;40:398–406.

31. Downs JH, Haffejee A. Nutritional assessment in the critically ill. *Curr Opin Clin Nutr Metab Care* 1998;1:275–279.

32. Morgan SL. Identification of indicators for improving the diagnosis of malnutrition. *Nutrition* 1995;11:202–204.

33. Kondrup J, Allison SP, Elia M, et al. ESPEN guidelines for nutrition screening 2002. *Clin Nutr* 2003;22:415–421.

34. Windsor JA, Hill GL. Weight loss with physiologic impairment. A basic indicator of surgical risk. *Ann Surg* 1988;207:290–296.

35. Matarese LE, Gottschlich MM. Contemporary nutrition support practice. In: Hommond K, ed. *History and physical examination*, 1st ed. Philadelphia: WB Saunders, 1998;25–26.

36. Ottery FD. Definition of standardized nutritional assessment and interventional pathways in oncology. *Nutrition* 1996;12:S15–S19.

37. Merritt RJ. ASPEN: Nutrition support practice manual. In: Pesce-Hammond K, Wessel J, ed. *Nutrition assessment and decision making*, 2nd ed. Silver Spring: ASPEN Publishers, 2005;3–26.

38. Charney P. Nutrition assessment in the 1990s: where are we now? *Nutr Clin Pract* 1995;10:131–139.

39. Jeejeebhoy KN, Detsky AS, Baker JP. Assessment of nutritional status. *J Parenter Enteral Nutr* 1990;14:193S–196S.

40. Boosalis MG, Ott L, Levine AS, et al. Relationship of visceral proteins to nutritional status in chronic and acute stress. *Crit Care Med* 1989;17:741–747.

41. Gabay C, Kushner I. Acute-phase proteins and other systemic responses to inflammation. *N Engl J Med* 1999;340:448–454.

42. Kudsk KA, Minard G, Wojtysiak SL, et al Visceral protein response to enteral versus parenteral nutrition and sepsis in patients with trauma. *Surgery* 1994;116:516–523.

43. Manelli JC, Badetti C, Botti G, et al. A reference standard for plasma proteins is required for nutritional assessment of adult burn patients. *Burns* 1998;24:337–345.

44. Sganga G, Siegel JH, Brown G, et al. Reprioritization of hepatic plasma protein release in trauma and sepsis. *Arch Surg* 1985;120:187–199.

45. Raguso CA, Dupertuis YM, Pichard C. The role of visceral proteins in the nutritional assessment of intensive care unit patients. *Curr Opin Clin Nutr Metab Care* 2003;6:211–216.

46. Kudsk KA, Tolley EA, DeWitt RC, et al. Preoperative albumin and surgical site identify surgical risk for major postoperative complications. *J Parenter Enteral Nutr* 2003;27:1–9.

47. Ferard G, Gaudias J, Bourguignat A, et al. C-reactive protein to transthyretin ratio for the early diagnosis and follow-up of postoperative infection. *Clin Chem Lab Med* 2002;40:1334–1338.

48. Klein CJ, Stanek GS, Wiles CE III. Overfeeding macronutrients to critically ill adults: metabolic complications. *J Am Diet Assoc* 1998;98:795–806.

49. Pomposelli JJ, Baxter JK III, Babineau TJ, et al. Early postoperative glucose control predicts nosocomial infection rate in diabetic patients. *J Parenter Enteral Nutr* 1998;22:77–81.

50. Pomposelli JJ, Bistrian BR. Is total parenteral nutrition immunosuppressive? *New Horiz* 1994;2:224–229.

51. Flancbaum L, Choban PS, Sambucco S, et al. Comparison of indirect calorimetry, the Fick method, and prediction equations in estimating the energy requirements of critically ill patients. *Am J Clin Nutr* 1999;69:461–466.

52. Chiolero R, Revelly JP, Tappy L. Energy metabolism in sepsis and injury. *Nutrition* 1997;13:45S–51S.

53. Barton RG. Nutrition support in critical illness. *Nutr Clin Pract* 1994;9:127–139.

54. Cutts ME, Dowdy RP, Ellersieck MR, et al. Predicting energy needs in ventilator-dependent critically ill patients: effect of adjusting weight for edema or adiposity. *Am J Clin Nutr* 1997;66:1250–1256.

55. Marik P, Varon J. The obese patient in the ICU. *Chest* 1998;113:492–498.

56. Ireton-Jones CS, Turner WW Jr, Liepa GU, et al. Equations for the estimation of energy expenditures in patients with burns with special reference to ventilatory status. *J Burn Care Rehabil* 1992;13:330–333.

57. Patino JF, de Pimiento SE, Vergara A, et al. Hypocaloric support in the critically ill. *World J Surg* 1999;23:553–559.

58. Grimble RF. Interaction between nutrients, pro-inflammatory cytokines and inflammation. *Clin Sci (Lond)* 1996;91:121–130.

59. Grimble RF. Genotypic influences on metabolic alterations during inflammation and the nutritional outcome. *Nestle Nutr Workshop Ser Clin Perform Programme* 2002;7:1–13.discussion 13–18.

60. Mendez C, Jurkovich GJ, Garcia I, et al. Effects of an immune-enhancing diet in critically injured patients. *J Trauma* 1997;42:933–940. discussion 940–931.

61. Krishnan JA, Parce PB, Martinez A, et al. Caloric intake in medical ICU patients: consistency of care with guidelines and relationship to clinical outcomes. *Chest* 2003;124:297–305.

62. McCowen KC, Friel C, Sternberg J, et al. Hypocaloric total parenteral nutrition: effectiveness in prevention of hyperglycemia and infectious complications-a randomized clinical trial. *Crit Care Med* 2000;28:3606–3611.

63. Dickerson RN. Hypocaloric feeding of obese patients in the intensive care unit. *Curr Opin Clin Nutr Metab Care* 2005;8:189–196.

64. Dickerson RN, Boschert KJ, Kudsk KA, et al. Hypocaloric enteral tube feeding in critically ill obese patients. *Nutrition* 2002;18:241–246.

65. Brady M, Kinn S, Stuart P. Preoperative fasting for adults to prevent perioperative complications. *Cochrane Database Syst Rev* 2003;CD004423.

66. American Society of Anesthesiologist Task Force on Preoperative Fasting. Practice guidelines for preoperative fasting and the use of pharmacologic agents to reduce the risk of pulmonary aspiration: application to healthy patients undergoing elective procedures: a report by the American Society of Anesthesiologist Task Force on Preoperative Fasting. *Anesthesiology* 1999;90:896–905.

67. Lennard TW, Shenton BK, Borzotta A, et al. The influence of surgical operations on components of the human immune system. *Br J Surg* 1985;72:771–776.

68. Thorell A, Nygren J, Ljungqvist O. Insulin resistance: a marker of surgical stress. *Curr Opin Clin Nutr Metab Care* 1999;2:69–78.

69. Hausel J, Nygren J, Lagerkranser M, et al. A carbohydrate-rich drink reduces preoperative discomfort in elective surgery patients. *Anesth Analg* 2001;93:1344–1350.

70. Hausel J, Nygren J, Thorell A, et al. Randomized clinical trial of the effects of oral preoperative carbohydrates on postoperative nausea and vomiting after laparoscopic cholecystectomy. *Br J Surg* 2005;92:415–421.

71. Ljungqvist O, Nygren J, Soop M, et al. Metabolic perioperative management: novel concepts. *Curr Opin Crit Care* 2005;11:295–299.

72. Melis GC, van Leeuwen PA, von Blomberg-van der Flier BM, et al. A carbohydrate-rich beverage prior to surgery prevents surgery-induced immunodepression: a randomized, controlled, clinical trial. *J Parenter Enteral Nutr* 2006;30:21–26.

73. Noblett SE, Watson DS, Huong H, et al. Pre-operative oral carbohydrate loading in colorectal surgery: a randomized controlled trial. *Colorectal Dis* 2006;8:563–569.

74. Nygren J, Soop M, Thorell A, et al. Preoperative oral carbohydrates and postoperative insulin resistance. *Clin Nutr* 1999;18:117–120.

75. Rombeau JL, Roldandelli RH. Clinical nutrition: enteral and tube feeding. In: McCamish MA, Bounous G, Geraghty M, ed. *History of enteral feeding: past and present perspectives*, 3rd ed. Philadelphia: WB Saunders, 1997.

76. King BK, Kudsk KA, Li J, et al. Route and type of nutrition influence mucosal immunity to bacterial pneumonia. *Ann Surg* 1999;229:272–278.

77. Kudsk KA, Croce MA, Fabian TC, et al. Enteral versus parenteral feeding. Effects on septic morbidity after blunt and penetrating abdominal trauma. *Ann Surg* 1992;215:503–511. discussion 511–503.

78. Fink MP. Gastrointestinal mucosal injury in experimental models of shock, trauma, and sepsis. *Crit Care Med* 1991;19:627–641.

79. Minard G, Kudsk KA. Nutritional support and infection: does the route matter? *World J Surg* 1998;22:213–219.

80. Kirby DF, Delegge MH, Fleming CR. American Gastroenterological Association technical review on tube feeding for enteral nutrition. *Gastroenterology* 1995;108:1282–1301.

81. Larson DE, Burton DD, Schroeder KW, et al. Percutaneous endoscopic gastrostomy. Indications, success, complications, and mortality in 314 consecutive patients. *Gastroenterology* 1987;93:48–52.

82. Wilmore DW. Postoperative protein sparing. *World J Surg* 1999;23:545–552.

83. Bengmark S. Immunonutrition: role of biosurfactants, fiber, and probiotic bacteria. *Nutrition* 1998;14:585–594.

84. Bengmark S, Jeppsson B. Gastrointestinal surface protection and mucosa reconditioning. *J Parenter Enteral Nutr* 1995;19:410–415.

85. Jensen GL, Mascioli EA, Seidner DL, et al. Parenteral infusion of long- and medium-chain triglycerides and reticuloendothelial system function in man. *J Parenter Enteral Nutr* 1990;14:467–471.

86. Stipanuk MH. Biochemical and physiologic aspects of human nutrition. In: Tso P, Crissinger, KD, ed. *Digestion and absorption of lipids*, 1st ed. Philadelphia: WB Saunders, 2000;125–140.

87. Hasselmann M, Reimund JM. Lipids in the nutritional support of the critically ill patients. *Curr Opin Crit Care* 2004;10:449–455.

88. Calder PC. Fatty acids and gene expression related to inflammation. *Nestle Nutr Workshop Ser Clin Perform Programme* 2002;7:19–36. discussion 36–40.

89. Serhan CN. Novel eicosanoid and docosanoid mediators: resolvins, docosatrienes, and neuroprotectins. *Curr Opin Clin Nutr Metab Care* 2005;8:115–121.

90. Ferrucci L, Cherubini A, Bandinelli S, et al. Relationship of plasma polyunsaturated fatty acids to circulating inflammatory markers. *J Clin Endocrinol Metab* 2006;91:439–446.

91. Kudsk KA. Immunonutrition in surgery and critical care. *Annu Rev Nutr* 2006;26:463–479.

92. Heller AR, Rossler S, Litz RJ, et al. Omega-3 fatty acids improve the diagnosis-related clinical outcome. *Crit Care Med* 2006;34:972–979.

93. Angerer P, von Schacky C. n-3 polyunsaturated fatty acids and the cardiovascular system. *Curr Opin Clin Nutr Metab Care* 2000;3:439–445.

94. Hasselgren PO. Pathways of muscle protein breakdown in injury and sepsis. *Curr Opin Clin Nutr Metab Care* 1999;2:155–160.

95. Plank LD, Hill GL. Sequential metabolic changes following induction of systemic inflammatory response in patients with severe sepsis or major blunt trauma. *World J Surg* 2000;24:630–638.

96. Wolfe RR, Martini WZ. Changes in intermediary metabolism in severe surgical illness. *World J Surg* 2000;24:639–647.

97. Rombeau JL, Roldandelli RH. Clinical nutrition: parenteral nutrition. In: Fukuchtl S, Bankhead R, Rolandelli RH, ed. *Parenteral nutrition in short bowel syndrome*, 3rd ed. Philadelphia: WB Saunders, 2001;282–303.

98. Wilmore DW, Shabert JK. Role of glutamine in immunologic responses. *Nutrition* 1998;14:618–626.

99. Avenell A. Glutamine in critical care: current evidence from systematic reviews. *Proc Nutr Soc* 2006;65:236–241.

100. Ziegler TR, Bazargan N, Leader LM, et al. Glutamine and the gastrointestinal tract. *Curr Opin Clin Nutr Metab Care* 2000;3:355–362.

101. Griffiths RD. Glutamine: establishing clinical indications. *Curr Opin Clin Nutr Metab Care* 1999;2:177–182.

102. Schloerb PR. Immune-enhancing diets: products, components, and their rationales. *JPEN J Parenter Enteral Nutr* 2001;25:S3–S7.

103. De Bandt JP, Cynober LA. Amino acids with anabolic properties. *Curr Opin Clin Nutr Metab Care* 1998;1:263–272.

104. Stehle P, Zander J, Mertes N, et al. Effect of parenteral glutamine peptide supplements on muscle glutamine loss and nitrogen balance after major surgery. *Lancet* 1989;1:231–233.

105. Houdijk AP, Rijnsburger ER, Jansen J, et al. Randomised trial of glutamine-enriched enteral nutrition on infectious morbidity in patients with multiple trauma. *Lancet* 1998;352:772–776.

106. Griffiths RD, Jones C, Palmer TE. Six-month outcome of critically ill patients given glutamine-supplemented parenteral nutrition. *Nutrition* 1997;13:295–302.

107. Ziegler TR, Young LS, Benfell K, et al. Clinical and metabolic efficacy of glutamine-supplemented parenteral nutrition after bone marrow transplantation. A randomized, double-blind, controlled study. *Ann Intern Med* 1992;116:821–828.

108. Anderson PM, Ramsay NK, Shu XO, et al. Effect of low-dose oral glutamine on painful stomatitis during bone marrow transplantation. *Bone Marrow Transplant* 1998;22:339–344.

109. Yoshida S, Matsui M, Shirouzu Y, et al. Effects of glutamine supplements and radiochemotherapy on systemic immune and gut barrier function in patients with advanced esophageal cancer. *Ann Surg* 1998;227:485–491.

110. Wischmeyer PE. Glutamine: the first clinically relevant pharmacological regulator of heat shock protein expression. *Curr Opin Clin Nutr Metab Care* 2006;9:201–206.

111. Singleton KD, Serkova N, Beckey VE, et al. Glutamine attenuates lung injury and improves survival after sepsis: role of enhanced heat shock protein expression. *Crit Care Med* 2005;33:1206–1213.

112. Ziegler TR, Ogden LG, Singleton KD, et al. Parenteral glutamine increases serum heat shock protein 70 in critically ill patients. *Intensive Care Med* 2005;31:1079–1086.

113. Barbul A, Lazarou SA, Efron DT, et al. Arginine enhances wound healing and lymphocyte immune responses in humans. *Surgery* 1990;108:331–336. discussion 336–337.

114. Evoy D, Lieberman MD, Fahey TJ III, et al. Immunonutrition: the role of arginine. *Nutrition* 1998;14:611–617.

115. Cynober L, Boucher JL, Vasson M-P. Arginine metabolism in mammals. *J Nutr Biochem* 1995;6:402–413.

116. Beale RJ, Bryg DJ, Bihari DJ. Immunonutrition in the critically ill: a systematic review of clinical outcome. *Crit Care Med* 1999;27:2799–2805.

117. Heys SD, Walker LG, Smith I, et al. Enteral nutritional supplementation with key nutrients in patients with critical illness and cancer: a meta-analysis of randomized controlled clinical trials. *Ann Surg* 1999;229:467–477.

118. Rombeau JL, Roldandelli RH. Clinical nutrition: parenteral nutrition. In: Ikizler TA, Hakim RM, ed. *Renal failure and parenteral nutrition*, 3rd ed. Philadelphia: WB Saunders, 2001;366–391.

119. American Society for Parenteral and Enteral Nutrition. Guidelines for the use of parenteral and enteral nutrition in adult and pediatric patients. American Society for Parenteral and Enteral Nutrition. *JPEN J Parenter Enteral Nutr* 1993;17:1SA–52SA.

120. Kopple JD. The nutrition management of the patient with acute renal failure. *JPEN J Parenter Enteral Nutr* 1996;20:3–12.

121. Barton RG, Wells CL, Carlson A, et al. Dietary omega-3 fatty acids decrease mortality and Kupffer cell prostaglandin E2 production in a rat model of chronic sepsis. *J Trauma* 1991;31:768–773. discussion 773–764.

122. Karlstad MD, DeMichele SJ, Leathem WD, et al. Effect of intravenous lipid emulsions enriched with gamma-linolenic acid on plasma n-6 fatty acids and prostaglandin biosynthesis after burn and endotoxin injury in rats. *Crit Care Med* 1993;21:1740–1749.

123. Mancuso P, Whelan J, DeMichele SJ, et al. Dietary fish oil and fish and borage oil suppress intrapulmonary proinflammatory eicosanoid biosynthesis and attenuate pulmonary neutrophil accumulation in endotoxic rats. *Crit Care Med* 1997;25:1198–1206.

124. Gadek JE, DeMichele SJ, Karlstad MD, et al. Effect of enteral feeding with eicosapentaenoic acid, gamma-linolenic acid, and antioxidants in patients with acute respiratory distress syndrome. Enteral Nutrition in ARDS Study Group. *Crit Care Med* 1999;27:1409–1420.

125. Nelson JL, DeMichele SJ, Pacht ER, et al. Effect of enteral feeding with eicosapentaenoic acid, gamma-linolenic acid, and antioxidants on antioxidant status in patients with acute respiratory distress syndrome. *JPEN J Parenter Enteral Nutr* 2003;27:98–104.

126. Pacht ER, DeMichele SJ, Nelson JL, et al. Enteral nutrition with eicosapentaenoic acid, gamma-linolenic acid, and antioxidants reduces alveolar inflammatory mediators and protein influx in patients with acute respiratory distress syndrome. *Crit Care Med* 2003;31:491–500.

127. Mayer K, Gokorsch S, Fegbeutel C, et al. Parenteral nutrition with fish oil modulates cytokine response in patients with sepsis. *Am J Respir Crit Care Med* 2003;167:1321–1328.

128. Sidery MB, Macdonald IA, Blackshaw PE. Superior mesenteric artery blood flow and gastric emptying in humans and the differential effects of high fat and high carbohydrate meals. *Gut* 1994;35:186–190.

129. Rombeau Jl, Roldandelli RH. Clinical nutrition: parenteral nutrition. In: Driscoll EF, Adolph M, Bristrian BR, ed. *Lipid emulsions in parenteral nutrition*, 3rd ed. Philadelphia: WB Saunders, 2001;35–39.

130. Peters AL, Davidson MB. Effects of various enteral feeding products on postprandial blood glucose response in patients with type I diabetes. *JPEN J Parenter Enteral Nutr* 1992;16:69–74.

131. Printz H, Recke B, Fehmann HC, et al. No apparent benefit of liquid formula diet in NIDDM. *Exp Clin Endocrinol Diabetes* 1997;105:134–139.

132. James JH, Ziparo V, Jeppsson B, et al. Hyperammonaemia, plasma aminoacid imbalance, and blood-brain aminoacid transport: a unified theory of portal-systemic encephalopathy. *Lancet* 1979;2:772–775.

133. Fraser CL, Arieff AI. Hepatic encephalopathy. *N Engl J Med* 1985;313:865–873.

134. Freund H, Dienstag J, Lehrich J, et al. Infusion of branched-chain enriched amino acid solution in patients with hepatic encephalopathy. *Ann Surg* 1982;196:209–220.

135. Proceedings from summit on Immune-enhancing enteral therapy. May 25-26, 2000, San Diego, California, USA. *Jpen J Parenter Rnteral Nutr* 2001;25:51–63.

136. Saffle JR, Wiebke G, Jennings K, et al. Randomized trial of immune-enhancing enteral nutrition in burn patients. *J Trauma* 1997;42:793–800. discussion 800–792.

137. Heyland DK, Novak F, Drover JW, et al. Should immunonutrition become routine in critically ill patients? A systematic review of the evidence. *JAMA* 2001;286:944–953.

138. Montejo JC, Zarazaga A, Lopez-Martinez J, et al. Immunonutrition in the intensive care unit. A systematic review and consensus statement. *Clin Nutr* 2003;22:221–233.

139. Waitzberg DL, Saito H, Plank LD, et al. Postsurgical infections are reduced with specialized nutrition support. *World J Surg* 2006;30:1592–1604.

140. Correia MI, Nicoli JR. The role of probiotics in gastrointestinal surgery. *Curr Opin Clin Nutr Metab Care* 2006;9:618–621.

141. Anderson AD, McNaught CE, Jain PK, et al. Randomised clinical trial of synbiotic therapy in elective surgical patients. *Gut* 2004;53:241–245.

142. Rayes N, Seehofer D, Muller AR, et al. Influence of probiotics and fibre on the incidence of bacterial infections following major abdominal surgery—results of a prospective trial. *Z Gastroenterol* 2002;40:869–876.

143. Cremonini F, Di Caro S, Nista EC,, et al. Meta-analysis: the effect of probiotic administration on antibiotic-associated diarrhoea. *Aliment Pharmacol Ther* 2002;16:1461–1467.

144. D'Souza AL, Rajkumar C, Cooke J, et al. Probiotics in prevention of antibiotic associated diarrhoea: meta-analysis. *BMJ* 2002;324:1361.

145. Quigley EM, Quera R. Small intestinal bacterial overgrowth: roles of antibiotics, prebiotics, and probiotics. *Gastroenterology* 2006;130:S78–S90.

146. Minard G, Kudsk KA. Postoperative nutrition in surgery for major trauma. *Curr Opin Clin Nutr Metab Care* 1998;1:35–39.

147. Matarese LE, Gottschlich MM. Contemporary nutrition support practice. In: Skipper A, ed. *Principles of parenteral nutrition*, 1st ed. Philadelphia: WB Saunders, 1998;227–242.

148. Rombeau JL, Roldandelli RH. Clinical nutrition: parenteral nutrition. In: Kinney JM, ed. *History of Parenteral Nutrition, with Notes on Clinical Biology*, 3rd ed. Philadelphia: WB Saunders, 2001;1–20.

149. Health and Public Policy Committee, American College of Physicians. Perioperative parenteral nutrition. Health and Public Policy Committee, American College of Physicians. *Ann Intern Med* 1987;107:252–253.

150. Wilmore DW, Dudrick SJ. Growth and development of an infant receiving all nutrients exclusively by vein. *JAMA* 1968;203:860–864.

151. Pillar B, Perry S. Evaluating total parenteral nutrition: final report and statement of the Technology Assessment and Practice Guidelines Forum. *Nutrition* 1990;6:314–318.

152. Sitzmann JV, Pitt HA. The Patient Care Committee of the American Gastroenterological Association. Statement on guidelines for total parenteral nutrition. The Patient Care Committee of the American Gastroenterological Association. *Dig Dis Sci* 1989;34:489–496.

153. Deitch EA. Simple intestinal obstruction causes bacterial translocation in man. *Arch Surg* 1989;124:699–701.

154. Kotani J, Usami M, Nomura H, et al. Enteral nutrition prevents bacterial translocation but does not improve survival during acute pancreatitis. *Arch Surg* 1999;134:287–292.

155. King BK, Li J, Kudsk KA. A temporal study of TPN-induced changes in gut-associated lymphoid tissue and mucosal immunity. *Arch Surg* 1997;132:1303–1309.

156. Li J, Kudsk KA, Gocinski B, et al. Effects of parenteral and enteral nutrition on gut-associated lymphoid tissue. *J Trauma* 1995;39:44–51; discussion 51–42.

157. Xu D, Lu Q, Deitch EA. Elemental diet-induced bacterial translocation associated with systemic and intestinal immune suppression. *JPEN J Parenter Enteral Nutr* 1998;22:37–41.

158. Heyland DK, MacDonald S, Keefe L, et al. Total parenteral nutrition in the critically ill patient: a meta-analysis. *JAMA* 1998;280:2013–2019.

159. Lipman TO. Grains or veins: is enteral nutrition really better than parenteral nutrition? A look at the evidence. *JPEN J Parenter Enteral Nutr* 1998;22:167–182.

160. Vernet O, Christin L, Schutz Y, et al. Enteral versus parenteral nutrition: comparison of energy metabolism in healthy subjects. *Am J Physiol* 1986;250:E47–E54.

161. Tappy L, Schwarz JM, Schneiter P, et al. Effects of isoenergetic glucose-based or lipid-based parenteral nutrition on glucose metabolism, de novo lipogenesis, and respiratory gas exchanges in critically ill patients. *Crit Care Med* 1998;26:860–867.

162. Moore FA, Moore EE, Jones TN, et al. TEN versus TPN following major abdominal trauma-reduced septic morbidity. *J Trauma* 1989;29:916–922; discussion 922–913.

163. Murry MJ. Parenteral Nutrition. *Curr Opin Gastroenterol* 1996;12:183–189.

164. Wolfe RR. Herman Award Lecture, 1996: relation of metabolic studies to clinical nutrition-the example of burn injury. *Am J Clin Nutr* 1996;64:800–808.

165. Koea JB, Wolfe RR, Shaw JH. Total energy expenditure during total parenteral nutrition: ambulatory patients at home versus patients with sepsis in surgical intensive care. *Surgery* 1995;118:54–62.

166. Brennan MF, Pisters PW, Posner M, et al. A prospective randomized trial of total parenteral nutrition after major pancreatic resection for malignancy. *Ann Surg* 1994;220:436–441. discussion 441–434.

167. Khaodhiar L, McCowen K, Bistrian B. Perioperative hyperglycemia, infection or risk? *Curr Opin Clin Nutr Metab Care* 1999;2:79–82.

168. Rosmarin DK, Wardlaw GM, Mirtallo J. Hyperglycemia associated with high, continuous infusion rates of total parenteral nutrition dextrose. *Nutr Clin Pract* 1996;11:151–156.

169. Lev-Ran A, Johnson M, Hwang DL, et al. Double-blind study of glycerol vs glucose in parenteral nutrition of postsurgical insulin-treated diabetic patients. *JPEN J Parenter Enteral Nutr* 1987;11:271–274.

170. Waxman K, Day AT, Stellin GP, et al. Safety and efficacy of glycerol and amino acids in combination with lipid emulsion for peripheral parenteral nutrition support. *JPEN J Parenter Enteral Nutr* 1992;16:374–378.

171. Abbott WC, Grakauskas AM, Bistrian BR, et al. Metabolic and respiratory effects of continuous and discontinuous lipid infusions. Occurrence in excess of resting energy expenditure. *Arch Surg* 1984;119:1367–1371.

172. Fan ST, Lo CM, Lai EC, et al. Perioperative nutritional support in patients undergoing hepatectomy for hepatocellular carcinoma. *N Engl J Med* 1994;331:1547–1552.

173. Bower RH, Muggia-Sullam M, Vallgren S, et al. Branched chain amino acid-enriched solutions in the septic patient. A randomized, prospective trial. *Ann Surg* 1986;203:13–20.

174. Cerra FB, Mazuski JE, Chute E, et al. Branched chain metabolic support. A prospective, randomized, double-blind trial in surgical stress. *Ann Surg* 1984;199:286–291.

175. Freund H, Hoover HC Jr, Atamian S, et al. Infusion of the branched chain amino acids in postoperative patients. Anticatabolic properties. *Ann Surg* 1979;190:18–23.

176. von Meyenfeldt MF, Soeters PB, Vente JP, et al. Effect of branched chain amino acid enrichment of total parenteral

nutrition on nitrogen sparing and clinical outcome of sepsis and trauma: a prospective randomized double blind trial. *Br J Surg* 1990;77:924–929.

177. Yu YM, Wagner DA, Walesreswski JC, et al. A kinetic study of leucine metabolism in severely burned patients. Comparison between a conventional and branched-chain amino acid-enriched nutritional therapy. *Ann Surg* 1988;207:421–429.

178. Furst P. New parenteral substrates in clinical nutrition. Part I. Introduction. New substrates in protein nutrition. *Eur J Clin Nutr* 1994;48:607–616.

179. Morlion BJ, Stehle P, Wachtler P, et al. Total parenteral nutrition with glutamine dipeptide after major abdominal surgery: a randomized, double-blind, controlled study. *Ann Surg* 1998;227:302–308.

180. Zheng YM, Li F, Zhang MM, et al. Glutamine dipeptide for parenteral nutrition in abdominal surgery: a meta-analysis of randomized controlled trials. *World J Gastroenterol* 2006;12:7537–7541.

181. Starker PM, LaSala PA, Forse RA, et al. Response to total parenteral nutrition in the extremely malnourished patient. *J Parenter Enteral Nutr* 1985;9:300–302.

182. Nutrition Advisory Group. Multivitamin preparations for parenteral use. A statement by the Nutrition Advisory Group. American Medical Association Department of Foods and Nutrition, 1975. *J Parenter Enteral Nutr* 1979;3:258–262.

183. Nutrition Advisory Group. Guidelines for essential trace element preparations for parenteral use. A statement by the Nutrition Advisory Group. American Medical Association. *J Parenter Enteral Nutr* 1979;3:263–267.

184. Forceville X, Vitoux D, Gauzit R, et al. Selenium, systemic immune response syndrome, sepsis, and outcome in critically ill patients. *Crit Care Med* 1998;26:1536–1544.

185. Driscoll DF. Total nutrient admixtures: theory and practice. *Nutr Clin Pract* 1995;10:114–119.

186. Ryan JA Jr, Abel RM, Abbott WM, et al. Catheter complications in total parenteral nutrition. A prospective study of 200 consecutive patients. *N Engl J Med* 1974;290:757–761.

CHAPTER 6

Wound Healing: Normal and Abnormal Mechanisms and Closure Techniques

Subhas Gupta and W. Thomas Lawrence

In the recent past, there has been a very significant expansion of knowledge relating to the underlying pathophysiology of the body's response to injury. This has provided an improved platform for understanding what needs to be done to heal wounds and minimize the problems of scarring. This chapter will review the mechanisms of normal wound healing and explore the alterations in this process that produces abnormal wound healing, including chronic wounds and abnormal scarring.

Records of the nature and treatment of wounds have existed since the earliest documents. Unlike less complex organisms, humans lack the ability to regenerate lost or damaged tissues. For man in the ancient world, the ability to heal a wound was indispensable to survival. One of the oldest manuscripts is a clay tablet that dates back to approximately 2200 BC. The tablet describes the three healing "gestures" from the opening quotation (1). The gestures appear in ancient records recovered from widely separated civilizations. Much of the history of wound healing and most major advances fall into the realm of one of these three interventions:

1. **Wash the wound**—cleansing the wound to remove debris and control bacterial colonization.
2. **Make plasters**—applying dressings to protect the wound from infection and enhance the healing environment.
3. **Bandage the wound**—covering the wound to protect it from reinjury and to prevent excessive bleeding.

To execute any of these interventions effectively requires a thorough understanding of the phases of wound healing and the factors that affect its progress.

PHASES OF HEALING

The healing process can be broken down into early, intermediate, late, and terminal phases. Specific biologic processes characterize each phase. The primary activities involved in the early phase of healing are inflammation and the creation of hemostasis. Mesenchymal cell proliferation and migration, epithelialization, and angiogenesis are the primary events of the intermediate phase. Central events of the late phase of healing include the synthesis of collagen and other matrix proteins and wound contraction. The terminal phase of healing is characterized by wound remodeling. Each of these phases will be discussed as a separate entity although the phases blend from one to another with no clear boundaries between them (Fig. 6.1).

Early Wound Healing Events

In all injuries that penetrate the epidermis, blood vessels are disrupted, resulting in hemorrhage. Hemostasis must be the first event achieved in the healing process. Cellular damage occurs with any injury, and this initiates an inflammatory

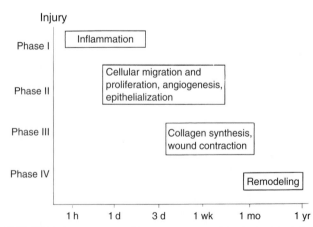

FIGURE 6.1 Sequence of events in wound healing. (Modified from Stevenson TR, Mathes SJ. Wound healing. In: Miller TA, ed. *Physiologic basis of modern surgical care.* St. Louis: CV Mosby, 1988:1011.)

response. The inflammatory response triggers events that have implications for the entire healing process.

Hemostasis is created primarily by aggregated platelets and fibrin. In normal blood vessels with intact endothelial linings, endothelial products such as prostacyclin as well as other proteins limit clot formation (2). However, when the endothelial lining is disrupted, platelet aggregation is stimulated by exposure to collagen (3,4) and other intravascular and extravascular proteins. Platelets adhere to collagen and release adenosine diphosphate (ADP), which, in the presence of calcium, stimulates further platelet aggregation. Thrombin produced by the coagulation cascade and fatty acids released by injured cells also contribute to continuing platelet aggregation (5). Platelet adhesion to other platelets and to subendothelial proteins is mediated primarily by fibrinogen and von Willebrand factor although other proteins such as thrombospondin, fibronectin, vitronectin and laminin may also be involved (2). These factors derive from both the serum and the α granules of platelets (6).

Platelet aggregation also leads to the release of cytokines that reside in the α granules. These include platelet-derived growth factor (PDGF), transforming growth factor (TGF-α), TGF-β fibroblast growth factor-2 (FGF-2) and platelet-derived epidermal growth factor (EGF). Cytokines are proteins that mediate cellular function by binding receptors located on cell membranes. Different cytokines have different biologic effects. Some cytokines can stimulate a variety of different cellular activities depending on their concentration and the cells to which they bind. They play critical roles in later aspects of healing.

The intrinsic and extrinsic coagulation cascades are triggered by separate events (7). The intrinsic coagulation pathway is initiated by activation of factor XII, and is not essential, in that individuals deficient in factor XII clot normally. The alternative extrinsic coagulation pathway is initiated by exposure to tissue factor, which binds factor VII or VIIa and is essential for normal clotting. Tissue factor is not found in vascular endothelial cells but is found in abundance on subendothelial cellular surfaces, particularly in adventitial fibroblasts. Both pathways result in the production of thrombin, which catalyzes the conversion of fibrinogen to fibrin. In addition to contributing to hemostasis, both thrombin and fibrin contribute to other aspects of wound healing. Thrombin contributes to the increased vascular permeability seen after injury and also facilitates the extravascular migration of inflammatory cells (7,8). It may also have a role in both epithelialization and angiogenesis.

Fibrin is one of the primary components of the provisional matrix that forms in a wound soon after it is created. Fibrin, along with fibronectin that becomes bound to it, forms a lattice that provides a scaffold for the migration of inflammatory, endothelial, and mesenchymal cells. Fibronectin is produced by fibroblasts and epithelial cells (9). It is found in plasma and in connective tissue, and it has a variety of functions. Primarily, it aids in cellular attachment and modulates the migration of various cell types

into the wound (10–12). Fibronectin includes approximately a dozen binding sites (13). These binding sites recognize integrins on the surface of different cells. The binding of cell surface integrins with fibronectin allows cells to attach to the lattice and subsequently pull themselves through the lattice as they migrate to sites where they are needed. The fibrin–fibronectin lattice also binds cytokines released at the time of injury and serves as a reservoir for these factors as healing progresses (14). In addition, fibrin has direct effects on inflammatory cells, and its breakdown products are a stimulus to angiogenesis.

Hunter described the physical signs of inflammation initially in 1794; they include erythema, edema, pain, and heat. These signs are largely a result of changes that occur in the microcirculation, particularly in the 15 to 20 μ in diameter micro venules. Immediately after injury, intense local vasoconstriction of arterioles and capillaries occurs, which contributes to hemostasis and produces blanching in the wounded area. This process is mediated by circulating catecholamines (epinephrine) and the sympathetic nervous system (norepinephrine) and prostaglandins released by injured cells. Vasoconstriction reverses after 10 to 15 minutes and is replaced by vasodilation. Vasodilation generates erythema and heat in the area of injury. Vasodilation is mediated by histamine, kinins, prostaglandins (15), and possibly additional factors such as leukotrienes (16) and endothelial cell products (17,18). Mast cells in connective tissue are the primary source of histamine (19), which directly increases vascular permeability and indirectly causes vasodilation through stimulation of prostaglandin synthesis (20). Mast cells also release heparin, several enzymes, and a tumor necrosis factor (TNF)-like peptide. The kinins are a family of peptides with nine amino acids that act predominantly as short-term vasodilators. They are released from protein-binding molecules by activation of kallikrein, another by-product of the clotting cascade. PGE_1 and PGE_2 are the prostaglandins that increase capillary permeability. Prostaglandins affect vasodilatation through activation of adenyl cyclase and production of cyclic adenosine monophosphate (cAMP) (21). Prostaglandins accumulate in injured tissue, probably from activation of phospholipases located on injured cell membranes. Phospholipase activity causes arachidonic acid release and the subsequent induction of prostaglandin synthetase.

As suggested earlier, several factors including histamine and prostaglandins are involved in stimulating both gap formation between endothelial cells resulting in increased vascular permeability and vasodilation. Other factors such as some neutrophil-derived factors only contribute to gap formation (22,23). Plasma passively leaks through the gaps from the intravascular space to the extravascular compartment (24–26). Plasma proteins such as albumin, and globulin bind to the provisional matrix forming in the wound. Leukocytes migrate into wounded tissues through an active phenomenon known as *diapedesis*. They initially loosely adhere to endothelial cells lining capillaries in a process mediated by selectins (27). They then roll along the capillary walls before finally becoming firmly adherent to endothelial cells through a process involving integrins on the leukocyte surface and intercellular adhesion molecules (ICAMs) on the endothelial cells. The cells then actively migrate between endothelial cells into the wounded tissues. Chemotaxis is the movement of an organism or cell in response to a chemical concentration gradient. A substance that can stimulate a cell to migrate in this manner is known as a *chemotactic agent* for that cell type. Chemotactic agents contribute to the migration of leukocytes into the extravascular space.

The migration of cells and fluid into the injured area generates edema. Alterations in pH resulting from breakdown products of tissue and bacteria, along with swelling and decreased tissue oxygenation from damage to the blood supply, produce the pain noted in areas of injury.

Neutrophils, macrophages, and lymphocytes are leukocytes involved in the inflammatory response to injury. Bacterial products (28), complement factors (29,30), histamine (31), PGE_2, leukotriene (32), and PDGF (33) are chemotactic for leukocytes. Neutrophils, also known as *polymorphonuclear* (PMN) leukocytes, are the first of the leukocytes to be found in wounded tissue in large numbers. Neutrophils function as defensive units that engulf foreign material and digest it through the action of hydrolytic enzymes. After phagocytosing damaged tissue or bacteria, neutrophils are either phagocytosed by macrophages or die, releasing oxygen radicals and destructive enzymes into the wound. The release of these inflammatory mediators further propagates the inflammatory response. Neutrophils do not appear to have a role in the subsequent events of healing in an uncomplicated wound.

As monocytes migrate from the capillaries into the extravascular space, they transform into macrophages in a process mediated by serum factors (34,35) and fibronectin (36). Chemotactic factors then stimulate the migration of macrophages throughout the wounded area (37–43). Macrophages are tremendously important in normal wound healing (44). Macrophages phagocytose bacteria and dead tissue and also secrete matrix metalloproteinases (MMPs) that break down damaged matrix (45,46). Macrophages are a primary source of cytokines that stimulate fibroblast proliferation, collagen production, and other healing processes. Macrophages may be the most important cells in the healing process.

Lymphocytes produce factors essential for normal healing (47) in addition to functioning as immunoreactants involved in cellular immunity and antibody production. Subsets of T lymphocytes appear to be most involved in the healing process (48). Heparin-binding EGF and a form of basic FGF may be the critical lymphokines (49,50) although a variety of other lymphokines are produced. Interleukin 2(IL-2) and other factors have been demonstrated to be chemotactic for lymphocytes (51,52).

In normal healing, changes that occur in tissue over time are extremely reproducible. After hemostasis has been accomplished, inflammatory cells migrate into the wound, with neutrophils initially predominating. At 48 to 72 hours, macrophages begin to outnumber neutrophils. Large numbers of macrophages remain in the wound for several days. This is critical in that macrophages (53), unlike neutrophils (54), are essential for normal healing. After 5 to 7 days, few inflammatory cells remain in normal healing wounds (Fig. 6.2).

Foreign material or bacteria can change a scenario of normal healing into one of chronic inflammation. Although the acute phases of inflammation are necessary, the persistence of inflammation can be deleterious to the host (55). As mentioned, neutrophils release destructive proteolytic enzymes and generate free oxygen radicals, which damage tissue. A fibrous capsule isolating the process eventually surrounds an area of foreign material and/or chronic bacterial infection. These encapsulated areas of chronic inflammation are known as *granulomas*.

Intermediate Wound Healing Events

Intermediate wound healing events include mesenchymal cell chemotaxis, mesenchymal cell proliferation, angiogenesis, and epithelialization. These processes predominate 2 to 4 days after wounding and are all mediated by cytokines.

Fibroblasts are the primary mesenchymal cell involved in wound healing, although smooth muscle cells are also involved. Fibroblasts normally reside in dermis and are

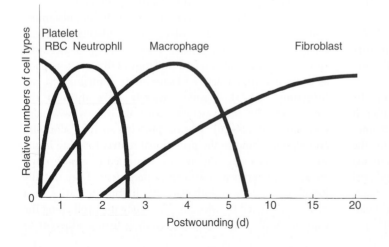

FIGURE 6.2 Cellular phase of wound healing. Relative concentrations of various cellular components versus time in the healing wound. RBC, red blood cell.

damaged by wounding. Undifferentiated mesenchymal cells in the area may subsequently differentiate into fibroblasts when stimulated by macrophage products secreted into the wound (56). Additional fibroblasts migrate to the wounded area under the influence of chemotactic factors. PDGF has been demonstrated to be chemotactic for both fibroblasts (57) and smooth muscle cells (58). Fibronectin (59–61), EGF (62), and other substances (63,64) have also been demonstrated to be chemotactic for fibroblasts. Fibroblasts have the capacity to secrete matrix MMPs including collagenase or (MMP-1), gelatinase (MMP-2) and stromelysin (MMP-3) when needed to break down matrix impeding their migration.

The mesenchymal cell population in a wound is augmented further by proliferation of both resident and newly arrived cells. PDGF is a potent mitogenic stimulant for both fibroblasts and smooth muscle cells (65,66). TGF-β is another important stimulant of fibroblast proliferation (67, 68). Mesenchymal cell proliferation can also be stimulated by additional cytokines including TNF, IL-1, lymphokines (69), insulin, and insulin-like growth factor (IGF) (70,71).

Angiogenesis reconstructs the vasculature in areas where it has been damaged by wounding and is stimulated by high lactate levels, acidic pH, and decreased oxygen tension in the tissue. Small capillary sprouts initially develop on venules at the periphery of the devascularized area (72). As capillary sprouts grow with endothelial cell proliferation, the cells develop a curvature that results in a lumen. The capillary sprouts continue to grow until they contact other sprouts growing from other directions. The sprouts then interconnect, forming a vascular loop, and the sprouting process begins anew.

Endothelial cell migration and tube formation are facilitated by changes in matrix (73,74). Cytokines directly and indirectly stimulate the endothelial cell migration and proliferation required for angiogenesis. Many of these are derived from macrophages (75–77). Basic FGF, also known as *Fibroblast growth factor-1* (FGF-1), is the most potent angiogenic stimulant identified (78); heparin is an important cofactor for this growth factor (79). Vascular endothelial growth factor (80) is becoming increasingly recognized as an additional critical angiogenic stimulant. TGF-α, TGF-β (81), wound fluids (82,83), prostaglandins, adipocyte lipids (84), and other factors (85–87) have also been demonstrated to stimulate angiogenesis. Stimulatory cytokines diminish in number when the wounded area is completely revascularized. This flux in angiogenic factors may stimulate maturation of the vascular system (88).

The epidermis provides a barrier between the external environment and internal milieu. It prevents the entry of hostile elements from the environment and the escape of fluid and electrolytes. Epithelial cells in the epidermis must constantly regenerate to survive continuing insults from the external environment. The gastrointestinal, genitourinary, and respiratory systems also have epithelial linings that serve a similar function.

The epidermis is composed of multiple layers of epithelial cells superficial to the dermis. The first layer above the dermis is the basal layer composed of more basaloid cells. The cells become more elongated as they progress through the different epithelial layers to the most superficial stratum corneum. The stratum corneum consists primarily of dead cells and keratin. After injury, the process of epithelial renewal is called *epithelialization*. Epithelialization is particularly important in the healing of partial thickness wounds, such as abrasions or superficial burns, although it plays a role in the healing of all wounds. Partial thickness wounds are those in which the epidermis and a portion of the dermis are damaged while some dermis is preserved. Epithelial cells involved in the closure of partial thickness wounds derive from both the wound edges and epithelial appendages, such as hair follicles, sweat glands, and sebaceous glands in the more central portions of the wound. These appendages extend into the underlying dermis and subcutaneous tissues and persist in partial thickness injuries (89). In contrast, epithelialization in an incisional wound involves cellular migration over a distance of less than a millimeter from one side of the incision to the other. Incisional wounds generally are re-epithelialized completely in 24 to 48 hours.

The sequence of events that comprise epithelialization include cellular detachment, migration, proliferation, and differentiation (90). In the first 24 hours after injury, thickening of the basal cell layer begins. Marginal basal cells then elongate, detach from the underlying basement membrane, and migrate into the wound. They migrate essentially as a monolayer across the denuded area. Migrating basal cells usually orient themselves along collagen fibers and exhibit what is called *contact guidance* (91). The cells generate a provisional basement membrane including fibronectin, vitronectin and collagens type I and V if the normal basement membrane has been damaged in order to facilitate migration (92). Laminin and type IV collagen, two normally important basement membrane components, are not seen during this migratory period. They can also produce matrix MMPs if needed to facilitate their migration. Basal cells at the edge of the denuded area begin to divide 48 to 72 hours after injury (93,94). Epithelial cell proliferation contributes new cells to the advancing epithelial monolayer. Cells migrate until they reach cells migrating from a different direction. At that point, "contact inhibition" is reestablished, and migration ceases. Cells of the monolayer then differentiate into more basal-like cells with hemidesmosomes that bind them more firmly to the basement membrane (95). Cellular proliferation continues in the new basal cells as a multilayered epidermis is reestablished (96). Subsequently, new surface cells begin to keratinize. EGF stimulates the migration and proliferation of epithelial cells (97,98). TGF-β stimulates epithelial migration, although it slows epithelial proliferation. Keratinocyte growth factor (KGF), also known as *fibroblast growth factor-7* (FGF-7), is another potent stimulant of epithelialization (99).

Unfortunately, regenerated epithelium does not retain all of the functional advantages of normal epithelium. There are fewer basal cells in regenerated epidermis, and the interface between epidermis and dermis is abnormal (90). Rete pegs, undulating projections of epidermis that penetrate papillary dermis, are not found on re-epithelialized surfaces (100). The epithelium is thicker at the wound edge than in the midportion of a re-epithelialized area.

Late Wound Healing Events

Fibroplasia is the production of fibrous protein in the wound. Collagen makes up 25% of all body proteins and more than 50% of the protein found in scar tissue (101). Collagen is synthesized primarily by fibroblasts in a complex process that begins 3 to 5 days after injury. The rate of collagen synthesis increases rapidly and continues at an accelerated rate for 2 to 4 weeks in most wounds. As more and more collagen is synthesized, it gradually replaces fibrin as the primary structural matrix element in the wound. After 4 weeks, collagen synthesis rates decline, eventually balancing the rate of collagen destruction by collagenase. Age, tension, pressure (102), and stress (103) affect the rate of collagen synthesis. TGF-β stimulates collagen synthesis (104), whereas glucocorticoids inhibit it (105).

At least 19 types of collagen have been described, with slight differences in their component polypeptide chains. Type I is most common. It can be isolated from virtually all tissues. Type I collagen makes up 80% to 90% of collagen in skin, with the remaining 10% to 20% being type III. Increased levels of type III collagen are seen embryonically and in early phases of wound healing. Type V predominates in smooth muscle. Types II and XI are seen primarily in cartilage, whereas type IV is seen predominantly in basement membranes. The remaining collagen types are found in small quantities in specific parts of the body.

The molecular inscription for type I collagen is found on chromosome 17 (106,107). Collagen consists of three polypeptide chains that are individually synthesized in a manner similar to other proteins. Each chain is twisted into a right-handed helix. The alignment of three of these chains into a triple helix is facilitated by nonhelical terminal peptide sequences. The chains align themselves in the characteristic triple helix configuration within the endoplasmic reticulum. The aggregate of three peptide chains is subsequently twisted into a left-handed superhelix (108). Most polypeptide chains used in collagen assembly are α chains. Every third amino acid residue of α chains is glycine, and this structure facilitates helix formation. The α chains are further subtyped into α_1, α_2, and $\alpha3$ according to variations in other residues.

Another critical component of collagen synthesis is the hydroxylation of lysine and proline moieties within the polypeptide chains. This process occurs in the endoplasmic reticulum. Hydroxylysine is required for covalent cross-link formation. Hydroxyproline is found almost exclusively in collagen and serves as a marker of the quantity of collagen in tissue. This hydroxylation process requires specific enzymes for lysine and proline and, in addition, requires as cofactors oxygen, vitamin C, α-ketoglutarate,

and ferrous iron. Deficiencies in vitamin C, oxygen, or suppression of enzymatic activity by corticosteroids may lead to underhydroxylated collagen, which is incapable of generating strong cross-links and is broken down easily.

After the collagen molecule is synthesized, it is secreted into the extracellular space. Galactosyl-glucose is linked enzymatically to hydroxylysine residues within the molecule and probably contributes to the transport of synthesized collagen across the plasma membrane (109). When collagen is secreted into the extracellular space, it appears in the form of procollagen. Procollagen can be identified by persistent nonhelical extensions of the α chains. This linear extension, or registration peptide, interferes with the subsequent aggregation of collagen molecules into fibrils. Successful cleavage of the registration peptide by specific enzymes yields a collagen molecule, which can aggregate into collagen fibrils. Fibril formation is facilitated by proteoglycans in the extracellular matrix.

A transverse section of a fibril generally demonstrates four to five molecules aligned in a staggered manner. Electron microscopy demonstrates a banding pattern in the fibrils with a bandwidth of 640 Å (110). This pattern is produced by the overlap of individual molecules in a specific manner determined by electrostatic bonds that form between charged areas of molecules. Approximately 25% of the length of consecutive molecules overlaps.

As mentioned, individual polypeptide chains within the collagen molecule are held together by intramolecular cross-links. Intermolecular cross-links form between separate collagen molecules. The initial bonds formed both between individual polypeptide chains and between molecules are electrostatic. These are replaced eventually by covalent bonds, which are formed as a Schiff base reaction (111). Covalent bonding of collagen molecules is initiated by lysyl oxidase, an enzyme that causes deamination of the terminal NH group on the side chain of lysine (112). Oxidation at this site forms an aldehyde group. Neighboring aldehyde groups from parallel peptide chains form a covalent bond through an aldol condensation (113). A Schiff base reaction can occur between residues of lysine to lysine, lysine to hydroxylysine, or hydroxylysine to hydroxylysine. The strongest cross-links are formed between two hydroxylysine residues. Therefore, the strongest collagen molecules are found where the density of hydroxylysine is the greatest (114).

Unaggregated collagen molecules are soluble in cold saline. Fibril formation decreases the solubility of collagen (31) as a result of these intermolecular bonds, and dilute acid is generally required to solubilize aggregated tropocollagen. Strong acid and high temperatures are needed to solubilize maturely cross-linked collagen.

The extracellular connective tissue matrix contains components other than collagen, including proteoglycans, attachment proteins such as fibronectin, and elastin. Proteoglycans consist of a protein core covalently linked to a glycosaminoglycan (GAG) (115). Proteoglycans are synthesized primarily by fibroblasts. Chondroitin sulfate, dermatan sulfate, heparin, heparin sulfate, keratan sulfate, and hyaluronic acid are the more common proteoglycans. The biologic functions of proteoglycans are less well understood than those of collagen. They generally anchor specific proteins in certain locations and affect the biologic activity of target proteins. These processes often involve interactions with cytokines whose function proteoglycans can potentiate. Heparin, for example, is an important cofactor for basic FGF during angiogenesis. Other GAGs may impact the healing process in a similar manner by modulating the effects of different cytokines. It may also directly influence cellular activity including the direct stimulation of cellular proliferation. Hyaluronan may be a particularly important GAG (116). It is a prominent component of both early and mature wound matrix. It contributes to skin viscoelasticity in that is extremely hygroscopic, and it modulates the migration of a variety of cell types.

Attachment proteins, such as fibronectin, are critical components of the mature matrix as well as the provisional matrix that initially forms after wounding. As mentioned, a variety of cell types synthesize it. Elastin is a third component of the connective tissue matrix; however, it is not synthesized in response to injury. Normal skin has elastic properties that scar lacks due to the lack of elastin in scar.

Wound Contraction

Wound contraction, lsuch as collagen synthesis, begins approximately 4 to 5 days after wounding. Wound contraction represents the centripetal movement of the wound edge toward the center of the wound. Maximal wound contraction continues for 12 to 15 days, although it will continue for longer periods if the wound remains open. The wound edges move toward each other at an average rate of 0.6 to 0.75 mm/d. The rate of contraction depends on tissue laxity with great variability among tissues. A wound in the buttock, where the tissue is loose, will contract much more than a wound on the scalp or pretibial area where the skin is tighter. The relative contribution of wound contraction to the healing process also varies depending on wound type. Wound contraction is a trivial component in the healing of a closed incisional wound, whereas it is a major contributor to the healing of a full thickness open wound.

Wound shape can also affect contraction. Wounds with square edges contract more rapidly than circular wounds. Forces of contraction in a circular wound cancel each other to some degree, preventing effective centripetal movement of the wound edge. It is important to create a circular wound for intestinal stomas to limit stenosis from wound contraction.

Wound contraction occurs to a greater extent in relatively immobile areas, such as the back, abdomen, and the midportion of extremities. Contraction of a large wound across a joint surface, however, can lead to a contracture. A contracture is a physical constriction limiting joint motion which results from wound contraction. Contractures are often seen as a result of burn wounds across the neck, axillae, and other joint surfaces that heal secondarily. Some animals have a separate anatomic layer, called the *panniculus carnosus*, which allows substantial wound contraction without contracture production. Humans do not have a well-defined panniculus carnosus, although the platysma muscle is an analogous structure.

Disagreement exists as to the mechanism by which wounds contract. Large numbers of myofibroblasts are found in wounds during wound contraction, and many feel they mediate the process. Myofibroblasts were first described by Gabbiani in 1971 (117). They can only be differentiated from other fibroblasts by electron microscopy. Their defining characteristics include microfilaments in their cytoplasm, a multilobulated nucleus, and abundant rough endoplasmic reticulum. They most likely derive from normal or undifferentiated primordial fibroblasts in the wound area. They first appear in wounds on day 3 after wounding and persist in large numbers until approximately day 21 postwounding (118). They are primarily found at the periphery of the wound, thereby generating the theory that they pull the wound edges together in a "picture frame" manner. The concept that the "picture frame" is the location of dynamic forces in contraction has been supported by experiments in which the central portion of healing wounds was excised in some wounds and the peripheral area in others (119). No effect on contraction was measured after central tissue excision, whereas wound contraction could be stopped completely by excising a peripheral picture frame strip.

Alternatively, experimental work in contracting collagen matrices has suggested that fibroblasts within the wound are primary contributors to wound contraction through interactions with surrounding matrix (120). Contraction in this model occurs as fibroblasts migrate through matrix and effectively retract collagen fibrils (121,122) in a serum-dependent process (123). Advocates of this theory suggest that myofibroblasts at the wound perimeter are merely fibroblasts with stress fibers in their cytoplasm. The stress fibers are prominent because the cells are in close proximity to each other at the wound edge where contraction has, for the most part, been completed and the cells are becoming apoptotic.

Additional work with collagen matrices suggests that fibroblasts exposed to mechanical stress elongate and demonstrate stress fibers in their cytoplasm, making them more myofibroblast-like. This observation may explain why more myofibroblasts or myofibroblast-like cells are seen in actual contracting wounds where there is more stress than in floating contracting lattices (124). As stress is relieved in contracting matrices, these cells differentiate to less active cells.

Contraction is a cell-directed process that requires cell division but not collagen synthesis. Radiation and cytolytic drugs delay contraction, adding further evidence that cellular activity is required. Collagen deposition may be involved in fixing the tissues in their final state, however. TGF-β can stimulate collagen lattice contraction and appears to be a mediator of wound contraction (125). It may also facilitate the transition of fibroblasts into myofibroblasts (126). PDGF can also stimulate contraction of matrices by a TGF-β

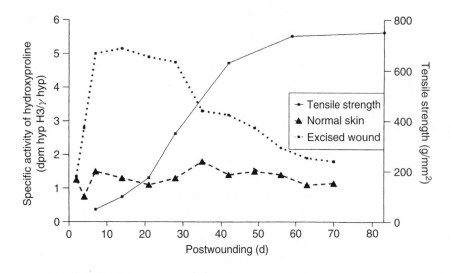

FIGURE 6.3 Graphs demonstrating collagen synthetic activity (specific activity of hydroxyproline) in healing wounds and unwounded skin at different time points and relating collagen synthetic activity to gain in tensile strength in wounds over time. (Reproduced with permission from Peacock EE Jr. *Wound repair*. 3rd ed. Philadelphia: WB Saunders, 1984:111.)

independent mechanism (127) whereas FGF (128) and interferon-γ (129) inhibit the process.

Although wound contraction cannot be eliminated, it can be limited. Full-thickness skin grafts (FTSGs) with a full complement of dermis can limit wound contraction to a greater degree than split-thickness skin grafts (STSGs) (130). Myofibroblasts disappear from the wound more quickly after a full-thickness skin graft than after an STSG. The timing of grafting is also important. Grafting early in the course of wound healing will prevent wound contraction to a greater degree than delayed grafting. Splints can temporarily slow wound contraction, although wound contraction will proceed at an accelerated rate after splint removal unless the splint is maintained until the wound healing process is essentially completed. Topical dressings may also delay wound contraction, although they will not prevent it. Pharmacologic manipulations to limit wound contraction have generally been unsuccessful, although in experimental models, smooth muscle antagonists have effectively inhibited wound contraction (131).

Terminal Wound Healing Event

Scar remodeling is the hallmark of the terminal period of healing. Approximately 21 days after injury, net accumulation of wound collagen becomes stable (132). Although collagen content is maximal at this point, bursting strength of the wound is only 15% of that of normal skin. The process of scar remodeling dramatically increases wound-bursting strength. The greatest rate of increase occurs between 3 and 6 weeks after wounding. By 6 weeks after wounding, the wound has reached 80% to 90% of its eventual strength (133) (Fig. 6.3). The bursting strength of scar never reaches that of unwounded skin, however, and it reaches a maximum of approximately 80% to 90% of skin breaking strength at 6 months.

During terminal wound healing, a continual turnover of collagen molecules occurs as old collagen is broken down by some of the matrix MMPs previously mentioned (134) and new collagen is synthesized in a denser, more organized

manner along stress lines (135). Other enzymes, such as hyaluronidase, are probably also involved in scar remodeling.

The matrix MMPs are a family of enzymes that break down proteins of different types. There are at least 25 different matrix MMPs (136,137). Different cell types produce slightly different enzymes and the different MMPs have different substrates. The activity of collagenolytic enzymes is modulated by one of four isoforms of tissue inhibitors of metalloproteinases (TIMPs) (138). The balance of MMP and TIMP activity is particularly important during the remodeling phase of healing (136).

During this period of scar remodeling, the number of intra- and intermolecular cross-links between collagen fibers increases dramatically. This increase in cross-linking is a major contributor to the increase in wound-breaking strength. As collagen matures during scar remodeling, the quantity of type III collagen decreases and is replaced by type I collagen. The quantity of water and GAGs in matrix decreases as well. The more mature matrix becomes less cellular through apoptosis of multiple cell types involved in the healing process. The mature matrix in the wounded area never obtains quite the level of organization that existed preinjury. Wound remodeling is visible to the surgeon as a change in the texture, thickness, and color of a healing wound. Remodeling continues over a period of approximately 12 months so that decisions regarding operative scar revision should not be made prematurely.

CYTOKINES/CHEMOKINES AND GROWTH FACTORS

Normal healing requires the successful completion of multiple coordinated biochemical and cellular functions that occur in a reproducible manner. Cytokines have emerged as primary mediators of most wound-healing events. The wound-healing process appears to be orchestrated by the carefully regulated release of specific cytokines at appropriate time intervals after injury. The term *growth factor* is often used interchangeably with cytokines, although technically, growth factors only stimulate cellular proliferation, whereas cytokines can mediate all types of cellular processes.

Cytokines can function in an endocrine, paracrine, autocrine, or intracrine manner. A factor functioning in an endocrine manner is released by a cell and affects a target cell at a distance. Endocrine factors are generally carried to the target cell through the bloodstream. Paracrine factors are released by one cell and affect a different cell in the same locale. Autocrine factors are released by a cell and affect the function of that same cell. Intracrine stimulation differs from the other modes of action in that it does not involve the extracellular release of the cytokine. The cytokine is released intracellularly and mediates function through internal binding (139). A given factor may mediate cellular activity in a variety of locations by acting on some cells in an endocrine manner and others in a paracrine or autocrine manner.

Cytokines have often been named for the cell of origin or a characteristic known about the factor when it was first described. Many of the names are misleading because they suggest that a polyfunctional factor has one function or that a factor is derived from only one cell type when many types of cells produce it. PDGF was named after the platelet from which it was originally discovered, although it has since been learned that multiple cell types produce it. TGF-β was named because *in vitro* studies suggested that the factor was capable of transforming normal cells into malignant ones, although it has since been learned that TGF-β is incapable of inducing malignant transformation.

Several factors determine whether a cytokine is involved in a particular cellular activity. First, it has to be released at the appropriate time and be available at the appropriate site in sufficient concentration. Second, the factor must not be broken down by proteolytic enzymes or bound to matrix. Third, affected cells must have receptors for the cytokine. Bound receptors primarily have direct kinase activity and facilitate the phosphorylation of proteins, which initiates a cascade of intracellular activities, eventually resulting in the stimulation of a cellular function. In some cases, the number of receptors bound is critical with a limited amount of binding producing one function, whereas a greater amount produces a different cellular function.

The functions of many of these cytokines have been discussed in previous sections. Growth factors that have been reasonably well characterized include EGF, PDGF, FGF, and TGF-β, although concepts regarding the relative importance of different cytokines have evolved with time. These factors will be discussed individually to clarify their sources, characteristics, and functions. Table 6.1 summarizes information regarding these factors and several additional ones.

Epidermal Growth Factor

EGF was the first cytokine described, and it was originally isolated from the salivary glands of mice. It is found in a wide variety of tissues, and most cells have its receptors (140).

Epithelial cells have the largest number of receptors, although large numbers are also present in endothelial cells, fibroblasts, and smooth muscle cells. EGF is a potent mitogenic stimulant for epithelial cells, endothelial cells, and fibroblasts, and it is chemotactic for epithelial cells and fibroblasts. It stimulates fibroplasia in wound chambers in addition to increasing collagenase activity (141), stimulating neovascularization (142), and fibronectin synthesis (143). TGF-α binds the same receptor as EGF and has similar biologic effects, as do other members of the EGF family such as heparin-binding EGF.

Fibroblast Growth Factor

FGF was originally discovered as a mitogen for mesenchymal cells and was secondarily found to be a primary stimulant of angiogenesis. The discovery of the molecule was followed by the identification of an acidic and basic form. Since then, it has been found that there is a family of FGF including at least 16 members (144). Acidic and basic FGFs have been renamed fibroblast growth factor-1 (FGF-1) and fibroblast growth factor-2 (FGF-2) respectively. FGF-1 and FGF-2 bind similar cellular receptors and have similar biologic effects. FGF-2 and, to a lesser degree, FGF-1 are extremely potent angiogenic stimulants. Endothelial cells both synthesize and respond to FGF-2 (145). FGF-2 stimulates endothelial cell migration and proliferation as well as differentiation into functional capillaries (146). In addition, topical FGF-2 can stimulate wound contraction in experimental wounds (147) although it has no effect in collagen matrix collagen models (128). It has also been shown to stimulate collagen synthesis, proteoglycan synthesis, fibronectin synthesis (148) and epithelialization (149).

The FGF family includes the protooncogenes *int-2* and *hst* as well as a number of other factors with little to no role in skin wounds (144). One additional member of the family, FGF-7, also known as *keratinocyte growth factor* (KGF) does play an important role in epithelialization and is a potent mitogen for epithelial cells (150). KGF is produced by mesenchymal cells such as fibroblasts and smooth muscle cells but not epithelial cells (151).

Platelet-Derived Growth Factor

The observation that PDGFs contribute to the healing process was made in the early 1970s. The initial factor identified was PDGF, which was localized to the α granules of platelets. Fibroblasts, keratinocytes, endothelial cells, macrophages, and a variety of other cell types also secrete PDGF-like factors (152). PDGF exists in AA, BB, and AB isoforms with slightly different activities (153). PDGF stimulates the chemotaxis of neutrophils and macrophages. PDGF stimulates the chemotaxis and proliferation of fibroblasts and smooth muscle cells as well as collagen synthesis and collagenase activity (154). It also stimulates fibronectin and hyaluron synthesis (155,156) and collagen matrix contraction. PDGF may influence the expression of TGF-β and influence cellular activity indirectly by that mechanism as well (157). The concentration of PDGF in an area

TABLE 6.1

Growth Factors in Wound Healing

Growth Factor	Cell Source	Function
PDGF	Macrophages Platelets Endothelial cells Epithelial cells Fibroblasts Others	Stimulates fibroblast and smooth muscle cell chemotaxis and proliferation, neutrophil and macrophage chemotaxis, collagen synthesis, proteoglycan synthesis, collagenase activity, fibronectin synthesis
TGF-β	Platelets Macrophages Lymphocytes Fibroblasts Keratinocytes Others	Stimulates fibroblast chemotaxis and proliferation (dose dependent), collagen synthesis, proteoglycan synthesis, fibronectin synthesis, angiogenesis, wound contraction
EGF	Macrophages Platelets Epithelial cells Others	Stimulates epithelial cell chemotaxis and proliferation, fibroblast chemotaxis and proliferation, endothelial cell proliferation
FGF-2	Macrophages Endothelial cells Fibroblasts	Stimulates fibroblast proliferation, epithelial cell proliferation, endothelial cell proliferation and migration, collagen synthesis, proteoglycan synthesis, fibronectin synthesis, angiogenesis, wound contraction
TGF-α	Macrophages Platelets Keratinocytes	Same as EGF
IL-1	Macrophages	Stimulates inflammatory cell chemotaxis, epithelial cell chemotaxis, fibroblast proliferation, collagen synthesis, collagenase activity
VEGF	Fibroblasts Macrophages Endothelial cells Epithelial cells	Stimulates endothelial cell proliferation and migration, angiogenesis
KGF (FGF-7)	Fibroblasts	Stimulates epithelial cell proliferation and migration
IGF	Fibroblasts Macrophages	Stimulates fibroblast proliferation, collagen synthesis, proteoglycan synthesis

PDGF, platelet-derived growth factor; TGF, transforming growth factor; EGF, epidermal growth factor; FGF, fibroblast growth factor; IL, interleukin; VEGF, vascular endothelium growth factor; KGF, keratinocyte growth factor; IGF, insulin-like growth factor.

(Modified from Peacock JL, Lawrence WT, Peacock EE Jr. Wound healing. In: O'Leary JP, ed. *The physiologic basis of surgery*. 1st ed. Baltimore: Williams & Wilkins, 1993.)

determines which cells are most attracted because different cells are attracted by different concentrations of PDGF. IGFs are synthesized primarily by hepatocytes and fibroblasts and act as cofactors with PDGF in stimulating fibroblast proliferation. IGF may also contribute to epithelial cell proliferation (158).

Transforming Growth Factor

TGF-β was discovered originally as a stimulant of anchorage-independent cellular proliferation in soft agar, and it has now been isolated from a number of tissues, including platelets, macrophages, lymphocytes, bone, and kidney (159). It has since been discovered that there is a superfamily of TGF-β molecules. More than 25 members of the superfamily have been described (160) including five isoforms of TGF-β itself, bone morphogenetic proteins (BMPs), activins, and a variety of other molecules. The three human isoforms of TGF-β, which have somewhat similar biologic activities, and particularly TGF-β_1, are primary participants in the wound healing process. Most studies have focused on the biologic activities of TGF-β_1 that has a wide variety of biologic effects. Like PDGF, TGF-β is found in high concentrations in the α granules of platelets and is released during platelet degranulation at the site of injury. TGF-β regulates its own production by macrophages in an autocrine manner. It also stimulates macrophages to secrete other growth factors, including FGF, PDGF, TNF, and IL-1. TGF-β stimulates fibroblast chemotaxis and proliferation. In different concentrations, it can either stimulate or inhibit cellular proliferation, and its effect may be modulated by other cytokines in the milieu. TGF-β may be the most potent stimulant of collagen synthesis, and it further contributes to collagen accumulation by decreasing protease activity. Specific antibodies to TGF-β can limit collagen accumulation in wounds (161). TGF-β has also been demonstrated to stimulate fibronectin synthesis, proteoglycan synthesis, and epithelial cell proliferation. In addition, it stimulates wound contraction, and it indirectly stimulates angiogenesis, although it has no stimulatory effect on endothelial cell proliferation (162).

As is apparent, many cytokines have similar functions. Which factors are the most critical stimulants of the various wound-healing functions is not altogether clear. Factors with similar functions may be acting at different time points in the wound-healing process.

DISTURBANCES OF WOUND HEALING

Wound healing does not always occur in the undisturbed manner as described. Both local and systemic factors have the capability of interfering with healing. Local and systemic factors producing abnormal wound healing are listed in Table 6.2. Several of these shall be considered in detail.

Local Factors

Infection

The body maintains a symbiotic relation with bacteria. Normal dry skin contains up to 1,000 bacteria per gram (163) and saliva contains 100 million bacteria per milliliter (164). The bacterial population is kept in control by several mechanisms. Bacterial invasion is mechanically limited by an intact stratum corneum in the skin and intact oral mucosa intraorally (165). In addition, sebaceous secretions contain bactericidal and fungicidal fatty acids which modulate bacterial proliferation (166). Edema dilutes these fatty acids rendering edematous areas more infection prone. Lysozymes in skin hydrolyze bacterial cell membranes and further limit bacterial proliferation (167). The immune system augments the local barriers to infection.

A difference between infection and contamination should be recognized. Contamination is the presence of bacteria from skin or other sources in a wound. Infection occurs when the number or virulence of bacteria has exceeded the ability of local tissue defenses to control them. Generally, infection exists when bacteria have proliferated to levels beyond 10^5 organisms per gram of tissue. At this level, bacteria overwhelm host defenses and proliferate in an uncontrolled manner. This number has been arrived at by studies done at the United States Army Institute of Surgical Research and elsewhere (167–171). Group B streptococci are the only bacterial species identified to cause infection at lower bacterial concentrations (172). Several factors can alter the

TABLE 6.2
Factors Impairing Wound Healing
Local infection
Foreign bodies
Ischemia/hypoxia
Cigarette smoking
Radiation
Previous trauma
Venous insufficiency
Devitalized tissues
Local toxins (e.g., spider venom)
Systemic
Connective tissue disorders
Ehler-Danlos syndrome
Systemic lupus erythromatosus
Inflammatory diseases
Polyarteritis nodosa
Crohn disease
Malnutrition
Protein deficiency
Vitamin and trace element deficiency or toxicity
Lathyrogen excess
Cancer and chemotherapy
Diabetes mellitus
Immune suppression
Pharmaceutical (e.g., corticosteroids)
Acquired (e.g., retroviral infection)
Uremia
Hepatic disease
Jaundice
Alcoholism
Advanced age
Atherosclerosis

balance point where infection develops, including foreign bodies or necrotic tissue in the wound. Hematomas function like foreign bodies as adjuvants promoting infection (173). Both local and systemic factors can compromise the ability of the host to defend against infection. Local factors such as impaired circulation or radiation injury increase the risk of infection. Systemic diseases such as diabetes, acquired immunodeficiency syndrome (AIDS), uremia, and cancer have all been shown to increase susceptibility to wound infection.

Operative procedures are classified as clean, clean–contaminated, contaminated, and dirty. Table 6.3 lists the characteristics of each classification (174). Classification of wounds allows the surgeon to predict the likelihood of wound infection and alter wound management accordingly. Predicting the chances of wound infection is important because the most cost-effective treatment of infection is prevention. Prevention requires meticulous surgical technique, judicious use of perioperative systemic antibiotics, and precise judgment as to which wounds should be closed primarily. Factors that should be considered in choosing to use prophylactic antibiotics are the condition of the patient,

TABLE 6.3

Classification and Infection Rates of Wound Contamination

Classification	Infection Rate (%)	Wound Characteristics
Clean	1.5–5.1	Atraumatic, uninfected; no entry of GU, GI, or respiratory tracts
Clean–contaminated	7.7–10.8	Minor breaks in sterile technique; entry of GU, GI, or respiratory tracts without significant spillage
Contaminated	15.2–16.3	Traumatic wounds; gross spillage from GI tract; entry into infected tissue, bone, urine, or bile
Dirty	28.0–40.0	Drainage of abscess; debridement of soft tissue infection

GU, genitourinary; GI, gastrointestinal.

the status of the host defense, the degree of wound contamination, and factors increasing the risk to the patient should an infection occur (e.g., prosthetic device). Once the decision for prophylactic antibiotics has been made, they must be administered preoperatively so that serum and tissue levels of antibiotics are maximal at the time of wounding.

Hypoxia and Smoking

Delivery of oxygen to healing tissues is critical for prompt wound repair. Oxygen is necessary for cellular respiration and for hydroxylation of proline and lysine residues. Adequate tissue oxygenation requires an adequate circulating blood volume (175), adequate cardiac function, and adequate local vasculature. Vascular disorders may be systemic because of peripheral vascular disease or they may be localized because of scarring from trauma or prior surgery. Anemia is not associated with impaired healing unless the anemia is severe enough to limit the circulating blood volume. The probability of healing wounds on the extremities can be predicted by transcutaneous oxygen measurements (176). Local tissue perfusion can sometimes be improved in compromised areas by treatment with hyperbaric oxygen. This treatment may have particular utility in diabetic patients with greater vascular compromise in smaller blood vessels.

Smoking can impair tissue oxygenation as it acutely stimulates vasoconstriction (177–179) and contributes to the development of atherosclerosis and vascular disease over time. It contains more than 4,000 potentially toxic compounds. Three percent to 6% of cigarette smoke is carbon monoxide, which binds to hemoglobin, producing carboxyhemoglobin. Smokers have carboxyhemoglobin levels between 1% and 20% (180). Carboxyhemoglobin limits the oxygen-carrying capacity of the blood and also increases platelet adhesiveness (181) producing endothelial changes (182,183). In a polytetra fluoroethylene (PTFE) tube model placed in human volunteers, smokers were noted to generate a significantly diminished amount of collagen at 10 days as compared to nonsmokers (184).

Radiation

Radiation damages the deoxyribonucleic acid (DNA) of cells in exposed areas. Some cells die, whereas others are rendered incapable of undergoing mitosis. When radiation is administered therapeutically, doses are fractionated and tangential fields are used to limit damage to normal cells and maximize tumor cell damage. In spite of such techniques, normal cells are damaged by radiation.

Radiation therapy initially produces inflammation and desquamation in a dose-dependent manner (185). After a course of radiation has been completed, healing ensues if surrounding normal tissues have not been irreparably damaged. Additional cells must migrate into the treated area for adequate healing to occur. Fibroblasts that migrate into irradiated tissue are often abnormal because of radiation exposure. These cells are characterized by multiple vacuoles, irregular rough endoplasmic reticulum, degenerating mitochondria, and cytoplasmic crystalline inclusion bodies. Increased levels of inflammatory mediators contribute to an abnormal healing response. Collagen is synthesized to an abnormal degree in irradiated tissue, causing a characteristic fibrosis. The media of dermal blood vessels in irradiated areas thickens and some blood vessels become occluded, resulting in a decrease in the total number of blood vessels. Superficial telangiectasias may be seen. The epidermis becomes thinned, and pigmentation changes often develop. Irradiated skin is dry because of damage to sebaceous and sweat glands, and it has little hair. The epidermal basement membrane is abnormal and nuclear atypia is common in keratinocytes.

In previously irradiated tissue, abnormal healing after wounding is predictable. The decreased vascularity and increased fibrosis limits the ability of platelets and inflammatory cells to gain access to wounds in the area. The quantity of cytokines released is therefore limited. This relative cytokine deficiency causes impairment of essentially all cellular aspects of healing. Damaged fibroblasts and keratinocytes in the area may not respond normally to stimulants. Because of its diminished blood supply, irradiated tissue is predisposed to infection, which can further slow the healing process.

Clinically, impairment in healing is manifested by a higher rate of complication when an operation is done in irradiated tissue (186). Vitamin A has been used to reverse the healing impairment induced by radiation therapy (187). Difficult wounds in irradiated tissue can often be managed surgically by bringing a new blood supply to the area with flaps from nonirradiated areas.

Systemic Factors

Malnutrition

Adequate amounts of protein, carbohydrates, fatty acids, vitamins, and other nutrients are required for wounds to heal. Malnutrition frequently contributes to suboptimal healing (188). Hypoproteinemia inhibits proper wound healing by limiting the supply of critical amino acids required for the synthesis of collagen and other proteins. Collagen synthesis essentially stops in the absence of protein intake (189), resulting in impaired healing (190,191). Arginine and glutamine appear to be particularly important amino acids. Cystine residues are found along the nonhelical peptide chain associated with procollagen, and in their absence, the proper alignment of peptide chains into a triple helix is inhibited (192).

Carbohydrate and fat provide an energy source for healing. Wound healing slows when carbohydrate or fat stores are limited. Protein is broken down as an alternative energy source instead of contributing primarily to tissue growth (193). Fatty acids are also vital components of cell membranes.

Several vitamins are also essential for normal healing. Vitamin C is a necessary cofactor for hydroxylation of lysine and proline during collagen synthesis. The ability of fibroblasts to produce new, strongly cross-linked collagen is diminished if Vitamin C is deficient. Clinically, existing scars dissolve because collagenolytic activity continues without adequate compensatory collagen synthesis. New wounds do not heal. In addition, Vitamin C deficiency is associated with an impaired resistance to infection (194). Vitamin A is essential for normal epithelialization, proteoglycan synthesis, and normal immune function (194–196). Vitamin A and thiamine deficiencies impair healing (197). Vitamin D is required for normal calcium metabolism and is therefore required for bone healing. Exogenous vitamin E impairs wound healing in rats, most likely by influencing the inflammatory response in a corticosteroid-like manner (198).

Certain minerals are necessary for normal healing as well. Zinc, a trace element, is a necessary cofactor for DNA polymerase and reverse transcriptase. Zinc deficiency can therefore result in an inhibition of cellular proliferation and deficient granulation tissue formation (199) and healing (200). Pharmacologic overdosing with zinc does not accelerate wound healing and can have detrimental effects (26).

Cancer

A cancer-associated wound healing impairment has been demonstrated experimentally (201) and is often noted clinically. Cancer-bearing hosts may have impaired healing for a variety of reasons, although severe impairment is generally only noted in terminal patients. Cancer-induced cachexia, which manifests itself as weight loss, anorexia, and asthenia, significantly limits healing. Cachexia is a result of either decreased caloric intake, increased energy expenditure, or both. Several other causes of cancer cachexia have also been proposed.

Decreased oral intake may be caused by anorexia or mechanical factors. Anorexia is mediated through, as yet, imperfectly defined circulating factors. Changes in taste perception, hypothalamic function, and tryptophan metabolism may contribute to anorexia. Tumors in the gastrointestinal tract can produce obstruction and/or fistulae that limit nutrient absorption. Other cancers generate peptides such as gastrin and vasoactive intestinal polypeptide (VIP) that alter transit times and interfere with absorption of nutrients.

Cancers can alter host metabolism in a detrimental manner as well. First, glucose turnover may be increased, sometimes leading to glucose intolerance. The effect of increased glucose use is higher energy needs (202). Second, protein catabolism may be accelerated. Protein breakdown in muscle is increased as is hepatic utilization of amino acids. Such changes in protein metabolism produce a net loss of plasma protein. Third, cancer patients may be unable to alter their metabolism to conserve energy by relying on fat for most of their energy needs. In tumor-bearing animals, fat has been shown to accumulate, whereas other more vital tissues are broken down for energy. Fourth, Vitamin C may be preferentially taken up by some tumors, limiting the vitamins availability for hydroxylation of proline and lysine moieties in collagen. All of these metabolic changes can contribute to a negative energy balance and inefficient energy use.

Cancer patients may be relatively anergic, most likely because of abnormal inflammatory cell activity. Macrophages do not migrate or function normally in cancer patients. Inflammatory cell dysfunction may limit the availability of cytokines required for healing and may also predispose to infection.

Impaired healing must be anticipated in cancer patients because of the many potential alterations in metabolism and immune function. It has been suggested that vitamin A can improve healing in tumor-bearing mice (203), but this effect has not yet been demonstrated in cancer patients.

Advanced Age

The elderly have been shown to heal less efficiently than younger individuals. DuNuoy and Carrell studied patients with war injuries in World War I and demonstrated that wounds in 20-year-old patients contracted more rapidly than those in 30-year-old patients (204). In a blister epithelialization model, younger patients healed more rapidly than older patients (204). In elderly subjects, wound disruption occurred with less force than in younger individuals (205).

Diabetes

Diabetes mellitus is also associated with impaired healing. The risk of infection in clean incisions was five times greater in diabetic patients than nondiabetic patients in a review of 23,649 patients (206). This diabetes-induced healing impairment has been experimentally demonstrated in several models as well (207–209). Diabetes is associated with impaired neutrophil chemotaxis (198) and phagocytic function (210–212). These changes predispose to infection. Diabetes is also associated with accelerated atherosclerosis rendering tissues relatively hypoxic, which impairs healing. Diabetic peripheral neuropathies can render an individual more susceptible to pressure-induced ulcerations. The diabetes-induced healing impairment may be improved by controlling hyperglycemia with insulin (213–215).

Steroids and Immunosuppression

Adrenocortical steroids inhibit all aspects of the healing process. Steroids slow the development of breaking strength in incisional wounds (216). In open wounds healing secondarily, steroids impede wound contraction (217,218) and epithelialization.

This healing impairment is a result of derangements in cellular function induced by steroids. A primary feature of wounds in steroid-treated individuals is a deficiency in inflammatory cell function. Inflammatory cells, particularly macrophages, mediate essentially all aspects of healing through cytokine release. By diminishing the supply of cytokines, steroids and other immunosuppressive agents profoundly impair all aspects of healing. Macrophage migration, fibroblast proliferation, collagen accumulation, and angiogenesis are among the processes diminished by steroid administration. The effects of steroids on healing are most pronounced when the drug is administered several days before or after wounding (219).

All aspects of steroid-induced healing impairment other than wound contraction can be reversed by supplemental vitamin A. The recommended dose is 25,000 IU/d. Topical vitamin A has also been found to be effective for open wounds (220). Anabolic steroids and growth hormone–releasing factor have reversed steroid-induced–healing impairments as well.

Chemotherapeutic Agents

Chemotherapeutic agents impair healing primarily through inhibition of cellular proliferation. Many agents have been examined in experimental models, and virtually all agents impair healing (221). Nitrogen mustard, cyclophosphamide, methotrexate, 1,3-bis-(2-chloroethyl)-1-nitrosourea (BCNU) (carmustine), and doxorubicin are the most damaging to the healing process. Most chemotherapeutic regimens use a combination of agents compounding their deleterious effects. Clinical trials with chemotherapeutic agents have not been associated with as high an incidence of complications as might be anticipated from experimental evidence. The timing of drug administration and the doses used may explain this apparent contradiction. Doxorubicin, for example, is a potent inhibitor of wound healing when delivered preoperatively but has a limited effect if initiated after healing has been initiated postoperatively (222).

CHRONIC WOUNDS

Any wound that is affected by compromising factors may become a chronic wound. Chronic wounds do not respond to standard care and remain substantially unhealed beyond the 6-week period typically required for normal wound healing. They are also characterized by slow progression of either re-epithelialization or contraction.

Although there are unifying etiologies for abnormal wound healing, specific pathologies related to chronic wounds include pressure ulcers, diabetic foot ulcers, venous insufficiency ulcers, lymphedematous extremity wounds, hematologic ulcers from sickle cell disease and polycythemia, infected wounds, neoplastic wounds, radiation ulcers, neoplastic wounds including Marjolin ulcers, Kaposi sarcoma, and metastatic lesions, and factitious ulcers. Progressive healing can be expected once treatable comorbidities have been treated.

ABNORMAL SCAR FORMATION

In normal healing, the events progress in an orderly, controlled manner producing flat, unobtrusive scars. Healing is a biologic process, and as in all biologic processes, there are cases where the process may vary. Healing disturbances with diminished healing have already been discussed. Excessive healing can result in a raised, thickened scar with both functional and cosmetic complications. If the scar is confined to the margins of the original wound, it is called a *hypertrophic scar* (223). In contrast, keloids extend beyond the confines of the original injury such that the original wound can often no longer be distinguished.

Certain patients and certain wounds are at higher risk for abnormal scarring. Dark-skinned individuals and patients between the ages of 2 and 40 are at higher risk for the development of hypertrophic scars or keloids. Patients who are in a rapid growth phase (e.g., puberty) are also more susceptible to keloid formation. Wounds in the presternal or deltoid area, wounds that cross skin tension lines, and wounds in thicker skin have a greater tendency to heal with a thickened scar. Some parts of the body rarely develop abnormal scars, such as the genitalia, the eyelids, the palms of the hands, and the soles of the feet.

Certain patient and wound characteristics increase the relative likelihood of developing a hypertrophic scar as opposed to a keloid (224). Keloids are more likely to be familial than hypertrophic scars. Hypertrophic scars are more likely to be seen in light-skinned individuals, although both occur more frequently in dark-skinned people. Hypertrophic scars may subside in time whereas keloids rarely do. Hypertrophic scars are more likely to be associated with a contracture across a joint surface.

Keloids and hypertrophic scars result from an overall net increase in the quantity of collagen synthesized by fibroblasts in the wound area. Recent evidence suggests that the fibroblasts within keloids are different than those within normal dermis in terms of their biologic responsiveness, and this may explain how the lesions develop. The reason why these aberrantly responding fibroblasts appear in certain wounds is unknown, however, although many theories have been suggested. Treatment of hypertrophic scars and keloids has included surgical excision, steroid injection, pressure garments, topical silastic gel, radiation therapy, and combinations of these modalities. The absence of a uniform treatment program accurately suggests that no modality of treatment is predictably effective for these lesions (225). A third type of abnormal scar is known as *widened-scar formation*. Found in regions of high-tension closure, these scars are characterized by an abnormally thin dermis and reduced amounts of collagen.

WOUND CLOSURE

The initial step in the management of a wound is a careful history and physical examination. It must first be assured that another more life-threatening problem does not require more immediate attention. In relation to the wound itself, it must be determined when and how the wound was created. The presence of coexisting problems that could interfere with wound management or wound healing must be ascertained. It should also be determined whether the patient smokes and if he or she is taking medications. The patient's nutritional status should be evaluated as well as their cardiac and vascular status.

The wound must be examined to assure that the injured tissue is viable and to determine whether foreign bodies are present. Dusky discoloration of tissue implies poor vascular supply. The possibility of injuries to nerves, ducts, muscle, or bones within the wound must be addressed; radiographic evaluation may be required. The patient's tetanus status should be considered. Antirabies treatment must also be considered for patients bitten by wild animals such as skunks, raccoons, foxes, and bats. The tissues missing from traumatic wounds should be enumerated.

Closure of any wound is evaluated with a reconstructive mindset that includes the following goals: closure of the wound, prevention of infection, provision of stable and robust coverage, minimization of the donor defect, and maximization of function. Taking those factors into account, surgeons use what is called the *reconstructive ladder*, shown in Table 6.4, which proceeds through the various levels of intervention used to close wounds. The ladder consists of basic principles of wound closure along with more complex closures such as using local, distant, and free flaps. As such, the reconstructive ladder is similar to an elevator. At some point along that elevator, clinicians must be able to make

TABLE 6.4	
The Reconstructive Ladder	

	High tech tools
• Healing by secondary intention	• Tissue engineering
• Direct tissue closure	• Tissue expansion
• Primary	• Hyperbaric oxygen
• Secondary	• Cytokine therapy
• Pedicled tissue transfer	• Xeno/allograft skin
• Local aps	• Negative pressure
• Distant aps	
• Free tissue transfer	
• Nonvascularized (skin, bone, tendon, nerve grafts)	
• Vascularized (skin, fascia, muscle, bone free flaps)	

"stops" to introduce the high-tech tools and devices now available, for example, negative pressure wound therapy with the wound vacuum assisted closure (VAC), which can be used at any level of the reconstructive elevator whether treatment is moving up or down levels of intervention.

Deciding which tools to use and how to adapt navigation of the elevator to each patient is critical to understand in wound closure. The patient's overall condition, including local wound conditions and systemic variables such as malnutrition, and immunosuppression, are all key to determining the ideal technique for wound closure treatment. The most important guiding principle remains the goal of "replacing like with like" in terms of tissue loss and replacement.

The first decision should be whether to primarily close the defect. Primary wound closure refers to closing the wound at the time of presentation and is preferred unless prevented by coexisting factors. Factors that might prevent primary closure include excessive or uncontrollable bleeding, significant quantities of necrotic and foreign material that cannot be removed easily from the wound, and excessive bacterial contamination. Excessive bacterial contamination is determined optimally by quantitative bacteriology, although this service is not always available. The level of bacterial contamination can be suggested by the time elapsed since injury and the mechanism of injury. The initial 6 to 8 hours after injury has been referred to as the *golden period*, in that closure can usually be accomplished without a markedly increased risk of infection. Experimental data suggest that bacteria trapped within the wound exudate cause infections seen in wounds closed after 6 to 8 hours and that the bacteria require that time period to reach levels of 10^5/g of tissue (226,227). Some mechanisms of injury are associated with excessive bacterial contamination. Human bites are a prime example in that saliva contains large quantities of bacteria. Human bites should rarely, if ever, be closed. Other mechanisms of injury, such as farm injuries, are associated with intermediate levels of bacterial contamination. The time and mechanism of injury have to also be considered in light of the location of injury and coexisting problems. Because of better vascularization, one can be more lenient in closing slightly older wounds that have a less favorable mechanism of injury in the head and neck than the foot. Malnourished or steroid-treated patients have less competent immune systems and may not be able to tolerate levels of bacteria that may accumulate in less than 6 to 8 hours. Another variable would be how aggressively the wound can be treated before closure. If a wound can be excised completely back to fresh tissue, one can be more aggressive in pursuing primary closure than in wounds where such aggressive debridement is not possible. Aggressive debridement may be contraindicated because of a lack of excess tissue or because adjacent structures must be preserved.

If primary closure is not feasible, then a period of wound management is initiated. Wounds initially left open may be closed in a tertiary manner once the original problem preventing primary closure has been corrected.

In some cases, the level of bacterial contamination is unclear, and a technique of wound closure known as *delayed primary closure* may be implemented (228). When this technique is used, the wound edges are left open at the time of injury or surgery, and the wound is examined 3 to 4 days later. If the wound appears healthy and uninfected at that point, the wound edges may be approximated with sutures or adhesive strips.

Wounds not closed primarily or in a tertiary manner may be allowed to heal secondarily. Secondary healing is healing through wound contraction and epithelialization. This method of healing may be preferable, not only for heavily contaminated wounds, but also for small or superficial wounds that will heal in a short period of time. The surgeon can estimate the ability of wound contraction to close most of the wounds simply by physically coapting the skin edges. If a great deal of force and tension is required to coapt the skin edges, then wound contraction itself will not cover the defect in a reasonable period of time. Conversely, if the skin edges coapt easily without a great deal of tension or contraction of surrounding joints, wound contraction will probably be successful in covering most of the wound surface.

Methods of Closure

If a wound is deemed adequate for closure, a decision must be made regarding the most appropriate method of closure. Options in order of complexity are (i) direct wound approximation, (ii) skin grafts, (iii) local flaps, and (iv) distant flaps (Table 6.4). The least complex method possible is generally used unless a more complex technique offers an advantage that outweighs the disadvantages of the added complexity. For example, it may be preferable to use a flap instead of a graft for a hand injury with damaged tendons, as a flap will better facilitate subsequent tendon reconstruction.

Direct Wound Approximation

The method used most commonly for incisional wounds is direct wound approximation. The steps involved in wound closure include (i) anesthesia, (ii) irrigation, (iii) shave and prep, (iv) debridement, and (v) wound closure. Anesthesia should virtually always be induced first and wound closure always last, although the order of the intermediate three steps sometimes varies. Local, regional, or general anesthesia may be chosen to facilitate wound closure depending on the wound and the patient.

A variety of local anesthetics are available, but for most limited injuries, lidocaine has traditionally been most commonly used at a concentration of 0.5% or 1.0%. Increased concentrations are not associated with improved anesthesia and have a higher risk of toxicity. Lidocaine's advantages include its rapid onset of action and its 2- to 3-hour duration of activity. In addition, few individuals are allergic to lidocaine. Epinephrine, in a concentration of 1:100,000 or 1:200,000, can be added in almost all locations. It aids in hemostasis, prolongs the duration of action of the anesthetic, and increases the volume of local anesthetic that can safely be injected by delaying absorption, thereby spreading out the metabolism of the agent over a longer period of time (229). Standard teaching is that epinephrine should not be used in the fingers and toes because it can induce vasospasm leading to digital loss. This concept has been questioned by a randomized prospective study that demonstrated no increase in morbidity when lidocaine with epinephrine was used for digital blocks (230). Maximum safe doses for lidocaine are 4 mg/kg without epinephrine and 7 mg/kg with epinephrine. This standard dictum has also been brought into question in that doses up to 35 mg/kg have been safely used for liposuction in 0.5% solutions with epinephrine at a 1:1,000,000 dilution (231,232). During liposuction, however, at least some of the anesthetic is aspirated with the fat so the actual dose to which the patient is exposed is less than that administered. Further studies need to be done before extrapolating this dosage to other cases.

Lidocaine, like all local anesthetics, causes pain when it is injected, both due to the injection itself and because of the acidity of the agent. Pain induced by the local administration of lidocaine can be minimized by using the smallest needle possible and minimizing the number of skin punctures. It is also helpful to inject the agent slowly. Subcutaneous injections are less painful than intradermal injections because the injected drug displaces fatty tissue more easily, although the anesthetic will take effect more slowly with subcutaneous administration (233). Injecting into a wound edge is less painful than injecting through intact skin. Warming the lidocaine and buffering it with sodium bicarbonate (8.4%) in 1:9 or 1:10 ratios to decrease its acidity also decreases the pain associated with its injection (234). Counterirritation by rubbing the skin may also interfere with pain transmission (235).

There has been increased interest more recently in topical anesthetics. tetracaine, adrenaline, and cocaine (TAC) (a solution of 0.5% tetracaine, 1:2,000 adrenaline and 11.8% cocaine) has been successfully used for inducing anesthesia in superficial lacerations before closure, particularly in the face and scalp (236,237). A number of other topical anesthetics have been evaluated in order to eliminate cocaine from the mixture. Topical 5% lidocaine with

1:2,000 epinephrine (238), topical 4% lidocaine with 0.1% epinephrine and 0.5% tetracaine (239), 0.48% bupivicaine with 1:26,000 norepinephrine (240) and 3.56% prilocaine with 0.10% phenylephrine (241) have been demonstrated to be equivalent to TAC in different studies. A eutectic mixture of lidocaine and prilocaine (EMLA) has been used to induce local anesthesia in intact skin, often before venous cannulation, (220 g) as well as open wounds (242). It is more effective in the lower extremity than TAC. It must be in contact with the skin for 1 to 2 hours in order to induce an adequate degree of anesthesia to be useful.

Surrounding hair may complicate closure of wounds in hair-bearing areas. In such areas, the hair may be clipped. Bacteria that reside within hair follicles are displaced if the area is shaved. This increases the risk of contamination of the wound and therefore wound infection (243). Shaving of the area should be avoided.

The wound should then be irrigated to decrease the number of bacteria and remove foreign material. High-pressure irrigation (>8 psi) is much more effective at diminishing bacterial concentrations than low pressure irrigation or scrubbing with a saline-soaked sponge (244–246). Pulsatile irrigation is the best mechanism for cleansing fragments of foreign debris from soft tissue. Pulsatile irrigation can help minimize the amount of sharp excision that is required to convert a contaminated wound into a clean-contaminated wound. Though a pressurized pulsatile irrigation device is optimal, such machines are rarely available in emergency departments. Alternative methods of providing irrigation with some force include the use of a 60-cc syringe and a 19-gauge angiocath or a flexible intravenous bag surrounded by a blood pressure cuff (244) and then attached to tubing and an angiocath. Though clearly of value in bacterially contaminated wounds, irrigation may not be necessary for clean wounds (247).

Clearly acceptable agents for irrigation include Ringers lactate solution, 0.9% saline, and fluids containing a surfactant (248–251). Various agents are often added to irrigation fluids, generally in efforts to kill bacteria. Any potential benefit in bacterial control must be weighed against the damage done to tissues by the antibacterial agent. One should avoid the use of surgical hand cleaning soaps in irrigation, as all of these agents have been demonstrated to impede healing (252–255). Alcohol is toxic to tissues and should not be placed on a wound (255). Dakin solution (0.5% sodium hypochlorite) is toxic to fibroblasts, impairs neutrophil function, slows epithelialization, and slows tensile strength development in incisional wounds (256,257). Similarly, 0.5% acetic acid is lethal to cultured fibroblasts, impairs epithelialization, and slows development of tensile strength in experimental models (258). Hydrogen peroxide may be useful for dissolving blood clots in the wound, but it has no antibacterial function. It has also been demonstrated to kill fibroblasts in culture and cause mild histologic damage to tissue (249). Even standard hand soap induces mild tissue damage (249). Solutions of some antibiotics such as 1% neomycin sulfate and 2% kanamycin sulfate, however, may

be safe in that they are nontoxic to cells in culture (248). There is some evidence that antibiotic supplements may more effectively diminish bacterial counts in contaminated wounds (259). A general guideline is that one should not irrigate an open wound with any solution that would not be comfortable in one's own conjunctival sac (260).

The skin around the wound itself should be prepared with an antibacterial solution. Skin preparation is carried out to limit cross-contamination of the wound from bacteria residing on surrounding skin. Povidone iodine is most commonly used; it has a broad spectrum of antibacterial activity and is tolerated by most individuals (261,262).

Wound debridement is carried out to remove foreign material and necrotic tissue that can contribute to wound infection (263). Wounds with perpendicular edges are more likely to heal with a fine scar than those with beveled or irregular wound edges. Unfavorable wound edges should be excised to create a more favorable wound.

The ideal wound closure method has not been identified. An ideal method would support the wound until it reaches near full strength (at least 6 weeks), would not penetrate the epidermis thereby predisposing to additional scars, would not impair any cellular function required for healing, and would not induce inflammation or ischemia. No method accomplishes all of these goals, and therefore all existing methods represent a compromise. Methods for direct wound closure include sutures, staples, tapes, and tissue adhesives.

Sutures of various types are probably used most commonly. One should choose the smallest caliber suture that is able to maintain the sutured tissues in approximation. This philosophy limits the quantity of foreign material placed in the wound. Sutures are classified as absorbable or nonabsorbable. Absorbable sutures include catgut, chromic catgut, and an increasing number of synthetic options. Catgut is derived from beef and sheep intestine. Chromic catgut is catgut treated with chromium salts to slow its absorption. Catgut is generally absorbed within a week, whereas chromic catgut persists for up to 2 weeks. Both catgut sutures incite a significant inflammatory response and are digested by proteolytic enzymes. Polyglycolic acid polymer sutures are synthetic absorbable sutures synthesized from organometallic compounds. They maintain substantial strength for 2 to 3 weeks, depending on location. They do not induce a significant inflammatory response. Newer synthetic materials such as polydioxanone and polyglyconate absorb even more slowly, producing more prolonged wound support. Absorbable sutures are useful for visceral wounds where healing is rapid, suture removal is difficult, and bacterial contamination makes a permanent suture a potential liability. They are also used for deeper tissues where permanent wound support is not required.

Nonabsorbable sutures include nylon and a variety of synthetic materials. Silk is also considered permanent, although it is absorbed slowly over a 2-year period. Nonabsorbable sutures are used in superficial locations where they can be removed and in deeper tissues where wound support is required for a long period of time.

Some sutures are monofilament and some are multifilamentous weaves. Monofilament sutures have the advantage of inducing a limited tissue reaction, although they have the disadvantages of being less easy to tie and manipulate and producing stiff, rigid knots. Multifilament suture are generally more pliable and easy to tie, although bacteria can multiply in the interstices of the multifilamentous weave and may induce a more severe reaction in the surrounding tissues.

Sutures are left in place until healing has created enough wound strength to allow their removal. Removal of sutures too early can result in widening of a scar or even disruption of a wound. However, an epithelialized tract will develop around a suture left in skin for longer than 7 to 10 days (264). The tract will fill with scar after suture removal, resulting in unsightly suture marks. Sutures should therefore be removed at or before 10 days if possible. The decision as to when to remove sutures from a particular wound necessitates developing a compromise between factors that require prolonged wound support and those that promote early removal. The factors involved include the age, site and type of wound, the general condition of the patient, and whether the wound is further supported by buried sutures. Skin wounds in most anatomic locations are generally not subjected to significant tension and can maintain satisfactory closure with 15% or less of the tensile strength of normal skin. Therefore, skin sutures can often be removed relatively soon after wound closure. Facial wounds are subjected to little stress, and healing in the head and neck is facilitated because of the excellent blood supply. A general rule is to remove sutures in the face at 4 to 5 days. Abdominal skin sutures are generally left in slightly longer and are removed at 7 to 10 days. Sutures on the lower extremity are left in longer (265). Wounds subjected to excessive tension, such as in skin overlying joints, or wounds in individuals with impaired healing due to diabetes, steroids, or other factors may require longer periods of suture closure to avoid disruption (Fig. 6.3). Any wound must be inspected carefully before sutures are removed. Evidence of undue tension or delayed healing may require that sutures be left in place longer than originally anticipated.

Closure with staples is more rapid than suture closure although tissue approximation may not be as precise (266). Additional sutures placed in the dermis can improve this. Like sutures, additional scars will result if staples are left in place too long. Tapes such as Steri Strips (3 M Health Care, St. Paul, MN) are easy to apply, comfortable for the patient, and leave no marks in the skin (267–269). However, they can be displaced inadvertently and may be less precise than sutures if used alone. In addition, wound edema tends to cause inversion of taped wound edges.

Tissue adhesives that have been used include cyanoacrylate and fibrin. Cyanoacrylate tissue adhesives slow healing by increasing wound inflammation and increasing the likelihood of infection if they are placed directly in the wound (270). They are not widely used in this manner clinically at this time. More recently, octylcyanoacrylate tissue adhesives have become available. This material is applied topically to skin edges that have been manually brought into apposition to provide an external sealant. The material has little to no contact with tissue below the stratum corneum. In wounds in low-tension areas such as the face, aesthetic results and complication rates have been equivalent to those achieved by traditional suturing (271). Wound closures can be accomplished in less time and with less discomfort to the patient. Octylcyanoacrylate tissue adhesives are not useful for extremely deep wounds involving fascia and in wounds subjected to high tension such as those overlying joints.

Fibrin glue has been used to improve the adherence and take of skin grafts (272,273), for sealing puncture wounds in blood vessels or in the lung, and for blepharoplasty closure along with the judicious use of sutures (274). Although a useful adjunct, fibrin glue does not produce a strong enough bond to allow its use alone for incisional wounds. Commercially produced homologous fibrin glue has been available in Europe for some time, and after achieving an excellent safety record, it has become available in the United States.

The old surgical dictum that dead space should be closed or obliterated seems to call for the use of stitches in subcutaneous tissues. However, this is not true; both laboratory and human studies have demonstrated that multiple layers of closure contribute to an increased risk of wound infection (275,276). Stitches in fat convey no additional strength to a wound closure and should be avoided; however, deeper fascial layers should be closed because they contribute to the structural integrity of the wound closure. Closed suction drains are preferable to subcutaneous stitches for the prevention of fluid collections beneath the skin. In addition to limiting the accumulation of blood and serum, suction drains aid in the approximation of tissues. Although most drains are relatively inert, all drains can potentiate infections and should be removed as soon as drainage is at an acceptable level.

Skin Grafts

Grafts or flaps are used in larger wounds when direct wound approximation cannot be accomplished without unduly distorting normal structures. Grafts are generally simpler to use than flaps. Skin grafts are taken at precise thicknesses that have traditionally been measured in thousandths of an inch. STSGs consist of epidermis and a portion of the underlying dermis. Thinner STSGs include less dermis, whereas thicker grafts include more dermis. FTSGs include the full thickness of dermis and epidermis. Full-thickness grafts can only be harvested from areas where skin is thin, or the graft will be too thick to survive. Thin and thick grafts have different characteristics, and the choice between them is based on the nature of the wound to be covered. Thin grafts take more readily and are preferred for less reliable recipient sites. Thicker grafts, especially full-thickness grafts, tend to maintain a more normal appearance than thin grafts. Thicker and full-thickness grafts are therefore commonly used in areas like the face where cosmesis is important. Full-thickness grafts also have the capability of maintaining hair growth when taken from hair-bearing areas.

Primary and secondary graft contracture is directly related to graft thickness. Primary graft contracture is the contraction noted after graft harvest, before placement on the wound bed, and is produced by dermal elastin. Only thicker grafts that include a significant amount of dermis undergo a large degree of primary contraction. Secondary graft contracture refers to the contraction that occurs after the graft is placed on a wound during healing. In secondary contracture, the wound is contracting, not the graft. Thicker grafts limit secondary graft contracture to a greater degree than thinner grafts (130). The critical variable is not the absolute thickness of the skin, but rather the amount of deeper dermis included in the graft. This is important because skin varies considerably in thickness from one part of the body to another, and a full-thickness graft from an area where the skin is thin (i.e., the upper eyelid) may be the same thickness as a split-thickness graft taken from the back where skin is thicker. The eyelid graft will be a more potent inhibitor of wound contraction.

Another consideration is whether to mesh the graft. Meshing involves rolling the graft through a device that places small incisions within it, allowing it to expand like a pantograph. Meshing provides several advantages but also produces some disadvantages. Meshed grafts can expand and cover more area than nonmeshed grafts, limiting the amount of graft required. Meshing provides drain holes that limit the possibility of blood or serum collecting beneath the graft. Meshed grafts may also conform to irregular contours better than nonmeshed grafts. Wounds closed with meshed grafts have a less aesthetic irregular contour than wounds closed with nonmeshed grafts, however. Wounds closed with meshed grafts may also contract more than wounds closed with unmeshed grafts because the interstices of meshed grafts must heal secondarily by wound contraction and epithelialization (277). Meshed grafts should therefore be avoided over joint surfaces.

Any reconstructive method has some cost associated with it. For skin grafts, the primary cost is the second wound at the donor site. The donor sites of split-thickness grafts will heal secondarily by epithelialization, whereas those of full-thickness grafts must be closed. Direct wound approximation is possible if the full-thickness donor site is small, although split-thickness grafting may be required if the donor site is large. Preferred donor sites for all grafts are from anatomic sites that are not easily visible. The buttocks and upper thighs, which are often covered by clothes, are the most commonly used donor sites for split-thickness grafts.

Skin harvested from the supraclavicular area and cephalad resembles facial skin more than skin from the back, abdomen, or extremities. For that reason, head and neck donor sites are preferred for grafts to the facial region. Commonly used donor sites include the postauricular area, the supraclavicular area, and the scalp. The postauricular area is commonly used for smaller full-thickness grafts.

Larger full- or split-thickness grafts can be harvested from the supraclavicular area. The scalp is an excellent donor site for split-thickness grafts. The donor site is hidden after hair regrowth, and split-thickness scalp grafts generally do not grow hair. The head must be shaved to take the graft, however, and this may not be acceptable to some patients.

Wounds closed with grafts are durable once the graft has healed. Full-thickness grafts grow predictably as the patient grows, although split-thickness grafts grow less predictably. Grafted skin, especially thinner grafts, tends to become more darkly pigmented after transfer. Only full-thickness grafts will grow hair. Sebaceous activity generally returns after several months in grafts, thick enough to include sebaceous glands. Sensation and sweating return after a variable period of months or even years. Sensation is most like that in the recipient area (278).

Skin Flaps

The decision whether to use a skin graft or a flap for the closure of a large wound is based on the nature of the wound and the desired aesthetic and functional result. Skin grafts will only take on a well-vascularized bed. Skin grafts cannot be used where the wound base includes relatively avascular tissue such as bone, cartilage, nerve, or tendon. Skin grafts also do poorly in areas rendered relatively avascular by radiation or chronic scarring. Such wounds require the use of a flap for closure.

Flaps may be used in place of skin grafts to provide either an improved aesthetic result or tissue with a specific desired characteristic. In general, local flaps are used if a flap of the appropriate dimension and type is available, and distant or free flaps are used when local tissue of the desired type is not available. The aesthetic and functional cost of any flap must be considered before flap transfer to ensure an appropriate cost/benefit ratio.

Flaps have been characterized in a variety of ways. The most meaningful categorization divides flaps into random-pattern and axial flaps (279) according to their blood supply. Random-pattern flaps are supplied by blood flowing through perforating vessels to the subdermal plexus proximal to the flap base. Generally, a large number of such small, unnamed perforating blood vessels exist. In random-pattern flaps, no single blood vessel is critical to flap survival, and their length is generally limited. Axial pattern flaps are based on a known, major blood vessel that has the capability of nourishing the entire flap. In many anatomic locations, axial vessels enter deep to muscle, allowing the elevation of muscle and skin as a single musculocutaneous flap. In other locations, axial vessels run adjacent to the fascia above the muscle, allowing the elevation of a fasciocutaneous flap. Most axial flaps have been defined by careful anatomic studies of the tissue supplied by a specific blood vessel, and many are large.

Flap tissue is unchanged in color, texture, thickness, hair-bearing characteristics, and sebaceous activity by the transfer process. Flaps will grow with the patient. Sensation and sweating will be maintained if a nerve supply is transferred intact. When a nerve supply is not maintained, some sensation usually returns to the flap over a matter of months. Flaps can be designed that allow the transfer of viable bone or specialized structures such as jejunum when such tissue is required for complex restorations.

Dressings

Different types of wounds have different needs and therefore require different dressings. Partial-thickness injuries where the epidermis and a portion of the dermis are lost heal primarily by epithelialization and are best treated by dressings that maintain a warm moist environment (280,281). A variety of dressings can meet this need, including biologic dressings such as allograft (282), amnion (283) or xenografts (284), synthetic biologic dressings (285), hydrogel dressings, and semipermeable or nonpermeable membranes (281). These dressings do not require changing as long as they remain adherent. Other types of dressing require frequent dressing changes (286).

Wet-to-dry dressings are preferred where the goal of dressing changes is debridement of necrotic tissue, foreign bodies, or other debris. Saline-soaked wide-meshed gauze dressings are applied, allowed to dry, and then changed every 6 to 8 hours. Granulation tissue and wound exudate, including necrotic tissue and other debris, become incorporated within the interstices of the meshed gauze as it dries, and therefore debridement is accomplished when the dressing is changed (287,288). Enzymatic agents, such as collagenase, may augment the debriding effect of wet-to-dry dressing changes (289).

The disadvantage of a wet-to-dry dressing change regimen is that viable cells are damaged by the desiccation and mechanical debridement. Wet-to-dry dressings should be discontinued when adequate debridement has been accomplished. Wet-to-wet dressing changes in which the gauze is not allowed to dry minimize tissue damage. Wet dressings can also be used to facilitate heat transfer, which decreases pain and increases capillary perfusion (260). Wet dressings can be harmful if the wounded area becomes overly moist and maceration occurs.

Virtually any type of dressing change regimen will lower the bacterial count in infected wounds (289). Regimens using antibacterial agents that directly affect the offending bacteria generally decrease the bacterial count in wounds more rapidly than other regimens. Silver sulfadiazine is a frequently used broad-spectrum antibacterial that has the secondary benefit of maintaining a moist environment and accelerating epithelialization (290–292).

For wounds with exposed tendons or nerves, it is particularly important that a moist environment be maintained to prevent desiccation. Options include biologic and membrane dressings, although they are both difficult to use in deep irregular wounds or if a wound drainage is present. Wet-to-wet dressings or dressings including creams such as silver sulfadiazine are particularly useful in these settings.

For incisional wounds, one option is to use a dressing including several layers with different functions. The layer immediately adjacent to the wound should be sterile and nonadhering and should not be occlusive. Fine meshed gauze impregnated with a hydrophilic substance is available and meets those needs. The layer over the contact layer should be absorptive and should wick exudate or transudate away from the wound surface. Wide-meshed gauze facilitates this capillary action and drainage (293). Such absorptive layers must not become saturated in that exudate will then collect on the wound surface and produce maceration. The outermost layer of the dressing is the binding layer that fixes the dressing in place. Tape is used most commonly, although wraps are useful on extremities. Dressings may generally be discontinued after 48 hours if no drainage occurs; the epithelial layer will have sealed the wound by that time. An alternative method of treating a minimally draining incisional wound is antibacterial ointment. The ointments are occlusive and maintain a sterile moist environment for the 48 hours required for epithelialization. The ointment prevents crusting and scab formation. Ointments, however, are washed away if drainage from the wound is excessive and can be easily inadvertently mechanically removed. This approach is best applied to the face. A third approach to incisional wounds is to use an occlusive dressing (294). Such an approach is primarily applicable to wounds where minimal drainage is expected, although in that setting, results have been excellent.

For small wounds in difficult areas, it may be easier not to dress the wound and to allow a scab to form. Scabs consist of fibrin, red blood cells, and exudate that protect the wound and limit bacterial invasion and desiccation. Epithelial cells advancing beneath the scab must break down the scab–wound interface as they migrate across the wound (295). Epithelialization is slower under a scab than under an occlusive dressing.

Newer techniques for wound management may have applicability to large open wounds. Skin substitutes have the capability of providing biologic elements to the wound, which the body may not need to replace. Some of these products such as Alloderm (Life-Cell Corp., Branchburg, NJ) and Integra (Ethicon Inc., Division of Johnson and Johnson Medical, Somerville, NJ) simply provide dermal matrix element and are acellular. Others like Apligraf (Novartis Pharmaceuticals, East Hanover, NJ) include cellular elements and provide both epithelial and dermal components. The cellular elements most likely do not persist over time but instead provide cytokines that may facilitate wound closure. Mechanical devices such as the VAC (KCI International, San Antonio, TX) have shown utility in facilitating the closure of large difficult wounds. The VAC device involves the application of negative pressure to a wound which may improve local blood flow and accelerate wound contraction as well as other aspects of the healing process (296).

Frontiers in Wound Healing

The focus for wound healing in the future will be to accelerate closure in both acute and chronic wounds. Molecular and biotechnology techniques to stimulate tissue regeneration through genetic manipulation and custom tissue prefabrication using stem cell technology are the future for wound healing. Such methodology could allow restoration of even complex damaged structures, such as hands or internal organs, instead of simply sealing the damaged areas with a scar. Recent advances in our understanding of the cellular and molecular basis of the wound healing process continue to bring us closer to this goal.

ACKNOWLEDGMENTS

The authors would like to acknowledge the original contributions of James L. Peacock and Erle E. Peacock from the first edition of this chapter in *The Physiologic Basis of Surgery*.

REFERENCES

1. Brown, H. The three healing gestures. In: Brown H, ed. *A brief history of wound healing*. Yardley: Oxford Clinical Communications, 1998:8–9.
2. Cines DB, Pollack ES, Buck CA, et al. Endothelial cells in physiology and in the pathophysiology of vascular disorders. *Blood* 1998;91:3627–3261.
3. Meyer FA, Fromjmovic MM, Vic MM. Characteristics of the major platelet membrane site used in binding collagen. *Thromb Res* 1979;15:755–767.
4. Santaro SA. Identification of a 160,000 dalton platelet membrane protein that mediates the initial divalent cation-dependent adhesion of platelets to collagen. *Cell* 1986;249:913–920.
5. Detwiler TC, Feinman RD. Kinetics of thrombin-induced release of calcium by platelets. *Biochemistry* 1973;12:282–289.
6. Plow EF, Ginsberg MH, Marguerie GA. Expression and function of adhesive proteins on the platelet surface. In: Phillips DR, Shuman MA, eds. *Biochemistry of platelets*. New York: Academic Press, 1986:226–256.
7. Esmon CT. Cell mediated events that control blood coagulation and vascular injury. *Annu Rev Cell Biol* 1993;9:1–26.
8. Tanaka K, Sueishi K. Biology of disease. The coagulation and fibrinolysis systems and atherosclerosis. *Lab Invest* 1993;69:5–18.
9. Hynes RO. Fibronectins. *Sci Am* 1986;254:42–51.
10. Oh E, Pierschbacher M, Ruoslahti E. Deposition of plasma fibronectin in tissue. *Proc Natl Acad Sci U S A* 1981;78:3218–3221.
11. Hynes RO, Yamada KM. Fibronectins: multifunctional modular glycoproteins. *J Cell Biol* 1982;95:369–377.
12. Grinnell F. Fibronectin and wound healing. *J Cell Biochem* 1984;25:107–116.
13. Clark RAF, Folkvord JM, Wertz RL. Fibronectin as well as other extracellular matrix proteins mediate human keratinocyte adherence. *J Invest Dermatol* 1985;84:378–383.
14. Postlethwaite A, Keski-Oja J, Balian G, et al. Induction of fibroblast chemotaxis by fibronectin. Localization of the chemotactic region of a 140,000 molecular weight non-gelatin-binding fragment. *J Exp Med* 1981;153:494–499.
15. Williams TJ, Peck MJ. Role of prostaglandin-mediated vasodilation in inflammation. *Nature* 1977;270:530.
16. Bisgaard H, Kristensen J, Sondergaared J. The effect of leukotriene C4 and D4 on cutaneous blood flow in humans. *Prostaglandins* 1982;23:797–801.
17. Cherry PD, Furchgott RF, Zawadzki JV, et al. Role of endothelial cells in relaxation of isolated arteries by bradykinin. *Proc Natl Acad Sci U S A* 1982;72:2106–2110.
18. Griffith TM, Edwards DH, Lewis MJ, et al. The nature of the endothelium derived vascular relaxant factor. *Nature* 1984;308:645–647.
19. Lewis T, Grant R. Vascular reactions of the skin to injury. Part II. The liberation of a histamine-like substance in injured skin; the underlying cause of factitious urticaria and of wheals produced by burning, and observations upon the nervous control of certain skin reactions. *Heart* 1924;11:209–265.
20. Hebda PA, Collins MA, Tharp MA. Mast cell and myofibroblast in wound healing. *Dermatol Clin* 1993;11:685–696.
21. Singfelder JR. Prostaglandins: a review. *N Engl J Med* 1982;307:746–747.
22. Ammeland E, Prasad CM, Raymond RM, et al. Interactions among inflammatory mediators on edema formation in the canine forelimb. *Circ Res* 1981;49:298–306.
23. Williamson LM, Sheppard K, Davies JM, et al. Neutrophils are involved in the increased vascular permeability produced by activated complement in man. *Br J Haematol* 1986;64:375–384.
24. Majno G, Schoefl GI, Palade G. Studies on inflammation. II. The site of action of histamine and serotonin on the vascular tree; a topographic study. *J Biochem Biophys* 1961;11:607–626.
25. Majno G, Shea SM, Leventhal M. Endothelial contraction induced by histamine type mediators. An electron microscopic study. *J Cell Biol* 1969;42:647–672.
26. McLean AEM, Ahmed K, Judah JD. Cellular permeability and the reaction to injury. *Ann N Y Acad Sci* 1964;116:986–989.
27. Ley K. Leukocyte adhesion to vascular endothelium. *J Reconstr Microsurg* 1992;8:495–503.
28. Marasco WA, Phan SH, Krutzsch H, et al. Purification and identification of formyl-methionyl-leucyl-phenylalanine as the major peptide neutrophil chemotactic factor produced by Escherichia coli. *J Biol Chem* 1984;259:5430–5439.
29. Snyderman R, Phillips J, Mergenhagen SE. Polymorphonuclear leukocyte chemotactic activity in rabbit serum and guinea pig serum treated with immune complexes: evidence for C5a as the major chemotactic factor. *Infect Immun* 1970;1:521–525.
30. Tonnesen MG, Smedly LA, Henson PM. Neutrophil-endothelial cell interactions: modulation of neutrophil adhesiveness induced by complement fragments C5a and C5a des arg and formyl-methionyl-leucyl-phenylalanine *in vitro*. *J Clin Invest* 1984;745:1581–1592.
31. Peacock EE Jr. *Wound repair*, 3rd ed. Philadelphia: WB Saunders, 1984.
32. Ford-Hutchinson AW, Bray MA, Doig MV, et al. Leukotriene B, a potent chemokinetic and aggregating substance released from polymorphonuclear leukocytes. *Nature* 1980;286:264–265.
33. Deuel TF, Senior RM, Huang JS, et al. Chemotaxis of monocytes and neutrophils to platelet-derived growth factor. *J Clin Invest* 1982;69:1046–1049.
34. Musson RA. Human serum induces maturation of human monocytes *in vitro*. *Am J Pathol* 1983;111:331–340.
35. Proveddini DM, Deftos LJ, Manolagas SC. 1,25-dihydroxyvitamin D3 promotes *in vitro* morphologic and enzymatic changes in normal human monocytes consistent with their differentiation into macrophages. *Bone* 1986;7:23–28.
36. Wright SD, Meyer BC. Fibronectin receptor of human macrophages recognizes sequence Arg-Gly-Asp-Ser. *J Exp Med* 1985;162:762–767.
37. Ishida M, Honda M, Heyashi H. *In vitro* macrophage chemotactic generation from serum immunoglobulin G by neutrophil neutral seryl protease. *Immunology* 1978;35:167–176.
38. Marder SR, Chenoweth DE, Goldstein IM, et al. Chemotactic responses of human peripheral blood monocytes to the complement-derived peptides C5a and C5a des arg. *J Immunol* 1985;134:3325–3331.
39. Norris DA, Clark RAF, Swigart LM, et al. Fibronectin fragment(s) are chemotactic for human peripheral blood monocytes. *J Immunol* 1982;129:1612–1618.

40. Postlethwaite AE, Kang AH. Collagen- and collagen peptide-induced chemotaxis of human blood monocytes. *J Exp Med* 1976;143:1299–1307.

41. Senior RM, Griffin GL, Mecham RP, et al. Val-Gly-Val-Ala-Pro-Gly, a repeating peptide in elastin is chemotactic for fibroblasts and monocytes. *J Cell Biol* 1984;99:870–874.

42. Snyderman R, Fudman EJ. Demonstration of a chemotactic factor receptor on macrophages. *J Immunol* 1980;124:2754–2757.

43. Wahl SM, Hunt DA, Wakefield LM, et al. Transforming growth factor induces monocyte chemotaxis and growth factor production. *Proc Natl Acad Sci U S A* 1987;84:5788–5792.

44. Diegelmann RF, Cohen IK, Kaplan AM. The role of macrophages in wound repair: a review. *Plast Reconstr Surg* 1981;68:107–113.

45. Huybrechts-Godin G, Peeters-Joris C, Vaes G. Partial characterization of the macrophage factor that stimulates fibroblasts to produce collagenase and to degrade collagen. *Biochim Biophys Acta* 1985;846:51–54.

46. Werb Z, Banda MJ, Jones PA. Degradation of connective tissue matrices by macrophages I. Proteolysis of elastin, glycoproteins and collagen by proteinases isolated from macrophages. *J Exp Med* 1980;152:1340–1357.

47. Peterson JM, Barbul A, Breslin RJ, et al. Significance of T-lymphocytes in wound healing. *Surgery* 1987;102:300–305.

48. Martin CW, Muir IFK. The role of lymphocytes in wound healing. *Br J Plast Surg* 1990;43:655–662.

49. Blotnick S, Peoples GE, Freeman MR, et al. T-lymphocytes synthesize and export heparin-binding epidermal growth factor-like growth factor and basic fibroblast growth factor, mitogens for vascular cells and fibroblasts: differential production and release by CD4$^+$ and CD8$^+$ T cells. *Proc Natl Acad Sci U S A* 1994;91:2890–2894.

50. Ross R. The role of T lymphocytes in inflammation. *Proc Natl Acad Sci U S A* 1994;91:2879.

51. Robbins RA, Klassen L, Rasmussen H, et al. Interleukin-2-induced chemotaxis of human T-lymphocytes. *J Lab Clin Med* 1986;108:340–345.

52. Van Epps DE. Mediators and modulators of human lymphocyte chemotaxis. *Agents Actions Suppl* 1983;12:217–233.

53. Leibovich SJ, Ross R. The role of the macrophage in wound repair. A study with hydrocortisone and antimacrophage serum. *Am J Pathol* 1975;78:71–100.

54. Simpson DM, Ross R. The neutrophilic leukocyte in wound repair. A study with antineutrophil serum. *J Clin Invest* 1972;51:2009–2023.

55. Baxter CR. Immunologic reactions in chronic wounds. *Am J Surg* 1994;167(Suppl 1A):12S–14S.

56. Ross R, Everett NB, Tyler R. Wound healing and collagen formation. VI. The origin of the wound fibroblast studied in parabiosis. *J Cell Biol* 1970;44:645–654.

57. Seppä H, Grotendorst GR, Seppä S, et al. Platelet-derived growth factor is chemoattractant for fibroblasts. *J Cell Biol* 1982;92:584–588.

58. Grotendorst GR, Chang T, Seppä HEJ, et al. Platelet-derived growth factor is a chemoattractant for vascular smooth muscle cells. *J Cell Physiol* 1982;112:261–266.

59. Gauss-Muller V, Kleinman HK, Martin GR, et al. Role of attachment factors and attractants in fibroblast chemotaxis. *J Lab Clin Med* 1981;96:1071–1080.

60. Postlethwaite AE, Keski-Oja J, Ballan G, et al. Induction of fibroblast chemotaxis by fibronectin. *J Exp Med* 1981;153:494–499.

61. Tsukamoto Y, Helsel WE, Wahl SE. Macrophage production of fibronectin, a chemoattractant for fibroblasts. *J Immunol* 1981;127:673–678.

62. Westermark B, Blomquist W. Stimulation of fibroblast migration by epidermal growth factor. *Cell Biol Int* 1980;4:649–654.

63. Postlewhaite AE, Snyderman R, Kang AH. The chemotactic attraction of human fibroblasts to a lymphocyte derived factor. *J Exp Med* 1976;144:188–1203.

64. Postlethwaite AE, Seyer JM, Kang AH. Chemotactic attraction of human fibroblasts to type I, II, and III collagens and collagen derived peptides. *Proc Natl Acad Sci U S A* 1978;75:871–875.

65. Grotendorst GR, Pencev D, Martin GR, et al. Molecular mediators of tissue repair. In: Hunt TK, Heppenstall RB, Pines E, et al. eds. *Soft and hard tissue repair: biological and clinical aspects.* New York: Praeger, 1984:20–41.

66. Rutherford RB, Ross R. Platelet factors stimulate fibroblasts and smooth muscle cells quiescent in plasma serum to proliferate. *J Cell Biol* 1976;69:196–203.

67. Roberts AB, Anzano MA, Wakefield LM, et al. Type-β transforming growth factor: a bifunctional regulator of cellular growth. *Proc Natl Acad Sci U S A* 1985;82:119–123.

68. Assoian RK, Grotendorst GR, Miller DM, et al. Cellular transformation by coordinated action of three peptide growth factors from human platelets. *Nature* 1984;309:804–806.

69. Wahl SM, Wahl LM, McCarthy JB. Lymphocyte-mediated activation of fibroblast proliferation and collagen production. *J Immunol* 1978;121:942–946.

70. Clemmons DR. Interaction of circulating cell-derived and plasma growth factors in stimulating cultured smooth muscle cell replication. *J Cell Physiol* 1984;121:425–430.

71. Ronning OW, Pettersen EO. Effect of different growth factors on cell cycle traverse and protein growth of human cells in culture. *Exp Cell Res* 1985;157:29–40.

72. Folkman J, Klagsbrun M. Angiogenic factors. *Science* 1987;235:442–447.

73. Sholley MM, Ferguson GP, Seibel HR, et al. Mechanisms of neovascularization. Vascular sprouting can occur without proliferation of endothelial cells. *Lab Invest* 1984;51:624–634.

74. Madri JA, Williams SK. Capillary endothelial cell cultures: phenotypic modulation by matrix components. *J Cell Biol* 1983;97:153–165.

75. Polverini PJ, Coltran RS, Gimbrone MA, et al. Activated macrophages induce vascularization. *Nature* 1977;269:804–806.

76. Polverini PJ, Leibovich SJ. Induction of neovascularization *in vivo* and endothelial cell proliferation *in vitro* by tumor-associated macrophages. *Lab Invest* 1984;51:635–642.

77. Koch AE, Polverini PJ, Leibovich SJ. Induction of neovascularization by activated human monocytes. *J Leukoc Biol* 1986;39:223–238.

78. Gospodarowicz D, Neufeld G, Schweigerer L. Fibroblast growth factor: structural and biologic properties. *J Cell Physiol Suppl* 1987;5:15–26.

79. Shing Y, Folkmann J, Sullivan R, et al. Heparin affinity: purification of a tumor-derived capillary endothelial cell growth factor. *Science* 1984;223:1296–1299.

80. Gospodarowicz D, Abraham J, Schilling J. Isolation and characterization of a vascular endothelial cell mitogen produced by pituitary-derived follicular stellate cells. *Proc Natl Acad Sci U S A* 1989;86:7311–7315.

81. Roberts AB, Sporn MB, Assoian RK, et al. Transforming growth factor type beta: rapid induction of fibrosis and angiogenesis *in vivo* and stimulation of collagen formation *in vitro*. *Proc Natl Acad Sci U S A* 1986;83:4167–4171.

82. Banda MJ, Dwyer KS, Beckman A. Wound fluid angiogenesis factor stimulates the directed migration of capillary endothelial cells. *J Cell Biochem* 1985;29:183–193.

83. Banda MJ, Knighton DR, Hunt TK, et al. Isolation of a nonmitogenic factor from wound fluid. *Proc Natl Acad Sci USA* 1982;79:7773–7777.

84. Castellot JJ, Karnovsky MJ, Spiegelman BM Jr. Differentiation-dependent stimulation of neovascularization and endothelial cell chemotaxis by 3T3 adipocytes. *Proc Natl Acad Sci U S A* 1982;79:5597–5601.

85. Teuscher E, Weidlich V. Adenosine nucleotides, adenosine and adenine as angiogenesis factors. *Biomed Biochim Acta* 1985;44:493–495.

86. Clemmons DR, Isley WL, Brown MT. Dialyzable factor in human serum of platelet origin stimulates endothelial replication and growth. *Proc Natl Acad Sci U S A* 1983;80:1641–1645.

87. Schott RJ, Morrow LA. Growth factors and angiogenesis. *Cardiovasc Res* 1993;27:1155–1161.

88. Ansprunk DH, Falterman K, Folkman J. The sequence of events in the regression of corneal capillaries. *Lab Invest* 1978;38:284–294.

89. Pang C, Daniels RK, Buck RC. Epidermal migration during the healing of suction blisters in rat skin: a scanning and transmission electron microscopic study. *Am J Anat* 1978;153:177–191.

90. Johnson FR, McMinn RM. The cytology of wound healing of body surfaces in mammals. *Biol Rev* 1962;35:364–412.

91. Odland G, Ross R. Human wound repair. I. Epidermal regeneration. *J Cell Biol* 1968;39:135–151.

92. Woodley DT, Chen JD, Kim JP, et al. Reepithelialization: human keratinocyte locomotion. *Dermatol Clin* 1993;11:641–646.

93. Dunlap MK, Donaldson DJ. Inability of colchicine to inhibit newt epidermal cell migration or prevent concanavalin-A mediated inhibition of migration studies. *Exp Cell Res* 1978;116:1519.

94. Sullivan DJ, Epstein WS. Mitotic activity of wounded human epidermis. *J Invest Dermatol* 1963;41:39–43.

95. Gipson IK, Spurr-Michaud SJ, Tisdale AS. Hemidesmosomes and anchoring fibril collagen appear synchronously during development and wound healing. *Dev Biol* 1988;126t:253–262.

96. Mackenzie IC, Fusenig NE. Regeneration of organized epithelial structure. *J Invest Dermatol* 1983;81:1895–1945.

97. Niall M, Ryan GB, O'Brien BM. The effect of epidermal growth factor on wound healing in mice. *J Surg Res* 1982;33:164–169.

98. Nanney LB, Magid M, Stoscheck CM, et al. Comparison of epidermal growth factor binding and receptor distribution in normal human epidermis and epidermal appendages. *J Invest Dermatol* 1984;83:385–393.

99. Werner S, Peters KG, Longaker MT, et al. Large induction of keratinocyte growth factor in the dermis during wound healing. *Proc Natl Acad Sci U S A* 1992;89:6896–6900.

100. Gillman T. Healing of cutaneous abrasions and of incisions closed with sutures or plastic adhesive tape. *Med Proc* 1958;4:751.

101. Nimmi ME. Collagen: its structure and function in normal and pathological connective tissues. *Semin Arthritis Rheum* 1974;4:95–150.

102. Caterson B, Lowther DA. Changes in the metabolism of the proteoglycans from sheep articular cartilage in response to mechanical stress. *Biochem Biophys Acta* 1978;540:412–422.

103. Weiss PH, Klein L. The quantitative relationship of urinary peptide hydroxyproline excretion to collagen degradation. *J Clin Invest* 1969;48:1–10.

104. Ignotz RA, Massaugue J. Transforming growth factor-beta stimulates the expression of fibronectin and collagen and their incorporation into the extracellular matrix. *J Biol Chem* 1986;261:4337–4345.

105. Cutroneo KR, Rokowski R, Counts DF. Glucocorticoids and collagen synthesis: comparison of *in vivo* and cell culture studies. *Coll Relat Res* 1981;1:557–568.

106. Sunder R, Church CV, Klobutcher LA, et al. Genetics of the connective tissue proteins. Assignment of the gene for human type I procollagen to chromosome 17. *Proc Natl Acad Sci U S A* 1977;74:4444–4448.

107. Church RL. Chromosome mapping of connective tissue proteins. *Int Rev Connect Tissue Res* 1981;9:99.

108. Madden JW, Arem AJ. Wound healing: biologic and clinical features. In: Sabiston DC Jr, ed. *Textbook of surgery.* 13th ed. Philadelphia: WB Saunders, 1986:193–213.

109. Fleischmajer R, Olsen BR, Kuhn K. Biology, chemistry and pathology of collagen. *Ann N Y Acad Sci* 1985;460:1–13.

110. Chapman JA, Kellgren JH, Steven FS. Assembly of collagen fibrils. *Fed Proc* 1966;25:1811–1812.

111. Petruska JA, Hodge AJ. A subunit model for the tropocollagen macromolecule. *Proc Natl Acad Sci U S A* 1964;51:871–876.

112. Siegel RC, Pinnel SR, Martin GR. Cross linking of collagen and elastin. *Properties Lysyl Oxidase. Biochem* 1970;9:4486–4492.

113. Tanzer ML. Cross linking of collagen. *Science* 1973;180:561–566.

114. Veis A, Averey J. Modes of intermolecular cross linking in mature insoluble collagen. *J Biol Chem* 1965;240:3899–3908.

115. Hassel JR, Kimura JH, Hascall VC. Proteoglycan core protein families. *Annu Rev Biochem* 1986;55:539–567.

116. Chen WYJ, Abatangelo G. Functions of hyaluronan in wound repair. *Wound Repair Regen* 1999;7:70–89.

117. Gabbiani G, Ryan GB, Majno G. Presence of modified fibroblasts in granulation tissue and their possible role in wound contraction. *Experientia* 1971;27:549–550.

118. McGrath MH, Hundahl SA. The spatial and temporal quantification of myofibroblasts. *Plast Reconstr Surg* 1982;69:975–983.

119. Rudolph R. Location of the force of wound contraction. *Surg Gynecol Obstet* 1979;148:547–551.

120. Ehrlich HP. The role of connective tissue matrix in wound healing. In: Barbul A, Pines E, Caldwell M, et al. eds. *Growth factors and other aspects of wound healing: biological and clinical implications.* New York: Alan R Liss, 1988:243–258.

121. Harris AK, Stopak D, Wild P. Fibroblast traction as a mechanism for collagen morphogenesis. *Nature* 1981;290:249–251.

122. Grinnell F, Lamke DR. Reorganization of hydrated collagen lattices by human skin fibroblasts. *J Cell Sci* 1984;66:51–63.

123. Guidry C, Grinnell F. Studies on the mechanism of hydrated collagen gel reorganization by fibroblasts. *J Cell Sci* 1985;79:67–81.

124. Farsi JMA, Aubin JE. Microfilament rearrangements during fibroblast-induced contraction of three-dimensional hydrated collagen gels. *Cell Motil Cytoskeleton* 1984;4:29–40.

125. Montesano R, Orci L. Transforming growth factor beta stimulates collagen-matrix contraction by fibroblasts: implications for wound healing. *Proc Natl Acad Sci U S A* 1988;85:4894–4897.

126. Ronnov-Jensen L, Peterson OW. Induction of alpha-smooth muscle actin by transforming growth factor-1 in quiescent human breast gland fibroblasts. *Lab Invest* 1993;68:696–707.

127. Clark RAF, Folkvord JM, Hart CE, et al. Platelet isoforms of platelet-derived growth factor stimulate fibroblasts to contract collagen matrices. *J Clin Invest* 1989;84:1036–1040.

128. Dubretet LF, Brunner-Ferber F, Misiti J, et al. Activities of human acidic fibroblast growth factor in an *in vitro* dermal equivalent model. *J Invest Dermatol* 1991;97:793–798.

129. Gillery P, Serpier H, Polette M, et al. Gamma-interferon inhibits extracellular matrix synthesis and remodeling in collagen lattice cultures of normal and scleroderma skin fibroblasts. *Eur J Cell Biol* 1992;57:244–253.

130. Rudolph R. The effect of skin graft preparation on wound contraction. *Surg Gynecol Obstet* 1976;142:49–56.

131. Madden JW, Morton D Jr, Peacock EE Jr. Contraction of experimental wounds. I. Inhibiting wound contraction by using a topical smooth muscle antagonist. *Surgery* 1974;76:1–8.

132. Madden JW, Peacock EE Jr. Studies on the biology of collagen during wound healing. I. Rate of collagen synthesis and deposition in cutaneous wounds of the rat. *Surgery* 1968;64:288–294.

133. Levenson SM, Geever EF, Crowley LV, et al. The healing of rat skin wounds. *Ann Surg* 1965;161:293–308.

134. Riley WB Jr, Peacock EE Jr. Identification, distribution and significance of a collagenolytic enzyme in human tissue. *Proc Soc Exp Biol Med* 1967;214:207–210.

135. Forrester JC, Zederfeldt BH, Hayes TL, et al. Wolff's law in relation to the healing skin wound. *J Trauma* 1970;10:770–779.

136. Parsons SL, Watson SA, Brown PD, et al. Matrix metalloproteinases. *Br J Surg* 1997;84:160–166.

137. Vu TH, Werb Z. Matrix metalloproteinases: effectors of development and normal physiology. *Genes Dev* 2000;14:2123–2133.

138. Brew K, Kinkarpandian D, Nagase H. Tissue inhibitors of metalloproteinases: evolution, structure and function. *Biochim Biophy Acta* 2000;1477:267–283.

139. Clark RAF. Growth factors and wound repair. *J Cell Biochem* 1991;46:1–2.
140. Cohen S. Epidermal growth factor. *Biosci Rep* 1986;6:1017–1028.
141. Laato M, Niinikoski J, Lebel L, et al. Stimulation of wound healing by epidermal growth factor. *Ann Surg* 1986;203:379–381.
142. Schreiber AB, Winkler ME, Derynck R. Transforming growth factor alpha: a more potent angiogenic mediator than epidermal growth factor. *Science* 1986;232:1250–1253.
143. Nishida T, Tanaka H, Nakagawa S, et al. Fibronectin synthesis by the rabbit cornea: effects of mouse epidermal growth factor and cyclic AMP analogs. *Jpn J Ophthalmol* 1984;196:196–202.
144. Werner S. Keratinocyte growth factor: a unique player in epithelial repair processes. *Cytokine Growth Factor Rev* 1998;9:153–165.
145. Gospodarowicz D, Neufeld G, Schweigerer L. Fibroblast growth factor: structural and biologic properties. *J Cell Physiol Suppl* 1987;5:15–26.
146. Baird A, Esch F, Mormede P, et al. Molecular characterization of fibroblast growth factor: distribution and biologic activities in various tissues. *Recent Prog Horm Res* 1989;42:143–205.
147. Klingbeil CK, Cesar LB, Fiddes JC. Basic fibroblast growth factor accelerates tissue repair in models of impaired healing. In: Barbul A, Caldwell MC, Eaglestein WH et al. eds. *Clinical and experimental approaches to dermal and epidermal repair: normal and chronic wounds.* New York: John Wiley and Sons, 1991:443–458.
148. McGee GS, Davidson JM, Buckley A, et al. Recombinant basic fibroblast growth factor accelerates wound healing. *J Surg Res* 1988;45:145–153.
149. Hebda PA, Klingbeil CK, Abraham JA, et al. Basic fibroblast growth factor stimulation of epidermal wound healing in pigs. *J Invest Dermatol* 1990;95:626–631.
150. Rubin JS, Osada H, Finch PW, et al. Purification and characterization of a newly identified growth factor specific for epithelial cells. *Proc Natl Acad Sci U S A* 1989;86:802–806.
151. Smola H, Thiekotter G, Fusenig NE. Mutual induction of growth factor gene expression by epidermal-dermal cell interaction. *J Cell Biol* 1993;122:417–429.
152. Heldin C-H, Westermark B. Mechanism of action and *in vivo* role of platelet-derived growth facto. *Phys Rev* 1999;79:1283–1316.
153. Heldin C-H, Westermark B. Platelet-derived growth factors: a family of isoforms that bind to two distinct receptors. *Br Med Bull* 1989;45:453–464.
154. Ross R. Platelet-derived growth factor. *Annu Rev Med* 1987;38:71–79.
155. Blatti SP, Foster DN, Ranganathan G, et al. Induction of fibronectin gene transcription and mRNA is a primary response to growth-factor stimulation of AKR-2B cells. *Proc Natl Acad Sci U S A* 1988;85:1119–1123.
156. Heldin P, Laurent TC, Heldin C-H. Effect of growth factors on hyaluronan synthesis in cultured human fibroblasts. *Biochem J* 1989;258:919–922.
157. Pierce GF, Mustoe TA, Lingelbach J, et al. Platelet-derived growth factor and transforming growth factor enhance tissue repair activities by unique mechanisms. *J Cell Biol* 1989;109:429–440.
158. Maciag T, Nemore R, Weinstein R, et al. An endocrine approach to the control of epidermal growth: serum-free cultivation of human keratinocytes. *Science* 1981;211:1452–1454.
159. Assoian RK, Komoriya A, Meyers CA, et al. Transforming growth factor-B in human platelets. *J Biol Chem* 1983;258:7155–7160.
160. O'Kane S, Ferguson MJ. Transforming growth factor-betas and wound healing. *Int J Biochem Cell Biol* 1997;29:63–78.
161. Shah M, Foreman DM, Ferguson MWJ. Neutralizing antibody to TGF-$\beta_{1,2}$ reduces cutaneous scarring in adult rodents. *J Cell Sci* 1994;107:1137–1157.
162. Ignotz RA, Endo T, Massague J. Regulation of fibronectin and type I collagen mRNA levels by transforming growth factor. *J Biol Chem* 1987;262:6443–6446.
163. Peebles K, Boswick JA, Scott FA Jr. Wounds of the hand contaminated by human or animal saliva. *J Trauma* 1980;20:383–389.
164. Kligman AM. The bacteriology of normal skin. In: Wolcott BW, Rund DA, eds. *Skin bacteria and their role in infection.* New York: McGraw-Hill, 1965:13–21.
165. Edlich RF, Rodeheaver GT, Morgan RF, et al. Principles of emergency wound management. *Ann Emerg Med* 1988;17:1284–1302.
166. Ricketts CR, Squire JR, Topley E. Human skin lipids with particular reference to the self sterilizing power of the skin. *Clinical Science* 1951;10:89–110.
167. Heggers JP. Natural host defense mechanisms. *Clin Plast Surg* 1979;6:505–513.
168. Lindberg RB, Moncrief JA, Switzer WE, et al. The successful control of burn wound sepsis. *J Trauma* 1965;5:601–616.
169. Teplitz C, Davis D, Mason AD, et al. Pseudomonas burn wound sepsis. I. Pathogenesis of experimental pseudomonas burn wound sepsis. *J Surg Res* 1964;4:200–216.
170. Kass EH. Asymptomatic infections of the urinary tract. *Trans Assoc Am Physicians* 1956;69:56–64.
171. Bendy RH, Nuccio PA, Wolfe E, et al. Relationship of quantitative bacterial counts to healing of decubiti: effect of gentamycin. *Antimicrob Agents Chemother* 1964;4:147–153.
172. Robson MC, Heggers JP. Surgical infection. II. The B-hemolytic streptococcus. *J Surg Res* 1969;9:289–292.
173. Krizek TH, Davis JH. The role of the red cell in subcutaneous infection. *J Trauma* 1965;5:85–95.
174. Cruse PJE. Wound infection. In: Howard RJ, Simmons RL, eds. *Surgical infectious disease.* East Norwalk: Appleton & Lange, 1988:319.
175. Hunt TK, Zederfeldt BH, Goldstick TK, et al. Tissue oxygen tensions during controlled hemorrhage. *Surg Forum* 1967;18:3–4.
176. Hauser CJ. Tissue salvage by mapping of skin transcutaneous oxygen tension index. *Arch Surg* 1987;122:128.
177. Roth GJ, McDonald JB, Sheard C. The effect of cigarettes and of intravenous injections of nicotine on the electrocardiogram, basal metabolic rate, cutaneous temperature, blood pressure, and pulse rate of normal persons. *JAMA* 1944;125:761–767.
178. Bruce JW, Miller JR, Hooker DR. The effect of smoking upon the blood pressures and upon the volume of the hand. *Am J Physiol* 1909;24:104–116.
179. Wright IS, Moffat D. The effects of tobacco on the peripheral vascular system. *JAMA* 1934;103:315–323.
180. Sackett DL, Gibson RW, Bross IDJ, et al. Relation between aortic atherosclerosis and the use of cigarettes and alcohol: an autopsy study. *N Engl J Med* 1968;279:1413–1420.
181. Birnstingl MA, Brinson K, Chakrabarti BK. The effect of short-term exposure to carbon monoxide on platelet stickiness. *Br J Surg* 1971;58:837–839.
182. Astrup P, Kjeldsen K. Carbon monoxide, smoking and atherosclerosis. *Med Clin North Am* 1973;58:323–350.
183. Kjeldsen K, Astrup P, Wanstrup J. Ultra-structural intimal changes in the rabbit aorta after a moderate carbon monoxide exposure. *Atherosclerosis* 1972;16:67–82.
184. Jorgensen LN, Kallehave F, Christensen E, et al. Less collagen production in smokers. *Surgery* 1998;123:450–455.
185. Fajardo LF, Berthong M. Radiation injury in surgical pathology: part III salivary glands, pancreas and skin. *Am J Surg Pathol* 1981;5:279–296.
186. Rudolph R. Complications of surgery for radiotherapy skin damage. *Plast Reconstr Surg* 1982;70:179–183.
187. Levenson SM, Gruber CA, Rettura G, et al. Supplemental vitamin A prevents the acute radiation-induced defect in wound healing. *Ann Surg* 1984;200:494–512.
188. Howes EL, Briggs H, Shea R, et al. Effect of complete and partial starvation on the rate of fibroplasia in the healing wound. *Arch Surg* 1933;27:846–858.

189. Haydock DA, Hill GL. Impaired wound healing in surgical patients with varying degrees of malnutrition. *JPEN J Parenter Enteral Nutr* 1986;10:550–554.

190. Thompson WD, Ravdin IS, Frank IL. Effect of hypoproteinemia on wound disruption. *Arch Surg* 1938;36:500–518.

191. Devereaux DF, Thistlewaite PA, Thibault LF, et al. Effect of tumor bearing and protein depletion on wound breaking strength in the rat. *J Surg Res* 1979;27:233–238.

192. Williamson MB, Fromm HJ. Effect of cystine and methionine on healing of experimental wounds. *Proc Soc Exp Biol Med* 1957;80:623–626.

193. Levenson SM, Seifter E. Dysnutrition, wound healing, and resistance to infection. *Clin Plast Surg* 1977;4:375–388.

194. Freiman M, Seifter E, Connerton C, et al. Vitamin A deficiency and surgical stress. *Surg Forum* 1970;21:81–82.

195. Shapiro SS, Mott DJ. Modulation of glycosaminoglycan synthesis by retinoids. *Ann N Y Acad Sci* 1981;359:306–321.

196. Cohen BE, Till G, Cullen PR, et al. Reversal of postoperative immunosuppression in man by vitamin A. *Surg Gynecol Obstet* 1979;149:658–662.

197. Alvarez OM, Gilbreath RL. Effect of dietary thiamine on intermolecular collagen cross linking during wound repair: a mechanical and biochemical assessment. *J Trauma* 1982;22:20–24.

198. Ehrlich HP, Tarver H, Hunt TK. Inhibitory effects of vitamin E on collagen synthesis and wound repair. *Ann Surg* 1972;175:235–240.

199. Fernandez-Madrid F, Prasad AS, Oberleas D. Effect of zinc deficiency on nucleic acids, collagen, and noncollagenous protein of the connective tissue. *J Lab Clin Med* 1973;82:951–961.

200. Chvapil M. Zinc and wound healing. In: Zederfeldt B, ed. *Symposium on zinc.* Lund, Sweden: AB Tika, 1974.

201. Lawrence WT, Norton JA, Harvey AK, et al. Wound healing in sarcoma-bearing rats: tumor effects on cutaneous and deep wounds. *J Surg Oncol* 1987;35:7–12.

202. Chlebowski RT, Heber D. Metabolic abnormalities in cancer patients: carbohydrate metabolism. *Surg Clin North Am* 1986;66:957–968.

203. Weingweg J, Levenson SM, Rettura G, et al. Supplemental vitamin A prevents the tumor-inducted defect in wound healing. *Ann Surg* 1990;211:269–276.

204. Dunuoy P, Carrell A. Cicatrization of wounds. *J Exp Biol* 1921;34:339–348.

205. Sandblom P, Peterson P, Muren A. Determination of the tensile strength of the healing wound as a clinical test. *Acta Chirurgica Scandinavia* 1953;105:252–257.

206. Cruse PJE, Foord RA. A prospective study of 23,649 surgical wounds. *Arch Surg* 1973;107:206–210.

207. Goodson WH, Hunt TK. Studies of wound healing in experimental diabetes mellitus. *J Surg Res* 1977;22:221–227.

208. Prakash A, Pandit PN, Sharma LK. Studies in wound healing in experimental diabetes. *Int Surg* 1974;59:25–28.

209. Arquilla ER, Weringer EJ, Nakajo M. Wound healing; a model for the study of diabetic microangiopathy. *Diabetes* 1976;25(suppl 2):811–819.

210. Bybee JD, Rogers DE. The phagocytic activity of polymorphonuclear leukocytes obtained from patients with diabetes mellitus. *J Lab Clin Med* 1964;64:1–13.

211. Nolan CM, Beaty HN, Bagdade JD. Further characterization of the impaired bactericidal function of granulocytes in patients with poorly controlled diabetes. *Diabetes* 1978;27:889–894.

212. Bagdade JD, Root RK, Bugler RJ. Impaired leukocyte function in patients with poorly controlled diabetes. *Diabetes* 1974;23:9–15.

213. Gottrup F, Andreassen IT. Healing of incisional wounds in stomach and duodenum: the influence of experimental diabetes. *J Surg Res* 1981;31:61–68.

214. Weringer EJ, Kelso JM, Tamai IY, et al. Effects of insulin on wound healing in diabetic mice. *Acta Endocrinol* 1982;99:101–108.

215. Yue DK, McLennan S, Marsh M, et al. Effects of experimental diabetes, uremia, and malnutrition on wound healing. *Diabetes* 1987;36:295–299.

216. Howes EL, Plotz CM, Blunt JW, et al. Retardation of wound healing by cortisone. *Surgery* 1950;28:177–181.

217. Hunt TK, Ehrlich HP, Garcia JA, et al. The effect of vitamin A on reversing the inhibitory effect of cortisone on the healing of open wounds in animals. *Ann Surg* 1969;170:633–641.

218. Stephens FO, Dunphy JE, Hunt TK. Effect of delayed administration of corticosteroids on wound contraction. *Ann Surg* 1971;173:214–218.

219. Sandberg N. Time relationship between administration of cortisone and wound healing in rats. *Acta Chir Scand* 1964;127:446–455.

220. Hunt TK, Ehrlich HP, Garcia JA, et al. Effects of vitamin A on reversing the inhibitory effects of cortisone on healing of open wounds in animals and man. *Ann Surg* 1969;170:633–641.

221. Shamberger RC, Devereaux DF, Brennan MF. The effect of chemotherapeutic agents on wound healing. *Int Adv Surg Oncol* 1981;4:15–58.

222. Lawrence WT, Talbot TL, Norton JA. Preoperative or postoperative doxorubicin hydrochloride (Adriamycin): which is better for wound healing? *Surgery* 1986;100:9–12.

223. Peacock EE, Madden JW, Trier WC, Jr. Biologic basis for the treatment of keloids and hypertrophic scars. *South Med J* 1970;63:755–759.

224. Brody GS, Peng STJ, Landel RF. The etiology of hypertrophic scar contracture: another view. *Plast Reconstr Surg* 1981;67:673–684.

225. Lawrence WT. In search of the optimal treatment of keloids: report of a series and a review of the literature. *Ann Plast Surg* 1991;27:164–178.

226. Edlich RF, Smith OT, Edgerton MT. Resistance of the surgical wound to antimicrobial prophylaxis and its mechanism of development. *Am J Surg* 1973;126:583–591.

227. Rodeheaver GT, Rye DR, Rust R, et al. Mechanism by which proteolytic enzymes prolong the golden period of antibiotic action. *Am J Surg* 1978;136:379–382.

228. Rodeheaver G, Bellamy W, Kody M, et al. Bacteriocidal activity and toxicity of iodine-containing solution in wounds. *Arch Surg* 1982;117:181–186.

229. Siegel RJ, Vistnes LM, Iverson RE. Effective hemostasis with less epinephrine: an experimental and clinical study. *Plast Reconstr Surg* 1973;51:129–133.

230. Wilhelmi BJ, Blackwell SJ, Miller JH, et al. Do no use epinephrine in digital blocks: myth or truth? *Plast Reconstr Surg* 2001;107:293–297.

231. Klein JA. Tumescent technique for local anesthesia improves safety in large-volume liposuction. *Plast Reconstr Surg* 1993;92:1085–1098.

232. Samdal F, Amland PF, Bugge JF. Plasma lidocaine levels during suction-assisted lipectomy using large doses of dilute lidocaine with epinephrine. *Plast Reconstr Surg* 1994;93:1217–1223.

233. Arndt KA, Burton C, Noe JM. Minimizing the pain of local anesthesia. *Plast Reconstr Surg* 1983;72:676.

234. Christopher RA, Buchanan L, Begalla K, et al. Pain reduction in local anesthesia administration through pH buffering. *Ann Emerg Med* 1988;17:117–123.

235. Adamson S, Menegazzi JJ, Paris PM, et al. A randomized controlled trial of the effectiveness of counterirritation on venipuncture associated pain. *Acad Emerg Med* 1997;4:425.

236. Anderson AB, Colecchi C, Baronoski R, et al. Local anesthesia in pediatric patients: topical TAC versus lidocaine. *Ann Emerg Med* 1990;19:519–522.

237. Hegenbarth MA, Allen MF, Hawk WH, et al. Comparison of topical tetracaine, adrenaline, and cocaine anesthesia with lidocaine infiltration for repair of lacerations in children. *Ann Emerg Med* 1990;19:63–67.

238. Blackburn PA, Butler KH, Hughes MJ, et al. Comparison of tetracaine-adrenaline-cocaine (TAC) with topical lidocaine-epinephrine (TLE): efficacy and cost. *Am J Emerg Med* 1995;13:315–317.

239. Schilling CG, Bank DE, Borchert BA, et al. Tetracine, epinephrine (adrenalin), and cocaine (TAC) versus lidocaine, epinephrine, and tetracaine (LET) for anesthesia in lacerations in children. *Ann Emerg Med* 1995;25:203–208.

240. Smith GA, Strausbaugh SD, Harbeck-Weber C, et al. Comparison of topical anesthetics without cocaine to tetracaine-adrenaline-cocaine and lidocaine infiltration during repair of lacerations: bupivicaine-norepinephrine is an effective topical anesthetic agent. *Pediatrics* 1996;97:301–307.

241. Smith GA, Strausbaugh SD, Harbeck-Weber C, et al. Prilocaine-phenylephrine and bupivicaine-phenylephrine topical anesthetics compared with tetracaine-adrenaline-cocaine during repair of lacerations. *Am J Emerg Med* 1998;16:121–124.

242. Zempsky WT, Karasic RB. EMLA versus TAC for topical anesthesia of extremity wounds in children. *Ann Emerg Med* 1997;30:163–166.

243. Alexander JW, Fischer JE, Boyajian M, et al. The influence of hair-removal methods on wound infections. *Arch Surg* 1983;118:347–352.

244. Madden H, Edlich RF, Schauerhamer R, et al. Application of principles of fluid dynamics to surgical wound irrigation. *Curr Top Surg Res* 1971;3:85–93.

245. Hollander JE, Richman PB, Werblud M, et al. Irrigation in facial and scalp lacerations: does it alter outcome? *Ann Emerg Med* 1998;31:73–77.

246. Gross A, Cutright DE, Bhaskar SN. Effectiveness of pulsating water jet lavage in treatment of contaminated crushed wounds. *Am J Surg* 1972;124:373–377.

247. Hamer ML, Robson MC, Krizek TJ, et al. Quantitative bacterial analysis of comparative wound irrigations. *Ann Surg* 1975;181:819–822.

248. Schauerhamer RA, Edlich RF, Panek P, et al. Studies in the management of contaminated wounds VII. Susceptibility of surgical wounds to postoperative surface contamination. *Am J Surg* 1971;122:74–77.

249. Branemark PI, Albrektsson B, Lindstrom J, et al. Local tissue effects of wound disinfectants. *Acta Chir Scand Suppl* 1966;357:166–176.

250. Rodeheaver GT, Smith SL, Thacker JG, et al. Mechanical cleansing of contaminated wounds with a surfactant. *Am J Surg* 1975;129:241–245.

251. Rodeheaver G, Turnbull V, Edgerton MT, et al. Pharmokinetics of a new skin cleanser. *Am J Surg* 1976;132:67–74.

252. Rodeheaver G, Bellamy W, Kody M, et al. Bacteriocidal activity and toxicity of iodine-containing solutions in wounds. *Arch Surg* 1982;117:181–186.

253. Custer J, Edlich RF, Prusak M, et al. Studies in the management of the contaminated wound V. An assessment of the effectiveness of pHisoHex and betadine surgical scrub solutions. *Am J Surg* 1971;121:572–575.

254. Mobacken H, Wengstrom C. Interference with healing of rat skin incisions treated with chlorhexidine. *Acta Derm Venereol* 1974;54:29.

255. Saatman RA, Carlton WW, Hubben K, et al. A wound healing study of chlorhexidine digluconate in guinea pigs. *Fundam Appl Toxicol* 1986;6:1–6.

256. Branemark PI, Ekholm R. Tissue injury caused by wound disinfectants. *J Bone Joint Surg Am* 1967;49:48–62.

257. Kozol RA, Gillies C, Elgebaly SA. Effects of sodium hypochlorite (Dakin's solution) on cells of the wound module. *Arch Surg* 1988;123:420–423.

258. Lineweaver W, Howard R, Soucy D, et al. Topical antimicrobial toxicity. *Arch Surg* 1985;120:267–270.

259. Dirschl DR, Wilson FC. Topical antibiotic irrigation in the prophylaxis of operative wound infections in orthopedic surgery. *Orthop Clin North Am* 1991;22:419–426.

260. Peacock EE Jr. Wound healing and wound care. In: Schwartz SI, ed. *Principles of surgery*. 5th ed. New York: McGraw-Hill, 1988:307–330.

261. Lowbury EJL, Lilly HA, Bull JP. Methods for disinfection of hands and operation sites. *Br Med J* 1964;2:531–536.

262. Saggers BA, Stewart GT. Polyvinyl-pyrrolidone-iodine: an assessment of antibacterial activity. *J Hyg* 1964;62:509–518.

263. Haury B, Rodeheaver G, Vensko J, et al. Debridement: an essential component of traumatic wound care. *Am J Surg* 1978;135:238–242.

264. Ordman LJ, Gillman T. Studies in the healing of cutaneous wounds: II the healing of epidermal, appendageal and dermal injuries inflicted by suture needles and by suture material in the skin of pigs. *Arch Surg* 1966;93:883–910.

265. VanWinkle N, Hastings JC. Considerations in the choice of suture material for various tissues. *Surg Gynecol Obstet* 1972;135:113–126.

266. George TK, Simpson DC. Skin wound closure with staples in the accident and emergency department. *J R Coll Surg Edinb* 1985;30:54–56.

267. Golden T. Non-irritating, multipurpose surgical adhesive tape. *Am J Surg* 1960;100:789–796.

268. Golden T, Levy AH, O'Connor WT. Primary healing of skin wounds and incisions with a threadless suture. *Am J Surg* 1962;104:603–612.

269. Conolly WB, Hunt TK, Zederfeldt B, et al. Clinical comparison of surgical wounds closed by suture and adhesive tapes. *Am J Surg* 1969;117:318–322.

270. Edlich RF, Thul J, Prusak M, et al. Studies in the management of the contaminated wound VIII. Assessment of tissue adhesives for repair of contaminated tissue. *Am J Surg* 1971;122:394–397.

271. Quinn J, Wells G, Sutcliffe T, et al. A randomized trial comparing octylcyanoacrylate tissue adhesive and sutures in the management of lacerations. *JAMA* 1997;277:1527–1530.

272. Saltz R, Sierra K, Feldman D, et al. Experimental and clinical applications of fibrin glue. *Plast Reconstr Surg* 1991;88:1005–1015.

273. Jabs AD Jr, Wider TM, DeBellis J, et al. The effect of fibrin glue on skin grafts in infected sites. *Plast Reconstr Surg* 1992;89:268–271.

274. Mandel MA. Minimal suture blepharoplasty: closure of incisions with autologous fibrin glue. *Aesthetic Plast Surg* 1992;16:269–272.

275. Ferguson DJ. Clinical application of experimental relations between technique and wound infection. *Surgery* 1968;63:377–381.

276. deHoll D, Rodeheaver G, Edgerton MT, et al. Potentiation of infection by suture closure of dead space. *Am J Surg* 1974;127:716–720.

277. Petry JS, Wortham KA. Contraction and growth of wounds covered by meshed and non-meshed split thickness skin grafts. *Br J Plast Surg* 1986;39:478–482.

278. Ponten HL. Grafted skin: observation on innervation and other qualities. *Acta Clin Scand Suppl* 1960;257:1–78.

279. McGregor IA, Morgan G. Axial and random pattern flaps. *Br J Plast Surg* 1963;26:202–213.

280. Gimbel NS, Farris W. Skin grafting. *Arch Surg* 1966;92:554–557.

281. Alvarez OM, Mertz PM, Eaglstein WH. The effect of occlusive dressings on collagen synthesis and re-epithelialization in superficial wounds. *J Surg Res* 1983;35:142–148.

282. Shuck JM, Pruitt BA, Moncrief JA. Homograft skin for wound coverage. *Arch Surg* 1969;98:472–479.

283. Robson MC, Krizek TJ, Koss N, et al. Amniotic membranes as a temporary wound dressing. *Surg Gynecol Obstet* 1973;136:904–906.

284. Bromberg BE, Song IC, Mohn MP. The use of pig skin as a temporary biologic dressing. *Plast Reconstr Surg* 1965;36:80–90.

285. Woodruff EA. Biobrane, a biosynthetic skin prosthesis. In: Wise DL, ed. *Burn wound coverings*. New York: CRC Press, 1984.

286. Salomon JC, Diegelman RF, Cohen IK. Effects of dressings on donor site epithelialization. *Surg Forum* 1974;25:516–517.

287. Noe JM, Kalish S. The problem of adherence in dressed wounds. *Surg Gynecol Obstet* 1978;147:185–188.

288. Noe JM, Kalish S. *Wound care*. Greenwich: Chesebrough-Pond's, 1976.

289. Varma AO, Bugatch E, German FM. Debridement of dermal ulcers with collagenase. *Surg Gynecol Obstet* 1973;136:281–282.

290. Kucan JO, Robson MC, Heggers JP, et al. Comparison of silver sulfadiazine, povidone-iodine and physiologic saline in the treatment of chronic pressure ulcers. *J Am Geriatr Soc* 1981;24:232–235.

291. Moncrief JA. Topical therapy for control of bacteria in the burn wound. *World J Surg* 1978;2:151–165.

292. Geronemus RG, Mertz PM, Eaglstein WH. Wound healing: the effects of topical antimicrobial agents. *Arch Dermatol* 1979;115:1311–1314.

293. Noe JM, Kalish S. The mechanism of capillarity in surgical dressings. *Surg Gynecol Obstet* 1976;143:454–456.

294. Thomas DW, Hill CM, Lewis MAO, et al. Randomized clinical trial of the effect of semi-occlusive dressings on the microflora and clinical outcome of acute facial wounds. *Wound Repair Regen* 2000;8:2358–2263.

295. Winter GD, Scales JT. Effect of air drying and dressings on the surface of a wound. *Nature* 1963;197:91–92.

296. Morykwas MJ, Argenta LC, et al. Vacuum-assisted closure: a new method for wound control and treatment: animal studies and basic foundation. *Ann Plast Surg* 1997;38:553–562.

SUGGESTED READINGS

Grove GL. Age-related differences in healing of superficial skin wounds in humans. *Arch Dermatol Res* 1982;272:381–385.

Lander J, Hodgins M, Nazarali J, et al. Determinants of success and failure of EMLA. *Pain* 1996;64:89–97.

Mowat AG, Baum J. Chemotaxis of polymorphonuclear leukocytes from patients with diabetes mellitus. *N Engl J Med* 1971;284:621–627.

CHAPTER 7

Basic Immunology for Surgeons

Richard J. Rohrer

We live in a dangerous world. Microbial invaders from without and defective cells from within present themselves continuously and stand ready to overrun us. Since the days of the first unicellular organisms in a primal "soup" more than 3 billion years ago, defense systems against these constant dangers have been critical to survival. Successful immune defense stratagems have been highly conserved over the course of evolution.

The immune response permeates all activities of surgical importance. In normal individuals, the immune response prevents many surgical conditions outright, especially infections and tumors. The immune response is an important aspect of the first phases of illness and injury. Finally, the immune response is central to the recovery process after surgical intervention, interdigitating with cardiopulmonary and nutritional homeostatic mechanisms.

As immunity (Latin *immunitas*) describes freedom from invasion, it follows that a review of immunology should first lay out the frontiers to be protected, that is, how "self" versus "nonself" are defined. The active components of the defense mechanism then may be described. Finally, the manner in which these components collectively function is sketched. Special attention is drawn to three major areas of surgical endeavor: shock and trauma, oncology, and transplantation.

The central dogma asserted in this construct is founded upon basic science efforts in many species of animal, especially rodents. Although there are many differences between human and other animals, in the interest of clarity, no attempt will be made to highlight them in this chapter.

As with the more commonly understood military defenses that protect whole societies, few actions of the immune system are "good" in the absolute, teleologically speaking. That is, virtually all defense mechanisms are "double-edged swords." The same agents that save us in one circumstance may harm us in another. Such circumstances of surgical significance will be highlighted as well.

COMPONENTS OF THE IMMUNE SYSTEM

Definition of Self

Before an organism can defend itself against invasion, it must know what turf it is protecting. This is relatively simple for a single-celled organism—the boundary in question is the cell membrane—but is more complex for individual humans. One boundary is made up of epithelial surfaces—skin, gastrointestinal, and respiratory. Another boundary is the endothelial surface that courses throughout the body—the vascular tree. Yet another boundary is apparent at the margins of individual organs or cohesive groups of cells. Finally, there are the boundaries of individual cells—their cell membranes.

Cell surface markers are fundamental to the staking out of turf as "self." Their presence may be purely for the sake of identification, or they may play critical functional roles. Some cell surface markers are unique to a species (xenospecific). Some markers are unique to a group of individuals within a species (allospecific). Some markers are completely unique to the individual itself (autospecific). Some cell surface markers are organ or function specific. Examples reach far from the immune system to include, for example, breast and gastrointestinal tissue markers. Even for a given individual, the cell surface markers expressed may change over time and, for that matter, during different phases of the cell cycle. This is best exemplified by surface molecule changes in many cells from fetal to adult life. Because cell surface markers may provoke an immune response in another individual or species (indeed, this is how they are most commonly discovered in the first place), they are often referred to as *cell surface antigens*.

Cell Surface Antigens

Cell surface antigens are generally glycoproteins that protrude through the lipid-rich cell membrane. They are coded for by deoxyribonucleic acid (DNA) in the nucleus of individual cells, constructed from messenger ribonucleic acid (mRNA) templates on ribosomes in the cellular cytoplasm, and transported to the cell surface. Under certain circumstances, they may detach and float through the interstitial or intravascular space. Therefore, the expression of cell surface molecules is universally a dynamic process, with new surface molecules being produced, expressed, and shed continually.

Easily understood are the familiar ABO markers on the surface of red blood cells. In humans, the A and B antigens, as well as a host of others (Lewis, Kell, etc.), protrude from the red blood cell membrane and define subgroups within the human species. A common proteinaceous moiety attached to the red cell membrane is coupled with a variable carbohydrate moiety. They are present in many other tissues as well, including vascular endothelium. This is an ancient system of self-definition; ABO glycoprotein antigens appear to be distant relatives of bacterial surface antigens. The development of anti-blood group antibodies (e.g., anti-A in a blood group O individual) early in life may be related to bacterial exposure in the neonate, with formation of cross-reactive antibody. Many primates share ABO antigens with humans.

Yet more specific are the major histocompatibility complex (MHC) antigens. In humans, they were first detected on white blood cells and therefore were termed *human leukocyte antigens* (HLA). They are present on many white blood cells and tissues. They are coded for on the short arm of chromosome 6. They constantly turn over and, like other cell surface molecules, may be bound or soluble.

For descriptive purposes, HLA antigens can be divided into two classes based on structure: class I and class II antigens (Fig. 7.1). Class I antigens are expressed on the surfaces of all nucleated cells. The known class I antigens in humans are labeled A, B, and C. Whereas class I antigens are largely just descriptive of "self," the class II HLA antigens are functional as well as descriptive. Class II antigens are accordingly more restricted in their distribution. Under normal conditions, they are present only on the surfaces of specialized immune cells. In humans, they are labeled as the D or D-related (Dr) antigens. In the immune response, the Dr antigens are thought to be the most important HLA participants, followed by HLA-B and HLA-A; HLA-C is relatively unimportant. Although class II antigen expression normally is restricted, all cells contain the genetic hardware for expression of this antigen. Under special circumstances, such as those involving tissue injury from ischemia, there may be "upregulation" of HLA expression, and class II antigen may be found on the surface of cells from which it is usually absent. This may best be viewed as part of the attempt of the viable cell to protect itself from "collateral damage" because of nonspecific inflammation about the nonviable cells.

Each of the HLA antigens has multiple variations. All are proteins that bear structural resemblance to

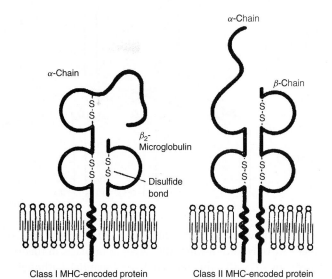

FIGURE 7.1   Molecular structures of the class I major histocompatibility complex (MHC)-encoded protein and the class II protein molecule are similar. The molecules also share similar sequences of amino acids. The molecules are characterized by loops made up of approximately 70 amino acids within each chain. Sulfur atoms at each end of the loop are joined by covalent bonds. Class I proteins are expressed on the surface of every nucleated cell in higher vertebrates, in association with the non–MHC-encoded protein β_2 microglobulin. Class II proteins are expressed only on the surface of selected cells, such as the β cells. The highly schematic diagrams are not drawn to scale. (From Marrach P, Kappler J. The T-cell and its receptor. *Sci Am* 1986;254:36 with permission.)

immunoglobulins (Igs; described later), but they differ functionally. Notably, class II antigen displays, at its outermost extent, a prominent fold that can be shown in three dimensions by radiographic crystallography. This fold is known as the *peptide-binding groove* and is critical for the functional capacity of this antigen (see "Macrophages"). A host of so-called "minor" histocompatibility surface antigens exist as well, but they are much less well defined.

HLA markers are passed from parent to offspring through standard mendelian genetics. For all chromosomes, including number 6, an individual inherits one maternal strand and one paternal strand. Each strand is referred to as a *haplotype*. Evidently, each offspring will share one haplotype with each of his or her parents. Among offspring from the same set of parents, one may calculate that the likelihood that any individual will share both haplotypes with a sibling is 25%, one haplotype 50%, and no haplotypes 25% (Fig. 7.2). By their nature, identical twins will share all cell surface markers, including HLA; fraternal twins will follow the inheritance previously described.

Given that every individual inherits a complete set (A, B, C, and Dr) of antigens from each parent and that there are numerous but finite variants of each, the HLA system confers on humans a high degree of individuality, which contrasts

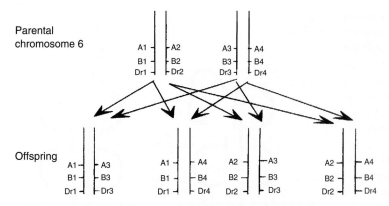

FIGURE 7.2 Two parents contribute one haplotype each to every offspring, yielding four possible outcomes.

with the individuality conferred by the ABO system. Whereas there are only four distinct ABO types in humans, in theory there are 3.7×10^{17} different HLA combinations (although, in reality, some are much more common than others).

In addition to HLA cell surface antigens, lymphocytes possess cell surface molecules that aid in lymphocyte functions and others that may not be functional in themselves, but serve to distinguish one functional subpopulation from another within the same individual. They are all glycoproteins and currently should be referred to by the "clusters of differentiation" (CD) nomenclature, although references persist to the older "T" and "B" terminology.

Defense against Nonself

Earth has always been a dangerous place to live. Defense against invasion is therefore an ancient, and highly important, evolutionary attribute. Some defense mechanisms are relatively primitive, whereas others are highly advanced. It appears that, in the evolutionary process, advanced host defenses appeared about the same time that the capacity for organ regeneration was lost, that is, around the time of evolution from amphibian to reptile.

Toxic Secretions

Perhaps the most ancient method of organismal defense is the secretion of substances that are chemically toxic to other organisms in the neighborhood. Secretion of penicillin by the *Penicillium* mold is a prominent example and may be thought of, loosely, as part of the immune defenses of the mold. The human commercial potential of such substances in the pharmaceutical industry has been, and still is, enormous.

In humans, secretion of directly toxic chemical substances by most organs and tissues is limited; the antibacterial acid environment of the stomach is a familiar example. Most other epithelial defense systems use mucous secretion and mechanical action to bolster the barrier function.

More recently, the formation of nitric oxide (NO) by cells not normally considered part of the immune system has attracted attention. NO has many effects, including smooth muscle relaxation (vasodilation) and neurotransmission. However, as a free radical, it also is a potent inhibitor of DNA synthesis. Its formation by vascular endothelial cells and hepatocytes has been offered as an example of nonspecific protection from microbial invasion. Neutrophils and macrophages (see later) also secrete NO as a direct attribute of their immune function.

Most of the human immune responses are derived from more specialized cellular functions and interactions.

Macrophages

Perhaps the most ancient cellular defense function is phagocytosis, which can be demonstrated easily in very primitive unicellular organisms. This function is performed in humans by the macrophage (or its monocyte counterpart). This cell is of mesenchymal origin and arises in any individual from an original bone marrow stem cell. It may be freely circulating in the intravascular compartment, migrating more slowly through the lymph and the interstitial space, or virtually stationary within tissues. Kupffer cells in the hepatic sinusoids, for example, are macrophages adapted to an important defensive role in the liver.

As nucleated cells, macrophages express class I MHC molecules on their surface; as highly specialized immune cells, they express class II MHC molecules. In addition, they express other recognition and function molecules, including the functional antigen B7-2 (CD80; see "T Lymphocytes").

As the pliable macrophage cell membrane encounters foreign substances in the local environment, it invaginates to surround and engulf the object. Once the invader is delivered in a cytosome to the cell cytoplasm, it is degraded by intracellular peroxidases and other enzymes, and neutralized. Macrophages have also been shown to contain the enzyme inducible NO synthase (NOS). This enzyme is able to mediate the oxidation of L-arginine to yield the gaseous free radical NO and the byproduct L-citrulline. Substrates and cofactors are necessary; in addition, the macrophage must be stimulated for enzyme activity to be induced (Fig. 7.3). The list of potent inducers is growing and includes endotoxin (lipopolysaccharide), malarial antigen, interferon γ (IFN-γ), tumor necrosis factor (TNF), and interleukin 1 (IL-1) (see "Cytokines"), alone or in combination. In the presence of these substrates, cofactors, and inducers, macrophages produce relatively large amounts of NO (in comparison to the NO produced in the vascular endothelium and in neurons). The half-life of this highly reactive substance (RS) varies from seconds to hours, depending on its association,

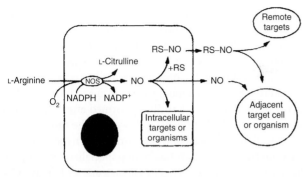

FIGURE 7.3   The synthesis and fate of nitric oxide (NO) in cells. NO is produced by the enzyme NO synthase (NOS). The nicotinamide adenine dinucleotide phosphate (NADPH) provides a source of electrons, and molecular dioxygen is incorporated into NO and citrulline, the coproduct of NO formation. Once formed, NO can diffuse to targets within the cell, in the extracellular space, or in adjacent cells or organisms. NO, which is normally short lived, may form stable adducts by interacting with thiol groups on carrier or storage proteins (RS). These stable RS–NO complexes then may have local or remote actions. (From Billiar T. Nitric oxide: novel biology with clinical relevance. *Ann Surg* 1995;221:339, with permission.)

or lack thereof, with a carrier substance. It is likely that NO acts intracellularly upon phagocytized particles, in the pericellular interstitium upon invading organisms, and at distant sites, when bound to one or more carrier proteins. Once present at the site of invasion, macrophage-derived NO has two major effects. Prominently, microvascular vasodilation occurs, thereby preserving local tissue perfusion. Subsequently, NO diffuses across the membrane of target cells, inhibiting that ribonucleotide reductase of the cell, the rate-limiting enzyme of DNA synthesis.

Beyond simple destruction of foreign particles or organisms, macrophages may specially reprocess certain breakdown products of phagocytosis. Fragments of foreign protein may be bundled together with a newly formed class II antigen molecule on its way to the macrophage cell surface. In the bundling process, fragments of degraded protein come to reside in the peptide-binding groove of the class II molecule. When the fragment is exteriorized with the new HLA molecule, it faces outward, where it may be recognized more easily as a foreign antigen by other elements of the immune system. This process is known as *antigen presentation*.

Macrophages also are important in that they secrete IL-1 (see later). Like the other interleukins, IL-1 is a polypeptide that, in hormonal manner, stimulates the immunologic function of responding cells that encounter it.

Natural Killer Cells

Another primitive line from the original bone marrow stem cell is a lymphocyte (non-T, non-B), the natural killer (NK) cell. NK cells are particularly active in the tumor cell response. They demonstrate spontaneous tumoricidal properties when exposed to tumor cells and, unlike T and B lymphocytes,

do not require recognition of MHC molecules or antigen processing. How they recognize tumor cells is unclear. They kill tumor cells by incorporating a lipophilic protein into the target cell membrane, which causes increased cell wall permeability, cell swelling, and, finally, cell destruction.

NK cells also produce a variety of cytokines, including IFN-α, IFN-γ, and B-cell growth factor.

Granulocytes

Granulocytes play an important, although relatively non-specific, role in immune homeostasis. Named for their histochemical staining properties, the three main lines are polymorphonuclear neutrophils, eosinophils, and basophils. All are derived from the same bone marrow stem cell. As nucleated cells, they express class I MHC molecules; however, they do not express class II antigens. In addition, they carry on their surface a number of molecules important for their functioning, including adhesion and interaction with other cells. The best known of these is the leukocyte function-associated (LFA) antigen (CD18). These white blood cells carry granules of toxic substances, such as peroxidases. They also contain chemotactic agents that attract cellular elements of the coagulation process, macrophages, and fibroblasts. Finally, granulocytes are also a source of kallikreins, enzymes that act upon free-floating kininogens in the plasma to produce kinins, the best known of which is bradykinin. Bradykinin and its kin have a pronounced histamine-like effect on tissues, leading to marked vasodilation and increased vascular permeability. When appropriately stimulated, granulocytes spill or secrete these substances, initiating local inflammation in a relatively indiscriminate manner.

B Lymphocytes

Named for their site of origin in the chicken, the bursa of Fabricius, these cells play an important intermediary role in immune defense. In humans, the bursa equivalent is likely the fetal liver or bone marrow. Once produced, they migrate to lymph nodes and spleen, where they appear to remain in residence. As nucleated cells, they express MHC class I molecules on their cell surface. As specialized cells of the immune system, they also express MHC class II molecules. In addition, they display a variety of B-cell–specific markers, known as *B*1 through *B*8, through which various lines of B cells may be identified immunohistologically. Finally, they display Ig on their surface.

When appropriately stimulated, B lymphocytes differentiate into plasma cells. These smaller cells, with cytoplasm containing abundant ribosomes on the endoplasmic reticulum, are "factories" with a single mission: to produce a specific antibody.

Immunoglobulins

Antibodies produced by B lymphocytes and plasma cells take the form of Igs, which are proteins of unique structure, composed of heavy and light peptide chains (Fig. 7.4). The "root" of the heavy chain complex is constant in its structure among individuals of the same species and is referred to

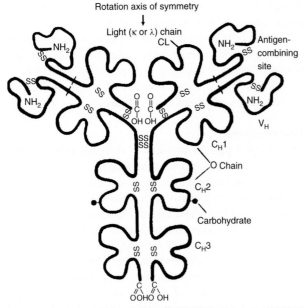

FIGURE 7.4 Schematic diagram of a molecule of human immunoglobulin G, showing the two light (κ and λ) chains and two heavy (γ) chains held together by disulfide bonds. The constant regions of the light (CL) and heavy (C_H1, C_H2, and C_H3) chains and the variable region of the heavy chain (V_H) are indicated. Loops in the peptide chain formed by intrachain disulfide bonds (C_H1, and so forth) form separate functional domains. (From Nossal G. Current concepts: immunology. The basic components of the immune system. *N Engl J Med* 1987;316:1320. with permission.)

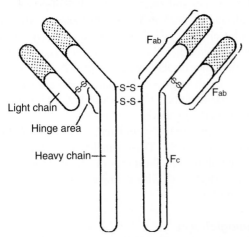

FIGURE 7.5 Representation of the characteristic Y-shape of a molecule of immunoglobulin G. The *dotted areas* indicate the variable regions of the molecule, and the *white areas* indicate the constant regions. F_{ab}, antibody-binding fragment; F_c, crystallizable fragment.

as the *crystallizable fragment* (F_c) (Fig. 7.5). The portion of an Ig molecule where light chains are complexed with heavy chains at the site where the antibody will bind to its target is designated the "antibody-binding fragment" (F_{ab}). A myriad of possibilities exists for antigen-specific antibody to be made, because the F_{ab} moiety is highly variable in its

discrete structure. More than 100 genes code for specific segments of the variable portions of heavy and light chains, leading to millions of potential Ig specificities. As complex and pluripotential as they are, it may come as a surprise to note their evolutionary antiquity: even worms produce Igs.

There are five general Ig classes: IgM, IgG, IgE, IgA, and IgD. IgM is the first antibody formed after exposure to common microbial antigens, followed by the more durable IgG. IgE figures prominently in immediate hypersensitivity reactions by binding to and activating specialized eosinophils, the mast cells. IgA is secreted in saliva, tears, and breast milk, thereby augmenting resistance to infection in these fluids. IgD is found on the surface of immature B lymphocytes; its function is uncertain. Igs may be soluble or bound to a surface of the cell.

The main functions of Igs are to provide opsonization and to activate complement. Opsonization occurs when the F_{ab} fragment of an Ig binds to its associated antigen, such as an invading organism. Subsequent macrophage and monocyte phagocytosis of the antibody-coated microorganisms is markedly enhanced. Complement fixation occurs when the antibody–antigen complex triggers the complement cascade (described later).

We are all born with certain natural xenoantibodies (antibodies against the MHC and other antigens of different species). In addition, we may acquire other antibodies through exposures later in life. As a result of bacterial exposures as a neonate, humans acquire a multitude of antimicrobial antibodies early in life. Many antigens may closely resemble one another. In these circumstances, cross-reactivity may occur between one antibody and multiple antigens. As noted previously, the carbohydrate moieties of ABO antigens closely resemble capsular carbohydrates of certain bacteria. This likely is the source of cross-reacting anti-blood group antibody (i.e., anti-A and anti-B in a blood group O individual, anti-B in a blood group A individual, etc.). When exposed to other human MHC antigens (through pregnancy, blood transfusion, or organ transplantation), antibodies may be formed against the HLA series as well.

Portions of Ig may, as specific proteins, serve as antigens for the formation of yet other antibodies (usually in a different species). When the constant (F_c) portion of an Ig serves as the antigen, the Ig formed against it is referred to as an *anti-isotypic antibody*. Because of the constancy of the F_c fragment, such an antibody will react with all Igs of the same class from the same species. When the variable (F_{ab}) portion of an Ig serves as an antigen, the Ig formed against it is referred to as an *anti-idiotypic antibody*. Anti-idiotypic antibodies are highly specific for the F_{ab} fragment against which it was formed.

Complements

The so-called "innate immunity" refers to the most ancient components of the humoral immune response. This is composed of a variety of individual proteins known collectively as *acute phase reactants* (heat shock protein, haptoglobin, C-reactive protein, fibronectin, and many

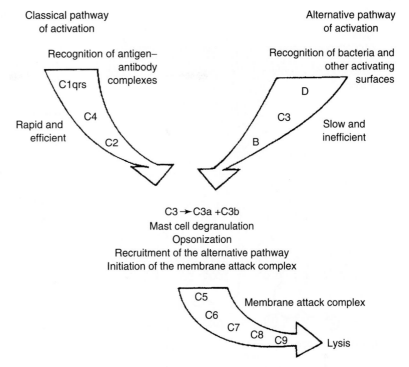

Classical pathway
of activation

Recognition of antigen–
antibody
complexes

Alternative pathway
of activation

Recognition of bacteria and
other activating
surfaces

C1qrs

C4

C2

Rapid and
efficient

D

C3

B

Slow and
inefficient

C3 → C3a + C3b
Mast cell degranulation
Opsonization
Recruitment of the alternative pathway
Initiation of the membrane attack complex

C5
C6
C7
C8 C9

Membrane attack complex

Lysis

FIGURE 7.6 The complement system consists of three families of proteins. Two of these, the classic pathway of activation and the alternative pathway of activation, cause cleavage of C3 into two fragments, C3b and C3a. These fragments have important biologic activities. In addition, C3b, together with elements of the classic pathway (C4b, C2a) or the alternative pathway (Bb, properidine), forms enzymes (C5 convertases) that cleave C5, the initial member of the terminal family of proteins. Cleavage of C5 leads to formation of the membrane attack complex that can cause osmotic lysis of cells. (From Paul W. The immune system: an introduction. In: Paul W, ed. *Fundamental immunology.* New York: Raven Press, 1984:3–22 with permission.)

others) as well as whole systems of proteins, such as the complement cascade.

An antigen–antibody complex may initiate the complement cascade through the "classic" pathway. In the absence of Igs, substances such as endotoxin may initiate the cascade through the alternate pathway (Fig. 7.6). Both pathways converge with the activation of C3. The sequential activation of proteases, which defines the complement cascade, eventually results in a tight cluster of proteins known as the *membrane attack complex* (MAC). The MAC is capable of adhering to the target cell membrane and rendering it porous, thereby causing osmotic cell rupture.

Aside from the directly cytotoxic MAC, the proteins of the complement cascade have a variety of other immunologic functions. These include vasodilation and chemotactic properties, which are of special importance with regard to neutrophil and eosinophil function in inflammation. The complement cleavage products with the greatest inflammatory activity are C3a (which opsonizes) and C5b (which is lytic). In addition, the complement cascade provides yet another source for both enzyme and substrate, leading to the production of bradykinin. In the normal host, this potent cascade is kept in check by a regulatory protein, C1 inhibitor.

Dendritic Cells

Derived from a bone marrow stem cell progenitor, dendritic cells are highly specialized antigen-presenting cells with no effector function. They reside primarily in the intercellular and interstitial spaces but, particularly after having encountered antigen, will migrate through lymphatics to lymph nodes and the spleen. There they migrate to T-cell–rich areas to present their antigen.

T Lymphocytes

The T lymphocyte is named for its site of origin, the thymus, and is one of the most sophisticated and important elements of the immune response. T cells derive from a fetal stem cell in the thymus and, before release from the thymus, undergo an extensive process of elaboration and deletion. Maturing T cells are "taught" to recognize "self" MHC antigens and become tolerant of them. Any T cells that fail to exhibit tolerance to self are eliminated in a process called *clonal deletion*. Failure of this system is one factor in autoimmune disease.

As a nucleated cell, the T lymphocyte carries MHC class I antigen on its surface. As a specialized immune cell, it also carries class II antigens. In addition, it expresses a variety of cell-specific and functional cell surface markers, several of the series CD1 to CD14, LFA (CD18), and CD28.

Three broad classes of T cells include helper T (Th) cells, which amplify the cellular immune response; cytotoxic T (Tc) cells, which effect target cell killing; and suppressor T (Ts) cells, which buffer the immune response. All T cells express CD3 on the cell surface. Tc and Ts cells express CD8, whereas Th cells do not. Conversely, Th cells expresses CD4, whereas Tc and Ts cells do not. Through quantitative analysis of lymphocytes bearing these antigens, indices of immunologic competency can be calculated, such as the absolute CD4 count (which is important in the management of human immunodeficiency virus) and the CD4/CD8 ratio.

The most important structure on its surface is the T-cell receptor (TCR). It is located on the cell surface geographically close to a CD3 antigen, and a CD28 antigen is not far away. The TCR has a relatively flat, outward-facing surface. This "antigen-recognition platform" of the TCR is the critical interface for peptide in the binding groove of macrophage

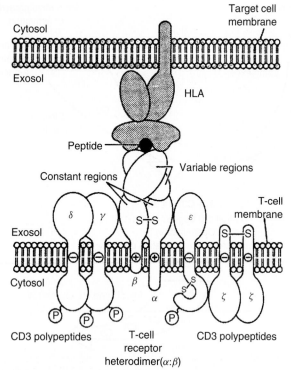

FIGURE 7.7 Interaction of human leukocyte antigen (HLA) and the T-cell receptor complex. The α and β polypeptide chains of the T-cell receptor form a heterodimer linked by a disulfide bond (S–S) and anchored in the T-cell membrane. The heterodimer recognizes and binds to peptide associated with an HLA molecule on the surface of a presenting cell. The monopolymorphic CD3 polypeptides (designated γ, δ, ε, and ζ) are assembled together with the T-cell antigen receptor and are probably involved in signal transduction. *P*, phosphorylation site. (From Krensky A, Weiss A, Crabtree G, et al. Mechanisms of disease: T lymphocyte–antigen interaction in transplant rejection. *N Engl J Med* 1990;322:510, with permission).

MHC class II molecules; indeed, the precise alignment of MHC class II antigen with a protein fragment in the peptide-binding groove is the signal event in antigen presentation (Fig. 7.7).

When appropriately stimulated through the TCR, a signal is transduced to the T-cell nucleus. Calcium fluxes and enzymatic phosphorylation figure prominently in this signal transduction. Messenger RNA is elaborated, coding for cytokines and cytokine receptors, which greatly amplify the immune response.

Cytokines

Various cytokines produced by T cells, macrophages, and other specialized cell lines include IL-1 through IL-18, TNF, IFN-α, and IFN-γ (Table 7.1). TNF and IL-1 appear to be phylogenetically ancient. Some of these original cytokines may have been cousins of pheromones, which are potent peptides that promote attraction between diverse insects. Cytokines have their intended effect when they reach a target cell with the appropriate cell surface receptor.

Clinically, the most important cytokines are IL-1, IL-2, and IL-6. The most important receptors produced are IL-2 receptors (IL-2R), which may be soluble or bound. Although they may derive from ancient and relatively simple peptides, cytokines as a group represent the modern communications hardware of the most advanced element of the immune system, the T cell. Prominent functions include the switching "on" of genes in target cells and chemotaxis of other effector cells.

IMMUNOPHYSIOLOGY OF SHOCK AND SEPSIS

Maintenance of homeostasis during the stress of injury is one of the most basic of bodily functions, strongly conserved in the evolutionary process. The initial response is dominated by cardiorespiratory and neurologic factors. Shortly after, however, metabolic and immunologic pathways become active.

Even in bland ischemic (hypotensive and/or hypoxic) or mechanical injuries, the tissue repair process recruits immunologic help. Acute-phase reactants are released, gaps in the microvascular endothelium appear, and white blood cells migrate into the interstitial space. As affected parenchymal cells die, they are liquefied in the process of sterile inflammation and are cleared by macrophages using phagocytosis and NO production. Surviving and regenerating cells, perhaps to avoid collateral damage in the inflammatory process, upregulate their expression of HLA antigens. As survivors wave "flags" of self-identity, macrophages are signaled that these are cells under repair and are not to be cleared away. In later phases of inflammation, depending on the tissue and severity of injury, fibroblasts are drawn by chemotactic factors and lay down collagen in the process of scarring.

However, injury frequently is not bland. Breaks in epithelial barrier function occur either intentionally (as in surgical interventions) or accidentally. Such breaks inevitably allow ingress of microbes. The front lines of the resistance are manned by macrophages and preformed antibodies. If the host has encountered an organism (or one like it) previously, specific (or cross-reacting) IgG antibody will bind to the capsule of the invader. The organism, thereby opsonized, will be cleared through lymphatics to the lymph nodes and spleen. In addition, local macrophages phagocytize and destroy invaders, processing their substructural elements and presenting them as antigens for further immune action. Therefore, a contaminated injury site may be kept free of infection and converted to a bland injury.

When tissue injury is extensive or the microbial inoculation great, local defenses may be overwhelmed, resulting in sepsis. Because of their broad interface with the outside world and potential for dense colonization, this is especially true for the pulmonary system and gastrointestinal tract; therefore, pulmonary alveolar macrophages and

TABLE 7.1

Cytokines

Cytokine	Major Sources	Major Functions
IL-1	Macrophages	Promotes phagocytic function and PMN adherence; lymphocyte activation; "endogenous pyrogen"
IL-2	Th cells	Stimulates T-cell proliferation and differentiation; stimulates B-cell proliferation
IL-3	T cells, myelomonocytes	Hematopoietic growth factor
IL-4	T and B cells, mast cells, macrophages	Induces differentiation of Th cells; induces differentiation of B cells
IL-5	T cells	Stimulates proliferation and differentiation of B cells and eosinophils
IL-6	Monocytes, macrophages, T cells	Stimulates epithelial cell, fibroblast, and B-cell proliferation, hepatocyte acute phase protein synthesis
IL-7	Stromal cells, thymus	Stimulates early B-cell production and thymocytes
IL-8	Monocytes, fibroblasts, endothelial cells	Stimulates granulocyte movement through vascular endothelium, and degranulation
IL-9	Lymphocytes, monocytes	T-cell growth factor; mast cell enhancing factor
IL-10	T cells, macrophages	Inhibits monocyte/macrophage function; suppresses inflammatory cytokines; enhances B-cell proliferation
IL-11	Lung fibroblasts, marrow stromal cells	Promotes several cell lines; inhibits adipocytes
IL-12	Macrophages, B cells	Stimulates differentiation of Th cells
TNF-α	Monocytes, macrophages, natural killer cells, Kupffer cells	Promotes PMN adherence to endothelium; stimulates fibroblast production of prostaglandin E$_2$; stimulates release of multiple other cytokines from lymphocytes
TNF-β	Monocytes, macrophages	Similar to TNF-α; in addition, stimulates B cell proliferation
IFN-γ	T cells	Promotes macrophage and monocyte differentiation
TGF-α	Fibroblasts, epithelial cells	Stimulates production of epithelial cells, endothelial cells, and fibroblasts
TGF-β	Lymphocytes, macrophages, fibroblast	Inhibits lymphocyte production and PMN adherence; stimulates fibroblast collagen synthesis
Platelet-derived growth factor	Endothelial cells, plts	Stimulates fibroblast and smooth muscle cell production
Platelet-activating factor	PMNs, endothelial cells	Promotes platelet degranulation, PMN function

IFN, interferon; IL, interleukin; PMN, polymorphonuclear neutrophil; TGF, transforming growth factor; Th, helper T; TNF, tumor necrosis factor.

Kupffer cells are frequently charged with a major defensive role in the seriously ill patient.

The release of vasoactive substances in the immune response, especially NO and TNF, is a double-edged sword. Although maintenance of tissue perfusion is cytoprotective, an excess of vasodilation may cause systemic hypotension and secondary deterioration of other organ functions. Although increased capillary permeability may allow greater access to the interstitium for leukocytes, concomitant edema may impair organ function and healing. Nonetheless, on balance, the effect of these substances appears to be beneficial. To date, blockade of the immune response in the sepsis syndromes has failed to show improvement in outcomes. Much current research involves the study of novel chemical (nonsteroidal anti-inflammatory drugs) and biologic agents (monoclonal antibodies) to blunt the adverse effects of the inflammatory response while sparing the beneficial effects. Anti-endotoxin, anti-TNF, and IL-1 receptor antagonist are examples. Although they are effective in laboratory models and show modest promise in clinical studies, none has been proved clearly effective in humans. Similarly, blockade of NO synthesis has thus far yielded adverse consequences when experimental animals are subsequently challenged with endotoxin. At this point, no agents have been shown to be capable of selectively blocking the adverse effects of vasoactive inflammatory substances whereas preserving the beneficial effects. More promising, at present, appears to be the exogenous administration of endogenous polypeptides, such as activated protein C.

Maintenance of nutritional parameters, especially in severe injury and sepsis, is critical for the ongoing immune response and may be looked upon as a true "immunoenhancement" tool at the clinician's disposal. For the sake of gastrointestinal mucosal integrity and Kupffer cell function, nutrition should preferably be maintained through the enteral route. From the immunologic perspective, antibiotics fill an important adjunctive role, without intrinsically enhancing immune activity.

IMMUNOPHYSIOLOGIC ASPECTS OF ONCOLOGY

In the process of DNA replication, mistakes are frequent. In the epithelial cell population, which experiences massive turnover during the course of a lifetime, it is particularly remarkable that errors in proliferation are not more common. Part of the answer lies at the surface of the abnormal cell. As cells are transformed from normal to malignant, a variety of changes in their cell surface marker population become apparent. If a virus is the causative agent, viral antigens may be expressed. If the DNA of the malignant cell operates at a more "primitive" level, a variety of fetal antigens may appear. Immune recognition of altered cell surface antigens may be extremely important in the tumor surveillance process. Indirect evidence for this may be afforded by the increased skin cancer and lymphoma rates in patients taking immunosuppressive medication. Diagnostically, generation of monoclonal antibodies against such tumor cell surface markers has allowed advances in detection and classification of tumors.

NK cells attack tumor cells directly (see "Natural Killer Cells"). Although first characterized *in vitro*, little is known of how this system functions *in vivo*.

In addition, T cells are involved in continuous tumor surveillance. When an abnormal (read "nonself") cell surface marker is encountered, the cell may be attacked as if it were an outside invader. In general, this response tends to be more pronounced at a primary tumor site than at a metastatic site. Tumors of viral origin appear to be more immunogenic than tumors that arise spontaneously. Many tumor surface antigens that are detected in laboratory assays may, in fact, elicit a humoral or cellular immune attack *in vitro*. Unfortunately, this is often associated with little or no immune response *in vivo*. One explanation for this may lie in the observation that one of the first cell lines to detect some tumors is the Ts cell. Tc cell function, in this circumstance, is suppressed before it can even begin. Experimentally, it is possible to selectively destroy Ts cell populations, in which case-enhanced host antitumor immunity becomes evident.

Macrophages, drawn to the scene by the abnormal tumor antigen, may mount an attack in which NO production is central. *In vitro* study of macrophage tumoricidal activity demonstrates that tumor killing is lost if NO production is inhibited.

Several lines of oncologic immunomodulation are being pursued. *Immunoenhancement* refers to the administration of agents, such as interferon (IFN), TNF, and various colony-stimulating or growth factors, in the hope of augmenting the native immune response to tumor. *Passive immunotherapy* refers to the administration of exogenous antitumor antibody. The antibody may be either directly active against the tumor cell or coupled with a more toxic substance. In the latter instance, the antibody uses its specificity to locate and adhere to tumor, whereas the toxic substance (e.g., ricin toxin, diphtheria toxin, or *Pseudomonas*

exotoxin) accomplishes the killing. *Active immunotherapy* involves the elution of tumor antigens from tumor specimens removed surgically, followed by their reintroduction to the host in hopes of eliciting a more productive immune response against any remaining tumor. Finally, *adoptive cellular immunotherapy* combines these technologies. NK cells (or Tc cells) are isolated from tumor specimens or peripheral blood, activated by lymphokines *in vitro*, and reintroduced into the host. Usually, supplemental IL-2 is administered to provide further immunoenhancement. To date, all such interventions are investigational.

Many tumor cells, especially lymphomas, express abundant, highly specific Ig on the cell surface. This has allowed the development of anti-idiotypic antibodies against the specific tumor Ig and therefore the cell line. Thus far, however, monoclonal antibody immunotherapy has only proved temporarily effective for patients with certain lymphomas. The most promising solid tumors for immunotherapy continue to be melanoma and renal cell carcinoma.

The mainstays of medical therapy for most cancers remain relatively nonspecific cytotoxic chemotherapy and radiation therapy. The host immune response is relegated to aiding in the healing after surgical therapy and cleaning up after medical therapy.

IMMUNOPHYSIOLOGY OF ORGAN AND TISSUE TRANSPLANTATION

Transplantation for end-stage organ failure has become a frequent event. Approximately 50,000 organ transplants are performed annually in the United States and Europe combined, with approximately 10,000 more in other parts of the world. Kidney transplants are the most voluminous, accounting for just over half of the total organ transplants completed. Liver and heart transplants, combined, account for one third. The remainder comprises pancreas, lung, small bowel, and various combination transplants. The limiting factor in organ transplantation is donor availability. Tissue transplants, including heart valves, blood vessels, corneas, skin, and a variety of bone and connective tissue products, do not require heart-beating donors and therefore have even greater growth potential.

The source of the donated organ has implications for subsequent recipient immunophysiology. Donors may be live or cadaveric. In the former, donors are considered "living related" if they are first-degree relatives (parent, sibling, offspring) of the recipient and "living unrelated" if anything else (generally spouses, relatives by marriage, and friends). For cadaveric donors, death may have been pronounced by neurologic criteria (brain death with persistent cardiac function and organ perfusion) or cardiac criteria (with cold preservation of organs as soon as possible after cessation of cardiac function).

With all donors, variable degrees of MHC matching are accomplished. Transplants between identical twins, the happiest immunologic circumstance, are rare for obvious reasons. One fourth of sibling transplants are between haploidentical individuals, who share all six of the most important (paired A, B, and Dr) MHC antigens, as well as an undetermined number of so-called "minor" histocompatibility loci. With computerized matching and a sharing arrangement, approximately 5% of cadaveric kidney transplants in the United States are now between unrelated individuals who just happen to share all six MHC antigens (so-called "six-antigen match" or "zero-antigen mismatch"). In these cases, although, there probably is little sharing of minor histocompatibility antigens.

The beneficial effect of matching donors and recipients is clear-cut in kidney transplantation for the combinations described. With lesser degrees of matching, the beneficial effects decline and may be quite secondary in importance to other factors, such as donor physiology and ischemic times. In situations where the patient to receive the organ is critically ill (i.e., heart and liver transplantation), logistical factors usually take precedence over matching considerations.

Before organ transplantation, attention must be paid to the potential for untreatable hyperacute (humoral) rejection caused by the presence of preformed antibodies. Rejection due to preformed xenoantibody is avoided by the simple expedient of using only human donors. Rejection due to preformed anti-ABO antibody is avoided through matching (with rare exception) donor and recipient blood groups by the rules of classic blood group compatibility. Finally, for all kidney transplants and some heart transplants, rejection due to preformed anti-MHC antibody is avoided by performing a lymphocyte (donor cells plus recipient serum) cross-match. Liver grafts appear to be rather tolerant of anti-MHC antibody; if a lymphocyte cross-match is done at all, the results are noted only retrospectively.

If an organ is transplanted in the face of preformed antibodies in the recipient, the expected result is immediate hyperacute rejection. The preformed antibody binds to its target antigen on the surfaces of vascular endothelial cells and graft parenchymal cells. Circulating complement is fixed. In the vascular compartment, the normally "anticoagulant" environment of the endothelium is changed to a "procoagulant" environment. Fibrin and platelets are attracted to the endothelium, and thrombosis occurs. The graft, momentarily pink and healthy, becomes violaceous, and infarction occurs within a few minutes. In the parenchyma, complement fixation initiates the complement cascade, culminating in the formation of an MAC. The parenchymal cell membrane is breached; there is unrestricted flux of anions and cations into and out of the cell; and it dies secondary to osmotic injury. No known treatment exists for hyperacute rejection, hence the emphasis upon prevention.

Hyperacute rejection remains the Achilles' heel of xenotransplantation. As the recipient immune reaction appears to be primitive and powerful, the most successful research efforts in this area center upon genetic manipulation of donor species–specific antigens to avoid complement fixation altogether, rather than simply dampen it.

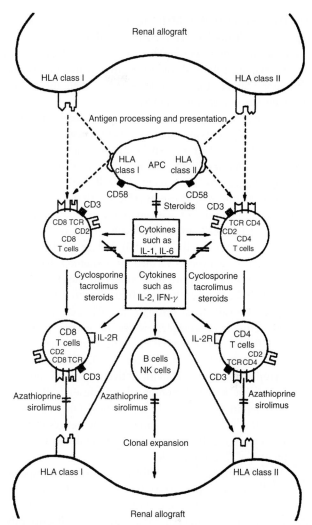

FIGURE 7.8 The anti-allograft response. Schematic representation of human leukocyte antigen (HLA), the primary stimulus for initiation of the anti-allograft response, shows the participation of cell surface proteins in antigenic recognition and signal transduction, the contribution of the cytokines and multiple cell types to the immune response, and the potential sites of action (*arrows with hatching*) of immunosuppressant agents. HLA class I includes the HLA-A, HLA-B, and HLA-C antigens. HLA class II includes the HLA-DR, HLA-DQ, and HLA-DP antigens. APC, antigen-presenting cell; TCR, T-cell receptor; IL, interleukin; IL-2R, interleukin 2 receptor; IFN-γ, interferon γ; NK, natural killer. (From Suthanthiran M, Strom T. Medical progress: renal transplantation. *N Engl J Med* 1994;331:365, with permission.)

Most transplant rejection, however, is cell mediated. In the unmodified host reaction, antigen recognition is the first step (Fig. 7.8). Any recipient Tc cells having prior exposure to donor class I antigen, or recipient Th cells having prior exposure to donor class II antigen, become activated at reexposure. More typically, in the absence of prior exposure to donor antigen, breakdown products of the injured and dying donor cells are recognized as foreign and are engulfed by macrophages. Engrafted organs undergo variable preservation injury and are therefore subject to both the shedding of MHC antigen from disrupted cell membranes and the upregulation of MHC antigens in cells undergoing repair and mitosis. Therefore, organs with relatively greater preservation injury—perhaps because of donor hypotension or hypoxia, or prolonged cold or warm ischemia times—are "brighter" targets for immune response than those with relatively less preservation injury.

As donor proteins are broken down in the macrophage cytoplasm, fragments are incorporated into newly assembled recipient class II (Dr) antigen bound for the macrophage cell surface. As described earlier, it binds to the peptide-binding groove. As a recipient Th cell draws near, the antigen-recognition platform interfaces with the Dr–peptide complex, and the donor antigen is presented. Simultaneously, the CD28 cell surface molecule of the recipient Th cell interacts with the B7-2 (CD80) surface marker of the macrophage in a process termed *costimulation*. Costimulation provides an important second pathway for Th cell activation and enhances the alloimmune response.

Signal transduction through the Th cell cytoplasm follows. This is a complex series of events involving calcium fluxes, phosphorylation, and enzyme activation (kinases, phosphatases, and isomerases). Because of its low cytoplasmic concentration, activation of the enzyme calcineurin (a serine–threonine phosphatase) is the rate-limiting step in Th cell signal transduction. Once the signal passes to the Th cell nucleus, however, the net result is the turning on of the IL-2 promoter gene and the resultant production of IL-2 and IL-2R.

Once Th lymphocytes are activated, the immune response enters a lymphocyte proliferation phase. IL-2 stimulates the proliferation of Tc cells and induces sensitized B cells to differentiate into plasma cells for production of alloantibody.

In the unmodified transplant immune response, graft destruction follows. Tc cells attack donor cells bearing the donor class I antigen, whereas antibodies may attack at any cell surface antigen. Apoptotic ("cell suicide") pathways in the donor cell may be switched on, leading to destruction of the cell. More granulocytes and macrophages are drawn by chemotactic factors, and the donor cell lytic process progresses.

If a humoral element to the otherwise predominantly cell-mediated rejection exists, as in so-called "accelerated" rejection, there may be vascular thrombosis and hemorrhage into the interstitium of the graft. On the other end of the rejection spectrum, chronic rejection refers to a slow but relentless inflammatory process. Also believed to be humorally mediated, it is characterized by low-grade histologic inflammation, microvascular injury and narrowing, and progressive graft fibrosis. There are no clearly beneficial treatments for chronic rejection at this time.

Because this sequence would occur in all cases except that of the identical twin donor–recipient combination, modulation of the immune response is essential for success. Whereas the historic transplant literature is replete with novel immunosuppressive attempts, from thoracic duct drainage to total lymphoid irradiation, modern immunosuppression rests largely upon the use of a variety of chemical and biologic agents.

Chemoimmunosuppression is the centerpiece of transplant management. Cyclosporine, tacrolimus, azathioprine, prednisone, and methylprednisolone are all commonly used agents. Mycophenolate mofetil and sirolimus are newer, more recently approved drugs (Table 7.2). Similar to combination chemotherapy for cancer, the simultaneous use of two or three agents for prophylaxis of transplant rejection is now routine. The fundamental principle is to use agents with different mechanisms of action to inhibit the immune response at several different steps. This allows for customization of dosage regimens, depending on the immunosuppressive

TABLE 7.2

Immunosuppressive Agents

Agent	Mechanism of Action
Cyclosporine (CSA)	Inhibits IL-2 production by Th cells
Tacrolimus (FK-506)	Inhibits IL-2 production by Th cells
Sirolimus (rapamycin)	Inhibits IL-2 action upon cells
Azathioprine	Inhibits DNA synthesis, lymphocyte proliferation
Mycophenolate mofetil	Inhibits DNA synthesis, lymphocyte proliferation
Glucocorticoids (prednisone, methylprednisolone)	Inhibit DNA and RNA production; inhibit nuclear factors that lead to cytokine production; decrease polymorphonuclear neutrophil and macrophage chemotaxis and function
Antithymocyte globulin (ATG)	Binds to surface of T cells, inhibiting proliferation and function
Monomurab (OKT3)	Binds to surface of T cells, inhibiting proliferation and function
Basiliximab and daclizumab	Bind to IL-2 receptor, preventing action of IL-2

DNA, deoxyribonucleic acid; IL-2, interleukin-2; RNA, ribonucleic acid; Th, helper T.
(Taken from O'Leary JP. *The physiologic basis of surgery*, 3rd ed. Philadelphia: Lippincott Williams & Wilkins, © 2002.)

needs of, and the toxicity experienced by, the individual patients.

Biologic agents also have a secure immunosuppressive role in the transplant recipient. Antithymocyte globulin (ATG) and c (OKT3) monoclonal antibody are among the most commonly used. Both are antibody (globulin) preparations produced by first immunizing nonhuman animals (usually horses, goats, rabbits, or mice) with human lymphocytes, then culling and purifying the Ig fraction of the serum. Whereas ATG is a polyclonal preparation containing antibodies with many different specificities, OKT3 is a very pure—monoclonal—preparation of murine IgG specific for the human CD3 (formerly T3) antigen. Both cause diminution in the circulating T-cell population and may be used either for "induction" immunosuppression or treatment of established rejection. In the former situation, the biologic agent is administered for 3 to 14 days immediately after transplant surgery in the hope of averting rejection altogether. In the latter, it is administered only after rejection has occurred and lymphocytes are in the proliferative phase. More recently, humanized monoclonal antibodies to IL-2R ("IL-2R antagonists") have secured an important immunosuppressive role. Basiliximab and daclizumab both have high affinity for IL-2R and thereby diminish the action of IL-2 without affecting its production. These agents appear to be well tolerated, are free of nephrotoxicity, and are most effective when used perioperatively.

Complications of over-immunosuppression include infection (especially with cytomegalovirus) and neoplasia (especially skin cancer and lymphoma). A host of potential individual side effects also exists for each agent, including tremor, leukopenia, cataracts, and avascular necrosis of long bones. Cyclosporine and tacrolimus are nephrotoxic, and they require close monitoring. However, in most transplant recipients, the quality of life is very good. With the best of surgical and immunosuppressive management techniques, 1-year graft survival rates are between 80% and 90%.

SUGGESTED READINGS

Abraham E, Jesmok G, Tuder R, et al. Contribution of tumor necrosis factor to pulmonary cytokine expression and lung injury after hemorrhage and resuscitation. *Crit Care Med* 1995;23:1319.

Beck G, Habicht GS. Primitive cytokines: harbingers of vertebrate defense. *Immunol Today* 1991;12:180.

Billiar TR. Nitric oxide: novel biology with clinical relevance. *Ann Surg* 1995;221:339.

Bone RC, Balk RA, Fein AM, et al. A second large controlled clinical study of E5, a monoclonal antibody to endotoxin: results of a prospective, multicenter, randomized, controlled trial. *Crit Care Med* 1995;23:994.

Brayman KL, Stephanian E, Matas AJ, et al. Analysis of infectious complications occurring after solid-organ transplantation. *Arch Surg* 1992;127:38.

Burns AT, Davies DR, McClaren AJ, et al. Apoptosis in ischemia/reperfusion injury of human renal allografts. *Transplantation* 1998;66:872.

Chang AE, Geiger JD, Sondak VK, et al. Adoptive cellular therapy of malignancy. *Arch Surg* 1993;128:1281.

Harvell CD. The evolution of inducible defense. *Parasitology* 1990;100:S53.

Hibbs JB, Taintor RR, Vavrin Z Jr. Macrophage cytotoxicity: role for L-arginine deiminase and imino nitrogen oxidation to nitrite. *Science* 1987;235:473.

Hoffman RA, Langrehr JM, Simmons RL. Nitric oxide synthesis: a consequence of alloimmune interaction. *Xenobiotica* 1994;2:5.

Kahan BD. Cyclosporine. *N Engl J Med* 1989;321:1725.

Murrach P, Kappler J. The T cell and its receptor. *Sci Am* 1986; 254:36.

Pannen BHJ, Robotham JL. The acute-phase response. *New Horiz* 1995;3:183.

Pinsky MR. A unifying hypothesis of multiple systems organ failure: failure of host defense homeostasis. *J Crit Care* 1990;5:108.

Robertson FM, Offner PJ, Ciceri DP, et al. Detrimental hemodynamic effects of nitric oxide synthase inhibition in septic shock. *Arch Surg* 1994;129:142.

Samuelsson BE, Breimer ME. ABH antigens: some basic concepts. *Transplant Proc* 1987;19:4401.Suthanthiran M, Strom TB. Renal transplantation. *N Engl J Med* 1994;331:365.

Takiff H, Cook DJ, Himaya NS, et al. Dominant effect of histocompatibility on ten-year kidney transplant survival. *Transplantation* 1988;45:410.

Theuer CP, Pastan I. Immunotoxins and recombinant toxins in the treatment of solid carcinomas. *Am J Surg* 1993;166:284.

CHAPTER 8

Oncology

John H. Stewart, IV and Edward A. Levine

Surgery has been, and will continue to be, the pivotal modality in the curative and palliative therapy of those with solid tumors for years to come. However, even technically perfect surgical procedures, in well-selected patients, may be followed by tumor recurrence. The limitations of surgical therapy for malignant disease have been well known to surgeons for more than a century. Increasingly aggressive and radical surgical procedures have not been the answer to most malignancies. Although our ability to pursue malignancy in the operating room now extends beyond our eyes and our hands, the efficacy of surgical procedures directed against a genetic disease, such as neoplasia, will always be limited. Why surgical therapy fails is inextricably linked to the genetic nature of the disease. Understanding this problem is the key to understanding the role of the surgeon in treating the patient with malignant disease.

An understanding of the clinically relevant biology of the oncologic process must support optimal surgical intervention. The biology of neoplasia is characterized by the uncontrolled growth of abnormal immortalized cells, which typically produces a tumor (mass) that invades and destroys normal tissues and spreads to other areas of the body through multiple routes (e.g., bloodstream, lymphatics, intracavitary direct invasion). Oncogenesis begins at a cellular level, in a process called *malignant transformation*. This may be either a single or, more often, a multistep process. A normal cell is transformed into a malignant one through a variety of mechanisms. The transformation events may occur as a result of exposure to certain viruses, chemicals, radiation and other physical agents, spontaneous random mutations, or genetic rearrangements. Considerable evidence exists that transformation occurs much more frequently than does clinical cancer. Transformed cells may undergo alterations in their surface composition, which is the basis for immunologic recognition. This chapter will review the normal molecular processes and the genetic changes underlying neoplastic growth and the techniques used to understand them.

Advancements in molecular biology and genetic techniques have provided a catalyst to address these fundamental problems. The process leading to neoplasia is now seen in terms of specific alterations in oncogenes and subsequent changes in the expression of growth factors or their receptors. Moreover, the process of metastasis formation is now known to be under similar genetic regulation. Further refinements in our knowledge should allow for the rapid diagnosis of the underlying genetic cause of malignancy, and provide for improved prognostication. Molecular characteristics of tumor are currently utilized clinically and in the future, surgical oncology will use molecular biology to an ever-increasing degree. Understanding these tools will enable surgeons to improve therapeutic decision making, interface with functional imaging, and perform less invasive procedures for earlier stage disease.

CELLULAR HOMEOSTASIS

The genetic constitution of a cell dictates its appearance and function. Our current understanding of molecular carcinogenesis is rooted in our appreciation for the role of genes in cellular homeostasis and the impact of genetic mutations on uncontrolled cell growth. Gregor Mendel discovered many of the basic principles of genetics in the 19th century. Mendel realized that genetic information was passed on from an organism to its offspring in discrete units that we currently label genes. The entire repertoire of genetic information carried by an organism is its *genome*. The human genome consists of approximately 22,000 genes packaged into 22 different pairs of chromosomes (autosomes) and 2 sex chromosomes, X and Y. The normal chromosomal constitution of the human somatic cell is a diploid state of 46 chromosomes. By convention, the short arm of the chromosome is designated p and the long arm is termed q. Chromosomes consist primarily of DNA, which associates with positively charged proteins termed *histones*. Nuclear DNA is configured in a double helix and composed of specific sequences of four nucleotides: the two purine bases, adenine (A) and guanine (G), and the two pyrimidine bases, thymine (T) and cytosine (C). In the complementary strands of the helix, A will pair (bond) only with T, and G only with C.

DNA is interpreted in groups of three bases or triples, known as a codon (e.g., ATT), on the DNA molecule which specifies a particular amino acid. Therefore, it is the precise order of the nucleotides or codons that determines the specificity of the genetic code. The integrity of the DNA code is necessary for cellular homeostasis.

Mitosis is the process of cellular division that apportions new chromosomes equally to daughter cells (Fig. 8.1). Normal mitosis is necessary to maintain the diploid state. Each individual inherits two copies of each gene, called *alleles*. The alleles are "expressed" when the DNA is *transcribed* into messenger RNA (mRNA) and subsequently *translated* into proteins which carry out the biologic activities.

The cell cycle involves two coordinated events: chromosomal DNA replication (synthetic or S-phase) and then division into daughter cells (mitotic or M-phase). These coordinated events are subdivided into four broad periods by gap periods (G-phases) that separate the S and M phases of the cell cycle. The G_1 (or gap) is the interval from the previous division to the beginning of DNA synthesis. Quiescent cells are recruited to G1 phase through mitogenic stimulation. At the restriction point (R), these cells either undergo cell cycle arrest or progress to the period of active DNA synthesis known as the *S-phase*. G_2 is the interval between DNA synthesis and nuclear division. The cell cycle is concluded with mitosis (M phase), during which chromosomes are separated into each daughter cell. The duration of the cell cycle and of each period is variable, depending on the cell type. The typical cycle takes 10 to 30 hours; S, G_2, and M take approximately 10 hours, and G_1 varies considerably (up to many days). Nondividing cells such as mature fibroblasts will exit the cell cycle after the M phase, stop further DNA synthesis and remain in the G_0 phase.

The cell cycle is tightly controlled by the interactions between retinoblastoma protein (pRb), cyclins and cyclin-dependent kinases (CDKs). Rb protein is the gatekeeper of the cell cycle. CDK-dependent phosphorylation of Rb, allows progression of cells through the cell cycle. Mitogenic stimulation causes increased expression of D cyclins (D1, D2, and D3) that assemble with CDKs 4 and 6 during G_1. This not only results in phosphorylation of the Rb protein at the restriction point in G_1, but it also results in activation of cyclin E/CDK2 complex leading to further phosphorylation of Rb and subsequent progression through the cell cycle. Other critical cyclin/CDK interactions during the cell cycle include cyclin A/CDK2 during S-phase and cyclins A, B/CDK1 during G_2 and M phases.

The flow of information in human cells is transferred from the DNA sequence to RNA, a process called *transcription*. RNA, unlike DNA, is a single-stranded moiety with ribose substituted for deoxyribose and uracil (U) substituted for thymine. Transcription of information coded in the DNA sequences is initiated by an RNA polymerase that uses the DNA strand as a template to build a complementary mRNA. Therefore, the DNA codon CTT would correspond to the mRNA triplet GAA. However, most eukaryotic genes are portions that are not translated. The DNA sequences that code for segments of the final protein product (exons) are interspersed with stretches of DNA that are transcribed but not translated (introns). Therefore, a gene is first transcribed into pre-mRNA, containing both introns as well as exons. The exons of this pre-mRNA are spliced together to generate a contiguous coding sequence of all exons to be translated into proteins. The 5′ and 3′ ends of the RNA are modified before being exported from the nucleus into the cytoplasm as mature mRNA. mRNA then migrates into the cytoplasm and binds to ribosomal RNA (rRNA) to act as a template for the translation of the original codon. To accomplish this, a continual wave of specific cytoplasmic transfer RNA (tRNA) binds to the mRNA triplet and then combines with the specific amino acid it coded for in a process known as *translation*.

Translation is a dynamic process. Because there are a limited number of pathways of response, there must be mechanisms of regulation that determine the appropriate types and amounts of proteins expressed. The genetic machinery must be flexible enough to alter its response to the requirements of wound healing or the catabolism of sepsis. What normally activates genes and what outside regulators are able to control cell behavior are areas of intense research. Regulation of gene expression is accomplished

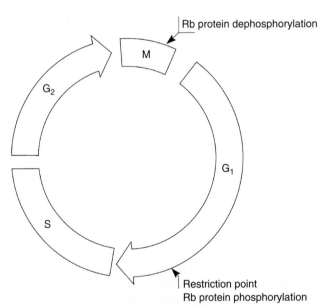

FIGURE 8.1 Homeostasis: Normal somatic cells proliferate, differentiate, and undergo apoptosis. An imbalance in this scheme causes cancer. Normal cell cycle consists of two distinct phases called M phase (mitotic phase) and the interphase, during which the DNA replication occurs. The gaps between mitosis and DNA synthesis are classified into G_1, and G_2. In G_1 phase, the RNA and proteins are synthesized, and under the permissive conditions, cells make a commitment to undergo chromosomal replication. After DNA replication, the commitment to undergo mitosis occurs in G_2 phase. After mitosis (M phase), cells enter a state called G_0 (not shown in the figure). At this point cells may remain quiescent and undergo further cell division under growth stimuli, or may withdraw from further division.

through four general categories. The first is regulation of RNA transcription. Certain genes become activated or deactivated, and this alters their availability for transcription. Methylation of the nucleotide (DNA methylation) is one mechanism proposed for this type of control. Another proposed mechanism is unwinding of the chromosome to uncover DNA, making it available for transcription. The second category of regulation is the control of mRNA processing. This includes alterations in the way mRNA is transported to the ribosome, as well as changes in the cellular environment that alter mRNA stability, and thereby change its half-life and availability for transcription. The third mechanism is translational regulation. These mechanisms are poorly understood but are suspected to involve the timing of translation and the rate of translation. Finally, posttranslational modification of proteins through the addition of biochemical function groups including acetate, phosphate, and carbohydrates.

Alterations in regulation of the cell cycle frequently allow for otherwise deleterious gene mutations to propagate through cancer cell progeny. Alteration of any portion of the cell cycle by oncogenic mitogens may cause mutations. Errors in mitosis may cause structural chromosomal changes and usually involve the exchange of material between two or more chromosomes (*translocation*), *deletions* of chromosomal material, or rearrangement of loci (*inversion*). Rearrangements, such as the Philadelphia chromosome, a marker for chronic myelocytic leukemia (CML), were one of the first abnormalities discovered. Understanding of the implications of such chromosomal translocation has substantial implications for therapy. For example, the bcr-*abl* oncogene is activated at the site of the translocation of the "Philadelphia chromosome" and codes for a tyrosine kinase. Study of this oncoprotein has led to the development of clinically useful specific inhibitor of this protein (STI-571 or Imatinib), which is active against not only CML but gastrointestinal stromal tumors as well.

TOOLS FOR ANALYSIS OF GENE EXPRESSION

The human genome project has shown the genome to contain approximately 22,000 genes. It is these genes that code for the proteins involved in cellular homeostasis. Because cancer actually represents the dysregulation of this homeostasis due to genetic dysfunction, a unique challenge in oncology is to recognize distinct molecular signatures associated with carcinogenesis. Such a molecular signature could not only classify patients according to the likelihood of response, but also guide therapeutic decision making and support the ongoing development of targeted therapy against cancer. Over the next decade, oncology will move toward a more predictive paradigm in which relevant molecular aspects of diseases will be applied to models that will assess the prognosis and likelihood of response to a broad range of specific therapies. Our challenge, then,

is to identify aberrant molecular profiles, understand the clinical implications of such changes and to develop specific "targeted" interventions.

In addition to well-established morphologic and immunohistochemical methods, several molecular and cell biologic techniques are being increasingly employed to analyze gene expression in tumor biology. Some of these techniques have quickly moved from the research laboratory to acceptance as clinical tools. The results of such analyses are now routinely used to decide what therapies may be appropriate for an individual depending on the expression of certain genes. These techniques include flow cytometry, nucleic acid hybridizations, polymerase chain reaction (PCR), microarrays, and proteomics.

Flow Cytometry

Flow cytometry is an optical-based technique that uses a fluorescent dye to stain cells so that specific fluorescent spectra can then identify unique categories of cells. For most cell kinetic studies, acridine orange or propidium iodide dye is used. The binding of these dyes is proportional to cellular DNA content. Once stained, single-cell suspensions are placed in the fluorescence-activated cell sorter (FACS). The cells are then directed into a single file and flow past a detector which measures the light scattered by each cell and the intensity of the fluorescence of the cell. Using an FACS, up to 1,000 cells per minute may be analyzed. FACS-directed analysis can determine ploidy status and the proliferative indexes of any population. Quiescent (G_1) cells will have a constant diploid amount of DNA (2N), whereas cells with increased DNA content (4N) must be in either S or G_2/M phase (Fig. 8.1). Most tumors will contain both diploid and aneuploid subsets. Aneuploidy is present if there is a second G_1 peak in addition to the normally seen G_1 peak. The ratio of DNA content of tumor to the normal diploid G_1 peak may then be determined; this is known as the *DNA index*. A normal DNA index is 1.0; therefore aneuploidy is any deviation from this.

The S-phase fraction (the proliferative index) is based on the ratio of S-phase cells to the total number of cells. A normal proliferative index is less than 10%. A higher S-phase fraction is associated with accelerated tumor growth. Currently, flow cytometry data have been used in prognostic estimation. That is, tumors with aneuploidy, an elevated S-phase, or an abnormal DNA index typically have poorer outcomes and therefore need additional therapy. Flow cytometry is also useful for determining receptor status on small amounts of breast tissue and has recently been shown to be reliable in diagnosing lymphoma on fine-needle aspirates. Higher levels of the S-phase fraction have been associated with poorer outcomes in a variety of neoplasms.

Immunologic phenotyping of lymphoma cell surface markers through flow cytometry is becoming increasingly important, not only for identification of progenitor cells, but also for evaluating the biologic potential of lymphocytes sharing common markers. Also, phenotyping is extremely valuable for evaluating the response to various modes of treatment and in analyzing changes that occur in a variety of histologically similar lymphomas. Immunologic phenotyping techniques reveal that approximately 75% of non-Hodgkin lymphomas are derived from T cells, 20% from B cells, and 5% from other cell types. The cells of origin in Hodgkin disease appear to have characteristics of B cells. Most cutaneous lymphomas (e.g., mycosis fungoides and Sezary syndrome) are shown by immunophenotyping to be helper–inducer T cells, whereas most patients with chronic lymphocytic leukemia have a clonal expansion of malignant B lymphocytes. Other immunodiagnostic tests have valuable prognostic information. Serial measurements of serum interleukin 2 (IL-2) receptors correlate with the disease activity in hairy cell leukemia, childhood non-Hodgkin lymphoma, and adult T-cell leukemia and lymphoma.

Nucleic Acid Hybridizations

The discovery that DNA can be specifically cut at defined positions by enzymes (restriction endonucleases) has contributed enormously to molecular biology. Restriction endonucleases, isolated from bacteria, recognize four to eight base pair sequences and cleave the DNA precisely at those positions, producing smaller DNA fragments consisting of ends with defined sequences. Some restriction enzymes produce cohesive overhangs that are generally compatible for ligating (joining) with a different fragment produced by the same enzyme. Some restriction enzymes, on the other hand, produce DNA fragments with "blunt" ends, without any overhanging bases. In either case, the DNA fragments can be fractionated based on size by agarose gel electrophoresis. The DNA fragments can then be denatured to open up the double stranded DNA, and transferred by "blotting" to a positively charged membrane (nylon or nitrocellulose). The membranes are then hybridized with a probe that is complementary to a given sequence. The probe is usually labeled with [^{32}P]-dCTP. After washing off the nonspecific interactions, the signal is visualized by autoradiography. This sensitive technique, originally introduced by Dr. Southern, is known as *Southern blotting* and can detect a single copy gene

in the human genome, and is routinely used in molecular cloning. Variations of this technique for the detection of RNA (Northern blotting), or protein (Western blotting) were named as a play on word of the name of Dr. Southern.

Northern blotting is used for detection of the expression of a given gene. In this method, RNA is isolated from the tissue or cultured cells, separated on denaturing agarose gels and transferred onto nitrocellulose or nylon filters. The detection of a specific mRNA is accomplished by using a DNA probe (as described in the preceding text) or by a RNA probe labeled with [^{32}P]-UTP by *in vitro* transcription. To quantify gene expression changes between two or more samples, the blot is stripped and reprobed for the expression of a housekeeping gene, such as actin or glyceraldehyde 3-phosphate dehydrogenase. The size of mRNAs can be also determined by Northern blotting.

Changes of the genome relating to chromosomal aberrations such as deletions, inversions, and translocations may be detected by restriction fragment length polymorphisms (RFLPs). Because restriction enzymes recognize specific DNA sequences, any mutations (variations) in their recognition sequences would result in altered sizes of the DNA fragments when digested with those enzymes. Because these variations are polymorphic, they may not alter the gene function. RFLPs can serve as useful markers for detection of inherited diseases and isolation of genes. For example, RFLPs have been used in the isolation and characterization of the retinoblastoma tumor suppressor gene (TSG).

A valuable tool in identifying chromosomal abnormalities is fluorescent *in situ* hybridization (FISH). FISH is useful in detecting gene amplifications, translocations, and deletions in tumor biopsies or cultured cells. DNA probes for a given chromosomal region/gene are generated by labeling with biotin-tagged nucleotides and are hybridized to denatured chromosome spreads. The probes bind to their targets and are visualized by incubation with avidin conjugated with a fluorochrome such as fluorescence isothiocyanate, rhodamine or Texas Red. As shown in the Figure 8.2, FISH detects human epidermal growth factor receptor-2 (HER2/*neu*) gene

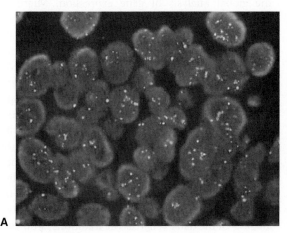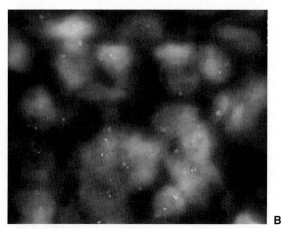

FIGURE 8.2 Amplification of HER2/*neu* gene in human tumors determined by fluorescence *in situ* hybridization. The HER2/*neu* gene is amplified in breast tumors (**A**) but not in other tumors. Melanoma (**B**) is used as an example for lack of amplification of the oncogene.

amplification in breast carcinoma. In 25% to 30% of the breast and ovarian carcinomas, HER2/neu growth factor receptor is amplified. The status of HER2/neu is of immense significance in the clinical management of the disease as a prognostic indicator and a marker of the potential utility of an antibody to the HER2/*neu* oncoprotein (Herceptin). However, HER2/*neu* is not amplified in all cancers, and therefore, HER2/*neu*-targeted therapies may not be relevant for all malignancies.

Polymerase Chain Reaction

The polymerase chain reaction is a simple, highly sensitive, and rapid technique, yet it represents a major technological leap in both laboratory and clinical research. The underlying principle is to utilize short sequences of DNA as primers (amplimers), one at the 5′ and the other at the 3′ ends, to amplify a given stretch of DNA. The sequence is replicated by a thermostable DNA polymerase called *Taq polymerase*, isolated from a bacterium that normally lives in hot springs, *Thermus aquaticus.*

A typical reaction involves "denaturation" (separation of DNA strands) of the template at 94°C, followed by annealing (primers bind to the single DNA strands) of the primers at 45°C to 60°C, and the synthesis of a new DNA strand at 72°C from the primers associated with the template DNA. The cycle is repeated approximately 25 to 30 times, resulting in amplification of several hundreds of thousands fold in a short span of 1 to 4 hours. The amplified product may be cloned and further analyzed. PCR amplification of target sequences has been demonstrated from single cells. This makes probes for single cancer cells in tissue or blood specimens possible, which has started the field of "molecular staging."

Two modifications of PCR have expanded the utility of PCR. In reverse transcriptase-PCR (RT-PCR or "expression" PCR), RNA isolated from the cultured cells or tissue specimens is first converted to cDNA by retroviral reverse transcriptase. The cDNA is then used as a template for PCR amplification. Because most mRNAs contain poly-A tail at their 3′ end, oligo dT primers are used in the reverse transcription; alternatively, a random hexamer combination is used. For PCR, gene-specific primers are used. Because RT-PCR can be made a semiquantitative method by comparing expression to that of a "housekeeping" gene (such as actin) which has relative steady levels of expression.

Because RNA is routinely isolated from blood or whole tissue samples, some analyses require determination of gene expression from a given subset of cells within the tumor specimen. For this purpose, tissue is microdissected by laser capture microdissection (LCM), RNA is isolated from the desired cells and RT-PCR is performed. Therefore, LCM makes analysis of tumor cells possible without potential contamination by nonmalignant stromal cells typically found in tumor specimens.

Sanger developed a method of DNA sequencing which has enabled us to decipher the genomes. The original method, known as *dideoxy chain termination method*, was used to sequence DNA cloned into a special M13 bacteriophage.

However, a number of technologic advances have improved and automated the technique, which enables sequencing of DNA fragments cloned in a variety of vectors. In principle, the template DNA is copied using a DNA polymerase in the presence of a mix of the four deoxynucleotides (dATP, dGTP, dCTP and dTTP), along with a small amount of each of the dideoxy nucleotides (e.g., ddATP) in four separate reactions: the four reactions will also contain a radioactive deoxynucleotide as a tracer and a short oligodexynucleotide fragment which will serve as a primer. The DNA polymerase normally incorporates only deoxynucleotides during polymerization. The polymerase can also incorporate a dideoxy nucleotide (present in the mix); however, it cannot extend the chain any further if a dideoxy nucleotide is incorporated instead of a deoxynucleotide. As a result, the chain is terminated, and that position indicates the presence of a respective deoxynucleotide in the DNA. Because incorporation of the dideoxy nucleotides is random, fragments of different lengths are generated. Because of the presence of a radionucleotide, the fragments can be visualized through autoradiography. Because four separate reactions are performed with each of the dideoxy nucleotides, a continuous sequence is generated. Owing to the advances in automation and the development of fluorescent nucleotides, DNA sequencing is routinely carried out by automated methods.

The techniques mentioned in the preceding text are primarily used to examine changes in the expression of one or two genes. However, to appreciate the numerous molecular events in a tumor, it is advantageous to have simultaneous insight into multiple genetic events. For example, the limited availability of tissue could limit the investigation of multiple genetic markers that may be of value in deciding on a certain course of treatment. Techniques such as differential display PCR and serial analysis of gene expression (SAGE) allow the profiling of several hundreds or even thousands of gene from a relatively small amount of cells/tissue in a single experiment.

The advent of microarray technology has revolutionized the global analysis of gene expression. Microarrays are assembled by using either unique oligonucleotide sequences of genes, or cDNA sequences on glass microscope slides. For example, cancer-related genes including oncogenes, TSGs, growth factors, and other key signaling intermediates are now available as microarrays. These arrays are hybridized with fluorescently labeled probes from different specimens. The kinetics of expression allows determination of relative expression levels. It is based on the ratio with which each probe hybridizes to a given DNA present on the array. Hybridization is assayed using a confocal laser microscope, which will allow simultaneous determination of the relative expression levels of all the genes represented in the array. Specially developed software programs facilitate further analysis of the data. Whereas the traditional studies analyzed expression of one or a handful of genes at a time, the array technology can offer insights into the expression of *thousands of genes* in a single experiment.

The current era of genomics provides substantial insight into the field of molecular oncology. Current studies have shown that gene-expression profiles can predict the behavior of a wide variety of malignancies. Although genetic events are the basis for carcinogenesis, cancer is also a disease of proteins and protein function. The dogma of "one gene equals one protein" is no longer tenable and the translation of the insights gained from genomics into truly meaningful clinical applications faces numerous challenges. Chief among these challenges is understanding the roles of split genes, RNA splicing, and posttranslational modifications in tumor biology. Consequently, real progress in the development of prognostic techniques in cancer will rely on new insights gained from the investigation of protein expression or proteomics. Immunoblotting or Western blotting has traditionally assessed changes in protein expression. In this method, protein extracts are prepared from fresh/frozen tissues or cells and separated by sodium dodecyl sulfate (SDS)-polyacrylamide gel electrophoresis, which resolves proteins based on their size. The proteins are then transferred electrophoretically to a nitrocellulose membrane and probed with a specific antibody. A second antibody, which recognizes the primary antibody, conjugated with horseradish peroxidase, is then added and incubated with a chemiluminescent substrate and the signal is recorded on an x-ray film or by a chemiluminescent detector.

Two-dimensional gel electrophoresis is a very powerful technique in proteomics. This technique can be used to generate a profile of total proteins expressed in samples. The resolution of proteins in the first dimension is based on the charge and in the second dimension is based on their size. Tissue culture cells are routinely labeled with $[^{35}S]$-methionine, although the tissues are directly homogenized and later visualized by staining with sensitive dyes. Because proteins are charged molecules, and at a certain pH, the positive and negative charges become equal and do not carry a net charge. This pH is defined as *isoelectric point*. The proteins are resolved in an electric field until they reach their respective isoelectric points. At the isoelectric point, the proteins do not carry a net charge and hence, do not migrate any further in an electric field. This process is called *isoelectric focusing* and constitutes the first dimension of 2-d gel electrophoresis. In the second dimension, the proteins are resolved based on their size, and it is usually carried out in the presence of SDS. As a result, the position of a protein on 2-d gels is unique. An advantage with the 2-d gel method is that posttranslational modifications, such as phosphorylations, may be detected. The desired protein spots may be cut out from the gels, digested with the protease trypsin, and resultant peptides can be analyzed by mass spectrometry (MS) to identify the protein.

Surface-enhanced laser desorption ionization-time of flight mass spectrometry (SELDI-TOF MS) and matrix-assisted laser desorption ionization mass spectrometry (MALDI MS) have been used extensively to identify protein profiles of a variety of tissues. Matrix assisted laser desorption ionization-time of flight mass spectrometry (MALDI-TOF MS) is a versatile method of studying a range of macromolecules from cells to tissues. Its ability to desorb high-molecular-weight molecules, its high accuracy and sensitivity, and its wide mass range make this a promising method for the identification of biomolecules in complex samples, including peptides and proteins. The technique employs the cocrystallizing of low-molecular-weight matrix and analyte on a target plate. Irradiation of these crystals by short pulses of ultraviolet (UV) or infrared light initiates desorption and ionization, where predominantly singly protonated intact molecular ions are produced. Because ionization is a pulsed process, it is easily compatible with a time of flight analyzer. MALDI-TOF MS is an extremely sensitive tool permitting the detection of sample molecules below the fentomole level with mass accuracies better than 10^{-4}. In addition, this technique has been used for comparative proteomics studies, examining the protein profiles generated from normal versus diseased tissues, or from nontreated control tissues versus drug-treated tissues. Differences in the protein profiles can be correlated to diagnostic or prognostic variables, leading to the generation of biomarker panels with analytical utility.

TOOLS FOR ANALYSIS OF GENE FUNCTION

Equally as important in understanding gene expression is the understanding of gene function. Given that genes are mutated in cancer, it is important to understand how mutations in these genes contribute to the behaviors associated with carcinogenesis. Currently, the two most common *in vitro* methods of defining gene function are *gene transfer* methods and *RNA silencing*. Transgenic mouse models are commonly used to dissect the functional implications of genetic mutations *in vivo*.

Gene transfer involves experimentally introducing genes into target cells. In addition, the idea of replacing defective genes holds promise for gene therapy of many diseases including cancer. A number of vectors to introduce genes and agents that transfer the DNA sequence of interest have been developed. Because many genes are interrupted with introns and many genes exceed the capacity of available vectors, cloned cDNAs are commonly used for gene transfer. Gene expression is dependent on several factors including positioning in the proper context of eukaryotic regulatory elements, such as the promoter to initiate transcription, sequences for optimal translation, and the polyadenylation signal for processing of the mRNA. In most gene transfer vectors, cytomegalovirus promoter sequences are used for their ability to direct strong expression of the inserted sequences, although different promoters have been employed. A very important feature of these vectors is that they also contain a drug selection marker, such as neo^r gene, which confirms resistance to neomycin. Drug selection ensures that the cells retain the introduced gene for many generations, although that, in itself, does not guarantee the expression of the introduced gene. For tissue culture experiments with a shorter time frame (transient transfection), drug selection is not necessary and the gene expression is transiently sustainable for 24 to 72 hours.

The expression vectors contain regulatory sequences to replicate in mammalian cells as well as those needed to grow in bacteria. The cDNAs encoding the gene of interest are ligated into the vector DNA fragment and the recombinant vectors are grown in sufficient quantities and then introduced into eukaryotic cells. A number of methods have been developed to introduce the recombinant plasmid vectors into mammalian cells. The earliest and still widely used method for cultured cells uses calcium phosphate to precipitate the recombinant DNA into large aggregates, which are taken up by the cells. A number of commercial liposomes are now available and generally yield higher transfection efficiencies.

The vectors may be broadly classified as plasmid and viral vectors (Table 8.1). Target cells are transfected with the plasmid vectors that either integrate into the genome of the target cells, or exist as self-replicating stable episomes. The viral vectors often produce a replication-defective particle that infects the target cells in a process referred to as *transduction*. To accomplish cloning into viral vectors, several kilobases of viral DNA that codes for viral structural proteins are substituted with the cDNA of interest. In most cases, the viral vectors are first generated as plasmids, and transfected into "packaging cells" which provide the necessary proteins for the assembly of an infectious particle. Then the recombinant infectious virus is used to infect the target cells. Currently, although retroviral vectors and adenoviral vectors are widely used, other viral vector systems are also used (Table 8.1). Each of the expression vectors has specific advantages and limitations. Therefore, the choice of the vector is primarily dictated by the experimental design.

Retroviral and adenoviral vectors are intensely investigated for human gene therapy. Retroviruses belong to the family of Retroviridae and consist of three widely studied subfamilies, Oncovirinae, Lentivirinae and Spumavirinae. The oncogenic retroviruses belong to the Oncovirinae subfamily, whereas the human immunodeficiency viruses belong to the Lentivirinae subfamily. All retroviruses contain a diploid RNA as a genome, ranging approximately 7 to 10 kb in size. The nondefective, replicating retroviruses generally contain *gag, pol* and *env* genes to code for the structural and catalytic proteins essential for replication, although viruses such as human immunodeficiency viruses code for additional proteins. Retroviral vectors integrate into the host genome and generally cannot exceed a total size of approximately 10 kb, and are therefore used to transduce smaller genes up to

TABLE 8.1

Mammalian Gene Expression Systems

Expression Vector Base	Features
Adenovirus	Broad mammalian host range; tropic for airways but infects other organs; generally a nuclear episome; high level of expression; high-titer recombinant virus stocks; used for gene therapy; immunogenic
Adeno-associated	Broad mammalian host range; requires adenovirus for packaging; wild-type virus integrates into specific site on human chromosome 19, but integration of recombinant expression virus is random; imited insert size (about 4–5 kb) for packaged recombinant virus; nonpathogenic; potential for gene therapy if transgene is small
Epstein-Barr virus	Retained as a nuclear epsome in human, monkey, and dog, but not generally in rodent; episome replicates autonomously; potential for gene therapy
Herpes simplex virus	Broad mammalian host range; lytic; caries large (>5 kb) fragments of exogenous DNA; packaged virion can accommodate 150-kb DNA; viral genomes are stable in serial propagation
Papilloma virus	Retained as a nuclear episome in rodent (BPV) or human and monkey (HPV); episomal nature of vector/transgene is unpredictable; must be empirically assessed for each transgene; used to study gene regulation and for high-level transgene expression
Polyoma virus	Broad mammalian host range; replicates best in murine cells; can integrate; will be episomal with polyoma ori and large T antigen in *cis* or *trans*
Retro virus	Host range dependent on virus coat—ecotropic (species from which wild-type virus was isolated) and amphotropic (broad mammalian); RNA virus; integrates into DNA as a reverse transcribed provirus; difficult to get high titer of recombinant virus; limited insert size approximately 8.5); used in gene therapy of small genes
SV40	Broad mammalian host range; replicated readily in simian cells; can integrate; will be episomal with SV50 ori and large T antigen in *cis* or *trans*
Vaccinia	Broad mammalian host range; viral infection shuts down host synthesis; lytic; used primary for transgene protein overexpression

This list represents some of the common viruses that are the basis for most mammalian expression systems. In BPV, bovine papilloma virus; HPV, human papilloma virus.

From Colosimo A, Goncz KK, Holmes AR, et al. Transfer and expression of foreign genes in mammalian cells. *Biotechniques* 2000;29:314–324, with permission.

approximately 4 kb. A major disadvantage is that it is often difficult to obtain high titer recombinant virus.

Adenoviruses are commonly found in healthy humans and are generally nonpathogenic viruses. Adenoviruses are DNA viruses which can accommodate larger genes and a high titer vector can be generated with a broad range of host specificity. Adenoviruses, on the other hand, can accommodate larger genes and can infect nonreplicating, quiescent cells as well, but they are immunogenic.

Direct injection of plasmid DNA into the target tissue has also been used for gene transfer. This method, known as *naked DNA inoculation*, may be suited for generating immune responses against tumor antigens, because a single injection in experimental animals can elicit immune responses that can last for several months. However, this and other gene transfer technologies are still in the developmental stages.

Antisense agents represent another class of techniques used to evaluate gene function. These molecules inhibit gene expression in a sequence-specific manner by binding to target RNAs. Once bound, these molecules induce target RNA dysfunction or degradation. The three major categories of antisense molecules include antisense oligonucleotide derivatives, ribozymes, and deoxyribozymes as well as small-interfering double stranded RNA molecules also referred to as *RNA interference* (*RNAi*).

Originally described in 1978, antisense oligonucleotides represent the original antisense technology. All antisense oligonucleotides, which are typically 10 to 25 nucleotides in length, hybridize to a host target RNA. Upon hybridization, these molecules either degrade the target mRNA through the cellular enzyme RNase H, inhibit translation by steric hindrance, or interfere with the splicing of pre-mRNA.

Ribozymes and deoxyribozymes are antisense molecules that catalyze chemical reactions without protein cofactors. These molecules bind directly to RNA substrates to specifically cleave target RNAs. RNAi has recently become a widely used technology for defining gene expression in mammalian cells. RNAi is an ancient cellular defense mechanism protecting plants and invertebrates from viruses and transposons. The introduction of synthetic small inhibitory RNAs (siRNAs), which are 20 to 25 bp in length through exogenous delivery or endogenous expression by RNA polymerase II and III promoters, has revolutionized our ability to modulate gene expression. siRNA molecules that engage a group of cellular proteins called *RNA-induced silencing complex* (RISC). The RISC guides the siRNA to its target messenger mRNA and proteins to destroy the mRNA. The process is extremely specific and enables siRNA to break up the mRNA associated with a disease-causing gene or virus.

Limited amounts of information can be gained by studying cells *in vitro*. However, the advent of transgenic mouse models allows investigators to define how mutations in genes associated with cancer affect tissues in the whole organism. Transgenic mouse models are genetically engineered by gene insertion, deletion, or gene replacement so that their cells express a genetic profile according to the tissue specificity of the associated regulatory DNA.

The generation of transgenic mouse models requires the insertion of a DNA fragment containing the desired gene fragment into embryonic stem cells. After a period of *in vitro* proliferation, cell colonies that have undergone homologous recombination are identified by PCR or Southern blotting. Cells from these colonies are then injected into early mouse embryos. The transfected embryo stem cells collaborate with host embryo cells to produce a chimeric mouse. Eventually, male and female mice, which are heterogenous for the gene replacement, are bred with the expectation that one fourth of their progeny will be homozygous for the gene of interest. Study of these homozygotes allow for the elucidation of gene function in molecular carcinogenesis.

MOLECULAR CARCINOGENESIS

Among the hallmarks of a malignant cell are hyperproliferation, diminished growth factor requirements, overexpression of growth factors, and loss of anchorage-dependent growth (Table 8.2). These changes are associated with malignancy and are the result of alterations in one or more of the feedback loop genes or regulator controls. Defects in the life cycle of a cell can occur either at the chromosome level, or within the cell cycle that ultimately results in the production of aberrant mRNAs. Such defective mRNAs are translated into mutated proteins, which affect the cell fate. Moreover, loss of any of a plethora of regulatory controls at posttranscriptional or posttranslational phases of gene expression would also impair normal gene function and ultimately alter the growth properties of cells. Alterations in the cell cycle by oncogenic mitogens may allow for otherwise deleterious gene mutations to propagate through cancer cell progeny. Errors in mitosis may also cause structural chromosomal changes and usually involve the exchange of material between two or more chromosomes (*translocation*), *deletions* of chromosomal material, or rearrangement of loci (*inversion*). Rearrangements, such as the Philadelphia chromosome, a marker for CML,

T A B L E   8 . 2
Some Properties of the Transformed Cells
Reduced cell-matrix and cell-cell interactions
Poorly organized actin microfilaments
Altered cell morphology
Anchorage-independent growth
Loss of contact inhibition and growth to high densities
Increased motility
Production of matrix-degrading enzymes
Loss or decreased growth factor dependence
Abrogation of hormonal control
Neovascularization
Immortalization
Tumor formation in susceptible animals
Resistance or failure to undergo apoptosis

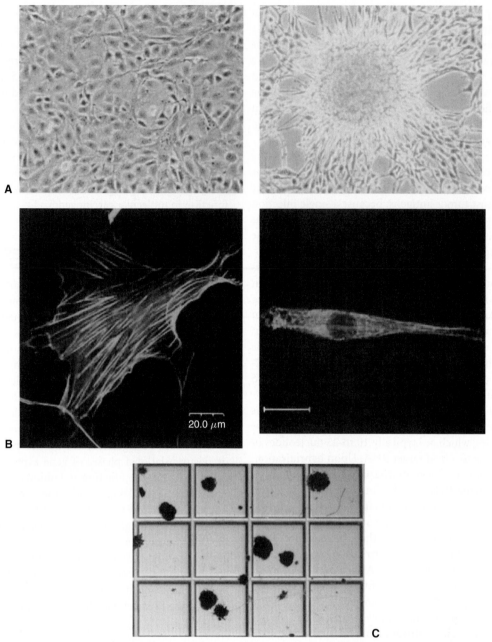

FIGURE 8.3   Some properties of the transformed cells. **A:** Mouse fibroblasts (NIH-3T3 cells; **left**) and those transformed by v-Ki-ras (**right**) oncogene are cultured in a monolayer. Normal cells stop growing at confluency but the transformed cells continue to grow on top of other cells, resulting in a multilayered growth. This phenomenon is called loss of contact inhibition. **B:** Normal (NIH-3T3 cells; **left**) and the v-Ki-ras–transformed cells (**right**) are stained for polymerized actin filaments (microfilaments) using fluorescently labeled phalloidin. The normal fibroblasts have well-developed filaments and grow as well-spread cells. The transformed cells, on the other hand, are spindle shaped, with little or no filaments. **C:** Transformed cells do not require normal cell–matrix interactions for growth. As an example, MCF-7 human breast carcinoma cells are grown under anchorage-independent conditions.

were some of the first abnormalities discovered. Understanding of the implications of such chromosomal translocation has substantial implications for therapy. For example, the *bcr-abl* oncogene is activated at the site of the translocation (9 → 22) of the "Philadelphia chromosome" and codes for a tyrosine kinase. Study of this oncoprotein has led to the development of clinically useful specific inhibitor of this protein (STI-571 or Imatinib), which is active against not only CML but gastrointestinal stromal tumors as well.

Functionally immature progenitor cells exit the cell cycle and differentiate under the influence of appropriate hormones, growth factors, cytokines, and other regulators. Additional factors, such as the microenvironment of the cells, polarity, position, cell-extracellular matrix and cell–cell interactions are also critical determinants of differentiation. The differentiated cells generally have a finite life span at the end of which they undergo programmed cell death. In cancer cells, however, this dynamic equilibrium is subverted to result in uncontrolled proliferation of undifferentiated or poorly differentiated cells that are resistant to apoptosis.

In sporadic cancers, which account for greater than or equal to 90% of human malignancies, accumulation of somatic mutations drive the clonal transformation of the progenitor cells to form neoplastic lesions. At the molecular level, a variety of genetic alterations including gene mutations and chromosomal abnormalities are demonstrated to be the causes of the neoplastic transformation. Additional genetic and epigenetic events either contribute to or expedite the tumor progression to culminate in invasion and metastasis. In hereditary cancers, like other genetic traits, the initiating mutation is inherited, and the genetic defect is present in the germ line as well as in all the somatic cells. As discussed later, multiple mutations or genetic "hits" are generally necessary for the malignant transformation. The initial mutations enhance the rate at which the subsequent ones occur, and with each mutation the cells acquire growth advantages over the neighboring normal populations. Therefore, the cumulative effects of these genetic alterations permit the tumor cells to escape normal restraints. The spectrum and pattern of these mutations define hormonal and growth factor requirements, and allow tumor cells to invade other tissues, and create a microenvironment that is permissive for metastatic growth. Some of the widely recognized properties of cancer cells include increased growth rates, loss of contact inhibition, loss of microfilaments and cell morphology, ability to grow under anchorage-independent conditions, increased motility, invasiveness, neoangiogenesis, and immortality. Some of these properties are illustrated in Figure 8.3.

Cancer-Critical Genes

Many genes that are repeatedly altered in cancer have been identified and termed *cancer-critical genes*. These genes can be broadly divided into two categories, according to whether the cancer arises from overactivity of the gene in which a gain-of-function mutation drives the cell to cancer, or too little activity in which a loss of function mutation results in carcinogenesis. Genes of the first class are referred to as *oncogenes*, whereas genes of the second class are called *TSGs*. The general properties of these cancer-critical genes are listed in Table 8.3. Both classes of tumor-critical genes can be classified into six categories based on their biochemical activities (Fig. 8.4).

Oncogenes

The activation of genetic elements has been associated with cancer. These genetic fragments (oncogenes) participate in key cellular pathways that regulate cell proliferation. The protooncogene is part of the normal cellular machinery of the host; the mutated overactive form is termed the *oncogene*. Dozens of viral and cellular oncogenes have been identified so far, some of which are described in Table 8.4. Activation of oncogenes abnormally stimulates the intracellular signaling pathways (or a *gain of function*) that culminate in malignant transformation.

Viruses have long been associated with oncogene transformation. Beginning with the discovery of the role of viruses in chicken sarcoma by Rous nearly a century ago, it is now well established that retroviruses and DNA viruses are associated with cancer in a viral oncogene model. In this model, viruses randomly acquire normal genetic material (the cellular protooncogene or c-*onc*) from their hosts (Table 8.4). A portion of the transforming virus genome is substituted with the cellular protooncogene in a process called *transduction*. During the transduction, a

TABLE 8.3

Oncogenes and Tumor Suppressor Genes

Property	Oncogenes	Tumor Suppressor Genes
Effect on growth	Positive	Negative
Differentiation	Generally block differentiation	Promote differentiation
Number of mutations required for a phenotype	One	Two
Nature of mutation	Gain of function	Loss of function
Somatic mutations	Yes	Yes
Germline mutations	Rare	Common, but not necessary
Altered function	Generally found in sporadic cancers	Sporadic and inherited cancers
Genetic alterations	Point mutations, gene rearrangements, amplifications, and truncations	Deletions and point mutations; epigenetic inactivation also occurs
Effect of gene transfer	Transform immortalized fibroblasts	Suppress malignant growth in a variety of transformed cells
Cooperation	Yes	Yes

Short list of the general properties of oncogenes and tumor suppressor genes (TSGs) is presented. The pathways regulated by oncogenes and TSGs are not mutually exclusive, and they regulate many cellular pathways in opposing manner. Some oncogenes and TSGs also interact and regulate each other's functions.

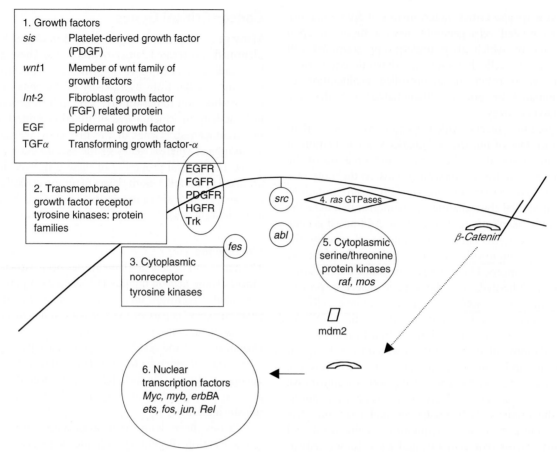

FIGURE 8.4   General outline of the classification of oncogenes based on their function. Oncogenes function in intracellular signaling pathways, and often there is cross-talk between different pathways. Two proteins (β-catenin and mdm-2) that exhibit transforming activity are discussed in the section on tumor suppressor genes. EGFR, epidermal growth factor receptor; FGFR, fibroblast growth factor receptor; PDGFR, platelet-derived growth factor receptor; HGFR, hepatocyte growth factor receptor.

significant portion of the retroviral genome may be lost to accommodate the acquired gene. These viruses are generally replication defective and classified as acute transforming viruses. As a result, acute transforming viruses usually require a helper virus to provide the structural components to produce an infectious particle. A second category of tumor viruses is referred to as *nondefective viruses* integrate in the host genome and upregulate one of the key cellular genes. These viruses do not carry a transforming gene of their own and contain their full complement of viral genes, and hence are replication competent. For example, mouse mammary tumor virus (MMTV) integrates and activates *wnt* genes resulting in the formation of breast tumors.

Protooncogenes may be either qualitatively or quantitatively modified by viral transduction to generate a viral oncogene (v-*onc*) that is refractory to normal growth controls. Because most cellular protooncogenes participate in key intracellular signal transduction pathways, the transforming retroviruses deregulate normal cell physiology to confer additional growth advantages to the infected cell. Therefore, conversion of the c-*onc* gene to v-*onc* represents a gain of

function. The three qualitative mechanisms include point mutations that result in small changes in the protooncogene sequence (e.g., *ras* oncogene), deletions in large segments of the protooncogene sequence (e.g., *src* oncogene) or chromosomal rearrangements which involve breakage and rejoining of the DNA helix (e.g., *bcr-abl* oncogene). Quantitative changes would result from the overproduction of the cellular oncogene due to either gene amplification or insertion of a powerful enhancer to drive the expression of a cellular gene. The *myc* and *erb-b* oncogenes are good examples of the activation of the oncogenes due to gene amplification.

A variety of gene transfer methods have been employed to discover mutations that differentiate cancer cells from their normal counterparts. In the gene transfer method, nontumorigenic, mouse embryonic fibroblasts (NIH-3T3 cells) are transfected with DNA extracted from malignantly transformed cells. The recipient cells are assayed for their growth phenotype in several ways:

Focus formation assays: Normal cells generally stop dividing once they reach confluent growth. Transformed cells do not exhibit this property known as *contact inhibition*, and continue to proliferate. As a result, they form

TABLE 8.4

Retroviral Oncogenes and the Corresponding Protooncogenes

Oncogene	Transducing Virus	Tumor	Function of the Protooncogene	Activation of the Protooncogene By
abl	Abelson leuemia virus	Pre–B-cell leukemia, sarcoma	Protein kinase (tyrosine)	Truncation
erb-A, erb-B	Avian erythroleukemia virus ES4	Erythroleukemia, fibrosarcoma	Transmembrane growth factor receptor kinase	Overexpression, truncation
fms	Feline sarcoma virus	Sarcoma	Transmembrane growth factor receptor kinase	Overexpression, deletion
fos	FBJ murine osteogenic sarcoma virus	Osteosarcoma	Transcription factor	Overexpression
myc	Avian myelocytomatosis virus-29	Carcinoma, myelocytoma, sarcoma	Transcription factor	Overexpression
raf	3611 murine sarcoma virus	Sarcoma	Protein kinase (serine)	Truncations
H-ras	Harvey murine sarcoma virus	Erythroleukemia, sarcoma	GTPase	Point mutations
K-ras	Kirsten	Erythroleukemia, sarcoma	GTPase	Point mutations
src	Rous sarcoma virus	Sarcoma	Protein kinase (tyrosine)	Truncation

Short list of representative oncogenes identified by their presence in the acute transforming retroviruses. Many of the oncogenes are overexpressed or present in human tumors.

multilayered cells. DNA can be extracted from these foci and the transforming oncogene may be isolated.

Anchorage-independent growth: Normal fibroblasts and epithelial cells require adherence to a substratum for their growth. Because of deregulation in their signaling pathways, transformed cells do not require such adherence-dependent growth cues, and hence can grow and form colonies in semisolid agar containing growth media (Fig. 8.2). This is an important attribute of most transformed cells.

Tumorigenesis: When inoculated into immunodeficient, athymic nude mice, a majority of tumor cells grow and form tumors in the host animal, whereas normal cells do not grow.

The above assays are also widely used techniques in assessing whether a given cell line is neoplastic or not. Although the studies on retroviral oncogenes have tremendously advanced our understanding of the biology of neoplastic transformation, human cancers seldom involve retroviruses. It should be noted that although each of the oncogenes have been shown to transform NIH-3T3 cells in culture, most oncogenes are by themselves weakly transforming when introduced into other cell types. "Cooperation" between oncogenes has been well documented. For example, transgenic expression of *myc* and *ras* together results in the formation of tumors with a much higher efficiency than with either oncogene, or sum of the rates at which both oncogenes form tumors.

Oncogenes are classified as growth factors, growth factor receptor tyrosine kinases (RTKs), nonreceptor protein tyrosine kinases, Ras GTPases, cytoplasmic serine/threonine kinases and nuclear transcription factors.

A common method by which oncogenes gain function to stimulate uncontrolled growth is through the production of growth factors. *Growth factors* are polypeptides that modulate cellular function and regulate cellular growth. These proteins are extremely potent, and in extremely small (picogram) quantities are able to induce a specific response. The actual response depends more on the type and conformation of the growth factor receptor present and the cellular environment than the specific growth factor itself. That is, a unique growth factor may induce several different responses in the same cell, depending on what receptors are available and what the current biochemical status of the cell is. Growth factor receptors are inactive until bound. When bound to a receptor, activation of the intrinsic enzymatic activity of the receptor occurs and signal transduction follows.

The growth factors function as autocrine or paracrine effectors to stimulate cell proliferation. The cellular homolog of *sis* oncogene was identified as the *B chain of platelet-derived growth factor* (PDGF). The PDGF receptor consists of heterodimers of A and B chains. Subsequent studies showed that enhanced expression of the A chain of PDGF receptor (PDGFR) could also induce cell transformation. Overexpression of v-*sis* and the cognate receptor PDGFR was found in several types of human tumors including sarcomas, lung carcinomas, and astrocytomas.

Epidermal growth factor (EGF) was identified in 1962 by its stimulatory action on epithelial cells. In the case of EGF, transformed cells will secrete EGF or EGF-like proteins that act as mitogens. Because these cells already have functional epidermal growth factor receptors (EGFRs) that bind to these peptides and possess the ability to make EGF, these cells possess an autocrine stimulatory feedback loop. Therefore, the transformed cells are capable of maintaining their transformed phenotype independent of other regulatory mechanisms. Mutation of the *erb* protooncogene results in a defective EGFR that can be activated without the action of EGF. Overexpression of HER occurs in a variety of human malignancies and is associated with a poor prognosis. EGFR expression in breast cancer is known to be inversely related to the presence of estrogen receptors and is associated with a poor prognosis. Blockade of the EGFR with a humanized monoclonal antibody (such as trastuzumab and cetuximab) is currently used clinically.

Other growth factors known to induce cellular transformation include EGF family members, fibroblast growth factor (FGF) and its related polypeptides, hematopoietic growth factors and the *wnt* gene family members. EGF and the related polypeptide, transforming growth factor alpha (TGFα) are secreted by many transformed cells. TGFα also acts through the EGFR. The *wnt* family of growth factors are implicated in a variety of growth processes and differentiation pathways. The Wnt-1 and Wnt-3 proteins are activated by insertional mutagenesis. Among the many hematopoietic growth factors, IL-2, IL-3, granulocyte-macrophage colony-stimulating factor (GM-CSF) and macrophage colony-stimulating factor (M-CSF) are known to induce cellular transformation. Activation of these genes is related to leukemias.

A second class of oncogenes is *growth factor receptor tyrosine kinases*. The prototypical oncogene of this family of oncogenes is EGFR. There are five different types of RTKs. They are EGFR-related proteins, PDGFR, FGF receptor, CSF-1R and hepatocyte growth factor/scatter factor receptor (HGF/SFR). All the RTKs have an extracellular domain, a transmembrane region, a cytoplasmic tyrosine kinase catalytic domain, and a carboxy terminal region that contains sites for tyrosine phosphorylation. The external amino terminal domains differ significantly among the different RTK subfamilies. For example, although EGFR has cysteine rich domains, the PDGFR has immunoglobulin-like motifs. Furthermore, the EGFR group comprises four related members designated HER1 through HER4, or c-*erb*-B1 through c-*erb*-B4. The general mode of activation of RTKs involves the ligand-induced dimerization that results in the stimulation of the tyrosine kinase activity associated with it, further leading to the activation of the downstream signaling activation. Aberrant activation either due to overexpression or the deletion of amino terminal extracellular ligand binding would lead to aberrant activation of the tyrosine kinase activity that produces a sustained stimulation for downstream effectors. The *HER2* gene is amplified in 30% of breast and ovarian cancers. *HER2* is a target for diagnosis and therapy by a recombinant antibody called *trastuzumab* (*Herceptin*). Trastuzumab has been shown to be efficacious in the treatment of *HER2* overexpressing breast cancers. It is now a standard part of therapy in stage II–IV disease when *HER2* is overexpressed.

A third class of oncogenes is the *cytoplasmic nonreceptor protein-tyrosine kinases*. A classic example of this class of oncogenes is *src*. *src* oncogene codes for a 60 kDa protein which has two domains, SH3 and SH2 domains that mediate protein–protein interactions, a catalytic domain and carboxy terminal–negative regulatory region. This carboxy domain is deleted in the viral oncogene, and consequently the kinase activity is constitutively activated. Both v-*src* and c-*src* are anchored to the plasma membrane on the cytoplasmic side through the amino terminus. There are at least nine other src-related tyrosine kinases. In addition, there are three other families of nonreceptor tyrosine kinases, which include the Abl, Fes, Csk families of proteins.

The fourth class of oncogenes referred to as *ras* GTPases has received significant attention as of late. The members of the Ras family and the heterotrimeric G protein receptors are GTPases which act as molecular switches that regulate a wide spectrum of signal transduction pathways. The *ras* genes code for a 21 kDa protein that is associated with the plasma membrane through carboxy terminus. Three mammalian Ras proteins, H-ras, K-ras and N-ras have been identified, and exist in active GTP-bound form and inactive GDP-bound state. A number of point mutations have been found at several positions in *v-ras* genes isolated from transforming viruses, and in mutated variants of *ras* found in spontaneous tumors. These mutations would either decrease the GTPase activity or increase the rate of exchange of bound GDP for free GTP. Both of these mutations would effectively increase the GTP-bound Ras, leading to activation of the *ras*-regulated signaling pathways.

Ras proteins activate the mitogen activated protein (MAP) kinase cascades to regulate gene transcription. In this pathway, Raf protein kinase is a central player and a direct downstream target of Ras. Ras proteins also integrate signals from the growth factor receptors. Ras regulates cytoskeletal organization through a subfamily of ras-related proteins called the *Rho proteins*. Rho proteins are critical mediators of Ras signaling pathways during normal growth and differentiation, and are required for ras-induced transformation. In normal cells, Ras activity is regulated by GTPase activating proteins (GAPs) and guanine nucleotide exchange factors (GEFs). The large family of *ets* transcriptional factors is one of the well-characterized targets of Ras signaling pathways.

The fifth oncogene class is *cytoplasmic serine/threonine kinases*. The most widely studied cytoplasmic serine/threonine kinase is *raf*. The *raf* oncogenes code for a protein kinase that phosphorylate target proteins at serine/threonine residues. There are three members of the *raf* family, c-Raf-1, A-Raf and B-Raf which range from 69 to 73 kDa in size. The three proteins share a related carboxy terminal domain and N-terminal regulatory domain. The viral transforming proteins differ from the c-Raf in that they lack the regulatory amino terminal domains, and contain a kinase domain that is constitutively active. Activated Raf phosphorylates MAP kinase kinase (MEK), which in turn phosphorylates extracellular regulated kinase (ERK). Activated ERK either enters the nucleus to activate gene transcription directly, or activate another kinase that ultimately upregulates gene expression.

The other members of this class of proteins are the protein kinase C (PKC) group of kinases and the *mos* oncogene. PKC is an intracellular target of tumor-promoting phorbol esters. In general, the several isoforms of PKC are activated by Ca^{2+}, diacylglycerol, and phospholipids, although the involvement of other second messengers and protein–protein interactions also needs to be considered. Structurally, the PKC isoforms consist of an amino terminal regulatory region and a carboxy terminal kinase domain, which can be constitutively activated by removal of the regulatory domain. Overexpression of PKC isoforms has been shown to cause cellular transformation. Given the central role of PKC in cell proliferation, PKC could contribute to the neoplastic transformation of cells.

The third member of the cytoplasmic serine/threonine kinases is *mos* oncogene. The expression of this oncogene is normally restricted to germ cells of both sexes. V-*mos* oncogene codes for protein kinase that lacks extensive regulatory domains, suggesting that overexpression or inappropriate expression could induce transformation.

The sixth class of oncogenes, *nuclear transcription factors*, directly alter the gene expression by binding to DNA to effect gene transcription. The retroviral oncogenes and the cellular protooncogenes regulate the expression of same set of genes. The transforming activity of the viral oncogenes may arise from either overexpression or by mutations. The mutated oncogenes may upregulate, act as dominant negative inhibitors to block the genes necessary for normal growth and differentiation, fail to respond normal regulation, or improperly localize into the nucleus and possibly interfere with the normal transcription program.

The thyroid hormone receptor was identified as the cellular homolog of *erb*A gene product and belongs to the steroid hormone receptor family. In the absence of the hormone, c-erbA binds to DNA, and suppresses the transcription. Upon binding to the hormone, the receptor becomes activated and transcribes genes necessary for normal growth and differentiation. Deletions at both the amino and carboxy terminal (hormone-binding domain) ends abolish hormone binding to v-*erb*A. As a result, v-*erb*A is insensitive to the hormone and blocks the transcription of essential genes that ensure normal growth and development.

Transcription factors encoded by the Jun and Fos families of the proteins are the components of transcription factor AP1. Jun and Fos proteins bind to DNA as hetero dimers and cooperatively activate genes as a complex. Although c-Jun is known to participate in cell proliferation by ERK signaling pathways and by integrins, it is also a key component of stress-regulated pathways. c-Jun is activated by a kinase called *Jun kinase* (JNK), which phosphorylates a serine residue in the N-terminal domain of c-Jun. Overexpression of c-Jun and c-Fos result in transformed growth. Additionally, deletion of the regulatory amino terminal region of c-Jun is required for the full oncogenic potential of c-Jun. Deletion of the 3′ untranslated regions of c-Fos enhances the stability of the mRNA, and also contributes to its transforming potential.

The members of the *myc* gene family including c-*myc*, N-*myc*, and L-*myc* are activated due to overexpression of the gene product. This overexpression is a consequence of insertional mutagenesis, chromosomal translocations, and gene amplification. Myc proteins dimerize with Max proteins and activate transcription. Overexpression of myc is used clinically as a prognostic marker for children with neuroblastoma.

Tumor Suppressor Genes

So far we examined a number of genes that promote growth and induce neoplastic transformation with a *gain of function*. There is another class of genes, known as *TSGs*, which normally suppress neoplastic growth. One definition of TSGs is the gene that sustains *loss of function* mutations in the development of cancer. Like the oncogenes, TSGs normally constitute key points in many complex cellular pathways that regulate proliferation, differentiation, apoptosis, and responses to DNA damage (Table 8.5).

The first evidence for the existence of TSGs came from the somatic cell fusion experiments in 1969. Somatic cell hybrids of normal and malignant cells were found to be normal, suggesting the presence of genes that suppress the transformed growth. An understanding of the function of TSGs came from the studies of a rare, childhood, inherited tumor, retinoblastoma. On the basis of the statistical analysis of the frequencies and age with which inherited retinoblastoma and the sporadic disease are developed, a "two-hit model" was proposed by Alfred Knudson. This model envisages that two mutations are required for the development of retinoblastoma. The first mutation is inherited, whereas the second is an acquired somatic mutation. Therefore, the inactivation of both alleles of the TSGs is necessary for tumor formation, and this model is generally valid for other TSGs as well. For those with an inherited mutation of one allele of a TSG, the probability of acquiring a second mutation is very high (approximately 90%), compared with those without a defective TSG allele. As a consequence, people with an inherited mutated TSG allele are at great risk of developing cancer because the inactivation of a single normal allele is all that is needed to initiate the transformation process.

However, studies by Fearon and Vogelstein suggest that, although inactivation of the two alleles of a TSG is necessary, additional mutational events are required to result in complete neoplastic transformation. The precise number of mutations may depend on the tumor and the genes involved in it. Perhaps the best known sequence of molecular genetic alterations in carcinogenesis is elucidated in colorectal cancer, as illustrated in Figure 8.5. Mutations in a TSG called *adenomatous polyposis coli* (APC) represent one of the early steps in the neoplastic transformation followed by activation of oncogenes and loss of other TSGs. Such a sequence of mutations results in the progression from hyperplastic colonic mucosa to polyp to colonic carcinoma.

TSG mutations are also commonly found in sporadic cancer and function as gatekeepers and caretakers. This has

TABLE 8.5

Hereditary Malignancy Associated with Mutated Tumor Suppressor Genes

Syndrome	Gene	Locus	Types of Tumor
Familial retinoblastoma	RB1	13q14	Retinoblastoma, osteosarcoma
Li-Fraumeni syndrome	p53	17p13	Soft tissue sarcomas, breast cancer, adrenocortical cancer
Familial adenomatous polyposis	APC	5q21	Colorectal polyps and cancer
Familial Wilms tumour	WT1	11p13	Wilms tumor
von Hippel-Lindau disease	VHL	3p2s	Renal cell carcinomas, central nervous system hemangioblastoma, retinal angioma, pheochromocytoma
Gorlin syndrome	PATCHED	9q22	Basal cell carcinoma, medulloblastoma, ovarian fibroma
Cowden syndrome	PTEN/MMAC1	10q23	Breast cancer, hamartomas
Tuberous sclerosis type 1	TSC1	9q34	Renal angiomyolipomas, rhabdomyoma
Tuberous sclerosis type 2	TSC2	16p13	Renal angiomyolipomas, rhabdomyoma
Neurofibromatosis type 1	NF1	17q12	Neurofibroma, neural sarcoma
Neurofibromatosis type 2	NF2	22q12	Acoustic neuroma, meningioma, schwannoma, neural sarcoma
Familial breast cancer	BRCA1	17q21	Breast cancer, ovarian cancer
	BRCA2	13q12	Female/male breast cancer, pancreatic cancer, prostate cancer
Familial juvenile polyposis cell	SMAD4	18q21	Gastrointestinal hamartomatous polyps and cancer
Familial gastric cancer	E-cadherin	16q22	Gastric cancer
Familial melanoma	CDKN2	9p21	Melanoma, exocrine pancreatic carcinoma
Multiple endocrine neoplasia type 1	MEN1	11Q13	Parathyroid hyperplasia, enteropancreatic tumors, anterior pituitary tumors
Peutz-Jeghers syndrome	STK11	19p13	Gastrointestinal hamartomatous polyps and cancer

From Teh BT, Larsson, C, Nordenskjold M. Tumor suppressor genes (TSG), *Anticancer Res* 1999;19:4715–4728.

important clinical implications. The status of TSG mutations can be very valuable in diagnosis and prognosis. Mutations in some TSGs, such as *BRCA1* and *BRCA2*, which are associated with hereditary cancers, are however, seldom found in sporadic cancers. Therefore, the TSGs appear to form two broad categories, gatekeepers and caretakers. The gatekeepers are those genes whose inactivation would be rate limiting in the initiation of a tumor, and both maternal and paternal alleles must be inactivated/altered for tumor development. The Rb, p53, APC and other proteins represent the gatekeeper proteins. Gatekeeper proteins inhibit growth and promote cell death.

Inactivation of the second group of proteins that belong to the caretaker category results in the genomic instability, and indirectly promotes mutations in all genes including gatekeepers. Inheritance of mutated caretaker gene allele results in a slow progression of subsequent mutations

(remaining one caretaker allele, and the inactivation of two gatekeeper alleles). In sporadic cancers, however, two alleles of the caretaker gene, and two alleles of the gatekeeper gene would be required, and that possibility is not very high. As a result, mutations of the caretaker genes are not high in sporadic cancers (Table 8.5). Proteins that maintain the genomic stability such as BRCA1 and BRCA2 belong to this category. The ability to genotype women with familial breast and ovarian cancer for the *BRCA1* and *BRCA2* genes, has changed the clinical approach to such patients, with many appropriately counseled patients choosing prophylactic surgery when mutations are found.

Unlike the oncogenes, TSGs are generally inactivated during the tumorigenesis by a variety of mechanisms. For example, one of the alleles of TSGs in a tumor cell may be deleted, resulting in a loss of heterozygosity (LOH), which almost invariably involves the normal allele, leaving

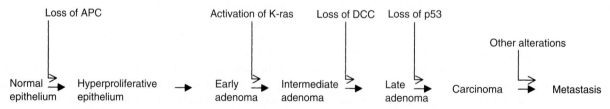

FIGURE 8.5   Genetic changes in the progression of colorectal cancer. APC, adenomatous polyposis coli; DCC, deleted in colorectal cancer. (Adapted from Alberts B. *Molecular biology of the cell*, 3rd ed. Garland Publishing, 1994:1289, with permission.)

the cell with a nonfunctional/dysfunctional gene. LOH can occur in several ways including chromosomal deletions and mutations, or methylation of their promoter sequences without chromosomal aberrations.

Because TSGs function in many interacting pathways, the loss of TSGs can have far reaching consequences. Inactivation of TSGs promotes cell proliferation and resistance to apoptosis. Because some proteins such as p53 and pRb are also involved in differentiation, loss of these proteins may impair the cell differentiation. In some tumors, the function of TSG may remain intact, but a key downstream effector of the TSG may be compromised, essentially achieving the same effect as the loss of TSG function. We will briefly consider the following TSGs.

Retinoblastoma Protein

pRb was the first tumor suppressor protein to be characterized, and served as a prototype for studying TSGs. Isolation of the retinoblastoma TSG (*RB*) was accomplished by RFLPs, linkage analysis, and molecular cloning. The *RB* gene was mapped to chromosome 13q14, and the 110 kDa pRb protein is coded by 4.7 kb DNA. Inactivation of *both RB alleles* is a distinctive feature of retinoblastoma (both inherited and sporadic). *RB* mutations have also been observed in small cell lung carcinoma, breast carcinoma, osteosarcoma, and glioblastomas.

The pRb is a critical regulatory protein of cell cycle control, apoptosis, and differentiation. Functionally, pRb is a nuclear protein that regulates the entry of cells into S-phase. The pRb undergoes cell cycle–dependent phosphorylations. In resting cells (G_0, or G_1), the protein is underphosphorylated. At this stage, pRb binds to E2F transcription factors and sequesters them thereby repressing transcription. The E2F transcription factors regulate the expression of several key proteins that are required during the S-phase, where DNA synthesis occurs. In late G_1 or at the restriction point (the stage at which the cell makes a commitment to undergo cell division), pRb is phosphorylated by CDKs. The phosphorylated pRb releases the transcription factor, which in turn, facilitates gene transcription and progression through the S-phase. pRb gets dephosphorylated at the end of the mitosis. Sequestration of E2F and regulation of cell cycle appear to be responsible for tumor suppression by pRb. Some of the transforming proteins produced by certain tumor viruses, such as simian virus 40 (SV40) T antigen and the product of adenoviral E1A, bind to pRb and impede its binding to E2F to generate free E2F which permits the progression of cell cycle. pRb binds to a large number of other cellular proteins as well, including the product of *mdm2* oncogene (discussed in the subsequent text) and c-Abl kinase (a protooncogene).

The p53 Protein

The p53 protein is perhaps the most frequently mutated protein in human cancers and often referred to as the *guardian angel of the genome* and the *ultimate tumor suppressor gene*. As the name implies, p53 is a 53 kDa protein with 393 amino acids that consists of several functional domains, which include transactivation domain, DNA binding domain, tetramerization domain, and a carboxy terminal regulatory domain. Through these domains, p53 interacts with a large number of proteins and regulates cell cycle, apoptosis, coordinates cellular responses to DNA damage repair, and other functions. Interestingly, p53 is not essential for normal growth and development, as shown from gene knockout experiments. However, the p53 null mice exhibit enhanced susceptibility to tumorigenesis.

Functionally, p53 is a nonspecific suppressor of transcription and a specific transcriptional activator. The tumor suppression by p53 is linked to its ability to regulate transcription. Because p53 regulates multiple pathways that affect cell fate, the pathway that gets stimulated, for example, cell cycle control or apoptosis, depends on the stimulus that activates p53. In general, p53 is a sensor of a variety of cellular stresses ranging from hypoxia to DNA damage by chemicals and radiation. Therefore, activation of p53 is very tightly controlled by several proteins, and the mechanisms of activation of p53 remain under intense scrutiny. The cellular levels of p53 are regulated at posttranscriptional level, and the protein is very rapidly turned over. Stress stimuli dramatically stabilize p53 and activate the protein; p53 also gets translocated to the nucleus. Inherited germ line mutations in p53 (the Li-Fraumeni syndrome) result in a variety of familial neoplasms including tumors of the breast, brain, adrenal, sarcoma, and leukemia.

A key protein that regulates p53 activity is Mdm2 protein. Mdm2 is transcriptionally induced by p53, and Mdm2 binds to p53 and targets for destruction by proteolysis. Under the conditions of stress, this autoinhibitory loop is broken by covalent modifications of p53 and Mdm2 that inhibits binding of Mdm2 to p53. The free p53 cannot be degraded and the protein is stabilized. The Mdm2 protein has been shown to possess transforming activity. Inactivation of *mdm2* by gene knockouts results in embryonic lethality due to deregulated activation of p53.

The p16 Protein

The p16 protein, which inhibits cell cycle progression by preventing the formation of an active cyclin D_1-Cdk4 complex, is also frequently deleted in melanoma and a subset of pancreatic cancers or silenced through methylation of its regulatory DNA in lung cancer. This gene has a role in familial melanoma.

E-Cadherin, β-Catenin and Adenomatous Polyposis Coli

E-cadherin is a structural protein involved in cell–cell adhesion, and is also referred to as *metastasis suppressor gene*. E-cadherin is a transmembrane protein involved in Ca^{2+}-dependent homophilic interactions to promote cell–cell adhesion. The cytoplasmic tail of E-cadherin binds to β-catenin, which binds to α-catenin. This complex is anchored to actin cytoskeleton through α-catenin, and strengthens cell–cell interactions and tissue architecture. Inactivation of E-cadherin, as in the case of tumors, results in poor cell–cell adhesion and contributes to metastasis. Similarly, inactivation of other components of the adhesion junctions also contributes to metastasis. Inactivating mutations of E-cadherin are found in gastric cancers, although transcriptional silencing of E-cadherin is reported in many different cancers—reduced expression of E-cadherin is considered to be associated with poor prognosis. Inherited E-cadherin mutations are related to a rare syndrome of familial gastric cancer.

β-catenin, in addition to its role in cell–cell adhesion, is also implicated in gene regulation as a transcription factor. Transcriptional targets of β-catenin include growth-promoting genes such as c-*myc*. Although β-catenin–mediated signaling is important during normal development in *wnt* signaling pathways, deregulation of these pathways leads to cellular transformation. It appears that β-catenin exists in several subcellular pools, including that found in association with E-cadherin and in cytoplasm as a soluble entity. The free cytoplasmic protein enters nucleus and upregulates transcription of mitogenic genes.

The tumor suppressor gene, APC, is involved in the regulation of the free pool of β-catenin. A multiprotein complex containing APC controls the levels of cytoplasmic β-catenin and targets β-catenin to proteolytic degradation. Inactivating mutations of APC, which impair the binding to β-catenin, raise intracellular β-catenin levels and stimulate cell proliferation resulting in colon cancer. The APC gene is implicated in familial colon cancers.

Tumor Viruses

The DNA tumor viruses may be grouped into six families: hepatitis B viruses, SV40 and polyoma viruses, papilloma viruses, adenoviruses, herpes viruses, and pox viruses. These viruses differ vastly in the size of their genomes ranging from 3 kb (hepatitis B viruses) to 200 kb (pox viruses). Viruses overtake the DNA replication machinery of the host cell to replicate viral genomes. On the one hand, this viral infection can result in host cell death. On the other hand, the virus can propagate its genome in parallel with the host genome. As previously stated, the virus can drive host cell proliferation that is independent of growth factors. Common gene products of the tumor viruses target tumor suppressor proteins p53 and Rb to drive the cell proliferation. For example, transforming proteins (known as *T antigens*) produced by SV40 and polyoma virus bind and inactivate p53 and Rb proteins. The human papilloma virus encodes two proteins, E6 and E7, which are routinely detected in cervical carcinomas. These proteins also degrade p53 and Rb proteins. Similarly, the adenoviral E1A oncoprotein interacts with Rb, and the E1B protein binds to p53 to promote transformed growth.

Programmed Cell Death

Tumor growth represents an imbalance between cell growth and death. To this point, we have discussed genetic mutations that drive cell growth. Genetic mutations not only drive cancer cells into rapid division, but they also can control or usurp programmed cell death or *apoptosis*. After receiving a death signal, normal cells propagate the death signal through the apoptotic cascade (Fig. 8.6). Cells undergoing apoptosis sustain profound changes, including the development of blebs on the cell membrane, volume contraction, nuclear condensation (pyknosis), and activation of an endonuclease that cleaves the DNA. Regulation of apoptosis continues to be defined. The *bcl-2* gene on chromosome 18 is characterized as a major repressor of programmed cell death at the mitochondria. Other genes, including *p53, Bax, myc,* and *abl,* have been shown to induce apoptosis. A variety of growth factors confer a death sparing effect on many normal and neoplastic cells *in vitro*. Because apoptosis is genetically controlled, defects in the control pathway or inappropriate production of apoptosis suppressing proteins will lead to situations where cells fail to die when they should and may well contribute to the induction of cancer. It is widely accepted that cancer cells that are resistant to conventional therapy overexpress antiapoptotic proteins such as bcl-2.

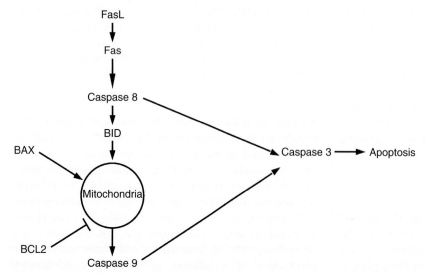

FIGURE 8.6 Apoptosis, or programmed cell death, is a complex process that occurs in many normal and altered cell populations. Apoptosis occurs through either an intrinsic pathway, in which activation of caspase 8 results in mitochondrial changes and ultimately cell death, or an extrinsic pathway in which the high production of caspase 8 leads directly to activation of caspase 3 and cell death.

Current efforts seek to either increase proapoptotic proteins such as Bax in cancer cells or inhibit the function of antiapoptotic proteins such as bcl-2. Because apoptosis mechanisms are better understood, many cancer types will be found to have defects in the molecular control of programmed cell death that can potentially be corrected.

Cell Immortalization

In the course of normal somatic replication, cells age in a process termed *replicative senescence*. This process is controlled by *telomeres*, which are the repetitive DNA sequences and associated proteins that cap the end of each chromosome. Telomeric DNA sequences are synthesized and maintained by the enzyme telomerase. During normal replication, telomeres become progressively shorter, resulting in chromosome instability and ultimately replicative senescence. In contradistinction to normal cells, the catalytic unit of telomerase is active in most malignant cells, therefore allowing them to constantly lengthen their telomeres, avoid replicative senescence, and divide without limit.

The role of telomerase in carcinogenesis is more complex than simple telomeric extension and subsequent immortalization. The role of telomerase in cancer cell propagation requires multiple mutations and the survival of these mutant cells is dependant on activation of the catalytic subunit of telomerase. This paradigm applies to many breast and colorectal cancers in which potentially catastrophic genetic mutations occur following the loss of p53. These cells reactivate telomerase to regain some genetic stability, continue to evolve and eventually metastasize. These findings have stimulated much discussion on the potential role of telomerase in the prevention, diagnosis, and management of cancer.

THE MOLECULAR BIOLOGY OF METASTASIS

Several avenues of research have demonstrated that the development of metastases is not the random event previously hypothesized, but is rather linked to genetic regulation. The process of metastasis is highly ordered, and consists of a series of sequential, interrelated steps. After the initial transformation and growth of cells, vascularization (angiogenesis) must occur if a tumor mass is to exceed 1 mm in diameter. The synthesis and secretion of several proangiogenic factors by tumor and host cells and the lack of antiangiogenic factors plays a key role in the initiation of a capillary network from the surrounding host tissues. Because of the enhanced expression of a series of enzymes (e.g., collagenase), tumor cells are able to invade target tissues. Once the invading cells penetrate the lymphatic or vascular channels, they may grow there or be transported (embolize) within the lymphatic and/or circulatory system. The tumor emboli must survive immune and other defenses as well as the turbulence of the circulation, before coming to rest in the capillary bed of receptive organs. After arriving in a recipient bed, cells must extravasate into the organ

parenchyma, and then proliferate, to form a micrometastasis. Growth of these microscopic lesions requires development of a vascular supply (angiogenesis) and evasion of host defenses. When the metastases grow, they, in turn, can shed tumor cells into the circulation, producing metastasis of metastases.

More than a century ago, Stephen Paget researched the mechanisms that regulate organ-specific metastasis. Paget questioned whether the organ distribution of metastases produced by human neoplasms was because of chance or an orderly process. He analyzed more than 700 autopsy records of women with breast cancer and found a nonrandom pattern of visceral (and bone) metastasis. This finding suggested that the process was not a random event, but that certain tumor cells (the seed) had a specific affinity for the milieu of certain organs (the soil). Metastases only resulted when the seed and soil were compatible.

Experimental data supporting the seed and soil hypothesis of Paget were derived from studies on the preferential invasion and growth of B16 melanoma metastases in specific organs. The successful metastatic cell must be viewed as a cell receptive to its environment. Signals, from endocrine or paracrine growth factors, could stimulate or inhibit tumor cell proliferation. For example, the implantation of human, colon carcinoma cells into the subcutaneous tissue (ectopic site) or the wall of the cecum (orthotopic site) results in locally growing tumors. However, metastasis to distant organs is produced only by tumors growing in the wall of the cecum. This key difference in production of distant metastasis directly correlates with the production of degradative enzymes by the tumor cells. These results suggest that factors in the cecal wall may stimulate the production of collagenases in colon cancer cells. In the subcutaneous tissue, a factor may be lacking, or potentially suppress production of the enzyme by the colon cancer cells.

Tumor growth, survival, and metastasis are dependent on an adequate supply of blood. The process of angiogenesis consists of multiple, sequential, and interdependent steps. It begins with the local degradation of the basement membrane surrounding capillaries. This is followed by invasion of the surrounding stroma by the underlying endothelial cells in the direction of the angiogenic stimulus. Endothelial cell migration is accompanied by the proliferation of endothelial cells at the leading edge of the migrating column. Endothelial cells then organize into three-dimensional structures to form new capillary tubes. The onset of angiogenesis involves a change in the local equilibrium between positive and negative regulatory molecules. The major proangiogenic factors include basic fibroblast growth factor (bFGF), vascular epithelial growth factor (VEGF), IL-8, and PDGF. In many normal tissues, factors that inhibit angiogenesis predominate.

The production of angiogenic molecules such as VEGF and bFGF is regulated by complex interactions with cells in the recipient tissue bed. The organ microenvironment also influences the expression of VEGF. Human gastric cancer cells were implanted into orthotopic (stomach) and ectopic (subcutaneous) organs of nude mice. Tumors in the stomach were highly vascularized, expressed high levels of VEGF, and grew more rapidly than the subcutaneous tumors. In addition, metastasis occurred only for the tumors implanted in the stomach. A similar finding was recently reported for a model of liposarcoma. This study by Dr. Judah Folkman's group found heterogenicity of the tumors in regard to angiogenic abilities, with rapidly proliferating cells at the periphery of lesions to be the most active. Substantial research on inhibiting angiogenesis is ongoing using agents such as angiostatin, thalidomide, and a variety of biologic response modifiers.

Although the problems of local control of malignancy are formidable, for most patients the outcome depends on metastasis. Clinical metastasis in turn depends on multiple interactions between metastatic cells and homeostatic mechanisms unique to some organ microenvironments. The microenvironment of the organ influences the biology of cancer growth, angiogenesis, and metastasis in several ways. Therefore, therapy of metastasis should be targeted not only against metastatic tumor cells, but also the homeostatic factors that are favorable to metastasis, growth, and survival of the metastatic cells. Therefore, while seeming to be a random event to physicians decades ago, metastasis does result from known, ordered processes.

SELECTED APPLICATIONS OF MOLECULAR BIOLOGY IN ONCOLOGY

Breast Cancer

Since the time of Halstead it has been known that tumor size and the presence of nodal metastasis are the most powerful prognostic indicators for cancer of the breast. However, evaluation of molecular parameters has led to the development of a "report card" of prognostic factors that may help decide which women will benefit the most from adjuvant therapies. It is now routine for breast tumor tissue to undergo analysis for estrogen and progesterone receptors, DNA content and S-phase fraction as well as HER2/*neu*. Each of these parameters has prognostic implications and expression of hormone receptors and HER2/*neu* suggest potential efficacy of hormonal or antioncoprotein therapies. Gene array panels are currently being utilized clinically to predict patients who will be better treated with hormone and chemotherapy, or hormonal therapy alone.

With the increased use of microarray technology, genetic profiles of breast cancers have been extensively evaluated. Clusters of coexpressed genes that have implications on clinical outcome have been identified through DNA microarray technology. Gene expression pattern analysis has broadly divided tumors into those that express genes characteristic of epithelial cells (i.e., estrogen receptor) and those that were negative for these genes. Further analysis has defined five breast cancer subtypes. The luminal epithelial-type tumors are subdivided into luminal subtype A, which expresses the highest levels of estrogen receptor cluster genes, and luminal subtype B, which showed low to moderate levels of

luminal/estrogen receptor cluster genes. In addition, a basal epithelial-type subtype of breast cancer has been shown to be completely negative for the luminal/ER cluster of genes. A fourth tumor subtype labeled ERB-B-2+ (HER2+) is characterized by high expression of genes that cluster with the HER2+/neu oncogene. A normal breast tissue–like group is defined by the highest expression of genes expressed in adipose and nonepithelial cell types. The specific expression patterns most likely reflect alterations in molecular pathways within the tumor cells. Interestingly, luminal type A cells rarely have mutations of the p53 TSG, whereas the other subtypes commonly have p53 mutations. Among genes highly expressed in tumors with wild-type p53, most of the genes are in the luminal/ER+ cluster.

The five breast cancer subtypes appear to identify clinically distinct groups of patients. Basal-like and ERBB2+ subtypes are associated with the shortest overall survival times. Interestingly, luminal subtype B tumors have poorer clinical outcomes than do luminal type A breast cancers although both of these subtypes have better outcomes than the basal-like and ERBB2+ subtypes.

The isolation of the breast cancer susceptibility genes *BRCA1* and *BRCA2* has added a new dimension to the health care of women. Together, these two genes account for approximately 80% of familial breast cancer. However, *BRCA2* causes a familial susceptibility to breast cancer but does not increase the risk of ovarian cancer as much as *BRCA1*. Currently, the detection of *BRCA1* and *2* has strong implications for counseling in high-risk women and is widely available. The BRCA genotyping is performed on a peripheral blood sample. More than 250 mutations in these two genes have been described, and most analyses sequence the entirety of the genes. Consultation with genetic counselors is frequently beneficial and thoughtful consideration of what will be done with a positive result is mandatory before obtaining the test. Because women who test negative for mutations remain at risk for breast cancer (although significantly less so than *BRCA1–2* carriers) they continue to require regular screening. Further, even bilateral mastectomy does not completely eliminate breast cancer risk. Therefore, careful counseling of women before and after genetic testing is mandatory.

Gastric Cancer

Mutation of p53 appears to play an early role in the development of intestinal types of gastric cancer. Recent studies have shown a mutation frequency of 41% in intestinal-type tumors, compared with 4% in diffuse types. Some authors believe that p53 is an early initiating event in gastric carcinogenesis. It appears that full expression of malignancy requires the mutation of other additional oncogene proteins, such as E-cadherin. Germ line mutations resulting in familial gastric cancer have been described. This is similar to the mechanism proposed for colon cancer and may represent a common pathway for the development of several epithelial malignancies.

Recent investigations of allelic losses lend some credence to this perspective. In some geographic areas, patients with familial adenomatous polyposis are at a significantly higher risk for developing gastric cancer. In one investigation, deletions occurred in one third of gastric cancers at the mutated colon cancer (MCC) and APC only in association with p53 mutations. The downstream accumulation of other oncogene products may also determine not only the degree of differentiation, but also impact on survival. Similar to breast cancer, expression of HER2/*neu* is associated with shortened survival in well-differentiated resected gastric cancers. Further elucidation of these findings may not only define therapeutic targets, but also provide a clearer understanding of gastrointestinal carcinogenesis.

Colorectal Cancer

The evaluation of clinically useful molecular prognostic factors for gastrointestinal tumors is not as well described as breast cancer. However, evaluation of mitotic index and ploidy status may provide additional prognostic power and guide decision making in the care of colorectal cancers. Patients with aneuploid tumors or with elevated S-phase have generally had a poorer prognosis.

Whereas *ras* oncogene mutations are common occurrences in diverse malignancies, overexpression of *ras* has been demonstrated in up to 60% of colon carcinomas, 40% of colonic dysplastic polyps, and 10% of adenomas. The degree of expression of *ras* has also been shown to correlate with the depth of bowel wall invasion. The *myc* oncogene is also overexpressed in colon cancer and is associated with deletion on the q arm of chromosome 5. *In vitro* activation of *ras* and *myc* often confers resistance to chemotherapeutics in standard assays. Errors in otherwise normal repetitive sequences of DNA (termed *microsatellites*) have been shown to be involved in the pathogenesis of genetic damage. Mutation of the microsatellite HRSAI has been shown to be significantly associated with colorectal carcinomas. Of interest is that HRSAI is juxtaposed closely to H-*ras,* suggesting that new mutations in HRSAI may disrupt the expression of proximity protooncogenes. This may explain the importance of *ras* in human colorectal carcinogens and underscore the importance of studies attempting to block the expression of *ras* with monoclonal antibodies. Further, microsatellite instability has been related to colorectal cancers, particularly in young patients.

Colorectal cancer has been shown to be the result of a clonal progression of hyperproliferation to polyps to carcinoma. This is most likely caused by the accumulation of mutated oncogenes rather than their actual order of appearance, although this certainly must have some significance as well. Allelic clones of specific tumor suppression genes are now known to occur. The multistep process of the development of colorectal cancer has been championed by the Vogelstein laboratory as shown in Figure 8.5.

This deletion on 18q is also a tumor-suppression gene designated DCC or deleted in colon cancer. DCC serves as a cell adherence molecule, and loss of cellular adhesion is a key step in the development of carcinogenesis. DCC is believed to underlie the development of Lynch syndrome II, which is an autosomal disorder. Reintroduction of cell surface adhesion molecules *in vitro* reduces the growth rate and tumorigenicity of colon cancer cells. Finally, the gene for familial APC has been mapped to 5q. Perturbation of APC not only results in familial adenomatosis polyposis (FAP) and frequent progression to colon carcinoma, but is also present in up to 60% of sporadic colon cancers and adenomas. Further loss of p53 abrogates tumor suppression and loss of regulatory control, which results in carcinoma. More recent epidemiologic studies have found that the DNA mismatch repair genes are also intimately involved in hereditary colorectal carcinoma. Commercial laboratories currently offer genetic testing for APC and DNA mismatch repair genes. Germ line mutations account for much of the familial colorectal cancer syndromes.

Multiple Endocrine Neoplasia

RFLP analysis was initially used to identify families at risk for familial medullary carcinoma of the thyroid and the MEN-2a syndrome. Determination of this mutation allowed for early intervention if evaluations for medullary thyroid carcinoma or pheochromocytoma were positive. The development and refinement of PCR has provided accurate and reproducible survival for MEN-2a kindreds. Detection of mutations in the RET protooncogene now predicts inheritance of MEN-2a. Noncarriers require no further evaluation, whereas carriers positive for RET undergo total thyroidectomy regardless of plasma calcitonin levels. Prophylactic thyroidectomy in children known to have RET mutations has frequently found C-cell hyperplasia, or medullary cancer during the first decade of life.

BIOLOGIC THERAPY FOR CANCER

Tumor Immunotherapy

Tumor immunology is the study of the antigenic properties of tumor cells, the host immune response to tumor cells, and the interaction between neoplastic cells and the host immune system. Despite a history exceeding 100 years, the science of immunology has only recently reached a point at which immunologic approaches to cancer diagnosis and treatment are feasible. Early attempts to study the immune response in both patients and animals showed the rejection of transplanted normal and tumor tissues in an unpredictable manner. This work led to the discovery of the major histocompatibility complex (MHC) and the development of multiple inbred mouse strains that have subsequently provided the foundation for many tumor immunology studies. The nature of immunoglobulins and immunoglobulin production was derived primarily from observations on multiple myeloma and other B-lymphocyte neoplasms.

Tumor Antigens

Tumor antigens are usually described as either unique or as tumor associated. Unique tumor antigens can be detected only on tumor cells and not on other cells of the host. These antigens appear to be highly specific and may be limited to a single tumor, or may be shared by certain other tumor cells. Tumor-associated antigens may be expressed on some normal cells but are expressed at their highest level on tumor cells. Some of these antigens are highly immunogenic, and their presence may induce an immune response, whereas others produce little or no immune response.

The recognition of specific unique tumor antigens is important for targeting the immune response to tumor cells. Unfortunately, few truly tumor-specific antigens or antibodies are currently available for diagnostic or clinical studies. Human tumors induced by specific viruses tend to share specific antigens. This finding has contributed to research to develop vaccines specific for the treatment/prevention of cancer. This approach has promise, but, despite decades of research, has had little clinical success to date.

Unlike tumor-specific antigens, tumor-associated antigens are found more frequently in patients with cancer. Table 8.6 lists some of the current clinically important tumor-associated antigens. The best-known tumor-associated antigens are the oncofetal antigens. These are generally not found in the adult or, if present, are at low levels. They are expressed at high levels *in utero*, where their functions are generally unknown. The best characterized of the oncofetal antigens are carcinoembryonic antigen (CEA) and α fetoprotein (AFP). CEA is found in the developing human colon but is not found in significant levels in the normal adult. It was first described in association with carcinomas of the colon, but has subsequently been found in most gastrointestinal carcinomas, lung, ovarian, and breast cancer. An elevated CEA before surgery indicates its value as a tumor marker. In such patients, a rising serum level of CEA after definitive surgery is a predictor of persistence or recurrence. Radiolabeled anti-CEA antibodies have been shown to be useful as a nuclear

medicine imaging agent as well as utility as a targeting probe used with an intraoperative gamma detector to find occult recurrences of CEA producing tumors in an experimental procedure known as *radioimmunoguided surgery*.

AFP is found in the developing fetus in the liver and yolk sac cells and is not found in normal adults. Certain patients with hepatocellular carcinoma and germinal tumors, such as nonseminomatous testicular carcinomas, will produce AFP; it can be used as a serologic marker of disease status and a predictor of recurrence. Other tumor-associated antigens include CA 125, neuron-specific enolase, prostate-specific antigen, CA 19-9, CA 27-29, chromogranin A, and CA 15-3. The utility of such tumor markers depends on the tumor type. However, the utility of tumor markers in breast cancer is quite limited. The utility of tumor markers for other sites of disease depends on the tumor and available therapy. Following a tumor marker when there is no further meaningful therapy is not of value.

Despite the large number of tumor antigens that have been characterized, none has proved to be a universal tumor marker. However, certain antibodies to tumor-associated antigens have been produced which are useful in the diagnosis of cancer and the monitoring of patients with cancer. Monoclonal antibody technology has provided a continually increasing array of important diagnostic antibodies. For the pathologist, monoclonal antibodies to a wide variety of antigens are useful to establish the cell lineage of some undifferentiated tumors and form the core of "special stains" used to characterize tumors.

Evidence for an Immune Response Against Tumors

Burnett hypothesized that a major role of the immune system was surveillance for the development of neoplastic cells which, when recognized, would be destroyed. This school of thought suggests that clinically apparent malignancy represents a failure of immunosurveillance. There is some evidence for a correlation between cancer occurrence and host immune deficiencies. For example, the frequency

TABLE 8.6

Tumor Antigens that Serve as Diagnostic Markers

Type	Antigen	Tumor
Oncofetal and lung carcinomas	α-Fetoprotein (AFP)	Hepatocellular and testicular carcinomas
	Carcinoembryonic antigen (CEA)	Colorectal, pancreas, gastric, breast, ovarian
Organ specific	Prostate-specific antigen (PSA)	Prostate carcinoma
	Tyrosinase	Melanoma
Proliferation antigen	Tissue polypeptide antigen (TPA)	Breast and gynecologic tumors
Thyroglobulin		Thyroid cancer
Oncogene product	HER2/*neu*	Breast, ovary, thyroid, lung carcinoma
Monoclonal antibody defined	CA 15-3	Breast carcinoma
	CA 19-9	Colorectal, gastric, pancreas carcinoma
	CA50	Colorectal, gastric, pancreas carcinoma
	CA125	Ovarian cancer

of malignant disease in patients with primary immunod-eficiency disorders and HIV disease have a frequency of malignant disease up to 1,000 times greater than the general population. This increased risk has also been found with HIV disease and in those receiving immunosuppressive treatment after organ transplantation. In these later groups the risk is greater than 100 times the general population and most of the tumors involve the lymphatics and skin. These data strongly support the preventative role of the immune system in tumor development.

Further evidence for immune system–tumor interaction comes from data on the spontaneous regression of both primary and metastatic tumors. A number of reports have shown regression of metastatic choriocarcinoma after removal of the primary tumor. This regression appears to be on an immunologic basis. Malignant melanoma is perhaps the most common tumor in which spontaneous regression has been noted (1 in 10,000 cases). Frequently, primary melanoma will have significantly large areas infiltrated with lymphocytes and may even undergo complete regression. In 3% to 5% of melanoma cases, the cutaneous primary is never found despite proven nodal metastasis. It is presumed that such "unknown primary" cutaneous melanomas have had the primary lesion destroyed on an immunologic basis.

Tumor infiltration with lymphocytes, when defined by strict criteria, may be associated with an improved prognosis compared with tumors that have no evidence of reactivity. This has been suggested in the case of melanoma, breast cancer, and several other tumor types. However, the prognostic value of this finding has not been uniformly found. Several studies have demonstrated the finding of circulating antibody reactive with autologous tumor, positive delayed hypersensitivity skin testing to tumor antigens and tumor cell extracts, and *in vitro* cell-mediated immunity against autologous tumor cells. These observations of tumor-specific immunity have formed the basis for many tumor immunotherapy protocols. Despite the observations that patients with cancer can develop humoral and cell-mediated immune responses to their tumors, there is no consensus that these responses play a significant role in the usual cancer patient. However, modulation of the immune response against tumors is an important potential treatment modality.

Mechanisms by Which the Immune System Kills Tumor Cells

Our understanding of the complexity of the immune response to tumors increases as newer studies reveal more details of this intriguing interaction. Tumor cells can be killed *in vitro* by antibody-mediated mechanisms, such as complement-mediated antibody cytotoxicity and antibody-dependent cell-mediated cytotoxicity. These methods of tumor killing are highly effective but are primarily limited to the plasma volume compartment. Cell-mediated cytotoxicity plays a more important role *in vivo*.

There are four different types of immune system cells that can kill tumor cells *in vitro* or *in vivo*: cytolytic T lymphocytes (CTLs), natural killer (NK) cells, lymphokine activated killer (LAK) cells, and activated macrophages. The ability of CTLs to kill tumor cells has strict limitations. The CTLs must be presensitized to the specific tumor antigen and only when the target antigen is present on cells that also carry MHC class I antigens. When these criteria are met, the CTL can interact with the tumor cell and produce lysis. Tumor killing can also take place by the induction of apoptosis (programmed cell death) that will be described later.

In humans, there is a group of large, granular lymphocytes that comprise 2% to 5% of peripheral blood lymphocytes. Within this subset are NK and LAK cells. The biologic role of NK cells has not been completely defined. NK cells appear to develop from progenitors under the influence of γ-interferon, and IL-2. *In vitro* studies of NK cells show a general lack of reactivity against normal cells and a varying but generally positive ability to kill a wide variety of tumor cells, even from diverse species. In contrast with CTLs, NK cells have a broad specificity and do not require the presence of class I MHC antigens on their target cells.

LAK cells are produced *in vitro* by incubating peripheral blood leukocytes with IL-2 in an incubator for at least 5 days. Such LAK cells can be grown from tumor infiltrating lymphocytes (TIL) cells that may be obtained from fresh tumor. The amounts of IL-2 used in the incubation far exceed biologic levels. The progenitors of LAK cells appear to be predominantly NK cells. LAK cells show a broader specificity than NK cells against a variety of freshly isolated solid tumors, which often lack NK reactivity. LAK cells also react with many cells in cultures with which NK cells react, generally at higher levels. LAK cells also lack cytotoxicity against normal cells. It is doubtful whether LAK cells as defined *in vitro* exist naturally *in vivo*. Such exogenously generated LAK/TIL cells have been evaluated for immunotherapy with some responses, but this technique remains a research modality at present.

Macrophages at rest have little cytotoxic ability, but, when activated, undergo biochemical and functional changes that permit them to kill and engulf bacteria, transformed cells, and other foreign material. Macrophages that have been activated can kill tumor cells in a manner that is neither antigen depen-dent nor MHC restricted. Macrophages can be activated by a number of agents, including lymphokines, antigen–antibody complexes, aggregated IgG, and endotoxin. Macrophages also appear to mediate a number of negative or inhibitory effects on various immune functions.

In addition to producing tumor cell death by cytotoxicity, apoptosis can be induced by a variety of immunologic mechanisms. Apoptosis is a genetic program of cellular self-destruction that involves many cells both within the immune system and at other sites to assure that cells die when they should. Cell death by apoptosis and cell proliferation maintains the homeostasis of cell numbers in normal tissues. In the thymus, the mechanism of removing autoreactive thymocytes is the induction of apoptosis triggered by the CD3/T-cell receptor complex. Both antibody-mediated and lymphocyte-mediated cell killing in many systems involves apoptosis in addition to direct porphyrin mediated killing.

Evasion of Immune Destruction by Tumor Cells

Despite the elaborate construction of the immune system with multiple components capable of killing tumor cells, transformed cells may escape destruction and go on to divide and eventually overcome the host. A number of factors have been observed in tumors that facilitate their eluding the immune system.

Sneaking through is a term that characterizes an ability some tumors have to elude the immune system by being poorly antigenic or reside in an area that does not have ready access to immune cells. Therefore, the host does not become sensitized to the tumor and allows the tumor to grow and escape detection. Even if the tumor later becomes more immunogenic, it may elude the immune system by virtue of its location and its size.

Induction of tolerance is the acquisition of nonreactivity toward particular antigens. Immunologic tolerance to foreign antigens is an extremely complex phenomenon and remains to be fully delineated. Tolerance may be complete or partial and may involve various components of the immune system. Multiple factors are contributory, and a single mechanism accounting for the generation and maintenance of the tolerance state has not been discovered. Tolerance may be induced by exposure of the antigen in embryonic life. High doses of antigen and particularly persistence of antigen in adult life leads to specific tolerance.

The immune system may be suppressed by *antigen overload*. A variety of tumors produce antigens that are shed from their cell surfaces. The circulating antigen produces a snowstorm effect in that it can bind to receptors on effector cells and prevent their interaction with tumor cells, as well as combining with circulating antibody to form antigen–antibody immune complexes. Some antibodies that bind to tumors are not cytolytic and actually prevent the attachment of the important cytolytic antibodies. These blocking antibodies have been shown in a variety of tumor models to actually enhance the growth of tumors by shielding them from the immune system.

Many tumors, particularly the more virulent types, have sufficient genetic diversity as a result of a high mutation rate that they may escape attack by the immune system. This phenomenon is called *antigenic modulation*. Nonreactive clones of tumor cells grow to replace those destroyed by the immune system, in effect constantly changing the surface antigens depending upon the immune reaction to them.

Some tumors possess the ability to produce host immunosuppression by inhibiting immune function through *specific tumor cell immunosuppression mechanisms*. This includes cytokine secretion, such as transforming growth factor-2, which inhibits CTL and NK cell activity, prostaglandin E_2 production, which inhibits macrophages, and multiple other mechanisms. In addition, the growing tumor may produce host metabolic effects, anorexia/cachexia, and immunosuppression on a nutritional basis.

Alteration of MHC antigens is another mechanism of immune system avoidance. Some tumors lack MHC antigens and cannot be killed by CTLs. Other tumors anomalously express MHC antigens, which again prevent their interaction with CTLs. MHC class I and class II induction is enhanced by certain factors used in immunotherapy, including interferons, IL-2, and tumor necrosis factor (TNF), and may serve to enhance CTL activity against tumors.

Clinical Immunotherapy

Immunotherapy is the term used for attempts to alter or enhance the immune system in an effort to bring about an immunologically mediated antitumor effect. Clinical immunotherapy for malignancy is divided into two major categories. *Active immunotherapy* consists of treatments that are designed to stimulate the immune system of the patient, either specifically against certain tumor antigens or nonspecifically with agents that tend to boost the overall immune response. *Passive immunotherapy*, often called *adoptive immunotherapy*, refers to the administration of immunologically active components (specific antibodies, activated cells, etc.), without any requirement for an immune response by the host.

In animal systems, active immunotherapy in the form of immunization with killed tumor cells or purified tumor antigens before tumor challenge has a significant therapeutic effect. However, immunization of patients with established metastatic tumors generally has been ineffective in causing tumor regression. This failure of translation from the animal model to humans can be attributable to the fact that most human cancer antigens are normal, nonmutated differentiation molecules or nonmutated proteins that are well tolerated by the immune system. This failure could also be due to the escape mechanisms of tumors. Although cytotoxic T lymphocytes generated by peptide immunization are long lasting, they are typically unable to home to and infiltrate tumor tissues. Moreover, tumors frequently lose antigen expression in the course of tumor proliferation.

An alternative approach to active immunotherapy is the use of passive immunotherapy through cell transfer techniques. This approach is particularly attractive because large numbers of selected cells can be delivered to the host. Furthermore, the recipient can undergo lymphodepletion before cell transfer. This allows for the elimination of host regulatory lymphocytes, thereby providing an optimal transfer environment. Recent studies have demonstrated promising results of this treatment modality for patients with metastatic malignant melanoma.

Cytokines, particularly IL-2 and interferon-α, have been utilized to stimulate the immune system. IL-2 is generated by activated helper/inducer T cells. It plays an essential role in promoting T-cell division and also potentiates B-cell growth and the activation of monocytes and natural killer cells. IL-2 treatment has significant toxicity, with patients having a syndrome resembling septic shock. It should currently be done only in an institution specializing in this form of treatment. The most significant responses to this form of treatment have been in patients with metastatic renal cell carcinoma and melanoma.

In recent years, clinical studies with IL-2 have shown more limited antitumor activity than was anticipated from earlier preclinical trials. IL-2 is approved by the U.S. Food and Drug Administration (FDA) for good performance status patients with metastatic melanoma and renal cell carcinoma. The overall response rate with melanoma and renal cell carcinoma is approximately 15%; however, a *complete tumor regression* is seen in 6% and 4%. A large number of trials have attempted to increase the efficacy and decrease the toxicity of IL-2 treatment by patient selection, modification of the dose and schedule, and the addition of other agents such as antitumor vaccines.

In patients with metastatic melanoma and renal cell carcinoma, the response rates with IL-2 treatment are not significantly higher than chemotherapy. However, the responses were durable, lasting considerably longer than would have been expected from responders to chemotherapy. Currently, the highest response rates reported in the treatment for metastatic melanoma are for regimens combining chemotherapy [usually cisplatin plus decarbazine (DTIC)-based regimens] with IL-2 alone or IL-2 plus interferon-α. Although some responses are durable, most responses last between 5 and 7 months and the toxicity of this regimen is formidable. IL-2 is clearly an active agent for cancer treatment, particularly for melanoma and renal cell carcinoma.

The interferons are a class of glycoproteins that have antiviral and immunomodulatory effects. There are three main types—α, β, and γ—each with multiple subtypes. The antitumor effects of the interferons include increased expression of class I and class II MHC proteins, which facilitate immune system recognition; activation of NK cells and macrophages and stimulation of B Lymphocytes; and direct inhibition of viral replication. Interferons α and β seem to exert antitumor activity principally by inhibition of cell growth and division. Interferons are produced by several cell types, particularly T cells and macrophages. γ-interferon is currently approved for use in the treatment of hairy cell leukemia. Interferon-α has activity against metastatic melanoma with response rates of 10% to 20% in metastatic disease. However, high-dose interferon has not consistently shown survival advantages as adjuvant therapy for resected node positive melanoma.

TNF is a third major class of cytokines that have antitumor activity. TNF is produced primarily by T lymphocytes and macrophages secondary to a variety of stimuli, including IL-1, γ interferon, lipopolysaccharide, viruses, and BCG. In animals receiving intravenous bacterial endotoxin and in patients in septic shock, large quantities of TNF (cachectin) are produced. TNF can induce hemorrhagic necrosis of malignant tumors. Human recombinant TNF has been tested on a variety of tumor cells and has been shown to have a cytolytic effect on approximately one third, a cytostatic effect on one third, and no effect on one third. The factors that make certain tumor cells susceptible to TNF, and the precise

mechanism of this effect, are not known. Unfortunately, TNF produces a profound cachexia and weight loss that severely limits its clinical applications. One way to avoid the substantial systemic toxicity of TNF is to use it as an adjunct to isolated limb perfusions. Because the limb is perfused beyond a tourniquet, systemic toxicity is avoided and trials have suggested that the addition of TNF to such a perfusion circuit has increased response rate.

Monoclonal Antibodies

After decades of research, therapy with monoclonal antibodies has finally reached oncology clinics. Cytotoxic monoclonal antibodies can be used directly to kill tumor cells, or high-affinity antibodies may be used to carry a variety of toxins, drugs, and radioisotopes to produce tumor imaging and killing. This methodology has been limited by the use of xenogeneic antibodies (primarily mouse and rat), which quickly induce an antibody immune reaction (through human antimouse antibodies or HAMA) and also are rapidly consumed by the reticuloendothelial system and concentrated in the spleen and liver. A successful approach is to "humanize" the murine antibodies by cleaving off antigenic portions of the Fc portion of the antibody. One such antibody to CD20 (rituxan) is currently used to treat B-cell lymphoma. At present, a number of monoclonal antibodies are used to treat a variety of malignancies (Table 8.7).

The *HER2 gene* encodes a 185-kDa transmembrane glycoprotein with tyrosine kinase activity that is a member of the EGFR family. HER2 overexpression has been found to contribute to oncogenic transformation, tumorigenesis, and metastatic potential. HER2 overexpression in women with breast and ovarian cancer is a negative prognostic factor, as several studies have found a correlation between HER2 overexpression and shorter disease-free and overall survival. This oncogene is overexpressed in 25% to 30% of human breast and ovarian cancers. The HER2 oncoprotein is an important antitumor target. The humanized anti-HER2 monoclonal antibody trastuzumab (Herceptin; Genentech, San Francisco, CA) has demonstrated activity in clinical trials in women with metastatic breast cancer overexpressing the gene. Response rate to the antibody given as a single agent have ranged from 12% to 27%. Clinical trials evaluating combination trastuzumab (Herceptin) and chemotherapy have resulted in higher response rates, significantly longer time to progression, and longer median overall survival compared with patients who had received chemotherapy alone. The addition of trastuzumab to adjuvant chemotherapy for the HER2 overexpressing breast cancer patient has cut the risk of recurrence approximately 50% when compared with chemotherapy alone.

EGFR, which is overexpressed in a variety of solid tumors, causes cell growth when stimulated by its ligand. Cetuximab (Erbitux; ImClone Systems Incorporated, New York, NY), and panitumumab (Amgen, Thousand Oaks, CA) are antibodies against the EGFR. These antibodies are both FDA approved and decrease receptor phosphorylation and ultimately result in cell growth inhibition. The addition

TABLE 8.7

Monoclonal Antibodies Approved by the U.S. Food and Drug Administration

Targeted Therapy	Type of Therapy	Cancer type	Approval Date
Bevacizumab (Avastin)	Monoclonal antibody, angiogenesis inhibitor	Colorectal cancer	2/26/04
Cetuximab (Erbitux)	Monoclonal antibody, EGFR inhibitor	Colorectal cancer	2/12/04
Ibritumomab (Zevalin)	Radiolabeled monoclonal antibody	NHL	2/19/02
Rituximab (Rituxan)	Monoclonal antibody	NHL	11/26/97
Panitumumab	Monoclonal antibody	Colorectal cancer	2006
Tositumomab (Bexxar)	Radiolabeled monoclonal antibody	Follicular lymphoma	6/27/03
Trastuzumab (Herceptin)	Monoclonal antibody	Breast cancer	9/25/98

EGFR, epidermal growth factor receptor; NHL, non-Hodgkin lymphoma.

of cetuximab or panitumumab to conventional therapy in colorectal cancer results in significantly improved clinical results relative to chemotherapy alone. Current trials are evaluating both agents with chemotherapy or each other. These data provide promise for the use of EGFR MABs in the treatment of metastatic colorectal cancer. Enzymatic inhibitors or EGFR erlotinib (Tarceva) and gefitinib (Iressa) have both been FDA approved. These agents have activity against lung cancer. Erlotinib has promise against pancreatic cancer as well.

Targeted agents against EGFR have become important agents recently. It is noteworthy that assays of EGFR have not reliably predated responses to therapy to date.

VEGF is a protein released by many tumors to stimulate proliferation of new blood agents. Bevacizumab (Avastin; Genentech, San Francisco, CA) is a monoclonal antibody that targets and blocks the VEGF receptor. Clinical trials comparing clinical outcomes of patients with metastatic colorectal cancer receiving standard chemotherapy with bevacizumab show a median survival of 20.3 months. This represents a substantial improvement for patients with metastatic colorectal cancer. Current trials are evaluating the potential of multiple targeted agents and the use of VEGF blockade in a variety of tumor systems.

THE EPIDEMIOLOGY OF CANCER

Cancer epidemiology is the study of the determinants of neoplastic disease and the frequency with which various types of cancers affect differing population groups. The primary thrust of epidemiologic investigation has been to identify specific cancer determinants in the hope that by eliminating them from the population at risk, subsequent tumor development may be prevented.

Epidemiologic observations related to cancer date back to 1700, when Ramazzini determined that breast cancer was more common among nuns than the general population, suggesting that celibacy was a risk factor. Paradoxically, in 1842, another Italian, Rigoni-Stern, concluded that endometrial cancer was significantly less common in convents than the general population, concluding in this case that celibacy played a protective role. In 1775, the British surgeon Pott surmised that scrotal cancer was an occupational hazard to chimney sweeps. Because of observations made by subsequent investigators, it was concluded that the combustion products of coal were a factor not only in the development of cancer of the scrotum but of all exposed skin. Hill made the first report suggesting a connection between tobacco use and the development of cancer in 1761 when he implicated the use of snuff as an etiology for the development of nasopharyngeal cancers. Von Soemmering, who in 1795 associated pipe smoking with carcinoma of the buccal mucosa, subsequently reaffirmed the role of tobacco as a carcinogen.

These early epidemiologic reports in large part depended on anecdotal observations by astute physicians who were dealing with groups of individuals with similar cultural or occupational backgrounds. As a result, quantitative data to support these reports were usually lacking. Until the development of the epidemiologic study incriminating tobacco as one of the precipitating agents in the development of lung neoplasms, cancer was commonly perceived as simply a manifestation of the degenerative processes associated with aging. These epidemiologic studies have been an impetus for not only the initiation of laboratory work to further define the causative agents involved in neoplastic development, but also for the designing of experimental studies in which the suspected cancer-producing agent is either introduced or eliminated from a population group. These experimental studies provide the most compelling evidence for implicating a particular determinant as a carcinogen. These experiments, however, are time consuming, expensive, and usually only justified after a causal relation has been established between a disease determinant and a population group by descriptive studies.

The wide fluctuations seen in the incidence of some cancers over time underscores the importance of this factor in the etiology of cancer. For example, in 1930, gastric cancer was the leading cause of cancer death among men in the United States. However, by 1985, although still a disease of significant impact, it had lost its dominant position. During the same period, the mortality rate for lung cancer in U.S. men had increased by a factor of 10, from sixth most common cause of cancer death to leading cause. This dramatic increase in the incidence of lung cancer is tied closely to the increased use of tobacco over the same time period. The incidence of pulmonary neoplasms among women has lagged behind their male counterparts. However, because of increased use of tobacco, lung cancer has surpassed breast cancer as the leading cause of cancer mortality among U.S. women.

The variable of place is defined by geographic or political boundaries. This factor has served to identify major international differences in both cancer incidence and mortality. The extreme international variation in the incidence of gastric cancer is an excellent example of the importance of this factor. The highest incidence rates for stomach neoplasms are found among Japanese men (90 per 100,000 per year). Latin American countries are intermediate at 45 to 50 per 100,000 per year, whereas rates for gastric cancer in the United States are among the lowest in the world (approximately 10 per 100,000 per year).

The study of migration patterns of population groups offers a unique epidemiologic opportunity to observe the roles genetic and environmental factors play in cancer development. In 1972, a study of Japanese natives who had immigrated to Hawaii demonstrated a continued excess risk for stomach cancer in their new homeland, but this risk factor was not passed on to their progeny born in Hawaii. However, although gastric cancer risk fell, the Japanese immigrants demonstrated an increased incidence of colorectal neoplasms similar to Native Americans. Because of the size and specificity of this population group, it was possible to make several observations: (i) the investigators noted that more bowel cancer patients than controls had abandoned the practice of eating at least one Japanese-style meal daily, and (ii) they also concluded that the frequency of beef ingestion correlates with an increased risk for the development of colorectal cancer.

In general, the incidence of cancer increases with age. Breast cancer demonstrates a steady increase in incidence with age, which plateaus in the sixth decade of life and is subsequently followed by a continued increase in frequency. This may be a result of cessation of estrogen production by the ovaries. Another exception to the general increase in frequency of cancers with age is the peak in incidence of Hodgkin disease in the third decade of life. There may be at least a subgroup of these patients who have an infectious etiology for their cancer.

The difference in the incidence of site-specific cancers between the sexes is certainly multifactorial. The preponderance of certain male cancers for a specific anatomic location may be attributed to exposure to carcinogenic factors within the workplace. Not all differences in sex-related incidence is related to the hormonal milieu. Additionally, commonly utilized medical therapy may be related to incidence of malignancy. Data suggesting that postmenopausal hormone replacement therapy increased the risk of breast cancer thereby led to a sharp decline in the use of such estrogen replacement near the turn of the century. This was shown by the end of 2006 to be related to an unprecedented fall in the rate of breast cancer.

Although environmental factors play a prominent role in cancer genesis, familial clustering suggests that genetic variations do expose the individual to increased susceptibility to specific types of cancer. However, a certain component of the risk that has been attributed to genetics may be the result of common environmental factors.

The Surveillance Epidemiology and End Results (SEER) Modality Data Program was started in 1973 and is a part of the National Cancer Institute. Early in its history, the SEER Program found variation in the incidence rates of cancers for different ethnic groups in the United States. Although the initial inclination is to implicate genetic factors to explain these differences, it is difficult to separate out the influences of environmental and cultural considerations as explanations for these trends. The latest SEER data is available at their website (*www-seer.cancer.gov*). The SEER database is a powerful tool for evaluation of trends and patient outcomes.

Descriptive Studies

The neoplastic process manifests itself in all human groups. Age, sex, race, geography, cultural norms, and sexual habits are but a few of the factors influencing the incidence of cancer. By defining the patterns of disease in population subgroups, descriptive epidemiology has provided insight into the etiology of many cancers. Descriptive epidemiologic studies measure three parameters—incidence, prevalence, and mortality.

Incidence describes the number of new cases of cancer occurring within a population group in a specified period of time. The unit of time is commonly defined as 1 year, and the rate usually is expressed per 100,000 individuals. The measurement of incidence may be crude (applying to all age groups) or age specific. Because the incidence of cancer within a specific population group varies greatly from young to old, age-specific incidence rates provide much more meaningful information than do crude rates.

Prevalence represents the number of cases, both old and new, existing within a given population at a specific point in time. Cancer prevalence depends not only on the incidence but also on the duration of the disease. For example, improvements in adjunctive or palliative management of breast cancer may increase the prevalence of disease although the incidence rate remains constant. Because of the difficulty in determining that nebulous point in time at which the patient may be considered "cured" of cancer, prevalence data are more difficult to ascertain than are incidence data.

The mortality or death rate expresses the frequency with which members of a population die of a cancer. Like incidence data, the mortality rate estimates the probability of an event. Cancer mortality rates are vulnerable to many inaccuracies. Death reporting data usually assign a single cause of death to each reported case. The cause of death of a terminally ill cancer patient may be incorrectly assigned to another condition. For many cancers, there may be an obvious disparity between incidence and mortality. For example, nonmelanoma skin cancers may have a case fatality rate less than 1%, whereas for other tumors (e.g., pancreas and lung), the case fatality rate, i.e., the proportion of cancer cases that terminate in death, may approach unity. In these latter examples, the mortality rate is a valid index of incidence.

Deciding which of these three descriptive measures (incidence, prevalence, or mortality rate) is most appropriate for a given situation is contingent on the nature of the specific problem under study. In studying causes of cancer, incidence data usually provide the most useful information. However, as a result of the widespread deployment of the death registration system, mortality data are usually more accessible than incidence rates. Mortality rates may be the data of choice in evaluating the efficacy of various treatment regimens. By combining incidence and mortality data, it is possible to determine the case fatality rate, which is the proportion of cancer cases resulting in death. Because of the difficulty in defining when a person may be considered "cured" of a cancer, prevalence data are the most difficult measurement to determine; yet this information is the most useful statistic in planning the long-term need for health care services.

Analytic Studies

Descriptive epidemiologic studies address the distribution of diseases within a population. Analytic studies, however, occupy an intermediate position between descriptive and experimental studies in studying cause and effect relations. In analytic studies, specific hypotheses are investigated by observation of population groups as opposed to experimental manipulation. Typically, the hypotheses being tested in analytical studies have evolved from observations made from earlier descriptive studies.

Analytic studies are classified as either being of the case–control (retrospective) design or cohort (prospective) design. In the case–control-type study, the population group is identified by disease. The population with a particular disease and a like disease-free group are studied to collect data on exposure to possible causative agents. An example is a study that attempted to associate estrogen use with the development of endometrial cancer. In that study, a group of women with endometrial cancer and a similar group of disease-free controls were interviewed to determine the incidence of the earlier use of estrogen in both groups. If the proportion of diseased individuals with exposure to the suspected agent exceeds that of the control group, then it can be surmised that an association may exist.

Because of its retrospective nature, a case–control study is particularly useful for studying uncommon disease states.

For a case–control study to arrive at accurate conclusions, the cases under study must be representative of all individuals with the disease process, and the control group must be representative of the nonaffected population. To put this in another way, the prevalence of the hypothesized carcinogen under study must be the same in the control group as it is in the general population. For this reason, hospital-based control studies are particularly vulnerable to the selection bias inherent in the differential probabilities of hospital admission for those individuals with and without the disease who may also have exposure to the risk factor under study. This potential for introduction of bias in selecting either the case group or the control group is one of the potential failings in the retrospective type of study. Case–control studies do have the advantage, however, of requiring a smaller study group and a shorter study time than does the cohort design (prospective) study.

The cohort design study differs from the case–control type, in that the population being studied is identified by exposure to a causative agent rather than the disease itself. An example of one such study involved identifying two groups of women who either had, or had not, been exposed to chest fluoroscopy. These women were followed for a number of years to determine if they eventually developed breast cancer. This study demonstrated a higher incidence of breast cancer in the fluoroscopy group, lending credence to the original hypothesis that fluoroscopy is the cause of breast cancer. When studies such as these are based on current exposures and followed for subsequent outcomes, they are termed *prospective cohort studies*. When they use information based on exposures that have occurred in the past, they are identified as retrospective cohort studies. Cohort studies are especially valuable in determining the risk of developing cancer associated with exposure to agents peculiar to a specific population subgroup (e.g., tobacco users and coal miners).

Cohort studies have the advantage of being able to measure incidence and mortality rates directly, whereas case–control studies cannot. Further, cohort studies are usually less susceptible to the selection bias associated with the case–control approach. However, cohort studies, especially those of the prospective design, are time consuming and expensive.

Experimental Studies

After analytic studies have suggested a causal relation between exposure to a suspected carcinogen and subsequent cancer development, experimental studies (referred to as *clinical trials* in humans) may be conducted to confirm these associations. Experimental studies are designed to either introduce or eliminate exposure to a suspected carcinogen followed by a period of observation to determine the impact, if any, on subsequent cancer development. Obviously, ethical considerations preclude the introduction of a carcinogen within a human population group for the sole purpose of detecting an increase in incidence rates. However, clinical trials are appropriate if they are designed to reduce exposure to a suspected carcinogen (e.g., tobacco and radiation) for the purposes of studying a favorable outcome. After experimental intervention, the follow-up data are analyzed using the cohort design.

An example of such designs relates to the role of *Helicobacter pylori* in gastric cancer. The high-risk areas for gastric cancer make focused studies possible with their high incidence/prevalence rates. Further, in one such area (Narino, Columbia) a trial of treatment for *H. pylori* or antioxidant therapy was found to cause regression of premalignant lesions in a very high-risk population. Such studies make significant progress in prevention strategies for malignancy, made possible by systematic epidemiologic research.

The study of cancer epidemiology has shown that nearly all cancers fluctuate in incidence, depending on the variables of person, place, and time, and that the variation is intimately associated with genetic and environmental factors. Historically, cancer epidemiologic studies have confined themselves to identifying the gross differences in cancer incidence existing among different subpopulations. The major task lying ahead for the epidemiologist is to expand efforts to identify the precise causes and mechanisms for these variations.

STAGING OF CANCER

Tumor staging was created to identify where a particular tumor is in its natural history. The ideal staging system should serve as a reliable prognosticator of patient outcome, aid in the therapeutic decision-making process, and be universally accepted so that it might be communicated readily to others. The first cancer staging system was developed for carcinoma of the uterine cervix in 1929 by the League of Nations. In 1932, Dukes, an English pathologist, proposed the staging classification for colorectal carcinoma, which bears his name. Dukes A cases were defined as limited to the rectal wall. Class B described spread to the extrarectal tissue, and class C were those tumors with lymph node metastases. Over the years, the Dukes staging system has undergone numerous refinements. The most widely accepted Dukes revision is the Astler-Collier modification (of 1954). Unfortunately, the numerous revisions made the system difficult to use and it has now been replaced by the TNM staging system.

In 1943, Denoix from the French Institute Gustave Roussy introduced the TNM classification system. The American Joint Committee on Cancer (AJCC) was organized in 1959 to develop staging systems for American medical professionals. The AJCC and the Union Internationale Contre le Cancer (UICC) have embraced the TNM system and expanded it to include a universal staging system specific for all anatomic sites. The American College of Surgeons Commission on Cancer, which accredits hospital tumor registries, endorses the TNM classification.

The TNM system is a classification scheme based on anatomic considerations. It is predicated on the supposition that tumor spread follows an orderly pattern, beginning with the localized tumor (T), which, after progressive growth and local invasion, spreads to regional nodes (N). Left untreated, the neoplasm eventually manifests itself at distant metastatic sites (M). Some tumor systems (such as soft tissue sarcoma) also use a G descriptor for Grade. Numbers are used after the T, N, and M to describe the extent of disease. Additional subscripts to the three components in the TNM system are used to further define the extent of spread of the tumor. Although descriptive numbers vary between anatomic sites, the following general rules can be made.

Tumor (T):	TX	Primary tumor cannot be assessed
	T0	No evidence of primary tumor
	Tis	Carcinoma *in situ*
	T1–T4	Numbers indicate increasing size and involvement of adjacent structures
Lymph Nodes (N):	NX	Regional lymph nodes cannot be assessed
	N0	Regional lymph node metastases
	N1–N3	Progressive involvement of regional nodes
Metastases (M):	MX	Presence of distant metastases cannot be assessed
	M0	No distant metastases
	M1	Distant metastases

The stage requires a T, N, and M for each tumor. Assignment of the TNM stage is the duty of the treating clinician.

Clinical staging of a tumor is based on information obtained before treatment. These data may come as a result of physical examination, imaging studies, or information gleaned at the time of surgical exploration. Such clinical staging may be abbreviated cTNM. *Pathologic staging* is based primarily on gross and microscopic histologic examination of the removed tumor and may be abbreviated as pTNM. Staging which occurs after an initial course of therapy (such as preoperative chemotherapy/radiotherapy for rectal cancer) is denoted by yTNM. If initial staging occurs at autopsy it is denoted by aTNM. Although the TNM classification system, because of its wide acceptance, is extremely useful, it is not the ideal classification system for all tumor sites. In soft tissue sarcomas, the histologic degree of cellular differentiation is clearly the single most important prognosticator, whereas for thyroid cancer, patient age is an important predictor of patient outcome. Further, as newer prognostic markers become available and more powerful, it seems clear that some of the old anatomic considerations of staging will give way to newer ones. As the specificity and sensitivity of biologic tumor markers increase and specialized techniques measuring the degree of cellular differentiation and mitotic activity evolve, these factors will certainly have to be incorporated in any staging system. This system is the common "language" by which patients are classified.

TABLE 8.8

Cooperative Oncology Groups Studying Malignancy

Acronym	Cancer Cooperative Groups	Chairman	Email Address
ACOSOG	American College of Surgeons Oncology Group	Samuel Wells, M.D., Chair	www.acosog.org
CALGB	Cancer and Leukemia Group B	Richard Schilsky, M.D., Chair	www.calgb.org
ECOG	Eastern Cooperative Oncology Group	Robert L. Comis, M.D., Chair	www.ecog.org
GOG	Gynecologic Oncology Group	Robert Park, M.D., Chair	www.gog.org
NSABP	National Surgical Adjuvant Breast and Bowel Project	Norman Wolmark, M.D., Chair	www.nsabp.ptt.edu
NCCTG	North Central Cancer Treatment Group	Michael J. O'Connell, M.D., Chair	www.ncctg.mayo.edu
RTOG	Radiation Therapy Oncology Group	Walter J. Curran, Jr., M.D., Chair	www.rtog.org
SWOG	Southwest Oncology Group	Charles Coltman, M.D., Chair	www.swog.org
COG	Children's Oncology Group	Gregory H. Reaman, M.D., Chair	www.childrensoncologygroup.org

CLINICAL TRIALS

One of the great advancements in clinical oncology over the last 50 years has been the enormous strides in clinical trials. Clinical trials for cancer patients are essentially experiments designed to evaluate the value of treatments. Such trials have generally been focused on medical therapy for oncologic problems, but surgical trials have changed the face of oncologic care forever. For example, it was the clinical trials from the National Surgical Breast and Bowel Project (NSABP) on breast cancer that have changed the treatment of cancer of the breast from radical mastectomy to breast conserving therapy. The importance of surgical therapy for cancer was recently underscored by the establishment of the American College of Surgeons Oncology Group (ASOSOG) specifically to study surgical issues related to cancer care.

Clinical trials are usually categorized into four phases. Phase I studies are essentially safety trials and when using new pharmacologic agents strive to reach the maximally tolerated dose of the drug and define the dose limiting toxicity, which can be used in later phases of study. Phase II trial evaluate the activity of the treatment against the tumor, with the response of the tumor to treatment being the critical endpoint. Phase III trials compare the effect of the new agent with standard therapy to guide practicing physicians on clinical decision making. The appropriate end points for phase III trials should be patient related such as survival or quality of life. Such phase III trials are prospective and randomized. It is crucial that they enroll enough patients (be appropriately powered) and take into consideration potentially confounding variables in the randomization (stratification). Trials comparing two well-established regimens of doses may also be referred to as phase IV trials. Although trials categorized into such phases works well for new drugs, it does not well describe experimental approaches to surgical or diagnostic procedures.

In an effort to enroll as many patients as possible onto important clinical trials, the National Institutes of Health through the National Cancer Institute support several cooperative oncology groups studying the gamut of malignancy (Table 8.8). Clearly, increased patient accrual onto such trials is one of the key measures of clinical progress. It is incumbent on any physician treating a patient with cancer to be familiar with available clinical trials and encourage patients to enter appropriate studies. Information on clinical trials is available through the National Cancer Institute at www.cancer.gov/clinicaltrials.

FUTURE DIRECTIONS

Advances in biotechnology continue to advance our knowledge of the molecular underpinnings of malignancy. The number of cytokines, growth factors, specific genes, monoclonal antibodies, tumor vaccines, and other active biologic agents continues to increase rapidly, almost beyond our ability to test their activities and evaluate them for clinical utility. Preclinical testing is extremely important to define which of the many promising biologicals should go into clinical trials for diagnosis, treatment, and imaging. Combinations of biologic treatments, together with standard approaches (surgery, chemotherapy, and radiation therapy) have significant benefit for cancer patients currently. Gene array analysis has become part of clinical evaluation and holds great promise. Our integration of newer technology with established treatments will clearly increase substantially in the future. The ability to genetically engineer human cells by restoring or blocking mutant genes to control cancer and other diseases is in its infancy and should soon be realized. Hopefully, this will lead to an age when genetic therapy will be available for the genetic lesions we know as cancer.

SUGGESTED READINGS

1. Adjei AA. Novel combinations based on epidermal growth factor receptor inhibition. *Clin Cancer Res* 2006;12(14 Pt 2):4446s–4450s.

2. Atkins MB, Lotze MT, Dutcher JP, et al. High-dose recombinant interleukin 2 therapy for patients with metastatic melanoma: analysis of 270 patients treated between 1985 and 1993. *J Clin Oncol* 1999;17(7):2105–2116.

3. Bruner DW, Jones M, Buchanan D, et al. Reducing cancer disparities for minorities: a multidisciplinary research agenda to improve patient access to health systems, clinical trials, and effective cancer therapy. *J Clin Oncol* 2006;24(14):2209–2215.

4. Dallas A, Vlassov AV. RNAi: a novel antisense technology and its therapeutic potential. *Med Sci Monit* 2006;12(4):RA67–RA74.

5. Gattinoni L, Powell DJ Jr, Rosenberg SA, et al. Adoptive immunotherapy for cancer: building on success. *Nat Rev Immunol* 2006;6(5):383–393.

6. Genovese C, Trani D, Caputi M, et al. Cell cycle control and beyond: emerging roles for the retinoblastoma gene family. *Oncogene* 2006;25(38):5201–5209.

7. Hahn WC, Weinberg RA. Rules for making human tumor cells. *N Engl J Med* 2002;347(20):1593–1603.

8. Hahn WC, Weinberg RA. Modeling the molecular circuitry of cancer. *Nat Rev Cancer* 2002;2(5):331–341.

9. Hanahan D, Weinberg RA. The hallmarks of cancer. *Cell* 2000;100(1):57–70.

10. Marshall J. Clinical implications of the mechanism of epidermal growth factor receptor inhibitors. *Cancer* 2006;107(6):1207–1218.

11. Smith L, Lind MJ, Welham KJ, et al. Cancer proteomics and its application to discovery of therapy response markers in human cancer. *Cancer* 2006;107(2):232–241.

12. Sorlie T. Molecular portraits of breast cancer: tumour subtypes as distinct disease entities. *Eur J Cancer* 2004;40(18):2667–2675.

13. Tinker AV, Boussioutas A, Bowtell DD. The challenges of gene expression microarrays for the study of human cancer. *Cancer Cell* 2006;9(5):333–339.

14. Greene FL, Page DT, Fleming ID, et al. eds. *AJCC cancer staging manual*, 6th ed. New York: Springer-Verlag New York, 2002.

CHAPTER 9

Surgical Infection

Donald E. Fry

Infection is the constellation of clinical manifestations caused by the local inflammatory response that is initiated by the proliferation of microorganisms in human tissues. Although perceived by clinicians to be a specific response to bacteria, fungi, viruses, or protozoans, the clinical signs and symptoms of the infected state are nonspecific inflammatory responses that are elicited with every wound and every injury. It is only because the stimulus of proliferating living microorganisms is so great and sustained over time, and the host response so prompt and vigorous, that one associates infection with most inflammatory responses. Indeed, every soft tissue contusion and every laceration elicits the same inflammatory response. However, when bacteria are present, the insult remains active and progressive because bacterial proliferation represents a substantial insult—a sustained injury that drives the inflammatory response until eradication of the microbial stimulus is achieved.

The probability of clinical infection when any anatomic site is contaminated by microorganisms is the biological summation of the numbers of organisms, the intrinsic virulence of the microorganism, and the microenvironment of the contaminated tissue. These proinfection variables are offset by the robustness and efficiency of the innate human inflammatory response. The effectiveness of the host defense response is modified or dampened by a number of acquired clinical conditions. An anatomic injury that introduces bacteria into the tissues, whether from a cutaneous laceration or a perforation of the gastrointestinal tract, will recover uneventfully or have clinical infection as a result, based on the summation of these variables. Although microorganisms have common features that permit discussion of the prototype bacterium or generic virus, the response from one area of the body to another is different with respect to host-response mechanisms. Likewise, environmental issues are different when examining the controlled trauma of a surgical wound compared to the biologic chaos of a perforated viscus. This chapter summarizes microbial, host, and microenvironmental factors that represent important basic issues in the evolution of clinical infection. With a better understanding of the fundamental variables of

infection, a more enlightened approach to therapy can be realized.

MICROORGANISMS

Bacteria

Bacteria are single-cell microbial flora that have a rigid cell wall that envelops the entire organism (Fig. 9.1). Like all cells, whether flora or fauna, the bacterium has a plasma membrane which envelops the organism. The cytoplasm has both a variable aqueous and a gel phase. Unlike higher classifications of plant and animal life, the bacterial cell does not contain a nuclear membrane, so the genetic material, while generally segregated in a specific area of the cell, is in immediate proximity to what would be ordinarily considered cytoplasmic components of the cell. Bacteria have deoxyribonucleic acid (DNA)-type genetic material and generally proceed through the translational and transcriptional processes for phenotypic expression, that is, protein synthesis. Unlike mammalian cells, bacterial DNA is a single circular structure rather than in strands. Bacterial DNA is attached to an invaginated segment of the plasma membrane, which is referred to as the *mesosome*.

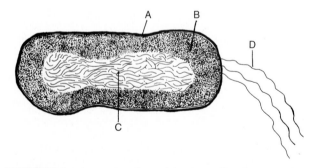

FIGURE 9.1 A prototype bacterial rod. *A*, cell wall; *B*, cytoplasm, which is rich in ribosomes used in protein synthesis; *C*, nuclear area (bacteria do not have a nuclear membrane); *D*, flagella, which are important in cell locomotion.

The cell wall-plasma membrane unit of the bacterial cell is an extraordinarily complex structure. Although customarily discussed as separate structural entities, the cell wall and plasma membrane are structurally and functionally integrated and should be discussed as a combined unit. There is a highly variable composition of the cell wall between species of bacteria, and a different physical relation between the cell wall and the plasma membrane of different strains of bacteria.

Gram-positive bacteria have a thick cell wall, which is located immediately on the external surface of the plasma membrane (Fig. 9.2). The cell wall is composed of peptidoglycan polymers that are cross-linked by polypeptides to form a rigid protective coat about the microorganism. The large amount of peptidoglycan is responsible for the blue coloration of the Gram stain. The cell wall is penetrated readily by solutes, nutrients, and ions. The cell wall serves primarily to protect against unfavorable osmotic changes that would otherwise cause cell swelling and lysis. The lipid bilayer of the plasma membrane contains the necessary enzymes and transport mechanisms that regulate ionic and nutrient access to the cell. The close apposition of the cell wall and the plasma membrane in gram-positive bacteria essentially provide for no periplasmic space between the two structures.

The gram-negative bacteria have a far more complex cell wall-plasma membrane structure (Fig. 9.2). These microorganisms have an outer and inner membrane that has the cell wall interposed in between. The cell wall is of a similar composition to gram-positive bacteria but is much thinner. The inner membrane is a characteristic lipid bilayer, and there is a periplasmic space between the cell wall and the inner membrane. Gram-negative bacteria have an outer membrane that makes the microorganism much less easily penetrated by drugs and other solutes than gram-positive bacteria. The outer membrane is a lipid bilayer that has a lipopolysaccharide (LPS) component known as *endotoxin*. Endotoxin is an important virulence factor for gram-negative bacteria. Endotoxin usually contains the lipid A moiety, which is an important component for virulence.

The outer membrane contains pores that have *porin* proteins that line these microbiologic passages. Porin proteins are different in different bacteria and may permit or exclude certain macromolecules, depending on the polarity and allosteric properties of both the porin proteins and the potential macromolecules. Because the outer membrane is principally lipid in structure, the porin proteins provide a hydrophilic avenue for access of nutrients, ions, and drugs into the microorganism.

An additional feature of the outer membrane is its immunogenicity, which allows the host to produce antibody specific to outer membrane antigens. Research attention has focused on the common immunogenicity of the lipid A component of endotoxin. This has resulted in the synthesis of antiendotoxin antibodies that have been studied in the treatment of gram-negative infection.

Certain strains of bacteria have a capsule that is external to, but contiguous with, the cell wall. The capsule may be composed of polysaccharide, glycoproteins, or complex protein structures. This capsular coat provides additional protection for the bacterial cell, and the capsule may retard phagocytosis by the host when the bacterial cell is part of an infection. The capsule may protect the bacterial cell from exposure of certain cell wall–surface antigens, and thereby prevent the formation of specific antibody by the infected host. Capsular material may actually serve as a virulence factor in facilitating the infectiousness of the bacterial cell.

The bacterial cell wall may have flagella and pili as external extensions. Flagella may be single and excentrically located at one end of the organism, or they may be multiple. The whip-like motion of the flagella provide the bacterial cell with a means of locomotion.

Sex pili are rigid protrusions from the bacterial cell and serve as a means for contact between different microorganisms. These specialized structures serve as conduits for the exchange of genetic material (e.g., plasmids) between bacterial cells and are important in the transfer of resistance among bacterial populations. Only gram-negative bacteria have sex pili.

Fimbriae and fibrillae are filamentous structures that protrude from the bacterial cell and primarily serve as adhesins to facilitate bacteria to bind to other cells. The adhesion of bacteria to epithelial cells is an important virulence factor, and fimbriae and fibrillae are important structures for that purpose. Fimbriae and fibrillae are found on both gram-positive and gram-negative bacteria. The

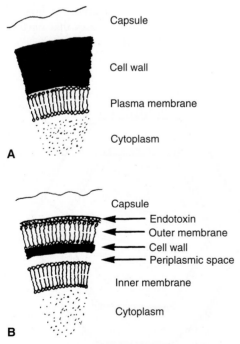

FIGURE 9.2 Differences between the cell wall–plasma membrane complex of gram-positive (**A**) and gram-negative (**B**) bacteria. The gram-positive organism has a much thicker cell wall. The gram-negative bacterium has both an inner and outer membrane around its relatively thin cell wall. Note the periplasmic space between the cell wall and the inner membrane in the gram-negative bacterium.

cytoplasm of the bacterial cell contains the necessary synthetic enzymes and energy-producing systems to maintain viability of the cell. Abundant ribosomes are present to provide the template for protein synthesis. These ribosomes are temperature sensitive and can be bound by specific antibiotics to inhibit protein synthesis. Bacterial cells do not have mitochondria but rather have the apparatus for oxidative phosphorylation on the cytoplasmic surface of the plasma membrane.

Fungi

The fungal cell has characteristics that are analogous to the morphology and structure of mammalian cells (Fig. 9.3). The fungal cells may be identified as single cells or may grow in a filamentous manner, which could be interpreted as a primitive effort at tissue formation because dividing cells actually maintain contact with one another. The continued presence of the cell wall about the fungal cell is the distinctive feature that makes these cells plant life.

Unlike bacteria, the fungal cell has a nuclear membrane. The genetic material of the fungus is in chromosomal strands rather than the circular configuration of the bacterial cell. Fungi have mitochondria for bioenergy processes. Like mammalian cells, sterols are component parts of fungal plasma membrane.

The cell wall of the fungi is structurally different from bacterial cells. The fungal cell wall does not contain peptidoglycans nor does it contain LPSs. The cell wall is usually composed of polysaccharide, which is commonly an *N*-acetyl-D-*glucosamine* polymer called *chitin*. Like bacteria, the cell wall may have a polysaccharide or polyprotein capsule on its external surface. The cell wall serves the role of osmotic control for the fungus in the same way that it serves bacteria.

Candida albicans is the most frequent clinical isolate and is usually identified in patients that are immunocompromised. Indeed, the fungi have fewer virulence factors when compared with the bacterial pathogens known to humans.

Fungal infections are increasing in frequency especially in the intensive care unit (ICU) patient. The suppression of normal bacterial colonization combined with the impaired host in critical illness has increased the frequency and the different types of fungal pathogens.

Viruses

Viruses represent the most primitive form of infectious pathogen. Viruses are distinctly simple in design and are extremely small in size. Viruses were discovered as putative living particles distinct from bacteria because they could not be filtered like bacterial cells. Viral particles are 0.02 to 0.30 μm in size, whereas the *Escherichia coli* bacterial cell is a 0.5 to 2.5 μm rod, the fungal cell is 2 to 3 μm in diameter, and the human erythrocyte is 8 μm in diameter.

Viruses are obligate intracellular parasites. They are unable to replicate outside of a host cell. They do not have any intrinsic capability to generate bioenergy and, therefore, must invade and exploit the energy-generating processes of other cells to be able to replicate.

The complete viral particle, known as the *virion*, has only two essential components (Fig. 9.4). The virus has a nuclear genetic material that is either DNA or ribonucleic acid (RNA), but not both. DNA viruses usually are double stranded, whereas the RNA viruses may be either single or double stranded. The genome is then encased within a symmetrical protein shell known as the *capsid*. The composite unit of the capsid with the DNA or RNA genome within is referred to as the *nucleocapsid*. The capsid serves the purpose of protecting the genome from environmental damage, and it also becomes the means for adherence to host cells that will be infected by the virion. Viruses that have only the nucleocapsid are called *naked viruses*. The nucleocapsid is

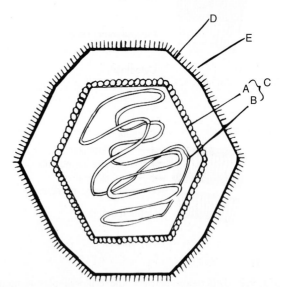

FIGURE 9.4 A prototype virus. *A*, capsid shell about the nuclear material; *B*, circular strand of genetic material, which is either RNA or DNA but not both; *C*, naked viruses; *D*, outer coat of the virus; *E*, viral spikes, which contain adherence receptors and other enzymes that may mediate virulence.

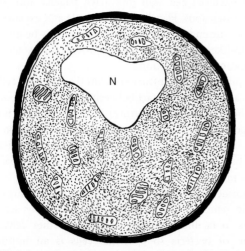

FIGURE 9.3 A fungal (e.g., *Candida albicans*) cell. Like bacteria, fungi have a cell wall, but unlike bacteria, fungi have a nuclear membrane and mitochondria in the cytoplasm. *N*, nucleus.

either a symmetrical icosahedron or helix. All DNA viruses are icosahedral in shape, but RNA viruses may be either icosahedral or helical.

Some viruses may have an additional envelope about the nucleocapsid. The protein component of this envelope is derived from the viral genome during the period of intracellular replication. However, the lipid and carbohydrate components are actually from the membranes of the infected cell because viral particles do not have genes for the production of enzymes that are necessary for synthesis of nonprotein structures. The protein components of the envelope structurally appear as spikes. These protein spikes, known in some viral species as *peplomers*, are analogous to the fimbriae of bacteria and may have specific enzyme activity that contribute to the virulence of the viral microorganism.

Infection of the host cell follows a generic pattern, although specific differences can be seen with different viruses. Adsorption to the plasma membrane of the cell to be infected occurs first. This is achieved by attachment from the spikes to specific receptor sites on the host cell. Because the envelope of the virus is made of plasma membrane, the fusion of the plasma membrane envelope with that of the host cell effects penetration of the nucleocapsid into the cytoplasm. Naked viruses presumably have binding sites on the capsid surface and are internalized into the infected cell by pinocytosis. Subsequent dissolution of the vacuole releases the nucleocapsid into the cytoplasm. The capsid shell around the viral genome is then digested by enzymes from the cytoplasm of the host cell. The viral genome is released, and depending on whether the genome is DNA or RNA, a specific series of events occur.

If the virus is a DNA virus, then the viral genome migrates into the nucleus of the infected cell where RNA polymerase of the host transcribes the viral DNA. Messenger RNA is similarly produced with translation of viral proteins in the cytoplasm of the infected cell. This leads to the synthesis of new viral particles, which are subsequently released with lysis and death of the infected cell. If the infecting virus is an RNA virus, then viral RNA within the host cell cytoplasm can directly become the template for translation of viral particles and the ultimate replication of new viruses.

An exception among RNA viruses is the retrovirus group. The retroviruses, the most notable being the human immunodeficiency virus (HIV), have the genetic information to produce reverse transcriptase, which then makes complementary strands of DNA from the viral RNA. The cDNA from the viral RNA then migrates into the infected cell nucleus, and the viral DNA is integrated into the host chromosomal complement. Viral proteins are then synthesized by the same process that provides transcription and translation for the host cell.

A brief summary of pertinent viral taxonomy for surgeons is provided in Table 9.1. Recently, viral infections have assumed increased interest, not only because of infections that are encountered in the surgical patient, but also because of potential occupational risks that may affect the surgeon.

The number of pertinent viruses of interest to the surgeon will continue to grow.

VIRULENCE FACTORS

Virulence factors intrinsic to bacterial microorganisms are essentially of three types (Table 9.2). They may synthesize and secrete biological products that attack cell populations of the host or attack other homeostatic mechanisms to produce clinical disease. The second group of virulence factors represents structural components of the normal bacterial cell. These structural components, when shed into the environment or when released following the death and lysis of the bacterial cell, have various toxic effects on the host. Finally, the bacterial cell may secrete enzymes, have cell-structure components, or develop mutational phenotypic changes that make them resistant to antimicrobial chemotherapy. This latter trend among microorganisms is the most important virulence factor currently seen in pathogens.

Exotoxins

Exotoxins are produced by many different strains of bacteria, but none are more notable or toxic than the clostridial exotoxins. Fulminant cellular necrosis of host cells can be seen with the cytotoxic exotoxins of *Clostridium perfringens*. The membrane toxicity of the *C. perfringens* cytotoxin may also provoke hemolysis of red cells. *Clostridium tetani* produces a potent neurotoxin, and *Clostridium botulinum* produces a neuromuscular toxin. Toxin A and Toxin B produced by *Clostridium difficile* have potent toxic effects upon the colonocyte and mediate the severe enterocolitis that has become the most common infection due to the Clostridium species in the United States.

Exotoxins are commonly produced by other gram-positive organisms. Pathogenic Group A streptococci are well known to secrete potent hemolysins. Staphylococci are also known to produce hemolysins. Selected Group A streptococci produce the so-called "super-antigens" which are extremely toxic and are associated with the severe necrotizing soft tissue infection of these organisms.

Staphylococcus aureus produces coagulase as a potent virulence factor. Coagulase provokes coagulation and the precipitation of fibrin within the microenvironment of infection. The resulting fibrin matrix serves to protect the pathogen from phagocytic elements of host defense. Coagulase also provokes intravascular coagulation of the blood supply around the area of infection. This thrombosis commonly leads to the central necrosis within the infectious milieu and results in the characteristic pyogenic character of *S. aureus* soft tissue infections. Although coagulase is identified most notably among staphylococcal species, *E. coli*, *Serratia* spp, and *Pseudomonas aeruginosa* may also produce coagulase.

Gram-positive organisms may actually produce toxins that directly affect phagocytic cells. These leukocidins are

TABLE 9.1

The Families of Viruses Known to Cause Infection in Humans

Family	Nuclear Material	Typical Virus	Disease Associations
Poxviridae	DNA	Variola	Smallpox
		Cowpox	Vaccinia
Herpesviridae	DNA	Herpes simplex	Cold sores
		Varicella/Zoster	Chickenpox, shingles
		Cytomegalovirus	Mononucleosis
		Epstein-Barr virus	Burkitt lymphoma
			Kaposi sarcoma
Adenoviridae	DNA	Adenovirus A–F	Respiratory infections
			Conjunctivitis
			Gastroenteritis
Papovaviridae	DNA	Human papilloma virus	Skin and genital warts
			Cervical cancer
Hepadnaviridae	DNA	Hepatitis B virus	Human hepatitis
Parvoviridae	DNA	Parvovirus 19	Childhood exanthem
Reoviridae	RNA	Rotavirus	Severe diarrhea of infants
			Gastroenteritis
Togaviridae	RNA	Equine encephalitis virus	Equine encephalitis
		Rubella	Measles
			Yellow fever
			Dengue fever
Coronaviridae	RNA	Infectious bronchitis virus	Common cold
			Viral pneumonitis
			Severe acute respiratory syndrome (SARS)
Paramyxoviridae	RNA	Parainfluenza viruses	Mumps, measles
		Respiratory syncytial virus	Bronchiolitis, pneumonia
Rhabdoviridae	RNA	Vesiculovirus	Vesicular stomatitis
		Rabies virus	Rabies
Filoviridae	RNA	Ebola virus	Hemorrhagic fever
Orthomyxoviridae	RNA	Influenza A, B virus	Influenza syndrome
Bunyaviridae	RNA	Hantavirus	Hemorrhagic fever
Arenaviridae	RNA	Lassa virus	Lassa fever
Retroviridae	RNA	Human immunodeficiency virus	AIDS
Picornaviridae	RNA	Poliovirus	Poliomyelitis
		Hepatitis A virus	Hepatitis
Caliciviridae	RNA	Norwalk virus	Gastroenteritis
Flaviviridae	RNA	Hepatitis C virus	Hepatitis C
Deltaviridae	RNA	Hepatitis D virus	Hepatitis D
Hepeviridae	RNA	Hepatitis E virus	Hepatitis E

DNA, deoxyribonucleic acid; RNA, ribonucleic acid.

seen most commonly as products from *Streptococcus* spp and *Staphylococcus* spp. A particularly potent leukocidin known as the *Panton-Valentine leukocidin* (PVL) is produced by community-associated methicillin-resistent *Staphylococcus aureus* (MRSA). PVL retards phagocytosis and provokes a fierce local inflammatory response that yields local tissue necrosis in soft tissue infections. Both gram-positive and gram-negative bacteria may produce a leukotoxin that is stimulated by the presence of hemoglobin, or the metabolism of hemoglobin by bacteria may produce the toxin. These products appear to be important in the pathophysiology of polymicrobial infections within the intra-abdominal cavity.

Selected bacteria may produce various enzymes that affect bacteriocidal mechanisms of phagocytic cells. Superoxide anion is produced and delivered into the phagosome after neutrophil phagocytosis of bacteria to effect killing of the ingested pathogen. Strains of *Bacteroides fragilis* produce superoxide dismutase, which converts superoxide anion to hydrogen peroxide. Selected strains of *E. coli* produce

TABLE 9.2

Summary of the Known Secretory Products of Bacteria That are Identified as Virulence Factors in Human Infection

Virulence Factor	Action	Microorganism
Exotoxins	Cytotoxicity	*Clostridium perfringens*
	Neurotoxin	*Clostridium tetani*
	Neuromuscular blockade	*Clostridium botulinum*
	Enteropathic	
Hemolysins	Lyses red blood cells	Group A streptococci
		Staphylococcus aureus
Coagulase	Activates coagulation	*S. aureus*
		Escherichia coli
		Serratia sp
		Pseudomonas aeruginosa
Leukocidins	Kills phagocytic cells	*Streptococcus* sp
		Staphylococcus sp
Superoxide dismutase	Neutralizes superoxide	*Bacteroides fragilis*
Catalase	Neutralizes hydrogen peroxide	*E. coli*
Collagenase	Hydrolyzes collagen	*Streptococcus* sp
		Staphyloccus sp
		Pseudomonas sp
Hyaluronidase/heparinase	Hydrolyzes intercellular matrix	*Streptococcus* sp
		Staphylococcus sp
		Clostridium sp

catalase, which then reduces the potentially toxic hydrogen peroxide to water. The combined effects of superoxide dismutase from *B. fragilis* with the catalase production of *E. coli* represents another potential synergistic relation that may facilitate the combined virulence of these two strains of pathogens in intra-abdominal infection and in selected polymicrobial soft tissue infections.

Enzymes secreted by certain strains of bacteria may aid the invasion of pathogens into adjacent tissues. Collagenase that is produced by streptococci, staphylococci, and certain *Pseudomonas* spp is thought to expedite invasion of infection along fascial planes. Elastase production similarly promotes microbial invasion. Hyaluronidase and heparinase enzymes are produced by streptococci, staphylococci, and certain clostridial species. These two enzymes may degrade the intercellular matrix and are of importance in bacterial cellulitis in which organisms are able to progress rapidly through otherwise normal tissues.

Another interesting virulence factor is the secretion of a polysaccharide product by certain strains of *Staphylococcus epidermidis*. This glycocalyx actually surrounds and encases the organism. It appears to facilitate the binding of the *S. epidermidis* to foreign surfaces, making it less vulnerable to phagocytic cells. This biofilm has been identified among isolates from infections of peripheral intravascular devices and vascular grafts. This matrix assumes a certain physical rigidity, which poses some serious problems in attempts to culture the organism.

Cell Structure Factors

Structural components of bacteria are clearly virulence factors. The M protein coat of streptococci appears to provide relative protection against phagocytosis. It appears to have features that help bind streptococcal pathogens to epithelial cells and may explain the difference in virulence of different strains. Mutant streptococci without M protein do not have virulence. Encapsulated bacteria such as *Streptococcus pneumoniae*, meningococcus, and *Haemophilus influenzae* also resist phagocytosis and require opsonization with antibody if hepatic reticuloendothelial (RE) clearance of these organisms is to occur. Of interest, opsonization is not a requirement for splenic clearance of blood-borne encapsulated bacteria, a function that is thought to be critically deficient in the patient who has undergone splenectomy but does not have specific immunity against the encapsulated pathogens.

The polysaccharide capsule of *B. fragilis* has been studied extensively and assumes considerable significance in the virulence of these organisms. Not all *B. fragilis* strains have this capsular component. If present, the organism has increased virulence as an abdominal infectious pathogen. The capsule retards phagocytosis and may actually be leukotoxic. It is clearly associated with the pathogenicity of intra-abdominal infections. If this purified polysaccharide capsular material is injected into the rat peritoneal cavity, abscesses result without any viable bacteria being present.

Perhaps the most important structural virulence factor of bacteria is endotoxin. This LPS component of the bacterial outer membrane is a common feature of essentially all gram-negative enteric bacteria. Different bacterial species may have chemical variations in the molecular detail of their own endotoxin, but the common lipid A component seems to provide similar biological actions and common virulence features. When the endotoxin molecule lacks the lipid A component, its virulence appears to be lost. Hence, *B. fragilis*, which lacks the lipid A moiety within its endotoxin does not produce any hemodynamic changes when administered intravenously to experimental animals.

Endotoxin has many biologic effects. It provokes macrophages to produce endogenous pyrogen, which causes fever. Endotoxin may directly stimulate the thermoregulatory center in much the same manner as interleukin 1 (IL-1), without needing the intermediary production of endogenous pyrogen by a macrophage cell. Endotoxin activates mechanisms in both the intrinsic and the extrinsic coagulation pathways and is experimentally and clinically associated with the development of disseminated intravascular coagulation. Endotoxin provokes platelet aggregation and the subsequent release of platelet-derived vasoactive compounds. Endotoxin is a potent activator of the complement cascade through the alternative pathway.

ANTIBIOTIC RESISTANCE

Antibiotic use has brought a major advance in the management of patients with bacterial infections. Antibiotics are designed to slow bacterial growth, thereby allowing the host defenses to eradicate the microorganism. Many antibiotics have bactericidal effects *in vitro*, although whether microorganisms are killed efficiently *in vivo* without the participation of the host response remains a point of debate. Nevertheless, antibiotics have significantly improved the outcome of many infections in terms of both survival and recovery time. Unfortunately, the effectiveness of many antibiotics has been seriously compromised by the development of resistance. It has been the generalized use of antibiotics that has led to antibiotic resistance.

Resistance is the loss of activity of an antibiotic against a microbe that was formerly inhibited or killed by the antibiotic. Resistance can evolve quickly and may even develop during the course of therapy in a given patient. Conversely, it can be the accumulative consequences of antibiotics in a specific environment. Therefore, antibiotic use in the ICU over time may cause the development of resistant pathogens. This resistance within a critical care unit then leads to these resistant species becoming the resident microflora of that environment. Subsequent nosocomial infections reflect these new resistance patterns. The generalized use of antibiotics in our society has resulted in even community-acquired infections that reflect resistance changes. The resistance patterns to penicillin and the semisynthetic penicillin derivatives that have occurred with

both hospital- and community-associated *S. aureus* over the last 30 years validates that the entire world of microbial resistance has been changed by antibiotic use.

Resistance may take several forms. It may be the consequences of the organism developing the synthetic capability to produce a neutralizing enzyme, or it may actually reflect structural changes of the microorganism that may eliminate access to the target site of activity for the drug. Resistance appears to be a likely problem that will continue to evolve and potentially threatens the use of antibiotic therapy for patients in the 21st century.

To understand the mechanisms of resistance, it is important first to understand how sensitivity determinations are made in the clinical laboratory. Standard, reliable, and reproducible methods to provide clinical determinations of sensitivity and resistance of a given organism to a given antibiotic have been the cornerstones of treatment in clinical infectious disease.

The most accurate quantitative method to determine sensitivity is the serial tube dilution method. The microbial isolate is inoculated into a series of tubes containing either agar or broth, each of which has a defined concentration of antibiotics. One is then able quantitatively to define the concentration of antibiotic at which microbial growth is inhibited or, conversely, the concentration at which bacterial activity is present. The minimum inhibitory concentration (MIC) is the drug concentration at which inhibition of bacterial growth occurs, and the minimum bacteriocidal concentration (MBC) defines the drug concentration at which the bacteria are killed. Although quantitatively more accurate, the determination of MIC and MBC are expensive for routine use in the clinical laboratory and are reserved largely for use in research. Newer automated microdilutional techniques have facilitated MIC determinations in the clinical microbiology laboratory when particularly problematic organisms are identified.

The disc-diffusion method is the commonly employed method in the clinical laboratory. In this method, a 6-mm disc with a threshold concentration of antibiotic is placed onto a freshly inoculated agar plate with the bacterial strain to be tested. The concentration of the antibiotic in the disc defines the break point for the determination of resistance and sensitivity. Because essentially all microorganisms may be inhibited by all available antibiotics if the concentration is high enough, the disc concentration of the drug must be defined in terms of clinically appropriate concentrations. If an antibiotic provides inhibition of bacterial growth at a concentration of 600 μg/mL but the achievable serum concentration is only 32 μg/mL, then in terms of clinical application, the organism is resistant to the antibiotic. Antibiotic strips are being used in some laboratories that have a gradient of antibiotic concentrations along the length of the strip. This modification of the disc-diffusion technique allows a more quantitative assessment of the sensitivity of the bacterial isolate across a range of antibiotic concentrations.

Another important consideration in antibiotic sensitivity is the inoculum effect. If antibiotic activity is governed by the

TABLE 9.3

The Effects of an Increased Inoculum of *Escherichia Coli* Bacteria on the Sensitivities of the Microorganisms to Commonly Employed Antibiotics

Antibiotic	Sensitivities of E. coli at Different Inocula[a]	
	10^5	10^7
Ampicillin	2	8
Carbenicillin	<4	32
Cephalothin	8	64
Amikacin	4	32
Gentamicin	1	16
Kanamycin	4	64
Tobramycin	1	16
Chloramphenicol	4	64
Tetracycline	1	32

[a]The sensitivities are expressed in micrograms per milliliter as determined by the tube dilution technique.

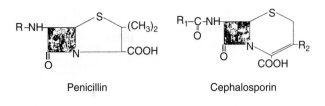

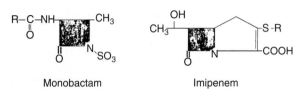

FIGURE 9.5   The four principal groups of β-lactam antibiotics. The shaded area in each prototype molecule reflects the common lactam ring.

ability of the drug to bind to a critical number of receptor sites on the microorganism, then the bacterial concentration within the environment is important. Therefore, an antibiotic that inhibits the growth of an organism when there are 10^5 bacteria per milliliter may not inhibit the growth when 10^7 to 10^8 bacteria are present. This concentration-dependent activity of an antibiotic is referred to as the *inoculum effect*. The impact of bacterial concentration on MIC is illustrated in Table 9.3.

Quantitative assessments generally have defined bacterial concentrations at 10^5 organisms per milliliter of fluid or per gram of tissue for most infections. The notable exceptions to this observation are infection with the presence of necrotic tissue and those infections with a pyogenic character. Concentrations in these settings reach 10^7 to 10^8 bacteria per milliliter. The need for surgical drainage and debridement of these types of infection is further amplified because concentration-dependent resistance for clinically reported sensitive organisms is a potentially contributing cause for antibiotic failure in these settings.

ANTIBIOTICS

Mechanisms of Action

Each class of antibiotics has different mechanisms of action that presumably exploit a metabolic or structural vulnerability of the sensitive organism. The vulnerability of the target site is different in different species, and therefore sensitivity to a given drug differs by species, depending on the presence or exposure of the target site.

Target Site: Cell Wall/Plasma Membrane

Antibiotics that attack the outer envelope of the cell are the most common drugs employed in the treatment of clinical

infection. These include the penicillins, cephalosporins, monobactams, and carbapenems, which are referred to collectively as β-*lactam antibiotics* because they have a common structural feature, illustrated in Figure 9.5.

The β-lactam group of antibiotics are bacteriocidal drugs that inhibit the synthesis of the bacterial cell wall. Because the actual enzyme system responsible for cell-wall synthesis lies within the plasma membrane, it is convenient to think of the actions of this group of antibiotics as involving the entire outer envelope of the cell wall and plasma membrane complex.

Knowledge of cell-wall synthesis is important to understanding the actions of β-lactam antibiotics. A critical component of the bacterial cell wall is a complex peptidoglycan. This peptidoglycan is vitally important to control intracellular osmotic regulation. In gram-positive organisms, the cell wall may be as much as 50 times thicker than in gram-negative species.

The synthesis of the peptidoglycan portion of the cell wall has three component features: (i) the monomer unit of the peptidoglycan is synthesized within the bacterial cytoplasm; (ii) the monomer is then transported across the plasma membrane, and the polymer is synthesized by the process of transglycosylation; (iii) the new polymer is cross-linked to the old cell-wall structure in the newly formed daughter cells. This cross-linking activity occurs after division of the parent bacterium by the process of transpeptidation.

The enzymes responsible for transglycosylation and transpeptidation are within the plasma membrane of the bacterial cell. These enzymes covalently bind penicillins and are collectively referred to as *penicillin-binding proteins* (PBP). Although initially described for penicillins, these binding sites are potential sites for all β-lactam antibiotics. The binding of antibiotics to these membrane enzymes neutralizes the synthetic activity. Therefore replicating bacteria in the face of antibiotics that can bind to PBPs cannot complete the cell wall after division into

TABLE 9.4

Morphologic Changes of *Escherichia Coli* Penicillin-Binding Protein (PBP) Sites When Bound by β-lactam Antibiotics

PBP	Molecular Weight	PBP-Associated Enzyme Activity	Morphology Seen with Binding
1A	92,000	Transglycosylation Transpeptidation	Cell lysis if 1B is also bound
1B	90,000	Transglycosylation	Cell lysis if 1A is also bound
2	66,000	Transpeptidation	Spherical daughter cells instead of rods
3	60,000	Transglycosylation	Filamentous daughter cells instead of rods
4	49,000	Carboxypeptidation	None known
5	42,000	Carboxypeptidation	None known
6	40,000	Carboxypeptidation	None known

daughter cells. Failure of the cell-wall synthesis results in loss of osmotic control and lysis of the new bacterial cells.

Each species of bacteria has a different constellation of PBPs. The affinity and the consequences of binding for each PBP are different between species. Therefore, the nomenclature and literature on PBPs can be confusing.

The PBPs for *E. coli* are identified in Table 9.4. Binding of an antibiotic to both PBP-1A and PBP-1B affects transglycosylation and transpeptidation; cell lysis is the consequence. Both sites must have threshold-level binding for the antibiotic effects to occur. Binding of only one site does not injure the microorganism. Mutants with the loss of either binding site become resistant to a previously effective drug. Binding of PBP-2 creates spherical instead of rod shaped bacterial progeny. *E. coli* mutants without the PBP-2 receptor grow as spheres as well. Spherical *E. coli* spontaneously lyse when fully mature for reasons that are not understood. Binding of PBP-3 causes filamentous growth. Filamentous growth also results in cell death. The binding of other *E. coli* PBPs is not identified as having any biological consequences.

Vancomycin is a non–β-lactam glycopeptide antibiotic that also has inhibition of cell wall synthesis as its primary biological activity. Vancomycin appears to bind to the plasma membrane, but not through the binding of PBPs. Instead, it interferes with the polymerization of normally synthesized monomer units of peptidoglycan. As with β-lactam antibiotics, vancomycin affects actively dividing cells and requires active cell replication to be effective. Unlike β-lactam antibiotics, vancomycin does affect the growth of protoplasts in culture, which reflects a second mechanism of antibacterial activity, which probably relates to impairment of RNA synthesis.

Two new lipoglycopeptide antibiotics of a similar class to vancomycin are likely to be clinically used. Telavancin and dalbavancin are potent bacteriocidal agents that attack cell wall synthesis like vancomycin and have similar gram-positive activity. These newer agents have a much longer half-life than vancomycin.

Polymyxin and colistimethate are seldom-used antibiotics that target the outer envelope of the cell membrane. Polymyxin appears to have a detergent effect on the bacterial cell membrane by interacting with the phospholipid component. Plasma membrane injury is thought to cause diffusional loss of intracellular enzymes. This mechanism of action affects resting cells and does not require metabolically active or dividing cells for effect. Binding to plasma membrane poses some toxicity problems because of similar receptor sites on normal tissue plasma membranes.

Daptomycin is a new lipopeptide antibiotic with exclusively gram-positive activity. This antibiotic actually binds to the plasma membrane of the gram-positive organism and results in membrane depolarization. This results in extravasation of cytoplasmic components of the cell and death of the bacterium.

The antifungal antimicrobial agents have activity against the cell wall/plasma membrane complex as a primary target. The antifungal imidazole derivatives affect plasma membrane synthesis and cause lysis of actively dividing cells. The imidazole group of drugs appears to inhibit a demethylation step in the synthesis of lanosterol by binding to one of the cytochrome P-450 enzymes. This inhibition results in reduced concentrations of ergosterol, which results in a defective plasma membrane. Synthetic manipulation of the basic imidazole ring has resulted in the compounds of ketoconazole, fluconazole, itraconazole, voriconazole and others.

Amphotericin B is another antifungal agent that has the plasma membrane as its primary target, but it does not affect the synthesis of the plasma membrane. Rather, this drug binds to ergosterol, fungisterol, and other sterols in the plasma membrane, which results in alterations of membrane permeability. Oxidative damage has also been identified as a potential mechanism of antifungal activity. The binding of amphotericin B to sterols poses some problems in that the sterols of mammalian membranes may also be bound, potentially causing some toxicity.

The echinocandins are the newest of the antifungal agents, which inhibit the enzyme 1,3-β-glucan synthase.

Inhibition of this enzyme blocks cell-wall synthesis. Caspofungin, micafungin, and anidulafungin are antifungal agents in this class of drugs.

Target Site: Protein Synthesis

Certain antibiotics inhibit protein synthesis. Inherent in the effect of such drugs is the ability either to diffuse or to be transported actively into the bacterial cell. The target of these antibiotics is the ribosome. The antibiotic binds to the ribosome and inhibits the transcriptional phase of protein synthesis. Chloramphenicol, clindamycin, lincomycin, erythromycin, and tetracycline are traditional drugs that inhibit protein synthesis, but they do not irreversibly bind to the ribosomal target. Newer agents that also bind to ribosomal receptors to inhibit protein synthesis include linezolid as a prototype oxazolidinone antibiotic, and tigecycline that is a glycylcline antibiotic with similarities to tetracycline. The reversible nature of binding makes these drugs essentially bacteriostatic in nature. Aminoglycosides irreversibly bind to the ribosome and, therefore, are bacteriocidal. This irreversible binding results in the postantibiotic effect for the aminoglycosides; that is, the action of the drug is present after the antibiotic has been cleared from the environment. The postantibiotic effect has been the basis upon which once-daily treatment of infections with the aminoglycosides has been based.

Target Site: Nucleic Acids

Several antimicrobial agents have the metabolism of nucleic acids as the primary target. Rifampin, the new quinolones, and metronidazole inhibit DNA synthesis by binding to the nucleic acid within the nucleus. Antiviral therapy is also targeted at nucleic acid synthesis. Acyclovir, which is the prototype antiviral agent, is a nucleic acid analog that is incorporated into the new viral genome and has the net effect of preventing new DNA synthesis. In addition, the uptake of acyclovir and related drugs also results in its intracellular phosphorylation, which inhibits viral DNA polymerases.

Target Site: Metabolic Pathways

Sulfonamides and trimethoprim represent the prototype of the antimetabolite group of antibiotics. The sulfonamide molecule is a competitive inhibitor of the incorporation of p-aminobenzoic acid into tetrahydrofolic acid (Fig. 9.6). This competitive inhibition is a reversible process (bacteriocidal). Trimethoprim is an inhibitor of bacterial dihydrofolate reductase, which is the enzyme step following the one blocked by sulfonamide in folic acid metabolism.

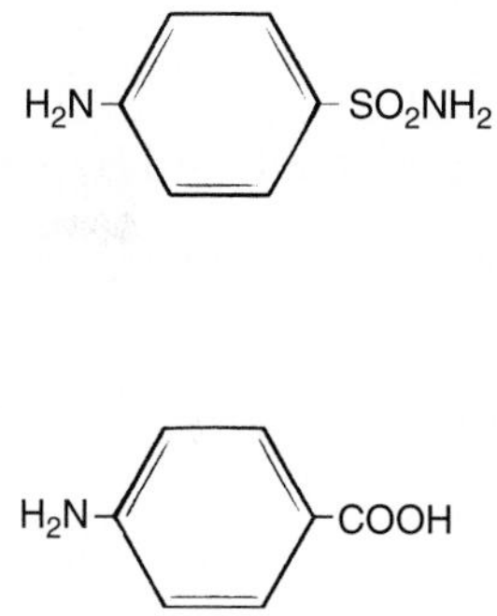

Mechanisms of Resistance

Resistance to antibiotics is the consequence of phenotypic differences between resistant and sensitive strains. The phenotypic changes are genetically mediated, although as will be discussed, the genetic material to mediate the phenotypic change can be acquired from the environment or from other bacteria even in the fully mature bacterial cell. The ability of

FIGURE 9.6 The structural similarities between sulfonamide and p-aminobenzoic acid (PABA). Competitive inhibition by sulfonamide of PABA metabolism can be appreciated from these similarities.

organisms to acquire resistance genes from the environment means that resistance can occur rapidly, even during therapy.

Intrinsic resistance becomes a characteristic of certain bacteria against certain antibiotics. These bacteria do not express PBPs for β-lactams and have always been resistant to these drugs. Certain bacteria have phenotypic traits that prohibit the diffusion or transport of an antibiotic across the cell wall–plasma membrane complex. In this latter group, antibiotics that have ribosomes or nucleic acids as their target sites will not be effective. Intrinsic resistance is constant over time and is commonly used in the clinical laboratory as a means to subspeciate organisms.

Acquired resistance may occur by a variety of different mechanisms. Spontaneous mutation may cause a structural or biochemical change that is permanent in the phenotypic expression of that bacterial cell and its progeny. Mutation may change cell wall–plasma membrane permeability or may change the presentation of plasma membrane receptor sites. Mutations may have metabolic sequelae, such as mutants that increase dihydrofolate reductase production and overcome the growth inhibition from trimethoprim.

Mutation is an infrequent event with a probability of 10^{-7} to 10^{-10} for any bacterial cell during a generation. Mutations that affect drug sensitivity are, fortunately, the least common genetic changes that occur spontaneously.

The consequence of a mutation that imparts drug resistance during a course of therapy means that sensitive strains will be eradicated, whereas the resistant strain will proliferate and soon become the predominant isolate. Fortunately, such mutations are infrequent in the management of a given patient; however, the accumulative effect of a mutation over time and the selection pressure created by extensive antibiotic use mean that resistance trends in specialty units with very ill patients is a virtual certainty.

Plasmids represent the most common mechanism for the acquisition of resistance by a bacterial cell. Plasmids are extrachromosomal genetic material that can be acquired by a number of different mechanisms and cause phenotypic changes in the bacterial cell. Phenotypic changes that can be acquired from plasmids are identified in Table 9.5. Antibiotic resistance from plasmids may give the bacterial

TABLE 9.5

Phenotypic Changes Mediated by Plasmids in Bacteria

Antibiotic resistance
Anabolic pathways
Bacteriophage resistance
Catabolic pathways
Detergent resistance
Gene transfer
Metal resistance
Radiation resistance
Replication changes

cell the capacity to produce neutralizing enzymes that reduce antibiotic effectiveness or may mediate structural changes.

Transduction is one means for a bacterial cell to acquire plasmids. Infection of a bacterial cell by a bacteriophage may bring entrapped plasmids with the viral particle. The new genetic material may actually be incorporated into the genome of the bacteria itself. Therefore, a bacteriophage either may confer resistance by carrying plasmids as new extrachromosomal resistance or may actually introduce a chromosomal change by insertion of its own genome into that of the infected bacteria.

Transformation is the process by which plasmids may be acquired from the environment about the bacterial cell. Plasmids are nonchromosomal segments of genetic material that can be internalized within the bacterial cytoplasm and change phenotypic expression of the cell. Death and subsequent lysis of bacteria cause the release of both chromosomal and extrachromosomal genetic material into the environment. Indeed, plasmids may have been derived originally from the release of chromosomal material that was then assimilated by other microorganisms but was not incorporated into the chromosomal configuration of the recipient microbe.

Direct cell-to-cell transfer of plasmids occurs through the process of conjugation. Sex pili of bacteria permit the transfer of genetic material from one bacterium to another and provide the means for plasmid transfer. This is a common mechanism for the transfer of resistance, particularly among the gram-negative Enterobacteriaceae.

Resistance to β-Lactam Antibiotics

Resistance to β-lactam antibiotics may occur by several mechanisms, but the predominant mechanism is either hydrolysis or enzyme-substrate binding by the enzyme β-lactamase. β-Lactamase production in some concentration has been identified in essentially every bacterial species. The enzymes generally work by hydrolysis of the amide bond on the lactam ring, which neutralizes the drug activity. Hundreds of different β-lactamase enzymes have been reported since the initial isolation in the 1940s.

The near ubiquitous nature of β-lactamase among all bacterial species is secondary to normal chromosomal genetic information. Because β-lactamase was actually identified before the use of antibiotics in clinical practice, its biological role may have been to protect the cell from naturally occurring β-lactam compounds produced by competing fungal species within the microenvironment. β-Lactamase may actually serve a biologic role in the polymerization process of peptidoglycans as part of the normal biosynthesis of the cell wall.

Each β-lactamase enzyme has unique features and activity. Some are active against only penicillins, whereas others are only active against cephalosporins. Of course, some β-lactamases have a more general scope of activity against both groups of drugs. Initially, the activity of β-lactamase enzymes was measured in terms of the rate of hydrolysis of a common substrate, either benzylpenicillin or cephaloridine. More sophisticated systems for classification and characterization of activity are employed, using isoelectric focusing, gene mapping, and other chemical analysis techniques.

Plasmids have resulted in formerly sensitive strains of bacteria to acquire resistance to β-lactam antibiotics. The plasmid mechanism for acquiring resistance through production of this enzyme is a much greater source of resistance than from naturally derived β-lactamase.

The identification of *Pseudomonas* spp that develop resistance from the production of β-lactamase, but produce a form that does not hydrolyze the antibiotic in question raises the issue of alternative mechanisms of antibiotic neutralization. The nonhydrolytic activity of β-lactamase may be the consequence of the nonreversible binding of the enzyme to the antibiotic with the subsequent formation of an enzyme-substrate complex that neutralizes the drug effect. The antibiotic bound with the enzyme may not be able to bind to the PBPs of the membrane or it may not have its customary effects when bound at the PBP.

Enzyme-antibiotic binding appears to occur from β-lactamases that are derived from the normal chromosome of the bacterial cell. Binding β-lactamase rather than the action of hydrolysis appears to be inducible by gene derepression and may be another mechanism for the evolution of resistance during therapy. Because gene expression and control of extrachromosomal plasmids is not thought to be under regulation by repressor genes, β-lactamase induction is believed to be of chromosomal origin. Enzyme-antibiotic binding activity of β-lactamase appears to be less specific than the hydrolysis activity of other β-lactamases. This cross-resistance mechanism can actually cause antagonism between two simultaneously used antibiotics, because the induction of β-lactamase by one can provoke resistance to the second.

β-lactamases of gram-positive bacteria are principally those that are identified from *Staphylococcus* spp. Staphylococcal β-lactamase is plasmid derived and has a relatively specific activity against penicillins. It does not have activity against the cephalosporin group of antibiotics. Chemical substitution around the β-lactam ring at the R_1 site in the semisynthetic penicillins of methicillin, oxacillin, and nafcillin has resulted in allosteric inhibition of β-lactamase

TABLE 9.6

β-Lactamase Enzymes are Presented in Broad Groupings

Activity Group	Molecular Class	Characteristics	Antibiotic Substrates
Broad-spectrum β-lactamases	A, D	Plasmid-mediated; inhibited by clavulanate (except OXA family)	Benzylpenicillin; ampicillin; piperacillin; cefazolin, cefuroxime; OXA[a] family: methicillin, oxacillin
Expanded-spectrum β-lactamases (ESBLs)	A, D	Chromosomal gene; inhibited by clavulanate (except OXA family)	All broad-spectrum substrates plus cefotaxime; ceftazidime; ceftriazone; aztreonam.
Amp C	C	Chromosomal or plasmid; inducible; no inhibition by clavulanate	Same as ESBLs plus cephamycins (cefoxitin, cefotetan)
Carbapenemases	A, B, D	Currently uncommon; Pplasmid-mediated No clavulanate inhibition (except KPC family)	Same as ESBLs plus cephamycins and carbapenems

Organization and classification of these enzymes is very difficult. This table is an attempt to make this vast area unstandable to the uninitiated.
[a]Named because the enzyme hydrolyzes oxacillin. KPC, Klebsiella pneumoniae carbapenemase

activity, causing the semisynthetic drugs to have anti-staphylococcal activity against those organisms that readily hydrolyze conventional penicillin.

The number of different β-lactamases that are active against gram-negative bacteria are vast in number and complexity. In Table 9.6 a summary of four functional groups of gram-negative β-lactamases is present. Virtually all β-lactam antibiotics will be affected by one or more of these groups of β-lactamases. The phenotype for the production of β-lactamase may be either chromosomal or plasmid mediated. The activity of β-lactamase inhibitors is highly variable. It can only be expected that the number of β-lactamases will increase and that continued changes in antibiotic sensitivities can be anticipated in future years.

A number of β-lactamase inhibitors have been added to existing β-lactam antibiotics to maintain antibacterial activity of the drug. Clavulanic acid is a competitive inhibitor that has been used with amoxicillin and ticarcillin to enhance activity particularly against B. fragilis. Sulbactam and tazobactam actually bind to the β-lactamase enzyme to negate activity. Unfortunately, these inhibitors are not active against all β-lactamase enzymes.

Finally, there are non–β-lactamase mechanisms that mediate resistance to β-lactam antibiotics. Particularly in gram-negative bacteria, mutation-mediated phenotypic changes may impede or prevent the antibiotic from penetrating the outer membrane and gaining access to the target proteins on the plasma membrane. The inability of the antibiotic to penetrate the outer membrane may represent changes in the porin proteins.

A particularly important non–β-lactamase mechanism of resistance is seen in MRSA. MRSA resistance is mediated by the protein product of the mecA gene. This PBP 2a has a low affinity for the β-lactam antibiotics. However, PBP 2a has the necessary functional effectiveness to achieve cell wall synthesis. MecA is found in many staphylococcal strains but it is only expressed in those with methicillin resistance. Therefore, a mutation involving the regulation and control of the mecA locus may be pivotal in the emergence of resistance.

The mecA gene is present within a staphylococcal chromosomal cassette (SCCmec). The SCCmec has four genotypes. Types I, II, and III are identified with the hospital-associated MRSA and carry resistance genes for many other non–β-lactam antibiotics within the cassette. The hospital-associated MRSA are routinely resistant to clindamycin, erythromycin, sulfa derivatives, and tetracycline. However, the type IV cassette has the mecA resistance gene but is a shorter cassette and does not carry the comprehensive non–β-lactam resistance pattern. This type IV cassette is most commonly seen in the community-associated MRSA, and accordingly these clinical isolates commonly demonstrate methicillin-resistance but sensitivity to many of the non–β-lactam antibiotics. The emergence of increasing numbers of MRSA within and outside of the hospital environment means that a heterogenous pattern of resistance to all of the non–β-lactam antibiotics will evolve over time.

Resistance to Aminoglycoside Antibiotics

Since 1970, the aminoglycoside group of antibiotics has been one of the most commonly used for the treatment of infections with gram-negative bacteria. Gentamicin, tobramycin, and amikacin are the aminoglycosides that are most commonly used intravenously. Neomycin is used as an orally administered, nonabsorbed drug for intestinal antisepsis. Streptomycin and kanamycin are parenteral aminoglycosides that are extinct because of toxicity.

The aminoglycosides are transported actively into the bacterial cytoplasm by a transport process that is adenosine triphosphate (ATP) dependent. This results in the concentration of the drug within the cell that is significantly greater than that which exists outside the cell. The absence of a transport mechanism excludes the aminoglycosides from the cytoplasm of human cells, except, unfortunately, for the proximal renal tubular and cochlear cells. Although the primary target of aminoglycoside activity is thought to be the irreversible binding to ribosomal sites, the marked bacteriocidal effects of these drugs suggests that other mechanisms of action may be operational.

Resistance to aminoglycosides can potentially occur by the three following mechanisms: (i) drug transport into the cell may be impaired by mutations that downregulate the active transport mechanisms. Fortunately, this mutation is infrequent, because all aminoglycosides apparently use the same transport mechanism, and loss of transport efficiency would cause comprehensive resistance against all aminoglycosides. (ii) A mutational loss of affinity for ribosomal binding sites would increase resistance. This mechanism has only been identified with aminocyclitols but looms as a potential source of resistance for aminoglycosides. (iii) Enzymatic conjugation of the aminoglycoside may occur. Unlike β-lactamase hydrolysis, which occurs external to the cell, aminoglycoside conjugation is an intracellular event mediated by enzymes, which are encoded on plasmids. These enzymes can cause N-acetylation, O-phosphorylation, or O-adenylation of the aminoglycoside and thereby neutralizes its intracellular effects. All aminoglycosides are vulnerable to this mechanism. Enzymes that are targeted to a specific aminoglycoside do not necessarily cross-react with others; however, because these conjugation enzymes are on plasmids, transfer of resistance to other bacteria is a real concern.

The aminocyclitol group of antibiotics has similar mechanisms of action as the aminoglycosides and should be considered here. The prototype drug of this group is spectinomycin. The aminocyclitol antibiotics bind to ribosomes in an irreversible manner and inhibit protein synthesis. Because there is no competitive inhibition between the aminocyclitols and the aminoglycosides, it would appear that they have different receptor sites on the ribosomes. The aminocyclitols are less toxic and may have a separate transport mechanism that excludes them from the cell populations in which the aminoglycoside display their toxicity. Resistance to aminocyclitol antibiotics is thought to be by the same mechanisms as the aminoglycosides.

Resistance to Tetracyclines

Tetracyclines are transported actively across the plasma membrane and bind to the 30s ribosome in a reversible and concentration-dependent manner. This binding blocks the important bonding of tRNA to the mRNA-ribosome complex. Resistance to tetracyclines appears to be through two plasmid-mediated mechanisms: (i) the active transport

of the drug is rendered ineffective; and (ii) the bacterial cell may develop the capability to actively eliminate the drug from the cytoplasm, thereby keeping the antibiotic concentrations within the cell suboptimal. No known enzyme systems exist to degrade or conjugate tetracyclines. Because mammalian cells do not have the transport mechanism for tetracyclines, the toxicity of this group of antibiotics in humans is minimal.

Resistance to Chloramphenicol

Chloramphenicol, with its highly publicized toxicity (aplastic anemia), has continued to have very limited use for the treatment of infections involving *H. influenzae,* meningococcus, and anaerobic pathogens. It is a small molecule and penetrates the central nervous system effectively. Like tetracycline, chloramphenicol is transported into the cell and then binds to the 50s ribosome. The binding is reversible. Resistance is primarily through the plasmid-mediated production of the enzyme chloramphenicol acetyltransferase. The acetylation occurs within the cell cytoplasm. Newer fluorinated chloramphenicol derivatives appear to resist acetylation by this enzyme. Mutant strains of bacteria may have a chromosomally mediated reduction in the transport efficiency of chloramphenicol, which also effectively excludes the fluorinated derivatives as well.

Resistance to Sulfonamide and Trimethoprim

Sulfonamide and trimethoprim are commonly employed together because they have a tandem effect on sequential steps of the biosynthesis of tetrahydrofolate. Sulfonamides inhibit the enzyme dihydropteroate synthetase by competitive inhibition of *p*-aminobenzoic acid, which reacts with aminohydroxy-tetrahydropteridine to form tetrahydropteroic acid. Trimethoprim then blocks the subsequent step by inhibition of the enzyme dihydrofolate reductase.

Resistance to sulfonamides and trimethoprim may occur by four separate mechanisms: (i) the bacterial cell may naturally or by chromosomal mutation exclude the antibiotics from penetrating the cytoplasm; (ii) plasmid-mediated alternative enzymes may bypass the sites of inhibition in folate metabolism; and (iii) induction of *p*-aminobenzoic acid synthesis may overcome the inhibition achieved by sulfonamide, and probably reflects derepression of chromosomal gene expression. (iv) enzymatic degradation of one or both of these antibiotics is suspected, but has not been proved.

Resistance to Erythromycin

Erythromycin is transported into the cell and binds to the 50s ribosome. Because there is competitive inhibition with chloramphenicol, these two antibiotics appear to have a common binding site. Binding to the ribosome is reversible.

Resistance is mediated by four mechanisms: (i) there appears to be both a plasmid- and chromosomal-mediated transformation in the ribosomal binding sites; (ii) chromosomal mutation may exclude the antibiotic from penetration of the cellular cytomatrix; (iii) some evidence suggests that enzymatic removal of the drug from the cell may be a chromosomally mediated mechanism for some resistant mutants; and (iv) an erythromycin esterase that hydrolyzes the drug has been identified.

Resistance to Clindamycin

The lincosamide antibiotics (which also includes lincomycin) have similar actions to that of erythromycin and chloramphenicol in that they too bind to the 50s ribosome and binding is similarly reversible. Resistance is mediated by both plasmid and chromosomal mutation and follows the same pattern as erythromycin.

Resistance to Vancomycin

The evolution of MRSA and *S. epidermidis* has rejuvenated the use of vancomycin. As noted earlier, it inhibits cell-wall synthesis but not through PBPs. Therefore, mutational changes that render the semisynthetic penicillins and cephalosporins ineffective do not neutralize the effects of vancomycin.

Unfortunately, resistance to vancomycin appears to be developing, especially among *Enterococcus* spp that are cultured from institutions with high vancomycin use. Intermediate levels of resistance to *S. aureus* is also being seen. A few strains of vancomycin-resistant *S. aureus* are reported, as are resistant *C. difficile*. Three mechanisms appear to contribute to this resistance. Drug penetration of a mutationally transformed and more complex cell wall seems to be one likely mechanism. A reduction in the affinity for the vancomycin receptor on the plasma membrane is another. A reduction in the role of peptidoglycan in the construction of the cell wall is a third mechanism. Resistance in the enterococcal species have been associated with the *VanA*, *VanB*, and *VanC* genes. *VanA* and *VanB* are inducible genes upon exposure to vancomycin, whereas *VanC*-associated resistance is constitutively expressed. The expanded use of vancomycin because of the increased problem of MRSA infection means that increased resistance to this drug can be anticipated.

Resistance to Metronidazole

Metronidazole penetrates the sensitive bacterial cell, is reduced to a short half-life, toxic intermediate, and then mediates damage to the DNA and other macromolecular structures within the cell. Resistance is rare but is probably the result of delayed bacterial cell penetration or alteration of the reduction process that produces the toxic intermediate. Resistance appears to be chromosomally mediated.

Resistance to Other Antibiotics

From the previous discussion, it should be possible to predict the mechanisms that are responsible for resistance among those drugs not discussed. Resistance to monobactams and carbapenems are mediated by β-lactamase. Resistance to the new quinolone antibiotics is likely to be the consequence of the inability of the drug to penetrate the cytoplasm of the bacteria or changes in the nuclear enzyme target. Acyclovir resistance is from changes in the viral thymidine kinase or changes in the DNA polymerase.

Environmentally Mediated Resistance

In vitro determinations of antibiotic resistance are made within the clinical laboratory under ideal conditions. A standardized inoculum of 10^5 bacteria per milliliter is used. The environment is well-oxygenated, and an optimal neutral pH is employed. There is no protein in the environment to bind the antibiotic and alter drug activity.

The microenvironment of acute bacterial infection is different from that in the clinical laboratory. The bacterial concentrations may be 10^7 to 10^8 organisms per milliliter. An increased concentration of bacteria means that an increased number of target sites are available for the antibiotic and an increased threshold of sites to be bound are necessary for the antibiotic effect. This antibiotic inoculum effect, as discussed previously, is one likely explanation for the clinical failures that are encountered when the cultured bacteria are sensitive to the antibiotics employed.

The microenvironment of suppurative infection is anaerobic and acidic. Those antibiotics that are transported actively into the bacterial cell (e.g., aminoglycosides) will not be transported during anaerobiosis by this oxygen-dependent mechanism. Similarly, the acid environment affects the proton gradient necessary for aminoglycoside activity. Because the microenvironment is rich in protein exudate from the inflammatory response, necrosis of tissue, and dissolution of phagocytic cells, protein binding is a major issue in neutralizing certain highly protein-bound antibiotics.

The description of high bacterial count, acid pH, anaerobiosis, and high protein concentrations is the environment of pus. Antibiotics in this environment will not be effective. For the surgeon, these considerations underscore that even in the high-tech environment of contemporary medicine, pus still needs to be drained.

DETERMINANTS OF INFECTION

Every wound and every epithelial surface is contaminated by bacteria and other microorganisms. Only a few actually get infected. Infection as an outcome is determined by the complex interaction of the bacterial contaminants and the host response. In Figure 9.7, a schematic is presented that represents the variables that interact to predict infection in a given clinical situation. Previous discussion has already addressed the important issues of inoculum and virulence. The additional variables that influence infection as an outcome is the microenvironment where contamination occurs, and the effectiveness of the host in combating potential pathogens.

The Microenvironment

Because every open soft tissue injury and every surgical wound has some degree of bacterial contamination, a critical

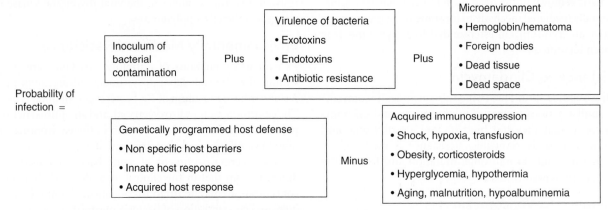

FIGURE 9.7   This figure illustrates a hypothetical equation that describes the numerous clinical variables that affect the probability of infection at the surgical site. The inoculum of bacteria, the virulence of the bacteria, and the microenvironment of the wound form the numerator of events that enhance the likelihood that infection will occur. The denominator of the host defense is the variable that prevents infection from occurring in every case. Our host response is compromised by acute physiologic perturbations and by chronic diseases.

threshold of bacterial contaminants must be exceeded to cause clinical infection. Most surgical and traumatic wounds do not become infected, although culturable bacteria can be isolated from the wound surface. For a given level of virulence, a specific density of bacteria must be present to create the clinical inflammatory response known as *infection*.

To produce a clinical infection in subcutaneous fat, the density of bacteria needed has experimentally been defined at approximately 10^5 colony-forming units (cfu) per gram of tissue. Therefore, even a poorly vascularized area, such as subcutaneous tissue, requires large numbers of bacteria to cause clinical disease. The presence of adjuvant factors in the wound may lower the number of necessary bacteria. Silk sutures reduce the threshold of bacterial density by 10^2 to 10^3 to cause infection. Bacteria with unusual and potent virulence factors may require relatively few bacteria to cause severe and even life-threatening situations. Such is the case with clostridial gangrene or tetanus following a puncture wound.

Because skeletal muscle is well vascularized, it rarely becomes the primary site for infection even in the face of massive contamination. Muscle tissues usually become the haven for bacterial infection when the blood supply is compromised or actual necrotic tissue is present. Therefore the toxin from *C. perfringens* results in necrosis of muscle, which in turn becomes the growth media for a host of other proliferating bacteria. In necrotizing fasciitis, the advancing line of bacteria moves through the relatively avascular plane of the fascia and only secondarily causes muscle necrosis as the blood vessels, which perforate the fascial layer and perfuse the muscle, are thrombosed.

The threshold of 10^5 bacteria is identified again in other areas. Greater than 10^5 cfu/mL of urine is considered diagnostic for urinary tract infection (UTI). Bronchoalveolar lavage or protected brushings are commonly employed in the diagnosis of pneumonia in the critical care unit and have

generally had a threshold of 10^3 to 10^4 employed for the diagnosis of pulmonary infection.

In other areas, the number of bacteria necessary to cause infection is uncertain. In the peritoneal cavity, the type of bacteria and the presence of adjuvant factors may be more important than the actual bacterial numbers. Because intravascular devices represent a direct conduit into the bloodstream, relatively small numbers of bacteria disseminated through these mechanisms are necessary to cause clinical sequelae. Therefore, there are additional adjuvant factors that need to be considered in clinical infection. When these factors are present, they result in fewer contaminates necessary for infection, and they amplify the virulence of the microbes that cause subsequent infection.

Work in the research laboratory clearly illustrates the importance of adjuvant factors. The peritoneal cavity of rodents is virtually impossible to infect without the use of lysed red cells, mucus, or foreign bodies to augment the infectious process. The role of these adjuvant factors is thought to be either stimulation of bacterial proliferation or impairment of host defenses.

Hemoglobin may be the most potent adjuvant factor. Clot or hematoma within the surgical or traumatic wound reduces the number of bacterial contaminants necessary to cause infection. The mechanism of the adjuvant effect of hemoglobin remains unclear. Evidence has generally favored that ferric ion derived from hemoglobin may be a potent growth factor for bacterial proliferation. In selected patients with hemolysis, hemoglobin may also be a systemic factor in the exacerbation of septic events.

Foreign bodies reduce the number of bacteria necessary to cause infection. Suture material, vascular grafts, heart valves, and other prosthetic materials increased infection rates in patients. Foreign bodies left in traumatic wounds will become the focus of infection. Perforations of the distal gastrointestinal tract are associated with foreign bodies such as fiber, exfoliated cells, and other debris from the gut to augment the probability of infection. The diapedesis of phagocytic cells in the extracellular matrix requires the presence of counter-receptors to effect movement. No such counter-receptors exist on foreign surfaces, and may be an important issue in the adjuvant effect of foreign bodies in the wound.

Dead tissue remains an important adjuvant. Dead tissue serves both as a substitute for bacterial proliferation and as a haven for bacteria growth, unencumbered by host defense mechanisms. Recently, it has become clear that necrotic tissue is a potent stimulus to the host's inflammatory responses. Therefore, clinical infection in wounds is likely to be the consequence of the additive effects of necrotic tissue and bacteria.

Fibrin represents another clinical variable that may be viewed as being either an adjuvant factor for bacterial growth or a positive nonspecific host defense variable. Studies in experimental peritonitis have shown that bacteria imbedded in a fibrin clot will cause abscess and death of experimental animals compared with intraperitoneal bacteria released free into the peritoneal cavity. Several publications have demonstrated a beneficial effect of heparin on animal models of peritonitis and have suggested that the salutary effects are secondary to the prevention of the fibrin matrix within the peritoneal cavity. In addition, because antibiotics generally penetrate the fibrin matrix poorly, the fibrin matrix could protect bacteria from the effects of these drugs. However, the localization effects of fibrin may serve to prevent dissemination of bacteria and in that respect have a positive benefit when bacterial concentrations within the peritoneal cavity are large.

Systemic factors may likewise affect local vulnerability to infection and may facilitate the dissemination of bacteria that lead to the septic state. Hypoxemia reduces the availability of oxygen at the interface between the host and the potential pathogens. Molecular oxygen is necessary for the oxidation burst of the neutrophil, which is necessary for the synthesis of reactive oxygen intermediates necessary for intracellular killing of bacteria by the phagocyte (Fig. 9.8). Hemorrhagic shock and hypovolemia likewise impair the delivery of oxygen and substrate to the area of injury and contamination. Ischemia may also contribute to local infection by impairment of the egress of acid end products of the host–pathogen interaction. Experimental and clinical data have implicated blood transfusion as being immunosuppressive and increasing infection rates in surgical patients.

Underlying conditions may be systemic variables in the enhancement of bacterial infection. Considerable clinical suspicion has focused on the increased incidence of infections in diabetic patients. Efforts to define specific abnormalities have been inconsistent, and the microvascular disease of diabetes may also contribute to this apparent predisposition to infection. Hyperglycemia has been implicated as a cause for increased frequency and severity of infection in the diabetic patient. Maintenance of core body temperature at normal

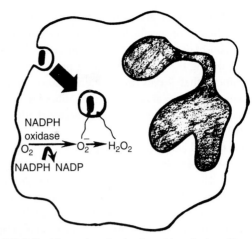

FIGURE 9.8 The reduced nicotinamide adenine dinucleotide phosphate (NADPH) oxidase pathway generates toxic oxygen intermediates from molecular oxygen with the neutrophil. NADP, nicotinamide adenine dinucleotide phosphate.

levels may similarly overcome increased infections associated with intraoperative hypothermia. Multiple-organ injury has been associated with increased infection morbidity and probably represents the added inflammatory potentiation of tissue necrosis plus bacterial contamination.

Malnutrition has been studied exhaustively and appears to affect all components of host responsiveness. A blunted inflammatory response, altered neutrophil functions, and adversely affected delayed hypersensitivity skin testing have all been recognized. What remains less clear is the degree of nutritional repletion necessary to reverse these adversarial parameters. Although delayed hypersensitivity skin tests and *in vitro* studies of immune function can be reversed by various formulations of nutritional support, clinical data showing improved patient outcome are difficult to identify.

Finally, drugs may represent a systemic variable predisposing to an increased risk of infection. Exogenous steroid use has a generalized dampening effect on all components of host responsiveness. Acute and chronic alcoholism has been identified as producing specific abnormalities of host responsiveness. This is important because a high frequency of alcoholism exists among the trauma patient population.

In summary, adjuvant effects amplify bacterial virulence or repress host responsiveness. The consequence is that fewer bacteria per gram of tissue or per milliliter of body fluid is necessary to trigger clinical infection. Indeed, adjuvant factors may be more important variables than the actual numbers of contaminating bacteria in the prediction of subsequent clinical infection.

HOST DEFENSE

The host defense can be subdivided into three distinct parts: (i) nonspecific barrier defense, (ii) innate host defense, and (iii) adaptive host defense. Each has an important role to play in the prevention of infection. Nonspecific barrier defenses are designed to prevent access of microorganisms to the tissues of the host. Nonspecific host defenses can include the glottis mechanism of the airway, which limits contamination of the lung during the process of eating or swallowing, or the integument that serves as a veneer against potential contaminants. Mucins and secretory antibodies become nonspecific mechanisms by preventing bacterial adherence to epithelial cells.

The innate and adaptive host responses have important and integrated roles in the prevention and eradication of infection. The innate host defense is a programmed generic response that behaves in a standardized and nonspecific manner to injury and to different potential pathogens. The response is the same for a cut, scrape, or burn, and the response is the same regardless of the composition of the bacterial contamination. The humoral and cellular responses are specific for the event with a biological memory

to have a sensitized and tailored response when a pathogen is visited upon the patient for a second time. Although the adaptive immune response is important in immunization and chronic infections, it is the innate response that is of critical importance in the prevention and control of bacterial infection in most surgical patients.

The events that characterize the innate host response are best examined from the events within a surgical or a traumatic soft tissue wound (Fig. 9.9). The wounding process transgresses the skin. A laceration or incision results in disruption of blood vessels and devitalization of tissues. Injury and blood vessel disruption result in the expression of tissue factor from subendothelial and fibroblast cells, exposed collagen, endothelial damage, release of adenosine diphosphate (ADP), and local bleeding. This activation event results in activation of the aggregation of platelets and activation of the coagulation cascade in what first appears

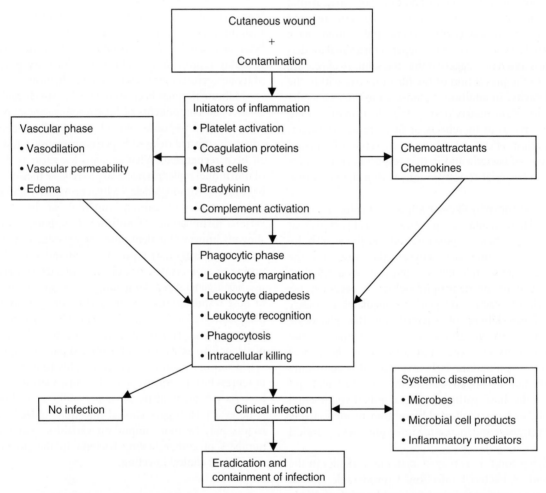

FIGURE 9.9 This figure illustrates the foundation of the innate inflammatory response. Injury and contamination lead to the initiation of inflammation. The initiator events result in signaling that causes the vasoactive phase of inflammation but also generates the abundance of chemoattractant signals that lead to the phagocytic phase of the response. Eradication of the contaminating microbe leads to resolution of the process. Severe infection that results in dissemination of microbes, microbial cell products, or excessive proinflammatory signaling then leads to disseminated inflammation and clinical sepsis.

to be hemostasis, but is also the first step in the activation of the inflammatory response. In a synchronous cascade of events, mast cells are activated for the release of histamine and other products, bradykinin is produced from high molecular weight kininogen, and the complement cascade is activated. The net effects of these initiators of human inflammation is vasodilation, increased microcirculatory permeability, and edema formation at the site of the wound. The microcirculatory vasodilation results in increased bulk flow to the area but also a reduction in flow velocity as the microcirculation is being prepared for arrival of circulating leukocytes. Vascular permeability increases as intercellular exit routes are prepared for leukocyte migration. Soft tissue edema creates aqueous conduits for leukocyte migration through what is ordinarily a dense extracellular matrix. This vasoactive phase of inflammation is also attended by the release of numerous chemoattractant signals which bind to endothelial receptors to upregulate important selectin and integrin proteins for leukocyte docking, and serve to provide direction for neutrophils toward the area of injury and would-be pathogens. Neutrophils are followed by mononuclear monocytes.

The various exotoxins, endotoxins, other structural elements of microbial cells, and metabolic microbial products serve an aggregate role in the expression of virulence, but they also become key elements in the recognition of infection by the infiltrating cells of innate host defense. These microbial products become ligands that bind to membrane receptors of host cells and provoke specific responses. Although the full scope of potential receptors are not fully defined, toll-like receptors (TLRs) have been the source of considerable interest.

Ten human TLRs have been identified. They have a broad array of cell populations for expression but are primarily found on endothelial cells, neutrophils, mononuclear cells, and dendritic cells. TLR-1, TLR-2, and TLR-6 form heterodimer complexes for certain ligands, but are generally receptors for gram-positive bacteria. TLR-4 is the priniciple receptor for gram-negative bacterial endotoxin, but requires co-receptor participation by MD-2 (an extracellular glycoprotein), LPS-binding protein, and CD14. The array of different TLRs and their specific ligands are identified in Table 9.7. TLRs result in activation of the primary transcription factor, nuclear factor κ B (NF-κB). NF-κB enters the nucleus of the host cell and results in gene expression for proinflammatory cytokines. The narrow specificity of many TLRs suggests that other receptors will likely be identified.

TABLE 9.7

This Table Identifies the Specific Ligands for Each of the Ten Toll-Like Receptors

Toll-Like Receptor (TLR)	Ligands	Comments
TLR-2	Lipoteichoic acid Lipoarabinomannan Zymosan Porins	Important in recognition of gram-positive bacteria, fungi, *Neisseria* sp, and others; TLR-2 may function as a homodimer or as heterodimer with TLR-1 or TLR-6.
TLR-1/TLR-2 heterodimer	Triacylated lipoproteins	Important in recognition of mycobacteria and meningococci
TLR-2/TLR-6 heterodimer	Diacylated lipoproteins Peptidoglycan	Important in recognition of mycoplasma and gram-positive bacteria
TLR-3	Double-stranded RNA	Ligand is likely to be important in recognition of viruses; stimulation of TLR-3 results in production of interferon in addition to proinflammatory cytokines
TLR-4	Lipopolysaccharide (LPS)	TLR-4 requires presence of CD14 and the glycoprotein MD-2 for LPS recognition
TLR-5	Flagellin	Ligand is protein component of the flagella of gram-negative bacteria
TLR-7	Single-stranded RNA	Ligand for recognition of viruses; produces interferon in addition to proinflammatory cytokines
TLR-8	Single-stranded RNA	Ligand for recognition of viruses; produces interferon in addition to proinflammatory cytokines
TLR-9	Bacterial DNA	Bacterial recognition
TLR-10	No defined ligand	Unknown

RNA, ribonucleic acid; DNA, deoxyribonucleic acid.

TABLE 9.8

Effects Stimulated by Interleukin 1 (IL-1)

Fever
Neutrophilia
Hypoferremia
Hypozincemia
Hypercupremia
Upregulation: hepatic acute phase reactants (e.g., C-reactive protein)
Downregulation: hepatic albumin synthesis
Stimulation of muscle proteolysis
Increase in amino acid oxidation
Stimulation of thymocyte proliferation
Stimulation of immunoglobulin synthesis
Modulation of T-helper/T-suppressor cells
Enhancement of natural killer cell activity
Stimulation of fibroblasts

A cascade of proinflammatory cytokine products follow which provide a large number of physiologic effects. Tumor necrosis factor (TNF), IL-1,(Table 9.8) and IL-6 are the most well studied and produce autocrine, paracrine, and endocrine events that are fundamental to the host response. (Table 9.9) Each has redundant and overlapping functions which lead to enhanced neutrophil phagocytic activity, the febrile response, and the production of acute phase proteins. The intensity of the response will be commensurate with the intensity of the aggregate chemoattractant and proinflammatory receptor recognition events dictate. Minimal contamination or effective eradication of potential pathogens by phagocytosis and intracellular killing results in the orderly retreat of the process and uneventful wound healing. Evolving infection from the unchecked proliferation of microbes at the site

of injury leads to a robust stimulation of the inflammatory cascade with all of the clinical sequelae of rubor, dolor, calor, and tumor at the site of clinical infection.

Intense local infection illustrates the second function of innate host defense beyond eradication of the pathogen and that is containment of infection locally. Intense chemoattractant and proinflammatory signaling results in continued infiltration of the phagocytic cells into the environment of the infection. Margination of large numbers of leukocytes within the microcirculation about the perimeter of the infected area combined with continued activation of platelets and coagulation proteins leads to thrombosis of the microcirculatory units. The central portion of the infection becomes functionally ischemic and egress routes through the microcirculation for bacteria and bacterial cell products have been sealed. The central portion of the infection becomes a proteinaceous semiliquid medium of dead leukocytes, inflammatory exudates, and bacteria known everywhere as *pus*. The abscessed collection is bounded on the perimeter by a wall of fibrin and sealed egress routes to contain the process locally.

As the discussion turns to other areas of infection in the host, it is important to emphasize that the wound scenario mentioned earlier is analogous to infection as it occurs at any anatomic site. With minor modifications, the innate host defense responds in this generic manner to eradicate and contain potential pathogens.

SPECIFIC INFECTIONS

Intra-abdominal Infection

Intra-abdominal infection begins as the process of peritonitis, or inflammation of the mesenchymal cell lining of the

TABLE 9.9

Defines the Types of Mediators That are Responsible for Cell-to-Cell Interactions

Class of Mediator	Definition of Class	Example of Class
Autocrine—intracellular	A mediator that is synthesized within a cell and has a target within that same cell	PgE is synthesized within muscle cells and then promotes proteolysis within that same cell
Autocrine—extracellular	A mediator that is synthesized and released external to that cell, which either has itself or the same cell population as its target	TNF is released by stimulated macrophages and then stimulates membrane receptors on its own membrane or other macrophage membranes
Paracrine	A mediator that is synthesized and released to target another cell population in the immediate vicinity	TNF is released by macrophages and stimulates receptors on adjacent neutrophils
Endocrine	A mediator that is synthesized and released to target another target site that is remote and requires the chemical signal to travel through the blood stream to reach the effector site	Interleukin 1 is released by macrophages and travels through the bloodstream to stimulate hypothalmic receptors to provoke the febrile response

While autocrine, paracrine, endocrine seem to be distinct classifications, a given mediator may fit into more than one category or may actually serve all three functions [e.g., (TNF)].
PGE, prostglandin E; TNF, tumor necrosis factor.

peritoneal cavity. The process of peritonitis has the distinct phases of contamination, dissemination, inflammation, and resolution or loculation. Peritonitis may occasionally be a primary process, but more commonly, it is secondary to another intra-abdominal disease.

Primary peritonitis is the consequence of peritoneal contamination arising from a remote source and without a fundamental intra-abdominal process. Microorganisms lodge within the peritoneal cavity through either hematogenous or lymphatic spread. Although primary peritonitis secondary to miliary tuberculosis was common in the past, in the modern era, it usually occurs in cirrhotics with ascites. Therefore, S. pneumoniae may be the most common pathogen causing primary peritonitis (from a pulmonary infection) but certainly other bacteria from a remote site can be the pathogens for this infection.

Secondary peritonitis is the usual scenario. The process customarily begins with perforation of the gastrointestinal tract and contamination of the peritoneal cavity. Perforation usually occurs secondary to inflammatory or neoplastic processes. Therefore, the peritonitis is a secondary process. The extent, severity, and outcome of the subsequent infection are consequences of multiple biologic factors.

An important consideration for predicting the severity of peritonitis is the size of the bacterial inoculum. The inoculum will generally reflect the density of bacteria from that segment of the gastrointestinal tract that perforates. Therefore, a perforated peptic ulcer will initially have relatively few organisms and will be more of a chemical peritonitis. Perforation of a gastric ulcer or a gastric carcinoma will commonly have a significant number of bacteria because of reduced or lost gastric acidity. The organisms will be primarily aerobic gram-negative rods. As perforations occur more distally in the gastrointestinal tract, the bacterial density will progressively increase. The perforated appendix will have 10^6 to 10^7 bacteria per gram of luminal content. The highest bacterial densities will be 10^{10} to 10^{11} bacteria per gram of content in the sigmoid colon. Anaerobic species become greater in number at the distal portion of the intestine, and anaerobic species exceed aerobes by 1,000-fold within the sigmoid colon. Blood and hematoma, foreign bodies (i.e., fecal material), and dead tissue are important adjuvant factors that enhance the infectious process.

Contaminants within the peritoneal cavity are disseminated throughout the abdomen by the natural forces of peritoneal fluid movement. Peritoneal fluid accumulates secondary to normal hydrostatic tissue forces. The upright position increases peritoneal fluid formation, whereas recumbent posture allows for fluid clearance. Accumulated peritoneal fluid in the recumbent position has a natural movement toward the diaphragm. With each exhaled breath, a pressure gradient is created that draws peritoneal fluid toward the diaphragm. The fluid is then cleared through the lymphatic fenestrations that are present across the diaphragmatic surface of the peritoneal cavity. The fluid then passes directly into the lymphatic system. Therefore, the human peritoneal cavity is, in reality, a giant lymphocele that communicates directly with the lymphatic system through the thoracic duct. The movement of peritoneal fluid becomes a normal force that disseminates bacteria throughout the peritoneal space.

Dissemination of intraperitoneal contaminants can be viewed as having positive nonspecific host defense consequences. Dissemination reduces the density of bacteria. Because the severity of bacterial infections has clearly been associated with the density of bacteria, dissemination is probably of some biologic importance. Dissemination increases the interface between the peritoneal pathogens and phagocytic host defenses. Finally, dissemination with movement of bacteria toward the diaphragm facilitates evacuation of bacteria from the peritoneal cavity.

With seeding of bacteria and other foreign particles into the peritoneal cavity, the inflammatory response is activated. The soft tissue response within the peritoneum is similar to that seen with the soft tissue wound described earlier. Resident peritoneal macrophages are activated and release the full array of inflammatory mediators, initiating the process. Complement and mast cell activation cause vascular permeability changes, edema, and recruitment of neutrophils from the systemic circulation into the area of injury. The generalized activation of inflammation results in activation of the coagulation cascade, which results in the formation of fibrin. Fibrin may entrap microorganisms, which has the potentially positive benefit of preventing bacterial invasion of soft tissues but may have the negative effect of insulating the entrapped organisms from phagocytic cells.

The bacterial contaminants within the peritoneal cavity are eliminated by two mechanisms. Bacteria are either ingested, killed, and digested by phagocytic cells or removed into the lymphatic system as part of the physiologic clearance of peritoneal fluid. When the density of bacterial contaminants exceeds clearance mechanisms, loculation of the contaminants occurs. Fibrin deposition about the perimeter of the dense bacterial collection matures with collagen replacement of the fibrin scaffolding to form the wall of the abscess. The fibrin–collagen barrier protects the host from the consequences of the bacterial dissemination but also shields the septic collection from phagocytic infiltration.

Infection within the peritoneal cavity is usually polymicrobial (Table 9.10). The synergism of aerobic and anaerobic organisms is a major contributor to the pyogenic nature of intra-abdominal infections. Gram-negative enteric organisms are particularly virulent, presumably because of the LPS component of the cell wall. B. fragilis does not have a potent LPS cell wall component and appears in most experiments to have minimal pathologic importance. However, a mixture of gram-negative enteric bacilli with the anaerobic B. fragilis yields synergism, and the resultant infection is considerably greater than would have been anticipated.

The synergism evolves because the aerobic pathogens not only express their own virulence but also consume the oxygen of the microenvironment and essentially produce an anaerobic condition for their anaerobic partner. Because bacteria like E. coli are facultative, they can proliferate

TABLE 9.10

Pathogens in Complicated Intra-abdominal Infection

Pathogen	Percentage of Positive Cultures
Aerobic gram-negative rods	
Escherichia coli	70–90
Klebsiella spp	10–15
Pseudomonas spp	5–10
Proteus spp	5–6
Enterobacter sp	5–6
Gram-positive organisms	
Streptococcus spp	30–40
Enterococcus faecalis	10–15
Enterococcus faecium	5–6
Other enterococci	5–10
Staphylococcus aureus	3–4
Anaerobic organisms	
Bacteroides fragilis	30–40
Other *Bacteroides* spp	50–60
Clostridium spp	20–25
Peptostreptococcus spp	10
Others	20–25

with or without oxygen. For *B. fragilis,* the anaerobic conditions permit full expression of its pathologic potential. Important among its virulence factors is the polysaccharide capsule that retards phagocytosis and promotes a pyogenic response (e.g., dead neutrophils) within the inflammatory environment. This polysaccharide capsule can be shed into the environment and provides protection for *B. fragilis'* facultative symbiont.

The location of abscesses within the peritoneal cavity tends to be the physiologic drainage basins of the abdomen (Table 9.11). The two forces that govern the site of the collections of pus are gravity and the movement of

TABLE 9.11

Identifies the Frequency with Which Abdominal Abscess Occurs at Different Locations within the Abdominal Cavity

Location of Abscess	Percentage of Patients
Subphrenic space	30–40
Pelvic space	30–35
Subhepatic space	20–25
Paracolic gutter	10–15
Subfascial space	10–15
Lesser sac	5–10
Multiple abscess	20–30

Abscesses tend to occur in the most dependent areas of the abdominal space.

peritoneal fluid. Dense collections of bacteria will occur in the subphrenic spaces, the pericolic gutters, and the pelvis because of their dependent locations. Because peritoneal fluid moves toward the diaphragm, obstruction of the egress route of fluid and microorganisms through the diaphragm, secondary to fibrin and other exudative debris, results in subphrenic collections and abscess.

Therefore, a complex interaction occurs between the invading microorganisms and nonspecific host defenses. The virulence of the infection process is dictated by the biologic summation of bacterial numbers, intrinsic bacterial virulence, and adjuvant factors within the environment. The summed virulence is pitted against the inflammatory response, which may have intrinsic inborn strengths or weaknesses and may also be compromised by certain systemic influences. Efficient host responsiveness in the face of minimal summed virulence results in resolution of the peritonitis. Overwhelming virulence factors with a compromised host results in fulminant peritonitis and death of the host. Not uncommonly, a biologic stand-off results in abdominal abscess. The inaccessibility of the abscess to host defense mechanisms allows for proliferation. Such abscesses require mechanical intervention to allow for resolution of the infection.

Postoperative Pneumonia

Postoperative pneumonia represents a common infection among surgical patients and is the most common infectious complication (if infections of the surgical site are excluded). The gas-exchange surface of the lung is approximately 150 m^2. Considering that such a large surface area of both tracheobronchial epithelial surface and alveolar surface are at risk for atelectasis, aspiration, and contamination from mechanical ventilatory systems, it is amazing that more postoperative patients do not have pulmonary infection. Postoperative pneumonitis assumes particular importance because of the reportedly high mortality rates (30%–50%), particularly among older patients.

Numerous host defense mechanisms exist to prevent infection in the lung (Table 9.12). The glottis serves as the primary barrier to bacteria or other substances that might provoke an inflammatory response. The endobronchial surface of the tracheobronchial tree is covered by ciliated epithelial cells, which become the target for binding and invasion by potential pathogens. A coating of mucus from goblet and bronchial gland cells becomes a primary barrier to prevent bacterial adherence to the epithelial cells. The coordinated motion of cilia in the lower airway results in the dynamic evacuation of bacteria-laden mucus into the larger proximal airways where it can be expectorated.

An additional mechanism to prevent bacterial adherence to epithelial cells is the normal secretion of IgA antibodies into the mucus that lines the luminal surface of the airway. These nonspecific antibodies bind to specific sites on the bacterial contaminants and appear to prevent bacterial adherence to the epithelial surface of the airway. Nonadherent bacteria are then evacuated through the mucociliary mechanism, or they may be eliminated distally at the alveolar level by macrophage

TABLE 9.12

Host Defense Mechanisms of the Lung

Host Defense	Mechanism of Action
Glottis/epiglottis	Prevents aspiration of oropharyngeal fluids and aspiration of ingested food and liquids
Ciliated epithelial cells	Coordinated ciliary motion constantly moves the "carpet" of mucus and other endobronchiolar fluids toward the proximal larger airways for subsequent expectoration by the host
Mucus	Produced by resident goblet cells within the tracheobronchial tree, mucus provides a vehicle for cilia to expel potential contaminants and also provides a protective layer to prevent bacterial binding to epithelial cells
Secretory IgA antibody	Binds to bacterial contaminants and prevents bacteria from then binding to epithelial cells
Secretory IgG antibody	Predominantly identified in the distal airways, this antibody serves as an opsonin to facilitate macrophage and neutrophil phagocytosis
Surfactant/fibronectin/C-reactive protein	All appear to have nonspecific opsonic functions that facilitate the phagocytic clearance of bacteria
Lactoferrin/transferrin	Binds iron within the microenvironment of the lung and prevent bacterial growth and proliferation
Alveolar macrophage	Represents the primary phagocyte of the alveolar area and becomes the important cell to signal neutrophil invasion of the lung when potential infection is initiated

Ig, immunoglobulin.

cells. These antibodies are elaborated continuously by submucosal plasma cells and resident lymphocytes within the epithelial lining of the lung. They become a part of the admixture of the mucus coat. IgA does not fix complement and therefore does not have cytotoxicity for bacterial pathogens. It does not appear to serve a role for microbial opsonization.

Several mechanisms do appear to serve primarily an opsonic function. IgG antibody has been identified in greater concentrations in the distally bronchoalveolar areas of the lung. It is probably associated with opsonization or even lysis of microorganisms through the activation of complement. Surfactant binding to the surface of microbes may facilitate phagocytosis. Similarly, fibronectin binding, particularly to *Staphylococcus* spp, may serve an opsonic function. Finally, C-reactive protein, and possibly other acute phase reactants that are upregulated through the proinflammatory response, may serve an opsonic function.

Bacteria have specific needs for certain trace elements and nutrients from their environment. Therefore, nonspecific host defenses that restrict the availability of these trace requirements can be effective in retardation of bacterial growth. Iron is a particularly important element facilitating bacterial growth. Many bacteria have their own siderophore mechanisms to bind iron from the microenvironment. Nonspecific host defenses of the lung restrict iron availability by the competitive chelation of iron by lactoferrin within the

mucosal secretions of the larger airways and the presence of transferrin within the alveolar secretions.

The final intrinsic host defense mechanism of the lung to be discussed is the alveolar macrophage. These phagocytic cells "patrol" the alveolar space for evidence of potential pathogens at the most distal portion of the airway. Putative pathogens within the alveolar space are phagocytosed promptly. Like other macrophages, bacterial growth and proliferation in this space elicits a prompt response of local cytokine release, which ushers the full forces of the inflammatory response. Neutrophils are likewise drawn into the area by the chemotactic signals synthesized upon activation of the macrophage. IL-8 appears to be a particularly important neutrophil chemoattractant that is released by the activated alveolar macrophage. In addition, IL-8 serves an important endocrine role in promoting systemic neutrophilia. Additional monocytes are mobilized into the evolving inflammatory focus by the production of monocyte chemotactic protein by the alveolar macrophage. Eradication of pathogens becomes the objective in this setting in much the same way that phagocytic cells respond to soft tissue contamination. Macrophage inflammatory proteins appear to be an important signal to stimulate neutrophil phagocytic activity in the evolving lung infection.

Pneumonia in the postoperative period occurs by three separate routes, each of which is discussed. The common feature of pneumonia, regardless of the clinical setting,

TABLE 9.13

Identifies the Most Common Pathogens that are Associated with Postoperative Pneumonia

Pulmonary Pathogens	Percentage of Isolates	Comments
Pseudomonas sp.	30–40	The most common ICU isolate with a resistant antibiotic sensitivity pattern
Klebsiella/Enterobacter spp	25–35	Have increased in frequency in many areas because of expanded-spectrum β-lactamase production
Staphylococcus aureus	25–35	Have increased as a cause of ventilator-associated pneumonia with 60% of isolates being MRSA
Escherichia coli	10–20	This organism is seen in both nonventilator and ventilator-associated infections. Generally seen in patients without antecedent antibiotic therapy
Enterococcus sp	<5	This pathogen is increasing in many areas as vancomycin-resistant E. faecium in particular is increasingly being identified
Streptococcus pneumoniae	5–10	Usually in nonventilator patients with short preoperative hospitalization and no prior antibiotics
Hemophilus influenzae	3–5	Nonventilator-associated pathogen, associated in patients with chronic lung disease

is that the host defenses of the lung are compromised, which renders the lung vulnerable to either endogenous colonization or externally introduced bacterial pathogens. The common pathogens of postoperative pneumonias are identified in Table 9.13.

Nonventilator-Associated Pneumonia

The nonventilator-associated pneumonia group consists of patients with an inadequate minute volume of ventilation. With an inadequate tidal volume per ventilatory cycle and without periodic "sigh" respirations, collapse of multiple segments of alveoli and small airways results in the clinical syndrome of atelectasis. With atelectasis, the normal movement of mucus through ciliary action is compromised, and those bacteria customarily expelled become entrapped in a confined space. Bacterial proliferation begins, and the alveolar macrophage responds by initiating the inflammatory response. Endogenous pyrogens from the alveolar macrophages elicit a systemic febrile response, and similarly the release of IL-1 and particularly IL-8 promote neutrophilia. Neutrophils migrate to the area of bronchoalveolar collapse and the evolving inflammatory response. Bacterial invasion into adjacent but previously uninvolved areas of lung results in clinical infection as the inflammatory response extends into larger segments of pulmonary tissue.

The postoperative patient has numerous reasons to have a reduced tidal volume. Anesthetic agents and analgesia employed in the immediate postoperative period reduce ventilatory drive and the minute volume of gas exchange. Painful thoracic and abdominal incisions cause "splinting,"

that is, patients avoid deep ventilatory activity. Splinting predisposes to atelectasis, compromised mucociliary function, and invasive infection.

The prevention of nonventilator-associated pneumonia is the correction of the fundamental pathophysiology. The airways and alveoli should be kept expanded by early ambulation, coughing, and deep breathing. Fever within the initial 24 hours of an operation will most commonly be atelectasis. A rapid response by the clinician to atelectasis will re-expand collapsed bronchoalveolar units and abort the evolving infection without the use of systemic antibiotics. Re-expansion of atelectatic segments of lung is associated with resolution of the postoperative fever.

When new infiltrates are identified on the chest roentgenogram, the inflammatory response has become severe enough to make a diagnosis of pneumonia. Treatment of established pneumonia requires continued efforts to restore reinflation of the collapsed airways. In severe or rapidly evolving cases, ventilator support may be necessary because the number of involved pulmonary units may actually compromise systemic oxygenation. Antibiotic therapy should focus on culture-proven bacterial pathogens.

Empirical drug therapy is necessary when culture data are pending or are not available. Although the magnitude and the composition of normal colonization of the healthy human airway remain unclear, the hospitalized surgical patient is certainly colonized. In older patients and in patients with elements of chronic lung disease, normal colonists of the airway include S. pneumoniae and H. influenzae. These become common pathogens for pneumonia in postoperative patients with a limited preoperative hospitalization and no antecedent antibiotic therapy. When preoperative hospitalization has exceeded several days or when patients have received a course of antibiotics, colonization of the respiratory tract will be with more resistant hospital-acquired bacteria. Culture data in this latter group become important in guiding subsequent antibiotic therapy.

It is important to draw the analogy of bronchopneumonia with a pyogenic process anywhere else in the body. The disease is the consequence of bacterial proliferation that arises from within the respiratory tract. The inflammatory response results in purulence that still requires mechanical drainage. In addition to antibiotic therapy, tracheobronchial toilet must be continued to facilitate recovery from postoperative pneumonia. Coughing, expectoration, suctioning, and postural chest physiotherapy remain necessary treatments that are designed to drain the infected lung of the retrained inflammatory exudate.

Ventilator-Associated Pneumonia

The use of mechanical ventilation in postoperative patients has become commonplace. The ventilator is necessary when patients have had lengthy procedures, massive blood and crystalloid volume administration, blunt chest trauma, or when preexisting lung disease is present. Ventilator support becomes important for the patient but represents a means for increased rates for postoperative pneumonia.

Unfortunately, the ventilator-assisted patient has virtually every host defense mechanism of the lung compromised either by the ventilation process or by the patient's underlying disease. The endotracheal tube eliminates the barrier defense of the glottis in the prevention of direct access of bacteria into the trachea. The balloon-tipped endotracheal appliance may cause abrasion or pressure necrosis of the tracheal epithelial lining. Edema of the pulmonary parenchyma may likewise interfere with mucociliary action, and loss of the cough reflex further compromises expectoration of bacteria-laden mucus. Pulmonary bacterial clearance appears to be compromised by pulmonary contusion, steroids, remote infection, shock, and probably by increased lung water. The combination of direct bacterial access through the airway appliance combined with the fundamental disease processes makes pneumonia an unfortunate outcome for many patients.

The prevention of ventilator-associated pneumonia requires efforts to reduce bacterial contamination and vigorous treatment of the underlying process responsible for the ventilator support. Adherence to conventional infection control practices in the placement and management of the endotracheal tube will minimize the early introduction of bacteria into the airway. Minimizing unnecessary volume administration may reduce the risks of tissue edema. Defined protocols that focus on early weaning and extubation may be the most important aspect for prevention of infection. Preventive antibiotics will only change the character of bacterial colonization, thereby changing the likely pathogens, but they will not affect the frequency of pneumonia.

The treatment of ventilator-associated pneumonia is difficult. Host defenses are compromised and bacterial pathogens are generally the most resistant organisms characteristic of the surgical ICU. *Pseudomonas* spp and resistant expanded-spectrum β-lactamase producing Enterobacteriaceae are the common pathogens of these pneumonias. Within the last decade, MRSA has increased in frequency and are the most common pathogen of pneumonia in the ICU in selected areas. Antibiotic therapy for the ventilator-associated pneumonia patient must be driven by culture and sensitivity documentation, although knowledge of the patterns of pathogens identified will permit the appropriate selection of empirical choices when culture results are not available. Frequent, effective suctioning of the large airways remains important. Tracheostomy may need to be done to facilitate the aggressive suctioning necessary for effective management of secretions.

The penetration of antibiotics into the pulmonary secretions of these patients is problematic. The inflammatory focus has a compromised blood flow secondary to the infection. Penetration of the antibiotics into the area is poor and usually requires high-dose therapy. Antibiotic therapy with one promising drug (daptomycin) failed in a clinical trial because of inadequate penetration of the drug into the lung fluid. Because of poor penetration of antibiotics and because of highly resistant pathogens, combination therapy is common for these pneumonias and dosing needs to be aggressive.

Aspiration-Associated Pneumonia

The third category of postoperative pneumonia is aspiration-associated pneumonia. This type of pneumonia may be the consequence of either vomiting and aspiration of gastric contents into the lung, or a more subtle, occult aspiration of oropharyngeal fluids that provide the bacterial inoculum, which may subsequently cause clinical infection.

Gross aspiration pneumonia is initially a chemical pneumonitis. Particulate matter becomes the foreign body adjuvant that fosters bacterial growth and proliferation. Aspiration of unbuffered gastric contents causes a severe chemical injury of the lung as a sterile inflammatory response is provoked. The chemical pneumonitis from aspiration means that the lung becomes extremely vulnerable to intercurrent bacterial contamination. If the chemical pneumonitis is sufficiently severe, the patient will require ventilatory support, and the scenario of ventilator-associated pneumonia will have been created. Pneumonia in such circumstances is often very severe.

Prevention of aspiration-associated pneumonia requires recognition of the patient at risk. Gross aspiration may be a consequence of altered sensorium and a distended stomach. The altered sensorium is commonly caused by head injury, persistent effects of anesthesia, or postoperative analgesic excess. Elderly postoperative patients may have sensorium changes independent of any of these clinical variables. Gastric distention may be from recently eaten food, as is seen in trauma cases, or it may be from gaseous distention of the stomach. Distention from swallowed air or from active insufflation, such as Ambu bag–associated ventilation, sets the stage for vomiting and aspiration. Nasogastric tube decompression in these clinical scenarios seems warranted. Preventive antibiotics given in a futile attempt to prevent bacterial colonization and infection after the aspiration event will only promote resistant bacteria. Treatment of aspiration-associated pneumonia becomes essentially the same as for ventilator-associated infection.

The aspiration of oropharyngeal fluids may occur in postoperative patients, patients who have had nasogastric tubes in place for a sustained period of time, and older patients with a loss in hypopharyngeal sensation. Subtle and occasional aspiration events probably affect all adults but are inconsequential because of the normal paroxysms of coughing that are usually provoked. In seriously ill patients, the cough reflex is suppressed.

The risk of subtle aspiration of oropharyngeal fluids is a problem, and for the seriously ill patient, the colonization of the upper aerodigestive tract may be with resistant hospital-acquired nosocomial pathogens. Prolonged hospitalization and attendant systemic antibiotic therapy increases the risk of resistant colonization.

Prevention of this subtle form of aspiration pneumonia has proved difficult. Oropharyngeal antibiotic pastes have been used and have been reported to be of value. Topical antibiotics invariably lead to enhanced microbial resistance; accordingly, long-term consequences of the routine use of oropharyngeal antibiotics should be suspect for induction of resistance.

Reduction in acid production by the stomach has been a goal of therapy in the critical care unit patient to prevent stress-associated gastritis and bleeding. H2-antihistamine blockers and proton-pump inhibitors are the most common drugs used for this purpose, but the effects of alkalinization of the stomach makes for a reservoir for resistant bacteria for the ICU environment. Migration and reflux of these resistant bacteria into the upper aerodigestive tract are thought to be aspirated and sources of pneumonia. Sucralfate as a nonalkalinizing agent has been employed to be a barrier to prevent stress gastritis but avoid acid reduction. Although considerable evidence points to as association between antiacid therapies and pulmonary infection, the benefits of prevention of stress gastritis has led to the continued use of antacid drugs.

Postoperative Urinary Tract Infection

UTI following surgical procedures is usually the consequence of Foley catheterization. The human urinary tract from the pelvis of the kidney to the proximal opening of the urethra at the bladder trigone is with reduced bacterial colonization. The urethra as the communicating channel to the outside is colonized with small numbers of bacteria at its distal most extent. Encroachment of the minimally contaminated area of the urinary bladder by the Foley catheter provides the avenue for bacterial colonization.

TABLE 9.14

Host-Defense Mechanisms that Prevent Infection within the Urinary Tract

Host-Defense Element	Mechanism of Action
Urine flow	Constant urine flow provides resistance to retrograde migration of bacteria either proximally in the ureters or retrograde within the urethra
Ureterocystic antireflux mechanism	The angulation and submuscular course of the ureters when entering the urinary bladder cause a function antireflux mechanism that prevents retrograde urine flow from the bladder
Transitional epithelium	The cellular lining of the urinary bladder is resistant to bacterial binding; injury to the epithelial layer secondary to the Foley catheter is a major factor in increased infection rates secondary to catheter utilization
Urethral mucus	Provides a physical barrier to bacterial binding to the mucosal cells of the urethra
Urethral IgA	Binds to putative bacterial pathogens within the urethra and prevents their binding to epithelial cells both within the urethra itself and potentially within the bladder.
Urethral length	The male urethra is of sufficient length that retrograde migration is infrequent in he absence of instrumentation

The host defense of the urinary tract is simple but generally effective (Table 9.14). The constant flow of urine from the kidney to the bladder combined with a functional ureterocystic antireflux mechanism prevents bacterial colonization of the upper tract. For most patients infection or colonization within the bladder does not result in ascending infection.

The urinary bladder and urethra have numerous host defense mechanisms that prevent infection. The bladder is lined by transitional epithelium, which resists bacterial binding. The mucus of the urethra has bacteriostatic properties and also secretes IgA to coat would-be pathogens and prevent their binding to epithelial cells. Voiding activity has the mechanical effect of "flushing" the system, and infection is generally an uncommon event. For male patients, the 20-cm length of the urethra makes UTI in the absence of bladder intubation unusual. The shorter female urethra (5 cm) makes retrograde bacterial colonization and community-associated UTI more common.

With placement of a Foley catheter, all host defense mechanisms are breeched. The catheter provides direct access to the lumen of the bladder through a patent tube for contamination from the external world. The catheter within the urethra erodes and inflames the urethral mucosa and neutralizes the mucin and IgA protective mechanisms. The space between the outer wall of the Foley catheter and the urethral mucosa is no longer subject to the cleansing effect of periodic urination. As a result, retrograde migration of bacteria within this biologic dead space sets the stage for proximal proliferation and migration of bacteria around the catheter and into the bladder. In addition, the inflated balloon of the Foley catheter erodes and abraids the transitional epithelium at the trigone and provides the portal of entry for bacteria into the bladder wall.

Finally, bacterial pathogens adhere to the catheter itself and by this means escape being eliminated by the normal process of voiding. Catheters seem to impair the normal function of phagocytic cells that would potentially rid the urinary tract of the unwanted colonization. As with other indwelling foreign devices, bacteria that colonize the catheter may produce a biofilm that protects the microorganisms from either being mechanically expelled or ingested through the host phagocytic cells.

The pathogenic bacteria that cause UTI are those that colonize the perineum of the patient. Surface colonization of the skin becomes the colonists of the catheter and the pericatheter space of the urethra. Despite the heavy colonization in the area with anaerobic bacteria, anaerobes are rare pathogens of the urinary tract. This probably reflects the unfavorable oxidation-reduction potential of the bladder lumen for anaerobic growth. Therefore *E. coli,* as the predominant aerobic organism of the perineum, is the most common pathogen causing UTI.

Owing to the duration of hospitalization and the use of antibiotics in patients with indwelling Foley catheters, *E. coli* is less predominant in the urinary tract than would ordinarily be expected (Table 9.15). The duration

of hospitalization results in competing colonization of the perineum with resistant nosocomial pathogens. Systemic antibiotics will almost invariably have activity against *E. coli* and other common enteric bacteria, which further affects the selection process to favor resistant organisms. Indeed, postoperative patients with greater than 48 hours of prior antibiotic therapy will have a statistically greater probability of having *Pseudomonas* spp or *Enterobacter* spp as urinary tract pathogens.

An understanding of the biology of UTI provides the basis for prevention strategies. Adherence to accepted infection control practices in placement of the catheter is obviously important. Anchoring the catheter in place after placement avoids erosion of the balloon on the epithelial lining of the bladder and reduces irritation of the urethra itself. To-and-fro movements of the unanchored catheter will have a sump action and will facilitate the migration of bacteria into the bladder. Obviously, removal of the catheter at the earliest possible time after its purpose has been served is the best way of preventing catheter-induced UTI. Although bladder irrigation with antimicrobial solutions is a common practice in an attempt to prevent UTI, such practices when studied prospectively do not reduce infection rates but certainly do increase the likelihood of resistant pathogens ultimately being cultured.

Treatment of established infection is with antibiotic therapy. Because hospital-acquired pathogens are characteristically more resistant to conventional antibiotic choices, culture and sensitivity data are important. Restoration of urine flow is an underdiscussed but important treatment for the patient with a postcatheterization UTI. Urine flow restores normal homeostasis for the bladder and the urethra by the evacuation of microorganisms. Indeed, the truly invasive

TABLE 9.15

Identifies the Bacterial Pathogens Identified in Surgical Patients with Foley Catheter–Associated Urinary Tract Infections

Pathogen	Percentage of Isolates	Comments
Escherichia coli	25–40	Although still most common, this is a much lower frequency than community-acquired urinary tract infection
Pseudomonas spp	20–25	Seldom seen pathogen in community-acquired infection, it occurs in ICU and with prior systemic antibiotic therapy
Enterobacter spp	10–20	This pathogen has really increased in hospitals with expanded-spectrum β-lactamase pathogens
Klebsiella spp	5–10	This second most common community-acquired bacteria is seen infrequently in hospitalized UTIs
Enterococcus spp	5–10	Has increased in frequency as the resistant enterococci are increasing
Candida spp	5	May be a marker for candidiasis; occurs in immunocompromised patients

ICU, intensive care unit; UTI, urinary tract infection.

TABLE 9.16

Factors that Promote Infection with Intravascular Device Use

Factor Favoring Infection	Comment
Penetration of skin	The skin is the most effective of the nonspecific host defense mechanisms for the prevention of infection; subsequent bacterial proliferation around the skin puncture site will readily lead to migration down the catheter tunnel
Contamination of catheter and/or tunnel	Despite careful cleansing of the puncture site, some bacteria are carried down into the soft tissue with placement; subsequent skin growth and migration down into the tunnel makes infection virtually inevitable and underscores the need for periodic changes of the catheter site
Foreign body effect	The catheter itself results in binding of bacteria; the foreign body also retards phagocytic function and facilitates bacterial proliferation
Intimal injury/clot formation	The placement of the catheter (not to mention other failed attempts in the immediate area) results in intimal injury of the vessel and clot formation; the clot is ideal for bacterial growth and serves as a ready source of iron
Hub/device secondary contamination	The constant manipulation of the device and with changes of intravenous tubing results in unavoidable contamination of the device at the site of tubing changes; this can lead to secondary migration of bacteria down into the catheter tunnel and resultant infection

nature of many so-called UTI in postcatheterization patients is disputable and may only reflect colonization of the urinary bladder. Urine flow following catheter removal appears to restore the single most important nonspecific host defense mechanism of the urinary tract.

Occasionally, an acute septic event can be encountered in patients following catheter removal. The septic event is most often in postoperative patients, and when it occurs, it is usually associated with acute urinary retention. Stagnant and heavily colonized urine within the urinary bladder after a period of catheterization will cause invasive infection and bacteremia especially if voiding is less than complete following removal of the catheter. The inability to void after catheterization, especially among male patients, may result from several sources; among these are underlying spasms from a mild bacterial infection or from obstructive outflow disease (e.g., prostatic hypertrophy). Replacement of the catheter to effect drainage of the infected bladder is an important treatment for these patients in the same way that draining pus is important at any anatomic location.

Intravascular Device Infection

The placement of indwelling devices directly into the vascular tree through percutaneous penetration of the skin has become extraordinarily valuable for the management and monitoring of surgical patients. Peripheral intravenous lines, central venous lines, arterial lines, and Swan-Ganz catheters have become standard and accepted parts of the management of surgical patients. However, the placement of a foreign body conduit into the intravascular compartment poses a major

breech to the epithelial barrier and provides a direct avenue for bacterial penetration and dissemination (Table 9.16).

An indwelling intravascular catheter is a wound in the skin that has a foreign body within it. This leads directly into the intravascular compartment. Soft tissue trauma is created by the percutaneous puncture, which activates all the elements of inflammation. With the percutaneous puncture, skin bacteria can be introduced into the percutaneous tunnel that represents the track from the patient's skin to the venous structure. Bacteria from the individual placing the catheter may actually be the microorganisms that contaminate the tract. These contaminating microorganisms are harbored in the pericatheter space between the external wall of the catheter and the adjacent soft tissue of the tract. The injury created by the trauma of catheter placement, the foreign body itself, and the contaminating bacteria about the catheter establish an inflammatory response in the microenvironment.

Another important pathophysiologic event occurs at the site where the catheter actually penetrates the vein. Intimal disruption of the vein and placement of a foreign body in a peripheral vein predispose to the formation of a platelet plug and clot formation. If multiple passes of the catheter were attempted before achieving successful catheterization, multiple areas of intimal injury may be present in proximity to the ultimate site of venous cannulation. The indwelling segment of the catheter may also damage the venous endothelium by to-and-fro movements created by normal patient activity. Finally, hypotonic, hypertonic, or otherwise noxious substances within the infusate may damage the venous endothelium and produce thrombosis of the vein. The net consequence of these variables of venous endothelial injury is clot, an ideal situation for bacterial proliferation.

A mechanism for catheter contamination involves the care of the puncture site. The skin about the site of percutaneous catheter placement is cleansed, albeit in a superficial and commonly haphazard manner, at the time of catheter placement. A porous dressing may be placed over the site. Commonly, the gauze dressing is assaulted by fluids. The hub of the catheter is usually handled by a different individual as each new infusion is begun. This results in bacterial contamination and proliferation about the site of the skin puncture and may lead to the migration and proliferation of bacteria down the catheter and into the pericatheter space. Like the Foley catheter infection, the pericatheter space serves as the reservoir for bacterial proliferation and a source for contamination of the intravascular component of the catheter. If an intravascular clot is present, it too becomes infected. Bacterial proliferation proceeds within this environment that is rich in nutrients (particularly iron), and bacteremia is the consequence.

Therefore, it should be no surprise that staphylococcal organisms are the most common bacteremic pathogen associated with intravascular device infections. *S. aureus* and *S. epidermidis* represent approximately two thirds of the pathogens from such devices. In the ICU, the patient who is exposed to the nosocomial pathogens and broad-spectrum antibiotic regimens frequently have a gram-negative rod contaminating their intravascular device. Central lines seem to have a certain predilection for being contaminated by *C. albicans* and other *Candida* species.

Prevention and treatment of this problem can then be formulated by understanding the biology of how infection occurs in this setting. Careful cleansing of the skin at the time of placement is of paramount importance. Continued care of the skin site, particularly for central lines and Swan-Ganz lines that will remain in place for a sustained period of time, is essential. Because the real culprit in peripheral catheter bacteremia is the foreign body within the soft tissue wound, removal and rotation of the catheter site every 48 to 72 hours for peripheral lines is of vital importance. Preventive systemic antibiotics will only change the pathogen that will ultimately colonize the puncture site and the catheter. Topical antiseptics and topical antibiotics about the puncture site have been used commonly, but objective evidence that bacteremic events are actually prevented is difficult to find. Impregnation of catheters with silver compounds and other antimicrobial agents are being explored for prevention of infection, but none have generally been accepted. Adherence to infection control practices in the placement and management, along with rotation of peripheral sites, appears to be the best recourse to prevent intravenous catheter bacteremia.

Treatment of intravenous device–related bacteremia requires a high index of suspicion that the catheter is the culprit. Infected catheters need to be removed and cultured by the semiquantitative technique. Appropriate antibiotic therapy needs to be started. The bacteremia associated with gram-negative organisms tends to be shortlived after removal of the catheter, and long-term drug therapy (>48–72 hours) is probably not justified. Because *S. aureus* may cause metastatic infection to heart valves, and because *C. albicans* may cause metastatic infection to the eye, a full 7- to 10-day course of antimicrobial chemotherapy is necessary for these organisms.

Customarily, the septic response that is triggered by the bacteremia from a device will defervesce promptly after catheter removal. Persistence of the bacteremia may mean that the patient has suppurative thrombophlebitis. The clot within the venous structures at the site of catheter placement can support bacterial growth even after removal of the foreign body. Such situations can develop into intravascular abscesses with continued bacteremia from the site. Excision of the infected vein may be necessary and must be pursued for the patient with persistent bacteremia. *S. aureus* device infections are notorious for this complication.

Clostridium Difficile Enterocolitis

C. difficile enterocolitis has become a major nosocomial pathogen in recent years. This bacterium, like all clostridial species, is an obligate anaerobe that exists in spore form in nature. Ingestion of the spores followed by ecologic change in the microflora of the colon, or ingestion of the spores after ecologic changes are already present, permits the transformation of the spore to the vegetative form of the organism. The vegetative form adheres to the colonocyte specifically where Toxin A and Toxin B are released. Enterocolitis is the consequence from the cytotoxic effects on the colon, which commonly gives an endoscopic picture of pseudomembranes from the local inflammatory response in the colon mucosa. With severe disease, usually among older patients who may have received antimotility drug treatments, impairment of colonic peristaltic activity leads to toxic megacolon and even full-thickness necrosis of the colon. Antimotility agents that may be significant in this clinical setting include codeine-based pain medications, loperamide HCL (Imodium), and diphenoxylate/atropine (Lomotil). The marked inflammatory response to the released toxins involves the colonic smooth muscle which leads to loss of normal peristalsis, and without effective elimination of the toxin by diarrhea, the toxic megacolon state is the consequence. In this latter scenario, the disease has often progressed beyond management with either oral metronidazole or oral vancomycin therapy and surgical subtotal colectomy may well be required.

At a pathophysiologic level, many changes have evolved with *C. difficile* over the last decade that has made it a major nosocomial pathogen. First, new strains of the bacterium are identified which produce 16 to 20 times the amount of toxin that was produced by the traditional pathogens. This results in a far more fulminate infection. This change has occurred because of the mutation of a gene that regulates synthesis. This production of larger amounts of the toxin results in rapid progression to toxic megacolon with patients having only a limited period of time with the actual clinical diarrhea syndrome. Second, resistance to conventional antimicrobial treatment is being reported and newer antibiotic agents are going to be needed. Finally, community-associated *C. difficile* enterocolitis is being identified in patients without prior hospitalization or prior antibiotic therapy. This is still likely spores from the hospital reservoir that have been transmitted by another person to the naïve host, but does reflect a change in the recognized pattern of the disease.

Other Infections

Although the infections discussed earlier clearly represent most of the infections that are encountered by the surgeon, there are, obviously, others that do occur. Posttraumatic meningitis, suppurative sinusitis, parotitis, and septic arthritis are but a few of the less common but significant infections that can be encountered in the surgical patient.

Posttraumatic meningitis is the consequence of injury that disrupts the bony encasement of the brain and results in contamination of the meninges by organisms. Basilar skull fractures are notorious for allowing microorganisms of the upper aerodigestive tract to contaminate the meninges and the subarachnoid space. Infection is often the result. Binding of bacterial cells to the meningeal cell, bacterial proliferation, and activation of the inflammatory response become the common features that make this infection similar to other infections.

Nosocomial sinusitis is another infection that can be clinically subtle in postoperative patients. Chronic nasogastric intubation, which inflames and potentially impairs free drainage from the sinus cavities, combined with antibiotic therapy, which alters the normal colonization, can cause a contamination of static sinus fluids and subsequent acute bacterial infection.

Suppurative parotitis may be seen as a consequence of all the same variables that provoke infection in other tissues. It is likely that suppurative parotitis is the consequence of retrograde migration of bacteria through Wharton duct into the parenchyma of the parotid salivary gland. It is an uncommon infection, and normal salivary flow possibly removes potential bacterial colonists in the same way that urine flow maintains the relatively sterile environment of the urinary tract. Secretory IgA within salivary secretions prevents binding of pathogenic bacteria to the ductal system of the salivary gland. Under conditions of severe illness, salivary production declines and IgA production may be inadequate. Unfavorable bacterial overgrowth in the mouth allows potential pathogens to infect the parenchyma of the salivary gland.

Septic arthritis can be a complication of an open fracture of any joint. Contamination, binding of bacteria to the surface epithelium, proliferation, and inflammation can cause an active infection. Septic arthritis can even be the consequence of blood-borne contamination and does not always require actual penetration of the joint space. Both *Staphylococcus* spp and occasionally Group A streptococci are well known for causing primary septic joints.

Open fractures can predispose to a major infectious event in trauma patients. An open fracture is a soft tissue injury that has a broken bone within its midst. The combination of devitalized tissue, hematoma, bone sequestra, and an open avenue for bacterial access creates an ideal environment for bacterial proliferation. Infection may be associated with nonunion of the fracture and, potentially, amputation. Hospital-acquired bacteria appear to be the most common pathogens of these infections and underscore the failure of long-term preventive antibiotics to prevent infections.

Regardless of the site, a common theme in postoperative infection of any location is injury and contamination. This commonly occurs in the compromise of host defense mechanisms and results in bacterial proliferation and inflammation. Although the clinical presentation of infection assumes the unique feature of the anatomic area affected, the interaction between the host and potential pathogens is generic.

SPECIAL CONSIDERATIONS IN SURGICAL INFECTION

Postsplenectomy Sepsis

Fulminant bacteremia and septic deaths in patients with prior splenectomy were identified as infrequent but serious problems in the 1970s. The association of these bacteremic deaths with splenectomy changed attitudes about the clinical indications for splenectomy, particularly in patients who had sustained splenic trauma. Conservation of the spleen became a desired objective. Diagnosis of splenic injury without operation and nonoperative therapy became goals of management, particularly for younger patients. Studies were undertaken to elucidate the pathophysiologic consequences of splenectomy.

The splenic RE system removes bacterial cells that gain access to the circulation without the requirement that the potential pathogen be opsonized. Bacteria that gain access to the bloodstream are generally cleared efficiently by the splenic or hepatic RE cells. Pneumococcus and *H. influenzae* are encapsulated bacterial strains that likely gain access to the blood through the respiratory tract. These encapsulated bacteria are difficult for the hepatic RE cells to clear if the bacteria have not been opsonized adequately. Without specific immunization against the polysaccharide capsule of the specific bacterial strain in blood, opsonization is poor and the spleen rather than the liver is necessary for clearance. Splenectomized patients may not have efficient clearance if the patient does not have specific antibody for the pathogen to permit hepatic Kupffer recognition.

Therefore, the capacity for removal of encapsulated bacteria is achieved most effectively by the spleen. An acute IgM response from the white pulp of the spleen after a bacterial challenge results in the release of opsonic antibody to facilitate bacterial clearance by both the liver and the spleen. Loss of the spleen compromises the acute immune production of IgM and is associated with decreased clearance by the RE system.

An additional host defense mechanism for the spleen is the production of two nonspecific opsonins. Tuftsin appears to facilitate the clearance of bacteria and may also serve as a stimulant to the generalized phagocytic functions of the host. The spleen is also thought to be a major source for the synthesis of properdin, a protein important in the initiation of the alternative pathway of complement activation. The true significance of the loss of tuftsin remains unclear. The physiologic reserve within the complement cascade is such that splenectomy is probably not that important in increasing the host vulnerability secondary to decreased levels of tuftsin.

Splenectomy compromises the host. If splenectomy occurs in a preteen or an adolescent, he or she is vulnerable to acute overwhelming sepsis. Despite efforts at conservation, splenectomy remains a necessity for many patients. Methods to prevent this relatively infrequent (<1%) but morbid (death rates of 60%–70%) complications have been explored. The use of preventive antibiotics has been attempted and remains largely of unproven value. Long-term compliance with the daily administration of preventive antibiotic is unlikely. If compliance is adequate, long-term antibiotic administration is associated with all the problems of modifying the patient's resident microflora and selecting out resistant strains.

The polyvalent pneumococcal vaccine has been employed effectively to reduce the frequency of postsplenectomy sepsis. This vaccine provides immunization of the host against the 23 most common polysaccharide serotypes of pneumococci. Obviously, it does not provide protection against those serotypes not represented within the vaccine, nor does it provide protection against other bacterial strains (e.g., *H. influenzae*) that are known to be agents of postsplenectomy sepsis. *H. influenzae* and meningococcal vaccines are available and are used in splenectomized patients as well. Nevertheless, a risk remains for the splenectomized patient. Patient cognizance of the risk is essential so that immediate antibiotic therapy can be initiated at the first sign of a clinical infection.

Preventive Systemic Antibiotics

Classic animal studies demonstrated that administration of systemic antibiotics before tissue contamination was necessary if prevention of infection was to be achieved. It has been demonstrated that infection could be prevented if antibiotics were given before or at the same time as bacterial contamination. Antibiotics given after contamination were progressively less effective. Antibiotics given more than 2 to 4 hours after contamination had no preventive effect upon the natural history of the infection.

The failure of preventive systemic antibiotics in the early trials stemmed from the fact that the antibiotics were not administered before the operative procedure. In the early patient trials that did not show a drug effect, the antibiotics were invariably not given until after the patients were in the recovery room. As a result, active antibiotic was not present within the surgical wound fluid at the time of bacterial contamination. The importance of preoperative administration of the preventive antibiotic requires an understanding of the unique features of the surgical wound.

A surgical incision activates all the biological mechanisms of inflammation that were discussed earlier. Tissue injury activates complement proteins, mast cells, and most important, coagulation of serum proteins to form a fibrin interface across the cut surface of the wound. The process is an active one and occurs continuously, as long as the wound remains open. During the entire period of the procedure, bacterial contamination assaults the wound edges from all potential sources. Bacteria from the patient's skin, the air of the operating room, the gloves of the surgeon, and endogenous sources are lodged into the wound and become incorporated into the fibrin matrix at the wound interface. With completion of the procedure, the opposite sides of the surgical wound are approximated with sutures to create a fibrin "sandwich," which has varying concentrations of bacteria, depending on the magnitude of intraoperative contamination. Adjuvant factors within the closed wound such as hematoma, dead tissue (e.g., excessive use of the electrocautery), and foreign bodies (e.g., silk sutures) will then amplify the potential virulence of the bacterial contaminants. If the sum of the bacterial numbers plus adjuvant effects exceed the phagocytic functional capacity of the host, then infection results.

If antibiotics are initiated after the wound is closed, they are destined to fail. The fibrin matrix with its entrapped bacteria is relatively impervious to antibiotics. The closed wound has sustained edema formation from the continued effects of the vasoactive phase of inflammation, which increases the hydrostatic tissue pressure within the surgical wound. A perimeter of relative ischemia develops in the area of the incision.

The key to successful systemic use of preventive antibiotics is to administer the drug before the surgical incision so that adequate antibiotic concentrations may be present within the fibrin matrix as it forms. Precise surgical techniques to minimize the quantity of contamination during the procedure, control of adjuvant factors within the wound, and adequate wound concentrations of antibiotic throughout the duration of the procedure will minimize the likelihood of a wound infection.

The premise that the drug must be present within the wound during the period of fibrin formation and bacterial contamination can be violated by the use of antibiotics that have extraordinarily short biologic half-lives. For example, previous studies with cephalosporin antibiotics have shown that the drugs are present for approximately two half-lives within the surgical wound following systemic administration. Antibiotics with short half-lives must be redosed at that interval to maintain drug concentration in the surgical wound. It is desirable to use longer half-life antibiotics to cover the complete duration of the operative procedures so that redosing will not be necessary. When lengthy procedures are contemplated, a schedule for antibiotic redosing should be planned in advance to minimize the risks of unprotected periods of contamination.

Unfortunately, there is the tendency of surgeons to give preventive antibiotics for prolonged periods of time after wound closure. The evidence is clear that prolonged administration beyond 12 to 24 hours following wound closure do not improve patient outcomes. Prolonged preventive antibiotics do change the patient's colonization to resistant forms of bacteria. Any nosocomial infection will be resistant to the preventive antibiotic used. Prolonged preventive antibiotics are a needless expense and they set the stage for *C. difficile* enterocolitis.

Antibiotic Pharmacokinetics

Another important factor that results in poor biologic effect of antibiotic therapy, even when the microorganisms are sensitive to the drug employed, is antibiotic pharmacokinetics. The presumption of all systemic antibiotic treatment is that the drug reaches the site of infection in concentrations adequate to achieve an antimicrobial effect. This goal of therapy assumes that the dosing schedule is appropriate. To understand dosing schedules, fundamental knowledge of the dynamics of drug distribution and elimination is essential.

When an antibiotic is administered intravenously, the drug is distributed rapidly throughout the central pool of extracellular body water. The central pool represents the plasma volume and the freely diffusible area of the extracellular fluid volume. The antibiotic then proceeds through a secondary equilibration phase as the drug is distributed into cells and into other less readily reached areas of body fluid. Drug distribution into different tissues varies, depending on extracellular water volume, intracellular water volume, percentage of body weight that is adipose tissue, and whether the drug is freely transported across cell membranes and tissue barriers. For example, certain drugs readily pass across the blood–brain barrier and others do not. Access of a drug to the cerebrospinal fluid has obvious consequences to the total volume of water into which a drug is distributed. The volume of distribution reflects the theoretically maximum volume of body water to which a given drug has access and is extrapolated from a kinetic clearance plot (Fig. 9.10). The volume of distribution may be low and approximates only the extracellular water volume when a drug is highly protein bound and is excluded from the intracellular compartment. Paradoxically, the volume of distribution may exceed total body water and reflects the binding of the drug to interstitial or intracellular sites that are not in equilibrium with the central pool.

When the equilibrated concentration is achieved, the antibiotic concentration in the central pool is at a steady rate. As drug elimination occurs either through excretion or metabolism, a reduction of central pool concentration results. The rate of concentration decline follows a semilogarithmic linear pattern (Fig. 9.10). Drug elimination is therefore described as the biologic elimination half-life. The half-life is the time required for the drug concentration to decline by 50% after it has achieved the equilibrium state within the patient. The dosing interval for an antibiotic is

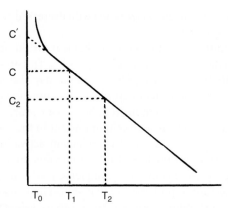

FIGURE 9.10 A standard antibiotic clearance curve from the serum of an adult patient. Drug concentration is measured to $\log_{10}$ on the ordinate and time is measured on the abscissa. At T_0, the peak antibiotic concentration is achieved, which rapidly enters the linear clearance curve. Extrapolation to the ordinate gives the serum concentration. This allows the computation of the volume of distribution. The time interval for the concentration to decline from point C to C/2 equals $T_2 - T_1$. The time it takes for the serum drug concentration to decline by 50% is the biologic elimination half-life.

determined by the number of half-lives that occur before the drug concentration declines below the target concentration required to achieve the desired effect.

Concern about the adequacy of drug dosing can cause surgeons to double the dose in an effort to get better therapeutic benefits. The consequence of doubling the dose is illustrated in Figure 9.11. Because the area under the

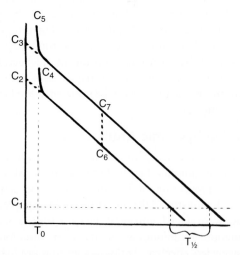

FIGURE 9.11 The effects on serum kinetics of an antibiotic caused by doubling its dose. Drug concentration is on the ordinate, and time is on the abscissa. Doubling the dose of the antibiotic doubles the peak concentration from C_4 to C_5 and the T_0-equilibrated concentration from C_2 to C_3. The drug concentration at any point in time is increased by one half-life, from C_6 to C_7. If C_1 represents the threshold of antibacterial action of the antibiotic, then doubling the dose increases antibacterial action by only one half-life.

elimination plot of an intravenously administered antibiotic represents the bioavailability of the drug, doubling the dose means that the area under the curve will be doubled. At most, the peak-equilibrated concentration of the antibiotic will be doubled. Because the elimination half-life is relatively constant across multiple drug doses, doubling the peak concentration will only extend the drug-dosing interval by one half-life. For long half-life antibiotics, the extended duration of drug presence about the threshold concentration might extend the dosing interval in a clinically relevant way. For short half-life drugs, doubling the dose not only tends to increase peak concentration, but also has minimal benefits for increasing the duration of drug presence in the central pool. The half-life of commonly employed β-lactam antibiotics are listed in Table 9.17.

Another concern about antibiotic use is whether the concentration at the target site, as opposed to the central pool, is adequate. Figure 9.12 illustrates the theoretical relations between the central pool and six other tissues. Tissue A might represent the biliary tract, where the drug in question

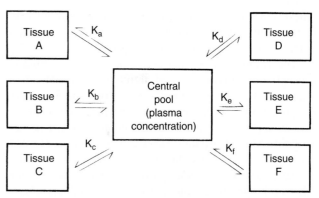

FIGURE 9.12 The relation between the central pool concentration and tissue concentrations. The variables that govern tissue penetration by a given antibiotic are complex. Tissue concentrations are not necessarily reflected by plasma measurements.

TABLE 9.17

Identifies the Different Biological Elimination Half-lives of Commonly Employed β-Lactam Antibiotics

β-Lactam Antibiotics	Elimination Half-Life
Penicillins	
Penicillin G	30 min
Ampicillin	1 h
Ticarcillin	70 min
Mezlocillin	55 min
Piperacillin	54–63 min
Cephalosporins	
Cephalothin	35 min
Cefazolin	1.7–2 h
Cefoxitin	41–59 min
Cefamandole	32 min
Cefuroxime	80 min
Cefonicid	4.5 h
Cefotetan	3–4.6 h
Cefotaxime	1 h
Cefoperazone	2 h
Ceftizoxime	1.7 h
Ceftriaxone	5.8–8.5 h
Ceftazidime	1.9 h
Cefopime	2 h
Monobactams	
Aztreonam	1.7 h
Carbapenems	
Imipenem	2–3 h
Meropenem	2–3 h
Ertepenem	4–5 h

Although much is made about the antimicrobial activity of antibiotics that are selected in patient care, only a limited amount of discussion is focused upon half-life. The half-life of the drug dictates the dosing schedule which may prove to be as important as the deoxyribonucleic acidantimicrobial activity.

is excreted into the bile and bile concentrations are actually higher than concurrent central pool concentrations. Tissue B might be the cerebrospinal fluid with essentially no identified concentration. Tissue C might be the subcutaneous tissue, and if the drug were lipophilic, antibiotic concentration might persist at significant concentrations long after the central pool concentration is zero. Tissue D might represent skeletal muscle, which is a well-vascularized tissue without intrinsic fat, and might have drug concentrations that will parallel those in serum. Tissue E might be bone, where the drug is slow to enter but is also slow to exit. Tissue F might represent infected lung tissue, where the inflammatory focus and the central area of the infection is somewhat remote from the nearest functioning microvascular units, with drug concentrations at a reduced level. Therefore, the rationale for increasing drug concentration in the central pool would theoretically increase the gradient of drug delivery into certain areas and might be of therapeutic benefit.

Unfortunately, drug-dosing schedules are designed for patients by trials in healthy volunteers. The critically ill surgical patient and the severely injured patient are not represented by healthy volunteers. First, the volume of distribution of most antibiotics will be dramatically increased in these patients. The so-called third space of injured patients and patients following major operations means that the functional interstitial space is increased dramatically. An increased volume of distribution means that peak concentrations will be less, and the duration of antibiotic concentration above the critical threshold target will be reduced. Second, the elimination half-life may be changed in the critically ill. Intrinsic failure of either kidney or liver function may prolong half-life. Patients with the septic response characteristically have an increased cardiac output and appear to have a corticomedullary redistribution of renal blood flow. The consequences of these changes are a loss of renal concentrating ability and increased secretory elimination of drugs that are eliminated by this mechanism (e.g., aminoglycosides) and a reduced elimination half-life. The net effect of physiologic changes mediated by critical illness is that adequate tissue antibiotic concentrations may be compromised. Suboptimal dosing schedules represent a potential problem for the severely ill patient.

The assumption here has been that sustained antibiotic concentration above the critical inhibitory threshold is important. For some antibiotics this is true, and for others it is probably not valid. Aminoglycosides bind irreversibly to ribosomal proteins. Saturation of binding sites means that a significant postantibiotic effect can be seen. Continued drug effect is identified for a period of hours after the central pool concentration approaches zero. However, for other antibiotics there is minimal or no postantibiotic effect. For example, cephalosporin binding to PBP, particularly in gram-negative bacteria is reversible. Reduced environmental concentration of the antibiotic results in dissociation of the antibiotic from the PBP. As a result, essentially no postantibiotic effect exists for cephalosporins against gram-negative bacteria.

Vascular Graft Infections

The use of prosthetic implants have become commonplace. The development and use of vascular prosthetic grafts have expanded enormously the surgical management options for patients with severe vascular disease. Prosthetic materials have even achieved a measure of popularity in the management of vascular trauma.

However, the vascular graft poses some special problems with respect to potential for the development of serious prosthesis-associated infections. The graft is a foreign body, which harbors adherent bacteria. The grafts are employed necessarily in ischemic tissues that are being revascularized. Revascularization is often attempted when open traumatic wounds or distal infection exists. Frequently, antecedent antibiotic therapy may have been necessary, which leaves the patient with resistant bacterial colonization.

The biology of graft infection is similar to wound infection in other settings with the exception that a large foreign body has been used. The surgically dissected wound will have a fibrin matrix, which develops like a film across the wound surface. Its quantity is a function of the procedure's duration. Bacteria may be entrapped into this fibrin matrix. When the vascular graft is placed, the activation of the coagulation cascade similarly occurs about the foreign body. A fibrin matrix develops around the entire graft's surface. Contamination during the placement of the graft is entrapped in this fibrin "cast." The foreign body effect reduces the number of bacteria that are necessary to cause clinical infection. Dead tissue about the graft from vigorous dissection or poorly perfused tissue also has a potent adjuvant effect. Retained blood clot augments the process. All the variables are present to favor infection.

It should be obvious that the biologic basis favoring an infectious complication in this setting is compelling. Effective infection control techniques aimed at reducing bacterial contamination during graft placement are vital. Reduction of other adjuvant factors such as clot, soft tissue ischemia, or dead tissue is equally important. The perioperative coverage of the wound with preventive antibiotics has been shown to reduce clinical wound infection and should reduce the probability of graft infection.

Graft infection is fortunately an uncommon event that complicates less than 1% of such procedures. The discharge of pus, thrombosis of the graft, and the development of pseudoaneurysms are common clinical indicators of infection. Graft infections are the consequence of operative contamination, even if the infection is not clinically identified for months or even years later. Although seeding of the graft from a secondary source of infection or bacteremia is clearly a possibility, and in patients with distal extremity infections is a real concern, operative contamination is by far the most common cause in prosthetic graft infection.

S. aureus has been the traditional pathogen of concern for graft infection. These bacteria are present on the patient's skin and in the environmental fallout in the operating room. MRSA have emerged as major problems in graft infections and the community-associated MRSA looms as yet another potential threat. Gram-negative bacteria can be a particular problem if the patient has had a prolonged preoperative hospitalization or has had a course of antecedent systemic antibiotics.

S. epidermidis has become a pathogen of considerable significance. The resistance of *S. epidermidis* to many antistaphylococcal antibiotics has resulted in colonization of patients in the hospital environment. This organism appears to be the primary pathogen for graft infections that are delayed in clinical presentation. The ability of these organisms to form a glycoprotein matrix about the foreign body surface results in protection of the pathogen from host phagocytosis. It also makes culturing the organism from delayed infections difficult. Sonication of the infected graft material appears to be an important means of disrupting the glycocalyx and permitting culture of the pathogen from the supernatant.

The biological basis for the treatment of graft infection is removal of the foreign body. It is generally unrealistic to think that antibiotics will sterilize infections of prosthetic material. Furthermore, immediate placement of a new prosthetic into the infected environment of the former graft bed seems to be destined for failure in most cases. The options for management require alternate routes to restore perfusion to the tissues that are served by the vascular graft. However, biologic lesions are commonly relearned time and time again. Infections of foreign bodies require removal of the foreign body. Antibiotics have yet to override this fact.

Hepatitis

Hepatitis has significance for surgeons because chronic hepatitis B virus (HBV)) and chronic hepatitis C virus (HCV) result in cirrhosis, end-stage liver disease, and portal hypertension. Of particular significance is the occupational risk for infection that these viruses pose to surgeons.

Six hepatitis viruses are currently identified (Table 9.18). Hepatitis A virus (HAV) and hepatitis E virus (HEV) are fecal–oral transmitted RNA viruses that cause an acute viral

TABLE 9.18

Identifies the Characteristics of the Six Recognized Viruses of Hepatitis

Hepatitis Virus	Transmission	Route of Chronic/Persistent Infection	Vaccine	Nucleic Acid	Occupational Risk
HAV	Fecal–oral	No	Yes	RNA	None
HBV	Blood borne;	Yes	Yes	DNA	30% with needle injury in unvaccinated host
HCV	Blood borne	Yes	No	RNA	2% with needle injury
HDV	Blood borne	Yes	No	RNA	None
HEV	Fecal–oral	No	No	RNA	None
HGV	Blood borne	Yes	No	RNA	None

HAV, hepatitis A virus; RNA, ribonucleic acid; HBV, hepatitis B virus; DNA, deoxyribonucleic acid; HCV, hepatitis C virus; HEV, hepatitis E virus; HGV, hepatitis G virus.

infection but do not cause chronic, persistent infection. Although the acute infection with HAV and HEV can be severe, deaths from infection are infrequent and the infections resolve completely with no chronic sequelae. Hepatitis D virus (HDV) is an incomplete viral pathogen that requires a coexistent infection (i.e., HBV) to cause infection. Occupational risk of infection from HDV is possible but not a likely event. Hepatitis G is seldom associated with acute infection and is not considered an occupational risk.

HBV is a DNA virus that is the cause of chronic infection in more than 1 million people in the United States. Infection is transmitted by percutaneous injury and sexual contact. Acute infection generates a prompt antibody response, and prior infection confers life-long immunity from reinfection. Approximately 5% of acute infection results in chronic infection. Chronic infection leads to a persistent stage of antigen positivity. Chronic infection leads to limited progression of disease for many individuals, although they remain infectious to others. Severe and progressive liver injury occurs for others with cirrhosis, portal hypertension, and hepatocellular carcinoma being the end result. The liver injury is likely due to the robust response of the host inflammatory response rather than specific cytotoxicity of the replicating virus. Vaccination against HBV is achieved with a highly immunogenic recombinant vaccine. A positive IgG antibody response should be documented after the three-dose schedule is complete because approximately 5% of individuals do not respond to the initial vaccination.

Patients (and infected surgeons) may be positive for the e-antigen for HBV. The e-antigen is a degradation product of the viral nucleocapsid and is a surrogate marker for high-viral DNA concentrations in the blood of the infected individual. An e-antigen–positive surgeon is a potential risk to patients with some evidence indicating that antigen may actually be shed into the surgical glove during operations from nonintact skin of the hand.

HCV is an RNA virus of six different serotypes that is a chronic infection in 3 to 4 million people in the

United States. Infection is transmitted by percutaneous injury with a contaminated device (e.g., needle, tattoo, etc). Acute infection yields a clinically occult infection in 75% of patients, but nevertheless results in 60% to 80% of infected individuals with chronic disease. The antibody response is delayed for up to 6 months following acute infection. A sustained positive antibody titer is evidence of chronic infection. Patients recovering from the acute infection do not have immunity against reinfection. Chronic HCV has an unpredictable natural history with many patients being antibody and antigen-positive but have no progression of disease, and selected patients spontaneously resolve the infection after years. Hepatocellular carcinoma and end-stage liver disease is a risk for those developing cirrhosis. HCV infection is the leading cause for liver transplantation. No vaccine is available and is very problematic for development when even acute HCV infection does not confer protective immunity against future reinfection. Surgeons are at risk for this infection with clinical evidence that 2% of percutaneous injuries of health care workers from infected patients result in occupational transmission. Four surgeons have been documented from the literature to have transmitted HCV infection to patients.

The pathophysiology of hepatitis viruses in human blood is an incomplete story. The old non-A, non-B hepatitis of 20 years ago was not fully explained by the identification of HCV and is currently replaced by non-A–G hepatitis. There remains evidence that additional transmissible hepatitis viruses are yet to be identified.

Human Herpesviruses

There are eight human herpesviruses that are recognized which cause infection (Table 9.19). The human herpesviruses infect host cells in a manner consistent with DNA viruses that was described earlier. Thymidine kinase, DNA polymerase, and other enzymes arise from the viral DNA to produce new viral particles. Each herpesvirus has a target cell population.

The unique feature of herpesvirus infection is latency. Although an active clinical state of infection is not present,

TABLE 9.19

Identifies the Chararcteristics of the Eight Human Herpesvirus Infections

Virus Type	Route of Transmission	Site of Latency	Clinical Disease
HHV-1	Saliva	Sensory nerve ganglia	Herpes simplex
HHV-2	Sexual contact	Sensory/autonomic ganglia	Genital herpes
HHV-3	Saliva/airborne droplets	Sensory ganglia	Chickenpox/herpes zoster
HHV-4	Saliva/intimate contact	Sensory ganglia/salivary glands	Mononucleosis; Burkitt lymphoma
HHV-5	Oral/genital secretions/blood transfusion organ transplantation	Monocytes/neutrophils	Cytomegalovirus infection
HHV-6	Saliva	Macrophages	Roseola infantum
HHV-7	Saliva	CD4$^+$ lymphocytes	Not understood
HHV-8	Genital secretions blood transfusion transplantation	Endothelial cells	Kaposi sarcoma

HHV, human herpesvirus.

the virus assumes a quiescent state only to be reactivated at a future time. Biological stress and immunosuppressive events are associated with reactivation of the clinical disease. More than 90% of the population has one or more latent human herpesviruses.

Surgical patients will demonstrate reactivation of latent herpesvirus infection following major procedures or during severe surgical illnesses (e.g., peritonitis). Reactivation disease may be perioral "cold sores" or "shingles." In transplant patients with immunosuppressive therapy, cytomegalovirus reactivation and loss of the transplant graft is a sufficient problem that inhibitors of viral DNA replication (e.g., acyclovir, ganciclovir) are used for suppression of the virus for many months following transplantation. Uncommonly, reactivation of cytomegalovirus infection can cause small intestinal perforation. Herpesvirus type-8 causes Kaposi sarcoma that is associated with acquired immunodeficiency syndrome (AIDS).

Bacteremia-Septic Response without Infection

Hemorrhagic shock and other potentially physiologic perturbations have been implicated in the release of bacteria or bacterial endotoxins into the systemic circulation from the reservoir of gut colonization. Although initially challenged and discredited, the concept of *bacterial translocation* has been identified and associated with potentially being of pathophysiologic significance in human sepsis and the multiple organ dysfunction syndrome. Because fungi (e.g., *C. albicans*) are also associated with dissemination from the gastrointestinal tract, this "escape" of microbes from the gut might more appropriately be termed *microbial gastrointestinal translocation*. As a potentially significant clinical event,

the dissemination of bacteria and bacterial cell products into the systemic circulation, without the provocation of inflammation at the primary site of entry, is bacteremia and the septic response without a primary focus of infection.

There are pathophysiologic requirements for microbial gastrointestinal translocation. First, there must be failure of the intricate gut barrier function that keeps gastrointestinal colonization from being disseminated throughout the body. Second, the hepatic Kupffer cells that ordinarily rid portal blood of all potential toxins and bacteria fail to perform this function. Some endotoxin or whole bacteria may leak into the portal circulation and may occur with normal defecation. Colonic endoscopy, proctoscopy, and intraoperative portal blood cultures have been identified to provoke bacteremia. Occasional portal bacteremia must occur. Access of portal endotoxins or whole organisms from the gut into the systemic circulation must mean that Kupffer cell function is impaired or that the capacity of these cells to clear organisms and toxins in certain circumstances can be saturated. Yet another pathophysiologic route is for translocating organisms to gain access to the regional lymph nodes. Bacteria or fungi could therefore gain access to the thoracic duct lymph and gain access to the systemic circulation. Complete failure of lymphatic RE function would be required for this to be a plausible event.

The barrier function of the human gastrointestinal tract has both functional and anatomic components. Motility of the intestine is certainly a component part of the intestinal barrier. Propulsion of contents through the intestinal lumen in a distal direction minimizes the period of time that microorganisms are in contact with the mucosa. The *in situ* proliferation and invasion of bacteria is simply retarded by movement. Loss of this motility function, either by intestinal obstruction or by gastrointestinal ileus, has been associated with bacteremia and the septic response in humans.

The anatomic barrier of the intestinal epithelium is obviously an important partition that keeps bacteria and bacterial cell products from entering the lymphatics or bloodstream. Atrophy of the epithelial cells or degradation of the intercellular matrix may be major contributing factors to intestinal microbial translocation.

Concern about cellular atrophy has raised new issues in the design and delivery of nutritional support systems in critically ill patients. Maintenance of the enterocyte and colonocyte appear to require specific nutrients under circumstances of hypermetabolism and stress. The enterocyte of the small intestine appears to prefer glutamine as an energy substrate, whereas the colonocyte appears to need short-chain fatty acids for oxidation. Failure of these two cell populations to receive critical nutrients may lead to epithelial atrophy with compromise of the barrier function of the gut. Because conventional solutions for parenteral nutrition of patients are deficient in both glutamine and short-chain fatty acids, compromise of the gut barrier is thought to be the result of selective nutritional deprivation. These observations have led to an enteral formulation with arginine, nucleic acids, and Ω-3 fatty acids. This "immunonutrition" is designed to enhance the gut barrier and enhance the effectiveness of the gut-associated lymphoid tissue. Prospective, randomized studies have demonstrated reduced rates of postoperative infection, but improved survival remains controversial. Other manipulations of enteral formulations can be expected.

The route of nutritional delivery to the critically ill patient may be as important as the specific composition of the nutrients. Gut epithelial cells access nutrients from the lumen of the intestine, and failure to have luminal nutrients results in gut atrophy. Preservation of the gut barrier function requires intraluminal delivery of proteins and other nutrient components. Loss of the barrier by gut atrophy may be important for translocation to occur. Intraluminal nutrients may also promote normalization of the gut microflora and diminish the emergence of nosocomial pathogens within the gastrointestinal reservoir. For these and other reasons, enteral feeding is the preferred route in the surgical patient when gastrointestinal function and integrity permit.

The intercellular matrix between the apposing cells of the intestinal epithelium is another important consideration in the gastrointestinal barrier. The composition of the intercellular matrix is complex; it is a dynamic structure that is constantly being degraded, resynthesized, and remodeled. Biological stress and protein-calorie malnutrition must certainly increase the porosity of the intercellular matrix and potentially create avenues for the invasion of intraluminal microorganisms. The colonization of the lumen by undesirable microorganisms, either from exogenous contamination or secondary to the influence of broad-spectrum antibiotics, may occur, and they may actually amplify enzymes that digest the intercellular matrix and facilitate the movement of microorganisms out of the lumen.

Another mechanism that reinforces the biologic barrier of the intestinal tract is retardation of bacterial (or fungal) adherence to the epithelial cells. Considerable evidence suggests that pathologic bacteria must bind to the epithelial cell to express virulence. Pathogenic bacterial cells that are kept from binding to the epithelium are simply propelled downstream by the normal peristaltic function of the gut.

Several mechanisms within the gut inhibit bacterial binding to the epithelium. Goblet cells are found throughout the gastrointestinal tract and produce a complex glycoprotein mucin that is constantly secreted into the lumen. This mucin has bacteriostatic properties that suppress excessive bacterial overgrowth, particularly within the small intestine. This mucin also provides a protective film over the surface of the intestinal epithelium that retards bacterial binding to the lining cells.

A second mechanism that retards microorganisms from binding to the epithelium is secretory IgA. The gastrointestinal tract has abundant submucosal lymphocytes and mature plasma cells that serve numerous biologic functions. One function is the synthesis of secretory IgA, which is constantly secreted into the lumen of the intestine. This secretory IgA is thought to bind to bacterial cells and block those receptors that mediate their binding to epithelial cells.

A final important barrier that retards binding of microorganisms to intestinal epithelial cells is the normal gastrointestinal flora. The normal colonization of the gut serves to provide antagonism to the growth of bacterial or fungal species that may be potentially injurious to the host. Bacteriocin produced by resident species suppresses the growth of potential pathogens. Short-chain fatty acids may be toxic to selected unwanted colonists of the intestine. Lactobacilli can produce hydrogen peroxide, which activates the peroxidase–halide mechanism that suppresses both viral and fungal pathogens.

Binding of normal microflora to the epithelial cells of the intestine prevents the binding of potentially pathogenic bacteria. The specificity of this binding by the intestinal colonization of certain animal species is remarkable. For example, the lactobacilli of rats can bind to rat intestinal epithelial cells and block the binding of pathologic organisms. The lactobacilli of birds can serve a similar function. What is truly amazing is that the avian lactobacilli are unable to bind to rat gut cells. Although the specificity of gut colonization in humans has not been characterized to the extent identified earlier, the loss of normal colonization because of the use of broad-spectrum antibiotic has led to considerable discussion about the need for selective decontamination of the human gut during critical illness. This technique attempts to eliminate aerobic bacteria and preserve anaerobic species. The assumption in selective gut decontamination is that preservation of anaerobic colonization is critical to the barrier function of the human gut.

The beneficial effects of normal gut colonization has stimulated interest in the potential value of recolonization of the intestinal tract as a therapeutic strategy. Probiotics are the idea of administering microorganisms to treat disease, instead of antibiotics designed to kill microorganisms. Lactobacilli and other strains of bacteria have been postulated to serve in this role. Even genetically engineered microbes are being investigated as potential treatments. Prebiotics are nutrients that are speculated to promote the proliferation of desired microbial strains within the gut that would foster a healthier condition for the host. Probiotics and prebiotics are being hypothesized as potential treatments for nosocomial infections, inflammatory bowel disease, irritable bowel syndrome, and other diseases. This area of investigation may have a role in the management of the patient at risk for *C. difficile* enterocolitis. As more information develops about the role of normal colonization upon the gut barrier, it is likely that innovative efforts will be made to restore microbes rather than killing them.

If the gut barrier is breached, the liver Kupffer cells ordinarily prevent these transient portal bacteremias from gaining systemic access to the host and provoking a septic event. The RE function of the liver is efficient and has been shown experimentally to remove 10^4 to 10^5 microorganisms per milliliter of portal blood flow. Hepatic RE function probably needs ample opsonic protein to facilitate the removal of blood-borne microorganisms. Therefore, exhaustion of opsonic proteins may be one mechanism of RE ineffectiveness that could lead to portal bacteremia. Other variables experimentally shown to alter hepatic RE efficiency include corticosteroids, exotoxins, and chemotherapeutic agents. Shock, hypoxemia, protein-calorie malnutrition, burns, and other perturbations not only affect the gut barrier but also impair hepatic Kupffer cell function.

Patients may have endotoxemia, bacteremia, or fungemia from the gastrointestinal reservoir. The diagnosis of this biologic event remains a diagnosis of exclusion. Despite some good data from human subjects to support bacteremia from the gut as an important event, the true clinical relevance and frequency of microbial translocation remains to be defined.

Prions

The germ theory of disease has generally been accepted for >100 years, and dictates that infectious diseases are the consequence of transmission of living microorganisms. However, recent evidence, especially surrounding the epidemic of "mad cow disease" in the United Kingdom has brought attention to prions. Prions represent proteins that behave as infectious agents. They do not have nucleic acid, but represent neuroproteins that have an amino acid chemical sequence identical to the normally occurring proteins. However, their secondary and tertiary protein configuration is at variance from normal structure and results in neurologic disease.

Prion disease in humans is associated with Creutzfeld-Jakob disease (CJD). CJD occurs from genetic predisposition or from sporadic events. However, it was the increase in the new-variant CJD that brought attention to transmission of prion disease from ingestion of contaminated beef. Transmission appears to occur with exposure to the abnormally configured protein, which then appears to serve as a template to reconfigure normal neuroproteins into the abnormal structure. Prion disease is being speculated to have a potential role in many degenerative diseases of the central nervous system.

Why then do prions have any interest for surgeons? Nosocomial transmission of prion disease has now been documented. Transmission has occurred with dura mater grafts, corneal transplantation, pericardial grafts, and the use of contaminated electroencephalographic electrodes. Human-derived hormones such as growth hormone and pituitary gonadotropin have been demonstrated to transmit CJD. Contaminated instruments used in central nervous system operations have been shown to transmit disease from patient to patient. Conventional sterilization processes do not eradicate the risk of transmission. The mechanism by which a protein can resist extreme heat sterilization defies current understanding and has led to speculation that even the residual cast of the former protein might convey the "template" necessary to reconfigure the host normal proteins to the pathologic structure. There is experimental and four case reports of human transmission of prion disease with blood transfusion. Therefore, the concept of a new form of transmissible disease is evolving. Our concept of the germ theory of infectious disease may be at the threshold for a major revision.

The Septic Response

The primary function of host defense mechanisms is to prevent and contain infection when tissues are contaminated by microorganisms. Unfortunately, severe invasive infections result in microorganisms gaining access to the circulation, or toxic products (e.g., endotoxin, exotoxins) from the bacteria gain access to the circulation. The intensity of the local inflammatory response leads to normal and beneficial proinflammatory signals being produced in large concentrations such that a systemic distribution of the cytokine proteins occur. This dissemination of bacteria, bacterial products, and/or proinflammatory signaling results in a generalized activation of the inflammatory cascade. Clinically, this syndrome is referred to as *sepsis* or *septicemia*.

This systemic inflammatory response syndrome (SIRS) is a generic response that can occur from any clinical event that activates the inflammatory cascade in a generalized manner. Hemorrhage, ischemia-reperfusion injury, extensive soft tissue injury, severe pancreatitis, and other insults have been associated with SIRS. SIRS that is activated by infection is sepsis.

The clinical syndrome of sepsis is usually described as fever, tachycardia, tachypnea, and leukocytosis when the process is driven by infection at a specific site. Although

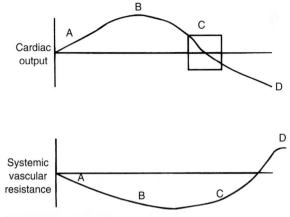

FIGURE 9.13 The four states of the septic response from the perspective of cardiac output and peripheral vascular resistance. In state A, the cardiac output is elevated modestly and peripheral vascular resistance is modestly diminished. In state B, cardiac output is increased dramatically, whereas vascular resistance is extremely diminished. In state C, cardiac output is in the range of the customarily identified normal values, but because of profound loss of vascular resistance, the patient is identified as in clinical septic shock. State D is congestive heart failure superimposed on the fundamental septic condition. Cardiac output is reduced and peripheral vascular resistance is increased.

septic events are customarily identified with these clinical signs, the reality is that these criteria would qualify every child with otitis media as having sepsis.

A more appropriate understanding of sepsis can be identified in the physiologic and biochemical responses that characterize the septic response. These responses of sepsis are (i) an increase in cardiac output, (ii) a reduction in peripheral vascular resistance, (iii) a narrowed arteriovenous oxygen difference, and (iv) the evolution of lactic acidemia before hypotension.

The extensive evaluation of injured and septic patients has permitted the design of a four- component staging system for the septic response (Fig. 9.13). State A is characteristic of the physiologic stress response. Patients experience a modest elevation of cardiac output and have a modest decline in peripheral vascular resistance. Oxygen consumption is increased and the arteriovenous oxygen difference is normal to slightly increased. Given appropriate volume resuscitation, they do not have increased serum lactate concentrations.

State B represents the exaggerated stress response. Cardiac output may be increased to twice normal levels. The peripheral vascular resistance is dramatically reduced. The arteriovenous oxygen difference is narrowed, reflecting the presence of defective peripheral oxygen utilization. Total oxygen consumption may be reduced or minimally elevated relative to the increase observed in cardiac output. Lactic acidemia (usually without lactic acidosis) is present.

State C represents the evolution of septic shock. The cardiac output is normal or slightly increased. However, the profound loss of peripheral vascular resistance means that cardiac output cannot meet peripheral demands, and

hypotension results. The peripheral abnormality of oxygen use is now compounded by the reduction in perfusion pressure. Marked lactic acidosis results.

State D is the low cardiac output–septic shock state. Left-ventricle failure occurs and is associated with increased peripheral vascular resistance. Patients have profound lactic acidosis. There is peripheral abnormality of oxygen consumption, reduced cardiac output, reduced perfusion pressure, and peripheral vasoconstriction. It is commonly a preterminal condition.

The state B patient can be sustained in this exaggerated stress response for a considerable period of time with current support technology. The sustained state B condition sets the stage for the evolution of multiple organ failure, as the peripheral abnormality of oxygen metabolism persists although cardiac output is elevated and the central perfusion pressure appears to be satisfactory.

Individual patients do not sequentially pass through each of the states of the septic response. The transition from state A to state B requires that the patient has the myocardial reserve to generate the elevated cardiac output to compensate for the loss of peripheral vascular resistance. In those patients that have intrinsic myocardial disease or in the elderly patient, the ability to generate the necessary cardiac output may be lacking. Therefore, older patients will commonly decompensate to a state C level with no apparent interval of a state B.

The mechanism to explain the extensive physiologic and metabolic changes of human sepsis continues to escape full definition. A simplified perspective of this very complex process is to draw analogies between inflammation as it unfolds at the local tissue level and to apply those processes to a systemic level of organization. As is illustrated in Figure 9.14, the activation of the systemic inflammatory response occurs with systemic dissemination of the microbe, the microbial cell products, the proinflammatory signals for the invasive infection, or more likely a systemic assault of all three components. The five initiators events of systemic inflammation are activated. Coagulation proteins are activated which results in disseminated coagulation, although not always with clinical bleeding. Platelets aggregate releasing an array of enzymes and a results thrombocytopenia occurs. Mast cells release histamine, neutral proteases, and presynthesized proinflammatory signals. Bradykinin is produced and nitric oxide synthase is induced. Complement proteins are activated. The vasoactive phase of the septic response is produced and is characterized by vasodilation, reduction in vascular resistance, increased vascular capacitance, and systemic edema. Reduced vascular resistance, reduced ventricular afterload, and an increased cardiac output is the pathophysiologic result. Hypotension is the result when cardiac output becomes inadequate to meet the lost of vascular resistance.

The microcirculatory phase of the process then follows. Neutrophils and monocytes are activated by the systemic domain of the numerous chemottractant signals that are released. Endothelial adhesion proteins are upregulated. Diffuse white cell sequestration within the microcirculation

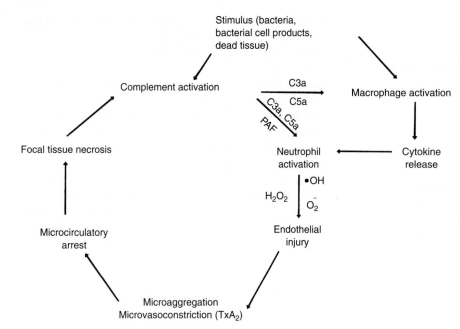

FIGURE 9.14 Theoretical relation of multiple variables to explain the microcirculatory hypothesis of multiple organ failure. The biologic stimulus leads to the activated neutrophil state. Adverse interactions between the neutrophil and the endothelial cell cause microvascular injury, which produces a necrotic focus. The focal ischemic injury then becomes the inflammatory focus to recycle the inflammatory process. PAF, platelet-activating factor.

follows. Reactive oxygen intermediates and acid hydrolases are released by the activated but sequestered white cells within the microcirculation. Within the microcirculation of the lung, liver, splanchnic vessels, and the kidney the aggregation of cellular elements and aggregated protein from inflammation creates a microcirculatory occlusion and arrest that leads to failure of microcirculatory units and focal ischemia. Focal necrosis of cells leads to the creation of an injury that serves as a stimulus to maintain continued and sustained activation of the inflammatory cascade. A point is reached where a self-energizing cycle of uncontrolled inflammation makes the progression of sepsis and organ failure a relentless and fatal process.

Although the mechanisms that are responsible for the septic response remain to be fully elucidated, many newer treatment modalities have been explored using current knowledge and using the model of the SIRS. These newer treatment strategies have been designed to neutralize or modulate the mediator and effector systems of human inflammation. Clinical trials of antibodies to bind endotoxin, antibodies to TNF, IL-1 receptor antagonists, bradykinin inhibitors, and many others have been attempted and have failed. Only activated recombinant protein C has shown promise of clinical improvement. The failure of these biological modulators resides in the fact that we still do not understand the regulation and control of inflammation and the other mechanisms that are likely to be involved in this complex disease process that we call sepsis.

Inflammation of local infections is down-regulated once the biological purpose of bacterial eradication has occurred. Drainage of a cutaneous abscess is promptly followed by resolution of the erythema, induration, and other features of inflammation by intrinsic mechanisms. It is likely that regulation and control of the systemic inflammatory

processes will be found in a better understanding of the counter-inflammatory mechanisms that we know exist when local infection is controlled.

Perhaps a more fruitful area of future investigation will be in exploiting the natural counter-inflammatory mechanisms of the host. When a cutaneous abscess is examined, all of the characteristic features of human inflammation can be recognized. When the abscess is drained, natural downregulatory processes cause curtailment of the inflammation. IL-4, IL-10, and IL-13 and others are currently recognized as being potential signals that are counter-regulatory to inflammation. Indeed, the use of naturally occurring biological signals to treat the septic condition may prove to be much more effective than all of the synthesized efforts with receptor antagonists and monoclonal antibodies.

SUMMARY

The complex interaction among the host, the microbial pathogen, and the microenvironment of infection is becoming better defined. Understanding the mechanisms of antibiotic action and microbial resistance has provided new drugs that are designed to block the resistance mechanism (e.g., clavulanic acid and sulbactam) rather than attack the microorganisms themselves.

Although surgical drainage, debridement, and antibiotic therapy are effective modalities, these treatments have probably reached a point of maximum benefit. Newer treatment modalities should address host modulation, either by facilitation of local containment or by downregulation of the systemic inflammatory response. These newer treatments will require the continued growth of basic information about surgical infection.

SELECTED READINGS

Besselink MG, Timmerman HM, van Minnen LP, et al. Prevention of infectious complications in surgical patients: potential role of probiotics. *Dig Surg* 2005;22:234–244.

Burke JF. The effective period of preventive antibiotic action in experimental incisions and dermal lesions. *Surgery* 1961;50:161–168.

Crum NF, Lee RU, Thronton SA, et al. Fifteen-year study of the changing epidemiology of methicillin-resistant Staphylococcus aureus. *Am J Med* 2006;119:943–951.

Deitch EA. Role of gut lymphatic systemic in multiple organ failure. *Curr Opin Crit Care* 2001;7:92–98.

Fry DE. Herpesviruses: emerging nosocomial pathogen? *Surg Infect* 2001;2:1221–1230.

Hoover L, Bochicchio GV, Napolitano LM, et al. Systemic inflammatory response syndrome and nosocomial infection in trauma. *J Trauma* 2006;61:310–316.

Jacoby GA, Munoz-Price LS. The new β-lactamases. *N Engl J Med* 2005;352:380–391.

Lin E, Calvano SE, Lowry SF. Inflammatory cytokines and cell responses in surgery. *Surgery* 2000;127:117–126.

McDonald LC, Killgore GE, Thompson A, et al. An epidemic, toxic gene variant strain of Clostridium difficile. *N Engl J Med* 2005;353:2433–2441.

Siegel JH, Cerra FB, Coleman B, et al. Physiological and metabolic correlations in human sepsis. *Surgery* 1979;86:163–193.

Turina M, Fry DE, Polk HC Jr. Acute hyperglycemia and the innate immune system: clinical, cellular, and molecular aspects. *Crit Care Med* 2005;33:1624–1633.

West AP, Koblansky AA, Ghosh S. Recognition and signaling by toll-like receptors. *Annu Rev Cell Dev Biol* 2006;22:409–437.

CHAPTER 10

Principles of Pharmacology

Wayne L. Backes and Joseph M. Moerschbaecher, III

DRUG–RECEPTOR THEORY

Drugs produce their effects through interplay with existing biochemical and physiologic systems within the body. For example, a drug that influences heart rate or blood pressure acts on that part of the autonomic nervous system that controls that process. Drugs themselves do not have inherent effects. Most drugs exert their effects by binding to specific macromolecules within the body. This interaction initiates a series of biochemical and physiologic changes that culminates in the observed drug response. These macromolecules are known as *receptors* and are the sites of the initial interaction for the drug. Normally, receptors interact with endogenous compounds in the body. Drugs act by altering the rate at which these normal bodily functions proceed. Drugs do not create novel effects but only modulate the rate of ongoing physiologic processes.

Most drug–receptor interactions fall into three general classifications: (i) an agonist is a compound that both binds to and produces an alteration in a receptor, which results in the observed pharmacologic response; (ii) an antagonist binds to the receptor but on binding does not alter the receptor. Antagonists act by inhibiting the effects of endogenous agonists; (iii) a partial agonist binds to and alters the receptor; however, the resulting response is not as great as that produced by a full agonist.

Most drugs bind to receptors in a reversible manner, which means that the drug can freely bind and dissociate from the receptor molecule. The chemical bonds that are important for reversible drug–receptor interactions include ionic bonds, hydrogen bonds, hydrophobic bonds, and van der Waals forces. Ionic bonds are electrostatic attractions between ions of opposite charge. These ionic bonds provide the initial interaction between the drug and receptor. Hydrogen bonds are weaker interactions that occur and further stabilize this initial ionic bond. They are produced by a reciprocal partial ionization of both the drug and the receptor molecules. Last, hydrophobic interactions and van der Waals forces provide the final stabilization of the complex. These bonds ultimately control the affinity and also the ability of that particular drug to produce the change in the receptor (1).

Drug–receptor interactions are governed by the law of mass action. In an attempt to describe these types of interactions, Clark (2) developed the basis for most of the theories of drug action. The treatment is analogous to the Michaelis-Menten treatment for enzyme kinetic data. The treatment is called the *occupancy theory* and is based on five assumptions: (i) the magnitude of the response is proportional to the number of receptors occupied, (ii) drug–receptor complex formation is rapid and freely reversible compared with the rate of response, (iii) one drug combines with one receptor, (iv) all receptors are identical and equally accessible to the drug, and (v) only a small portion of the drug is involved in forming complexes with the receptor molecules (3).

$$\text{Drug} \rightleftarrows \text{Receptor Drug} \rightarrow \text{Receptor Response} \qquad (10.1)$$

According to this model, the drug combines with the receptor, producing a drug–receptor complex. Formation of this complex is the initial interaction that eventually culminates in the pharmacologic response. According to the occupancy theory, the amount of drug–receptor complex is directly proportional to the magnitude of the response; therefore, if the occupancy theory holds and 100% of the receptors are occupied, the maximal response will be attained. In a similar manner, if only 50% of the receptors are occupied, then only 50% of the maximal response will be observed.

Drugs differ in their ability to bind to receptors. This binding is characterized and quantified by use of the dissociation constant (K_d), which is described by Equation 10.2.

$$\frac{[\text{Drug}][\text{Receptor}]}{[\text{Drug} - \text{Receptor}]} = K_d \qquad (10.2)$$

The K_d is a measure of the affinity of the drug for the receptor. A tighter drug–receptor complex will have a smaller K_d. Rearrangement of Equation 10.2 yields Equation 10.3, which predicts the pharmacologic effect as a function of

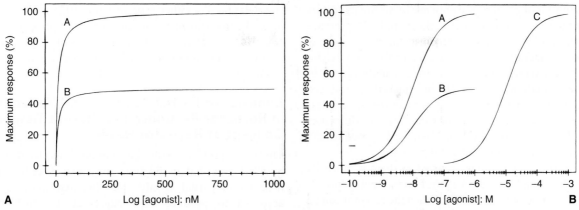

FIGURE 10.1   The effect of agonist concentration on pharmacologic response. **A:** Linear plot. Curve *A* represents a full agonist, whereas curve *B* represents that of a partial agonist. Both drugs in this figure have the same K_d value. **B:** Semilogarithmic plot. Curves *A* and *C* represent full agonists that differ in their potencies, whereas curve *B* represents that of a partial agonist.

drug dose.

$$\text{Response} = \frac{E_{\max}[\text{Drug}]}{K_d[\text{Drug}]} \qquad (10.3)$$

The relation between drug dose and response is depicted in Figure 10.1. At the lowest drug doses, a small increase in drug concentration leads to a large increase in the observed pharmacologic effect; however, further increases in drug concentration will lead to a proportionately smaller increase in the drug effect.

Pharmacologists frequently plot such data as the response or the effect observed against the log (dose) as shown in Figure 10.1B. A wide range of concentrations are easily displayed with such a plot, which is particularly useful when drugs that have different affinities for their receptor site are being compared. Two important pieces of information that can be gained from a dose–response curve are the maximal effect ($E_{\max}$) and the ED_{50}. The $E_{\max}$ is the maximum possible effect produced by a particular drug as measured on the y-axis. As shown in Figure 10.1B, the maximal effect shown

for a partial agonist (curve *B*) is less than that shown for the full agonist (curve *A*). The ED_{50} is that dose at which 50% of the maximal effect is observed. Determination of the ED_{50} is shown in Figure 10.1B for the full agonist (curve *A*) and the partial agonist (curve *B*).

Antagonism

There are two types of antagonists: (i) irreversible antagonists, for which the drug covalently binds to the receptor site, and (ii) reversible antagonists, which are the most common type for therapeutically useful agents. Reversible antagonism can be further subdivided into competitive, or surmountable, antagonism and noncompetitive antagonism. As stated previously antagonists do not act by producing an effect on the receptors themselves, but act by inhibiting the interaction of endogenous agonists with the receptor molecule. Competitive antagonism occurs when both the antagonist and the agonist compete for the same binding site on the receptor molecule. As shown graphically in Figure 10.2, the response

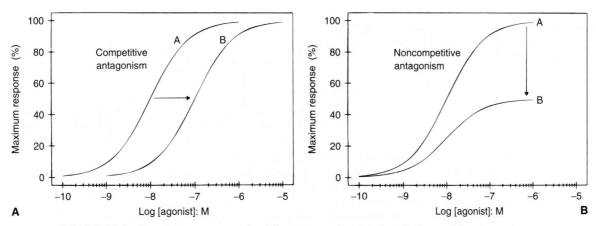

FIGURE 10.2   Dose–response curves for different types of antagonism. **A:** Competitive antagonism. Agonist dose response in the absence (curve *A*) and presence of a fixed concentration of competitive antagonist (curve *B*). **B:** Noncompetitive antagonism. Agonist dose response in the absence (curve *A*) and presence (curve *B*) of a fixed concentration of noncompetitive antagonist.

to an agonist is affected by the presence of the antagonist by shifting the dose–response curve to the right. In the presence of higher concentrations of antagonist, the dose–response curve for the agonist will be shifted even further to the right, resulting in an increase in the apparent ED_{50} of the agonist in the presence of the antagonist. The maximal effect produced by an agonist, such as morphine, is not affected by the presence of an antagonist, such as naloxone. The only difference is that a higher dose of morphine is required to produce the maximal response when naloxone is present.

Competitive interactions occur when there is mutually exclusive binding between an agonist and an antagonist. If the agonist is bound to the receptor, then the receptor can be altered, resulting in the pharmacologic response. However, because the antagonist cannot produce such an alteration in the receptor as does an agonist, it acts by blocking agonist binding to the receptor (Fig. 10.3A). Therefore, to overcome the effects of the antagonist, higher concentrations of agonist would be required to produce an equivalent response.

With simple noncompetitive antagonism, both agonist and antagonist can freely bind to the receptor; however, each compound must bind to its own site (Fig. 10.3B). In the absence of antagonist, an agonist will be able to bind to the receptor site and produce its pharmacologic response. However, antagonist binding to a separate site will inactivate a certain proportion of the receptors, depending on the affinity of the antagonist for the receptor site and the antagonist concentration. The binding of agonist to the receptor in the presence of antagonist will neither affect the binding of the antagonist to the receptor nor permit a pharmacologic response to be produced in those receptors where the antagonist is present (even if agonist is present). As a result, the presence of the antagonist will inactivate a certain percentage of the receptors. Further addition of agonist will not overcome the effects of a noncompetitive antagonist. A graphic representation of the effects of a noncompetitive antagonist is shown in Figure 10.2B.

Irreversible antagonism occurs when the antagonist molecule covalently binds to either the active site or a second site. Graphically, either type of irreversible inhibition can look like that shown for simple noncompetitive inhibition (Fig. 10.2B). Differences between irreversible inhibition and noncompetitive inhibition can be identified by more detailed examination.

Behavior of Partial Agonists and Variations in Receptor Response in Different Tissues: Concept of Receptor Reserve

The basic problem with the simplified model described by Clark was that it did not adequately describe (i) the behavior of partial agonists and (ii) that some agonists appeared to produce their effects at less than 100% receptor occupancy. Such results are obtained because the drug–receptor interaction does not directly lead to the pharmacologic response. Formation of the drug–receptor complex is the initial interaction triggering a series of events that will eventually culminate in the pharmacologic response. This process is known as *signal transduction*. The most common mechanisms for signal transduction involve G proteins, phosphoinositide hydrolysis and calcium mobilization, and alterations in the activities of certain regulatory enzymes after phosphorylation by protein kinases. As shown in Equation 10.4, formation of the drug–receptor complex produces an initial response (R_1).

$$\text{Drug} + \text{Receptor} \rightleftarrows \text{Drug-Receptor} \rightarrow R_1 \rightarrow \text{Response} \tag{10.4}$$

As an example, let us assume that the initial response is the mobilization of calcium ion. The initial effect (R_1) subsequently leads to the observed pharmacologic effect.

Now let us examine the effect of a drug in three different tissues that have differences in receptor density. Drug X produces its pharmacologic effect by binding to the receptors in each of the tissues A, B, and C by a process mediated by Ca^{2+} mobilization. Drug X, therefore, produces its effect by binding to the receptors and mobilizing calcium. The released Ca^{2+} then produces the pharmacologic response. Drug X requires a receptor density of ten receptors per unit

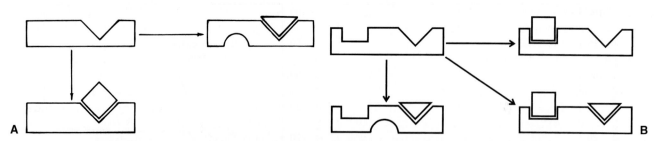

FIGURE 10.3 Antagonist action. **A:** Competitive antagonism. The receptor molecule can be bound by either agonist (∇) or antagonist ($\diamond$), both of which bind to the same site on the receptor molecule. Agonist binding results in a modification of the receptor molecule in such a manner as to elicit the pharmacologic response. The antagonist cannot produce such a change in the receptor but acts by preventing binding of agonist. **B:** Noncompetitive antagonist. In this case, the receptor has two sites, one that binds agonist and one that binds antagonist. Binding of antagonist ($\square$) does not alter the ability of agonist (∇) to bind; however, when antagonist is present, the agonist cannot produce the modification of the receptor. As a result, the antagonist effectively inactivates a certain proportion of the receptors, and the magnitude of the inhibition depends on the concentration of antagonist present.

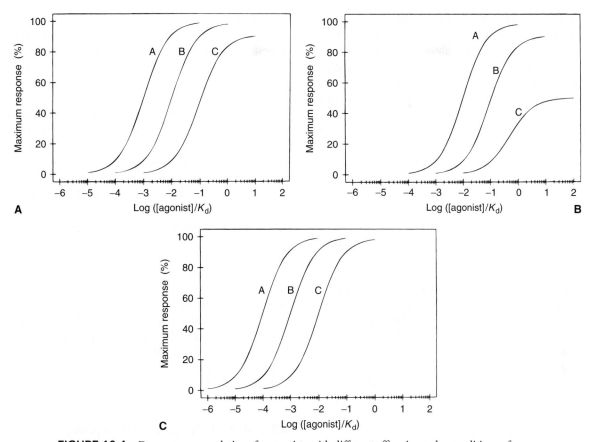

FIGURE 10.4 Dose–response relations for agonists with different efficacies under conditions of different receptor densities and reserves. **A:** Curves A, B, and C represent the dose–response curves for agonist X in three tissues with different receptor densities. Drug X obeys the assumptions of occupancy theory in tissue B (where 100% of the receptors are occupied, producing a maximal response) and behaves as a full agonist. In tissue C, which has a lower receptor density, drug X cannot produce as large of a response and behaves as a partial agonist in that tissue. In tissue A, a maximal response is obtained with less than 100% tissue occupancy. **B:** Behavior of drug Y in tissues A, B, and C. Because of the decreased ability of drug Y to modify the receptor (intrinsic efficacy), this drug does not exhibit receptor reserve. It behaves as a full agonist in tissue A and a partial agonist in tissues B and C. **C:** Agonist Z appears to behave as a full agonist in each tissue, because of its larger intrinsic efficacy. The drug exhibits increasing receptor reserve in tissues B and A.

area to mobilize sufficient calcium to produce this maximal response. In tissue B (having ten receptors per unit area), drug X is capable of producing its maximal response by binding to all of the receptors per unit area. However, if drug X is placed in tissue C, where there are only five receptors per unit area, sufficient calcium cannot be mobilized to produce the same response seen in tissue B. Drug X behaves as a partial agonist in tissue C, but in tissue B it behaves as a full agonist. On the other hand, in tissue A, where the receptor density is twice that found in tissue B, there are more than enough receptors to mobilize the Ca^{2+} required to produce the maximal response. In fact, in tissue A the maximal response will be observed when only half the receptors are occupied. Therefore, to produce an equivalent response in tissue A compared with tissue B, lower concentrations of drug X would be required. The presence of the receptor reserve found in tissue A will cause a shift in the dose–response curve to the left with respect to the response in tissue B

(Fig. 10.4A). This example demonstrates how a drug can behave as a partial agonist in one tissue and a full agonist in another tissue and exhibit receptor reserve in a third tissue (3).

Because agonists differ both in their affinity for receptor site and in their ability to produce the change in the receptor, which results in the pharmacologic response, different drugs could produce different responses in these tissues although they are binding to the same receptor sites. As an example, drug Y can produce its effects in a manner similar to drug X but may require a receptor density of only five receptors per unit area to produce its maximal response. Therefore, drug Y would behave as a full agonist in tissue C (where a receptor density of five is observed), and exhibit increasing degrees of receptor reserve in tissues B and A, respectively (Fig. 10.4B). Drug Z, which requires 20 receptors per unit area bound to mobilize sufficient calcium to produce its maximal response, would behave as a full agonist only in tissue A and would behave as a partial agonist in tissues B and C (Fig. 10.4C). These results indicate that the response to a drug depends on both the affinity of the drug for the receptor site and the ability of that drug to stimulate the signal transduction mechanisms. Furthermore, the response of a drug depends on the receptor density present in a particular tissue.

Two terms are generally used to describe drug behavior: potency and efficacy. *Potency* is simply the concentration of drug necessary to produce a response. When less of a drug is required to produce a particular response, it is said to be more potent. A number of factors can affect potency of a drug. The first factor is the affinity of the drug for the receptor. If a drug has a higher affinity (i.e., lower ED_{50}), it is said to be more potent. The potency of a drug can also be affected by the functional relation between the receptor and response. As described earlier, the same drug in different tissues has different potencies owing to the presence of receptor reserve in some of the tissues. Additionally, drugs having different abilities to elicit the initial response (R_1) could have different potencies. The final factors that will affect the potency of a drug are pharmacokinetic parameters: absorption, distribution, metabolism, and excretion. Each of these factors will affect the concentration of drug that will get to the receptor site and could therefore affect the drug dose required to produce a particular pharmacologic response.

Differences in *efficacy* can be manifest as either differences in the apparent effect of a particular agonist or changes in the apparent potency of a drug. When comparing a full agonist that does not exhibit receptor reserve with a partial agonist, the changes in their efficacy will be reflected by a change in the maximal effect seen with each drug. However, when comparing a drug that exhibits receptor reserve to that same drug in another tissue where receptor reserve is not found (but the drug still behaves as a full agonist), no changes in the maximal effect will be found, although the drug has a different efficacy in the different tissues. These changes will be manifest as a difference in the apparent potency of the drug in these tissues.

Therefore far dose–response curves have been discussed for a single subject. These dose–response curves show a measured change in the magnitude of response from a subject who is administered different doses of a drug. This type of representation is referred to as a *graded dose–response curve*. Because such dose–response curves are for individual subjects, comparisons of the curves among subjects show biologic variation; no two individuals produce exactly the same response at all drug concentrations.

Another method for expressing dose–response data is to classify an individual based on whether the administration of a particular drug dose leads to a response of a predetermined magnitude. An individual is then said to either respond or not to respond. Populations of individuals are treated with a particular dose of the drug and categorized as either responders or nonresponders. As the concentration of drug is increased, the total number of individuals responding

to that drug will also increase. A plot of the log of the drug concentration against the total number of individuals responding will generate a dose–response curve that is called a *quantal dose–response curve*. A quantal dose–response curve can be used to describe the relative effectiveness of a drug in a population of individuals.

No drug produces a single response. For example, aspirin has analgesic effects, anti-inflammatory effects, and a variety of toxic effects. Each of these effects would have its own dose–response curves. Finally, at high enough doses, the drug would be lethal. Quantal dose–response curves can be used to estimate the relative safety of a particular drug. A term used to estimate the relative safety of a drug is the *therapeutic index*. This is equal to the LD_{50} (the dose that produces lethality in 50% of the subjects) divided by the ED_{50}. The larger the therapeutic index the greater the relative safety of a drug. For example, the barbiturates have a much smaller therapeutic index than do the benzodiazepines making the latter compounds preferred in general for clinical use. A more practical relation for human subjects can be derived by dividing the TD_{50} (the dose that produces a particular toxicity in 50% of the subjects) divided by the ED_{50}. This relation would provide an estimate of the drug to produce an adverse effect.

ABSORPTION, DISTRIBUTION, METABOLISM, AND EXCRETION OF DRUGS

The pharmacologic response to a drug depends on its concentration at the receptor site; however, the ability of a drug to get to its receptor can be influenced by a number of factors (Fig. 10.5). Once a drug is administered to an organism, it can do a number of things. First, it must be absorbed into the circulation. After absorption, the drug will be distributed. Once in the circulation the drug can bind to plasma proteins, accumulate in various tissue reservoirs, or associate at the receptor site where it will produce its pharmacologic effect. The unchanged drug can be excreted or can be converted by the drug metabolizing enzymes to metabolites, which may be active or inactive. These metabolites can then be excreted (4,5).

Mechanisms of Drug Transport

Drugs differ in their rates of accumulation and elimination from the body because of differences in their physical properties. To reach their sites of action, drugs must cross one or more biologic membranes, which are composed largely of lipid. These membranes act as primary barriers to drug transport. Therefore, for a drug to get to its site of action, it must either pass around or through these membranes. The body uses a number of different mechanisms for transport of endogenous compounds from one site of the body to another. These processes include passive diffusion, filtration, endocytosis, and carrier-mediated transport. These same mechanisms are used for the transport of drugs to their sites

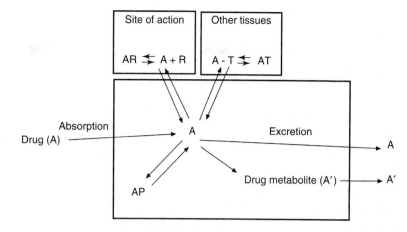

FIGURE 10.5 Fate of a drug after entering an organism. (Adapted from Yagiela JA. Pharmacokinetics: the absorption, distribution, and fate of drugs. In: Neidle EA, Yagiela JA, eds. *Pharmacology and therapeutics for dentistry*, 3rd edn. St. Louis: Mosby, 1989:17–47.)

of action and are also involved in their removal from the body (5).

Passive Diffusion

The most common mechanism for drug transport is passive diffusion. This process can be further subdivided into passive diffusion of nonelectrolytes and passive diffusion of weak acids and bases. Passive diffusion occurs when there is a high concentration of drug on one side of a membrane and a low concentration on the other. The drug will then passively transfer directly through the membrane, a process that will continue until the concentration of drug on both sides of the membrane is equal. Most drugs can transfer across membranes by passive diffusion at least to some extent; however, the rate of transfer by this mechanism differs for different drugs. The major factor that controls the rate of passive diffusion of nonelectrolytes is the lipid solubility of the drug. A term used to estimate the lipid solubility of a drug is the *partition coefficient* (K_p), which is simply the ratio of the concentration of drug in the lipid phase divided by its concentration in the aqueous phase. Therefore, highly lipid-soluble drugs will have larger K_p values. The addition of carbon and hydrogen atoms to a particular drug molecule will have a tendency to increase the partition coefficient for the drug, whereas the addition of polar groups such as hydroxyl, carboxyl, and amino groups will have a tendency to decrease the partition coefficient. Such modifications in the structure of a drug compound alter the rate at which the compounds can transfer by passive diffusion across membranes, where an increase in the partition coefficient will lead to a more rapid transfer of drug across a membrane. This can affect the drug concentration at the receptor and, as a result, the pharmacologic response to a drug.

If all drugs were nonelectrolytes, then the rate of drug transfer would simply depend on the drug's lipid solubility. However, most drugs are electrolytes and have a tendency to ionize in solution. The ability of drugs to ionize has a profound impact on their rate of transfer across biologic membranes. Electrolytes are categorized as either acids or bases. For the sake of this discussion, an acid is a compound that is uncharged when it is in a complex with a hydrogen ion (Equation 10.5).

$$HA \rightleftarrows H^+ + A^- \tag{10.5}$$

The types of functional groups that behave as acids are carboxyl, sulfhydryl, and hydroxyl groups. Drugs that behave as bases exhibit ionization characteristics as illustrated in Equation 10.6.

$$BH^+ \rightleftarrows H^+ + B \tag{10.6}$$

In this case, when the drug is in a complex with the hydrogen ion, the complex has a positive charge. The main functional group that undergoes this type of ionization is the amino group that will ionize to $-NH_3^+$.

Different drugs, whether they are acids or bases, will differ in their ability to ionize. For example, some drugs will readily give up their additional hydrogen ion, whereas other drugs will do so less readily. The relative ability of a drug to ionize is defined by its pK. The term pK is defined in the Henderson-Hasselbalch equation as the pH at which a drug would be 50% ionized. For example, a weak acid drug with a pK of 4 is 50% ionized (and 50% unionized) in a solution of pH 4. Likewise, a weak acid with a pK of 10 would have equal amounts of ionized and unionized species if it were in a solution of pH 10. It is important to remember that the pK indicates the pH at which ionization occurs. Weak acids can have pK values greater than 7, and bases can have pK values that are smaller than 7. As the pH of the solution is decreased (the hydrogen ion concentration is increased), the amount of acid in the "HA" complex will increase as a result of the law of mass action (Equation 10.6). Because pH and pK are logarithmic functions, each pH unit difference between the pH and pK represents a 10-fold difference in the concentrations of the ionized and unionized species. Therefore, if the pH is 3 units lower than the pK value, there is a 1,000-fold higher concentration of the unionized complexed form of the acid compared with the ionized uncomplexed species. An analogous situation occurs with a base. For example, in a base with a pK of 4 in a solution of pH 2, there will be a 100-fold excess of the ionized complexed species over that of the unionized uncomplexed form (Equation 10.6).

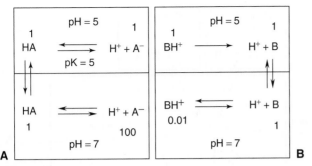

FIGURE 10.6 Examples of passive diffusion of electrolytes across membranes. **A:** Passive diffusion of a weak acid (pK = 5), when a pH difference exists between the solutions on opposite sides of the membrane. The drug has a tendency to accumulate in the compartment where the drug is most ionized, in this case where the pH = 7 (101:1 for pH 7/pH 1). **B:** Passive diffusion of a weak base (pK = 5) across a membrane with an existing *pH* differential. The drug accumulates in the compartment where the pH is 1, again where the drug is most ionized.

The reason that ionization is important with regard to drug transfer across membranes is that only the unionized species can transfer by passive diffusion. For a weak acid, the HA species will be the one that transfers by passive diffusion, and for a weak base, the uncomplexed species (B) will transfer by passive diffusion. Figure 10.6 illustrates how ionization can alter the transfer of a drug across biologic membranes. In this case, drug A is a weak acid with pK 5 transferring from a solution of pH 1 into a solution of pH 7 (Fig. 10.6A). The figure shows the relative amounts of each species after transfer has occurred. As previously mentioned, passive diffusion occurs until equal concentrations of the unionized species are attained on both sides of the membrane. As a result, the relative amounts of HA on both sides of the membrane will be 1. Because, in this example, the drug has a pK equal to 5 and is in a solution of pH 5, there are equal amounts of ionized and unionized species on that side of the membrane. Once the drug transfers into the pH 7 side of the membrane, it will have a greater tendency to ionize. The 2 pH unit difference between the pK of the drug and the pH of the solution will produce a 100-fold difference between A^- and HA. As a result, the total amount of drug on the pH 5 side of the membrane will be 2 and the amount of the pH 7 side of membrane will be 101. This illustrates that the ionization of a drug can have a profound influence on the ability of that drug to transfer across a biologic membrane by passive diffusion (remember that equal amounts of a nonelectrolyte would be on each side of the membrane at equilibrium). This process is called *ion trapping*. An example of the effect of ionization on the transfer of a weak base is shown in Figure 10.6B. The conditions are identical to those shown in Figure 10.6A; the only difference is that the drug is a base rather than an acid. These results show that a weak base under the same conditions as a weak acid will have a greater tendency to accumulate on the side where the pH is lower.

It is important to keep in mind that the ionization characteristics of a drug will affect its rate of transfer across a biologic membrane by controlling the relative amount of unionized species that are present. Therefore, a drug that is highly ionized will transfer more slowly because there is a lower concentration of the readily diffusible unionized species. There are, however, cases in which two drugs can have the same pK values and be transferred at very different rates; the reason for this occurrence is due to differences in the lipid solubility of these drugs. The more lipid-soluble drug will be transferred more rapidly. In summary, the rate of transfer by passive diffusion depends on (i) the lipid solubility of the drug, (ii) whether the drug is an acid or a base, (iii) the pK of the drug, and (iv) the pH of the surroundings.

Filtration

Filtration is the transfer of drugs either between or into cells through pores. The process depends on the existence of a pressure gradient and on the relative size of the compounds with respect to the size of the pore through which filtration is occurring. In general, compounds will pass through or be excluded from the membrane according to their molecular size. If the compound and the pore are similar in size then there will be resistance to transfer; however, if the compound is much smaller than the pore, then transfer of the drug simply depends on the magnitude of the pressure gradient. Sites at which filtration is important include the glomerulus and capillaries (with the exception of capillaries in the central nervous system).

Endocytosis

Endocytosis is the process whereby a drug molecule is engulfed by invagination of a membrane and internalized to produce a vesicle. This process can mediate the transfer of a drug molecule from one side of a membrane to the other. Endocytosis can be divided into pinocytosis and phagocytosis. Many examples of endocytosis have been shown to be receptor-mediated processes for which a ligand binds to the receptor in an area called a *coated pit*. The coated pit is lined by the protein clathrin. The coated pit invaginates and is pinched off to form a vesicle called an *endosome*. The endosome contains an adenosine triphosphate (ATP)-dependent proton pump, which will maintain a pH of 5 inside the endosome. Once in the endosome, the receptor and ligand can undergo different fates: (i) the ligand can be internalized and the receptor can be returned to the surface, (ii) both the receptor and ligand can be internalized and targeted for degradation, (iii) both the receptor and ligand can be transported to the opposite surface of the cell.

Active Transport and Facilitated Diffusion

Active transport and facilitated diffusion represent two receptor-mediated transport systems. Active transport is an energy-dependent movement of compounds against the concentration gradient. It is a receptor-mediated process whose primary function is the transport of endogenous compounds, usually compounds that are charged at physiologic pH. Drugs that are structurally similar to the endogenous compounds can also associate with the transport proteins and can be transported by active transport. Active transport is a uni-directional process in which the drug can accumulate on one side of the membrane. Because a transport protein is required for transfer of the compound, the process is also saturable and requires energy, usually in the form of ATP. As a result, active transport can be inhibited either by structural analogs of the drug or by ATP inhibitors.

Facilitated diffusion is similar to active transport in that it is a receptor-mediated transport process. Facilitated diffusion is also saturable, and drugs can be transported by this process if they can properly associate with the transport protein. Facilitated diffusion differs from active transport in that energy is not required to mediate this process, and facilitated diffusion only occurs down a concentration gradient. Therefore, a drug cannot accumulate on one side of a membrane.

Routes of Drug Administration

There are a number of routes whereby drugs can be administered. Oral administration is the most common route. It is generally the safest, most convenient, and most economical way to administer drugs. However, oral administration cannot be used in all circumstances. Some drugs are irritating to the gastric mucosa or are destroyed by digestive enzymes or low gastric pH. There are also problems of irregularities with absorption of particular drugs. For example, in some individuals the absorption of phenytoin is negligible, whereas other patients absorb the drug readily. Many drugs are inactivated after metabolism by liver or intestinal enzymes. Drugs that are metabolized by hepatic and intestinal enzymes before their distribution throughout the body are said to undergo a first-pass effect. After absorption from the intestine, the blood supply empties directly into the hepatic circulation. Because the liver and, to a lesser extent, the intestine are primary locations of drug-metabolizing enzymes, drugs that undergo extensive metabolism can be largely destroyed before distribution to their sites of action. In compounds that are extensively metabolized, the first-pass effect can be quite large. For example, the standard oral dose of morphine is approximately six times larger than a standard intramuscular dose because of first-pass metabolism.

Parenteral administration usually refers to intravenous, intramuscular, or subcutaneous injection of the drug. The rate of absorption of drugs after intramuscular or subcutaneous injection is generally controlled by a filtration process in which the rate of absorption will be affected by the surface area of the capillaries at the injection site and the solubility of the drug in the interstitial fluid. The major advantage of both intramuscular and subcutaneous injection is to bypass the first-pass effect of the liver. Subcutaneous administration can be used for drugs that are not irritating to the tissue; it will provide a slow, constant absorption the rate of which can be intentionally altered. The rate of absorption after subcutaneous administration is fastest if the drug is in aqueous solution. It can be slowed by suspension of the drug in oil and can be further slowed by implanting a solid pellet under the skin. Intramuscular administration provides a more rapid absorption than does the subcutaneous route. The rate of absorption from muscle can also be slowed by suspending the drug in oil.

When drugs are administered intravenously, the absorption process is bypassed. Intravenous administration has several advantages: (i) a desired drug concentration in the blood can be attained immediately and accurately; (ii) the doses can be adjusted according to the patient's response; and (iii) irritating solutions can be administered, particularly if they are administered slowly. There are, however, disadvantages to intravenous drug administration: (i) once a drug has been injected, there is no absorption process that can be manipulated in the event of overdose; (ii) drugs cannot be dissolved in oily vehicles; (iii) drugs cannot be administered that may precipitate constituents of blood; and (iv) a patent vein must be maintained for continuous injections. In general, intravenous administration must be performed slowly with constant monitoring to avoid drug toxicities.

Absorption of Drugs

Absorption is the rate at which a drug leaves its site of administration and enters the general circulation. Anything that affects absorption will affect the drug concentration in the blood and consequently the efficacy and toxicity of a particular drug therapy. There are a number of factors that modify absorption. The first is drug solubility, which is particularly important for orally administered drugs; the drug is generally administered as a tablet. The more rapidly the drug dissolves, the more rapidly it will be absorbed because it can mix more readily with the aqueous phase at the absorptive site. The second factor that will modify absorption is the concentration of drug at the absorptive site. The rate of transfer by most transport processes depends on the concentration difference between the two sides of the membrane. Therefore, the higher the concentration at the absorptive site, the more rapidly absorption will occur. Blood flow will also affect the rate of absorption by transporting the newly absorbed drug away from the site, thereby maintaining the concentration gradient. Another factor that will affect the absorption of a drug is the area of the absorbing surface. Increases in the absorbing surface lead to an increased rate of absorption. The fifth factor that will affect the absorption of a drug is the route of administration, which has already been discussed (6).

Sites of Absorption through the Gastrointestinal Tract

When drugs are administered orally, they can be absorbed from a number of sites. The first potential site is the mouth. The mouth has a small surface area and a pH of approximately 6. Drugs absorbed from the mouth must be highly lipid soluble and must be potent. Because of the pH of the mouth, certain weak bases can be better absorbed from this site than from the stomach. One of the primary advantages of absorption of drugs from the mouth is that drugs can directly enter the general circulation, avoiding the first-pass effect of the liver. An example of a compound that is absorbed by this mechanism is nitroglycerin, which is often administered sublingually.

The stomach is primarily a digestive organ. It has a rich blood supply and a reasonable amount of surface area. Therefore, the stomach can be a site of absorption for some drugs, particularly weak acids. The pH of the stomach ranges from around 1 to 2 and this low pH can affect the degree of ionization of many drugs and consequently affect the rate of absorption of drugs from this site. In general, weak acids will be more readily absorbed from this site than weak bases. Furthermore, weak bases can be found to accumulate in the stomach even if they are intravenously administered.

The small intestine is the major site of absorption for most orally administered drugs, primarily because of its extremely large surface area. Although absorption is usually mediated by passive diffusion, it can occur by facilitated diffusion, active transport, endocytosis, or filtration. The pH of the small intestine ranges between 5 and 8; however, in the proximal jejunum, where most of the absorption occurs, the pH is approximately 5. It is important to note that both weak acids and weak bases are better absorbed from the intestine than from the stomach, principally because of the extremely large surface area of the small intestine compared with the stomach.

The large intestine has a smaller surface area than the small intestine. Owing to the solid nature of the intestinal contents and its smaller surface area, the large intestine is not thought to be a significant site for drug absorption; however, the rectum can be used as a site of administration for some drugs. Rectal administration can be used for local conditions such as hemorrhoids, or it can be used for introducing compounds into the systemic circulation. The primary dosage forms are solutions or suppositories. This route is used most often in patients who have nausea or vomiting. Rectal administration also has the advantage that 50% of the blood supply bypasses the liver and can, at least partially, circumvent the first-pass effect (6,7).

Drug Absorption Outside the Gastrointestinal Tract

The lung can be used as the site of administration for both local effects, as with albuterol, or for systemic effects, as with general anesthetics. The lung has a large surface area and a high rate of blood flow, which makes it a particularly good site for drug absorption. Drug absorption occurs by simple diffusion, endocytosis, or active transport and avoids the first-pass effect of the liver. There are certain disadvantages: (i) administration through the lung is cumbersome, (ii) there are difficulties in dosage regulation, and (iii) there can be irritation to the pulmonary epithelium.

Drugs can be administered through the skin, usually to take advantage of their local effects (e.g., benzocaine for minor burns). In addition, the use of transdermal patches permits the cutaneous absorption of drugs into the systemic circulation for prolonged action (scopolamine patches for motion sickness and nicotine patches for tobacco dependence). Most drugs enter the skin by passive diffusion, which means that the partition coefficient of the drug and its pK will be important in controlling the rate of its absorption. The outer layer of the skin, the stratum corneum, forms a barrier against rapid penetration of most drugs. This is primarily the result of the low degree of hydration of the cells in this layer, which usually ranges from 5% to 15% but can be increased up to 50% by use of occlusive dressings. The increase in hydration will increase the absorption of drugs from this site. Lipid-insoluble drugs can enter through hair follicles, sweat glands, and sebaceous glands.

Drug Distribution

Drug distribution is the transfer of a drug from the circulation to the interstitial fluid and finally to the tissues of the body. After absorption, drugs will be distributed throughout the vasculature within approximately 2 to 3 minutes. There are a number of factors that affect further distribution into the tissues. One factor affecting distribution of drugs is regional blood flow. Different tissues have different rates of perfusion. The heart, liver, and brain are highly perfused tissues; muscle and skin are moderately perfused; and finally, adipose tissue is slowly perfused. The differences in perfusion rates are particularly important for the distribution of lipid-soluble drugs. Because drugs that are extremely lipid soluble are rapidly absorbed by passive diffusion, they will first be distributed into the highly perfused tissues and then are rapidly reabsorbed from that site. An example of a drug that follows such a distribution pattern is thiopental, which rapidly produces anesthesia because it arrives at the brain in large concentrations and is then rapidly absorbed. However, as the drug continues to distribute into muscle, skin, and fat, the drug concentration in the plasma decreases. The drug will then transfer back out of the highly perfused tissues (e.g., brain) and into the blood. This causes a decrease in the drug concentration in the brain and permits the patient to regain consciousness within a few minutes.

Drug distribution is also affected by the permeability of capillaries. After transport throughout the vasculature, the drug reaches the capillaries and can be transferred either by filtration, passive diffusion, or endocytosis. A drug will be transferred across the capillary membranes, primarily by ultrafiltration on the arterial side and by osmotic pressure on the venous side. As a result, the pressure gradient driving the ultrafiltration and the molecular size of the drug will be major determinants controlling the distribution into the interstitial fluid. The sizes of the capillary fenestrations vary in different tissues and affect the rate of drug transfer. If the drug is lipid soluble, it can be transferred by passive diffusion despite fenestration size. In this case, the degree of ionization and lipid solubility will be important factors controlling the rate of transfer (6).

Once the drug has been transferred across the capillary membranes into the interstitial fluid, it can then be taken up into the tissues. The mechanism of uptake into tissues depends on the physical characteristics of the compound and/or the ability to utilize receptor-mediated transport mechanisms.

The extent of drug distribution can be restricted by binding to plasma proteins, because such binding decreases the free drug concentration in the plasma. The bound portion of the drug cannot reach the receptor site and, therefore, cannot produce its pharmacologic effect. However, the bound drug also cannot be distributed, metabolized, or excreted. The bound drug therefore acts as a drug reservoir, which will delay the onset of a drug effect on its initial administration and can prolong drug action once administration of drug is discontinued. These effects depend on (i) the affinity of the drug for plasma proteins, (ii) the drug concentration in the plasma, (iii) the degree of saturation of the plasma protein-binding sites, and (iv) the potency of the drug. There are three principal plasma proteins that are involved in drug distribution. Albumin is a plasma protein with a molecular weight of approximately 68,000; it has one or two high-affinity sites for acidic compounds. Additionally, albumin normally carries fatty acids, so it can also bind lipid-soluble drugs to a lesser extent. This protein also has many sites for the binding of bases; however, these are low-affinity sites.

Lipoproteins comprise the second major group of plasma proteins and have the ability to bind highly lipid-soluble drugs. In general, the binding depends on the lipid content; very low-density lipoproteins have a greater ability to bind lipid-soluble drugs than do the low-density and high-density lipoproteins.

The third major plasma protein is α_1-acid glycoprotein, which has one high-affinity binding site for basic drugs. This protein is inducible by trauma, injury, or stress, and the protein has a biologic half-life of approximately 5.5 days. The inducibility of this protein can have a profound effect on the pharmacologic response to a drug. For example, suppose an individual is taking a basic drug that binds to α_1-acid glycoprotein at a level that produces an adequate therapeutic response. If this individual experiences some form of trauma, the level of α_1-acid glycoprotein will be increased, leading to a decreased level of free drug and a diminished therapeutic effect. Maintenance of the proper therapeutic effect under these conditions may require an elevated drug dose. On the other hand, suppose a patient is injured (and therefore has an elevated α_1-acid glycoprotein level) and is administered a basic drug at a concentration that produces a desired therapeutic response. When the level of α_1-acid glycoprotein decreases 10 to 20 days later (after the injury or stress is no longer present); the decrease in the protein level could lead to an increase in the free drug concentration to the point where toxic effects may be observed. These examples illustrate how alterations in the level of this plasma protein influence the therapeutic response to a drug (6,7).

Drugs bind to plasma proteins and they can also accumulate in tissues (which also serve as a reservoir for drugs). There are three basic mechanisms for accumulation in tissues. The first is ion trapping owing to pH differences. For example, cellular pH is approximately 7, whereas plasma pH is approximately 7.4. This pH difference can cause the accumulation of certain drugs (i.e., weak bases) within the cells, if they are more ionized at 7 than at 7.4. Drugs can also accumulate by binding to intracellular components. For example, iodine can accumulate in the thyroid gland, metals can accumulate in the kidney by binding to metallothionein, and lead can compete with calcium in the bone. The third mechanism for drug accumulation in tissues is partitioning into lipid. Individuals who have been administered a lipid-soluble drug for a long period of time will have a tendency to accumulate such a drug in their adipose tissue. This accumulation is relatively slow because of the low amount of perfusion of this tissue; however, over protracted periods of time, large amounts of a drug can accumulate at that site, particularly if it is extremely lipid soluble. Despite the mechanism, the major consequence of drug accumulation in tissues will be a delay in the onset of drug action after its administration; or a prolongation of the drug effect after termination of its administration.

Physiologic Barriers to Drug Distribution

The capillaries in most organs contain fenestrations that permit the transfer of drugs by filtration. In the brain, however, the capillary endothelial cells and the glial cells are joined by tight junctions, which will prohibit the transfer of drugs by this process. Generally, for drugs to enter the brain, they must passively diffuse through the cells or utilize some receptor-mediated transport process rather than be filtered among them. Therefore, factors that control passive diffusion of drugs will control whether a drug can be transported into the brain.

Under some conditions, the placenta also provides a barrier to the transfer of compounds. It is important to note that in general the placenta does not prevent transport. Molecular size is an important determinant for the transfer of water-soluble drugs; those that have molecular weights less than 600 freely transfer across the placenta. Compounds having molecular weights larger than 600 cross with increasing difficulty, until the molecular weight exceeds 1,000 kDa. Such large compounds will not transfer across the placenta. If the compounds are lipid soluble, they will be readily transferred from the mother to the fetus by passive diffusion regardless of molecular size. The rate of transport of such compounds therefore depends on the drug's pK, its partition coefficient, and whether it binds to plasma proteins.

Excretion of Drugs

Drugs can be excreted from a number of different sites including the kidney, liver, skin, and lungs; however, most excretion occurs from either the kidney or the liver. Renal excretion is the primary route of excretion for most drugs, especially water-soluble drugs. The three major processes are glomerular filtration, passive reabsorption, and tubular secretion.

Glomerular Filtration

Drugs transfer from the glomerulus into the renal tubules by filtration of the blood. This process permits the filtration of substances with the appropriate molecular size, charge, and shape. If the drugs have a molecular weight between 5,000 and 75,000 kDa, filtration will be increasingly restricted with increasing molecular weight. Compounds with molecular weights greater than 75,000 kDa will not be filtered. For drugs with molecular weights in the restricted filtration range (between 5,000 and 75,000 kDa), both charge and shape will have an influence on glomerular filtration. Charged substances are filtered more slowly than uncharged substances, and globular proteins are filtered more slowly than proteins of random coil. If the drugs are bound to plasma proteins, they generally will not be filtered because of the high molecular weight of the protein–drug complexes.

Passive Reabsorption

Approximately 20% of the blood volume is filtered into the renal tubules as the blood passes through the kidney. Because plasma proteins and other high molecular weight compounds are not filtered through the glomerulus, an osmotic gradient is produced between the blood and the fluid in the renal tubules. As a result, water will have a tendency to transfer from the renal tubules into the blood. Drugs in the renal tubules will then have a tendency to transfer back into the blood by passive reabsorption. Like other passive-diffusion processes, passive reabsorption is controlled by the lipid solubility of the drug, its degree of ionization, and the pH of both the blood and tubular filtrate. If the compound is unionized, it will have a greater tendency to be reabsorbed. If the compound is charged, it will tend to be excreted. The pH of the renal tubules can be therapeutically manipulated to increase the excretion of drugs. For example, in the case of overdose from the weak acid phenobarbital, increasing the pH of the urine will cause an increase in the rate of excretion of the drug. This process is called *forced alkaline diuresis*. The excretion of weak bases can sometimes be increased by acidification of the urine, using ammonium chloride.

Active Tubular Secretion

Strong organic acidic and basic drugs can use the two active secretory systems that are present in the renal tubules for the excretion of certain endogenous compounds. Through these systems, drugs are actively transferred from the blood to the lumen. These systems are not particularly selective, but they do fall into two categories: one for anions and one for cations. The system can exhibit saturation when a high concentration of a drug is present. As with other active-transport processes, the system also requires energy and can be inhibited by competition with other acidic or basic compounds that are eliminated by this mechanism.

Hepatic Excretion

The other major excretory organ is the liver. The hepatic blood capillaries have extremely large fenestrations, which will permit the transfer of most drugs into the interstitial fluid surrounding the hepatocyte. These compounds can be readily taken up into the hepatocyte by either passive diffusion or carrier-mediated transport. Once in the hepatocyte, the parent drug can either be excreted into the bile canaliculus

or metabolized by the hepatic drug-metabolizing enzymes. Some of the products of drug metabolism can also be taken into the bile canaliculus and excreted in bile. Uptake into the bile is mediated by active-transport systems capable of transporting the following classes of compounds: anions, cations (both of which are similar to those found in renal tubules), bile acids, and neutral organic compounds. After concentration in the bile, the drugs are then released into the intestine. If the drugs are ionized, they tend to be eliminated in the feces; however, if the drugs are lipid soluble, they can be reabsorbed back into the circulation. This process of drug transfer from the circulation into the hepatocyte, uptake and concentration into the bile, release into the intestine, and reabsorption back into the circulation is called *enterohepatic cycling*. This process can prolong the pharmacologic action of some drugs (7–9).

In general, the liver excretes larger compounds than does the kidney. Compounds with molecular weights less than 400 are usually excreted by the kidney; however, as the molecular weight increases, biliary excretion becomes more important.

Although renal and hepatic excretion are the primary routes for excretion of drugs, other sites can be involved. Drugs can be excreted through the lungs. The primary types of compounds that are excreted by this mechanism are gases and volatile liquids. Excretion occurs by simple diffusion across the alveolar membranes and is a major mechanism for excretion of the inhalational general anesthetics. Drugs can also be excreted into sweat and saliva and expressed in breast milk. The primary transport mechanism for their excretion is passive diffusion, for which the partition coefficient, its pK, and the pH of the tissue are important. Excretion into the saliva has been shown to be responsible for the drug taste that is frequently observed after intravenous injection of a drug. Drugs can also be excreted into breast milk. Generally, drugs will transfer by passive diffusion, and because the pH is approximately 6.5, weak bases have a tendency to be ion trapped within milk. If the drug binds to plasma proteins, the concentration of the drug in the milk will be decreased, and highly lipid-soluble drugs will have a tendency to accumulate in milk fat.

Drug Metabolism

Most drugs are lipid-soluble substances that are partially ionized at physiologic pH. As a result of their high lipid solubility, large amounts of these drugs can be reabsorbed into the general circulation after transport into either the renal tubule or the bile. In fact, some lipid-soluble drugs could not be eliminated effectively within the lifetime of a human if the body had to rely solely on renal excretion for elimination. Therefore in addition to normal excretory processes, drug metabolism is a major mechanism by which drug action can be terminated. The process of biotransformation has certain general characteristics. First, it causes a chemical change in the drug, which usually produces more water-soluble metabolites. As a result, the partition coefficient of the drug is altered, causing the metabolites to be excreted more readily. In some cases, the metabolites can be actively secreted by transport systems in the kidney or in the liver. Finally, the pharmacologic activity of a drug is usually terminated by biotransformation reactions.

Oxidation Reactions

Biotransformation reactions can be broken into two general categories: (i) nonsynthetic, or phase 1 reactions, including oxidation, reduction, and hydrolysis reactions, and (ii) synthetic, or phase 2 reactions, including conjugation of the drug or its metabolite to endogenous compounds (5). The major enzyme systems involved in biotransformation are found in the liver, but others are found in the kidney, lung, and gastrointestinal tract as well as other tissues. The major enzyme involved in the oxidative reactions of drug metabolism is called *cytochrome P-450*. This enzyme is quite nonselective and can catalyze the metabolism of compounds having widely diverse chemical structures. Cytochrome P-450 cannot act independently, but it is part of an electron-transport chain found in the endoplasmic reticulum, which is required for catalysis. Cytochrome P-450 generally catalyzes the hydroxylation of the substrate molecule by inserting one atom from molecular oxygen into the substrate and the other atom issued to form water (Fig. 10.7). Reducing equivalents required for this reaction ultimately originate from reduced nicotinamide adenine dinucleotide phosphate (NADPH) and are transferred through the flavoprotein NADPH-cytochrome P-450 reductase. The electrons are then transferred to cytochrome P-450. Cytochrome P-450 can catalyze a number of reactions in addition to simple hydroxylations, including epoxidation reactions; N-, O-, and S-dealkylation reactions; oxidative deamination; sulfoxide formation; and desulfuration reactions (10,11).

Cytochrome P-450 has a broad substrate selectivity. It can hydroxylate compounds of widely varying structure, including simple hydrocarbons such as benzene and naphthalene up to endogenous compounds such as steroids, fatty acids, and some vitamins. It is responsible for the metabolism of many drugs. The enzyme can also hydroxylate the same substrate at different positions.

There are two basic reasons for the broad substrate selectivity of cytochrome P-450. The first is that the enzyme has a relatively nonselective active site, which can accommodate a wide variety of different compounds as long as they possess a degree of lipid solubility. The other factor controlling the nonselectivity of the enzyme system is that cytochrome P-450 exists in multiple forms, with each enzyme having its own substrate selectivity. This leads to a system

that is capable of metabolizing a compound to many different metabolites, with the levels of metabolite production being dependent on the relative levels of expression of specific P-450 enzymes.

Although cytochrome P-450 is generally thought of as a detoxifying enzyme system, it is important to keep in mind that the system simply catalyzes a wide range of oxidation reactions. Most of these reactions lead to products that are pharmacologically inactive, more water soluble, and consequently more rapidly excreted from the body. However, some of these oxidations produce reactive intermediates capable of binding to deoxyribonucleic acid (DNA), ribonucleic acid (RNA) and important proteins within the cell. The covalent binding of reactive metabolites to these critical macromolecules can lead to toxicity, mutagenesis, carcinogenesis, and teratogenesis (11).

A unified nomenclature was established in 1988 for naming members of the superfamily of P-450 enzymes. This nomenclature was based on sequence similarity of the different P-450 (CYP) enzymes (e.g., CYP1A2), with each form given a number (to identify the family), followed by a letter (to identify the subfamily), and then a number (to identify the individual proteins). P-450s with the same first number are at least 40% similar, and those having the same letter being 59% similar.

Identification of the P-450 enzymes present in humans has become an area of intensive investigation. These studies have led to the characterization of several P-450s of clinical importance, including CYP1A2, CYP2A6, CYP2Cs, CYP2D6, CYP2E1, and CYP3A4/5. Generally, there is a large degree of interindividual variability in the levels of these proteins as well as their activities. Reasons for the variability of these P-450 enzymes will be discussed subsequently. Quantitatively, CYP3A4 and CYP3A5 is the most abundant subfamily of the P-450 superfamily, representing approximately 30% of the total P-450. These forms are responsible for the metabolism of approximately 50% of the drugs commonly encountered by humans. CYP2C comprises approximately 20% of the total P-450, including CYP2C8, CYP2C9, CYP2C18, and CYP2C19. CYP2C9 levels are elevated by treatment with barbiturates and rifampicin. CYP1A2, CYP2E1, CYP2A6, and CYP2D6 make up approximately 13%, 7%, 4%, and 2% respectively of the P-450 (12).

A number of noncytochrome P-450 oxidations can also occur. For example, alcohol dehydrogenase is a soluble enzyme that can convert ethanol to acetaldehyde. Aldehyde dehydrogenase is another soluble enzyme that further

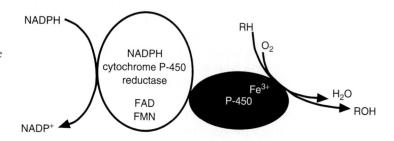

FIGURE 10.7   The cytochrome P-450 monooxygenase system. NADPH, reduced nicotinamide adenine dinucleotide phosphate; NADP, nicotinamide adenine dinucleotide phosphate; FAD, flavin adenine dinucleotide; FMN, flavin mononucleotide; RH, substrate; ROH, product (oxidised substrate).

converts acetaldehyde to acetic acid. Tyrosine hydroxylase and monoamine oxidase are enzymes that are involved in catecholamine metabolism.

There are three basic types of reduction reactions: azoreduction, nitroreduction, and ketoreduction. Enzymes catalyzing these reactions are found either in the endoplasmic reticulum or in the cytosol and in some cases in anaerobic microorganisms found in the ileum and colon.

Practically all organs contain hydrolytic enzymes. They are found in the highest concentrations in the liver, kidney, brain, and plasma. Both esterases and amidases are found in plasma and other tissues and are located primarily in the endoplasmic reticulum of those tissues. Epoxide hydrolase, an enzyme that is involved in the cleavage of the epoxide to a dihydrodiol, is found primarily in the liver with forms found in the endoplasmic reticulum and the cytosol (13).

Conjugation Reactions

Conjugation reactions involve the chemical combination of a drug with an endogenous compound. In general, the drug must have a reactive group or be metabolized to a compound containing a reactive group. Generally, conjugation reactions produce compounds with a reduced pharmacologic activity and a substantially increased rate of excretion. The most common conjugation reaction is the formation of glucuronides, owing to the high availability of glucose, which can form uridine diphosphate (UDP)-glucuronic acid. The drug combines with UDP-glucuronic acid through a reaction that is catalyzed by UDP-glucuronyl transferases. This conjugation occurs primarily in the liver but can also occur in the kidney, intestine and lung and, to a lesser extent, in other tissues. UDP-glucuronyl transferases are found in the microsomal fraction. These conjugates can be transferred to the bile and released into the intestine. Once in the intestine they can be excreted in the feces or, if the glucuronide is susceptible to catalysis by intestinal β-glucuronidase, the compound can be hydrolyzed. In some cases, the action of the β-glucuronidase can regenerate the parent drug. Consequently, the regenerated drug can be reabsorbed into the circulation (enterohepatic cycling). Generally, glucuronides are more water soluble and are usually stronger acids than the parent drug, which accounts for a relatively rapid excretion of the compounds. Glucuronide formation usually abolishes pharmacologic activity.

A primary characteristic of UDP-glucuronyl transferase activity is that it is either low or absent in the fetus and early infant. After birth, these activities increase until they attain their adult levels. Because of the low levels of these enzymes in newborns, drugs or endogenous compounds that require glucuronidation for elimination can accumulate to toxic levels. A syndrome called *kernicterus* is found in newborn infants, especially in those who are premature, and is the result of the inability of the liver to conjugate bilirubin to its glucuronide. Bilirubin is normally excreted in the bile as the glucuronide or bound to plasma proteins. However, in infants, the low level of UDP-glucuronyl transferase activity

leads to a high level of free bilirubin in the plasma; the bilirubin, in turn, can diffuse across the blood–brain barrier and result in irreversible damage to the central nervous system. Another condition called the *gray baby syndrome* is a toxicity resulting from the inability of infants to conjugate chloramphenicol.

Sulfate conjugation is catalyzed by sulfotransferases, which are located in the cytosol of the liver. Sulfate conjugation requires an active sulfate in the form of 3-phosphoadenosine-5′-phosphosulfate (PAPS). Sulfate conjugates are quite polar and easily excreted. They require ATP for the formation of activated sulfate. One of the primary characteristics of this system is its saturability, which is caused primarily by the depletion of PAPS. In the event that sulfate conjugation is saturated, many compounds usually eliminated by this process are eliminated by other routes (e.g., glucuronides).

The enzymes involved in *N*-acetylation reactions are called *N-acetyltransferases* and can combine acetate to the drug molecule. The activated endogenous substrate is acetyl-coenzyme A (CoA). Genetic studies have demonstrated that there are both slow and fast acetylators. Slow acetylators are homozygous for a recessive gene. These individuals are susceptible to dose-dependent toxicity from drugs that are eliminated through *N*-acetylation, such as isoniazid.

Methylation reactions are catalyzed by methyltransferases and use *S*-adenosylmethionine as the activated methyl donor. Methyltransferases are found in the cytosol of many organs including the liver, lung, and kidneys.

Many drugs can be conjugated with glutathione, a tripeptide that is extremely important for the detoxification of environmental pollutants and chemical carcinogens. The enzymes catalyzing these reactions are called *glutathione sulfotransferases*. Found primarily in the cytosol of the liver, they can also be found at lower levels in lung, kidney, and other tissues. There are multiple forms of glutathione sulfotransferases, which have overlapping substrate specificities (11,13).

Factors Affecting Drug Metabolism

Age

Age is a primary factor affecting drug metabolism; greater sensitivity to drugs is observed in the very young and very old. Although a number of factors change with age, the rate of biotransformation is probably the most important age-related effect (13). Overall drug-metabolizing activity is low in newborns and increases with age. This results in a greater sensitivity to toxicities to drugs in newborns. The elderly are also more sensitive to drugs than are young adults. There are several factors that contribute to this sensitivity. In elderly patients, the rate of absorption of drugs is decreased because of a decrease in gastrointestinal motility and blood flow. Distribution is also altered because of increases in the amount of body fat, decreases in muscle mass, hyperalbuminia, and decreases in total body water. Metabolism may also decrease due to decreases in the activity of the drug-metabolizing enzymes as well as decreased blood flow to the liver. Excretion in the elderly can be substantially altered. This is primarily caused by a decrease in renal function as an individual ages (13).

Enzyme Induction

A number of the drug-metabolizing enzymes have been demonstrated to be inducible. Induction of glucuronyltransferases and glutathione sulfotransferases has been shown; however, the drug-metabolizing enzymes most susceptible to induction are those of the cytochrome P-450 system. As mentioned previously, there are multiple forms of cytochrome P-450, with the level of each enzyme under genetic control. Exposure to a number of drugs, carcinogens, and other foreign compounds has been shown to increase the levels of particular cytochrome P-450 enzymes. Induction of these enzymes will not only accelerate the metabolism of the inducing compound but will also increase the metabolism of other compounds. Some compounds that have been shown to induce cytochrome P-450 include phenobarbital, other drugs, polycyclic aromatic hydrocarbons, and alcohol. In individuals who are exposed to such compounds, the metabolism of certain therapeutically administered drugs could be accelerated, leading to lower plasma levels, and a decreased therapeutic response (11).

Polymorphisms in Drug-Metabolizing Enzymes

Large variations in drug-metabolizing activities have been found among individuals. These variations are not only due to differences in expression of the drug-metabolizing enzymes because of dietary factors and induction status, but also genetic differences in the function of particular drug-metabolizing enzymes. These genetic differences are known as *polymorphisms*. A polymorphism is a mutation in the gene that confers either a difference in the activity or the expression of that protein. The mutations are inherited, and have been found to be expressed differentially in particular populations. Most of the polymorphisms identified thus far affect the structural gene, which can alter the activity of a protein. Commonly, polymorphisms in the drug-metabolizing enzymes lead to enzymes that have lower activities than the wild-type protein; however, some polymorphisms lead to higher enzyme activities, generally by the production of larger amounts of protein.

Not all mutations in the drug-metabolizing enzymes lead to polymorphisms that alter enzyme activities. Some changes in the region of the structural gene do not result in a change in the amino acid sequence for the protein, whereas other modifications lead to conservative changes in the protein. Neither of these alterations would be expected to affect the function of the drug-metabolizing enzyme. However, for those mutations affecting function or expression of an enzyme, alterations in enzyme activity can have a significant influence not only on the activity of an enzyme, but also on the products produced.

Several common polymorphisms in the drug-metabolizing enzymes are shown in Table 10.1. Generally, polymorphisms that decrease the metabolic activity of an enzyme would be expected to result in higher plasma concentrations of the parent compound and a greater pharmacologic effect. This can lead to life-threatening conditions as seen with succinylcholine apnea, where an abnormal plasma cholinesterase does not permit the inactivation of the muscle relaxant succinylcholine. This condition is found in approximately 1 in 3,000 patients. Another drug sensitivity due to a polymorphism in CYP2D6 is debrisoquine 4-hydroxylase deficiency. Patients with this polymorphism

TABLE 10.1

Polymorphisms in Drug Metabolizing Enzymes of Clinical Importance

Enzyme	Susceptible Group	Clinical Manifestation/Risk	Clinical Test for Polymorphism
CYP1A1	Rapid metabolizers	Increased association with lung cancer	
CYP1A2	Rapid metabolizers	Elevation in covalent adducts	Caffeine metabolism
CYP2A6	Slow metabolizers	Decreased risk for nicotine dependence	Nicotine metabolism
CYP2C19	Slow metabolizers	Increased association with lung cancer	
CYP2D6	Slow metabolizers	Lower risk for lung cancer	Dextromethorphan metabolism
	Extensive metabolizers	Higher risk for lung cancer	
CYP2E1	Wild type	Increased risk for lung cancer	Chlorzoxazone metabolism
Glutathione-S-transferase	Null genotype	Increased risk for lung cancer (when linked to CYP1A1 polymorphism)	
	Null genotype	Increased risk for bladder cancer	
N-acetyltransferase	Slow acetylators	Isoniazid-induced toxicity	
	Slow acetylators	Drug-induced lupus	
	Rapid acetylators	Isoniazid-induced hepatitis	
	Slow acetylators	Arylamine-induced bladder cancer	
Esterase	Slow metabolizers	Succinylcholine apnea	Dibucaine number

have very low metabolism of the antihypertensive drug debrisoquine and consequently an unexpectedly large hypotensive response. Other polymorphisms leading to an enhanced drug effect are listed in Table 10.1. Some polymorphisms have been associated with an increase in toxicity of drugs. Isoniazid-induced neurotoxicity results from a polymorphism in *N*-acetyltransferase activity, with the toxicity being associated with slow acetylators. Other conditions associated with acetylator status are mentioned previously and shown in Table 10.1.

Polymorphisms in several drug-metabolizing enzymes have been associated with risk for carcinogenesis. There is a polymorphism in the *glutathione-S-transferase* (GSTM) gene that has been associated with lung and bladder cancer. Individuals with this polymorphism are devoid of the GSTM1, and have been shown to be at increased risk for lung and bladder cancer (14). Increased cancer risk has also been associated with polymorphisms in CYP1A1, CYP2D6, and *N*-acetyltransferase (15).

It is important to keep in mind that many of the associations between polymorphisms and disease states are made from epidemiologic data. Frequently, an association in one study is not always found in other studies. Many of the differences are due to differences in the populations examined, the sample sizes of the studies, and the end points measured. Taken together, these studies can point to an increased susceptibility to contracting cancer or other diseases in groups possessing particular polymorphic genes.

Several other disease states have been associated with polymorphisms in drug metabolizing enzymes. For example, there have been reports of a polymorphism in CYP2A6, which leads to decreased metabolism of nicotine. Individuals having this polymorphism appear to have a decreased risk for nicotine dependence (16). Additionally, slow acetylators have been more susceptible to contracting drug-induced lupus erythematosus (17). There are reports of associations between polymorphisms in drug-metabolizing enzymes with Parkinson (18,19), Alzheimer (19,20) and even periodontal disease (21). Additional studies are required to determine if the reported associations are causal or coincidental.

Other Factors Affecting Drug Metabolism

The drug-metabolizing enzymes have also been expressed in a tissue-dependent and species-dependent manner. Tissue-dependent variations in drug metabolism are the result of differential expression of cytochrome P-450 enzymes in different tissues. Different P-450 enzymes have also been expressed in different species. In most cases, similar enzymes are expressed across species lines; however, these orthologous P-450s may possess different substrate selectivities. Both tissue- and species-dependent differences in expression of these drug-metabolizing enzymes can result either in differences in the rates of metabolism of particular drugs or differences in the metabolic products produced. Such differences may lead to toxicity to a drug in a particular tissue (because of differences in metabolism in a particular tissue)

and to difficulty in extrapolating metabolic data obtained in animals to humans.

A number of nutritional factors have also been shown to decrease drug metabolism. Protein deficiency, fat-free diets, and a deficiency in essential fatty acids can all decrease overall drug metabolism. Certain vitamin and nutrient deficiencies have also been shown to decrease drug metabolism, including deficiencies in vitamins A, C, and E; riboflavin; and calcium and magnesium ions. A number of hormones have been implicated in the regulation of drug metabolic activities. Thyroxine and insulin appear to increase drug metabolic activities, and glucocorticoids and testosterone have been shown to alter drug metabolism. Growth hormone appears to increase the activities of some drug-metabolizing enzymes and to decrease the activities of others in experimental animals.

The clinical importance of the drug-metabolizing enzymes is that when a patient is being treated with drugs, there may be substantial individual variation in drug metabolism. These differences may be due to genetic variability, differences in exposure to environmental toxicants, or the result of prior drug exposure. It is important to remember that individuals previously exposed to different compounds will not deal with drugs in a similar manner. As can be seen in cases of metabolic tolerance, prolonged exposure to some drugs alters their metabolism, thereby decreasing the steady-state levels for that drug. These variations in drug metabolism can also lead to drug interactions, for which the presence of one drug or environmental agent can alter the metabolism not only of the parent drug but also of any other drug eliminated by these enzymes. Toxicity from a drug as a result of lower levels of expression of certain drug-metabolizing enzymes or induction of isoforms capable of producing toxic metabolites can also occur (11,13,22).

CLINICAL PHARMACOKINETICS

Ultimately, the magnitude of a pharmacologic response is related to the drug concentration at the receptor site. As has been described, the ability of a drug to get to the receptor site is influenced by each of the pharmacokinetic parameters: absorption, distribution, metabolism, and excretion. Clinical pharmacokinetics permits a quantitative description of the behavior of drugs once they enter the body. It is useful in determining the dosage adjustments that may be required by altered physiologic states such as aging, or renal or hepatic impairment.

Compartmental Modeling

The fate of a drug in the body can be described by treating the body as a series of compartments into which drugs can transfer. This treatment is called *compartmental modeling*. In the simplest case, the entire body is treated as a single homogenous compartment (Fig. 10.8A). The drug enters the body at a certain rate, which is determined by the rate constant k_a, known as the *absorption rate constant* (there is

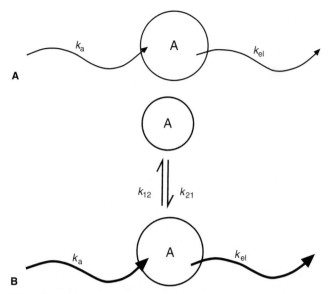

FIGURE 10.8 Compartmental modeling. **A:** One-compartment model. **B;** Two-compartment model.

no absorption occurring after intravenous administration). Once the drug enters the body, it is eliminated as governed by its elimination rate constant k_{el} (9,23).

The behavior of many drugs cannot be explained by a simple one-compartment model. In these cases, the body can be treated as two compartments, a central compartment and a peripheral compartment (Fig. 10.8B). The drug first enters the central compartment controlled by the absorption rate constant k_a. It can then be distributed into the peripheral compartment (governed by the rate constant k_{12}) and can be eliminated, as determined by the elimination rate constant k_{el}. Both the elimination of the drug and its distribution from the central to peripheral compartments will continue until the drug achieves a steady state between these compartments. Once the steady state is attained, the drug will continue to be eliminated from the central compartment (controlled by k_{el}). Because of the decreased drug concentration in the central compartment, the drug will begin to transfer back from the peripheral compartment into the central compartment until elimination of the drug is complete (9).

The physiologic volumes that are represented by the central and peripheral compartments depend on the physical characteristics of the drug. For example, if the drug has a higher molecular weight and is water soluble, it will have a tendency to be slowly transferred from the blood into the interstitial fluid. In this case, the blood would represent the central compartment and the remainder of the body would represent the peripheral compartment. In the event that the drug is small and water soluble, it could readily transfer by filtration into the interstitial fluid but would not be rapidly absorbed into the tissues. For this type of drug, the blood and interstitial fluid would represent the central compartment and the remainder of the body would represent the peripheral compartment. If the drug were very lipid soluble, then passive diffusion into the tissues will occur rapidly. For this type

of drug, the blood, the interstitial fluid, and those highly perfused tissues that would first encounter the drug would represent the central compartment, whereas the more slowly perfused tissue would make up the peripheral compartment. Actually, the body is a multicompartmental model, with each organ or tissue making up its own compartment. However, many of these organs are typically grouped together, and one- or two-compartment models can usually describe the behavior of most drugs.

One-Compartment Model

As a drug undergoes the processes of absorption, distribution, metabolism, and excretion, the drug concentration in the blood changes with time. The characteristics of the blood concentration versus time curves are different for different drugs and can be described by the various compartmental models. When a drug that follows a one-compartment model is administered by a single intravenous injection, the drug concentration found at early times is high and continues to decline as shown in Figure 10.9. The reason for the decrease in drug concentration is the elimination of the drug by either metabolism and/or excretion. As is shown in Figure 10.9, when the drug concentration in the blood is high there is a more rapid rate of elimination, which will tend to level off with time as the drug disappears from the body. The rate of elimination of most drugs depends both on the drug concentration in the body and on the inherent ability of the body to eliminate that drug as described in Equation 10.7.

$$v = -k_{el}[A] \qquad (10.7)$$

where v represents the rate of disappearance; k_{el}, the elimination rate constant; and [A], the concentration of drug A. Therefore, the elimination rate constant is a characteristic of the particular drug, with higher drug concentrations leading to more rapid elimination. For drugs that follow a first-order disappearance, a plot of the logarithm of the drug concentration in the blood versus time will produce a linear relation (Fig. 10.9B). The elimination rate constant for a drug can be calculated from the slope of the line from the natural log of the drug concentration versus time (Fig. 10.9B inset). The biologic half-life is the time required to produce a 50% decrease in the drug concentration in the body. This is also a characteristic of the drug and can be determined graphically. The half-life is related to the elimination rate constant as follows: $t_{1/2} = 0.693/k_{el}$.

When drugs are administered by an extravascular route, the drug must first be absorbed into the circulation. During and after absorption of the drug, elimination will occur, usually by a first-order process. Initially, while the absorption process is occurring, the drug concentration in the blood increases, reaches a plateau, and finally, decreases. This can be seen as the *broken curves* in Figure 10.9. The elimination rate constant can be calculated from this plot in a manner similar to that shown for intravenous administration. The absorption rate constant can also be calculated, but this determination is outside the scope of this discussion. It is important to realize that the elimination rate constant is a

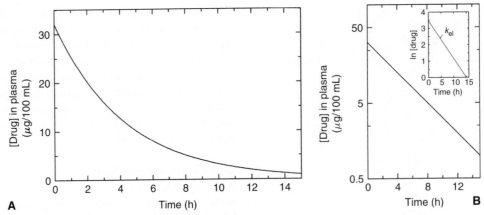

FIGURE 10.9   Change in drug concentration with time for a drug following one-compartment kinetics. **A:** Linear plot. The *solid line* represents the change in drug concentration with time after intravenous administration of the drug; the *dotted line* depicts extravascular drug administration. **B:** Semilogarithmic plot. This graph shows the drug concentration plotted against time where the y-axis represents a base 10 logarithm. **Inset**—In order to properly calculate the k_{el} from the slope, the natural log of the drug concentration needs to be used. The inset shows the natural log of the data in panel *A*.

characteristic of the drug and is independent of its route of administration. In other words, a drug given intravenously or by an extravascular route will have the same half-life and the same elimination rate constant (9).

Most drugs are eliminated according to a first order process. This means that the rate of drug elimination is proportional to the drug concentration in the blood as described in Equation 10.7. However, some drugs are not always eliminated in this manner. This is because some process governing elimination of this drug has become saturated. Once saturation is attained, further increases in the plasma drug concentration cannot lead to a more rapid elimination of the drug. These drugs are called *zero-order drugs* and have a constant rate of elimination once the elimination process is saturated. A comparison of drug elimination by first-order and zero-order drugs are shown in Figure 10.10. Zero-order drugs will eventually be eliminated by a first-order process once the plasma concentration

decreases sufficiently so that its elimination is no longer saturated. At intermediate drug levels, "concentration-dependent" elimination will be observed.

Two-Compartment Model

If a drug follows a two-compartment model and has been administered intravascularly, the curve is no longer linear when plotted on a first-order plot. There are now two phases. Initially, the drug concentration in the blood will be high and will rapidly decrease. Later, the drug concentration will decrease at a slower rate (Fig. 10.11). After the intravenous administration of drug A in (Fig. 10.8B) into the central compartment, a high concentration of the drug will be present. The drug will then be transferred from the central to the peripheral compartment at a rate determined by the rate constant k_{12} times the concentration of drug A in the central compartment. Early in this process, the drug concentration in the central compartment is high;

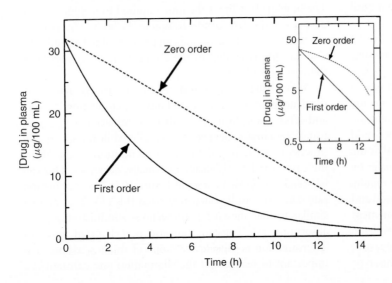

FIGURE 10.10   Comparison of a drug eliminated by first-order and zero-order processes. First-order elimination (*solid line*), zero-order elimination (*dashed line*). **Inset**—replot of the data on a semilogarithmic (first order) plot.

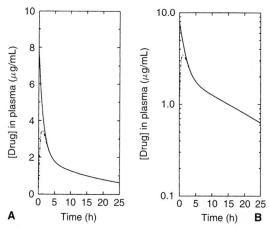

FIGURE 10.11 Change in drug concentration with time for a drug following two-compartment kinetics. **A:** Linear plot. The *solid line* represents the change in drug concentration with time after intravenous administration of the drug; the *dotted line* depicts extravascular drug administration. **B:** Semilogarithmic plot.

therefore, the rate of transfer from the central to peripheral compartment will also be high. As this process continues, the drug concentration in the central compartment becomes lower, decreasing the rate of accumulation in the peripheral compartment. In addition, because the drug concentration in the peripheral compartment will continue to increase, the rate of transfer back into the central compartment will depend on the concentration of drug A in the peripheral compartment times its rate constant k_{21}. A steady state will eventually be achieved between the drug in the central and peripheral compartments. While the distribution process is occurring, the drug is eliminated as governed by its elimination rate constant (k_{el}) times the concentration of the drug in the central compartment. Once the steady state is achieved between the central and peripheral compartments, the drug will continue to be eliminated; the rate depends on the drug concentration in the central compartment. As the drug continues to be eliminated from the central compartment, it can then be transferred from the peripheral into the central compartment. This process continues until the drug is completely eliminated. A graphical representation of what occurs is shown in Figure 10.11. During the early phase, which is called the *distribution phase* (α), the drug concentration rapidly decreases with time. At later times, the drug concentration decreases at a slower rate, which will continue until the drug is completely eliminated from the body. The second phase is called the *disposition phase* (β). It is calculated in the same way as the elimination rate constant is calculated for a one-compartment model and can be determined from the half-life of the drug (which can be estimated from the graph after the rapid distribution phase is complete). The disposition rate constant differs from the elimination rate constant in that the drug is not only being eliminated during this phase but also being redistributed from the peripheral to the central compartment. During the α-phase, the primary process responsible for the rapid

decrease in drug concentration in the blood is the distribution of the drug from the central to the peripheral compartment. However, during this phase, both the elimination and the redistribution of the drug also are occurring. If a drug following a two-compartment model is administered extravascularly, the absorption process is interposed on the pharmacokinetic plot (Fig. 10.11, *broken line*) (9).

Volume of Distribution

Once a drug is administered, it will be distributed as determined by its physical characteristics. Some drugs may have a tendency to stay in the plasma, others will transfer to the interstitial fluid, and still others will uniformly distribute throughout the body. Furthermore, some drugs have a tendency to accumulate in particular tissue reservoirs. The total volume into which a drug appears to distribute is known as its *apparent volume of distribution* (V_d). The calculation of volume of distribution is based on the assumption that the drug concentration in the blood is inversely proportional to how extensively the drug is distributed throughout the body. For example, if drug transfer to the rest of the body is restricted, it will be retained in the plasma and a higher drug concentration will be found in the blood. On the other hand, if the drug distributes throughout the body, then a lower drug concentration will be found in the blood. The apparent volume of distribution for a drug can be calculated by intravenous injection of a known amount of drug into an individual. The disappearance of drug with time is then plotted on a semilogarithmic plot. One then extrapolates back to time zero to determine what that concentration would have been in the blood if elimination did not occur (Fig. 10.12). The volume of distribution can be calculated as described in Equation 10.8.

$$V_d = \frac{X}{[A]_{t=0}}$$ (10.8)

where X represents the total amount of drug injected and $[A]_{t=0}$ is the drug concentration in the body extrapolated to time zero. A drug that tends to stay in the plasma has

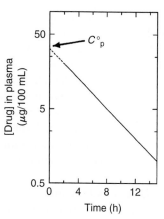

FIGURE 10.12 Determination of the initial plasma concentration (C°_p) for calculation of the apparent volume of distribution (V_d)

a volume of distribution of approximately 5 L. A drug that transfers into the interstitial fluid and the plasma has a volume of distribution of approximately 15 L, and a drug that uniformly distributes throughout the body has a volume of distribution of approximately 40 L.

Some drugs have very large volumes of distribution. In fact, these volumes can even be larger than the total fluid volumes of the body. For example, digoxin has an apparent volume of distribution greater than 700 L and the antimalarial drug quinacrine has a volume of distribution of approximately 50,000 L. The reason for these extremely large volumes is the binding of the drugs to tissue components. If a drug binds tightly to tissue components, it will tend to accumulate in that tissue, leading to lower drug concentrations in the blood. Because the volume of distribution depends on the amount of drug administered divided by the concentration that is measured in the blood, anything that decreases the concentration in the blood leads to a larger apparent volume of distribution. On the other hand, small volumes of distribution are observed if the drug has a tendency to stay in the blood. For example if a drug binds extensively to plasma proteins, a smaller volume of distribution might be expected (9,23).

Clearance

Clearance is the theoretic volume of blood from which a drug is completely removed in a given time period. In terms of whole organisms, it may be thought of in relation to the elimination rate constant or in terms of a particular organ such as the liver or the kidney. When referring to the whole organism, the term *total clearance* (Cl_T) is used. One of the simplest ways to calculate the total clearance is shown in Equation 10.9.

$$Cl_T = k_{el} \cdot V_d \qquad (10.9)$$

When clearance is controlled by first-order processes, it is additive. Therefore, the total body clearance is equal to the clearance from the kidney plus the clearance from the liver plus clearance from all other sites.

Multiple Dosing Schedules

In many therapeutic situations, there is a need to maintain a particular steady-state level of a drug. For a drug to be therapeutically effective, a certain minimum concentration must be maintained. Administration of a single dose of the drug may be therapeutically effective for a short time; however, as soon as the drug is administered, ionization begins, leading to a decreased concentration in the blood. Eventually, drug concentrations will drop below the minimum effective concentration. Maintaining therapeutic levels requires continuous administration of the drug.

Continuous Intravenous Infusion

Drugs are sometimes administered by constant intravenous infusion when sustained and carefully regulated drug concentrations must be obtained (Fig. 10.13). In this case, the drug is administered at a constant rate, and the drug is

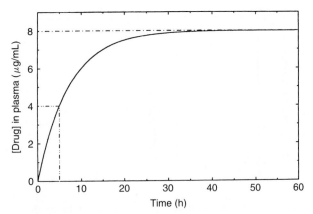

FIGURE 10.13 Change in plasma–drug concentration after intravenous infusion. This drug follows one-compartment kinetics, has a $t_{1/2}$ of 5 hours, and a steady-state concentration of 8 μg/mL.

eliminated according to a first-order process. In other words, the rate of elimination of a drug is proportional to the drug concentration in the body. On the initiation of infusion, the drug concentration in the plasma rapidly increases as a result of the slow rate of elimination (Equation 10.7); however, as the infusion continues, the drug concentration in the plasma increases, leading to an increase in the rate of its elimination. As a result, the concentration will reach a plateau (Fig. 10.13). Eventually, the rate at which the drug is being eliminated is equal to the rate of drug going into the body. At this point, the drug has achieved steady state. As shown in Equation 10.10, the steady-state concentration (C_{ss}) is equal to the dose rate divided by the total body clearance.

$$C_{ss} = \frac{\text{Dose/Time}}{Cl_T} \qquad (10.10)$$

Therefore, if both the total clearance and the desired steady-state concentration for a drug are known, the infusion rate (dose/time) can be readily calculated.

The time that it takes to achieve a steady state is a characteristic that depends on the half-life of the drug. It takes four to five half-lives to achieve a steady-state concentration after multiple drug administration. For example, a drug with a half-life of 5 hours would take approximately 20 to 25 hours to attain a steady-state concentration. If there is a change in the dose rate, then it will take another four to five half-lives from the point of the change in infusion rate before the steady state is again reached (Fig. 10.14). Therefore, the time required to achieve a steady state depends on the half-life of the drug, whereas the steady-state concentration that is achieved depends on the total body clearance of that drug and the dose rate at which the drug is administered (5,23).

Multiple Dosing

In general, repeated dosing is required to achieve and maintain a desired therapeutic effect. However, intravenous infusions are usually not necessary and in most cases impractical. Therefore, under some circumstances drugs can be administered by multiple intravenous injections. As is shown in Figure 10.15A drug being administered according

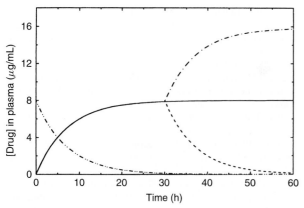

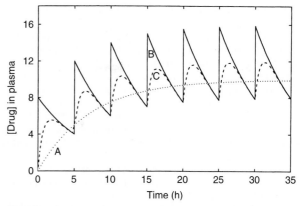

FIGURE 10.14 The effect of changes in infusion rate on the time required to attain a steady state. The drug depicted has a $t_{1/2}$ of 5 hours and achieves its C_{ss} after 20 to 25 hours (— • —), or four to five half-lives. Another four to five half-lives are required to attain a new steady state after a change in the infusion rate (—). Because the $t_{1/2}$ controls the elimination of a drug after either infusion (— —) or intravenous bolus (— •• —), the curves are complementary. At one $t_{1/2}$, either 50% of the C_{ss} is attained (after infusion) or 50% of the drug is eliminated (intravenous bolus)

FIGURE 10.16 Continuous administration of a drug by continuous intravenous infusion (curve A), multiple intravenous injections (curve B), and multiple extravascular administration (curve C)

to schedule *A* will be injected once every four half-lives. In this case, the drug concentration almost approaches zero before the next injection. Consequently, there would be very little accumulation of drug, and large fluctuations between the maximum and minimum serum drug concentrations are seen. However, if the drug is administered more frequently (schedule *B* Fig. 10.15), the drug concentration accumulates to a higher steady-state level and the fluctuations (on a percentage basis) are smaller. The rate of accumulation depends on the frequency of dosage administration relative to the half-life of the drug. The magnitude of the fluctuations depends on the frequency of administration with respect to the half-life of the drug. In other words, administration that

is more frequent leads to smaller fluctuations in plasma drug concentrations. As stated previously, the time taken to reach a steady state depends solely on the half-life of the drug. Therefore, if a drug with a long half-life were administered according to the same dosage schedule as a drug with a short half-life, the drug with the long half-life would have a higher degree of accumulation and smaller fluctuations.

In the case in which drugs are administered extravascularly, the drug must first be absorbed into the circulation. Because a finite time is required for absorption to occur, there will be a change in the shape of the curves corresponding to the absorption process (Fig. 10.16). The absorption process actually blunts the sharp changes in drug concentration caused by multiple intravenous injections. The same factors that control selection of a proper dosage schedule for intravenous administration also pertain to extravascular administration of these drugs. Therefore, increasing the frequency of administration will lead to accumulation of the drug and a decrease in the magnitude of the fluctuations. The half-life of the drug still controls the time that it takes for the drug to achieve its steady state (5,23).

In summary, an understanding of pharmacologic principles is important for the rational use of therapeutic agents. Not only is it important to understand the mechanism of action of particular drugs, their therapeutic and adverse effects, but also it is important to understand the factors that may influence the drug concentration at that receptor site. Such information is essential for selection of a therapeutic agent, choice of the proper route of administration and dosage regimen as well as to be alert to idiosyncratic reactions resulting in individual patients.

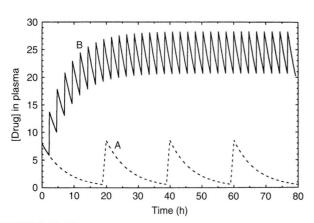

FIGURE 10.15 The change in plasma–drug concentration with time after repeated intravenous injections. The drug was administered once every four half-lives (schedule A) or twice every half-life (schedule B) by intravenous injection. The drug has a $t_{1/2}$ of 5 hours. More frequent administration (as in schedule B) permits accumulation of the drug and decreases the magnitude (on a percentage basis) of the variations.

REFERENCES

1. Yagiela JA. Pharmacodynamics. In: Neidle EA, Yagiela JA, eds. *Pharmacology and therapeutics for dentistry*, 3rd edn. St. Louis: Mosby, 1989:5–16.
2. Clark AJ. The antagonism of acetylcholine by atropine. *J Physiol (London)* 1926;61:547–556.

3. Ruffolo RR Jr. Review important concepts of receptor theory. *J Auton Pharmacol* 1982;2:277–295.

4. Yagiela JA. Pharmacokinetics: the absorption, distribution, and fate of drugs. In: Neidle EA, Yagiela JA, eds. *Pharmacology and therapeutics for dentistry*, 3rd edn. St. Louis: Mosby, 1989:17–47.

5. Benet LZ, Mitchell JR, Sheiner LB. Pharmacokinetics: the dynamics of drug absorption, distribution, and elimination. In: Gilman AG, Rall TW, Nies AS, et al., eds. *The pharmacological basis of therapeutics*, 8th edn. New York: Pergamon Press, 1990:3–32.

6. Gram TE. Drug absorption and distribution. In: Craig CR, Stitzel RE, eds. *Modern pharmacology*, 3rd edn. Boston: Little, Brown and Company, 1990:21–38.

7. Pratt WB. The entry, distribution, and elimination of drugs. In: Pratt WB, Taylor P, eds. *Principles of drug action*, 3rd edn. New York: Churchill Livingstone, 1990:201–296.

8. Berndt WO, Stitzel RE. Excretion of drugs. In: Craig CR, Stitzel RE, eds. *Modern pharmacology*, 3rd edn. Boston: Little, Brown and Company, 1990:59–67.

9. Ritschel WA. *Handbook of basic pharmacokinetics*. Hamilton: Drug Intelligence Publications, 1976.

10. White RE, Coon MJ. Oxygen activation by cytochrome P-450. *Annu Rev Biochem* 1980;49:315–356.

11. Alvares AP, Pratt WB. Pathways of drug metabolism. In: Pratt WB, Taylor P, eds. *Principles of drug action—the basis of pharmacology*, 3rd edn. New York: Churchill Livingstone, 1990:365–422.

12. Lin JH, Lu AY. Inhibition and induction of cytochrome P450 and the clinical implications. *Clin Pharmacokinet* 1998;35:361–390.

13. Gram TE. Metabolism of drugs. In: Craig CR, Stitzel RE, eds. *Modern pharmacology*, 3rd edn. Boston: Little, Brown and Company, 1990:39–58.

14. Bell DA, Taylor JA, Paulson DF, et al. Genetic risk and carcinogen exposure: a common inherited defect of the carcinogen-metabolism gene glutathione S-transferase M1 (GSTM1) that increases susceptibility to bladder cancer. *J Natl Cancer Inst* 1993;85:1159–1164.

15. Bartsch H, Nair U, Risch A, et al. Genetic polymorphism of CYP genes, alone or in combination, as a risk modifier of tobacco-related cancers. *Cancer Epidemiol Biomarkers Prev* 2000;9:3–28.

16. Sellers EM, Tyndale RF. Mimicking gene defects to treat drug dependence. *Ann N Y Acad Sci* 2000;909:233–246.

17. Nebert DW, Weber WW. Pharmacogenetics. In: Pratt WB, Taylor P, eds. *Principles of drug action—the basis of pharmacology*, 3rd edn. New York: Churchill Livingstone, 1990:469–531.

18. Tan EK, Khajavi M, Thornby JI, et al. Variability and validity of polymorphism association studies in Parkinson's disease. *Neurology* 2000;55:533–538.

19. Bon MA, Jansen Steur EN, de Vos RA, et al. Neurogenetic correlates of Parkinson's disease: apolipoprotein-E and cytochrome P450 2D6 genetic polymorphism. *Neurosci Lett* 1999;266:149–151.

20. Stroombergen MC, Waring RH. Determination of glutathione S-transferase mu and theta polymorphisms in neurological disease. *Hum Exp Toxicol* 1999;18:141–145.

21. Meisel P, Timm R, Sawaf H, et al. Polymorphism of the N-acetyltransferase (NAT2), smoking and the potential risk of periodontal disease. *Arch Toxicol* 2000;74:343–348.

22. Gonzalez FJ. The molecular biology of cytochrome P450s. *Pharmacol Rev* 1989;40(4):243–288.

23. Gwilt PR. Pharmacokinetics. In: Craig CR, Stitzel RE, eds. *Modern pharmacology*, 3rd edn. Boston: Little, Brown and Company, 1990:68–81.

CHAPTER 11

Biostatistics

Alan T. Davis

ASSUMPTION

The student believes that the study of statistics constitutes the lowest form of academic masochism and, unless under extreme coercion, would not touch it with a 20-ft pole.

INTRODUCTION

Statistics, as defined by Steel and Torrie (1), is "the science, pure and applied, of creating, developing, and applying techniques such that the uncertainty of inductive references may be evaluated." Definitions of this nature send most residents hurtling through plate-glass windows or launching into violent esophageal reflux. In this same vein, one observes that Webster's definition of sadistic is to receive pleasure from inflicting physical or psychological pain on another or others. Hence the term *sadistics teacher*. (The reader is referred to the glossary at the end of this chapter for other useful terms.)

A far less threatening and more palatable definition is that statistics is "logic or common sense with a strong admixture of arithmetic procedures" (1). This develops an important concept, in that statistics does not involve throwing your good common sense right out the window anytime someone incants in a publication $p < 0.05$. Contrary to common belief, this is not a signal to run up the white flag, plead shameful ignorance of your former method of conducting surgery, and swear obeisance to the new, statistically verified way. When used correctly, statistics is a powerful tool for the analysis of data. However, it is strictly a mathematic argument for the determination of significance. Depending on how the study was designed, statistical significance does not necessarily imply clinical significance. This will be a basic tenet throughout the following discussion. In addition, no attempt will be made in this chapter to show the mathematic origins of the tests. You probably do not know how to make an electric drill, but you should know how to use one. Similarly, the emphasis in this text will be on the application of tests, and not on derivation.

Scientific investigations, in general, develop through the following ways (1):

1. A review of facts, theories, and proposals
2. Formulation of a logical hypothesis, subject to testing by experimental methodologies
3. Objective evaluation of the hypothesis on the basis of experimental results

Somewhere between steps 2 and 3, you develop your research design (more on that later). The research design is developed with the intent of using the strongest statistical analysis available. In other words, research design and statistical design are developed concurrently and are plotted and written before one sample is ever taken, be it blood, sweat, or 50-lb chart. If statistics has a bad name, it is from people deciding after the study is over that "oh, my gosh, my golly, this test would be good, but I bet that I can find a really big difference if I massage the data (read: mangle) and use this other test over here." Pretty tempting, eh? Forget it. The path to invalid conclusions is paved by researchers who allow their data and improperly chosen statistics to lead them around by the nose. Besides, if you have your statistics chosen ahead of time, you do not have to worry about what to do when the time comes to analyze the data. This applies, I might add, to proposals in general—once written, they provide a convenient cookbook for your study.

RESEARCH DESIGN

There are a wide variety of research designs to choose from, so only the more common types will be identified here. The first four are retrospective designs, whereas the remainder are prospective designs.

Chart Reviews

A chart review implies that the major source for the acquisition of data for a research project is from information recorded in a patient's chart. Therefore, the data were acquired in the past, which is why these studies are collectively known as *retrospective studies*. These studies are also known as *historical studies* or *prospectively impaired studies*.

When designing or writing these studies, the time period must be specified, as well as all inclusion and exclusion criteria, that is, who was allowed into the study, who wasn't, and why. Oftentimes the results of a published study will be of little value to you because the study sample is so different from the patient population that you normally see. The major criticism of retrospective studies is the lack of random allocation of patients to study groups. When reviewing data from a retrospective study, either your own or someone else's data, ask yourself, are the differences shown caused by the treatments, or caused by the patient allocation? For example, perhaps a percutaneous endoscopic gastrostomy (PEG) would appear to be superior to surgical gastrostomy (GAST) or surgical jejunostomy (JEJ), relative to incidence of wound infections. Further analysis, however, may reveal that the PEG was a new procedure during the time period of the study, and therefore only the lower risk patients were given PEGs. This question of allocation is the major point to consider for all retrospective studies. However, some studies can only be accomplished retrospectively. A blanket condemnation of retrospective studies is not intended, but rather a caution as to the limitations of these designs.

Case Report

The case report is the simplest type of study in the literature. It involves the discussion of a finding concerning a single individual. It is primarily a device to draw attention to the readership that the condition in question, although rare, does exist. An improper use of a case report would be to advocate sweeping changes in therapy or treatment of a given condition based on one subject.

Case Series

The case series is similar to the case report but it involves more than one individual. The case series may involve the documentation of a rare disorder in a group of people or may actually be a how-we-do-it study, wherein a given procedure that has been done on a certain number of patients is described and, commonly, advocated. Once again, a study of this type is of informational value only and must not be confused with studies in which treatments are compared with one another. Although the reader may decide that a new procedure is worth trying after reading a case series, the caution remains that no proof was documented in the study to demonstrate superiority of one method over another.

Case–Control Study

In this retrospective design, patients with two outcomes are compared, relative to some previously acquired risk factor(s). An example would be a review of hospital records to determine the ideal long-term enteral feeding procedure. The question might be whether the type of enteral feeding procedure is a risk factor for aspiration. We could use a case–control design by dividing the patients into those who aspirated (the cases) and those who did not (the controls).

Then we could look at various feeding procedures as risk factors, such as PEG, JEJ, and GAST. This research design is one of the best for the study of rare diseases or conditions. One of the major disadvantages of this design, however, is that the cases and controls have to be drawn from two different populations.

Retrospective Cohort Study

In the previous example, the subjects were grouped according to outcome. What if we had wanted to group the patients according to the feeding procedure (i.e., PEG, JEJ, and GAST) and determine the frequency of various complications, such as the incidence of aspiration, tube failure, wound complications, and the like? If the study was designed as a retrospective study, this would be a retrospective cohort study. It is worth repeating that in a case–control study, the subjects are grouped according to outcome, whereas in the cohort study, the subjects are grouped according to risk factor. One of the major advantages of this design is that it takes less time to run than a prospective study, which becomes particularly important for studies which require extensive follow-up periods. A major disadvantage is that the researcher has no control over the quality or quantity of the data available in the charts for review. Most residents who have been sent off on a glorious chart review have realized quickly that some or all of the variables of interest in present day surgery weren't very interesting at all 10 years ago, as evidenced by their dearth in the charts. Missing data have altered the variables of interest in many a retrospective study, a problem which is avoided easily in the prospective study designs.

Cross-Sectional Survey

For a cross-sectional survey, a sample of subjects who fit the defined entry criteria (i.e., inclusion and exclusion criteria) are interviewed. An example is a group of 50- to 70-year-old men who are asked whether they have seen a physician or been hospitalized over the last 12 months concerning chest pain. They would also be asked if they exercise 3 or more days a week for at least 30 minutes a day. The objective, obviously, is to link lack of exercise and heart problems. The difficulties, particularly with this study, should also be obvious. Because the study depends totally on subject recall, the accuracy of the recollection is open to question. The influence of confounding variables, such as diet or previous medical history, must also be considered before using this type of design. Depending on the questions being asked, researchers may find that sample size in one group could be absurdly low. Another problem with the cross-sectional survey is that deaths caused by heart disease, even in the age-group under study, will not be observed. On the plus side, the study is relatively inexpensive and easy to conduct.

Prospective Cohort Study

In this design, patients are nonrandomly assigned to treatments (as in a retrospective cohort study), and prospectively monitored. An example would be the study of the effectiveness of percutaneous contact cholecystolithotripsy (PCCL).

Patients could be selected on a volunteer basis to either receive PCCL, or opt for cholecystectomy. Therefore, the assignment would be nonrandom. Complications could be compared between the two groups. Again, whenever there is nonrandom assignment, the question arises as to whether differences noted in the study are caused by differences between the treatments, or between the patients. Another complicating factor may be that, if one treatment is sufficiently less palatable than the other, the more palatable treatment may be selected much more frequently. It would be like trying to enroll patients into a study on brain tumors. The choice could be between taking a magic, horseshoe-shaped capsule ten times a day, or undergoing brain surgery with a renowned (or maybe even not so renowned) neurosurgeon. There could be a wee tad of bias in treatment selection. An advantage of using this prospective design is the ability to match patients for age and gender. Another advantage over a retrospective design is that all of the data which are of interest can be recorded.

Randomized Controlled Trial

It seems as if there should be a little halo above the words randomized controlled trial (RCT) with, perhaps, a choir in the background, doesn't it? So, what is the big deal about these studies anyway? Most important, as opposed to all of the designs listed earlier, the subjects are randomly allocated to treatments, that is, each subject has an equal chance of receiving any treatment. This allows the experimenter to allocate patients, by use of appropriate inclusion and exclusion criteria, such that the groups are as similar as possible, so that any effects noted in the study can be attributed to differences between treatments and not between subjects. This is the preferred situation, in which the experimenter is in control of as much of the study as possible. It is the ideal study design. One of the disadvantages of this design is the expense. Another is that to run the study you must expose subjects to treatments that are possibly either much more harmful than the other treatment or much less beneficial. In some situations, the RCT may be logistically feasible but totally unethical. For these reasons, cohort and case–control studies will continue to have value in the medical literature.

VARIABLES AND RANDOMIZATION

Every experiment needs a hypothesis. For example, let us state that "carnitine is a required nutrient in the diet of the premature infant receiving total parenteral nutrition (TPN)." How would you go about testing this? You could measure weight gain, incidence of cholestasis, plasma and urinary ketones, fatty acid oxidation, respiratory quotient, or urinary dicarboxylic acid output. These are characteristics that can show variability or variation and have been cleverly designated as variables. Variables can be either qualitative or quantitative. It is important to differentiate between these types of variables because they require different types of statistical tests.

Quantitative variables are described as being continuous or discrete. A continuous variable is a value that is only limited by the accuracy of the instrument being used to measure the variable. An example is weight: a person's weight usually is listed as an integer in kilograms or pounds, but the accuracy could be extended to several decimal places if the researcher so desired. A discrete variable is one for which only certain values are possible. An example of this is the number of people in a hospital, which, obviously, cannot be a fraction of a number. Similarly, the spots on a die are discrete numbers. A variation of the continuous and discrete variable is the ratio variable, which is the ratio of two quantitative variables, such as the plasma insulin:glucagon ratio.

Qualitative variables are divided into nominal and ordinal variables. A nominal variable is nothing more than a named category. An example is an individual's favorite ice cream flavor (chocolate, vanilla, or rocky road). In the clinical setting, one often sees this broken down into a yes or no answer, as in survival of the patient or the presence or absence of a complication. When a nominal variable consists of only two categories (such as yes and no), it is also referred to as a *dichotomous variable*. An ordinal variable usually is seen in ranking scales, such as in injury severity scores. An example is how miserable an individual feels on a particular day, measured on a scale of 1 to 10; 1 might be not miserable at all and 10 could be low-down, dragged-out, dead-duck miserable. Another type of ordinal variable is a visual analog scale, wherein a patient is asked to mark on a line his or her reaction to pain, scar healing, etc. An example is shown in Figure 11.1.

At first glance, this would appear to be similar to a continuous variable. The only difference is that with continuous variables, the value 10 is 10 times greater than 1. On an ordinal scale, although, this may not be the case. For example, in a pain survey, if 1 means great and 10 means jackhammer headache, 10 obviously means something different than 10 times 1. Therefore, the strict mathematical relation is lacking, which is why a quantitative, continuous variable is different from a qualitative, ordinal variable, and it is also why different statistics are used to analyze these two disparate types of variables.

Back to the original hypothesis. Let us assume that the variable to be measured is plasma ketone body concentration. The original question asks whether there is a carnitine requirement in the premature infant given TPN. The treatment groups, at the very least, will involve one group of babies receiving TPN with carnitine, and one group receiving TPN without carnitine. Now one must determine which babies will receive which treatment. If the researcher wishes to run an RCT, babies must be randomly assigned to treatment groups.

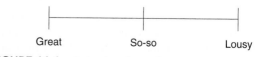

FIGURE 11.1 A visual analog scale.

Why do we bother with all this junk? The primary reason for randomization is to make sure that treatments are distributed over the entire range of the subgroup so that conclusions can be made concerning a larger population. And that is what it is all about. After our study of infants is completed, we will be able to say whether carnitine should be used if any of these little people get premature or need TPN again. What we really want to do, however, is to make a broad statement about any premature infant anywhere in the world who requires TPN. Therefore we want our sample—our study group—to be representative of the population, that is, all premature infants who require TPN.

The process of randomization is normally done using a random number table or a computerized randomization scheme. Either of these techniques will be sufficient to allocate individuals randomly to treatment groups, with the added advantage of being able to assure equal numbers of subjects in each treatment. Another acceptable technique, known as *sampling with replacement*, is to draw numbers from a suitable receptacle, such as an expensive but woefully out-of-fashion tennis shoe. For example, let us say that you have three treatments. You write the three numbers on three pieces of paper and drop them into the shoe. When a patient comes into the unit that matches your inclusion and exclusion criteria, you first obtain informed consent. Then, you reach into the shoe and pull out number three. Your patient will be on treatment three. The number is then put back into the shoe. This ensures that each patient has an equal chance of being entered onto each treatment. The major disadvantage of this technique is that, unless you have a very large sample size, it is unlikely that you will have equal numbers of patients in each group. Therefore, this method should be reserved for a large sample size study or for studies in which having equal numbers of subjects per group is not a concern.

The treatment allocation described in the preceding text is called *simple random sampling*. Let us throw another curve ball into our study, though. Let us assume that the gender of the baby could have an impact on our results. If true, it would be very important to make sure that we have equal numbers of men and women in each group. Now, if we were dealing with a really huge sample size, with a few thousand in each sample, our randomization technique described in the preceding text would be able to do the job. More often, however, the researcher deals with far smaller sample sizes for a study. With a smaller sample size, it is more likely that we will have differences in the male:female ratio in our two groups. Stratified random sampling is one solution to this problem. In terms of the randomization scheme, instead of randomizing into two groups, we would now randomize into four groups: men receiving carnitine, women receiving carnitine, men not receiving carnitine, women not receiving carnitine. Suggestions on how to analyze an experiment such as this will be described later.

Randomization using a random number table, computerized randomization, or sampling with replacement is the only legitimate means for randomly allocating subjects to treatment groups. In practical terms, when reading a prospective, randomized study that uses improper randomization, what are the concerns? The same as those listed for any retrospective study or for the cohort analysis. If a treatment effect is denoted, is it the result of differences in the treatments or between the subjects that comprise the treatments? Therefore, improper randomization is not, in and of itself, a reason to trash a study, but it should be a warning flag.

A word about blinding. If you have just devised this randomization scheme, you are no longer blinded. And heaven only knows, only wimp studies are not blinded. Actually, blinding is something that has to be considered on a case-to-case basis. For example, the babies in our study are probably more interested in their critical mass diapers than in placebo effects, and we can safely tell them which treatment group they are in, that is, the babies will not be blinded. Their sneaky parents are somewhat smarter and should be kept in the dark. However, if the subject is capable of differentiating between treatments, then the subjects need to be blinded. From the investigators' point of view, if our measures of interest (i.e., variables) are all objective (i.e., do not depend on an observer), then the researcher does not need to be blinded. If subjective measures are to be used by the researchers to evaluate the effectiveness of the treatments, then the researchers need to be blinded. If both the subjects and the researchers need to be blinded, you have a double-blind study. In this case, a person outside the study must prepare the randomization scheme. The ultimate study design, applied with one's tongue planted firmly in one's cheek, is the triple-blind study, in which the subjects do not know what they are getting, the residents do not know what they are giving, and the researchers do not know what they are doing (2).

SUMMARIZATION OF DATA

So, we have established our design, isolated our variable, and specified the treatment groups—it looks like a good time to hand out some definitions. Let us say that we have decided to sample 50 babies. Another way of putting this is to say that out of all the premature infants on the earth who have been, are, or will be receiving TPN (the population), we are taking a representative sample of 50 (the sample). Somewhere back in your misspent youth, you have no doubt encountered the celebrated and highly renowned bell-shaped curve (Fig. 11.2). The curve, also referred to as the

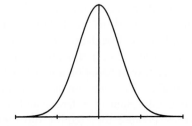

FIGURE 11.2   The normal distribution.

normal distribution, implies that the variable being studied is symmetrically distributed throughout the population. Populations of quantitative variables that are distributed normally are described by parameters. When we study a sample from this population, we use statistics to describe the sample. A statistic is a guess of the true value of the parameter. Statistics that are used to make reasonable guesses of the true values of parameters are known as *parametric statistics*. The two primary assumptions for the use of parametric statistics are that the variables in question are quantitative and that the population from which the sample is drawn is distributed normally. The reason for using samples and statistics is that populations, for the most part, are too large to study conveniently.

The center of the bell-shaped curve, which divides the distribution into two symmetric halves, is called the *mean*, designated $\overline{\mu}$ (parameters are always designated by Greek letters). In the sample, the population mean $\overline{\mu}$ is estimated by the sample mean $\overline{x}$. Occasionally, you will see a mean designated as $\overline{y}$, or some other letter with a bar on top, but $\overline{x}$ is the usual representation. The sample mean is calculated by adding up all of the numbers, and dividing by the sample size.

For example, consider the following data set:

67.1, 69.0, 65.0, 68.5, 66.9, 69.3; $n = 6$

$\overline{x} = (67.1 + 69.0 + 65.0 + 68.5 + 66.9 + 69.3)/6 = 67.6$

(11.1)

The assumption was made beforehand that the population from which the sample was derived had a normal distribution (Fig. 11.2). What if the population was distributed non-normally, as shown in Figure 11.3? In this situation, we note that the population is not described by parameters, and therefore, guesses as to the nature of this population must be made using nonparametric statistics. Ordinal and nominal variables are also analyzed by nonparametric statistics. The two most commonly used descriptors of central tendency in populations not described by parameters are the mode and the median. Consider the following set of data: 1, 2, 3, 4, 7, 7, 7. The mode is the value that occurs most often, which in this case is 7. If we list our values in increasing magnitude, the median is the value that divides the distribution exactly in half, which in this case is 4. Let us look at another example: 1, 1, 1, 1, 2, 6, 7, 7, 7, 7. In this case, we count four 1s and four 7s. This is a bimodal distribution. The median value lies between 2 and 6, so we add these two values and divide by 2 to arrive at a median of 4. In a normally distributed

population, the mean, median, and mode are all equal. The nature and use of nonparametric descriptors and statistics will be discussed later.

For now, let us consider the ramifications of the central limit theorem. Well, actually, it is not as bad as it looks. Basically, it means that you can assume normality of the sampling distribution (and the ability to use parametric statistics on your data), if your sample is sufficiently large. This holds true even if your population distribution is unknown or non-normally distributed. So, the question becomes, how large is large? Marks (3) notes that with a sample size of 30, almost any distribution—whether it be skewed, rectangular, uniform, or dinosaur shaped—will be amenable to parametric statistics because of the central limit theorem. With this as a premise, let us return to our discussion of descriptors of parameters and statistics.

Reconsider the exemplary data set. The mean for parametric samples defines the midpoint of the data. However, observe the following data:

73.0, 55.2, 66.1, 71.9, 59.2, 80.2; $n = 6$; $\overline{x} = 67.6$ (11.2)

These data have the same mean as the previous data, but here there is a wider spread about the mean (55.2–80.2 versus 65.0–69.3). Therefore, other measures dealing with the variability of the sample are needed. The two most commonly used parametric descriptors of variability are σ^2 and σ, called the *variance* and *standard deviation* (SD). The SD is the square root of the variance. The corresponding statistics are s^2 and s.

The SD for the first set of data was 1.6, whereas for the second set of data it was 9.3. We can express these data as $\overline{x} \pm$ SD. For our two examples, the data are expressed as 67.6 ± 1.6 and 67.6 ± 9.3. Therefore we can tell at a glance which sample is more variable. Figure 11.4 depicts the distribution of three normally distributed populations, all with the same mean, but with different variances. A functional definition is that the range from $(\overline{x} -$ SD$)$ to $(\overline{x} +$ SD$)$ encompasses 68% of the sample data, the range $(\overline{x} \pm 2$SD$)$ encompasses 95%, and the range $(\overline{x} \pm 3$SD$)$ encompasses 99% (Fig. 11.5).

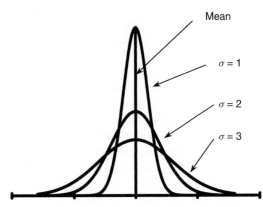

FIGURE 11.4 Effect of differing variance on the shape of normally distributed populations with the same mean.

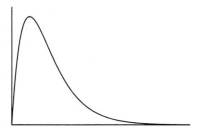

FIGURE 11.3 Distribution skewed to the right.

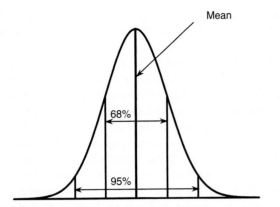

FIGURE 11.5 Percent of a normally distributed sample encompassed by $\bar{x} \pm$ SD and $\bar{x} \pm$ 2SD.

Another term used to describe sample spread is the *standard error of the mean* (SEM), also called the *standard error*. The parameter is $\sigma_{\bar{x}}$, and the statistic is $s_{\bar{x}}$. The parameter $\sigma_{\bar{x}}$ is the SD of means of all possible groupings of size n from a parent population with SD of σ. The kicker here is that the actual determination of statistically significant differences in parametric statistics involves the use of $s_{\bar{x}}$. We also use $s_{\bar{x}}$ to determine the confidence interval about a mean. For example, for large sample sizes, a 95% confidence interval equals $\bar{x} \pm (1.96 \times s_{\bar{x}})$. In plain English, this means that we are 95% confident that the population mean lies within this interval. Confidence intervals can be described for a wide variety of data.

Data are usually expressed as $\bar{x} \pm$ SD or $\bar{x} \pm$ SEM. The SEM is derived from the SD, as follows: SEM $=$ SD$/\sqrt{n}$. Therefore, the SEM will always be less than the SD. When presenting data, you should always make very clear which measure of variability you are reporting. Note also that a wide data range in a sample can appear very small if the SEM is used. For example, consider $\bar{x} \pm$ SD of 100 ± 120. For a variable such as plasma taurine, this might cause a concern because $\bar{x} \pm 1$ SD should encompass 68% of the sample, meaning either some poor slob has negative plasma taurine, or your distribution is skewed impressively to the right. However, if your sample size is 100, then your SEM $= 120/\sqrt{100}$, or 12. Therefore, $\bar{x} \pm$ SEM is 100 ± 12. Careful observation of which measure of variability is being used will help you gauge the true range of values observed. As an aside, because of the central limit theorem, even samples as variable as this are amenable to parametric statistics.

What of ordinal data or non-normally distributed quantitative data? Because we cannot use parameters to describe these data, the variance, SD, and SEM cannot be used. Data must be described as the median or the mode, followed by the range in parentheses. The data set {1, 2, 3, 4, 10, 18, 19}, using the median as our measure of central tendency, would be described as 4 (1 − 19). Another technique is to provide the interquartile range in parentheses. This would provide the range between the 25th and 75th percentiles of the data. This is a nice technique for describing the range of the central 50% of the data.

This also brings up the question, how do you know if your sample is non-normally distributed? Any time that you are dealing with all non-negative or all nonpositive values, and your SD is greater than half of the mean, you should begin feeling uncomfortable about the assumption of normality. Non-normally distributed quantitative data samples should never be analyzed using parametric statistics, unless the sample size is 30 or greater.

One other form of data description used in the literature is to express data as a percentage. For nominal variables, this might be the percentage of wound infection or percentage of intensive care unit (ICU) patients with adult respiratory distress syndrome (ARDS). For quantitative variables, it may involve expressing the value of one treatment as a percentage of another. Although this is a fairly common occurrence, when reading reports, you should remember that 1 of 2 is 50%; of course, so is 2,000 of 4,000. Sometimes, intentionally or unintentionally, a percentage can obscure the true sample size. When reading a report, make sure that you know the values from which the percentages are calculated. Similarly, when writing, make sure that you provide your readers with the same information. A measure of variability for percentage data is the 95% confidence interval. It is worth noting that a 95% confidence interval can also be calculated for the mean and the median, if it is desired.

SIGNIFICANCE TESTING

Back to our hypothesis: premature infants on TPN require carnitine. Our variable is plasma ketones. First, some perspective. Plasma ketones are a normal byproduct of fatty acid oxidation. Abnormal fatty acid use has been hypothesized to be indicated by lowered plasma ketone bodies. Therefore, in the proposed study, two possibilities exist. The first is that the mean plasma concentration of ketone bodies in infants not given carnitine (let us call this $\bar{x}_1$) will be the same as the plasma concentration of ketone bodies in infants receiving carnitine ($\bar{x}_2$). That is, $\bar{x}_1 = \bar{x}_2$. For this study, this is the null hypothesis, which is usually abbreviated H_0. Every study has a null hypothesis, and the null hypothesis always means either that there is no treatment effect or that the effect is of no interest to the researcher. This would be the meaning of the null hypothesis, whether we had 2 or 2,000 treatments.

For every experiment, there is always one, and only one, other hypothesis. This is called the *alternate hypothesis*, and is abbreviated H_A, or H_1. The alternate hypothesis always implies that there is a treatment effect, that something is happening, that the effects of the different treatments are not the same. For the present study, we have three choices for an alternate hypothesis: $\bar{x}_1 \neq \bar{x}_2$; $\bar{x}_1 > \bar{x}_2$; or $\bar{x}_1 < \bar{x}_2$. The choice of the alternate hypothesis will have some impact not only on the wording of the null hypothesis but also on the mechanics of the statistical test. This latter point, related to one-tailed and two-tailed testing, will be discussed later in this section. For the present, let us choose the alternate hypothesis to be

$\bar{x}_1 \neq \bar{x}_2$. The two hypotheses are usually presented in the following form:

$$H_0 : \bar{x}_1 = \bar{x}_2$$
$$H_1 : \bar{x}_1 \neq \bar{x}_2 \qquad (11.3)$$

Now we are presented with two diametrically opposed hypotheses. We use statistics to test these hypotheses and, in particular, to test the null hypothesis. This process is called *significance testing*. By accepting the null hypothesis, we have not proved conclusively that it is true, but rather that the evidence acquired in the study is insufficient to reject its validity. Similarly, by rejecting the null hypothesis, we have not proved the alternate, but have accepted the alternate hypothesis by process of elimination. Therefore all significance tests are based on H_0, and H_1 is accepted or rejected by default. One added note. The word significant is now one of the official buzzwords of authors everywhere. Its use always implies that significance testing has occurred. If this is not the case, then the word significant should not be used in the report.

Significance testing involves setting limits to protect against two types of error. One is called *Type I error*. Recall again that we have used a sample to make guesses about the population. A Type I error occurs when we reject the null hypothesis incorrectly. What is done to protect against Type I error is to set a probability of acceptable error. This probability, named α, is commonly set at 0.05. This, then, is the origin of the fabled $p < 0.05$. So what does it mean? Simply put, if I say that I reject the null hypothesis at $p < 0.05$, it means that there is less than a 5% chance that I am mistaken. Another way of putting this is to say that the probability that the differences between means is a result of random chance is less than 5%. In addition to its use in significance testing, the α-level is also used before the study begins, in the determination of sample size.

The second type of error is mysteriously called the *Type II error*. Type II error occurs when the null hypothesis is accepted incorrectly. Once again, a probability of acceptable error is designated. This probability, called β, is usually set at a low level, but higher than α, usually approximately 0.20. This means that, if we accept the null hypothesis, there is less than a 20% chance that we will be wrong. The β-level is used in sample size determinations. Another term associated with the β-level is power. The power of a study, that is, the ability to reject the null hypothesis, is equal to $1 - \beta$.

Sharp minds in the reading audience will note that the chance of a Type II error is commonly set at four times the chance of a Type I error. In other words, we are willing to accept four times the chance of making a mistake in accepting the null hypothesis as opposed to rejecting it, that is, significance testing is slanted toward accepting the null hypothesis. Because of this, only true differences in the data will lead to a rejection of the null hypothesis. If statistics has a bad name, it is through inappropriate application. When the statistical design and experimental design are selected before the study is begun (hint, hint), the statistics at the end of the study provide you with a powerful tool for determining the worth of your data.

Just a little bit longer on the soapbox. I have rather glibly referred to the usual values for α and β that is, 0.05 and 0.20, respectively. One can almost discern a radiant aura about these values, as if they had somehow become blessed from above and etched into the fabric of the space-time continuum. Actually, these levels are entirely under the control of the researcher. A word to the wise, however. If you propose to use less stringent α- and β-levels in your study, be prepared to defend those levels, not only in the acquisition of your grant but also when it comes time to present and publish your data.

It was mentioned previously that statistical significance does not always mean clinical significance. However, if you are designing a study, you can set your α-level at such a point that statistical significance does imply clinical significance. For example, in a proposed study of the efficacy of bupivacaine in open wound healing, you determine before the study that for the sample size you will use, if you can determine a significant difference at $p < 0.001$, this will also be clinically significant. Similarly, you can set stringent α- and β-levels to determine a sample size to find a clinically significant result.

To recap: a Type I error involves an error in the testing of the null hypothesis. Type II error means that you have accepted the null hypothesis incorrectly because your sample size was too small. How is sample size determined, anyway? The following, purely for your viewing enjoyment, is a formula to determine sample size in a study of two treatments with nominal variables, such as incidence of wound infection (4).

$$n = (2.8/(P_1 - P_2))^2 \times (P_1(100 - P_1) + P_2(100 - P_2)) \qquad (11.4)$$

where n is the sample size; P_1, the rate of infection in patients given placebo; and P_2, the rate of infection in patients given the drug. The factor 2.8 is related to the fact that α- and β-levels were chosen to be 0.05 and 0.20, respectively. Therefore, the formula will generate a number that delivers the sample size you will need to see a significant difference between groups at $p < 0.05$. Wow, pretty easy, huh, kids? Just plug in P_1 and P_2 and you are off to the races, right? Now is when it would be helpful to have some sinister background music building up. Think about it. All you need to do to figure out your sample size in a study to determine the percentage of people who get wound infections on either drug or placebo is to plug in the values for the percentage of people who get wound infections on either drug or placebo. Hey, if you know the answer to that one, why run the study?

Oooh, good point. So how do you set up a sample size with this formula? Remember, if you are using this formula, you have not begun the study yet, because you are still designing the study. One way of using this formula is to look over the literature, which you needed to review to write that proposal. Maybe someone has written about a study using a different age-group or different gender, or maybe he or she has looked at the same drug in a different surgical procedure or used a different drug in the same procedure. In all of these cases, percentages of wound infection were most likely provided. By plugging in the most relevant information into the formula given earlier, you can arrive at an estimate for your study. Another possibility is to run a pilot study and determine percentages for the larger study based on the pilot. Alternatively, maybe you do not believe the published results from someone else's study, so you want to reproduce the experiment using similar sample subjects and the same sample size. Yet another suggestion would be to use the rate of wound infection currently obtained with the standard of care at your institution. You could then declare a difference in terms of percent improvement, based on what you think would constitute a clinically significant difference.

This is, however, the real world. And just because someone else has published results does not mean that yours will be the same. In addition, the results from the pilot study may not bear any resemblance to the results in your big study. The fact is, however, you have based your estimate of sample size on the best information you had before the start of your study. Only one sample size formula is shown here, but there are others. All of these formulas have the same limitation, that is, some prior knowledge or educated guess concerning the outcome of the study, whether it be percentage wound infection or variability of plasma ketone bodies, is required.

So let us set up the following scenario. You are at a big national meeting, presenting some data of which you are particularly proud. You have concluded that there is no difference in percent wound infection after biliary surgery between groups treated with antibiotic prophylaxis with either a cephalosporin with a long half-life or a broad-spectrum ureidopenicillin. You are handling the questions in the discussion period quite well, when suddenly, there looms before you a deranged misanthrope with an evil, leering grin. It is obviously a Ph.D. with a hate complex for MDs, but before the guards can throw him or her out, this person slithers to the microphone and sneers, "It appears to me, Doctor, that you have committed a Type II error!" So what has this person said and why has he or she said it to you? Again, a Type II error implies that you have incorrectly accepted the null hypothesis. Because the Type II error rate is set by the β-level and because the β-level is only used to determine sample size, you interpret the twisted little misanthrope's remark to mean that your sample size was too small.

What does a poor resident do? You could (i) fix him or her with your evil eye and char the person to foul smelling cinders right on the spot, (ii) beg for mercy and swear you will never use a small sample size again, or (iii) stand tall in the saddle, defend your study, and win the acclaim of millions. Although choice i has the advantage of ego-inflating gratuitous violence, it might not sit well with your Hippocratic oath. Choice ii is loathsome and should be avoided at all costs. Choice iii is obvious. Your sample size was chosen for a good reason, and all you have to do is defend your reasons. Let's face it, folks, if you don't have confidence in the validity of your data, you shouldn't be presenting the stuff in the first place. The ultimate answer may lie in the fact that the experimental treatment or drug just is not as effective as you (or some people in the audience) would like for it to be.

What if it is not your study, but someone else's? When the authors of studies accept the null hypothesis, are you really going to take the time to calculate sample size formulas for every article you read to determine whether a Type II error has been committed? For most of you, it will be a pretty frosty day in Brownsville before that happens. That is why for you quick-and-dirty types it is more important to evaluate the α-level and the sample size. In this sense, if the null hypothesis is accepted (at $p > \alpha$), it is up to the reader to determine if the sample size is sufficiently large to warrant the conclusions. That is to say, although the null hypothesis was accepted, do you believe that the differences noted are clinically significant and would have been statistically significant if a larger sample size had been used?

Some authors have interpreted the preceding statement to indicate that clinically significant events are not always statistically significant. It is preferable to state that if a Type II error has been committed and a clinically significant event may have been obscured, the null hypothesis should be retested. To enact a change in clinical practice based on the presumption that the treatment would have been effective if not for Type II error is asinine. If you believe that there was a Type II error made in a study important to your work, either wait for a better study to be published or conduct the study yourself.

Let us look at the other end of the scale. Suppose someone has presented you with a statistically significant difference at $p < 0.05$. How does that change with sample size? Look at the data in Table 11.1. The variable is diastolic blood pressure, and the values represent the point at which for a given sample size $p < 0.05$. In this example, the variance is held constant for all of the sample sizes. As you can see, the larger the sample size, the smaller the difference required for significance. By the time you get out to 500 individuals in

---

TABLE 11.1

Depiction of the Effect of Sample Size on the Difference Required to Show a Significant Depression in Diastolic Blood Pressure at $p < 0.05$, Using a One-Tailed, Unpaired t Test[a]

Sample Size	Control Blood Pressure (mm Hg)	Treatment Blood Pressure (mm Hg)	Difference (mm Hg)
5	108	96.3	11.7
10	108	100.3	7.7
20	108	102.7	5.3
30	108	103.7	4.3
40	108	104.3	3.7
50	108	104.7	3.3
100	108	105.7	2.3
500	108	107	1.0
1000	108	107.3	0.7

[a]Standard deviation is held constant at 9.9.

each arm of the study, you can achieve a whopping 1 mm Hg difference and be significant at $p < 0.05$. And you know what the ads say: "Clinically tested by doctors to cause a significant decrease in blood pressure." There is significance and there is significance. Statistics, when applied properly, give you the framework on which to base your clinical decision, using your clinical judgment. Statistics are not an excuse to check your brain at the door.

Let us go back to our original null and alternate hypotheses. Our null hypothesis was that the treatments were equal, whereas the alternate hypothesis stated that they were not equal. Therefore, if treatment 1 is either much less or much greater than treatment 2, we will reject the null hypothesis. Mathematically, it can be shown that treatment 1 must be at least 1.96 pooled standard errors greater or less than treatment 2 to see a significant difference. This would be an example of a two-tailed test. The pooled standard error refers to the estimated standard error of the difference between the two-sample means. What if the hypotheses had been worded differently? For example, $H_0 : \bar{x}_1 \leq \bar{x}_2$ and $H_1 : \bar{x}_1 > \bar{x}_2$. To disprove the null hypothesis in this case, treatment 1 would only have to be 1.64 pooled standard errors greater than treatment 2. This constitutes a one-tailed test. Therefore, use of a one-tailed test requires a smaller difference to demonstrate statistical significance. There are two catches to this pleasant little scenario. The first is that the decision to use a one-tailed or two-tailed test must have been made as part of the design of the study, that is, while the proposal was being written. The second catch is that for this particular pair of hypotheses, if treatment 1 is less than treatment 2, the null hypothesis is accepted and no analysis need be done. Before selecting a one-tailed test, you should be sure that you have no interest in results being significant in the reverse direction to your alternate hypothesis. If any doubt exists on this point, a two-tailed test is more appropriate. The most common uses of one- and two-tailed tests are for the t test, Fisher exact test, and Pearson r (the correlation coefficient), all of which will be discussed later.

PARAMETRIC STATISTICS

Enough, already! Which tests do you use? Let us first concern ourselves with cases for which we want to determine differences between treatments as in our original hypothesis with the two TPN solutions, observing that eminently quantitative variable, plasma ketone body concentration. Let us assume that we are dealing with normally distributed data. Okay, we have a quantitative variable that is normally distributed and we have two treatments—this looks like a job for (dramatic pause) the t test! The t test (also known as *Student's t test*) is used to determine if differences exist between one or two (but no more than two!) samples of quantitative data. A one-sample t test involves testing a distribution against some known standard. An example would be to compare the resting energy expenditures (REEs) of the next 30 patients with closed head injuries to a standard

feeding protocol of 1,500 cal/d. A two-sample t test compares the means of two treatments with one another. The two-sample t test will be the focus of the following discussion.

There are three types of t tests: (i) paired observations, equal variance; (ii) unpaired observations, equal variance; and (iii)) unpaired observations, unequal variance. For example, paired observations in the present example would be to let each infant, at different time points, have each of the two TPN solutions. This is also called letting each infant be his or her own control. Another use would be with age- and sex-matched individuals, such as in the comparison of bone mineral content in female patients with primary or secondary parathyroidism versus age-matched female control subjects. An example of unpaired observations would be the testing of one cancer therapy in one group of patients and another therapy in another group of unmatched patients. In the third type of t test, you assume unpaired observations and unequal variance. Normally, unless there is a wide difference in the variance, one assumes equal variances.

What are the differences between the three tests? The differences lie in the power of the test. In this regard, a paired t test has the most power and an unpaired t test with unequal variance has the least power. This is based on the fact that, because each subject is his or her own control, there is a reduction in the variability of treatment response. Therefore, for a given set of paired data, a t test for paired observations will lead you to reject the null hypothesis more often than a t test for unpaired observations. In addition to being a more powerful analysis, the paired test also needs less than half the sample size required by an unpaired analysis, when each person is his or her own control. These advantages point out the wisdom of using a paired design and emphasize the importance of creating the research design and statistical design before the study begins. It will not always be possible to use a paired design, but when applicable, its advantages are great. But overall, no matter how great the temptation, no matter what the circumstances, the t test can only be used to compare one or two means of normally distributed, quantitative data, that is to say, no more than two!

What if we had wanted to compare more than two TPN solutions? Let us say that we had decided to expand our study, so that we would be testing a control (TPN without carnitine) and two formulas containing two levels of carnitine. Well, we know that a t test can be used to compare no more than two means. With more than two means, for parametric data, we use an analysis of variance (AOV or ANOVA). Simply put, the AOV analyzes the variance between the treatments and within each treatment to determine statistical significance. Variance between the treatments refers to the width of the spread between the treatment means. The greater the spread (i.e., the greater the variance), the more likely it is that a significant difference will be seen, leading to rejection of the null hypothesis. Variance within each treatment refers to the spread within each treatment group. The greater the spread, the more likely that values between treatments will overlap, leading to acceptance of the null hypothesis. Therefore, a significant AOV will have a high between-group variance and a low within-group variance. The ratio of these two variances, called the *F ratio*, is the basis for the test. The relevant hypotheses are shown in the subsequent text.

$$H_0 : \bar{x}_1 = \ldots = \bar{x}_n, \text{where } n \geq 2$$

$$H_1 : \text{inequality; all means are not equal} \quad (11.5)$$

You should note that the AOV can be used for two or more treatments. A small light clicks on in the dusty recesses of your neuronal vault, and you think, "In that case, why do we even mess with the *t* test then?" Mathematically, the statistical test for the *t* test relies on the *t* statistic, whereas the AOV relies on the *F* statistic. For two treatments, for a two-tailed *t* test, $t^2 = F$. However, the AOV is not applicable for one tailed, two treatment analyses. Also, the *t* test is far easier to calculate, hence the preference for the *t* test for two treatments.

So what is this big deal about not using a *t* test for more than two treatments? Is this more statistical flim-flammery, or is there some hard evidence to deter the restive masses? Take a peek at Table 11.2. The table describes the postulated significance level and the actual significance level for multiple mean comparisons. The more treatments you have, the more pair-wise comparisons there are, and the more likely it is that you will make a Type I error, that is, reject the null hypothesis incorrectly. For example, with 5 means, you would need to run 10 *t* tests to compare all of the means with one another. By rejecting the null hypothesis at the 0.05 level, you would in actuality be taking a 40% risk of making a Type I error among those 10 *t* tests. Why is this? Remember, the default α in most studies is 0.05. This means there is a 1 in 20 chance of making a mistake. But what happens to that 1 in 20 if we make repeated tests on the same set of data? Try this example. A good goal-tender in hockey will stop approximately 90% of the shots on net. Therefore, for any given shot, the odds are fairly high that he or she will stop the puck. However, during a hockey game, after facing 30 shots on goal, the odds are high that at least one goal will be scored. The same is true with multiple *t* testing. A similar argument holds for multiple testing of two samples for a large number of variables. The more tests you make, the more likely it will be that you make a Type I error. The only problem is that you will not know when or where the error lies. Hence the use of the AOV test, to avoid such uncertainties.

Back to those two hypotheses. Notice that if you reject the null hypothesis, you are accepting the alternate, which only tells you that an inequality exists somewhere. Maybe $\bar{x}_1 = \bar{x}_2 \neq \bar{x}_3$ or $\bar{x}_1 \neq \bar{x}_2 = \bar{x}_3$ or $\bar{x}_2 \neq \bar{x}_3 = \bar{x}_1$ or $\bar{x}_1 \neq \bar{x}_2 \neq \bar{x}_3$. Which is right? Do you, as numerous other researchers have done, use multiple *t* tests to find the inequality? Well, good, you just do that, and meanwhile why don't you take the rest of this chapter and paper train your new Doberman? Come on, folks, use of a *t* test after an AOV makes no more sense than using it beforehand. The argument described in the paragraph earlier still applies. You need to use a fully approved mean comparison procedure.

There are numerous techniques available for this purpose. If the author wishes to make all possible comparisons between treatments, then a multiple range test such as the Fisher Protected Least Significant Difference or the Tukey ω test should be used. If the author only wishes to make a select few comparisons, then the use of contrasts, such as Bonferroni *t* statistic, should be used. If the only comparisons to be made are between each treatment and a control, the use of Dunnett test is warranted. Finally, if a comparison needs to be made that was not planned before looking at the data, the low powered Scheffé test should be used. By low power, we mean that a comparison that would have shown a significant effect using contrasts may no longer be significant when a Scheffé test is used.

The preceding has been an overview of what is known as a *one-way AOV*, followed by a multiple comparison procedure. The AOV, however, can be used for any number of treatment comparisons. To make a simple example, suppose that instead of just looking at three TPN solutions containing varying levels of carnitine, we also want to look at differences in plasma ketone body concentrations between men and women. So we have one set of treatments (called *Factor A*) concerning the TPN solutions and another set of treatments (called *Factor B*) concerning the gender of the subjects. Any type of AOV involving more than one factor is called a *factorial AOV*. This particular case is called a *two-factor*, or *two-way*, *AOV*. The AOV generated by these data would determine whether there were effects caused by gender or TPN carnitine concentration. In addition, the test would provide information as to whether an interaction between the two factors occurred during the study. Interaction is best depicted graphically, as shown in Figure 11.6. The upper graph shows the effect on plasma ketone bodies for men and women as a function of carnitine content of the TPN. The slopes for the two curves are very similar. An AOV for this data would show that no interaction existed. The lower graph in Figure 11.6 shows a case in which the lines intersect. This would be a highly significant interaction. In simple terms, it means that the effect of carnitine addition to the men was the opposite of that seen in the women, that is, the addition of carnitine had a different effect on the two genders. Although not frequently referred to in reports, the interaction analysis can at times be more revealing than the analysis of the factors themselves.

TABLE 11.2

Evaluation of the Effect of Multiple Testing on the True Chance of Type I Error[a]

Number of Treatments	Number of Tests Required	True p Value[b]
2	1	0.05
3	3	0.14
4	6	0.26
5	10	0.4
10	45	0.9
20	190	1.0

[a]Modified from Marks RG. *Designing a research project*. Belmont: Lifetime Learning, 1982.

[b]Assuming a target α level of 0.05.

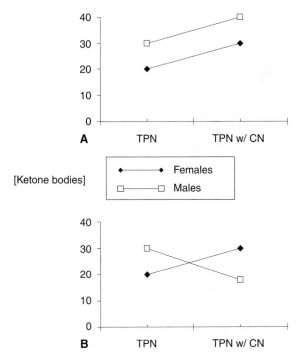

FIGURE 11.6 **A:** Depiction of a factorial analysis of variance with a nonsignificant interaction effect. **B:** Depiction of a factorial analysis of variance with a significant interaction effect. TPN, total parenteral nutrition; CN, carnitine.

This concept of factors can be expanded to many levels. For the study defined earlier, a third set of factors could be age of the child. Therefore the AOV is fairly open ended and can accommodate a wide variety of experimental designs. Three other variants of the AOV deserve mention here. When dealing with the *t* test, we spoke of a paired analysis, in which each child would receive each treatment and each subject is his or her own control. The same technique is available in the AOV, and the term for this is *blocking*. Blocking, as it is used in a clinical study design, means that each subject will receive each treatment. As in the *t* test, when properly used, the use of blocking increases the power of the analysis.

Repeated measures is a buzzword that is found in many clinical studies. For example, imagine a study designed to determine changes in total urinary nitrogen after blunt trauma, using two different drugs designed to decrease muscle protein catabolism. You want to measure urine nitrogen every 24 hours for a 5-day period, and you will obtain the urine from the same patients each day. Therefore, you will be taking repeated urine measurements from each subject. This is a design for a repeated measures AOV. You will note that only two treatments are proposed here, so that initially it appears that a *t* test would be appropriate. The key term is repeated measures. The AOV will be a much more appropriate, not to mention more powerful, test to use compared with the *t* test.

Let us take yet another popular design, the cross-over study, and apply it to the original study: two groups of infants, receiving TPN with or without carnitine. We know

that a paired design will give more power to the study, but we are concerned that time may be a factor. That is, as the babies age, their response to TPN with or without carnitine may differ. One solution may be a cross-over study. In this design, half of the babies would be randomized to receive TPN with carnitine, whereas the other half would receive the control solution. The study would proceed and samples would be collected until, at some predesignated time point, the babies would be switched to the other solution. This is the cross-over. Once again, we are only dealing with two treatments, so it looks like a *t* test. However, the correct and more powerful choice is the AOV.

The *t* test and AOV are called *univariate statistics* because they determine differences between treatments based on a single outcome variable. When one wants to measure two or more outcome variables that are dependent variables, multivariate statistics are used. With two treatment groups, Hotelling T^2 is used, and for more than two treatments, a multivariate analysis of variance (MAOV or MANOVA) is appropriate. The reader is referred to a more detailed text for additional information concerning these tests. Norman and Streiner (5) recommend the text by Tatsuoka (6), with the proviso that the reader should be familiar with matrix algebra.

The discussion up to this point has centered on the determination of differences between treatment groups. What if you have quantitative, normally distributed data, and you do not want to look at differences, but at relations? This is a case for linear regression. As you recall from that hellish year in algebra I that your parents forced you to take back when you were too young to know better, $y = mx + b$. The rest, of course, is history. The x is the independent variable, y is the dependent variable, b is the y intercept, and m is the slope.

How is regression analysis used? In the laboratory, it is the basis of the notorious standard curve, by which readings of glucose or free fatty acid concentration can be derived from spectrophotometer readings of optical density of samples. Clinically, it may be used to determine the amount of drug necessary to obtain a desired response. Therefore, regression can be used to predict the value of a variable based on the value of another variable or other variables. An example taken from the arena of lithotripsy involves the dependence of fragmentation time of gallstones on gallstone weight. As the weight of the gallstone increases, so does the fragmentation time. The equation for the line that describes this relation is derived by linear regression.

The coefficient of determination is r^2, and r^2 is the proportion of variability that is attributable to the independent variable. The quantity r^2 can vary between 0 and 1. An r^2 approaching 1 indicates that the linear regression equation is a good estimate of the relation between the points, whereas an $r^2 = 0$ indicates that your data resemble a cluster nebula.

Regression analysis can also be used to demonstrate the degree of association between independent variables. A typical example that has received close scrutiny in the literature in recent years is the relation between the volume of colonic methane gas and the blood insulin concentration 2 hours after a bolus dose of frijoles (refried beans). Such data could have very important social and political ramifications, so linear regression is used. However, because we are dealing with two independent variables (as opposed to an independent and a dependent variable), we can now test to see how closely the variables are correlated. Pearson correlation coefficient r is used. The range is $-1 \leq r \leq 1$. Negative numbers infer inverse correlation, that is, $x \propto 1/y$. Values close to 1 or -1 indicate a good fit, and values close to 0 indicate the opposite. The value r can be tested statistically, where the null hypothesis is $r = 0$ (no correlation between x and y) and the alternate hypothesis is $r \neq 0$ (correlation between x and y). The test would be two-tailed for these hypotheses. If set up properly when designing the study, the hypotheses can be restated to test for a one-tailed test: $r > 0$ or $r < 0$.

Now, here is an important point. If you accept the null hypothesis (there is no correlation), the regression line should not be drawn. Furthermore, and especially, the regression line should not be displayed in a presentation or a publication, because the line, in and of itself, implies correlation. The usual comeback is, "But my computer drew a line!" That's right, it did. Computers, and their software, are wonderfully obedient little marvels. They will do every stupid little thing you tell them to do, and do it very quickly. In this case, a program will gleefully take data that have an r value of 0, and whip out a mighty fine line, complete with coefficients and exponents, suitable for framing. However, just because a computer can do something does not make it right. A computer will also crunch nominal data into a t test, but that is not correct either. The weak link in this whole operation is that maniac at the keyboard. If Dr. Loon puts garbage in, most assuredly garbage will come out.

Just to beat it to a miserable, pulsating, pulpy mass, is it legitimate to display the regression line if you also show that the r value is not significant? My personal opinion is no. The visual image has strange, seductive powers, and a picture of a graph showing a line relating two independent variables will always carry more weight than some r value tucked away in the text. If there is no correlation, there should not be a line.

Now, it is a curious circumstance that Pearson correlation coefficient, when squared, equals r^2, the coefficient of determination. And although r^2 can be used whether you are dealing with two independent variables or an independent and a dependent variable, r can only be used when dealing with two independent variables. Well, that was pretty smooth. Okay, smart guy, how do you know what kind of variable you've got? For the most part, there are two instances when we know that we are dealing with independent and dependent variables. The first occurs when the independent variable is assigned by the researcher. Examples are varying levels of lysine in the diet, varying drug dosages, or even some time interval. The second case is where a known relation exists between the two variables, such as between blood insulin and glucose concentrations. If the researcher has not assigned one of the variables, and a large body of evidence does not exist to suggest a dependent relation of one variable on another, then one can safely presume that one is dealing with two independent variables.

That brings us to two very important points. If you are looking at data dealing with two independent variables and the correlation has been shown to be significant, that's great! But, remember that this is still a mathematic argument. With a sufficient sample size, one could show variables to have significant correlation at $p < 0.05$ with an $r = 0.1$ (this is similar to the argument shown in Table 11.1). Squaring this number, to form r^2, gives a value of 0.01. Interpretation of this figure implies that the equation for the line can only account for 1% of the variability associated with the line, that is, it does a smashingly lousy job of describing the data. This is where your clinical judgment needs to kick in and say that although the correlation has statistical significance, it has little or no clinical significance. In general, if there is any doubt as to the clinical significance of an r value, square it. The value r^2, as mentioned previously, tells you what percent of the variability is accounted for by the line. By this logic, even a seemingly reasonable r value of 0.7 means that the line only accounts for 49% of the variability of the data.

A second major point involving interpretation of correlations deals with the relation itself. A significant correlation merely implies that the response of two variables, in relation to each other, is predictable. It does not, never has, and never will imply a cause-and-effect relation. It does not matter if $r^2 = 1.000000$, there is still no cause-and-effect relation. That is for other experiments and other pieces of data to demonstrate.

So far, we have been talking straight lines. Do not let your mind be constrained by the restrictive linearity that is linear regression. Curvilinear, or nonlinear, regression also exists, and r and r^2 values can be generated just as for linear regression. Therefore, although your data are nonlinear, a function (quadratic, cubic, logarithmic, etc.) may yet exist to connect the dots, with the help of our friend, Mr. Computer.

The final type of regression up for discussion is called *multiple regression*. Multiple regression is yet another type of multivariate statistical test. This technique is indicated if you feel that several independent variables (several different x's) can be used to predict the outcome of another independent variable (y). An example would be the prediction of REE (the y variable) in males, based on age, weight, serum albumin, and a 24-hour total urinary nitrogen excretion (the x variables). Multiple regression not only has an r value for the entire equation but individual r values for each of the component x variables. These give the researcher some indication as to which are the most important in terms of predictive value.

Multiple regression equations can also be formulated using a mixture of qualitative and quantitative variables. However, to use multiple regression, the y variable must be quantitative. One example would be to have gender, or presence or absence of sepsis, in our equation for REE. Because these are nominal variables, dummy variables will have to be ascribed to them. Therefore, women can arbitrarily be assigned a value of 1, and men a value of 0. Similar assignments could be given for the presence or absence of sepsis, and the multiple regression equation, complete with r values, can be described.

Another procedure, which is best described as a combination of the AOV and regression analysis, is the analysis of covariance (AOCV or ANCOVA). AOCV is used to test for differences between several treatments, in terms of some quantitative, normally distributed variable. The added twist is that the AOCV can correct for some confounding factor, called a *covariate*. In the presence of a covariate, the use of AOCV provides additional precision and power to the analysis, relative to AOV. For example, look at those babies from our TPN versus TPN plus carnitine study. It was mentioned previously that the age of the infant may have an impact on how he or she responds to supplemental carnitine. One technique that was mentioned to control for this was the cross-over AOV. Another technique that could be used, however, is the AOCV; the covariate is age. Multiple covariates can also be controlled by this procedure.

NONPARAMETRIC STATISTICS

You should know, and I certainly do know, that the preceding has not been an exhaustive list of parametric procedures. However, they are the ones that you will run across most often. What about nonparametric procedures? Let us look at the tests for nominal variables first. Those are the categorical variables (type of organism, presence or absence of wound infection, etc.). For these, there will be no means or SDs, only totals in a group. The typical case found in the literature would be a comparison of two treatments. For example, what if, instead of measuring ketone bodies in our premature infant study, we had used incidence of fatty liver as our measure of the usefulness of carnitine? That is, the babies were recorded as having or not having cholestasis. These types of yes/no data (enumeration data, nominal variables) are handled by the use of χ^2 (chi-squared) analysis. Another name for this type of test is a contingency table analysis. The null hypothesis for χ^2 is independence, and the alternate hypothesis is dependence. Do not be misled, the hypotheses really mean the same thing as the hypotheses discussed under parametric statistics. Rejection of the null hypothesis means that there are differences in treatment effect. The most common form of χ^2 analysis is the 2×2 table. This form of χ^2 (2×2 table) is usually expressed as a corrected χ^2, using the Yates correction for continuity.

For example, consider a study of patient-controlled analgesia (PCA) compared with epidural-catheter-injection (EPI) analgesia. An observation of the complications revealed that pruritus occurred in 17 of 22 patients receiving PCA and in only 5 of 19 patients receiving EPI. The 2×2 table is shown in Figure 11.7. The analysis would reveal that significant differences did exist between treatment groups.

A 2×2 table is by no means the only form of χ^2 analysis, however. We could just as easily have had a more complex

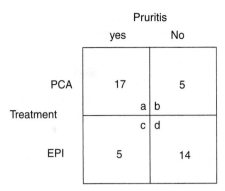

FIGURE 11.7 An example of a χ^2 2×2 contingency table. PCA, patient-controlled analgesia; EPI, epidural-catheter-injection.

design such as the incidence of nosocomial infections over a 12-month period in five different ICUs in various parts of the country. Another example would be to identify which of three different techniques for gallbladder removal are preferred among surgeons from eight different hospitals in a five-state area.

One special note for χ^2. The calculated χ^2 is just an estimate, and as your sample size becomes smaller and smaller, your estimate becomes less accurate, leaving you open to making invalid decisions for rejection or acceptance of the null hypothesis. In a 2×2 table, we speak of the four cells in the table. If the expected value(s) for any particular cell in a 2×2 table is less than 5, then the χ^2 method will not be accurate. The formula is as follows:

$$e_s(\text{expected value}) = (\text{smallest row total}$$
$$\times \text{ smallest column total})/\text{sample size}$$
$$(11.6)$$

From the analgesia example cited in preceding text, $e_s = (19 \times 19)/41 = 8.8$. For this example, the χ^2 is appropriate. For the case of a 2×2 table in which e_s is less than 5, Fisher exact test should be used. Fisher exact test is accurate for all sample sizes for a 2×2 design but usually is reserved for those cases for which a χ^2 test is not advisable. In larger χ^2 designs, such as 3×5 or 7×3, the general rule of thumb is that if 20% of the cells have an $e_s < 5$, the χ^2 will not be accurate for the analysis. In cases like these, the researcher only has two choices. The first is to eliminate the offending treatment group, and the second is to use good judgment and combine similar treatments.

So here we go again. In the case of Fisher exact test, the advice is to use an entirely different test than was proposed originally, whereas in the second case, we are advocating serious *post facto* data manipulation. Fisher exact test is acceptable because it is actually more accurate than the χ^2 test. The reason it has not been used routinely for the large sample sizes in 2×2 tables is because the analysis involves a great deal of excited numbers (factorials, for you sophisticated types, like 5!, 10!, and 457!), and when you are doing these puppies by hand, it tends to give you caution. Granted, with the use of a computer, this caveat no longer carries the weight it once did, but Fisher exact test is still generally reserved for a 2×2 table with small sample size.

An additional concern with Fisher exact test involves the difference between one-tailed and two-tailed tests. Because of the nature of the calculations involved, the χ^2 is always calculated as a two-tailed test. Fisher exact test, however, can be calculated as a one- or two-tailed test. Therefore, whenever Fisher exact test is being used in place of the χ^2 owing to small sample size, a two-tailed Fisher exact test should be used. Conversely, if the original alternate hypothesis called for one treatment to be higher than another treatment in a given direction, nominal variables are involved, and the experimental design is amenable to a 2×2 table, a one-tailed Fisher exact test should be indicated in the proposal as the test to be used.

In the other case, for which the choice is to eliminate data or combine cells, it appears that we are saying that *post facto* data manipulation is okay. The reality is that the χ^2 test has limitations. Certainly, no one would predict a large proportion of cells with $e_s < 5$. This is, however, real life, and things like this happen. We research types just despise going to all the trouble of data gathering and then finding out we have to vaporize some of it. Therefore, combining similar treatments under these special circumstances is acceptable. Please, when placed in this situation, use good common sense to make your decision. This has been a repeated theme in this chapter, but it bears restating: numbers, data, and statistical tests are wonderful things, but if you insist on being out to lunch, it's all rather a waste.

Other, more specialized analyses of nominal variables are available. One type of χ^2 analysis is the McNemar test. This is analogous to working with a paired sample. In this situation, a before-and-after determination is made on the same group of subjects. For example, suppose you cornered 100 people and asked them whether they use seat belts. After getting their responses, you herd them into Grand Rounds on a day when a series of horrific automobile accidents, featuring individuals who did not use their seat belts, is going to be presented. After the presentation, you now ask your 100 individuals whether they will use seat belts. The data would then be fitted into a 2×2 table and analyzed for significance.

Another specialized χ^2 is the Mantel-Haenzel, which is a nonparametric equivalent of controlling for a single nominal covariate. It can be used to control for a confounding variable while discerning the difference between two treatments. If more than one covariate is present, logistic regression is used. Logistic regression requires that the y variable be nominal. The x variables can be either nominal or quantitative. Logistic regression can be used to determine risk factors for conditions such as cancer or heart disease. One additional advantage from the use of logistic regression is that odds ratios can be derived from the coefficients for the nominal x variables. A form of regression analysis in which all of the variables (x and y) are nominal is log-linear regression. Log-linear regression would be used to predict a nominal variable such as survival, if all of the x variables were nominal, such

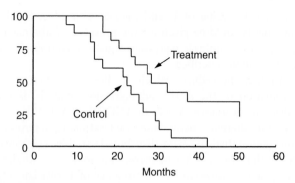

FIGURE 11.8   Survival curves, generated using the Kaplan-Meier technique.

as gender, smoker/nonsmoker, incidence of previous heart disease, or presence or absence of sepsis.

Yet another type of analysis for nominal variables that is used frequently in the literature is the life table. Essentially, the life table is a device to determine whether there are differences between treatments in patient survival over time. The analysis takes into account varying factors, such as patients entering the study at different times, patients who leave the study before the end of the study period, and patients who are still survivors by the end of the study. A pair of typical survival curves, using the Kaplan-Meier technique, are shown on Figure 11.8. The null hypothesis is that the two curves are the same, which is the same thing as saying that no treatment effect exists. A variety of statistics are available to analyze these data, depending on how many distributions are to be compared. When the effect of several covariates on survival time is to be assessed, the Cox proportional hazards model is often used. From this analysis, hazard ratios, similar to the odds ratios generated from logistic regression, can be derived from the coefficients for the nominal x variables.

When comparing treatments in a life table, however, keep in mind that the larger the sample size, the smaller the difference that is required to achieve statistical significance. With a sufficiently large sample size, you could have two curves that are virtually identical, and yet the treatments will be statistically significantly different at the $p < 0.05$ level. Therefore, having satisfied yourself that there is mathematic significance, you must now use your good clinical judgment to determine if there is also clinical significance.

Ordinal variables are also tested with nonparametric statistics. Nonparametric statistics for ordinal variables are also applicable to non-normally distributed, quantitative data for small data sets. Ordinal data are commonly referred to as *ranked data*, that is, describe your excitement about popular spawning aids for fish, such as fish ladders, on a scale from 0 (least) to 5 (hysterically excited). For most of the more common parametric tests, there is a corresponding nonparametric test. The major disadvantage of the use of the nonparametric tests is that they are not as powerful as the corresponding parametric test. In other words, with the same set of data, you may detect differences with the latter, but not necessarily with the former. Another disadvantage is that, for

TABLE 11.3

Common Statistical Tests

Study	Quantitative Variables	Nominal Variables	Ordinal Variables[a]
One sample[b]	t test	χ^2	Kolmolgorov-Smirnov
Two unpaired treatments	t test, equal variances	χ^2	Mann-Whitney U test
	t test, unequal variances	Fisher exact test	Wilcoxon rank sum test
			Kolmolgorov-Smirnov
			Median test
Two paired treatments	Paired t test	McNemar test	Wilcoxon signed rank test[c]
			Sign test
Three or more treatments	AOV	χ^2	Kruskal-Wallis AOV
	AOV with blocking		Friedman AOV w/blocking
	Factorial AOV		
Analysis adjusted for covariates	AOCV	Mantel-Haenzel	
Regression	Linear regression	Logisitic regression	Cumulative odds
	Nonlinear regression	Log-linear regression	Continuation ratio
	Multiple regression		
Correlation	Pearson r	Contingency coefficient	Spearman rank correlation
			Kendall rank correlation
			Kendall coefficient of concordance

[a]These tests are also appropriate for non-normally distributed quantitative data of small sample size.
[b]This refers to the comparison of treatment data to some recognized norm or distribution, such as the January to December monthly incidence of cesarean delivery compared with the average of the last 20 years.
[c]This test has more power than the sign test.

some of the more complex AOV designs, no nonparametric equivalents exist. One solution to this dilemma is the use of rankits. Conversion of ranked data, or non-normally distributed quantitative data that have been converted to ranks, allows the use of parametric statistics on the data. The procedure is described briefly by Gill (7). Yet another solution, similar to the rankits, is the transformation of ranks to fit a normal distribution. An example of this is fitting intelligent quotient (IQ) scores to a normal distribution with a mean of 100.

In general, the nonparametric tests that you will encounter most frequently are the following:

1. The Mann-Whitney *U* test, also known as the *Mann-Whitney*, for testing differences between two unpaired treatments
2. The Wilcoxon signed rank test, for testing differences between two paired treatments
3. The Kruskal-Wallis AOV, for testing differences between more than two treatments
4. The Spearman rank correlation, for testing the strength of relation between two variables

Occasionally, you will read a paper and note that the author has used parametric and nonparametric statistics on the same set of data. When you see this, you should consider that the author knows little or nothing about statistics. Data cannot be both normal and non-normal, ranked and nonranked. Choose one or the other, not both! What of the case for which you determine, before the experiment has begun, to use parametric statistics, and you have non-normal data? In this situation, it is perfectly legitimate to use

the corresponding nonparametric test. A brief rundown of the more popular statistical tests is shown in Table 11.3. The nonparametric tests for ordinal data are also listed.

CONTINGENCY TABLES IN DIAGNOSTIC TESTING

As mentioned previously, the χ^2 test is also known as a *contingency table analysis*. The contingency table has other uses besides the χ^2, however. The specificity and sensitivity of a test are derived from a 2×2 table. The sensitivity is the ability of a test to detect a disease, and the specificity is the ability of a test to determine if no disease is present. The calculations for a 2×2 table for sensitivity and specificity are shown in Figure 11.9. An example is the use of ultrasonography in the detection of gallstones. Obviously, the test would only be used if indicated by other signs and symptoms noted on examination. The data are shown in Figure 11.10. Here, the sensitivity and specificity of the test are quite high, at 95% and 97%, respectively. Another term that occurs in the literature is accuracy, which is the sum of the true positives (TP) and the true negatives (TN), divided by the total sample.

Unfortunately, you do not always have the luxury of knowing exactly how many people have the disease of interest. Therefore, an even more useful pair of parameters are the positive predictive value and the negative predictive value. The positive predictive value is the chance of having the disease, if the test results for the disease are positive. Conversely, the negative predictive value is the chance of not

Condition

Present   Absent

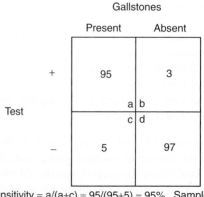

+	a	b
−	c	d

Test

Sensitivity = a/(a+c)   Sample size = a+b+c+d
Specificity = d/(d+b)   Prevalence = (a+c)/(a+b+c+d)
Positive predictive value (PV+) = a/(a+b)   Accuracy = (a+d)/(a+b+c+d)
Negative predictive value (PV−) =d/(d+c)

FIGURE 11.9   Calculations for sensitivity, specificity, accuracy, positive predictive value, and negative predictive value.

having the disease, if the test results are negative. Calculations for these two values are shown in Figure 11.9. Sample values for the ultrasound example are shown in Figure 11.10.

How are the predictive values and specificity and sensitivity related? In the example in Figure 11.10, ultrasonography has a high probability of detecting the disease and a high positive predictive value. However, this is in a carefully screened group of patients, who would be expected to have a high frequency, or prevalence, of the disease. What about the opposite case? Let us assume that you, in an inexplicable fit of frenzy, begin ordering ultrasonographies to test for gallstones on everyone in the greater metropolitan area. Innocent bystanders, small children, household pets—no one is safe from your bout of ultrasonophilia. Upon your recovery 12 months later, you notice a preponderance of very sleek sports cars in the radiologists' parking lot, in addition to reams of data. The results might appear as shown in Figure 11.11. Note that the specificity and sensitivity, which are independent of disease prevalence, are the same as in Figure 11.10. However, the positive predictive value is now low (3.1%), whereas the negative predictive value has increased to 99.99%. These changes have occurred because of the change in the prevalence of the disease. Although the prevalence of gallstones in the first example was high as a result of the way that patients were selected, the prevalence was extremely low in the second example. Therefore, the positive predictive value has a direct relation with the prevalence, that is, as the prevalence increases, the positive predictive value increases. The negative predictive value is indirectly related to the prevalence, that is, as the prevalence increases, the negative predictive value decreases. Therefore, from Figure 11.10, a negative result would indicate no disease was present, and a positive result, owing to its low predictive value, would require additional work to determine if gallstones were present.

There is one other piece of information, derived from the precepts of evidence-based medicine, which is also extremely helpful in determining the practical utility of a test. This is the likelihood ratio (LR). This can be expressed as LR+ or LR−. The LR for a test compares the likelihood of that result in patients with disease to the likelihood of that result in patients

without disease. A large LR+ implies that a positive test is strongly associated with the presence of disease, whereas a small LR- implies that a negative test is strongly associated with the absence of disease.

Using the contingency table from Figure 11.9, LR+ = (a/a+c)/(b/b+d), whereas LR- = (c/a+c)/(d/b+d). Using these formulas for the data from Figure 11.10, the LR+ would be 31.7, wheraes the LR- would be 0.05. Alternatively, the LR+ could be calculated as the TP divided by the false positives (FP), and the LR- could be calculated as the false negatives (FN) divided by the TN. Both the LR+ and LR− are insensitive to changes in the prevalence. Table 11.4 gives some guidelines for the interpretation of LRs.

RELATIVE RISKS AND ODDS RATIO

Two other concepts that appear in the surgical literature are relative risks and odds ratios. In particular, these values are used often in discussions of cancer and heart disease.

Gallstones

Present   Absent

+	95	3
−	5	97

Test

a b
c d

Sensitivity = a/(a+c) = 95/(95+5) = 95%   Sample size = 200
Specificity = d/(d+b) = 97/(97+3) = 97%   Prevalence = 50%
PV+ = a/(a+b) = 95/98 = 96.9%   Accuracy = 96%
PV− = d/(d+c) = 97/102 = 95.1%

FIGURE 11.10   Use of ultrasonography as a diagnostic test for gallstones when the suspected prevalence of gallstones is high.

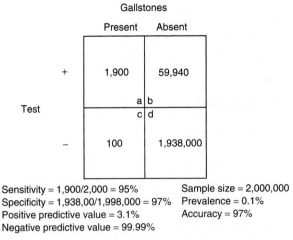

Sensitivity = 1,900/2,000 = 95%   Sample size = 2,000,000
Specificity = 1,938,00/1,998,000 = 97%   Prevalence = 0.1%
Positive predictive value = 3.1%   Accuracy = 97%
Negative predictive value = 99.99%

FIGURE 11.11 Use of ultrasonography as a diagnostic test for gallstones when the suspected prevalence of gallstones is low.

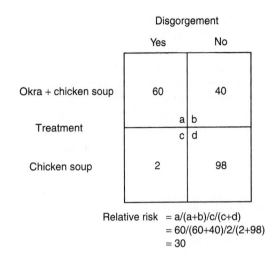

Relative risk = a/(a+b)/c/(c+d)
= 60/(60+40)/2/(2+98)
= 30

FIGURE 11.12 Determination of the relative risk.

Relative risk can be applied in most commonly used designs, with the exception of the case–control study. Relative risk computes the possibility of disease when exposed to a certain agent, relative to the risk of disease when not exposed to the same agent. For a relatively benign example, let us compare a delightful bowl of chicken soup to a bowl of chicken soup that has been tainted with okra, without a doubt the most baneful vegetable ever to photosynthesize. These two treatments will be compared, relative to their ability to initiate the disgorgement of gastric material. Subjects will be randomly assigned to both treatments and their responses noted. The results and calculations are shown in Figure 11.12. The risk of disgorgement after ingestion of okra-chicken soup, relative to the chicken soup, is (60/100):(2/100), or 30 times greater. Valuable data for 6-year- olds growing up in the South!

These calculations, however, are not applicable to case–control designs. This is because a much lower incidence of cases exists in the population, relative to the proportion of cases to controls in the study. The odds ratio (also known as *relative odds*) is used as an estimate of the relative risk. An example of the use of the odds ratio is provided by Hurwitz et al. (8) in their study of the relation between aspirin usage and Reye syndrome. The data are provided in Figure 11.13. Note that the calculations for the odds ratio are different from those for the relative risk. The odds ratio indicates that

the risk of having Reye syndrome after salicylate exposure relative to no salicylate exposure was (28/2):(67/78), or 16.3 times greater.

Odds ratios can also be derived from meta-analyses and from logistic regression equations. In these two situations, the odds ratios are interpreted similarly to relative risks. This enables us to make further statements about the data, encompassing concepts such as the number needed to treat (NNT), discussed in more detail in subsequent text. An odds ratio generated from a case–control study, however, cannot make those same assumptions, beacause the proportion of cases to controls in the study is always far less than the proportion of cases to controls in the general population.

It was noted previously that it is insufficient to report a mean without also showing some measure of variability, such as the SD. Similarly, it is inappropriate to report a relative risk or an odds ratio without some measure of variability. In the clinical literature, this usually means that a 95% confidence interval must be calculated. In this context, a 95% confidence interval about a relative risk or odds ratio means that you can state with 95% confidence that the true relative risk or odds ratio lies within that interval.

TABLE 11.4		
Evaluation of Likelihood Ratios		
Likelihood Ratio	*Interpretation*	
LR+ >10 or LR- <0.1	Large changes in likelihood	
LR+ = 5–10 or LR- = 0.1–0.2	Moderate changes	
LR+ = 2–5 or LR- = 0.2–0.5	Small changes	
LR+ <2 or LR- >0.5	Tiny changes	
LR = 0	No changes in likelihood	

LR, likelihood ratio.

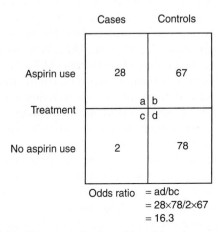

Odds ratio = ad/bc
= 28×78/2×67
= 16.3

FIGURE 11.13 Determination of the odds ratio.

When interpreting relative risks or odds ratios, it is important to remember that a relative risk or odds ratio greater than 1 means that the outcome is more likely in the experimental group, whereas an outcome less than 1 means that the outcome is more likely in the control group. The kicker for these arguments is that if the confidence interval includes 1 within its range, then there is no difference between the control and experimental groups. Another way of thinking about this is to say that the data are so variable we cannot exclude the possibility that there is no difference between the two groups.

For example, if you saw that the relative risk for mortality using the wonder drug Aricene was 0.167, you might be very impressed. This would indicate that a subject would be six times more likely to die if they weren't given Aricene. But what if I then told you that the confidence interval was from 0.03 to 6? Despite the impressive relative risk, since the range for the confidence interval includes the value of 1, we would conclude that the effect seen was not statistically significant.

Let's try a different example, where the use of Aricene gives us a relative risk of 0.95, and a confidence interval from 0.94 to 0.98. Because the confidence interval does not include the value of 1, we would have to conclude that the effect was statistically significant. More than likely, however, you would have strong concerns over the clinical significance of such a marginal relative risk. Once again, it is worth noting that if your sample size is sufficiently large, any relative risk, no matter how questionable, will show statistical significance.

Another concept which has become popularized through the use of evidence-based medicine is the NNT. This is defined as the number of subjects who have to be treated with a particular technique or medication to prevent one bad outcome. It is very useful in helping to evaluate whether the benefits of a treatment outweigh the potential harms and complications of a procedure.

Let's revisit our wonder drug Aricene, only now let's assume that the relative risk of mortality, 0.167, is statistically significant. One could say that mortality was reduced 83.3% through the use of Aricene, and could come to the potentially incorrect conclusion that if you gave Aricene to 100 patients, you would save 83 lives. What is the problem? The problem is that, unless the disease is ordinarily 100% fatal, you are overestimating the usefulness of the drug. The figure of 83.3% is called the *relative risk reduction* (RRR). What we need to know now is the absolute risk reduction (ARR). The ARR is the risk of death for patients receiving the control treatment, minus the risk of death for patients receiving Aricene. In this hypothetical case, the risk in the control group is 0.06%, whereas the risk in the Aricene group is 0.01%, which gives us an ARR of 0.05%, or 0.0005.

Now that we know the ARR, we can calculate the NNT. The NNT is nothing more than the reciprocal of the ARR. So, for this example, the NNT equals 1/0.0005, which is 2,000. Therefore, for every 2,000 people treated, we would save 1 life. Quite a far cry from the original thought that we would save 83 lives for every 100 people treated. The NNT

is an easily calculated value which helps to glean additional meaning from relative risks and, in certain instances, from odds ratios. However, the NNT cannot be calculated from odds ratios generated from case control studies.

CONCLUSION

You should realize, of course, that you will not become an expert in statistics after reading this chapter. If you believe that, then you are a living proof of the statement, "A little knowledge is dangerous." Some very complex topics, such as logistic regression or MAOV, were mentioned in a few sentences, whereas others, such as discriminant function analysis, have been ignored entirely. The emphasis in this chapter was focused on those experimental designs and techniques that you are most likely to encounter in the literature. What are the major points to remember?

1. Given a sufficiently large sample size, any two treatment groups can be shown to be statistically significantly different. The same holds true for significance in correlation.
2. Statistical significance does not necessarily imply clinical significance.
3. If treatment A versus treatment B has $p < 0.05$, and treatment C versus treatment D has $p < 0.0001$, it does not follow that the difference between C and D is of greater magnitude or importance than between A and B, merely that we are more sure that the difference between C and D is real.
4. When dealing with percentages, remember that 1 of 2 looks the same as 500 of 1,000.
5. Correlation between independent variables is indicative of association, not of a cause-and-effect relationship.
6. A t test is only used for normally distributed, quantitative variables, with one or two treatments.
7. When evaluating relative risks and odds ratios, if the 95% confidence interval contains the value of 1, we must conclude that there is no significant effect
8. A well-designed paper with poorly designed statistics is far superior to a poorly designed paper with well-designed statistics.

Just a few words on that last point. After taking a course in statistics, one usually looks at articles with a different eye. The usual response is to rend papers with slavering jaws and razor-sharp nails, shredding everything to bits, all in the name of improper statistics. Although a great deal of improvement in the proper choice of statistics in journal articles has occurred over the last few years, instances of improper uses of statistics still abound. Nevertheless, if the study design is good, it is a simple matter to disregard invalid p values and to evaluate the means and SDs (or nominal or ordinal variables) and still come to your own best guess. Logic and common sense, remember? However, if the experimenter has chosen the wrong control or if the treatment groups have tremendous underlying differences in the patient samples that, in your judgment, are sure to obscure the treatment effects, then it does not matter how beautiful the statistics are. Repeated measures AOV that uses an ingenious cross-over design with standard errors so low they bring tears to your eyes is not worth a slab of dung if the study design rots. It brings to mind the Condon concept of Type III error—the conclusions are not supported by the data represented (9).

As a closing note, I would like to dissuade the reader from the notion that the purpose of this chapter was to belittle the value of statistics. On the contrary, statistical analysis is an important tool in the ordering and interpretation of data. Its frequent application in the medical literature is a testament to widespread agreement among researchers and reviewers alike as to the importance of statistics. If anything, the purpose of this chapter was to demystify statistics and reinforce the concept that statistics is a tool to assist you in the determination of clinical significance.

GLOSSARY

95% confidence interval   a measure of variability, which states that you are 95% confident that the population value for your statistic, such as the relative risk or odds ratio, lies with the interval. For the relative risk or odds ratio, if the 95% confidence interval includes the value of 1, the effect is not statistically significant ($p > 0.05$).

Accuracy   the total number of true positive and true negative values for a test, divided by the total number of tests.

Alternate hypothesis   in hypothesis testing, the alternate hypothesis always implies that there is a treatment effect, that is, that the effects of the different treatments are not the same. It is abbreviated H_A or H_1.

ANOVA   see AOV.

AOV   analysis of variance test, used for testing differences between three or more treatments, if the variable is quantitative and if the samples are normally distributed. The AOV is also abbreviated ANOVA.

Case–control study   a retrospective comparison of treatments for which the subjects are not randomly assigned.

Coefficient of determination   used in regression analysis of quantitative variables and abbreviated r^2, the coefficient of determination is the percent of the variability of the data that can be accounted for by the equation for the regression line. The value r^2 can vary between 0 and 1.

Cohort analysis   a prospective or retrospective comparison of treatments for which the subjects are not randomly assigned.

Continuous variable   a quantitative variable whose measurement is only limited to the detection limits of the instrument; see discrete variable.

Cox proportional hazards model   uses a multiple regression model to look at the effect of a treatment on the probability of the occurrence of a dichotomous outcome over time, while controlling for confounding variables.

If the independent variables are dichotomous, a hazards ratio can be calculated, which is interpreted similarly to a relative risk or odds ratio.

Discrete variable   a quantitative variable whose values are limited to discrete numbers. For example, the spots on a die can only be described by whole numbers between 1 and 6 and the number of patients on a floor can only be described by positive whole numbers; see continuous variable.

F   statistic generated by the AOV, for determination of statistical significance.

Hazards ratio   see Cox proportional hazards model.

Hotelling T^2   a multivariate t test used when differences between two treatments in an analysis of more than one dependent, quantitative, normally distributed variable are desired.

Intention to treat   at the time of data analysis, subjects are analyzed according to the group in which they were randomized, as opposed to the treatment that they may have received. Example: In a study of laparoscopic versus open surgery, even if some of the lap patients are converted to an open procedure, they are still analyzed as lap patients. The purpose of intention to treat is to preserve the randomization of the subjects.

Kaplan-Meier curves   also known as *survival curves*, these give a visual representation showing the probability of an event, such as survival, over time. The Kaplan-Meier curves can be used to look at the probability of any dichotomous outcome over time.

MAOV   a multivariate analysis of variance used when differences between more than two treatments in an analysis of more than one dependent, quantitative, normally distributed variable are desired. The MAOV is also abbreviated MANOVA.

Mean   a population parameter; the arithmetic average of the quantitative variable in question. The sample mean is commonly abbreviated x. This should not be calculated for ordinal, nominal, or non-normally distributed quantitative variables.

Median   in a ranking, from lowest to highest, of all values in a distribution, the median is the middle value, or the average of the two middle values. In a normal distribution, the median is equal to the mean. It is primarily used as a variable descriptor for ordinal or non-normally distributed quantitative variables.

Mode   the value in a distribution that occurs most often; in a normal distribution, the mode equals the mean.

Multivariate statistics   required to determine differences between treatments when two or more dependent variables are analyzed; see Hotelling T^2 and MAOV. When associations between a single "y" variable and multiple "x" variables are required, multiple regression and logistic regression are commonly utilized multivariate tests.

Negative predictive value   the chance that an individual will not have the characteristic of interest if the test for that characteristic is negative: $d/(d + c)$.

Nominal variable   a qualitative variable that falls into one of several groups, or categories. Yes/no responses are nominal variables, that is, wound infection and survival.

Nonparametric statistic   used for the analysis of ordinal variables and non-normally distributed quantitative variables, assuming a small sample size.

Null hypothesis   in hypothesis testing, the null hypothesis always means that there is either no treatment effect or that the effect is of no interest to the researcher. It is abbreviated H_0.

One-tailed test   used in hypothesis testing for a t test or for Fisher exact test, the alternate hypothesis states that one treatment is greater than another treatment. For Pearson correlation coefficient, the alternate hypothesis can be either $r < 0$ or $r > 0$.

Ordinal variable   a qualitative variable involving scores or ranks, for example, Acute Physiology and Chronic Health Evaluation (APACHE) scores, injury severity scores, and pain scales.

$p<0.05$ chance that a true difference between treatments or a relation between variables does not exist is less than 5%. In this context, 0.05 is equal to α, the Type I error rate.

Parametric statistics   used for the analysis of quantitative, normally distributed variables; non-normally distributed variables may also be analyzed with parametric statistics, providing the sample size is sufficiently large.

Pearson correlation coefficient   in regression analysis, this is used to determine the strength of association between independent variables. The value for the coefficient r can vary between -1 and 1.

Population   all of the subjects in the world who possess the characteristics that are to be studied.

Positive predictive value   the chance that an individual will have the characteristic of interest if the test for that characteristic is positive: $a/(a + b)$.

Power   the ability to detect differences between treatments or relations between variables; mathematically, power $= 1 - \beta$.

Prevalence   the frequency of occurrence of the characteristic of interest in the sample tested.

Primary outcome variable   the most important outcome variable in the study, and the one which was used to determine the sample size.

Qualitative variable   an ordinal (ranks, scales, etc.) or nominal (categoric, yes/no, etc.) variable.

Quantitative variable   a continuous (weight, plasma amino acid concentration, etc.), discrete (patients in a hospital, spots on a die), or ratio (insulin:glucagon) variable.

Randomized controlled trial   a prospective comparison of treatments for which the subjects are assigned randomly.

Randomized sampling   a sampling scheme for which any experimental subject has an equally likely chance of being entered into any of the treatment groups.

Rankits   a technique to fit ranked data to a normal distribution for analysis by parametric statistics.

Ratio variable   a ratio of two quantitative variables.

Regression analysis   used to determine relations between variables; tests such as the t test and the AOV are used to determine differences between treatments.

Sample   a subset of the population that will be tested in a study; a good sample is an accurate reflection of the population from which it is drawn.

Sensitivity   the ability of a test to detect the characteristic of interest, given that the characteristic of interest is present: $a/(a + c)$.

Significance   a statistically significant event occurs when the null hypothesis can be rejected with a probability of error lower than the set significance level.

Specificity   the ability of a test to detect the absence of the characteristic of interest, given that the characteristic of interest is not present: $d/(d + b)$.

Standard deviation   a population and sample parameter; the square root of the variance. The sample standard deviation is commonly abbreviated SD. The SD is a useful means of expressing variability for a normally distributed, quantitative variable.

Standard error of the mean   a population and sample parameter; the standard deviation divided by the square root of the sample size. The sample standard error of the mean is commonly abbreviated SEM. The SEM is a useful means of expressing variability for a normally distributed, quantitative variable.

Statistics   a field of mathematics used to determine if differences between treatments or relations between variables exist, beyond a reasonable doubt.

Stratified random sampling   this is also known as *blocking*. It means that instead of randomizing all of your subjects into control and treatment groups, you are breaking your subjects into subgroups, and randomizing study entry in each of those subgroups. Example: In a multicenter trial, each enrollment site is blocked, so patients are equally randomized in New York, San Antonio, and Hudsonville. It is commonly used to ensure that the sample reflects the population and that the subject mix of each treatment group is similar.

t test   used for testing differences between two treatments, if the variable is quantitative and if the samples are normally distributed; also called *Student's t test*.

Two-tailed test   used in hypothesis testing. For a t test or for Fisher exact test, the alternate hypothesis states that one treatment is not equal to another treatment; for Pearson correlation coefficient, the alternate hypothesis states that $r = 0$.

Type I error   the chance that the null hypothesis has been rejected incorrectly; the probability of a Type I error is designated as α, which is used for hypothesis testing and sample size estimation.

Type II error   the chance that the null hypothesis has been accepted incorrectly; the probability of a Type II error is designated as β, which is used for sample size estimation and power determination.

Type III error   described by Condon (9); occurs when the conclusions are not supported by the data. Although not a true statistical entity, its existence can be verified by careful literature review.

Univariate statistics   required to determine differences between treatments when one variable is analyzed; see *t* test and AOV.

χ^2 chi-squared; used to determine differences between treatments, if the variables are nominal.

REFERENCES

1. Steel RGD, Torrie JH. *Principles and procedures of statistics*, 2nd ed. New York: McGraw-Hill, 1980.
2. RF. The triple blind test. In: Scherr GH, ed. *The best of the Journal of Irreproducible Results*. New York: Workman, 1983:96.
3. Marks RG. *Designing a research project*. Belmont: Lifetime Learning, 1982.
4. Evans M, Pollock AV. Trials on trial. *Arch Surg* 1984;119:109–113.
5. Norman GR, Streiner DL. *PDQ statistics*. Philadelphia: BC Decker, 1986.
6. Tatsuoka MM. *Significance tests: univariate and multivariate*. Champaign: Institute for Personality and Ability Testing, 1971.
7. Gill JL. *Design and analysis of experiments in the animal and medical sciences*, Vol. 1. Ames: Iowa State University Press, 1978.
8. Hurwitz ES, Barrett MJ, Bregman D, et al. Public health service study on Reye's syndrome and medications: report of the pilot phase. *N Engl J Med* 1985;313:849–857.
9. Condon RE. Type III error. *Arch Surg* 1986;121:877–878.

SUGGESTED READINGS

Feinstein AR. *Clinical biostatistics*. St. Louis: Mosby, 1977.
Hulley SB, Cummings SR, eds. *Designing clinical research*. Baltimore: Williams & Wilkins, 1988.
Ingelfinger JA, Mosteller F, Thibodeau LA, et al. *Biostatistics in clinical medicine*. New York: Macmillan, 1987.
Marks RG. *Analyzing research data*. Belmont: Lifetime Learning, 1982.
Michael M, Boyce WT, Wilcox AJ. *Biomedical bestiary: an epidemiologic guide to flaws and fallacies in the medical literature*. Boston: Little, Brown and Company, 1984.
Sackett DL, Haynes RB, Tugwell P. *Clinical epidemiology: a basic science for clinical medicine*. Boston: Little, Brown and Company, 1985.
Streiner DL, Norman GR, Blum HM. *PDQ epidemiology*. Philadelphia: BC Decker, 1986.

CHAPTER 12

Female Reproductive Biology

Keith A. Hansen

Medical care of the female patient requires a thorough understanding of the normal development and physiology of the reproductive system. The purpose of the human female reproductive tract is to maintain our species by producing oocytes, allowing for fertilization and development of the embryo and fetus. The reproductive system is under a complex series of regulatory mechanisms involving autocrine, paracrine, hormonal, and neuronal systems. Perturbations in any of these systems can result in abnormalities which can mimic or complicate pathophysiologic processes in other organs. This chapter will explore the normal development, growth, and function of the female reproductive system and how it applies to medical care of the female patient.

EMBRYONIC DEVELOPMENT

The Ovary

Genetic sex is determined at the time of conception when a spermatozoa fuses with the oocyte in the ampullary segment of the fallopian tube. The spermatozoa has a haploid number of chromosomes with either an X or Y sex chromosome. If the spermatozoa that fertilizes the oocyte has an X chromosome, then the fetus will usually develop along female lines; whereas, if the spermatozoa has a Y chromosome, then the fetus will develop into a male. The human fetus at 4 to 5 weeks' gestation is sexually undifferentiated and has the potential to develop into a normal male or female.

The fetal gonad begins as a thickening along the urogenital ridge overlying the mesonephros consisting of coelomic epithelial cells and underlying mesenchyme. The primordial germ cells begin development in the yolk sac at 4 weeks' gestation and migrate by ameboid type movement and differential growth to the urogenital ridge (Fig. 12.1). In the developing ovary, these primordial germ cells undergo a remarkable, exponential increase in numbers through mitosis from a few thousand in early development to more than 6 million at 20 weeks' gestational age (Fig. 12.2).

The primordial germ cells continue active development during gestation. Not only are the numbers of cells exponentially increasing by mitosis, but they also enter meiosis where they arrest in prophase of the first meiotic division. At this stage, the primordial germ cells become surrounded by a single layer of mesenchymal cells from the urogenital ridge (the future granulosa cells) and form a primordial follicle.

At 16 weeks' gestational age, the process of atresia begins to affect germ cells, significantly reducing their total number. By birth, the total number of oocytes has been reduced to approximately 1 to 2 million. The fetal ovary is active throughout gestation and follicles will be stimulated to varying degrees of development during latter stages of gestation, including preantral and antral follicles. However, ovulation does not occur until maturation of the hypothalamic pituitary axis at puberty.

The Uterus

The uterus begins development as two longitudinal infoldings of the coelomic epithelium just lateral to the mesonephros (Fig. 12.3). This forms two tubular structures known as the *mullerian ducts*, which later fuse to form the uterine body. The distal ends of the mullerian ducts remain unfused to form the fallopian tubes (Fig. 12.4).

The undifferentiated human embryo at 5 to 6 weeks' gestational age has both mesonephric ducts (potential to develop into male internal genitalia) and müellerian ducts. Alfred Jost, in a classic series of experiments, demonstrated the dependence of ductal differentiation on gonadal secretions. In the developing male gonad, Sertoli cells produce anti-müellerian hormone, and the Leydig cells secrete androgens. Anti-müellerian hormone is a paracrine hormone that causes ipsilateral regression of the müellerian ducts. Testosterone acts on the developing mesonephric ducts in a paracrine manner to stimulate their differentiation into epididymis, vas deferens, and seminal vesicles. Anti-müellerian hormone in the male fetus may be involved in descent of the testis into the scrotum. In contrast, the developing female gonad does not produce significant

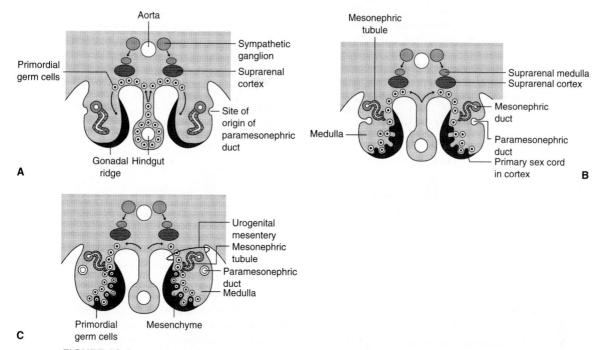

FIGURE 12.1 **A:** Transverse section through 5-week embryo at level of suprarenal glands. This diagram illustrates migration of primordial germ cells from yolk sac to gonadal ridge. **B:** Transverse section through 6-week embryo. Demonstrating continued migration of primordial germ cells and development of mesonephric duct. **C:** Infolding of paramesonephric (mullerian duct) ducts starting. (Reprinted with permission from Moore KL. *The developing human: clinically oriented embryology*. Philadelphia: WB Saunders, 1988.)

quantities of anti-müellerian hormone, and the müellerian ducts continue development into fallopian tubes, uterine body, and the upper part of the vagina. Low levels of androgens produced by the developing ovary are not sufficient to maintain the mesonephric ducts, and they

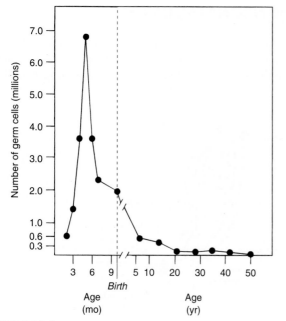

FIGURE 12.2 Ontogenetic development of human oocytes. (Reprinted with permission from Baker TG, Wai Sum O. Development of the ovary and oogenesis. *Clin Obstet Gynecol* 1973;3:3.)

undergo regression. Male development requires the active secretion of steroidal and nonsteroidal molecules from the gonad, whereas female development has always been referred to as the default pathway of sexual differentiation. Recent studies suggest that female development requires the coordinated expression of a number of different genes, including *HOX* and *WNT* genes.

Müellerian system development is intimately dependent on normal development of the renal system. Kidney development occurs in stages, and each stage is dependent on normal differentiation of the previous stage. The stages of renal development include the pronephros, mesonephros, and metanephros. The close association between renal and genital differentiation explains the association of kidney abnormalities with genital tract abnormalities.

External Genitalia

The external genitalia of male and female embryos is undifferentiated at 5 to 6 weeks with the potential to develop into the external genitalia of either sex, depending on the hormonal milieu. In the male fetus, the testes begin to produce testosterone by 8 to 9 weeks' gestational age. Masculinization of the external genitalia can be detected as early as 1 week later, and is completed by 14 weeks' gestational age. Masculinization of the external genitalia relies on the conversion of testosterone to dihydrotestosterone by 5-α reductase. Dihydrotestosterone results in (i) enlargement of the genital tubercle which ultimately forms the penis; (ii) fusion of the folds of the urogenital sinus which form the

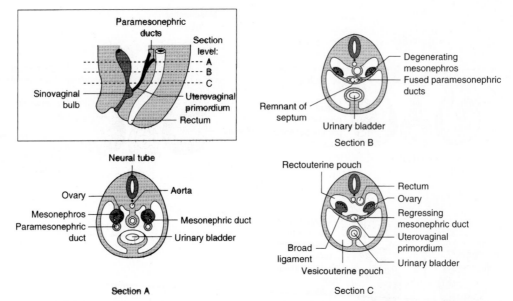

FIGURE 12.3 Eight-week female fetus. Transverse sections at various levels through müllerian ducts, showing their fusion into a single uterine cavity. Mesonephric ducts undergoing degeneration. (Reprinted with permission from Moore KL. *The developing human: clinically oriented embryology*. Philadelphia: WB Saunders, 1988.)

penile urethra; and (iii) fusion of the labioscrotal folds to form the scrotum.

The female fetus lacks adequate androgen levels, resulting in (i) the genital tubercle forming the clitoris; (ii) the folds of the urogenital sinus forming the labia minora; (iii) the urogenital sinus contributing to formation of the lower vagina; and (iv) the labioscrotal folds forming the labia majora (Fig. 12.5). If the female fetus is exposed to androgens during development, it can result in variable degrees of masculinization depending on dose, duration, and timing of exposure.

Normal external genitalia development in the male and female fetus depends on appropriate timing and level of exposure to the respective sex steroids. In a male fetus, reduced levels of androgens, either testosterone or

dihydrotestosterone, will result in inadequate virilization, resulting in a male pseudohermaphrodite. The degree of genital ambiguity will correlate with the level of androgen to which the fetus is exposed during development. In the female fetus, elevated levels of androgens can result in masculinization of the external genitalia. Similarly, the degree of virilization of the female genitalia correlates with the intensity and length of androgen exposure.

THE NEONATAL OVARY

The total endowment of germ cells has been reduced from 20 million to 1 to 2 million by birth. The neonate is separated from the maternal environment at birth, resulting in a fall in

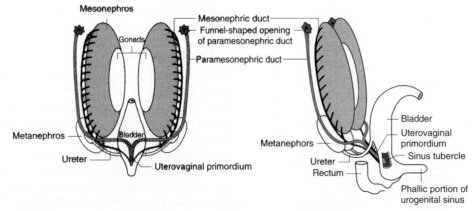

FIGURE 12.4 Schematic frontal view of 7-week embryo. Illustrating relation of undifferentiated müllerian and mesonephric ducts to the developing gonad. (Reprinted with permission from Moore KL. *The developing human: clinically oriented embryology*. Philadelphia: WB Saunders, 1988.)

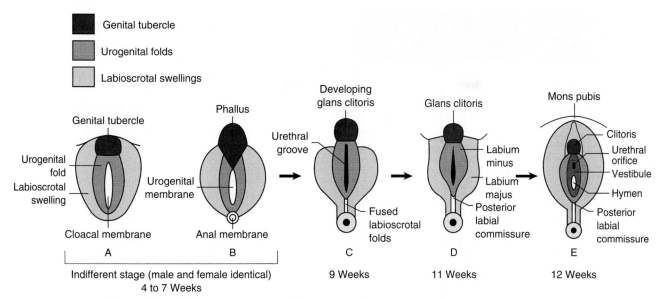

FIGURE 12.5 External genitalia development from undifferentiated stage to complete development. A and B are at 4 to 7 weeks' gestation. C, D, E are at 9, 11, and 12 weeks respectively. (Reprinted with permission from Moore KL. *The developing human: clinically oriented embryology.* Philadelphia: WB Saunders, 1988.)

circulating steroid levels. This decrease in maternal steroids results in decreased negative feedback on the fetal pituitary gonadotrope with resultant release of gonadotropins, follicle-stimulating hormone (FSH), and luteinizing hormone (LH).

In the female fetus, there are increased levels of pituitary and circulating levels of FSH with increased pituitary levels of LH. The male fetus has lower levels of gonadotropins, probably related to androgen and inhibin production by the developing testes. Inhibin is a dimeric polypeptide hormone secreted by Sertoli cells, producing a negative feedback effect on FSH secretion by the pituitary gland. After birth, the female neonate has a larger rise in FSH than LH, and this rise will remain for 12 to 24 months. This rise in gonadotropins can stimulate follicular development in the neonatal ovary, resulting in formation of cysts. One of the common causes of abdominal masses in the female neonate is ovarian cysts resulting from gonadotropin stimulation.

Gonadotropin levels remain elevated for 12 to 24 months in the female before reaching a nadir in early childhood which lasts until puberty. These low levels of gonadotropins result from a highly sensitive negative feedback mechanism coexisting with a nonsteroidal central inhibitor of gonadotropin secretion. Despite a quiescent hypothalamic pituitary gonadal axis, the ovary continues to show evidence of follicular development and atresia.

PUBERTY

Puberty is a time of transition from immaturity to a sexually mature adult. This results in numerous physical, hormonal, and psychological changes in an individual. Puberty is usually heralded by onset of a growth spurt, followed by breast budding (median age 9.8 years). The development of the breast usually follows a well-defined sequence of events which characterizes the stages of pubertal development (Tanner stages) (Fig. 12.6). The development of axillary and pubic hair followed by menarche at an average age of 12.8 years are the usual sequence. The development of the ovulatory mechanism with positive feedback is a late event in normal puberty. The usual length of time to complete the pubertal process is 4.5 years for a healthy European girl. Any abnormality in the timing (age at onset or length of time) of puberty may be a sign of a serious underlying disease and needs to be evaluated with a thorough, systematic approach.

The timing of puberty is primarily genetic with significant environmental influences such as nutrition and psychological stresses. Recent studies show a reduction in the mean age of onset of menarche in developing countries, reflecting an improvement in nutrition and general health. A critical weight for the onset of puberty has been hypothesized and probably reflects a shift in body composition to a higher percentage of fat in the premenarchal female. The percent body fat has an important role in initiation and maintenance of normal menstrual function during the female's reproductive life. Perturbations (high or low) of the percent fat may disturb ovarian function, resulting in oligo-ovulation or anovulation with an accompanying disturbance in menstruation.

Adrenarche results from increased secretion of adrenal androgens as manifested by the appearance of pubic and axillary hair. These androgens include dehydroepiandrosterone (DHEA), its sulfate, and androstenedione. This increase in androgens first appears at approximately 6 to 7 years of age and continues to increase into midadolescence (~age 13—15), correlating with an increase in size of the zona

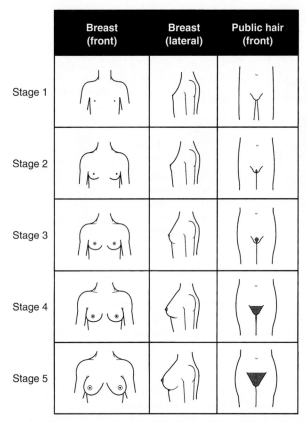

FIGURE 12.6 Tanner stages of breast and pubic hair in pubertal female. (Reprinted with permission from Lee PA. Physiology of puberty. In: Rebar RW, Bremner WJ, eds. *Principles and practice of endocrinology and metabolism.* Philadelphia: JB Lippincott Co., 1990.)

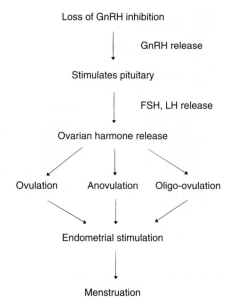

FIGURE 12.7 The release of the hypothalamus from inhibition both by a decease in sensitivity of negative feedback by steroid hormones and a reduction in the central nonsteroidal inhibitory factor results in gonadotropin-releasing hormone (GnRH) production and secretion. The consequence of this process is maturation of the productive axis. FSH, follicle- stimulating hormone; LH, luteinizing hormone.

reticularis of the adrenal cortex. Adrenarche usually occurs 2 years before the onset of pubertal changes, but is not felt to be a "trigger" for other pubertal changes. The exact initiating event for onset of adrenarche is unknown. This "trigger" mechanism does not appear to involve ACTH or cortisol because these hormones remain stable through the pubertal period of time. Recent evidence supports another pituitary molecule as a possible initiating "trigger," a posttranslational cleavage product of pro-opiomelanocorticotropin (POMC).

Puberty is heralded by activation and maturation of the hypothalamic pituitary gonadal axis, which culminates in sexual maturity. During early childhood, pituitary gonadotropins are suppressed to very low levels, thought to be the result of a highly sensitive negative feedback mechanism and an intrinsic central inhibitory influence. Puberty is marked by an orderly decline in the negative feedback mechanism and release from the central inhibitory influence.

The release of the hypothalamic pituitary axis from these suppressive influences releases gonadotrophin-releasing hormone (GnRH) from the hypothalamus, which stimulates the release of gonadotropins from the pituitary which interact with the gonad, resulting in production and release of sex steroids (Fig. 12.7). GnRH acts on gonadotrope cells in the anterior pituitary where it induces production of GnRH

receptors. By upregulating the GnRH receptors it acts as a "self-primer" and stimulates the synthesis and release of gonadotropins by the gonadotropes. As the gonadotropin levels rise, they increase the production and release of sex steroids by the ovary. This release of sex steroids by the gonad results in the development of secondary sex characteristics in a well-described sequence.

Both sexes have the onset of GnRH pulses initially during sleep. Sleep associated GnRH pulses (measured as LH pulses) are an initial sign of puberty which concurs with onset of LH release in response to exogenous GnRH. The GnRH responsiveness of LH correlates with "awakening" of the hypothalamic gonadotrope axis in the early stages of puberty. As puberty progresses and sex steroids rise, the GnRH pulses extend through the day.

An initial event in puberty is the reduction of negative feedback of estrogen on the hypothalamic pituitary axis resulting in increasing gonadotropin and estrogen levels. This change in hormonal milieu is marked by the onset of secondary sexual characteristics. The development of estrogen-induced positive feedback on the hypothalamic pituitary axis is a late manifestation of puberty and correlates with ovulation. Positive feedback is necessary for normal ovulation to occur and results when the mature pituitary is exposed to elevated levels of estrogen for a prolonged time. A surge of gonadotropins occurs, known as the *LH surge,* and is responsible for inducing ovulation.

The onset of menses is usually followed by irregular cycles for a few years consistent with oligo-ovulatory cycles. The menses do not become regular until maturation of the positive feedback mechanism and onset of regular, ovulatory cycles. The onset of positive feedback in the hypothalamic pituitary gonadal axis heralds the onset of regular, ovulatory cycles with the resultant potential for pregnancy.

Precocious Puberty

Precocious puberty is defined as pubertal changes before the age of 8 years and demands a thorough, systemic evaluation. Recent studies suggest that the age of pubertal maturation may be occurring earlier, especially in African American girls, however, a thorough evaluation is still important in the girl who presents with precocious pubertybefore age 8. The causes of precocious puberty can be divided into GnRH-dependent and -independent groups. GnRH-dependent precocious puberty is associated with premature maturation of the hypothalamic pituitary axis with the onset of GnRH pulses resulting in gonadotropin and steroid release. GnRH-dependent precocious puberty can result in ovulation with the potential for pregnancy. GnRH-independent precocious puberty does not result in maturation of the GnRH pulse generator, but is dependent on a peripheral source of gonadal steroids that result in secondary sexual characteristic development (Table 12.1).

Precocious puberty is seen five times more frequently in girls than boys. In 75% of girls, no etiology can be found and is known as *idiopathic*. The diagnosis of idiopathic precocious puberty is one of exclusion and requires a thorough evaluation. In girls, the younger the patient is on presentation, the more likely she has a pathologic condition. The most common diagnosis in girls with GnRH-dependent precocious puberty is idiopathic. Approximately 7% will

TABLE 12.1

Etiologies of Precocious Puberty

GnRH-dependent precocious puberty
   Idiopathic
      Sporadic
      Familial
   CNS disorders
GnRH-independent precocious puberty
   Gonadal tumors and hyperfunctioning disorders
      Ovarian
         Granulosa cell tumors
         Granulosa-luteal cell cysts
      Ovarian hyperfunctioning syndromes
         McCune-Albright syndrome
         Peutz-Jeghers syndrome
      Adrenal tumors and disorders
         Adrenal disorders
            Congenital adrenal hyperplasia
         Adrenal tumors
            Adrenal adenomas
            Adrenal carcinomas
   Exogenous sex steroids
   Primary hypothyroidism

have central nervous system (CNS) lesions that require further evaluation and treatment. Because of activation of the GnRH pulse generator, these patients can ovulate, and reports of early pregnancy document their sexual maturity. The onset of sexual development, however, does not require activation of the GnRH pulse generator with ovulation. Some examples of GnRH-independent causes of sexual precocity include ovarian tumors, adrenal tumors, McCune-Albright syndrome, and ectopic gonadotropin producing tumors.

McCune-Albright syndrome is characterized by café au lait spots, polyostotic fibrous dysplasia of bone, and hyperfunction of a number of endocrine systems. One of the most commonly affected endocrine systems in females is ovarian, resulting in precocious development. Other systems that are frequently affected include the thyroid, adrenal, pituitary, and parathyroids. Molecular diagnosis reveals that McCune-Albright syndrome is caused by an activating mutation of a G protein.

The workup of precocious puberty should focus on defining the etiology and eliminating the possibility of serious illness. The initial evaluation includes a thorough history and physical examination with detailed historic evaluation of growth and the development of secondary sexual characteristics. Evidence of heterologous sexual development caused by excess androgen secretion in the female should be sought; it may be the first sign of an adrenal tumor or congenital adrenal hyperplasia (CAH). A thorough neurologic, abdominal, and pelvic examination is important to discover signs of tumors involving these organ systems. The patient should also be examined for any signs of systemic illnesses that could result in precocious puberty (McCune-Albright syndrome).

Laboratory evaluation of patients should include serum gonadotropins and steroid levels [estradiol, progesterone, 17-hydroxy progesterone, dehydroepiandrosterone sulfate (DHEAS), and testosterone]. A GnRH test can be extremely helpful in determining pituitary gonadotropin reserve. Patients with early maturation of the hypothalamic pituitary gonadal axis demonstrate release of gonadotropins on stimulation with GnRH. Important radiologic tests include bone age, imaging of the head with computed tomography (CT) or magnetic resonance imaging (MRI), CT imaging of the adrenals, and pelvic ultrasonography. This series of tests can help distinguish GnRH-dependent from GnRH independent causes of precocious puberty. Once categorized to the GnRH-dependency group, the previously described tests can further characterize the nature and localize the site of excess hormone secretion.

Pubertal Delay

Lack of sexual development may also be a sign of serious illness. The following presentations are signs of potentially serious pathology and demand a rapid, thorough evaluation: (i) lack of onset of menses by age 14 with no signs of secondary sexual characteristics; (ii) lack of menses by age 16 regardless of secondary sexual characteristics; or (iii) prolonged duration of puberty (>4.5 years). Lack of pubertal development is rare in females and requires an evaluation directed toward abnormalities, including genetic, hypothalamic pituitary, and anatomic (Table 12.2).

The initial evaluation should include (i) signs of past poor health; (ii) evidence of excess exercise or abnormal eating habits; and (iii) chronologic height and weight records. The physical examination should include accurate height and weight measurements as well as Tanner staging. Short stature may be the first clue that the subject suffers from: (i) an isolated growth hormone deficiency; (ii) global pituitary hormone deficiency; or (iii) gonadal dysgenesis. Intracranial disease should be considered, and a detailed neurologic examination is essential.

The laboratory evaluation of patients with delayed puberty includes thyroid function tests, prolactin, gonadotropins, and steroid levels (both gonadal and adrenal). A bone age and skull imaging is important if the patient has low gonadotropins. Patients with high gonadotropins require cytogenetic testing to evaluate for sex chromosome privations.

TABLE 12.2

Etiologies of Delayed Puberty Dependent on Gonadotropin Levels

Elevated serum gonadotropins
  Chromosomally incompetent ovarian failure
    Turner syndrome
      45,X
      45,X mosaics (46,XX or 46,XY)
      X structural abnormalities
  Chromosomally competent ovarian failure
    Congenital adrenal hyperplasia
    17 α-hydroxylase deficiency
    Autoimmune oophoritis
    Iatrogenic
      Oophorectomy
      Radiation therapy
      chemotherapy especially alkylating agents
    Galactosemia
    Idiopathic (vanishing testis syndrome)
    Resistant ovary syndrome
Normal or Decreased Gonadotropin Levels
  Constitutional delay
  Hypopituitarism
    Panhypopituitarism
    Isolated gonadotropin deficiency (Kallmann)
  Hypothyroidism
  Chronic systemic illness
    Anorexia nervosa
    Sickle cell disease
    Thalassemia
  Chronic exercise
  Hyperprolactinemia
  Müllerian anomalies
    Müllerian agenesis
    Müllerian segmental anomalies
  Complete androgen insensitivity

Gonadotropin levels will help direct the evaluation. Elevated gonadotropin levels are consistent with gonadal deficiency. The most common cause of gonadal deficiency is gonadal dysgenesis caused by a privation of the X chromosome. These patients can vary from a complete absence, mosaic condition, or structural abnormality of the X chromosome. Many patients with gonadal dysgenesis will have a normal 46, XX karyotype. A number of etiologies exist for their gonadal failure, including torsion, inflammation, sickle cell disease, and enzymatic deficiencies. An example of an enzymatic deficiency is 17-hydroxylase deficiency, which results in a sexually infantile patient with hypertension and hypokalemia.

Low gonadotropins can be caused by constitutional delay of puberty or to pathologic conditions. Pathologic conditions include hypothalamic amenorrhea, Kallmann syndrome, and hyperprolactinemia. In this group of patients, panhypopituitarism and tumors of the pituitary or hypothalamic region should be ruled out. The most common neoplasm is craniopharyngioma, which is a tumor of Rathke pouch. The treatment for a craniopharyngioma is surgery with possible radiation therapy.

Eugonadal subjects most commonly have müellerian segmental abnormalities such as a transverse vaginal septum, complete müellerian agenesis, or androgen insensitivity. Patients with müellerian abnormalities will have 46, XX karyotypes with functional ovaries and a normal distribution of female pubic and axillary hair. Serum testing will show evidence of ovarian function with normal gonadotropins, estrogen and progesterone levels, and female testosterone levels. Subjects with müellerian abnormalities have an increased frequency of renal and skeletal abnormalities. Subjects with complete androgen insensitivity will present with 46,XY karyotypes, functional intra-abdominal testes, and sparse or absent pubic and axillary hair. Serum testing will reveal male levels of testosterone.

Treatment of subjects with delayed puberty is determined by the etiology. Constitutional delay should be treated by reassurance and counseling. If an XY cell line is discovered, gonadectomy is necessary to prevent ovarian neoplasms (most commonly dysgerminomas and gonadoblastomas). Delayed puberty should be treated with hormone replacement therapy to stimulate development of secondary sexual characteristics.

THE OVARIAN CYCLE

The ovary serves important roles in production of gametes and ovarian steroids. The ovary is under complex regulatory mechanisms, with both positive and negative feedback control, resulting in the production of usually one egg per cycle. The human menstrual cycle is divided into three phases: follicular, luteal, and menstrual. The menstrual cycle is a continuum of follicular development, ovulation, and luteinization (Fig. 12.8).

The follicular phase is characterized by a series of events involving feedback mechanisms which allow for the

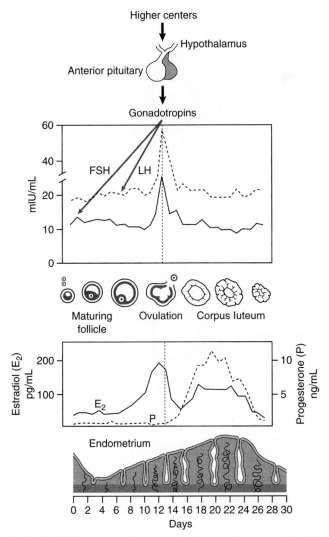

FIGURE 12.8 Cyclic changes during normal menstrual cycle involving the pituitary, ovary, and uterine endometrium. FSH, follicle-stimulating hormone; LH, luteinizing hormone. (Reprinted with permission from Danforth DN, Dignam WJ, Hendricks CH, eds. *Obstetrics and Gynecology*. Philadelphia: Harper & Row, 1982.)

sequential development of a follicle, usually resulting in the release of a single ovum at ovulation.

Primordial follicles are formed initially during embryonic and fetal development from germ cells which arise in the endoderm of the yolk sac. A primordial follicle consists of an oocyte, arrested in the prophase of the first meiotic division, surrounded by a single layer of cells. These will subsequently become functional granulosa cells. The primordial follicle complement is formed by mitotic expansion, reaching maximal numbers in the second trimester of pregnancy. Continual reduction of the number of follicles occurs during the life of the ovary. This process of initiating growth and atresia of follicles continues without interruption until the ovary is completely devoid of follicles (the menopause).

The number of primordial follicles that begin growth in each cycle is unknown, but are related to the total number of follicles remaining in the gonads. Most follicles

that begin development eventually undergo atresia. The dominant follicle, that follicle which is destined to ovulate, is selected in the first few days of the follicular phase and is dependent on elevations in FSH in the early follicular phase.

Elevation of FSH follows the late luteal phase reduction in steroids and inhibin. This rise in FSH in the early follicular phase is accompanied by morphologic changes in the follicle, including an increase in the size of the oocyte and a change from flat to cuboidal granulosa cells. Gap junctions also form between the granulosa cells and the oocyte and serve as a mechanism of communication between these cells (allowing for effective paracrine actions). Under the continued stimulatory effect of FSH, the granulosa cells begin to proliferate and transform the primordial follicle into a primary follicle. Stromal development is also occurring under gonadotropin stimulation resulting in the differentiation of two layers, theca interna and externa, in the primary follicle (Fig. 12.9).

FSH binding to gonadotropin receptors on the developing primary follicle results in proliferation of granulosa cells and steroidogenesis. As the primary follicle continues to enlarge, a membrane develops around the oocyte, the zona pellucida, changing the follicle into a preantral follicle. The preantral follicle depends on continued FSH production, stimulating cell growth, and steroidogenesis.

Granulosa cells contain an enzyme with aromatase activity. This activity is stimulated by FSH binding to receptors on granulosa cell membrane. The aromatase enzyme converts androgens into estrogens, thereby maintaining the estrogenic environment of the follicle. Estrogen and FSH combine to increase the FSH receptor number on granulosa cell membranes, thereby increasing the cellular sensitivity to FSH. This increase in FSH sensitivity allows the cells to continue to respond as FSH levels fall in the latter follicular stage.

The aromatase enzyme is also sensitive to androgen production by thecal cells. A low level of androgens stimulates aromatization, whereas higher levels suppress this process. This combination of follicular phase events results in most follicles becoming atretic, with one or a few growing to maturity. Continued growth of the follicle is accompanied by the appearance of fluid around the granulosa cells, eventually forming a cavity within the follicle, transforming the preantral follicle into an antral follicle. The follicular fluid contains FSH, estrogen, and other granulosa cell metabolites in relatively high concentrations that bathe the developing oocyte.

Follicular development is a highly integrated process involving effective communication between various compartments of the follicle. A two-cell model has been proposed to explain granulosa cell dependence on thecal cells. In this model, granulosa cells are predominantly FSH dependent, as reflected by FSH receptors on their surface, whereas thecal cells are predominantly LH dependent, as reflected by LH receptors on their surface. Thecal cells under the influence of LH convert cholesterol into androgens. The androgens then diffuse to the granulosa layer where they are aromatized into estrogens, thereby maintaining the estrogenic milieu of the follicle.

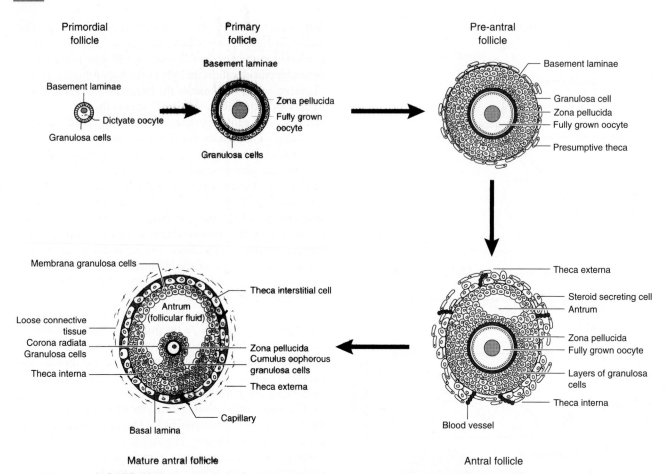

FIGURE 12.9 Morphologic changes in a developing follicle during a normal follicular phase. (Reprinted with permission from Erickson GF, Magoffin DA, Dyer CA, et al. The ovarian androgen producing cells: a review of structure/function relations. *Endocr Rev* 1985;6:371.)

Conversion from an androgen-dependent to estrogen-dependent environment marks the selection of the follicle destined to ovulate. This process depends upon the interaction of FSH and estrogen within the follicle and the pituitary gland. Within the developing follicle, FSH and estrogen function to increase FSH receptor number, increasing the gonadotropin sensitivity of the follicle. The increased circulating concentration of estrogen exerts an inhibitory effect upon the pituitary, thereby decreasing circulating concentrations of FSH (classic negative feedback). This combination of events, an increased sensitivity of the dominant follicle and decreased concentration of FSH, selects the follicle destined to ovulate. The ovary supporting the dominant follicle can be distinguished from its counterpart by the fifth day of the follicular phase. In nondominant follicles, the fall in circulating FSH causes atresia (Fig. 12.10).

The increase in number of granulosa cells in the maturing follicle is accompanied by an increase in vascularity of the theca. The increase in vascularity results in preferential delivery of FSH to the follicle with the greatest blood flow, which can be detected by day 9 of the follicular phase.

Granulosa cells develop LH receptors, which allow them to respond to the LH surge at midcycle with completion of development and ovulation. LH receptors first appear in large antral follicles at time of falling FSH levels and increasing intrafollicular estrogen levels. LH receptors form in response to the estrogenic environment and local paracrine events.

Production of GnRH by the hypothalamus serves an obligatory role in stimulating release of gonadotropins. Feedback of follicular derived growth factors and hormones "fine tune" the secretion of gonadotropins required to stimulate ovulation. Estrogen, the primary steroidal hormone released from the developing follicle, has both positive and negative feedback effects on the hypothalamic pituitary axis. Estrogen decreases gonadotropin secretion by reducing the secretion and response to GnRH in pituitary cells. The exact mechanism of this negative feedback is unknown. When estrogen reaches adequate concentrations for an extended period of time, a positive feedback mechanism results in robust release of gonadotropins from the pituitary gland. This positive effect involves both the hypothalamus and the pituitary gland. In the hypothalamus, estrogen increases the amount of GnRH that is released with each GnRH pulse. In the pituitary gland, estrogen increases the number of GnRH receptors, which results in more gonadotropins being released with each GnRH pulse.

FSH is sensitive to negative feedback, even at low levels of estrogen. LH has a variable response to estrogen; suppression

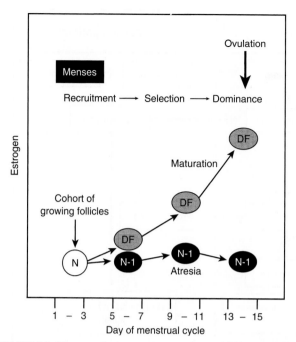

FIGURE 12.10 Development of a dominant follicle. Illustration of dominant follicle selection during the follicular phase. DF, dominant follicle; N, number of developing follicles in the developing cohort. Reprinted with permission from the American Society for Reproductive Medicine (The American Fertility Society) from Hodgen GD. The dominant ovarian follicle. *Fertile Steril* 1982;38:281–300.

at low levels and stimulation at higher levels. The change from suppression to stimulation occurs when estrogen levels reach an adequate value for a sustained period of time.

The preovulatory follicle responds to different hormones and locally acting growth factors. In the preovulatory follicle, FSH promotes luteinization of the granulosa manifested by enlargement and appearance of lipid inclusions in the cells. Thecal cells simultaneously develop inclusions and become richly vascular. These morphologic changes in the follicle are accompanied by increased production of estrogen and progesterone. Midcycle progesterone production facilitates the LH surge and has a dominant role in production of the FSH surge. The LH surge results after adequate estrogen priming and provides the ovulatory stimulus for the dominant follicle.

Ovulation with the release of a mature oocyte occurs after the LH surge. Ovulation occurs 10 to 12 hours after the LH peak and 34 to 36 hours after the start of the LH surge. Resumption of meiosis and stimulation of a number of proteolytic enzymes, which digest the walls of the follicle, allow the oocyte to release; this occurs after the gonadotropin surge. Ovulation is not an "explosive" event, and studies have shown no increase in intrafollicular pressure before ovulation.

After ovulation, granulosa cells continue to enlarge and develop a vacuolated appearance while becoming the corpus luteum. Thecal cells also contribute to the formation of the corpus luteum. The postovulatory follicle accumulates a

yellow pigment known as lutein, hence the name of the corpus luteum. A rapid period of vascularization with ingrowth of capillaries into the granulosa cells occurs immediately after ovulation. The vascularity of the corpus luteum ensures the continued supply of substrates to the metabolically active cells.

The corpus luteum produces ovarian steroids, primarily progesterone and estrogen. The secretion of sex steroids is episodic during the luteal phase and correlates with the pulsatile release of LH. Adequate production of sex steroids depends on adequate follicular growth and gonadotropin receptor formation during the follicular phase. The combination of estrogen and progesterone function to transform the endometrium into an environment which will accept and nurture the developing embryo. A normal menstrual cycle luteal phase is approximately 14 days (range is 11–17 days). The luteal phase is the most constant part of the menstrual cycle in terms of length. The corpus luteum is programmed to undergo involution in 9 to 11 days after the LH surge, unless rescued by human chorionic gonadotropin (hCG), which is secreted actively by the developing fetoplacental unit. If implantation occurs, hCG maintains the corpus luteum until the ninth to 10th week of gestation.

Leptin

Leptin is a polypeptide hormone produced by the adipocyte, which plays an important role in energy homeostasis, feeding, and reproduction. Leptin was first identified in the ob/ob mouse, which carries a mutated leptin gene resulting in an obese, hypogonadal mouse. This hormone is felt to bind to hypothalamic centers and serve as a satiety factor. Increased levels of leptin have been identified in obese as compared to lean individuals, and in females compared to males. Congenital leptin deficiency in humans, due to a frameshift mutation, has been reported and results in a severely obese individual with hypogonadism. Leptin may play a role in the initiation of puberty and in normal and abnormal menstruation.

PREGNANCY

Pregnancy is a unique time in ontogeny of the human. A semiallograft thrives in the center of a potentially hostile maternal immune system. The exact mechanism for this apparent paradox of classical transplant immunology is unknown. Proposed mechanisms include such theories as: (i) the uterus as an immunologically privileged site; (ii) production of maternal blocking antibodies; (iii) idiotype anti-idiotype antibody networks, and multiple other mechanisms.

Pregnancy is also a unique situation in terms of steroidogenesis when three different interacting systems exist: mother, placenta, and fetus. Each of these units contributes essential nutrients and metabolites to the other while allowing the conglomerate to function as an integrated whole (Fig. 12.11).

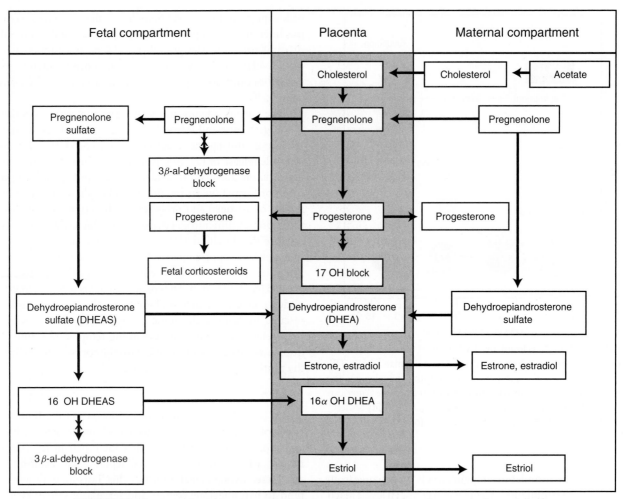

FIGURE 12.11   Steroidogenic pathways during pregnancy. Interrelation of maternal-placental-fetal compartments. (Reprinted with permission from Reece EA, Hobbins JC, Mahoney MJ, et al. eds. *Medicine of the fetus and mother.* Philadelphia: JB Lippincott Co., 1990.)

Progesterone is synthesized from cholesterol from any source: (i) conversion of acetate to cholesterol; (ii) hydrolysis of stored cholesterol esters; or (iii) from low density lipoprotein (LDL)-cholesterol. Maternal blood LDL-cholesterol is the usual source for progesterone synthesis during pregnancy.

During pregnancy, progesterone is produced initially by the corpus luteum that has been rescued by HCG from the syncytiotrophoblast. The developing pregnancy depends entirely on the corpus luteum for progesterone until the seventh week of gestation. From 7 to 10 weeks, both the placenta and corpus luteum are producing progesterone. After 10 weeks, the placenta is the primary source of production. Early miscarriage occurs if the corpus luteum is removed before 7 weeks' gestational age, unless the pregnancy is "rescued" with exogenous progesterone.

Progesterone plays a number of important roles in pregnancy, including preparation and maintenance of the uterine endometrium. The endometrium is thought to suppress maternal immune response to the fetal allograft. Progesterone also supplies the fetus with precursors for the production of glucocorticoids and mineralocorticoids.

Estrogen concentrations are also elevated during pregnancy, but unlike progesterone, estrogen synthesis depends on the production of adequate precursor steroids by the developing fetus. There are three main categories of estrogen produced during pregnancy: estrone, estradiol, and estriol. Estrone and estradiol concentrations in the blood are approximately 100-fold greater in pregnancy than in the nonpregnant state, whereas estriol is more than 1,000-fold greater.

Estrogens depend primarily on the 19-carbon steroid precursors, androgens, for their production. The placenta has a deficiency of P-450 17-hydroxylase enzyme activity, which contains both 17-hydroxylase and 17–20 desmolase activity. Therefore, placental synthesis of estrogen depends on 19-carbon steroid precursors from both maternal and fetal sources. In early pregnancy, androgen precursors come primarily from the mother, whereas later in pregnancy, most 19-carbon precursors come from the fetal adrenal.

The thin outer definitive zone of the fetal adrenal can be differentiated from the thick inner fetal zone by 7 weeks' gestation. The inner fetal zone is proportionately larger than the adult adrenal gland, rapidly undergoing involution after delivery (Fig. 12.12). Initially, the fetal adrenal develops

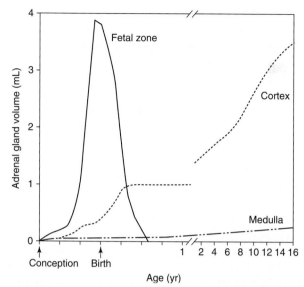

FIGURE 12.12 Ontogenetic development of adrenal glands. Note large size of fetal zone during intrauterine life. (Reprinted with permission from Reece EA, Hobbins JC, Mahoney MJ, et al. eds. *Medicine of the fetus and mother*. Philadelphia: JB Lippincott Co., 1990.)

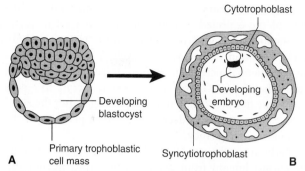

FIGURE 12.13 **A:** Human blastocyst. Demonstrating inner cell mass which will develop into the placenta and membranes. **B:** Early embryo illustrating the differentiation of trophoblast into cytotrophoblast and syncytiotrophoblast. (Reprinted with permission from Reece EA, Hobbins JC, Mahoney MJ, et al. eds. *Medicine of the fetus and mother*. Philadelphia: JB Lippincott Co., 1990.)

under the control of HCG, independent of ACTH. After midgestation, the secretion of fetal ACTH by the developing hypothalamic pituitary axis assumes greater importance. ACTH is felt to play an obligatory role in steroidogenesis and development of the fetal adrenal but may not be the only control mechanism. Previous studies have suggested a role for prolactin.

DHEAS is the primary 19-carbon precursor secreted by the fetus. The large quantities of estrogen produced during pregnancy inhibit 3 β-hydroxysteroid dehydrogenase isomerase activity in the fetal adrenal. This inhibition of 3 β-hydroxysteroid dehydrogenase isomerase results in the fetal adrenal, producing large quantities of delta-5 steroids, DHEA, and DHEAS.

DHEAS secreted by the fetal adrenal may be 16-hydroxylated by the fetal liver to form 16-hydroxy-DHEAS. DHEAS and 16-hydroxy-DHEAS are transported to the placenta, which has an active sulfatase enzyme encoded on the short arm of the X chromosome that will cleave the sulfate moiety from the 19-carbon precursor. DHEAS will then be converted into estrone and estradiol by the placenta, whereas 16-hydroxy-DHEAS will be converted to estriol. Hence, the production of estrogens by the placenta depends intimately on 19-carbon precursors from the fetus transferred to the placenta.

A number of clinical conditions exist in which alterations in fetal adrenal androgen production result in reduced estrogen production. In an anencephalic fetus, the adrenal is small and ill-developed. This does not produce adequate quantities of estrogen precursors, resulting in low estrogen levels. In situations where the fetus is under chronic stress, there will be a lowering of fetal adrenal androgen production resulting in low estrogen production. In the past, estriol was

used as a method of determining fetal well-being; however, because of a lack of sensitivity and specificity, this test has been abandoned. Fetal biophysical testing, nonstress test, and ultrasonography are the best predictors of fetal well-being.

The major protein hormones of pregnancy are produced by the placenta. The cytotrophoblast cell layer of the placenta is composed primarily of single, mononuclear cells that are precursor cells to the syncytiotrophoblast. The syncytiotrophoblast is a syncytium with multinuclei and is most active in hormone production (Fig. 12.13). The placenta releases a number of hormones similar to those produced by the hypothalamus and pituitary, leading to speculation that the placenta has a system of feedback control mechanisms. Hypothalamic hormones expressed in the placenta include corticotropin-releasing hormone, GnRH, thyrotropin-releasing hormone, and others.

HCG is a glycoprotein hormone produced by the syncytiotrophoblast of the placenta. The protein HCG is a dimer composed of an α and β chain. The α chain of HCG is the same as the α chain of a number of pituitary glycoproteins including LH, FSH, and thyroid-stimulating hormone (TSH). The β chains of these molecules are different in structure and presumably are the functional protein moieties. The β chain of HCG is similar to the β chain of LH, which accounts for the clinical use of HCG as a substitute for the LH surge in stimulated cycles.

Structural differences in β subunits of the various glycoprotein hormones have allowed development of highly specific and sensitive immunoassays. The development of a radioimmunoassay for the β subunit of HCG allows earlier detection of metabolically active placental tissue and pregnancy. Recent developments have included a sensitive radioimmunometric assay directed against the entire HCG molecule, with specific antibodies raised against the α and β subunits. One antibody can be fixed on a solid surface like a microsphere and the other tagged with a detection device, such as a radioactive label for detection.

The concentration of HCG is 10 mIU/mL at the time of the expected missed menses. This level increases exponentially during early pregnancy until approximately 10 weeks' gestation, when it reaches levels of 100,000 mIU/mL. The exponential increase in HCG levels has led to the clinical axiom that the HCG level should double every 2 to 3 days during the first weeks of a normal gestation. After the HCG level reaches its peak, it decreases and then plateaus for the remainder of pregnancy.

Early in pregnancy, HCG plays a vital role by rescuing the corpus luteum from demise. The corpus luteum will continue to produce progesterone to maintain the uterine endometrium and maintain pregnancy. The developing fetus depends on HCG for stimulation of the fetal testes to produce androgen and stimulation of the fetal adrenal gland.

A number of pathologic conditions exist where HCG concentration can help establish the diagnosis. In early pregnancy, determination of serial HCG levels can predict pregnancy viability. If HCG levels do not increase in a normal progression, then the possibility of an abnormal pregnancy, such as an ectopic gestation or spontaneous abortion, should be considered.

Determinations of HCG are helpful in arriving at a correct diagnosis in a patient suspected of having an ectopic gestation. Ectopic gestation occurs when the pregnancy implants outside the normal intrauterine location, most commonly in the fallopian tube. A negative HCG determination essentially eliminates the possibility of a viable trophoblast and pregnancy. Approximately two thirds of ectopic pregnancies will have an abnormal rise in serial HCG titers obtained in early pregnancy. The other third will have normal rising titers but may fall or plateau later in gestation.

Pelvic ultrasonography has added an important dimension to diagnosis of an abnormal gestation. A "discriminatory zone" is the HCG level where an intrauterine gestational sac should be detected in a normal gestation. With abdominal ultrasonagraphy, the "discriminatory zone" is at 6,000 to 6,500 mIU/mL, whereas vaginal sonography has a discriminatory zone of 1,000 to 1,500 mIU/mL. The combination of serum HCG level and ultrasonography has proved helpful in the diagnosis of ectopic gestation.

Human placental lactogen (HPL) is also secreted by the syncytiotrophoblast and is composed of a single polypeptide chain with two disulfide bonds. This polypeptide hormone belongs to a group of hormones that also includes growth hormone and prolactin. HPL is produced throughout pregnancy, but tends to increase to high levels in the latter stages of gestation where it correlates with fetoplacental weight. HPL functions by inducing insulin resistance (carbohydrate intolerance) along with increasing insulin-like growth factor (IGF-I) levels.

Glucose is the primary carbohydrate fuel for the developing fetus and is transported actively by the placenta. The placental hormones, including the sex steroids and HPL, induce a state of insulin resistance in the mother. When glucose levels are elevated (fed state), free fatty acids are stored as triglycerides. When glucose levels fall (fasting state), HPL levels increase, resulting in the mobilization of free fatty acids in the mother. By mobilizing free fatty acids, HPL maintains glucose levels for the developing fetus. Prolonged fasting results in mobilization of maternal adipose tissues and a rise in serum ketone levels. These ketones can be used by the developing fetus but, if persistent, may result in abnormalities in certain developing tissues.

α-Fetoprotein is produced primarily by the fetal liver and has no known fetal function. α-Fetoprotein is a glycoprotein that resembles albumin and reaches high levels in the fetal circulation. This similarity to albumin has led to hypotheses that it may function as a carrier molecule in the fetal circulation much as albumin does in the adult.

Maternal serum levels of α-fetoprotein may be abnormal in a number of abnormal pregnant conditions. Elevated levels of maternal serum α-fetoprotein are seen with open neural tube defects, anterior abdominal wall defects, congenital nephrosis, fetal death, multiple pregnancy, fetal maternal hemorrhage, and other less common causes. Data suggest that elevated levels of α-fetoprotein of unknown etiology are associated with poor pregnancy outcome. Low maternal serum α-fetoprotein levels have been useful in diagnosis of fetal aneuploidy, especially Down syndrome.

Prolactin is a polypeptide hormone belonging to the growth hormone family that is secreted actively in pregnancy. Prolactin is synthesized and secreted into three compartments during pregnancy: (i) the fetal blood stream; (ii) amniotic fluid; and (iii) maternal blood stream. Circulating prolactin, whether maternal or fetal, is produced and secreted from the respective pituitary glands and maintains its regulatory pathways, primarily under negative control by dopamine.

Prolactin is also synthesized by decidua and is detected initially soon after decidualization of the endometrium. Prolactin in amniotic fluid is secreted primarily by the decidua that is not under the same control mechanisms as the pituitary. This conclusion results from no change in amniotic fluid prolactin in a patient on dopamine agonist therapy. Amniotic fluid prolactin may play an important role in fluid and electrolyte hemostasis.

A number of polypeptide hormones are produced by the placenta, including human chorionic growth hormone, human chorionic thyrotropin, and human chorionic adrenocorticotropin. These hormones, along with a number of growth factors, play important roles in maternal fetal physiology during pregnancy.

Pregnancy results in a number of hormonal changes in fetal, amniotic fluid, and maternal compartments that help to initiate and maintain pregnancy. These hormonal alterations play an important role in each stage of pregnancy and its successful outcome.

LABOR AND DELIVERY

The embryo and fetus are nurtured within the uterine cavity until the developing human reaches maturity and can exist in the extrauterine environment. During the latter stages of gestation, the human uterus begins to episodically contract. These contractions can occur for a period of time but are characterized by a lack of uterine effacement or dilatation. Labor occurs only when the contractions become sufficiently coordinated to cause cervical effacement and dilatation. This change in the cervix allows for the presenting part of the fetus to pass through the pelvis.

The exact mechanism that initiates labor is unknown; however, there are a number of theories that potentially explain it. One intriguing possibility is progesterone withdrawal. In sheep, the withdrawal of progesterone is felt to play a major role in the onset of labor. In humans, systemic progesterone levels do not change before the initiation of labor. The possibility remains of a local decrease in progesterone at the uteroplacental interface resulting in the start of uterine contractions. Another potential etiology for labor is an increase in oxytocin. Oxytocin (or Pitocin) has been used for a number of years to induce and augment labor, so it is a natural extension to consider it as a cause of labor. In normal labor and delivery, Pitocin levels are only found to significantly increase in the second stage of labor, and hence probably do not play an active initiation role. Investigators have found an increased concentration of oxytocin receptors in the mature uterus. This data supports oxytocin as having a role in labor but not initiating the process.

A unifying concept for the initiation of labor involves communication between the fetal membranes and uterine decidua. The components of this communication network could function together to signal maturity of the fetus and trigger labor. One potential signaling mechanism is prostaglandins, which are formed actively by the decidua and are increased in concentration during normal labor.

Labor is characterized by an increase in the number of oxytocin receptors in the myometrium, increase in myometrial gap junctions, and cervical effacement and dilatation. These changes allow for rhythmic, propulsive uterine contractions that propel the fetus through the bony pelvis.

Labor can be divided into three stages: (i) Stage 1, which involves effacement and dilatation of the cervix; (ii) Stage 2, which involves propulsion of the fetus through the bony pelvis; and (iii) Stage 3, which starts after delivery of the fetus and ends with delivery of the placenta. Some authors describe a fourth stage that occurs for the first hour after delivery of the placenta.

The first stage can be divided into the latent and active phases. When one analyzes cervical dilatation, it is found to follow a sigmoid curve. The latent phase is that period of time when the cervix is dilatating slowly and ends when it enters the phase of rapid dilatation, which is usually at 4 or 5 cm. The active phase is the linear portion of cervical dilatation and extends from 4 or 5 cm until the cervix is dilated completely at 10 cm. During effacement and dilatation of the cervix, the fetal presenting part will descend slowly into the bony pelvis. Only when the cervix is fully dilated will the second stage of labor begin. This stage of labor is marked by active pushing; the presenting part negotiates the bony pelvis and

is delivered. The second stage concludes with the clamping and cutting of the umbilical cord.

The third stage involves the time from delivery of the baby until delivery of the placenta and fetal membranes. This stage usually lasts between 15 and 30 minutes. Some authors describe a fourth stage which is the hour after delivery of the placenta and is marked by a number of physiologic changes, including contraction of the uterus (which reduces blood loss) and a rapid redistribution of maternal circulation.

The average amount of blood lost after a vaginal delivery is approximately 500 mL and 1,000 mL after a cesarean section. A number of etiologies exist for excess blood loss after delivery, the most common include uterine atony, retained placental fragments, and reproductive tract injuries. Less common causes of postpartum hemorrhage include uterine inversion, abnormalities of placentation (placenta accreta), and bleeding diathesis.

MENOPAUSE

Menopause is a retrospective diagnosis marked by the cessation of menses for 12 months due to follicular exhaustion. Menopause occurs at an average age of 52 years in the United States and this age has remained constant over time. The climacteric is that period of time marked by waning ovarian function and culminating in hypogonadism. Menopause correlates with the morphologic finding of few gonadotropin-resistant follicles in the ovaries. This lack of follicles and low gonadal steroids results in elevated gonadotropin levels especially FSH.

Owing to increased life expectancy, a woman from a developed country can expect to live one third of her life in the hypogonadal state of menopause. The loss of ovarian follicles results in a number of important physiologic changes. First, lack of responsive follicles results in sterility. Second, is loss of gonadal steroids, both estrogen and progesterone. This hypogonadism increases the risk of vasomotor symptoms, urogenital atrophy, osteoporosis, heart disease and possibly Alzheimer disease. The vasomotor symptoms, urogenital atrophy, and bone loss respond positively to estrogen therapy. Findings from the Women's Health Initiative have altered the indications for menopausal hormone therapy.

Vasomotor Symptoms

The hot flush/flash is the most common reason that perimenopausal and menopausal women consult a physician during this time of their life. The prevalence of hot flushes varies across the world with women of European origin experiencing these symptoms 60% to 80% of the time. Asians complain of vasomotor symptoms only 10% to 20% of the time and Mexican Mayans rarely complain of hot flushes. There are a number of theories to explain these differences of hot flash prevalence including social and cultural reasons and ingestion of variable amounts and types of phytoestrogens. Hot flushes typically occur in the years 1 to 5 following the menopause before disappearing.

The hot flush is described as a hot, flushing feeling occurring in the face, head, neck, and upper chest with a typical duration of 1 to 5 minutes. Before the flush there is a small but significant increase in core temperature followed by peripheral vasodilatation. This vasodilatation results in increased blood flow to the skin, a rise in temperature, and sweating.

The loss of estrogen production has an important role in the genesis of hot flushes. The faster and larger decline in estrogen equates with more severe and prevalent hot flashes. In premenopausal women after oophorectomy more than 90% will experience vasomotor symptoms. However, estrogen loss does not totally explain the presence of these symptoms. CNS neurotransmitters such as catecholamines especially norepinephrine, dopamine, and serotonin may play important roles.

Estrogen replacement therapy is the most efficacious therapy for vasomotor symptoms. Recent results suggest that one should use the lowest dose of estrogen for the shortest duration to control vasomotor symptoms. If the patient has a uterus one should add progesterone to the regimen to avoid the development of endometrial hyperplasia and cancer. This progesterone can be added in a cyclic manner or continuously. Before initiating therapy with estrogen one needs to individualize treatment with the patient after reviewing the benefits and risks. If estrogen is not an option, other agents used include progestins, clonidine, veralipride, bromocriptine, and the selective serotonin reuptake inhibitors.

Urogenital Atrophy

Loss of estrogen can also result in urogenital atrophy. This can result in recurrent vaginitis, painful intercourse, pruritus, and even vaginal stenosis. Other events can include dysuria, recurrent urinary tract infections, and possible urinary incontinence.

The treatment for urogenital atrophy is the local delivery of estrogen or the use of lubricants. The classic therapy has been the application of estrogen cream to the affected area. An area of concern with locally applied estrogen cream is consistency of serum levels and the potential of variable estrogen absorption. A new, novel therapy is the use of Estring, which is an estrogen-impregnated ring delivering a low-dose of estrogen to the vagina for a period of 3 months. Once again, the lowest dose of estrogen for the shortest period of time should be used to minimize the risk of adverse events.

Bone Loss

Bone is a metabolically active tissue that is constantly undergoing remodeling, which is the removal of old and laying down of new bone. This process is normally under tight control to maintain the integrity of bone. Remodeling is important for repairing injury, renewing aging, and maximizing flexibility and strength of bone. Any interference with the tightly coupled process of the osteoclast/osteoblast unit results in weakened bone and increased fracture risk.

Humans achieve peak bone mass between age 25 and 35. This peak bone mass is multifactorial with both strong genetic and environmental components. After achieving peak bone density, both men and women experience a gradual decline with advancing age. Estrogen loss at menopause results in an accelerated osteoclast mediated breakdown of bone without an increase in calcium deposition. This breakdown with decreased deposition may result in up to 3% loss of bone for the first 5 to 8 years following onset of menopause. If allowed to continue unabated, this loss of bone structural integrity results in clinically significant osteoporosis and an increased risk of fractures.

Osteoporosis is defined by the World Health Organization as "a disease characterized by low bone mass and microarchitectural deterioration of bone tissue, leading to enhanced bone fragility and a consequent increase in fracture risk." Osteoporosis has been defined in terms of bone mineral density as a bone mineral density that is more than 2.5 standard deviations below the peak bone mineral density. Not all postmenopausal women will develop osteoporosis. A number of risk factors exist which increase a woman's chance of developing osteoporosis. These include being thin, Caucasian, a smoker, and having a family history of osteoporosis. However, no risk factor or test exists that can be used to absolutely predict which woman will develop osteoporosis.

Three major types of tests are used to determine bone health including biochemical tests, radiologic detection, and bone biopsies. Biochemical tests include bone formation markers such as serum alkaline phosphatase, serum osteocalcin, type I collagen peptides. Tests of bone resorption include hydroxyproline, the pyridinoline cross-links, and tartrate-resistant acid phosphatase. These tests may be beneficial in determining which patient will respond to therapy and in monitoring adherence to therapy. At this time these tests are limited in their usefulness because they cannot differentiate between focal and systemic disease. These tests also do not quantitate or significantly differentiate between resorption and formation, and are affected by a number of other factors such as liver uptake.

Radiologic evaluation of bone density remains the gold standard for determining bone health or disease for osteoporosis. The test most commonly used for evaluating bone density is Dual x-ray absorptiometry (DEXA) scanning. DEXA uses two energy peaks with the lower-energy wave primarily absorbed only by soft tissue whereas the high-energy wave is absorbed by soft tissue and bone. The differential absorption by bone and soft tissue allows calculation of bone mineral density for an individual. The bone density report will give both a z-score and t-score. The z-score compares a patient's bone density to individuals of the same age, sex, and race. The t-score compares a patient's bone density to the expected peak bone mineral density. Other tests of bone density include the quantitative computed tomography (QCT) scan and quantitative ultrasonography. Quantitative ultrasonagraphy is increasing in use because of its speed, ease of administration, less radiation, and good detection of decreased bone mineral density.

The prevention and treatment of osteoporosis is multifactorial including dietary intervention by increasing calcium and insuring adequate vitamin D intake, weight bearing exercise, reducing risk factors such as discontinuing smoking and excess caffeine, and pharmacologic therapy consideration. The use of exogenous estrogen can markedly retard osteoporosis and improve bone mineral density in postmenopausal women. Estrogen replacement epidemiologic studies demonstrate a 5% to 6% increase in vertebral and a 2% to 3% increase in femoral neck bone mineral density. The Women's Health Initiative demonstrated a statistically significant decrease in osteoporosis-related fractures. The minimum dose of estrogen needed to improve bone mineral density is equivalent to 0.625 mg of conjugated equine estrogens or 0.3 mg of conjugated equine estrogens with calcium and vitamin D supplementation. Although estrogen is a helpful therapy for the prevention and treatment of osteoporosis, most authors suggest using other medical therapies as first-line treatment due to the significant adverse effects of estrogen.

Raloxifene (Evista) is the first selective estrogen receptor modulator (SERM) approved by the U.S. Food and Drug Administration (FDA) for the prevention and treatment of osteoporosis in menopausal women. Raloxifene is an estrogen with variable activities in different tissues. Studies show raloxifene use improves bone mineral density as well as a beneficial effect on serum lipids. Raloxifene, however, does not stimulate the uterine endometrium or breast. The Multiple Outcomes of Raloxifene Evaluation (MORE) trial was a prospective, randomized, double-blind, multi-institutional trial evaluating the effect of raloxifene versus placebo on bone mineral density. This study demonstrated an increase in bone mineral density in the lumbar spine and femoral neck with a 55% reduction in fractures in women with no previous fractures and 30% reduction in women with previous fractures. Raloxifene improved total and LDL cholesterol and did not increase the incidence of vaginal bleeding, endometrial hyperplasia, or endometrial cancer. Raloxifene demonstrated a 65% reduction in the incidence of breast cancer. The decrease in breast cancer was in estrogen receptor positive cancers. This finding has led to a National Cancer Institute trial comparing raloxifene to tamoxifen for prevention of breast cancer in high-risk women.

Other pharmacologic agents with benefit in osteoporosis include bisphosphonates and calcitonin. All of these current agents (SERMs, bisphosphonates, and calcitonin) are antiresorptive and despite differences in bone mineral density gain with their use, all reduce the incidence of fractures by approximately 50%. The similar reduction in fracture risk among the currently available antiresorptive agents is most likely due to bone architecture improvement by agents with similar effects on bone. Exciting new research is under way evaluating anabolic agents such as parathyroid hormone, androgens, growth hormone, and statins that may improve bone strength through different mechanisms.

Cardiovascular System

Heart disease is a significant cause of morbidity and the most common cause of mortality in the postmenopausal women. There are a number of cardiovascular risk factors that increase with advancing age and the hypogonadal state of the menopausal woman. As a woman ages there is a general increase in body weight, central obesity, insulin resistance, and elevated blood pressure all of which predispose to the development of heart disease. The loss of estrogen at menopause is felt to play a role in the development of cardiovascular disease. Epidemiologic studies demonstrate an increase in cardiovascular disease in women after the menopause and the male-to-female ratio of disease rates decrease after this time.

Epidemiologic studies have shown estrogen replacement therapy to be beneficial for primary prevention of cardiovascular disease. The effects of hormone replacement therapy on cardiovascular disease were challenged with the publication of the Heart Estrogen/Progestin Replacement Study (HERS). The HERS trial was a secondary prevention trial in which women with a history of heart disease were randomized to placebo or estrogen and progesterone. At the end of the trial, the relative risk of having a cardiac event was not significantly different between the two groups. Temporal analysis demonstrated that the women on estrogen/progesterone therapy had a higher incidence of events in the first year of the study, which slowly decreased over time. This suggests an immediate prothrombotic or preischemic effect of estrogen/progesterone therapy, with long-term benefit from improvements in lipids.

The Women's Health Initiative was a prospective, randomized study performed by the National Institutes of Health and designed to evaluate the effect of hormone replacement therapy and dietary modification on cardiovascular disease. In the estrogen and progesterone arm of the Women's Health Initiative there was a nonsignificant increase in the incidence of coronary heart disease with a hazards ratio of 1.24 (95% confidence interval, 1.00–1.54). In the estrogen only arm there was no change in coronary heart disease, with a hazards ratio of 0.91 (95% confidence interval of 0.75–1.12). This data suggests that one should not use estrogen therapy as primary or secondary therapy for coronary heart disease and that other methods such as weight loss, exercise, smoking cessation, and statins are more effective. One concern with the data from the Women's Health Initiative was the age of the patients who were analyzed, with a large number initiating therapy approximately 10 years after the menopause. There are a number of observational studies that suggest the early start of estrogen therapy after menopause may be cardioprotective.

Hormone Therapy

Recommendations for estrogen therapy during menopause have substantially changed with results from new studies, especially the Women's Health Initiative. Menopausal hormonal therapy should be individualized with the lowest dose of estrogen used for the shortest duration to control menopausal symptoms. This treatment should only be initiated after a thorough discussion of risks and benefits.

Estrogen replacement during menopause is the treatment of choice for vasomotor symptoms and urogenital atrophy. Conventional therapy includes estrogen alone in the patient without a uterus, but estrogen combined with a progestin if she still has a uterus. Unopposed estrogen has been shown to stimulate the endometrium and may result in endometrial carcinoma if used for a prolonged time. In postmenopausal women, the addition of progestin to estrogen therapy reduces the risk of developing endometrial cancer to baseline risk.

The Women's Health Initiative demonstrated improvement in bone health in patients on estrogen. However, due to potential adverse events associated with estrogen therapy most authors suggest using other beneficial treatments in these patients. Estrogen therapy should not be used to prevent or treat heart disease. The Women's Health Initiative did demonstrate an increase in the incidence of stroke in patients using estrogen therapy as compared to placebo.

Previous studies have suggested a beneficial impact on prevention of dementia in patients on estrogen therapy. In the Women's Health Initiative, for women older than 65 there was an increased hazards ratio for the development of dementia (2.05 with 95% confidence interval of 1.21–3.48).

Breast cancer is a significant cause of morbidity and mortality in menopausal women. The risk factors for breast carcinoma suggest that the longer a woman is exposed to estrogen the higher her risk of developing cancer. Studies suggest that women on hormone replacement therapy may have an increased risk of developing breast cancer especially after greater than 5 to 10 years. In the Women's Health Initiative the risk of breast cancer was increased in the estrogen and progesterone arm, but decreased in the estrogen only arm of the study. This suggests that one should caution the patient with a uterus with a need for progesterone supplementation during estrogen therapy about this risk before initiating therapy.

Other adverse events associated with hormone replacement therapy include irregular vaginal bleeding, breast tenderness and pain, venous thromboembolism, and cholelithiasis. The risk of venous thromboembolism is three to four times greater in women on hormone replacement therapy than menopausal controls but this is still a low incidence of events. This risk of venous thromboembolism is greater in patients who are older, obese, or have factor V Leiden mutations.

CONCLUSION

The primary purpose of the reproductive tract is to allow for reproduction of the species. Many pathophysiologic processes can affect the reproductive system, and the reproductive system may modify the presentation of these same disease processes. Alterations of the reproductive system may also mimic or adversely affect other organ systems, especially intraperitoneal organs. An understanding of the reproductive system is vital to all health care providers caring for women.

This chapter reviews the development, function, and final cessation of the activity of the female reproductive system. This entire process culminates in female reproductive maturity with the ability to carry a pregnancy to successful completion. After approximately 40 years of ovulatory competence, the ovaries cease functioning. This cessation of function not only results in lack of gamete production but also substantially reduced hormone production. This loss of hormones, specifically estrogen and progesterone, results in menopause and the attendant risks of osteoporosis, heart disease, genitourinary atrophy, and the menopausal syndrome.

GLOSSARY

Cytotrophoblast single mononuclear cells of the developing placenta which fuse and form syncytiotrophoblast.

Diploid karyotype 2(n) condition where a cell contains two complete sets of chromosomes. In humans 46 chromosomes.

Ectopic pregnancy implantation of a pregnancy outside of the normal intrauterine environment, most commonly in the fallopian tube.

Follicle-stimulating hormone (FSH) a dimeric glycoprotein composed of an α and β chain produced by gonadotrophs in the adenohypophysis. Important during folliculogenesis and ovulation.

Human chorionic gonadotropin (HCG) a dimeric glycoprotein produced by the syncytiotrophoblast of the placenta which "rescues" the corpus luteum in early pregnancy.

Haploid karyotype (n) condition where a cell contains one complete set of chromosomes. In the human, 23 chromosomes.

Hirsutism androgen-induced excess body and facial hair growth.

Luteinizing hormone (LH) dimeric glycoprotein produced by gonadotrophs in adenohypophysis.

Meiosis cell division occurring in germ cells that reduces chromosome number to the haploid state (2n–n).

Menopause cessation of menstrual cycles.

Menstrual cycle cyclic hormonal and anatomic changes that occur in preparation for ovulation and pregnancy. Can be divided into follicular, luteal, and menstrual phases.

Mitosis cell division in somatic cells that maintains a diploid set of chromosomes (2n–2n).

Syncytiotrophoblast multinucleated, syncytium of cells of the placenta that function in the production and secretion of a number of placental hormones.

Virilization signs of pronounced hyperandrogenemia including temporal balding, deepening of voice, increased muscle mass, and clitoromegaly.

SUGGESTED READINGS

Aloia JF, Vaswani A, Yeh JK, et al. Calcium supplementation with and without hormone replacement therapy to prevent postmenopausal bone loss. *Ann Intern Med* 1994;120:97.

Baker TG, Sum OW. Development of the ovary and oogenesis. *Clin Obstet Gynaecol* 1976;3:3.

Bartlemez GW. The phases of the menstrual cycle and their interpretation in terms of the pregnancy cycle. *Am J Obstet Gynecol* 1957;74:931.

Calle EE, Miracle-McMahill HL, Hunb MJ, et al. Estrogen replacement therapy and risk of fatal cancer in a prospective cohort of postmenopausal women. *J Natl Cancer Inst* 1995;87:517.

Cohen HL, Eisenberg P, Mandel F, et al. Ovarian cysts are common in premenarcheal girls: a sonographic study of 101 children 2?12 years old. *Am J Roentgenol* 1992;159:89.

Delmas PD, Bjarnason NH, Mitlak BH, et al. Effects of raloxifene on bone mineral density, serum cholesterol concentrations, and uterine endometrium in postmenopausal women. *N Engl J Med* 1997;337:1641.

Erickson GF, Magoffin D, Dyer CA, et al. The ovarian androgen producing cells: a review of structure/function relationships. *Endocr Rev* 1985;6:371.

Ettinger B, Black DM, Mitlak BH, et al. Reduction of vertebral fracture risk in postmenopausal women with osteoporosis treated with raloxifene: results from a 3-year randomized clinical trial. *JAMA* 1999;282:637.

Gambacciani M, Spinetti A, Taponeco F, et al. Bone loss in perimenopausal women: a longitudinal study. *Maturitas* 1994;18:191.

Jost A, Vigier B, Prepin J, et al. Studies on sex differentiation in mammals. *Recent Prog Horm Res* 1973;29:1.

Knobil E. The neuroendocrine control of the menstrual cycle. *Recent Prog Horm Res* 1980;36:53.

Manolio TA, Furberg CD, Shemanski L, et al. Associations of postmenopausal estrogen use with cardiovascular disease and its risk factors in older women. *Circulation* 1993;88:2163.1.

McKinlay SM, Brambella DJ, Posner NG. The normal menopausal transition. *Maturitas* 1992;12:102.

Midgley AR Jr, Jaffe RB. Regulation of gonadotropins. IV. Correlations of serum concentrations of follicle-stimulating and luteinizing hormones during the menstrual cycle. *J Clin Endocrinol Metab* 1968;28:1699.

Mikhail G. Hormone secretion by the human ovaries. *Gynecol Obstet Invest* 1970;1:5.

Mittwoch U, Mahadevaiah S. Comparison of development of human fetal gonads and kidneys. *J Reprod Fertil* 1980;58:463–467.

Molnar GW. Body temperatures during menopausal hot flashes. *J Appl Physiol* 1975;38:499.

Noyes RW, Hertig AW, Rock J. Dating the endometrial biopsy. *Fertil Steril* 1950;1:3.

Oerter KE, Uriarte MM, Rose SR, et al. Gonadotropin secretory dynamics during puberty in normal girls and boys. *J Clin Endocrinol Metab* 1990;71:1251.

Rabinovici J, Jaffe RB. Development and regulation of growth and differentiated function in human and subhuman primate fetal gonads. *Endocr Rev* 1990;11:532.

Reindollar RH, Tho SPT, McDonough PG. Delayed puberty: an updated study of 326 patients. *Trans Am Gynecol Obstet Soc* 1989;8:146.

Riggs BJ, Jowsey J, Kelley PJ, et al. Role of hormonal factors in the pathogenesis of postmenopausal osteoporosis. *Isr J Med Sci* 1976;12:615.

Schreiber J. Current concepts of human follicular growth and development. *Contemp Obstet Gynecol* 1983;26:125.

Simpson ER, MacDonald PC. Endocrine physiology of the placenta. *Annu Rev Physiol* 1981;43:163.

Sturdee DW, Wilson KA, Pipili E, et al. Physiological aspects of menopausal hot flush. *Br Med J* 1978;2:79.

The Writing Group for the PEPI (Postmenopausal Estrogen/Progestin Inverventions) Trial. Effects of hormone therapy on bone mineral density: Results from the postmenopausal estrogen/progestin interventions (PEPI) trial. *JAMA* 1996;276:1389.

Tulchinsky D, Hobel CJ. Plasma human chorionic gonadotropin, estrone, estradiol, progesterone and 17 alpha-hydroxyprogesterone in early normal pregnancy. *Am J Obstet Gynecol* 1973;117:884.

Wilson JD, George FW, Griffin JE. The hormonal control of sexual development. *Science* 1981;211:1278.

Yen SSC. The biology of menopause. *J Reprod Med* 1977;18:287.

Yen SSC, Vela P, Rankin J, et al. Hormonal relationships during the menstrual cycle. *JAMA* 1970;211:1513.

CHAPTER 13

The Breast

Mary Morrogh and Patrick I. Borgen

Breast cancer is a complex family of genetic diseases. It is one of the world's most important public health threats and is the most expensive component of our cancer health care delivery system in the United States. Significant progress has been made in elucidating carcinogenic mechanisms for various subtypes of the disease. Currently, it is essential that clinicians endeavoring to prevent, diagnose, or treat breast cancer possess a fundamental understanding of the basic physiologic precepts that are the foundation of our knowledge base. Many biologic mechanisms have found expression in preventative and/or therapeutic strategies. This chapter represents a survey of the current wisdom and understanding in a field that is changing rapidly. In an effort to make this presentation accessible and usable, the authors have included a summary of clinical applications for many of the salient biologic observations in each subsection.

ANATOMY

Gross Anatomy

The breast tissue lies within the superficial fascia (the hypodermis) of the anterior thoracic wall and is separated from the skin by a layer of subcutaneous fat. It consists of approximately 15 to 20 ductolobular units that open individually onto the nipple areolar complex. The retroareolar space contains smooth muscle, but no subcutaneous fat. The suspensory ligaments of Cooper are fascial bands that run from the deep layer of the superficial fascia to the skin between the ductolobular units to the skin, and support the weight of the breast. There is no distinct fascial compartmentalization of the breast parenchyma. The deep layer of the superficial fascia is separated from the pectoral fascia by a distinct space known as the *retromammary space*. Both the suspensory ligaments and the retromammary space contribute to the mobility of the gland. The glandular portion of the peripubertal, nulliparous breast lies almost entirely over the pectoralis muscle, extending into the axilla as the "tail of Spence." At this stage of development, the breast assumes the classical, hemispheric shape. Increasing age, variations in body weight, pregnancy, and lactation alter the consistency and density of the breast significantly; the mature breast becomes more lax and extends inferolaterally, assuming a somewhat flattened, pendulous shape. (Fig. 13.1) (1,2).

Clinical Relevance

- The subcutaneous fat separating the breast tissue and the skin is a relatively avascular plane. Dissection through this subdermal plane preserves the blood supply to the skin flaps and minimizes blood loss.
- In cancer surgery, removal of the pectoralis fascia along with the deep layer of the superficial fascia is recommended to optimize clearance at the posterior margin.
- Tumors involving or adjacent to the suspensory ligaments may shorten the ligaments, pulling on the skin and resulting in skin dimpling or *peau d'orange*.

The inferolateral extension of the breast with age means that the upper-outer quadrant of the breast has the greatest proportion of glandular tissue, and this may explain the increased incidence of breast cancer in this quadrant.

Blood Supply to the Breast

The breast is a highly vascular organ deriving its blood supply from three principal sources: the internal mammary artery (IMA), the axillary artery, and the costocervical trunk and thoracic aorta.

The IMA. Ventral branches of this artery (anterior rami mammarii) penetrate the intercostal muscles of the second to the fifth intercostal spaces, approximately 1 to 2 cm lateral to the parasternal border (upper-inner quadrant) entering the breast.

The axillary artery. The lateral thoracic artery (*a. thoracalis lateralis; long thoracic artery; external mammary artery*) branches off the axillary artery between the subscapularis anteriorly, and the cords of the brachial plexus posteriorly. It follows the lower border of the pectoralis minor to the side of the chest, supplying the serratus anterior and pectoralis muscles, and sends branches across the axilla to the axillary

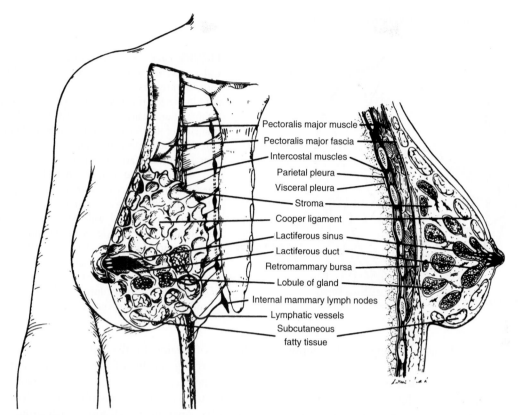

Pectoralis major muscle
Pectoralis major fascia
Intercostal muscles
Parietal pleura
Visceral pleura
Stroma
Cooper ligament
Lactiferous sinus
Lactiferous duct
Retromammary bursa
Lobule of gland
Internal mammary lymph nodes
Lymphatic vessels
Subcutaneous
fatty tissue

FIGURE 13.1   A tangential view of the breast on the chest wall and a cross-sectional (sagittal) view of the breast and associated chest wall. The breast lies in the superficial fascia just deep to the dermis. It is attached to the skin by suspensory Cooper ligaments and is separated from the investing fascia of the pectoralis major muscle by the retromammary bursa. Cooper ligaments form fibrosepta in the stroma that provide support for the breast parenchyma. Between 15 and 20 lactiferous ducts extend from lobules composed of glandular epithelium to openings located on the nipple. A dilation of the duct, the lactiferous sinus, is present near the opening of the duct in the subareolar tissue. Subcutaneous fat and adipose tissue distributed around the lobules of the gland give the breast its smooth contour and, in the nonlactating breast, account for most of its mass. Lymphatic vessels pass through the stroma surrounding the lobules of the gland and convey lymph to collecting ducts. Lymphatic channels ending in the internal mammary (or parasternal) lymph nodes are shown. The pectoralis major muscle lies adjacent to the ribs and intercostal muscles. The parietal pleura, attached to the endothoracic fascia, and the visceral pleura, covering the surface of the lung, are shown. (From Romrell L, Bland K. Anatomy of the breast, axilla, chest wall, and related metastatic sites. In: Bland KI, Copeland EM, eds. *The breast: comprehensive management of benign and malignant diseases*, 2nd ed. Philadelphia: WB Saunders, 1991:18(3). Reprinted by permission.)

glands and subscapularis. It supplies an external mammary branch, which turns around the free edge of the pectoralis major to supply the breast.

The costocervical trunk and the thoracic aorta through the lateral branches of the posterior intercostal arteries.

Other arteries that supply nutrients to the breast include the thoracoacromial, subscapular, upper thoracic, and thoracodorsal arteries. Extensive collateralization occurs between these vessels within the breast tissue (1,2).

The venous drainage of the breast follows the primary arterial supply. The superficial veins form an extensive anastomotic network and assume a circular configuration around the nipple, known as the *circulus venosus*. The deep veins drain almost entirely into the axilla. The principal deep veins include (1,2) the perforating branches of the internal thoracic vein, the tributaries of the axillary vein, and the perforating branches of the posterior intercostal veins (Fig. 13.2).

Clinical Relevance

- The internal mammary nodes (IMN) run along the course of the IMA, which lies between the superficial parietal pleura and the intercostal muscles, and are found in the intercostal spaces. IMN biopsy may be helpful to identify the subset of patients who would receive systemic therapy on the basis of "negative axillary nodes, but positive IMN." The location of the nodes is such that the approach does not necessitate interruption of the costal cartilage; however, the IMA is an important potential graft for coronary artery

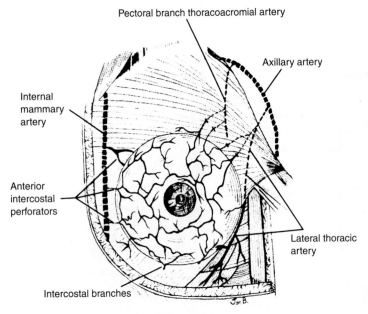

FIGURE 13.2 Arterial distribution of blood to the breast, axilla, and chest wall. The breast receives its blood supply through three major arterial routes: (i) medially from anterior perforating intercostal branches arising from the internal thoracic artery, (ii) laterally from either pectoral branches of the thoracoacromial trunk or branches of the lateral thoracic artery (the thoracoacromial trunk and the lateral thoracic arteries are branches of the axillary artery), and (iii) from lateral cutaneous branches of the intercostal arteries that are associated with the overlying breast. The arteries indicated with a *dashed line* lie deep to the muscles of the thoracic wall and axilla. Many of the arteries must pass through these muscles before reaching the breast. (From Romrell L, Bland K. Anatomy of the breast, axilla, chest wall, and related metastatic sites. In: Bland KI, Copeland EM, eds. *The breast: comprehensive management of benign and malignant diseases*, 2nd ed. Philadelphia: WB Saunders, 1991:26. Reprinted by permission.)

bypass, and care must be taken during an IMN biopsy to protect this vessel (3).

- The major perforators (anterior rami mammarii) are located in the upper-inner quadrant. They are branches of the IMA, a high-pressure vessel, and are the most frequent source of "bring-back" bleeding.
- The pectoralis major derives its blood supply through two branches (medial and lateral) of the lateral thoracic artery. Injury to both will result in atrophy of the muscle.
- The thoracodorsal branch of the subscapular artery contributes little to the blood supply of the breast, but is a key vessel when considering breast reconstruction. Not only does this vessel supply blood to the latissimus dorsi muscle (an ideal choice for myocutaneous pedicle flap reconstruction), but it is also the first choice for recipient vessels of free flaps. The central and scapular lymph nodes lie adjacent to this vessel, so it is essential that during axillary procedures, the surgeon identifies and protects this artery. In addition, the long thoracic and thoracodorsal nerves lie in close proximity to the vessel and may be injured during dissection.
- Knowledge of the blood supply of the breast is fundamental to understanding the pattern of metastasis in breast cancer. Not only does breast cancer metastasize through the venous system, but the lymphatic vessels (the principal conduit of metastasis) follow the course of the blood vessels. In addition, the Batson plexus (a valveless, venous plexus surrounding the vertebrae extending from the base of the skull to the sacrum) is in direct communication with the posterior intercostal arteries. This connection provides a potential pathway for metastasis to the vertebral column and central nervous system (CNS).

Lymphatic Drainage of the Breast

All four quadrants of the breast drain as a unit to a few common nodes in the axilla. A small proportion of

the breast drains to the IMN. The lymphatics of the skin overlying the breast are in direct contact with the underlying deeper lymphatics. There are many classification systems to describe the distribution of lymph nodes in the axilla. Anatomists categorize each group by virtue of their route of drainage and anatomic relations (axillary vein/lateral, external mammary/anterior, scapular/posterior, central and subclavicular/apical). Surgeons define each group with respect to their relation with the head of the pectoralis. Clinically, the most relevant description is by "level," determined by the relation of the nodes to the pectoralis muscle:

- Level I: Lateral to the lateral border of the pectoralis minor muscle
- Level II: Beneath the pectoralis minor muscle
- Level III: Infraclavicular, medial to the pectoralis minor muscle

There are two other groups of nodes that have clinical relevance: the interpectoral nodes (Rotter node) that lie between pectoralis major and minor, and the IMN that run alongside the IMA (Figs. 13.3 and 13.4) (1,2).

Clinical Relevance

- Sentinel lymph node biopsy (SLNB) is based on the hypothesis that that the breast drains as single unit to a few common nodes in the axilla, thereby disseminating tumor cells colonize one or a few lymph nodes before involving others. This hypothesis has been validated by prospective trials that have consistently reported sensitivity of SLNB in the range of 90% to 98%, and false-negative rates of 2% to 4%. Axillary node status is the most significant prognostic indicator in breast cancer patients, and systemic therapy is based on the presence of nodal disease. Traditionally, axillary dissection was required to assess the nodal status of

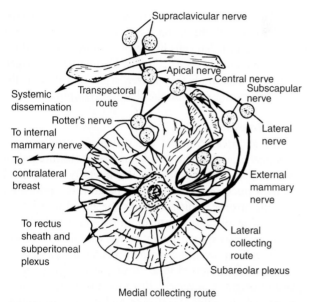

FIGURE 13.3 Schematic drawing of the breast identifying the position of lymph nodes relative to the breast and illustrating routes of lymphatic drainage. The clavicle is indicated as a reference point. Level I lymph nodes include the external mammary (or anterior) group, the axillary vein (or lateral) group, and the scapular group; level II, the central group; and level III, the subclavicular (or apical) group. The *arrows* indicate the routes of lymphatic drainage. (From Romrell L, Bland K. Anatomy of the breast, axilla, chest wall, and related metastatic sites. In: Bland KI, Copeland EM, eds. *The breast: comprehensive management of benign and malignant diseases*, 2nd ed. Philadelphia: WB Saunders, 1991:28. Reprinted by permission.)

the patients, but SLNB can spare patients axillary dissection by accurately sampling the axilla (4,5).

- Axillary dissection [axillary lymph node dissection (ALND)] is an important component of locoregional control. Residual disease may have the potential to seed further

distant metastatic disease, and uncontrolled axillary disease can substantially affect quality of life. Although we await the results of randomized control trials to determine the effect of axillary dissection after SLNB on disease-free and overall survival [National Surgical Adjuvant Breast and Bowel Project (NSABP) 32], standard procedure is to perform an ALND on all patients with clinically positive axillary nodes or positive SLNB. ALND involves clearance of nodes in Levels I and II. Intraoperative palpation of the Level III nodes and Rotter nodes determines whether or not dissection needs to be extended (6).

- The axillary nodes are the common route of lymphatic drainage for the breast and the upper limb. Lymphedema is an unfortunate complication of ALND, affecting up to 10% to 15% of patients (7).
- The IMN receive the lymphatic drainage from the posterior third of the breast. When considering the utility of IMN biopsy, it is important to consider the location of the suspicious lesion (3).

Innervation of the Breast

The retroareolar space lacks subcutaneous fat, but contains a layer of smooth muscle. This layer consists of two rings containing smooth muscle fibers that run perpendicular to one another (radial and circular). Excitation (somatic and autonomic) leads to contraction of these fibers in two opposing planes, resulting in erection of the nipple and a decrease in the diameter of the areola. Sensory innervation of the breast is limited to the overlying skin and is derived primarily from the lateral and anterior cutaneous branches of intercostal nerves II–VI, and in part from the supraclavicular nerve.

Clinical Relevance

- Skin incisions will interrupt the small cutaneous nerves and cause numbness, which may be temporary or permanent. All patients need to be counseled about altered sensation

FIGURE 13.4 Schematic drawing illustrating the major lymph node groups associated with the lymphatic drainage of the breast. The Roman numerals indicate three levels or groups of lymph nodes that are defined by their location relative to the pectoralis minor. Level I includes lymph nodes located lateral to the pectoralis minor; level II, lymph nodes located deep to the muscle; and level III, lymph nodes located medial to the muscle. The *arrows* indicate the general direction of lymph flow. The axillary vein and its major tributaries associated with the pectoralis minor are included. (From Romrell L, Bland K. Anatomy of the breast, axilla, chest wall, and related metastatic sites. In: Bland KI, Copeland EM, eds. *The breast: comprehensive management of benign and malignant diseases*, 2nd ed. Philadelphia: WB Saunders, 1991:32. Reprinted by permission.)

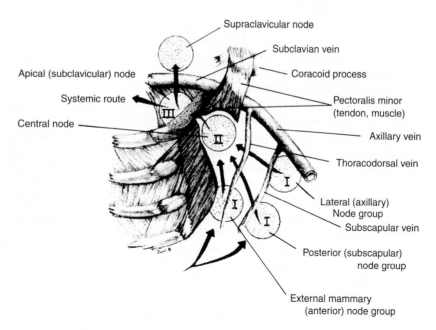

after surgery. Interruption of the retroareolar space during duct excision or nipple-sparing mastectomy may damage the layer of smooth muscle. Patients undergoing such procedures must be aware that not only may they notice altered sensation, but they may also suffer loss of erectile function of the nipple.

Contents of the Axilla

The axilla is a complex, unforgiving pyramidal compartment between the thoracic walls and the upper limb. A thorough understanding of the axillary anatomy is essential for any surgeon treating patients with breast cancer.

Clinical Relevance

- The initial approach to the axilla begins with identification of the axillary vein, followed by the medial pectoral nerve. Paradoxically, the medial nerve is found lateral to the lateral nerve. Both supply the pectoralis muscle, and injury would result in difficulty in adduction of the upper limb.
- The next nerve to be identified is the intercostobrachial. This is a sensory nerve only, supplying sensation to the upper, inner aspect of the arm. Attempts are made to preserve it; however, it is sometimes sacrificed, leading to cutaneous anesthesia or pain syndromes of the arm.
- The long thoracic nerve of Bell comes off the upper roots of the brachial plexus and enters the axilla deep to the axillary vein. Within the axilla, the nerve always runs posterior to the intercostobrachial nerves, and runs perpendicularly along the lateral border of the serratus anterior, beneath a layer of superficial fascia. It innervates the serratus anterior muscle, and injury results in "winging of the scapula."
- The thoracodorsal nerve arises from the posterior cord of the brachial plexus, runs in the lateral aspect of the axilla, and supplies the latissimus dorsi muscle. The latissimus dorsi is innervated from a number of sources, so sacrificing the thoracodorsal nerves rarely causes complications.

Microscopic Anatomy

The breast is composed of glandular epithelium, fibrous stroma, connective tissue, and fat. The relative contribution of these tissues is under the control of circulating hormones (namely estrogen, progesterone, and prolactin) and as such, varies according to age, menstrual cycle, pregnancy, parity and breast feeding. The glandular epithelium forms a complex branching system (ducts) that radiate outward from the nipple [10–20 primary ducts, 30–40 segmental ducts, and 10–100 subsegmental ducts that terminate in a lobular unit]. Each lobular unit consists of clusters of ductules and acini (milk-producing units).

The breast epithelium is made up of three different cell types with distinct morphologic features; the superficial (luminal) A cells, the basal (B) cells, and the myoepithelial cells. The A cells are characterized by dark nuclei and are thought to be responsible for milk production. The B cells (the most common cell type) have large, clear nuclei with distinctive intracellular filaments. Finally, the myoepithelial cells contain contractile myofilaments and are most abundant during lactation. Together, these cells assume a bilayered configuration, with the A and B cells in the innermost layer and the myoepithelial cells in the outermost layer. A thick basement membrane (BM) composed primarily of collagen and laminin surrounds this bilayer, separating it from the stroma. The stroma contains the blood and lymphatic vessels.

Clinical Relevance

- Almost all breast cancers are malignant proliferations of *epithelial* cells. The most important feature when describing a breast cancer is the integrity of the BM (on light microscopy). The BM separates the epithelium from the stroma, which contains the blood and lymph vessels. The primary route of breast metastasis is the lymphovascular system. An intact BM contains the cancer cells, thereby preventing lymphovascular invasion. Such a carcinoma is referred to as *in situ*, as it remains in its place of origin. Conversely, disruption of the BM allows cancer cells to enter the stroma and come into contact with the lymphovascular system. This type of cancer is called *invasive* and carries a much worse prognosis than *in situ* disease.
- *Nonepithelial* tumors of the breast include sarcomas, lymphoma, and phyllodes tumor (PT).
- Mammography (MG) can be limited by density of the breast tissue. Younger women tend to have more glandular or stromal breasts, limiting the sensitivity of MG in this age-group.

NORMAL BREAST DEVELOPMENT AND PHYSIOLOGY

Embryology

The breast is a modified sweat gland of ectodermal and mesodermal origin. The fetal stage of breast development is modulated primarily by local factors (8). During the fifth week of development, two ectodermal ridges (milk lines) appear along the ventral surface of the embryo, extending in parallel from the primitive axilla to the inguinal region. By week 9, these paired ectodermal ridges begin to disappear; however, they are preserved in the pectoral region, forming a pair of "primary buds" (Fig. 13.5). These primary buds divide into many (15–20) smaller "secondary buds" that individually extend into the underlying, vascularized connective tissue mesoderm. Over time, these ectodermal extensions branch, epithelialize, and develop lumens and terminal pouches (acini), thereby acquiring the classical "ductal and lobular" structure that typifies the mammary gland. At birth, there are no differences (morphologic or physiologic) between the sexes (9) (Figs. 13.6 and 13.7).

Clinical Relevance

- Failure of the milk line to undergo normal regression results in the formation of accessory nipples (polythelia or "supernumerary nipples") or accessory breasts (polymastia). Similarly, regression of the primary bud will

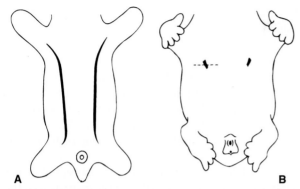

FIGURE 13.5 The mammary ridges and their regression. **A:** Ventral view of an embryo at the beginning of the fifth week of development (∼28 days), showing the mammary ridges that extend from the forelimb to the hindlimb. **B:** A similar view of the ventral embryo at the end of the sixth week, showing the remains of the ridges located in the pectoral region. (From Bland K, Romrell LJ. Congenital and acquired disturbances of breast development and growth. In: Bland KI, Copeland EM, eds. *The breast: comprehensive management of benign and malignant diseases*, 2nd ed. Philadelphia: WB Saunders, 1991:69. Reprinted by permission.)

result in a congenital absence of breast tissue (amastia) and nipple (athelia). Such anomalies occur not only as single phenotypes, but also in combination with others (such as ulnar-mammary syndrome), suggesting that genes affecting breast development are prone to epigenetic modification.

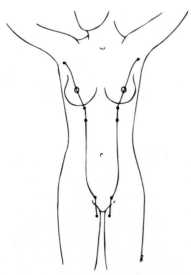

FIGURE 13.6 Mammary milk line. After development of the milk buds in the pectoral area of ectodermal thickening, the milk streak extends from the axilla to the inguinal areas. At week 9 of intrauterine development, atrophy of the bud has occurred except for the presence of the supernumerary nipples or breast. (From Bland K, Romrell LJ. Congenital and acquired disturbances of breast development and growth. In: Bland KI, Copeland EM, eds. *The breast: comprehensive management of benign and malignant diseases*, 2nd ed. Philadelphia: WB Saunders, 1991:70. Reprinted by permission.)

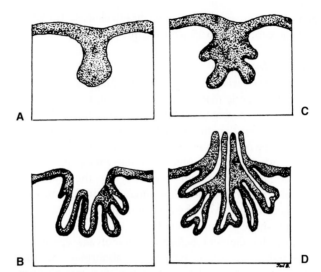

FIGURE 13.7 Sections through evolutionary development and growth of the mammary bud. **A–C:** Similar sections showing the developing gland at successive stages between the 12th week and birth. The mammary pit develops, and major lactiferous ducts are present at the end of gestation. **D:** A similar section showing the elevation of the mammary pit by proliferations of the underlying connective tissue forming the nipple soon after birth. (From Bland K, Romrell LJ. Congenital and acquired disturbances of breast development and growth. In: Bland KI, Copeland EM, eds. *The breast: comprehensive management of benign and malignant diseases*, 2nd ed. Philadelphia: WB Saunders, 1991:71. Reprinted by permission.)

- Cystosarcoma phyllodes (PT) is the most common breast tumor of nonepithelial (mesenchymal) origin.

Puberty

The human breast is a dynamic organ which is continuously remodeled under the influence of hormones and growth factors. In contrast to the fetal stage of breast development, growth and development of the adult breast is chiefly modulated by autocrine (systemic hormones) and paracrine (growth factors, cytokines) pathways. *Thelarche* marks the onset of adult (female) breast development. The release of gonadotropin-releasing factor (GnRH) from the hypothalamus stimulates and controls the release of pituitary hormones, follicle-stimulating hormone (FSH), and luteinizing hormone (LH). The early menstrual cycles are anovulatory and so the effects of estrogen are unopposed. This "ductal growth phase" involves ductal elongation, epithelial thickening, and an increase in stromal density (10). The most significant change that occurs during the perimenarchal period is the addition of lobular units to the rudimentary ductal system. Growing terminal end buds form new small ductules (alveolar buds) that branch and become smaller and more numerous (ductules). A type 1 lobule (lob 1) is a terminal duct with 10 to 12 associated alveolar buds and is the characteristic feature of a perimenarchal breast. These lobules continue to develop for 10 to 15 years until they are slowly replaced by more mature lobules. In the adult breast, cyclic changes occur during the menstrual cycle, increasing the rate of proliferation, especially during the luteal phase. Breast size may increase by up to 15% during this phase (11).

Clinical Relevance

- Such is the variation in epithelial proliferation during the menstrual cycle that it can alter the efficacy of magnetic resonance imaging (MRI) as a breast-imaging tool (12).
- It is thought that the intrinsic dynamic ability of breast cells to be continuously influenced and remodeled makes them especially susceptible to carcinogenesis.
- In women younger than 30 years of age, the stroma and lobules may respond to hormonal stimulus in an exaggerated manner with the development of fibroadenomas (FAs) (single or multiple) (13).
- Breast development before 8 years of age (premature thelarche, precocious puberty) is abnormal and most likely due to dysregulation of the hypothalamic-pituitary-adrenocortical axis. Conversely, lack of estrogen may result in failed development of the ductal system. There are many causes of estrogen insufficiency, namely, absence of ovarian tissue (Turner syndrome, Kallman syndrome), malnutrition, or injury (chemotherapy, radiation).
- Fibrocystic change represents a wide range of clinical and histologic findings. First presenting at menarche and typically resolving after menopause, it is believed to reflect an exaggerated response to circulating hormones and their effect on breast proliferation. Fibrocystic change is not associated with an increased risk of breast cancer.
- Gynecomastia (see "Breast Cancer") describes enlargement (hypertrophy) of the male breast. "Physiologic gynecomastia" refers to bilateral enlargement of breast tissue within 1 year of the onset of testicular development and is a normal finding in up to two thirds of men. Nonphysiological gynecomastia is typically a result of estrogen excess, androgen deficiency, or drug effects. A direct relation between gynecomastia and male breast cancer remains to be seen.

Pregnancy and Lactation

During pregnancy, autocrine and paracrine factors work to prepare the breast for lactation. The first phase of growth (*adenosis of pregnancy*) focuses on proliferation of distal ducts and lobular units, and is driven primarily by progesterone. During the second phase, these new lobular units mature by differentiating into secretory units (acini). Toward the end of the pregnancy, the secretory/A-cells become engorged with colostrum; the fat and connective tissue of the breast become almost entirely replaced by glandular epithelium.

Lactogenesis occurs in two stages and is dependent on prolactin and glucocorticoids. It begins with synthesis of the milk components by the basal/B-cells, engorgement of the acini with colostrum, and proliferation of the myoepithelial cells. The second stage (occurring at or just after parturition) is the initiation of milk secretion and is marked by a rise in oxytocin, and a fall in placental hormones (progesterone), citrate, and A-lactalbumin. Mature milk production usually begins at 36 to 48 hours postpartum, and the rate of lactation is more or less constant for the first 6 months. Weaning

results in a decrease in size and number of lobules and acini; the ducts are not involved.

Clinical Relevance

- Women who complete their first pregnancy in their 20s have a statistically significant reduction in breast cancer risk compared with those whose first pregnancy is during their 30s. Paradoxically, women with the BRCA1/BRCA2 mutation are at increased risk of developing a cancer during pregnancy.
- Lactational disorders include failure to lactate, and delayed onset of lactation, or galactorrhea (inappropriate secretion of milky discharge in the absence of pregnancy/breast feeding for more than 6 months). An important cause of delayed onset of lactation is retained placenta. Retained placenta will result in continued secretion of progesterone that will suppress lactation and may lead to a life-threatening postpartum hemorrhage. Lactational failure has been an interesting first presentation of Sheehan syndrome.
- A galactocele is a milk-filled cyst that usually occurs at the cessation of lactation and is thought to be the result of thickened, blocked fluid. Examination reveals a well-circumscribed, fluctuant mobile mass that typically resolves with aspiration.
- Pregnancy-associated fibroadenomas (FA) is a common finding. In this setting, fine-needle aspiration (FNA) frequently reports atypical cells. Caution must be used when interpreting FNA results in this setting.

Menopause

Menopause is described by cessation of ovarian function and withdrawal of steroid hormones. Involutional changes become evident approximately 20 years after menarche and are quite extensive by the time menopause is reached. This results in involution of breast epithelium (ductal and lobular) and connective tissue. Although there is an increase in fat deposition, the overall volume of the breast decreases.

Clinical Relevance

- The incidence of breast cancer increases with age, and most breast cancers are seen in postmenopausal women.
- Exogenous hormones [hormone replacement therapy (HRT)] may result in the persistence of epithelium. Epidemiologic studies have shown a statistically significant increased risk in developing breast cancer in women who took combined (estrogen and progesterone) HRT compared with women who took estrogen only, or placebo.
- In postmenopausal women, the principal source of circulating estrogen (primarily estradiol) is conversion of adrenally generated androstenedione to estrone by aromatase in peripheral tissues with further conversion of estrone to estradiol. Treatment of breast cancer has included efforts to decrease estrogen levels by ocphorectomy premenopausally, and by use of antiestrogens and progestational agents both pre- and postmenopausally; these interventions lead to decreased tumor mass or delayed

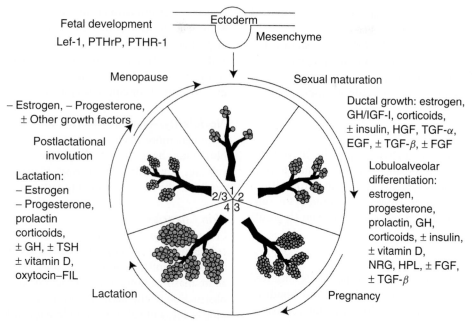

FIGURE 13.8 Regulatory influences on breast development. Numbers (*1, 2, 3,* etc.) correspond to lobule type (*1, 2, 3,* etc.). Ectoderm invaginates into mesenchyme during fetal development. Sexual maturation begins with the onset of puberty through periods of ductal and lobuloalveolar growth and is reflected in the formation of lobules type 1 and 2. Pregnancy initiates the formation of lobule type 3. Lactation, which follows, is associated with lobule type 4. Postlactational involution follows, with regression of lobules. Menopause is characterized by a majority of lobules type 1 and 2, similar to the virgin state. Lef-1, transcription factor Lef-1; PTHrP, parathyroid hormone-related peptide; PTHR-1, PTH/PTHrP receptor type 1; GH, growth hormone; IGF-1, insulin-like growth factor 1; HGF, hepatocyte growth factor; TGF-α, transforming growth factor α; EGF, epidermal growth factor; TGF-β, transforming growth factor β; FGF, fibroblast growth factor; GH, growth hormone; TSH, thyroid-stimulating hormone; FIL, feedback initiator of lactation; NRG, neuregulin; HPL, human placental lactogen; FGF, fibroblast growth factor. (Modified from Russo IH, Dickson R, Russo J. Biochemical control of breast development. In: Harris J, et al. eds. *Diseases of the breast.* Philadelphia: Lippincott, Williams and Wilkins, 2000.) (From Bland K, Kass, R, Mancino AT, Rosenbloom AL, et al. Breast Physiology: Normal and Abnormal Development and Function. In: Bland KI, Copeland EM, eds. *The breast: comprehensive management of benign and malignant diseases,* 3rd ed. St. Louis: Saunders, 2004:48. Reprinted with permission.)

progression of tumor growth in some women. Aromatase inhibitors (AIs) inhibit the peripheral conversion of androgens to estrogen and have been shown to be effective in treating hormone receptor–positive, postmenopausal breast cancer. Figure 13.8

DIAGNOSIS OF BREAST DISEASE

An estimated 212,920 American women were diagnosed with breast cancer in 2006, of whom over 40,900 died of the disease. Excluding skin cancer, breast cancer is the most common female cancer in the United States, the second most common cause of cancer death, and the main cause of death in women age 45–55. Excluding skin cancer, breast cancer is the most common female cancer in the United States, the second most common cause of cancer death in women, and the main cause of death in women aged 45 to 55. However, despite increasing incidence rates, there has been a decline in mortality rates (2.3% per year from 1990–2002).

Screening MG has contributed to this decline, allowing for the detection of earlier stage, smaller cancers (14). Although most breast cancers are diagnosed as a result of an abnormal mammogram, not all mammographic findings represent a cancer. Clinical history, examination, and MG are the cornerstones of breast cancer evaluation.

Clinical Evaluation

Most benign breast diseases (BBDs) are related to normal processes of reproductive life, and few breast cancers occur in the absence of risk factors. There are a number of established and potential risk factors for breast cancer. Many mathematic models (modified Gail model, Claus model) exist to quantify breast cancer risk based on certain established risk factors. These models have inherent limitations and, although validated, they can only be used as a guide. The following are the "established" risk factors: gender, age, family history, hormonal factors, BBD, and previous history of irradiation. There are many other potential modifiers of breast cancer risk (smoking, alcohol, body mass index, diet, etc.), but these remain controversial and so are of limited importance in clinical practice.

In addition to determining the risk factor status, it is important to assess breast-related symptoms and, if cancer is suspected, constitutional symptoms. Presenting complaints can include breast pain (mastalgia), nipple discharge, or a breast mass.

Breast Pain

Mastalgia is a common complaint, especially in younger women, due to normal physiologic changes related to hormonal fluctuation, and is typically cyclical in nature. It is a rare feature of breast cancer. However, adenoid cystic cancer (a rare form of breast cancer) can cause pain (typically noncyclical).

Nonbreast Pain

Pain arising from the chest wall may be falsely localized to the breast. Underlying causes include costochondritis (Tietze syndrome), ischemic heart disease, cholecystitis, or radiculopathies.

Nipple Discharge

Nipple discharge is a common complaint and, in the absence of an underlying mass (on examination or mammography), it is an uncommon presentation of breast cancer. However, unilateral bloody nipple discharge in a woman older than age 40, with or without an underlying mass, should be evaluated to rule out an underlying carcinoma (15,16). Preoperative galactography may be helpful in the localization of underlying pathology and treatment planning for patients presenting with spontaneous nipple discharge (17).

Breast Mass

Both benign and malignant breast disease may present as a lump in the breast. Ninety percent of new lumps in premenopausal women are benign. A tumor is more likely to be hard and immobile with irregular edges. However, physical examination alone is unspecific and all masses should be evaluated in context of history, examination, and investigations.

Constitutional Symptoms

Symptoms that may suggest metastatic disease include weight loss, bone pain, shortness of breath, headaches, and dizziness.

The clinical breast examination (CBE) is an integral component of screening and diagnosis, and should be a part of a periodic health examination approximately every 3 years for women aged 20 to 30, and annually for those aged 40 and older. Beginning with inspection and palpation of the breast and lymph nodes (axillary, cervical infraclavicular, and supraclavicular), it should also incorporate a general examination to assess for any evidence of distant disease. There are five frequently reported clinical findings.

Dominant Breast Mass

Dominant breast masses should be evaluated in context of age, clinical history, menstrual cycle, risk factors, and features on examination (mobility, pain, consistency, edges). Management options include observation and repeat CBE, or further investigation with mammography, sonography, and/or tissue sampling. Sonography is particularly helpful in younger women and can help to determine whether a breast mass is a simple or complex cyst, or a solid tumor.

Nodularity/Asymmetric Thickening

Although more likely to represent a benign condition or fibrocystic change, this finding must be evaluated further to rule out any underlying disease. Management approach is similar to that of a dominant breast mass.

Skin Changes

"Peau d'orange" describes the appearance of skin edema accompanied by erythema. Associated warmth and tenderness is typical of inflammatory carcinoma. It may be mistaken for acute mastitis; however, it is most often due to cancer cell obstruction of the dermal lymphatics. A single benign skin biopsy does not rule out an underlying inflammatory cancer as skip lesions are a common feature.

Nipple Changes

Inversion of the nipple can be congenital or acquired. Acquired unilateral nipple inversion should raise the suspicion of an underlying cancer. Direct invasion of the skin of the nipple with carcinoma results in eczematoid dermatitis, a hallmark of Paget disease of the nipple.

Lymphadenopathy

Lymphadenopathy is an element of many nonmalignant diseases, and so clinically suspicious axillary nodes comprise a wide spectrum of pathologic findings. Clinical examination of the axilla is unreliable for evaluating nodal status in breast cancer patients. Even intraoperative examination is challenging as malignant nodes may appear completely normal, and reactive adenopathy may be indistinguishable from gross metastasis. The high false-positive rate associated with clinical examination means that clinically positive nodes alone are not a clear justification for full lymph node dissection, suggesting a wider role for SLNB (18,19).

Imaging

Imaging is performed to detect occult cancer or to evaluate clinically evident disease.

MG is the most sensitive and specific imaging tool available. It cannot always accurately distinguish benign from malignant, however, missing 10% to 20% of clinically palpable breast cancers. If a suspicious lump is felt on clinical examination, a negative mammogram should not stop further investigation, and abnormalities should be followed by supplemental views and/or tissue sampling. Screening MG is performed on asymptomatic women to identify any clinically occult disease. Current recommendations include annual screening and clinical breast exams for asymptomatic women older than 40, and earlier screening for those with a strong family history. Digital MG and its applications, such as dual-energy subtraction mammography, subtraction angiography, and tomosynthesis allow for improved quality of imaging and possibly lower radiation doses. Initial results show that the overall diagnostic accuracy of digital and film MG as a means of screening for breast cancer is similar, but digital MG is more accurate in women younger than 50 (premenopausal or perimenopausal women) with radiographically dense breasts (20).

Clinical Relevance

- Suspicious mammographic findings include increased density, irregular margins, speculation, and accompanying clustered irregular microcalcifications. The degree of abnormality seen on the initial screening mammogram is categorized using the standardized Breast Imaging Reporting and Data System (BI-RADS) system (21). MG is limited by the density of the breast; for that reason, its efficacy in women younger than 35 is questionable.
- "Density" is a mammographic finding that suggests a high proportion of stromal and glandular tissue. Dense breasts have been found to have more ductal hyperplasia (normal and atypical). As such, breast density on screening MG is a risk factor for BBD and possibly breast cancer (22).
  - *Sonography.* The use of sonography in evaluating breast disease is controversial. It is most commonly used to determine whether a breast mass is a simple or complex cyst, or a solid tumor. It is particularly useful in patients younger than 35 with an impalpable screen-detected lesion, or a palpable lesion with a nonsuspicious mammography. Studies have shown a negative predictive value of up to 97% for cancer in patients with a palpable mass, but with negative MG and sonography (23).
  - *MRI.* The role of MRI in the evaluation of breast disease is continually evolving. Although it has a high sensitivity, specificity is low, costs are high, and it is subject to much interinstitutional variability (24). As a screening tool, studies have shown that using dual imaging (i.e., MRI and mammography) increases cancer yield in high-risk patients such as the BRCA1/BRCA2 populations (25). For patients presenting with N1 or M1 occult breast cancer, MRI has proved to be a powerful tool when MG has failed to identify the primary cancer (26). In addition, MRI can accurately predict those patients suitable for breast-conservation surgery following neoadjuvant chemotherapy and should be the imaging modality of choice in assessing the response of patients with primary breast carcinoma to neoadjuvant chemotherapy (27). Recent advances in technologies such as MR spectroscopy have been shown to improve the positive predictive value of standard MRI-detected lesions, suggesting that MR spectroscopy is a promising technique that may decrease the number of benign biopsy results generated with MR imaging (28).
  - *F-2-Fluoro-2-Deoxy-D-Glucose Positron Emission Tomography.* The role of positron emission tomography (PET) scanning in patients with breast cancer remains undefined. In terms of local disease, PET can detect lesions as small as 5 mm, but lacks the sensitivity of MG for microscopic disease. Similarly, PET cannot reliably detect microscopic nodal disease and therefore cannot reliably stage the axilla (29). However, PET is as sensitive as conventional imaging in detecting metastatic disease in patients with high-risk, operable breast cancer, and, importantly, is associated with fewer false positives (30).
  - *Technetium-99 Sestamibi scintimammography* Increased uptake of Tc-99m sestamibi is preferential in tumor cells compared with normal cells. Experimental studies have suggested a role for this technology in staging the axilla (31), preoperative assessment of breast lesions (32), and drug resistance (33), but findings have not proved significant. The technology is limited by the low resolution of the scanner used; however, dedicated scanners are being developed that may improve the efficacy of this technology.

Image-Guided Biopsy

Screening MG has resulted in an increased incidence of nonpalpable lesions, of which up to 30% are found to be malignant. Accurate assessment of such lesions is particularly challenging, requiring concordance between histopathology and imaging, and often necessitating follow-up procedure. The role of image-guided biopsy (IGB) [core needle biopsy (CNB), +/− vacuum assistance, and FNA] is to optimize treatment planning and reduce unnecessary procedures. Although there are clear benefits of IGB, there are some technical considerations (needle size, number of cores, type of biopsy device, specimen handling) that can compromise accuracy; certain histopathologic entities are difficult to identify with IGB and necessitate an excisional biopsy.

Clinical Relevance

In broad terms, underestimation is the primary consideration when determining the accuracy of IGB. Strict concordance between clinical, radiologic, and histopathologic findings is the goal of IGB; discordance should be prompt reevaluation. The following are notable diagnostic challenges encountered with IGB.

- *In situ or invasive?* FNA cannot accurately distinguish between *in situ* and invasive disease, but CNB can.
- *Lobular carcinoma in situ* (LCIS) *or ductal carcinoma in situ* (DCIS)? LCIS may have pathologic features that overlap with DCIS. The immunostain e-cadherin (lost in lobular pathology) may be useful in distinguishing between the two entities. As both entities have a very different prognosis, any suspicion warrants further evaluation.
- *Atypical ductal hyperplasia* (ADH)? The finding of ADH at stereotaxic core breast biopsy is an indication for surgical biopsy because of the high prevalence of ductal carcinoma in these lesions.
- *FA or PT?* Less than 1% of FA detected by CNB may represent an underestimated PT. If CNB of an FA shows

features such as stromal cellularity, mitosis, and stromal atypia, PT should be ruled out with excisional biopsy.

- *Papilloma or papillary carcinoma?* A recent study of percutaneously diagnosed papillomas in surgery revealed cancer in 14% and high-risk lesions in 17%, suggesting that lesions yielding a benign papilloma at percutaneous biopsy may warrant surgical excision (34).

BENIGN BREAST DISEASE

BBD represents a spectrum of clinical and pathologic changes that are typically related to normal processes of reproductive life. The breast is a dynamic, hormone-sensitive organ with a wide range of "normal" histologic features. Such changes may give rise to pain, heaviness, or lumpiness, all of which are normal responses to normal changes and do not constitute a disease. When managing BBD, it is fundamental to understand the difference between a "normal" change, a disorder (slight change of normal functioning), and a disease (abnormal functioning). The Aberrations of Normal Development and Involution (ANDI) classification of BBD (Table 13.1) addresses the fact that inaccurate terminology does not recognize this wide spectrum of "normal" by providing a framework that allows precise definition of an individual patient problem in terms of pathogenesis, histology, and clinical implications.

Clinical observations suggest that hormones are potential causal factors in BBD. Postmenopausal women taking HRT (estrogen +/− progestins) were shown to have an increased prevalence of proliferative BBD [relative risk (RR) 1.7, 95% confidence interval (CI) 1.06–2.72] (35). This is further supported by the finding that antiestrogens (tamoxifen) used in primary prevention are associated with a decreased prevalence of BBD (RR 0.72, 95% CI 0.65–0.79) (36).

Because most BBD does not carry an increased risk of breast cancer, attributing risk to the broad spectrum of

TABLE 13.2

Relative Risk of Developing Breast Cancer Associated with Benign Breast Disorder (BBD)

Lesion	RR of Breast Cancer (95% CI)
Nonproliferative lesions • Apocrine metaplasia • Cysts • Calcifications • Duct ectasia • Fibroadenoma • Mild ductal epithelial hyperplasia (DEH)	1.27 (95% CI 1.15–1.41)[a]
Proliferative lesions, without atypia • Florid DEH • Sclerosing lesion (adenosis, radial scars, complex) • Intraductal papilloma	1.88 (95% CI 1.66–2.12)
Proliferating lesions, with atypia • Atypical ductal hyperplasia (ADH) • Atypical lobular hyperplasia (ALH)	4.24 (95% CI 3.26–5.41)

[a]Data from Hartmann LC, Sellers TA, Frost MH, et al. Benign breast disease and the risk of breast cancer. *N Engl J Med* 2005;353(3):229–237. CI, confidence interval.

BBD has been problematic, compounded by inaccurate and inconsistent terminology. A classification system developed by Page et al. categorizes BBD into three clinically relevant groups based on histologic findings: nonproliferative lesions, proliferative lesions without atypia, and proliferative lesions with atypia (Table 13.2) (37,38).

TABLE 13.1

Aberrations of Normal Development and Involution (ANDI) Classification of Benign Breast Disease

	Normal	*Disorder*	*Disease*
Early reproductive years (age 15–25)	Lobular development Stromal development Nipple eversion	Fibroadenoma Adolescent hypertrophy Nipple inversion	Giant fibroadenoma Gigantomastia Subareolar abscess/mammary duct fistula
Mature reproductive years (age 25–40)	Cyclical changes of menstruation Epithelial hyperplasia of pregnancy	Cyclical mastalgia Nodularity Bloody nipple discharge	Incapacitating mastalgia
Involution (age 35–55)	Lobular involution Duct involution/dilation/sclerosis Epithelial turnover	Macrocysts Sclerosing lesions Duct ectasia Nipple retraction Epithelial hyperplasia	 Periductal mastitis/abscess Epithelial hyperplasia with atypia

From Beenken SW, Bland K. Evaluation and treatment of benign breast disorders. In: Bland K, Copeland EM III, eds. *The breast*, 3rd ed. Philadelphia: WB Saunders, 2004:225. Permission to use this table is pending.

Clinical Relevance

- Fibrocystic disease is a misnomer. The histologic changes associated with "fibrocystic disease" are normal variants that alone do not carry an increased risk of breast cancer. The term was used to explain a number of symptoms and rationalize a broad spectrum of biopsy findings, and carried no clinical relevance in terms of breast cancer risk. Because up to 60% of women without breast disease may have the histologic features of "fibrocystic disease," the preferred term is now *fibrocystic change*. The severity of fibrocystic change does *not* increase breast cancer risk; however, it may make it more difficult to detect a cancer.

- FA are well-circumscribed mobile masses present in approximately 5% to 10% of women with increased prevalence in younger women (2%–23%), and are benign tumors of epithelial and stroma origin. There is little or no increased risk of malignant disease; standard management is CNB followed by observation. However, tumors are often removed to alleviate patient concern. Difficulty arises if a PT is suspected, as less than 1% of FA detected by CNB may represent an underestimated PT. If CNB of an FA shows features such as stromal cellularity, mitosis, and stromal atypia, PT should be ruled out with excisional biopsy.

- Intraductal papillomas (IDPs) are proliferative lesions without atypia and, as such, carry a small increased risk of malignancy. However, multiple IDPs (often peripheral and bilateral) appear to have a higher risk of breast cancer (39). Many pathologists believe that is it difficult to accurately distinguish intracystic papillary carcinoma (IPC) from papillary carcinoma on core biopsy. A recent study of percutaneous image-guided biopsy, followed by surgical excision, revealed cancer in 14% and high-risk lesions in 17% (34), suggesting that benign papilloma at percutaneous biopsy may warrant further evaluation.

- The diagnostic criteria for ADH are the presence of atypia in the absence of the cytologic or architectural criteria for DCIS. Atypia diagnoses on CNB, FNA, and directional vacuum-assisted needle devices are problematic as they are associated with a significant false-negative rate of up to 56% (40). It is recommended that the presence of atypia on biopsy should be followed by surgical excision.

- Not unlike ADH, atypical lobular hyperplasia (ALH) is histologically similar to LCIS. ALH carries a fourfold increased risk of breast cancer, and LCIS is associated with a 10-fold increase. Unlike ductal carcinoma, LCIS is not a proven obligate precursor for invasive disease; however, women with a family history of breast cancer and a diagnosis of ALH have an increased risk of invasive disease twice that of women with ALH and no family history. The same issues of sample underestimation exist with ALH as with ADH; therefore, biopsy-proven ALH should be followed by surgical excision to rule out *in situ* disease.

- A radial scar is a complex sclerosing lesion characterized by a central scar with spiculations. Although they are not independent risk factors for breast cancer, they may be associated with atypical, preinvasive, or invasive pathology; therefore, excision may be warranted.

THE BIOLOGY OF BREAST CANCER

Breast cancer is a heterogeneous family of diseases associated with a broad spectrum of genotypic and phenotypic entities. A popularly embraced model of breast cancer tumorigenesis has been based on the Vogelstein model of colon carcinogenesis involving a progression from hyperplasia to metastatic carcinoma through an intermediate precursor (Table 13.3) (41). Although there is evidence to support that the colon-cancer hypothesis may hold true for breast cancer, it is challenged by two key findings. First, the seminal work by Vogelstein et al. (41) was based on the finding that dysplastic lesions were obligate precursors of invasive disease; however, dysplastic/atypical lesions of the breast are *not* obligate precursors (in fact, more than 85% of atypical breast lesions will never develop into a cancer, and some breast lesions may arise independent of the preceding stage). Second, in contrast to the *adenomatosis polyposis coli* (APC) gene deactivation in colon cancer, no gatekeeper gene has been proposed for breast cancer.

So, although some breast cancers may arise from mammary epithelium through a well-defined, albeit nonobligatory, sequence of histologic changes, this classical model of tumorigenesis appears oversimplified. The development of accurate tissue sampling (laser capture microdissection), sophisticated technologies of molecular analysis, and immunohistochemistry (IHC) has enhanced our knowledge of breast cancer biology. For example, previous distinctions between "ductal" and "lobular" pathways are now being questioned (42), and histologic variants of lesions, such as basal/luminal/nonbasal/nonluminal, poorly differentiated/well-differentiated DCIS, and classical/pleomorphic LCIS and invasive lobular carcinoma (ILC), have been identified. Such new information complicates the classical model and indicates that genetic, epigenetic, molecular, and biological events are far more complex than previously understood (43).

Our understanding of breast tumorigenesis is continuously evolving. The ultimate goal is to provide a comprehensive model that combines molecular and genetic analyses to explain the pathways in the progression of invasive disease, and define the relations between histologic variants in a manner that can be translated into practical clinical applications. For the purposes of this chapter, we will individually discuss some of the proposed mechanisms of tumorigenesis that may have putative clinical relevance. However, while it is not unreasonable to suggest that some tumors have a greater association with one mechanism than another, we remind readers that the process is extraordinarily complex and that the contribution of each mechanism should not be considered *individually*, but rather as part of a bigger picture.

TABLE 13.3

Evidence (Direct and Indirect) to Support the Application of Vogelstein Model of Carcinogenesis to Breast Cancer

Direct	Transfection of cells with murine mammary tumor virus into the 3CH mouse models transforms normal epithelium into hyperplastic nodules. Transplantation of the nodules into mammary fat pads leads to the development of tumors[a]
Indirect	Genetic: Fifty percent of hyperplastic lesions and almost 80% of DCIS lesions that coexist with invasive disease show loss of heterozygosity, suggesting a precursor/product relation between these lesions and the cancers they accompany[b]
	Cellular: Autopsy studies showed that women who died of breast cancer were more likely to have ductal hyperplasia (typical and atypical) and DCIS than women who died of other causes.[c] Other studies have reported an increased incidence of ADH in cancerous vs. noncancerous breasts,[d,e] and that synchronous invasive and "precursor" lesions are commonly found adjacent to, and often continuous with, one another.[f] In addition, studies suggest that up to 28% of women treated with biopsy-only for DCIS presenting as an incidental histologic finding will develop invasive carcinoma (follow-up period of approximately 15 years).[g,h]
	Epidemiologic: Benign breast disease (proliferative +/− atypia) and noninvasive lesions are established risks for breast cancer.

[a]Data from DeOme KB, Faulkin LJ Jr, Bern HA, et al. Development of mammary tumors from hyperplastic alveolar nodules transplanted into grand-free mammary fat pads of felame C3H mice. *Cancer Res* 1959;19(5):515–520.
[b]Data from O'Connell P, Pekkel V, Fuqua S, et al. Molecular genetic studies of early breast cancer evolution. *Breast Cancer Res Treat* 1994;32(1):5–12.
[c]Data from Bartow SA, Pathak DR, Black WC, et al. Prevalence of benign, atypical and malignant breast lesions in populations at different risk for breast cancer. A forensic autopsy study. *Cancer*, 1987;60(11):2751–2760.
[d]Data from Karpas CM, Leis HP, Oppenheim A, et al. Relation of fibrocystic disease to carcinoma of the breast. *Ann Surg* 1965;162:1.
[e]Data from Kern WH, Brooks RN. Atypical epithelial hyperplasia associated with breast cancer and fibrocystic disease *Cancer*, 1969;24:668.
[f]Data from Lakhani Sr. The transition from hyperplasia to invasive carcinoma of the breast. *J Pathol* 1999;187:272–278.
[g]Data from Page DL, Dupont WD, Rogers LW, et al. Intraductal carcinoma of the breast: follow-up after biopsy only. *Cancer* 1982;49(4):751–758.
[h]Data from Betsill WL Jr, Rosen PP, Lieberman PH, et al. Intraductal carcinoma: long-term follow-up after treatment by biopsy alone. *JAMA*, 1978;239(18):1863–1867.
DCIS, ductal carcinoma *in situ*; ADH, atypical ductal hyperplasia.

Molecular Genetic Bases of Breast Cancer

Fundamentally, breast cancer is a genetic disease. Like other cancers, specific germ-line or somatic mutations are required for malignant transformation, and it is likely that the accumulation of multiple genetic mutations, rather than their sequence, is what determines the biological behavior of the tumor. Sequential molecular changes result from these underlying genetic or epigenetic aberrations, and hormonal stimuli potentiate tumor development. Although some genetic changes have been linked to specific stages of differentiation (44), others seem to appear more stochastically (45), and little is known of the timing of critical mutations in early tumor development. Most tumors are heterogeneous, containing many subpopulations of cells that have accumulated varying mutations, causing each subpopulation to diversify phenotypically. The overall biological behavior of the tumor is determined by the ability of a particular subpopulation to survive and overtake other more genetically stable cells to the extent that the metastatic potential of a tumor is thought to be directly proportional to genetic instability (46).

The intrinsic ability of normal breast epithelium (particularly at the terminal ductolobular unit) to be continuously influenced and remodeled makes it especially susceptible to genetic alterations. Chromosomal abnormalities have been demonstrated in histologically normal tissue distant from the site of the tumor (47) ("field defects"), and the degree of instability is inversely proportional to the distance from the

tumor (48). Although little is known of the importance of such genetic changes in histologically normal tissue, we do know that genomic instability is an important contributor to inherited and acquired mutations associated with malignant transformation (49).

Oncogenes

There are two principal types of genes that are now recognized as playing a role in cancer: oncogenes and tumor suppressor genes (TSGs). Oncogenes refer to those genes whose alterations contribute to malignant progression by a *gain of function*. Common alterations include amplification, overexpression, point mutations, and chromosomal translocation. Oncogenes are mutations of certain normal genes of the cell called *protooncogenes*. The transformation of a protooncogene to an oncogene is irreversible. Oncogenes frequently interact with other genetic or epigenetic (nongenetic) changes. Numerous oncogenes have been described in breast cancer; some represent major mechanisms of carcinogenesis, whereas others are of unknown significance. A proposed classification model of oncogenes is based on their gene products and consists of five classes: growth factors; growth factor receptors [embryonic growth and development factor (EGDF)], signal transducer proteins (Ras), transcription regulators MYC and programmed cell death regulators. Of these, epidermal growth factor receptor (EGFR2) [human epithelial receptor (*HER2/neu*)] holds the most clinical relevance.

Epidermal Growth Factor Receptor or Human Epithelial Receptor

One of the most significant and frequent cellular effects of oncogene activation is the interaction with downstream cell-signaling systems, shifting the balance between cell proliferation and death. The epidermal growth factor (EGF) receptors are transmembrane, ligand-bound tyrosine kinase receptors. There are four homologous members in the family (HER1–4), all of which have two functional domains (cytoplasmic tyrosine kinase domain and an Src-homology domain, SH-2 and SH-3). Interaction between the receptor, the ligand, and intracellular proteins is regulated by phosphorylation of the C-terminal tyrosine kinase residues. Activation leads to multiple transduction cascades through a wide variety of kinase pathways, namely Src kinase, Ras, reception activation factor (RAF), mitogen-activated protein (MAP) kinase, mTOR, and 3-kinase (P13K)/Akt, resulting in apoptosis-resistance, proliferation, altered intercellular adhesion/motility, angiogenesis, and metastasis (50).

HER-2/neu (EGFR-2) is a 185-kDa transmembrane tyrosine kinase growth factor receptor encoded by a gene on chromosome 17q. Discovered in 1984 and cloned 2 years later (51,52), this molecule has been the subject of intense research for over two decades. A spliced variant of HER-2/neu messenger ribonucleic acid (mRNA) has been identified, and this remains the only identifiable HER-2/neu mutation in the human gene; its exact role in carcinogenesis is unclear (53). Also, the true HER-2/neu receptor ligand has yet to be identified. Its activity is modulated by association with other EGFR family members (54), and so the oncogenic effects of HER-2/neu overexpression are dependent upon the activation of other signaling pathways (55). HER-2/neu gene amplification and overexpression in primary breast cancer was associated with a more aggressive phenotype and a worse prognosis (56).

The other members of the epidermal growth factor response (EGFR) family (HER-1, HER-3, and HER-4) have yet to prove significant in breast carcinogenesis.

Clinical Relevance

- The American Society of Clinical Oncology (ASCO) recommends evaluation of HER-2/neu status in all primary breast tumors, either at the time of diagnosis or upon recurrence (57). Several methods for assessing the HER-2/neu status of tumors exist, and the two most common methods of measuring HER-2/neu levels in the clinical setting are IHC and fluorescent in situ hybridization (FISH).
- The expression of HER-2/neu varies by histologic subtype. BBD is not associated with amplification. Preinvasive lesions of lobular origin (LCIS) are negative for HER-2/neu, whereas most high-grade DCIS lesions appear to be positive for HER-2/neu amplifications (58). Of the invasive subtypes, only invasive ductal cancer demonstrates HER-2/neu amplification (59). Interestingly, high-grade DCIS lesions have a higher prevalence of HER-2/neu amplification compared with invasive ductal lesions (>90% versus <30%), suggesting that HER-2/neu signaling may have a greater role in induction as opposed to progression of tumorigenesis.
- Numerous studies have reported a high rate of recurrence in node-negative breast cancer with HER-2/neu overexpression, and that HER-2/neu status may be a predictor of treatment response/resistance (60). However, such findings are biased by short follow-up time and lack of standardization in HER-2/neu assessment.
- Trastuzumab is a humanized recombinant monoclonal antibody directed against the extracellular portion of the HER-2/neu receptor that modulates the transmission of growth signals. Phase II trials revealed an overall response rate of up to 35% for patients with HER-2/neu overexpression treated with trastuzumab monotherapy (61). Combination trials in patients with stage IV breast cancer, randomizing patients to receive either adriamycin cyclophosphamide (AC) or paclitaxel chemotherapy alone, or in combination with trastuzumab, revealed a statistically significant increase in overall response (50% versus 32%) and overall survival (25.1 versus 20.3 months) on those who were randomized to the trastuzumab arm (62). Cardiomyopathy was noted to be associated with anthracycline-based chemotherapy, but not with paclitaxel. As a result, trastuzumab, either alone or in combination with paclitaxel, is a standard therapeutic regimen for patients with HER-2/neu-positive stage IV breast cancer. HER-2/neu overexpression is found both in the primary tumor and in metastatic sites, indicating that anti-HER-2/neu therapy may also be effective in all disease sites (63). However, despite an initial response, most patients will experience disease progression within 1 year. Currently, trastuzumab is the only HER-2/neu-targeted therapy approved by the U.S. Food and Drug Administration (FDA) for the treatment of metastatic breast cancer. Novel strategies for targeting HER-2/neu and combination therapy with agents such as Src kinase inhibitors may increase the magnitude and duration of response (64).
- In addition to receptor blockade, targeting the downstream mediators may prove effective. For example, the Src kinase family regulates intercellular contact dynamics facilitating proliferation, migration, and invasion of tumor cells. Src kinase activation is associated with a reorganization of epithelial adhesion systems (adhesion-switch), giving rise to a more migratory phenotype and a reacquisition of a mesenchymal morphology, and is often increased during epithelial carcinogenesis. This and other downstream, centrally acting proteins (mTOR, Ras) are being investigated for possible therapeutic effect.

Topoisomerase II

Topoisomerases are enzymes that catalyze the transient breaking and rejoining of deoxyribonucleic acid (DNA) strands, thereby regulating for transcription. The TOP2A gene is located at chromosome band 17q12-21, close to the HER2/neu gene, and is a target for various chemotherapeutic agents such as anthracyclines, which inhibit TOP2A by trapping the DNA strand break intermediates, leading to persistent DNA cleavage. The protein expression status of TOP2A has been implicated in the prediction of clinical outcome and response to chemotherapy in breast cancer (65).

Fibroblast Growth Factor Family, Transforming Growth Factors α and β, cMyc Oncogene, Ras Oncogene, and Insulin-like Growth Factor Receptor

These have all been implicated in mammary carcinogenesis, suggesting that their associated genes may in fact be oncogenes. Preliminary results are interesting, but inconclusive.

Tumor Suppressor Genes

In contrast to oncogenes, whose alterations result in a gain of function, genetic alterations in TSG lead to loss of function. TSGs are normal genes that slow down cell division, repair DNA damage, or control apoptosis. TSG mutations that recognize and repair DNA damage are thought to contribute indirectly to tumorigenesis by allowing the mutation of one gene, which may lead to genetic instability in another; therefore, TSGs have been classified as either "caretakers" [maintaining genomic stability, e.g., ataxia telangiectasia mutated (ATM)], "gatekeepers" (directly inhibiting cell growth or promoting apoptosis, e.g., p53), or both (e.g., BRCA1/BRCA2) (66). Approximately 30 TSGS have been found to be associated with breast cancer, including p53, *BRCA1*, *BRCA2*, *ATM*, *check point kinase* (CHK), *and retinoblastoma* 1 (RB1). An important difference between oncogenes and TSGs is that oncogenes result from the *activation* of protooncogenes, but TSGs cause cancer when the protooncogene is *inactive*. Another major difference is that while the overwhelming majority of oncogenes develop from acquired mutations in protooncogenes, abnormalities of TSGs can be inherited as well as acquired. Knudsen 2-hit model of tumorigenesis dictates that dominantly inherited predisposition to cancer necessitates a germ-line mutation, and subsequent tumorigenesis requires a second (somatic) "hit" mutation. A nonhereditary cancer of the same type also requires two "hits," but in contrast, they are both somatic (67). Genetic alterations associated with TSG include deletions, insertions, or methylations of the gene promoter region.

Hereditary Breast Cancer

An estimated 5% to 10% of all breast cancers are hereditary in origin (68). A "hereditary cancer syndrome" is defined by the presence (over several generations) of multiple cases of cancer that are associated with a mutated gene in the germ-line (69). Most hereditary cancer syndromes are associated with loss of function of a TSG, and at least 40% of hereditary breast cancers are explained by germ-line mutations in the *BRCA1/BRCA2* genes (70). Approximately half of breast/ovarian families evaluated in a high-risk cancer evaluation clinic may have a BRCA1/BRCA2 germ-line mutation (71). Families with a strong history of breast cancer, but that are negative for BRCA1/BRCA2 mutation, have led to the exciting search for "BRCA3." To date, no

linkage analysis has identified other major genes associated with breast cancer susceptibility, and so this "BRCA3" stone remains unturned. The current understanding is that the *BRCA* genes do not play a role in sporadic breast cancer (72,73). Other breast cancer susceptibility conditions include Li-Fraumeni syndrome, Cowden disease, Ataxia-Telangiectasia, and Peutz-Jeghers syndrome (PJS), which are caused by mutations in the *p53/CHEK2*, *PTEN*, *ATM* and *LKB1/STK11* genes, respectively. The "founder effect" refers to the unusual prevalence of specific genotypes among a particular population. One of the most famous and most studied founder effects is that of BRCA1/BRCA2 mutations seen in individuals of Ashkenazi Jewish descent. In this population, the frequency of mutations is almost 10 to 50 times greater than that seen in the general population (1%–5% compared with 0.1%) (74).

BRCA

Both BRCA1 and BRCA2 are located on chromosomes 17 and 13, respectively (17q21, 13q12-13) (75,76). Inherited *BRCA* gene abnormalities are inherited in an autosomal dominant manner and have a high penetrance (77). However, penetrance is family-specific, not gene-specific, and may vary according to the specific mutation and other genetic or environmental factors (78,79). Accurate penetrance estimates are an important component in the process of clinical risk assessment. Initial penetrance estimates for BRCA1 and BRCA2 mutations have been generated from high-risk families, but the penetrance of "non–Ashkenazi" BRCA1 and BRCA2 mutations has yet to be determined directly. Most cancers that develop in BRCA1/BRCA2 mutation carriers exhibit loss of heterozygosity (loss of the wild-type allele), and so both BRCA1 and BRCA2 fulfill the criteria for a TSG. However, despite the ubiquitous loss in tumor-suppressor function, cancer is site specific, suggesting that other genetic events or local factors may be necessary for tumor development, and questioning the overall impact/role of haploinsufficiency.

The *BRCA1* gene occupies a 100-kb region on chromosome 17q21. It contains 22 coding and 2 noncoding exons. The coding region containing the *BRCA1* gene has been sequenced completely; Exon 11 (3,427 bp) is exceptionally large and contains over half of the coding region of the gene. BRCA1 contains an amino-terminal RING finger domain, a carboxy-terminal BRCA1 C-terminal (BRCT) domain, an SQ cluster domain (SCD), and multiple functional domains with associated binding proteins. The BRCA1 N-terminal RING domain interacts with BRCA1-associated ring complex protein-1 (BARD1), and this BRCA1/BARD-1 complex is thought to mediate ubiquitin ligase activity, which is important for tumor suppression (80). The C-terminal transcription activation domain of BRCA1 contains a 95-amino acid tandem repeat (BRCA1-associated C-terminal domain, BRCT) that is homologous to domains contained in some cell cycle checkpoint and DNA-repair proteins. The BRCA1 gene product is a 220-kDa nuclear phosphoprotein. Expression varies according to the cell cycle (maximal during the

S-phase) and by estrogen through the estrogen-response element (ERE).

BRCA1 and BRCA2 have no significant sequence similarity with each other, and neither resembles any proteins with known function in the sequence databases. The *BRCA2* gene covers approximately 80 kb and is thought to contain 27 coding exons. Exon 10 is 1,116 bp in length and exon 11 is 4,933 bp. A 1,000-residue C-terminal region follows the repeat domain and is thought to contain approximately 27% of the tumor-derived missense mutations associated with breast cancer. The BRCA2 gene product is a 3,418-amino acid protein that shares no sequence homology with any other protein (81).

Since their discovery, numerous studies have established functional roles of BRCA1 and BRCA2 in DNA repair, cell-cycle checkpoints, and apoptosis, and suggest that the *BRCA* genes function as "caretakers," preserving the integrity of the genome. Most of the BRCA-related biological actions are mediated through regulation of transcription. However, while a wide variety of data support the role of BRCA1 and BRCA2 as "caretakers," it does not explain the predilection for tumor types.

Despite the ubiquitous presence of a BRCA1 mutation amongst heterozygotes (BRCA1 carriers), the tissue-specific pattern of carcinogenesis clearly implicates a role for local factors in BRCA1-related tumorigenesis. All tissues susceptible to BRCA1-related cancer express steroid hormone receptors that are sensitive to circulating hormones. The observation that the highest incidence of BRCA1-related tumors occurs during the premenopausal years suggests that ovarian steroid hormone–induced mammary proliferation is particularly susceptible to proliferation-acquired mutations. It is estimated that the lifetime risk (by age 70) of developing breast cancer for BRCA1 mutation carriers ranges from 55% to 85%, and over half of carriers will be diagnosed with breast cancer before the age of 50 (82). Bilateral risk-reducing salpingo-oophorectomy results in a significant reduction (~50%) in breast cancer risk among BRCA1 carriers (83). Reproductive factors have been implicated in BRCA tumorigenesis: the BRCA1 population appears to benefit from a protective effect of pregnancy before the age of 30 and breast feeding. In contrast, early pregnancy increases the risk of BRCA2-related cancer, and breast feeding does not modify risk (84–87). Epidemiologic studies suggest BRCA1 carriers who used oral contraceptives (OC) for a minimum of 5 years had a small but significant increase in breast cancer risk (88).

Several molecular associations between BRCA1 and steroid hormone receptors have been established, suggesting that BRCA carcinogenesis may be hormone dependent.

- Estrogens play a crucial role in the growth of both normal and cancerous tumor cells. Estrogen exposure is an important determinant of breast cancer risk, and treatment of breast cancer has included efforts to decrease estrogen levels. Wild-type BRCA1 (wtBRCA1) inhibits the transcription of ER-α directly through the activation function (AF2) activation domain, and indirectly by

downregulation of nuclear receptor (NR) coactivator p300. Evidence of a functional interaction between wtBRCA1 and ER-β is evolving. By inhibiting cross talk with growth factor receptors, wtBRCA1 may inhibit estrogen-stimulated cell proliferation.

- The role of progesterone in mammary carcinogenesis is unclear. Although BRCA1 tumors are typically progesterone receptor (PR)-negative, it has been shown that the normal epithelium surrounding a BRCA1-related tumor has a higher expression of PR as compared with non-BRCA1 related tumors (89). A recent publication has suggested that BRCA1 functions as a coregulator of the PR and that loss (or partial loss) of wtBRCA1 derepresses the PR, leading to downstream transcription activation of progesterone response genes, cytokines, and growth factors. The overall biological effect may be an increase in cell growth and proliferation, which, in the absence of functioning wtBRCA, has the potential to escape cell-cycle control mechanisms and progress into a cancer.
- The androgen receptor (AR) exhibits genetic polymorphism in the number of polyglutamine cytosine-adenine-guanine (CAG) repeats in its AF1 domain. An association between an early age of BRCA breast cancer and long CAG repeat lengths has been suggested, but results have been controversial (90).
- Members of the steroid hormone receptor (p160) superfamily (SRC-1, AIB-1, GRIP-1) have been implicated as mediators of BRCA tumorigenesis (91). The growth regulatory effects of steroid hormones may be modulated by inherited mutations in genes such as CYP1A1, CYP3A4, CYP17, and CYP19 (92).

The wide variation in cancer risk among women with BRCA mutations can be explained by other factors that modulate risk. Suggested modifiers include the following:

- Different mutations. Certain mutations may predispose to ovarian over breast cancer (93,94), or may be associated with disease severity (95) [185delAG (also known as *187delAG*), 5382insC, 617delT, etc.].
- Steroid hormone receptor expression and hormone (endogenous and exogenous) exposure.
- Environmental carcinogens. Genes involved in the metabolism of carcinogens may modify risk by exposure to potentially mutagenic events.
- Other genes involved in DNA repair (RAD51) may also be involved in cancer risk modification in the BRCA population (96). This hypothesis was inferred from the discovery that the *BRCA1* gene colocalized with the RAD51 protein (97), and has been supported by others that suggest both BRCA1 and BRCA2 proteins are involved in the same biochemical pathway of DNA repair that is mediated by RAD51 (98).

Clinical Relevance

- Up to 10% of breast cancers are due to a hereditary syndrome (35% BRCA1, 25% BRCA2, 5% breast cancer susceptibility syndromes, and 35% unknown). Deleterious

BRCA mutations carry a 50% to 80% lifetime risk of female breast cancer, a 6% lifetime risk of male breast cancer (BRCA2), and a 15% to 25% lifetime risk of ovarian cancer. BRCA1 mutation carriers are more likely to present with breast cancer at a lower age than BRCA2 mutation carriers (peak incidence at 45–49 years and 65–69 years, respectively). It is important to understand these statistics when considering either genetic testing or prevention strategies in a known BRCA mutation carrier.

- There is no clear consensus on, or guidelines for, consideration of genetic sequencing. Many risk models exist that attempt to compute the likelihood of a mutation within a population (Claus, BRCAPRO), but these have considerable inherent limitations. Genetic testing assesses the "susceptibility to develop a cancer" and consists of sequence analysis of more than 17,500 base pairs of the protein-coding and adjacent noncoding regions of the *BRCA1* and *BRCA2* genes, or sequence analysis for three specific founder mutations prevalent in Ashkenazi Jewish individuals. DNA sequencing test results may inform individuals regarding their cancer risks, thereby influencing decisions regarding screening and prevention. Such tests have significant implications on both patients and their families. In the United States, all testing is done at the same center. Full-length sequencing of the protein-coding and adjacent noncoding regions may not detect large rearrangements of the genes, and such chromosomal rearrangements may account for as many as 15% of abnormalities. As a result, a negative test result can be of limited value. A negative genetic test result is most informative if a mutation has first been established in a family member.
- There are distinct pathologic variations between BRCA1 and BRCA2 cancers that infer a different clinical outcome. BRCA1 tumors are typically high-grade, invasive ductal lesions that are ER/PR-negative and exhibit the basal phenotype. As such, they are associated with a relatively worse clinical outcome. In contrast, BRCA2 tumors can be either ductal or lobular, are of a moderate to high grade, and are likely to be associated to a degree with *in situ* disease. They are not unlike sporadic cancers in that they are typically ER/PR-positive and exhibit the luminal phenotype. Another common feature of BRCA-associated cancers is a high expression of p53, S-phase fraction (SPF), and aneuploidy.
- Most studies report equivalence between BRCA-associated and sporadic cancers in terms of stage. However, selection, screening, and ascertainment biases may confound this information.
- Cancer risks in women with an inherited predisposition to breast cancer need to be considered on many levels:
  - *Breast cancer risk in the unaffected BRCA1 or BRCA2 mutation carrier.* Deleterious BRCA mutations carry a 50% to 80% lifetime risk of female breast cancer (6% male breast cancer, BRCA2). BRCA1 mutation carriers are more likely to present with breast cancer at a lower age than BRCA2 mutation carriers (peak incidence 45–49 years, and 65–69 years, respectively).

- *Modifiers of breast cancer risk in the unaffected BRCA1 or BRCA2 mutation carriers,* through, hormonal exposure and reproductive factors, notably, age at menarche, first-term pregnancy and nulliparity, pregnancy, and endogenous estrogen exposure.
- *Ovarian cancer risk in the unaffected BRCA1 or BRCA2 mutation carrier.* Ovarian cancer risk varies widely. The lifetime risk is thought to be 15% to 25%; however, it can be as high as 60% by age 70.
- *Other cancer risks for families with a predisposition to breast and ovarian cancer.* BRCA mutations are associated with colon, prostate, pancreas, gallbladder cholangiocarcinoma, and melanoma. The levels of risk are ill-defined, however, and are not of the frequency associated with either breast or ovarian cancer.
- *Risk of ipsilateral recurrence after breast-conservation therapy* (BCT) *for BRCA-associated cancer.* A recent multi-institutional study reported equivalent ipsilateral local recurrence rates at 10 years for BRCA1 or BRCA2 carriers compared with controls (99).
- *Risk of contralateral breast cancer in women with a BRCA-associated cancer.* The same multi-institutional study reported a significant increase in contralateral cancer in BRCA patients compared with sporadic controls (26% versus 3%). This group also found that tamoxifen use significantly reduced the risk of contralateral cancers in mutation carriers [hazard ratio (HR) 0.31, $p < 0.05$].

- Primary prevention for BRCA mutation carriers includes intense surveillance, chemoprevention, risk-reducing mastectomy, and oophorectomy.
- Surveillance incorporates CBE and imaging. Optimal methods are continuously evolving. MG is confounded by the fact that the BRCA surveillance population is likely to be young, with dense breasts that reduce the sensitivity of mammography. As such, false-negative rates among BRCA heterozygotes range from 30% to 40% (100). The role of ultrasonography is undetermined in these populations (101). Studies have shown that less than half of cancers in this population are identified by conventional screening (mammography and CBE), whereas MRI detects more than 77% of lesions (101), clearly documenting the benefits of breast MRI screening in women at the highest levels of hereditary risk. MRI is now recognized as a routine test for BRCA mutation carriers.
- The efficacy of tamoxifen or selective estrogen receptor modulators (SERMs) is unknown in the BRCA population. To date, all chemoprevention trials were not designed to look specifically at the BRCA population. However, the following inferences can be made: The NSABP-P1 trial that assessed the use of tamoxifen versus placebo as a chemopreventative agent reduced the incidence of ER-positive tumors, but not ER-negative tumors. Most BRCA1 tumors are ER-negative, thereby suggesting a limited role of tamoxifen for prevention in BRCA1 mutation carriers (102). Another "tamoxifen for prevention" trial focused specifically on patients with a strong family history of breast cancer (but unknown

BRCA status) and failed to demonstrate a beneficial effect from tamoxifen (103). Another controversy exists over OC. OC are known to decrease the risk of ovarian cancer in the general population, and there is evidence to suggest that they may have a similar effect in women with a familial predisposition (104). However, epidemiologic studies suggest BRCA1 carriers who used OC for a minimum of 5 years had a small but significant increase in breast cancer risk (88). In summary, BRCA mutation carriers should be aware of all limitations when considering either tamoxifen or OC for risk reduction.

- Risk-reducing mastectomy. No prospective trials have assessed the efficacy of prophylactic surgery for risk reduction, and so we rely on anecdotal retrospective evidence. Subgroup analysis of the Hartmann series that followed up more than 630 women who had bilateral subcutaneous mastectomies because of a family history of breast cancer identified 18 patients with a BRCA mutation. At a mean follow-up of 16 years, none of the 18 mutation carriers had developed a cancer. Contralateral risk-reduction surgery is a consideration for patients with a BRCA-associated cancer. As discussed, the risk of a contralateral cancer is significantly higher in this population compared with sporadic breast cancers. Although the mortality risk of a contralateral cancer is thought to be low (<2%) (105), contralateral risk-reducing surgery should be discussed with all women with hereditary breast cancer.
- Risk-reducing oophorectomy. Small, largely retrospective cohort studies have demonstrated a decreased incidence of breast cancer among BRCA mutation carriers associated with oophorectomy, with HRs ranging from 0.32 to 0.53 (83,106,107). However, although the benefits seem substantial and the procedure is low risk, there have been some reports of postoophorectomy peritoneal cancer (108).
- BCT. This may be an appropriate treatment for patients with BRCA mutations, and for those who have undergone a risk-reducing oophorectomy, BCT is associated with ipsilateral local recurrence rates equivalent to those seen in sporadic cancers. However, whether postconservation radiation therapy alters the risk of contralateral cancer in this population is unknown. Mastectomy is a reasonable option for women who may be concerned about a second primary.

p53 TSG/Li Fraumeni Syndrome

The *p53* gene is located on chromosome 17p and encodes a 393-kDa phosphoprotein. The *p53* gene product has multiple functions, acting primarily as a regulator of cell division. It exerts its effect either directly by regulating DNA transcription, or indirectly by forming complexes with other signaling proteins such as cyclins, MDM2, S-locus receptor kinase (SRK/INK4), and mitogen-activated protein kinase (MAPK), triggering cell-cycle arrest or apoptosis. The expression and function of p53 is controlled by a wide variety of mechanisms. p53 mutations are found in more than half of all cancers and up to 30% of breast cancers (109).

Clinical Relevance

- Overexpression of p53 may be associated with many poor prognostic features, such as grade and *HER2/neu* amplification, and disease-free or overall survival (110–112). To date, available data does not support a prognostic or predictive role for p53 in breast cancer.
- Li-Fraumeni syndrome is a breast cancer susceptibility condition associated with a high incidence of leukaemia, lymphoma, osteosarcomas, and adrenocortical carcinomas that is thought to be due to a point mutation of the *p53* gene (113).

PTEN TSG/Cowden Syndrome

Cowden syndrome is a rare autosomal dominant condition caused by germ-line mutations in the *PTEN* gene (a TSG). It is characterized by multiple hamartomatous lesions (skin trichilemmomas, oral mucosal papillomas, acral skin keratosis, intestinal hamartomas), and an increased risk of early-onset breast and thyroid cancer (114). Most affected individuals develop the syndrome's characteristic skin lesions by age 20. Most women with Cowden syndrome have benign breast conditions; malignant tumors are usually ductal in origin and often surrounded by densely collagenous hamartomatous lesions. An increased incidence of bilaterality has been observed for both benign and malignant breast disorders.

SKT11 TSG and Peutz-Jeghers Syndrome

PJS is another rare autosomal dominant condition associated with germ-line mutations in a serine threonine kinase (STK11) located on chromosome 19p13.3. The characteristic clinical features include hamartomatous polyps in the gastrointestinal tract, and mucocutaneous melanin deposits in the buccal mucosa, lips, and digits. Carriers are at increased risk for both gastrointestinal and extraintestinal cancers. The absolute risk of breast cancer has been estimated to be 55% and, interestingly, ovarian cancer has also been observed in many affected patients (estimated risk: approximately 20%) (115).

HORMONES AND BREAST CANCER

The concept that hormones play an important role in mammary carcinogenesis is not a novel one. More than 100 years ago, George Beatson proposed a relation between breast cancer and ovarian function. This landmark observation led others to discover that steroid hormones act as "initiators," "promotors," and "potentiators" of carcinogenesis, concluding that breast cancer is a steroid-dependent cancer. Many epidemiologic studies have supported this hypothesis by showing that hormones are key determinants of cancer in several hormone-sensitive tissues.

Biosynthesis and Metabolism

The biosynthesis of steroid hormones occurs *de novo* by pathways in the adrenals and ovaries (and testes in men).

In addition, circulating precursor cells that originate from the endocrine glands may produce steroid hormones in the peripheral tissues (e.g., liver, kidney, breast, skin). Most circulating steroid hormones are bound to proteins; the nonprotein-bound forms are "free" to bind to steroid hormone receptors and are therefore considered "bioavailable." Such "bioavailable" hormones may, if activated, exert a biological effect; alternatively, they are metabolized and excreted. The biosynthesis of steroid hormones is extraordinarily complex. A detailed description is beyond the scope of this chapter and so shall be discussed in brief.

Although the enzymatic pathways of steroid hormone biosynthesis have been known for quite some time (Fig. 13.9), we have only recently come to appreciate how these enzymes are controlled by genes. For example, the rate-limiting step of steroid hormone biosynthesis involves the conversion of cholesterol to pregnenolone and is converted by a cytochrome P-450 enzyme (CYP) encoded by the *CYP11A1* gene. Expression of the *CYP11A1* gene is regulated by many factors, namely FSH and LH in the ovary, and angiotensin II in the circulation. Pregnenolone is then converted to either progesterone or 17α-hydroxypregnenolone by the enzyme 3β-hydrozysteroid dehydrogenase (3β-HSD). 3β-HSD is expressed in the gonads, adrenal glands, placenta, liver, and kidney, and has two functional genes (type 1 and type 2). Both compounds (progesterone and 17α-hydroxypregnenolone) then undergo hydroxylation at carbon-17, followed by cleavage of a carbon-side chain (carbons 20 and 21), forming androstenedione and dehydroepiandrosterone (DHEA), respectively. These obligatory reactions of estrogen and androgen biosynthesis are catalyzed by a single protein, P-450c17, encoded by the *CYP17* gene. Next, the enzyme 17B-hydroxysteroid dehydrogenase-1 (HSD17B1) converts androstenedione and DHEA to testosterone, 5-Androstene-3B, and 17B-diol. The final step of estrogen biosynthesis involves *aromatization* and occurs through the action of complex aromatase cytochrome P-450, encoded by the *CYP19* gene (**Fig. 13.9**).

Circulating steroid hormones are primarily "protein bound." Steroid-binding proteins, such as sex hormone binding globulin (SHBG), corticosteroid binding globulin (CBG), and albumin play an important role in the availability of endogenous and exogenously administered steroid hormones.

Steroid hormones undergo extensive metabolism in a variety of peripheral tissues, the liver being the primary site. Steroids are excreted through the kidney and intestine in a water-soluble (conjugated) form. Steroid metabolism involves a complex interplay of reductases, methyltransferases, conjugation, and hydroxylases. The predominant reaction in estrogen metabolism is hydroxylation. The enzymes involved include members of the CYP P-450 family and the enzyme catechol–O–methyltransferase (COMT). The latter is found in large amounts in the circulation, liver, kidneys, mammary glands, and endometrium.

Clinical Relevance

- Many epidemiologic studies have repeatedly shown that postmenopausal women who develop breast cancer have a higher mean serum estradiol concentration than unaffected women (116). In the preventative setting, estrogen receptor blockage (tamoxifen) reduces the incidence of breast cancer by 50% in women at high risk of the disease (102), and endocrine therapy reduces the risk of local recurrence in the adjuvant setting. Studies evaluating a significance between low-serum SHBG levels and breast cancer risk have been inconsistent and therefore inconclusive (117).

- Although there is evidence that hormonal secretion and metabolism can be influenced by external factors such as diet and exercise, hormonal regulation is largely genetic. It has been hypothesized that polymorphisms in genes involved in estrogen biosynthesis and intracellular binding can predispose individuals to cancer (118). The proposed model suggests that such functional polymorphisms would act together and in combination with established risk factors to define a high-risk profile for breast cancer.

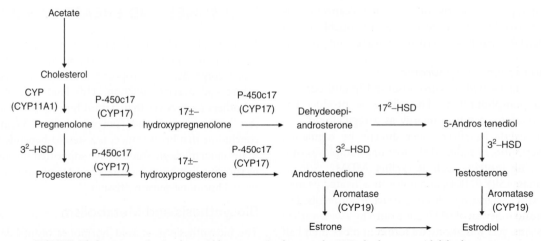

FIGURE 13.9 Biosynthesis of steroid hormones in the gonads. HSD, hydrozysteroid dehydrogenase.

The genes originally proposed included CYP17, CYP19, CYP1A1, HSD17B1, and COMT.

- The *CYP17* gene is located on chromosome 10. Its gene product mediates both steroid 17α hydroxylase and 17, 20 lyase activities. There is a compelling body of evidence to support a role for CYP17 in breast cancer. To date, studies have shown an association between *CYP17* gene polymorphism and use of age of menarche (119), HRT (120), estrogen metabolites in the urine (121), serum hormone levels in pre- and postmenopausal women, and breast cancer risk (122).

- The *CYP19* gene is located on chromosome 15q and encodes a steroid aromatase that catalyzes the conversion of C19 androgens to estrogens. Seven alleles have been reported ranging from 7 to 13 repeats. The available evidence of any functional significance between any known CYP19 polymorphism, aromatase activity, and breast cancer is conflicting. Investigators conclude that although it may be possible that an association between a CYP19 polymorphism and breast cancer risk exists, it is more likely that such polymorphisms of the *CYP19* gene are in linkage disequilibrium with other functional alleles in the *CYP19* gene.

- The *HSD17B1* gene encodes the 17HSD1 enzyme that catalyzes the conversion of estrone to a more biological active form, E2. Several polymorphisms of the *HSD17B1* gene have been identified. A recently published comprehensive analysis failed to identify any association between breast cancer and 17HSD1 polymorphisms common in Caucasians. However, among a subset of Caucasians with ER-negative tumors, they found evidence of an association between four of the known polymorphisms and the corresponding haplotypes that carry all high-risk alleles or all low-risk alleles.

- COMT polymorphism alleles are considered high or low activity. Studies on the association between COMT and breast cancer risk have been contradictory (123,124).

- In postmenopausal women, androgens are produced in the adrenal gland, and adipose tissue is the principal site for aromatization. Normal adipose tissue uses promoter I.4 of the *CYP19* gene to stimulate aromatase production; however, breast tumors and their surrounding adipose tissue activate promotor II of the *CYP19* gene, and the result is a greater expression of aromatase. AIs can reduce estrogen production by more than 90% and are classified according to the specificity, potency, and reversibility with which they inhibit the aromatase enzyme. Third-generation AIs (i.e., anastrozole, letrozole, and exemestane) are the most potent, most selective, and least toxic, and are the only three AIs with FDA approval. In the preventative setting, tamoxifen remains the gold standard, but in the adjuvant setting, the use of AIs as single agents, or sequentially with tamoxifen, has been approved. However, we await longer follow-up in trials to determine which treatment approach is better. In the neoadjuvant setting, the use of AIs resulted in better overall response rates and a more conservative surgery rate than tamoxifen. For patients with metastatic disease, in the first-line setting, large phase III trials have shown that AIs are equivalent or superior to tamoxifen. Finally, we caution that the side effects profile of the drugs differ (most notably in osteoporosis), and should be tailored as such.

- The liver is the principal site of estrogen metabolism. There is little available data to suggest an association between breast cancer risk and gynaecomastia. However, male breast cancer is more common in Egypt, representing 6% of all breast cancers, and in Zambia, where it represents 15% of all breast cancers. This may be due to the higher prevalence of liver diseases (from schistosomiasis or malnutrition), with resulting increases in endogenous estrogens.

Nuclear Receptor Superfamily

Steroid hormone action depends on the presence of highly specific intracellular receptors, known as the *NR superfamily*. Ligand-activated NRs are transcription factors that are essential for normal cellular growth, differentiation, function, and development; they initiate or enhance transcription of genes containing specific hormone response elements (HREs). All members of the NR superfamily share several conserved structural elements and contain up to six functional domains (denoted AF-1), including the zinc finger deoxyribonucleic acid-binding domain (DBD) (the most highly conserved element, sharing >90% homology); a hinge region; the amino-terminal transcriptional AF-1 domain; and a carboxyl-terminal ligand binding domain that overlaps with a second transcriptional AF-2 domain. The amino-terminal domain is highly variable in size and sequence, and contains a ligand-independent activation domain (AF-1) and a ligand independent domain (AF-2). NRs are classified by their DNA-binding and dimerization properties (homodimers, monodimers, heterodimers, etc.); estrogen, progesterone, and ARs are all homodimers and are class I NRs.

The estrogen receptor gene, located on chromosome 6q, codes for the two isoforms of the ER: ERα and ERβ. The ERα gene product is a 66 kDa, 595-amino acid protein that is separated into six functional domains, two of which are functional (AF-1 and AF-2). The AF-2 region is a ligand-dependent domain and is located along with the hormone-binding domain and heat-shock protein 90 region in the E domain. Estrogen diffuses into the nucleus when it binds to the ER, causing dissociation of hsp90 (heat-shock protein), leading to homodimerization and binding of the ER to EREs present in the promotor region, facilitating gene transcription. Transcription results in formation of mRNA that activate cytoplasmic ribosomes to produce specific proteins. ERβ differs from ERα in the structure of the ligand-binding domain, where they have only 55% homology. Their functional differences have yet to be elucidated.

Similar to the ER, there are two isoforms of PR-A and PR-B, both of which are coded for by the same gene located on chromosome 11q22. The isoforms differ in molecular weight. PR function/activation is similar to that of the ER; however, it is dependent on estrogen as an upstream transcription activator. The ratio of PR-A to PR-B is critical for normal mammary development.

There is only one active form of the AR coded for by a gene located on chromosome Xq11-12. The AR is most closely related to the PR and it functions as a transcription activator in a manner similar to both ER and PR. One of the known target genes of AR activation is insulin-like growth factor 1 (IGF-1).

Transcriptional activation by NRs is a complex process. Current understanding is that common transcriptional intermediary cofactors (coactivators or corepressors) that process intrinsic enzymatic activity as well as a variety of interaction motifs are required for transcriptional activity by NRs. The list of members of NR-cofactor members is ever expanding. The most well known coactivators are the p160 family. The p160 steroid coactivator gene family contains three homologous members (SRC-1, SRC-2, SRC-3/AIB) that serve as transcriptional coactivators for steroid receptors such as the ER, PR, and AR. Found in many cell types, their expression levels are tissue- and cell-type dependent and, by virtue of their relative concentrations, they act as control mechanisms of the steroid receptor. NR corepressors include silencing mediator for retinoid receptors (SMRT), NR corepressor *N-CoR* and the small unique NR corepressor (*SUN-CoR*). In addition to NR cofactors, NRs are regulated by epigenetic modification. Chromatin is a complex, high-order structure that contains the cellular DNA wrapped around an octamer of histones (nucleosome), and is an important epigenetic modulator of NR activity. Such "packaging" of DNA into chromatin presents a barrier for transcription factors, such as NRs, to access their target DNA sites. However, unlike many transcription factors, some NRs are capable of binding to their hormone-response DNA elements (HRE) embedded in chromatin. Upon ligand activation, NRs bind to HRE and recruit many transcriptional cofactors, including chromatin-remodeling factors, to the target gene promoters. The chromatin-remodeling activities recruited by NRs alter the local chromatin structure and allow other essential transcription factors to bind and activate or repress transcription. As well as this direct interaction with the HRE complex, NR cofactors are thought to interact with histone acetylases (HATs) and histone deacetylases (HDACs) to generate "open" chromatin formation, thereby allowing the NRs access to their target DNA sites. NRs can also influence the activity of other transcription factors [nuclear factor-kappa B (NFkB), STAT5] in a positive or negative way through protein kinase signaling pathways, such as the MAPK. In addition to the extensively studied genomic pathways of steroid hormone action, there is a growing body of information about physiologic events on the cellular level initiated by steroids. This "nongenomic pathway" is the subject of intense research.

Clinical Relevance

- Breast cancer is a steroid-responsive cancer. Both ER and PR have prognostic and predictive significance in breast cancer management; their predictive value is most

significant. The role of the AR is less clear. It is important to note that there is no standard protocol for determining receptor status, which is relevant when considering a cutoff between a negative and a positive reading, as a "false-negative" label could have significant therapeutic and outcome implications. Prognostic factors assess outcome, independent of treatment.

- ER/PR-positive tumors are more likely to be well differentiated with a low proliferative index, and are therefore associated with lower rates of local recurrence and better survival than ER/PR-negative cancer.
- DNA microarray studies have characterized breast cancer in terms of steroid receptor status, the most important of which is the luminal (ERα-positive) and basal (ERα-negative) differentiation, or more specifically, luminal-A, luminal-B, basal, normal, and ERBB2 (125). A recent microarray study has divided mammary tumor cells into three groups based on steroid receptor activity: luminal (ER-positive, AR-positive), basal (ER-negative, AR-negative) and molecular apocrine (ER-negative, AR-negative). This "molecular apocrine" group is androgen receptor-positive (AR-positive) and includes all the *nonbasal* ER-negative tumors. It has been suggested that this "molecular apocrine" group may represent up to 14% of breast cancers (126). "Pleomorphic lobular carcinoma (PLC) of the breast," a recently recognized aggressive variant of ILC with higher rates of recurrence then ILC, exhibits apocrine differentiation. PLC is typically AR-positive and exhibits "molecular apocrine" differentiation. An underlying androgen physiology of these cancers may explain their aggressive biology (127).
- Increased expression of PR-B may be indicative of a functional polymorphism of the PR promoter, which is associated with an increased risk of breast cancer (128).

By definition, "predictors" assess treatment-based outcome; ER and PR status are strong predictors of response to endocrine therapy.

- In the preventative setting, tamoxifen appears to prevent only ER-positive breast cancers (importantly, tamoxifen did not increase incidence of ER-negative tumors). The NSABP-P1 prevention trial did not assess the effect of chemoprevention on PR-positive tumors.
- In the adjuvant setting, 5 years of tamoxifen therapy reduces local recurrence rates by 50% and mortality by 28% for ER-positive tumors. Furthermore, there appears to be an association between outcome and degree of ER-positivity (129), but interestingly, there appears to be a response in tumors with as few as 1% of cells positive for ER by IHC (130). The role of PR as a predictor of response to hormonal therapy is more controversial. Conventional wisdom attributes its predictive value to the relative activity of the ER. Patients with ER-negative/PR-positive tumors benefit from endocrine therapy, suggesting that PR-positivity is an indicator of an active, intact estrogen pathway. In contrast to ER-positive breast cancer, patients with ER-negative/PR-negative tumors derive little or no

benefit from antiestrogen therapy. Although the Oxford overview analysis did not support a role for PR as an independent predictor of endocrine response, recent studies have shown that PR status predicts outcome to SERM therapy, showing that PR-negative tumors are more aggressive than PR-positive cancers (131).

- In advanced breast cancer, more than 70% of ER-positive/PR-positive tumors will respond to endocrine therapy, compared with less than 10% of ER-negative/PR-negative tumors. Those with discordant receptor status (ER-positive/PR-negative, ER-negative/PR-positive), have response rates ranging from 25% to 45%, respectively (132).
- ER-negative/PR-negative breast cancer represents approximately 25% to 30% of all breast cancers and generally has a more aggressive clinical course. In contrast to ER-positive breast cancer, patients with ER-negative/PR-negative tumors derive little or no benefit from antiestrogen therapy, and targeted therapies remain elusive (62). One notable exception has been the successful use of antibodies targeting the tyrosine kinase receptor *HER-2/neu* (ERBB2), which is disproportionally overexpressed in ER-negative breast cancer.

The value of ER and PR status is influenced by a number of factors. Postmenopausal women are more likely to have well-differentiated, ER-positive tumors compared with premenopausal women. Some studies have shown that ER expression correlates with tumor grade and size in postmenopausal women (133). There is a strong inverse relation between ER status and tumor grade; therefore, the lack of ER expression in a low-grade tumor is unusual and may represent a false negative. Both endogenous and exogenous hormones may yield a false-negative assay. This is relevant when a patient develops a local recurrence on tamoxifen, as tamoxifen may occupy the ER, yielding a false-negative assay.

- Many studies have investigated possible associations between AR status and other clinicopathologic features or measures of outcome. However, the mechanisms by which the AR contributes to the initiation and progression of breast cancer, and its functional relation to the ER, remain unknown.
- An interesting concept of breast cancer biology is the genetic and histopathologic status of normal breast tissue. One group has analyzed the ER expression in a variety of benign breast lesions and has found a wide range of expression levels. The most notable finding was that patients who subsequently developed a cancer had a greater proportion of cells that showed ER and Ki67 expression in the hyperplastic lesions than patients without cancer at 20 years' follow-up (134).

The Microenvironment

The microenvironment plays an essential role in breast cancer biology as all tissues require a functioning extracellular network to facilitate intercellular signaling and provide structural support. The extracellular matrix (ECM)/stroma contains a wide variety of molecules [matrix metalloproteases (MMPs), collagen 1, elastin, fibroblasts, laminin, fibronectin] that regulate homeostasis. The BM is a highly organized, bilayered, "specialized" ECM. The functional integrity of the breast is dependent upon the organization and architecture of the breast, which in turn depends on "normal" communication between genomically stable, functioning epithelium, and surrounding stromal cells (135).

Genetic alterations, such as loss of heterozygosity, have been reported to exist within normal tissue stroma, which suggests a protective effect of the ECM. Normal fibroblasts, an essential component of the ECM, have been shown to prevent transformation of initiated epithelial cells and to correct the malignant behavior of neoplastic epithelial cells. However, carcinoma-associated fibroblasts behave very differently from those in "normal" EMC as they are highly proliferative and enhance malignant epithelial-mesenchymal proliferation. Similarly, myoepithelial cells, the principal component of the BM, produce molecules such as collagen, laminin, fibronectin, MMPs, and growth factors, thereby facilitating the construction of new BM. The mechanisms behind destruction of the BM are unclear. Normal myoepithelial cells have been shown to exhibit tumor-suppressor activity, such as G2/M cell-cycle arrest, inhibition of invasion, and endothelial cell chemotaxis and proliferation. Interestingly, the myoepithelial cells associated with in-site lesions differ from "normal BM" in terms of gene-expression profile, cytokines produced (CXCL14 and CXCL12), and ability to polarize. These findings suggest that while normal myoepithelial cells may *suppress* tumorigenic activity, cancer-associated myoepithelial cells may *support* growth, differentiation, invasion, and migration of cancer cells. In summary, there are many lines of evidence to suggest that alterations in epithelial–ECM interactions can initiate, potentiate, or facilitate changes in the histologic or cellular characteristics of the tissue. The role of the microenvironment in tumorigenesis is now an intense area of scientific research.

In addition to its role in tumorigenesis, we must also consider the "environmental" conditions associated with metastasis. In 1889, British surgeon Stephen Paget published the "seed and soil" theory of cancer metastasis (136), hypothesizing that the potential of a tumor cell (seed) to metastasize depends on its interactions with the homeostatic factors of its microenvironment (soil) that promote tumor-cell growth, survival, angiogenesis, invasion, and metastasis (137). Animal models have proved that not all the cells in a primary tumor have the same potential to metastasize (seed), and clinical observations have shown that different tumor types have a tendency to metastasize to specific organs independent of mechanical factors (138). More recently, studies have suggested a molecular genetic explanation for the pattern of metastatic spread. Gene-expression profiling of cells from a primary lesion showed high expression of chemokines CXCR4 and CCR7, and increased expression of their respective receptors (CXCL12/SDF-1α and CCL21/6Ckine) was found in the corresponding regional lymph nodes and lung metastasis. Antibody-mediated receptor blockade resulted in a significant reduction in metastasis to these sites, suggesting that chemokines and their receptors may play a critical role in determining the metastatic destination of tumor cells (139). Similarly, others have identified a set of genes that, by providing growth advantages in the both the primary tumor and lung microenvironment, marks and mediates breast cancer metastasis to the lungs (140).

Clinical Relevance

- The BM separates the epithelium from the stroma, which contains the blood and lymph vessels. An intact BM (on light microscopy) contains the cancer cells, thereby preventing lymphovascular invasion. Therefore, the carcinoma is referred to as *in situ* as it remains in its place of origin. Conversely, disruption of the BM allows cancer cells to enter the stroma and come into contact with the lymphovascular system. This type of cancer is called *invasive* and carries a much worse prognosis than *in situ* disease.
- Cathepsin D is a lysosomal proteolytic enzyme associated with protein catabolism and tissue remodeling. As it is thought to play a critical role in the degradation of the BM, there has been considerable interest in the prognostic value of this protein. However, the lack of standardized assays and the wide range of results from clinical studies have led ASCO to conclude that the prognostic value of cathepsin D remains investigational (57).
- Therapeutic targeting of the tumor microenvironment has been developed. Most of these agents are in phase I or II clinical trials, but one has been approved by the FDA. Imatinib, initially named signal transduction inhibitor-571 (STI-571), targets pericytes and stromal fibroblasts, and is a specific blocker of *bcr-abl* kinase, c-KIT tyrosine kinase, and the platelet-derived growth factor (PDGF) tyrosine-kinase receptor. Initially approved for use in patients with chronic myeloid leukemia, currently a Phase II clinical trial is investigating the affect of docetaxel plus imatinib in metastatic breast cancer. Such agents hold promise in a multimodal approach to treatment.

Angiogenesis

Angiogenesis is a complex process that results in new vessel formation. Its central role in local tumor growth and metastatic spread is now well established. In their initial stages of growth, cancer cells remain separated from the host microvessels by a BM and derive their nutrients by a process of diffusion from nearby capillaries. During this "prevascular" phase, lesions exist in a steady state of proliferation and apoptosis. However, like all cells in the body, tumor cells cannot remain viable beyond the effective 100 to 200 μm oxygen diffusion distance from the vasculature; therefore angiogenesis is required for the tumor to grow beyond a small size.

The onset of angiogenesis is known as the *angiogenic switch* and is accompanied by rapid primary tumor growth and local invasion. Hypoxia-induced factors (HIF1 and HIF2), proangiogenic [fibroblast growth factor (βFGF), vascular endothelial growth factor (VEGF)] and antiangiogenic factors (thrombospondin, angiostatin, endostatin, interferon-α and interferon-β) contribute to the angiogenic switch. The governing factors of angiogenic growth-factor expression in tumor cells are largely unknown, but dominantly acting oncogenes seem to be implicated. For example, the p53 TSG appears to control thrombospondin, a potent angiogenesis inhibitor. The BM acts as a physical barrier and a source of tumstatin, a potent inhibitor of endothelial cell migration and proliferation, suggesting that the angiogenic phenotype appears after the expression of the malignant phenotype. The loss of endothelial cell inhibition and a rise in angiogenic stimulators (VEGF) recruits circulating progenitor endothelial cells from local and distant (bone marrow) sources to the vascular bed of tumors. Mast cells and macrophages are important sources of proangiogenic factors such as VEGF, βFGF, and metalloproteases.

The angiogenic switch causes budding of the preexisting capillaries, which elongate and develop into new capillaries. Concentric rings of tumor cells form around these vessels, and microscopic examination reveals a fine vascular network interspersed with tumor cells. Growth factors such as IGF-1, platelet derived growth factor-β (PDGF-BB), and herparin-binding (HB)-EGF-like growth factor that are released from the endothelial cells potentiate the growth and invasion of tumor cells into their microenvironment, and subsequent metastasis.

In addition to tumor growth, invasion, and metastasis, angiogenesis has been implicated as a putative factor in "tumor-dormancy," one of the classic models of breast cancer biology (141). "Dormant" tumor cells are micrometastatic cells that have a balanced rate of growth and apoptosis, but maintain the potential to infiltrate and invade if stimulated (142). This model hypothesizes that the increase in angiogenic stimulators (VEGF) and growth factors "wakens" these dormant cells, interrupting their equilibrium, thereby potentiating growth and proliferation (143).

Clinical Relevance

- Increased microvessel density (MVD, a pathologic marker of angiogenesis) is suggested to be associated with high-grade (versus low-grade) DCIS (144), shorter relapse-free and overall survival in node-negative patients (145), and, finally, invasive disease and increased metastatic potential (146). Such findings await validation.
- Numerous antiangiogenic agents have been developed and tested in the preclinical setting. Bevacizumab (avastin) is an antibody to VEGF-A ligand and is the first antiangiogenesis agent to be approved by the FDA. It has been tested in all solid tumors, and results suggest that response is tumor-dependent. Its effect as single-agent therapy in breast cancer appears to be limited. However, preliminary results from a Phase III clinical trial (ECOG 2100) have shown that bevacizumab combined with chemotherapy improves progression-free survival for patients with advanced breast cancer (147). Importantly, its

use is an absolute contraindication to a surgical procedure due to the potential effect on wound healing.

Tumor Growth Kinetics

The cell cycle is a multistep process with many checkpoints that govern its progression. Disruption in cell cycle control is a common finding in breast cancer. For example: p53 plays a key role in mediating cell response to various stresses, mainly by inducing or repressing a number of genes involved in cell cycle arrest, senescence, apoptosis, DNA repair, and angiogenesis. Bcl-2 protein is also an important molecule in the control of apoptosis; P16 protein inhibits cyclin-dependent kinase (cdk-4) and cdk-6 complexes to interrupt cell cycle progression, and pRB (the activated form of the RB gene product) increases cell-cycle transit. Furthermore, cyclins (-D1, -D2, -E) and cdks are complex cell-cycle control molecules that act primarily at the G1-S phase transition point of the cell cycle. In the normal state, they complex with one anther to initiate the S phase; Cdk-inhibitors cause G1-cycle arrest. Neoplasia may result from disruptions in the normal interaction between these molecules. All of these factors are interrelated.

The growth rate of a tumor is determined by the balance between cell gain and loss. Cell survival depends on a vascular supply and cell cycle control. Mathematic models have provided a greater understanding of the complexity of breast cancer growth kinetics, and current understanding is that growth patterns vary according to the stage of tumor development (148), demonstrating the *Gompertzian* pattern of growth. The discovery that many genes are associated with the biology of metastasis, and that the microenvironment plays a key role in tumorigenesis, has led some researchers to believe that the primary tumor is in fact a "conglomerate of small, Gompertzian tumors. . .each component of which can be considered a small metastasis that forms around a seed from the tumor to itself." In other words, the primary tumor is composed of multiple selfmetastases that form around a seed from the tumor to itself (149).

Clinical Relevance

- p53 mutations are associated with an increased risk of progression to breast cancer in women with BBD and are the most common mutations associated with Li-Fraumeni syndrome. Overexpression of the mutated *p53* gene is a feature of approximately half of sporadic cancers. This overexpression seems to be independent of age, size, and nodal status, but has been associated with poor nuclear grade, *HER-2/neu* overexpression and aneuploidy. Conflicting evidence exists as to a correlation between p53 status and disease-free or overall survival (110–112). Others have proposed a role for mutant p53 as a predictor of response to therapy. Despite numerous studies, available data does not support a prognostic or predictive role for p53 in breast cancer.
- Bcl-2 protein expression is associated with ER-positivity, low proliferation index, and a good response to anthracycline-based chemotherapy, and it has been suggested that overexpression of p16 may be indicative of a more undifferentiated, malignant phenotype (150) and acceleration proliferation (151). Once again, such findings await further study.
- Over 35% of breast cancers exhibit loss of heterozygosity of the *RB* gene; however, immunohistochemical assessment of the expression of Rb protein has no prognostic significance in clinical breast cancer over already-established prognostic factors.
- Cyclin D1 is encoded by an estrogen responsive gene *CCND1*, and is overexpressed in more than half of invasive breast cancers. Current data suggests that cyclin D1 merits further investigations as a marker of response to tamoxifen (ER-positive tumors) and prognosis (152). The clinical relevance of the overexpression of cyclins A and E in breast cancer is less clear. However, it appears to correlate with a poor prognosis (153,154).
- The targeting of cell-cycle regulation is ongoing. Cdk inhibitors have been developed and tested in mono and combination therapy. Preliminary results seem to be associated with a high rate of side effects (155,156).
- It has been suggested that deoxyribonucleic acid index (DI, the degree of "aneuploidy") and SPF, evaluated by flow cytometric analysis, may have prognostic significance. In other words, "diploid" tumors with low proliferative activity have a better clinical outcome compared with aneuploid tumors of high proliferative index. This technique has not been accepted universally for a number of reasons. First, as all tumors are aneuploid cells, diploidy is likely to represent a dilution of the sample with normal tissue rather than a more favorable tumor. Second, because the centers that support the role of flow cytometry use different software with loose definitions of S-phase duration, their results are not parallel and cannot validate one another. In all, we lack definitive evidence for the efficacy of such techniques.
- The natural history of breast cancer is such that uncontrolled disease is lethal, with most patients dying within a couple of years, but with many living for some years longer. Local control with surgery alone (radical mastectomy) reveals a 30-year overall survival rate of 38% (70% for node-negative patients, and 0% for patients with tumors larger than 5 cm or level III nodes) (157). The advent of screening MG has increased the number of asymptomatic cancers diagnosed, lengthening the associated lead-time bias and improving prognosis (158). Interval breast cancers are defined as tumors diagnosed in the interval between scheduled screenings and are thought to represent tumors with a short "doubling time" (159). Importantly, the results of two large randomized trials [the Health Insurance Plan (HIP) and the Swedish two-county study] confirm that when compared with the unscreened population, interval cancers in the screened population are not associated with a greater risk of systemic dissemination and death (160,161). Identification of those at greatest risk of an interval cancer is fundamental for optimal breast cancer screening.

Mechanisms of Breast Cancer Metastasis

"The best work in the pathology of cancer now is done by those who…are studying the nature of the seed. They are like scientific botanists, and he who turns over the records of cases of cancer is only a ploughman, but his observations of the properties of the soil may be useful." Wise words from renowned British surgeon Stephen Paget that still hold true some 100 years later. The pathogenesis of metastasis is one of the most rapidly evolving fields of surgical science. The process is sequential, involving cellular proliferation, neovascularization, and interruption of intercellular adhesion, facilitating motility and subsequent invasion through the ECM. The cells may then permeate the lymphovascular system, leading to dissemination throughout the body, followed by extravasation at a particular site and finally, growth and proliferation at the site. Although the above steps are interrelated, the process is primarily dependent on two factors: the host microenvironment, as discussed previously in this section, and the genetic stability of the disseminating cell. Most tumors are heterogeneous, containing many subpopulations of cells with specific germ-line or somatic mutations. It is the accumulation of multiple, varying mutations in the cells that populate a tumor that determines its overall biological behavior such that metastatic potential is directly proportional to genetic instability (46).

Clinical Relevance

- Up to 6% of newly diagnosed patients will present with stage IV (metastatic) disease, and despite advances in systemic treatments, up to 30% of patients with potentially curable disease (stage 0–III) will develop distant metastases (162). Metastatic breast cancer is an incurable disease with a median overall survival of 2 to 3 years.
- Does the risk of metastatic disease depend on the genotype of the disseminating cell or the genotype/phenotype of the microenvironment? Why is bone the most common site of metastatic breast cancer and why do we rarely see splenic or intestinal metastases? Although many prognostic and predictive factors have been established to identify those patients with local disease that may go on to develop metastasis, nodal status remains the most reliable. That the identification of signatures of site-specific metastatic capabilities may have a prognostic or predictive role, and that they identify therapeutic targets of therapy to likely sites of metastasis as well, is one of the hottest topics in molecular oncology. Certain genes (e.g., nm23, pS2, MMP1, CXCL1, and PTGS2) have been implicated as predictors of metastatic potential; however, their value remains investigational (140).
- Although there are more systemic agents available for the treatment of stage IV breast cancer than any other cancer, there is little direct evidence to suggest that progress has been made toward improving survival outcomes. The underlying presumption that objective response to chemotherapy can be used as a surrogate end point of survival awaits validation. Only recently have we seen evidence to suggest that modern agents (e.g., taxanes, trastuzumab) may have a meaningful survival benefit for patients with stage IV disease (163). Combination therapy with agents that target the microenvironment and angiogenesis holds considerable promise.

Stem Cells

A detailed discussion of stem cells in relation to breast cancer is beyond the scope of the chapter. In brief, stem cells have the remarkable potential to develop into many different cell types in the body. Serving as a sort of repair system for the body, they can theoretically divide without limit to replenish other cells. When a stem cell divides, each new cell has the potential to either remain a stem cell or become another type of cell with a more specialized function. The clonal nature of most malignant tumors is well established. Data from both hematologic malignancies and solid tumors have suggested that there are only minor populations of cells in each malignancy that are capable of tumor initiation. These tumor-initiating cells have the functional properties of a tumor stem cell. The promise of tumor stem cells in cancer is they may be used as a tool to study the disease and, more importantly, for the development of the next generation of targeted therapies. The last 30 years of basic science have witnessed a fascinating evolution in our understanding of breast cancer biology; landmark discoveries include the identification of the *BRCA1* and *BRCA2* genes. There is substantial evidence to support the existence of one or more pluripotent mammary epithelial stem cells (164); we eagerly await their discovery, which will undoubtedly carry profound implications.

BREAST CANCER

Epidemiology

Excluding skin cancer, breast cancer is the most common malignancy and the leading cause of cancer-related deaths among women worldwide. However, the burden is not evenly distributed and, according to the best available data, there are large variations in its incidence, mortality, and survival between different countries and regions (165). The last half century has witnessed an interesting shift in the breast cancer population: the incidence of DCIS has increased dramatically (28% per year between 1982–1988), reflecting a shift in stage of disease at diagnosis; death rates have decreased steadily (1.8% per year since 1989); tumor size distribution of incident breast carcinomas in Surveillance, Epidemiology and End Results (SEER) has shifted toward smaller tumors (166,167); and more recent data suggest that the incidence of ER-negative and/or PR-negative breast cancer is declining, whereas that of ER-positive/PR-positive disease is increasing (168). Furthermore, an interesting disparity is seen in breast cancer incidence and mortality rates in the United States between Caucasian and African-American women (169,170).

Established breast cancer risk factors have been mentioned briefly in Diagnosis of Breast Disease. Although the prevalence of risk factors in the general population ranges from 10% to 15%, some are associated with large RRs (e.g., BRCA mutation carriers) (171). Appreciating relevant risk factors for breast cancer is central to any preventive and control program aimed at reducing the burden of the disease. Established breast cancer risk factors include the following:

- **Gender.** A woman's lifetime probability of developing breast cancer is one in six (one in nine for invasive breast cancer) compared with men, who are more than 100 times less likely to develop breast cancer (172).
- **Age.** The incidence of sporadic breast cancer ranges from 0.39% for a 30-year-old woman to 4.01% for a 70-year-old woman (173).
- **Family History.** Breast cancer is a genetic disease; women with a family history of breast cancer are at an increased and fixed risk of developing cancer. This risk can be stratified according to the relation of the individuals (monozygotic twins, first-degree relative, etc.) and the age at diagnosis (pre/postmenopausal). In a meta-analysis using data from more than 50,000 women with breast cancer and 100,000 controls, the risk of breast cancer for a woman with one affected first-degree relative was increased 1.80-fold compared with a 2.93-fold increase with two affected first-degree relatives. The risk ratios were highest for women with young affected relatives (174). Between 5% and 10% of breast cancers are found to be associated with a BRCA1 or BRCA2 mutation. Carriers of a BRCA1/BRCA2 mutation carry a 50% to 80% lifetime breast cancer risk. Identification of such patients with thorough history taking and appropriate genetic testing is a key step in primary prevention.

- **Hormonal factors** (see "Hormones and Breast Cancer")
- **BBD** (see "**Benign breast disease**")
- **Previous history of irradiation.** There is a well-established association between exposure to ionizing radiation at a young age and breast cancer. The greatest risk is during the prepubertal years, but excess risk is seen in women exposed as late as 45 years of age.

Epidemiologic studies have identified a number of sociodemographic, socioeconomic, dietary, lifestyle, and environmental factors that may modify breast cancer risk. Their value in the clinical setting has not been established.

Pathology and Staging

More than 95% of breast malignancies arise from the breast epithelial cells. Epithelial carcinomas represent a diverse group of lesions which differ in cell type (ductal or lobular), microscopic appearance, and biologic behavior. Clinically, breast cancers are described in terms of their cell of origin (ductal or lobular) and the integrity of the BM on light microscopy (in situ or invasive). The World Health Organization (WHO) classification of breast tumors is listed in the table in the subsequent text (Table 13.4).

In situ Carcinoma
Ductal Carcinoma In situ
DCIS is defined as a malignant proliferation of the epithelial cells that line the lactiferous ducts in which the malignant cells remain confined within the duct when examined under light microscopy. Arising in the terminal ductolobular unit, it extends out to involve the extralobular units and is an obligate precursor to invasive disease. An estimated 20%

TABLE 13.4

ªThe World Health Organization (WHO) Classification of Breast Tumors/Adapted from the WHO and Systemized Nomenclature of Medicine Morphology Fields

Epithelial/benign	Intraductal papilloma; adenoma of the nipple; adenoma (-tubular, -lactating)
Epithelial/malignant	DCIS; LCIS
Noninvasive	Invasive ductal carcinoma; invasive lobular carcinoma; invasive
Paget	ductal with predominant intraductal component; mucinous
Invasive	carcinoma; medullary carcinoma; papillary carcinoma; tubular carcinoma; adenoid cyctic carcinomal; secretory (juvenile) carcinoma; apocrine carcinoma; carcinoma with metaplasia (-squamous, spindle cell, -cartilagenous and osseous; -mixed); others
Mixed connective tissue and epithelial tumors	Fibroadenoma; phyllodes; carcinosarcoma
Miscellaneous	Soft tissue; skin tumors; tumors of the hematopoietic and lymphoid tissues
Tumor-like lesions	Duct ectasia; inflammatory pseudotumors; hamartomas; gynecomastia; others
Unclassified	

ªData from http://www.who.int/topics/cancer/en/ and Tavassoli FA. *World Health Organization Classification of tumours: Pathology and genetics of tumours of the breast and female genetial organs.* Lyon: IARC Press, 2003.

of all newly diagnosed breast cancers are DCIS. Oftentimes it can be difficult to distinguish from ADH or LCIS, and specialized stains such as E-cadherin can sometimes help distinguish between ductal and lobular lesions (175).

DCIS has variable histologic features, such as comedo necrosis, cribriform, microacini, papillary structures, and pleomorphic nuclei, which imply different biology. The advent of BCT has shown that not all DCIS lesions have the same risk of local recurrence and, as a result, there has been intense interest in developing a classification system that reflects the potential of the lesion to recur within the breast or progress to invasive breast cancer. It seems that nuclear grade and the presence of necrosis define most of the risk associated with DCIS (176–178); however, certain architectural patterns may impact outcome independent of nuclear grade (179–181) and so the available data is conflicting (176,182).

For patients who undergo BCT, the risk of an in-breast recurrence depends not only on histologic features but on the age of the patient, clinical features such as a palpable (or mammographic) mass, margin status, lesion size, and whether the patient receives radiation therapy or hormonal therapy; none of these factors are independent of one another. The relative merits of these various classification systems with regard to their interobserver reproducibility and clinical utility remain controversial. Ultimately, a classification system that includes both histologic features and molecular markers of biological behavior is necessary to provide the most clinically meaningful information about DCIS lesions.

Clinical Relevance
- In the current era of screening mammography, the most common presentation is an abnormal mammogram with clustered microcalcifications. DCIS is an obligate precursor of invasive disease and so synchronous invasive disease must be suspected in all patients with DCIS (especially those with a palpable and/or mammographic mass, and/or histologic features as discussed). A synchronous invasive cancer may be detected in approximately 20% of DCIS cases (range: 2%–46%).
- Pathologic diagnosis is limited in its ability to rule out synchronous invasive disease as not all the specimens will be examined. DCIS with "microinvasion" is defined by a predominantly *in situ* lesion that has less than 100 μm of malignant cells beyond the BM of the involved duct on light microscopy. The clinical significance is unclear; however, it has been shown that the presence of microinvasion increased the likelihood of positive nodal disease on SLNB (183). The role of SLNB in the setting of DCIS is controversial. However, it can be used as a surrogate for identifying those with an invasive component.
- The prognostic significance of molecular markers such as *HER2/neu*, Ki67, and p53 in DCIS remains unproven.

Lobular Carcinoma In situ

The morphologic definition of LCIS is a proliferation of generally small and often loosely cohesive cells originating in the terminal duct-lobular unit, with or without pagetoid involvement of the terminal ducts. The term *ALH* is used when the lumina are not completely obliterated or when the terminal ductal units (TDUs) are not fully distended. LCIS encompasses a group of entities with distinctive histologic features, of which "classical LCIS" is the most common (184). Other subtypes of LCIS have been described (signet ring, apocrine, pleomorphic, etc.), and there is evidence to suggest that pleomorphic LCIS carries a worse prognosis than classical LCIS. However, all data is retrospective. All subtypes are associated with ER and PR expression, and classical LCIS typically does not show *HER2/neu* amplification or p53 expression. Pleomorphic LCIS, however, shows a higher Ki67 index, more frequent expression of both p53 and *HER2/neu*, and apocrine differentiation, which may explain its more aggressive phenotype.

The true incidence of LCIS is unknown as there are no specific clinical abnormalities associated with the lesion and there are no characteristic macroscopic features that could guide tissue sampling. The diagnosis is made as an incidental finding in breast biopsies performed for other indications. Classically, LCIS is associated with a high rate of multifocal disease (up to 50%), and up to 30% may have contralateral disease (185–187).

Clinical Relevance
- Unlike DCIS, LCIS not an obligate precursor for invasive disease. It is considered a "high-risk factor" that confers an increased rate of developing invasive disease (approximately 1%–2% a year, and 30%–40% lifetime) (188). Both invasive-ductal and lobular cancer can occur with LCIS. The risk can persist for up to 30 years; however, studies report that most of the cancers occur between years 15 and 30 postdiagnosis. The increased risk of invasive disease is bilateral, and while the common belief was that this risk was equal for both breasts (185,189,190), there is recent evidence to suggest that cancer is up to three times more likely in the ipsilateral breast (190,191). Although conventional wisdom teaches that LCIS is *not* an obligate precursor for invasive disease, there is a growing body of scientific data that suggests that some variants of LCIS may act as precursors (192).
- In general, LCIS is identified as an incidental finding following assessment of a coexisting symptomatic or screen-detected abnormality (e.g., calcifications). However, radiology may have a role in the surveillance of patients following a diagnosis of LCIS.
- It can be very difficult to distinguish between LCIS and ALH, ADH, DCIS, and ILC on FNA, and CNBs are considered more reliable. However, CNB may be subject to similar challenges, and therefore underestimation should always be considered. Therefore, it is reasonable that biopsy-detected LCIS should be followed by surgical excision. Margin status of excisional biopsy for LCIS alone is controversial.
- There is no role for radiotherapy (RT) in the management of patients with LCIS. The role of adjuvant hormonal therapy for patients with LCIS and will be discussed in part 5 of this section under the heading "Management/Hormonal therapy."

Infiltrating Ductal Carcinoma

Infiltrating ductal carcinoma (IDC) is a malignant proliferation of ductal cells that have broken through the BM and have the potential to disseminate locally and enter the lymphatic channels or blood vessels. It accounts for up to 80% of invasive lesions and is also called *infiltrating carcinoma of no special type*, or *infiltrating carcinoma not otherwise specified* (NOS).

Macroscopically, these lesions are typically hard, gray/white masses. They are characterized microscopically by cords and nests of tumor cells with varying amounts of gland formation. The malignant cells induce a fibrous response as they infiltrate the breast parenchyma and are divided into three grades based on a combination of architectural and cytologic features. A variable amount of associated DCIS is present in most cases.

Infiltrating Lobular Carcinoma

Infiltrating lobular carcinomas are the second most common type of invasive breast cancer, accounting for approximately 5% to 10% of invasive lesions. In many cases, no mass lesion is grossly evident, and the excised breast tissue may have a normal or only slightly firm consistency. Some infiltrating lobular carcinomas have a macroscopic appearance identical to that of infiltrating ductal cancers; however, infiltrating cells are usually small and are found in a characteristic single-file manner. They often proliferate in a target-like configuration around normal breast ducts, frequently inducing only minimal fibrous reaction. Associated LCIS is present in approximately two thirds of cases; however, DCIS may also accompany ILC.

Compared with IDC, ILC is associated with a higher frequency of bilaterality and multicentricity. Although older series report a similar prognosis for infiltrating lobular cancers and invasive ductal lesions, more recent reports suggest that the outcome may be more favorable for lobular cancers (193). Furthermore, ILCs tend to metastasize later than invasive duct carcinomas and spread to unusual locations, such as the peritoneum, meninges, and gastrointestinal tract (194). Variants of infiltrating lobular carcinoma exist, some of which have a poorer prognosis (pleomorphic ILC) (127).

Less-Common Variants of Invasive Carcinoma

All are variants of IDC and, with the exception of medullary carcinoma, are well differentiated and generally have a better prognosis than IDC.

Medullary carcinomas (1%–10%). Macroscopically, these lesions are well circumscribed and are often associated with areas of hemorrhage or necrosis. The tumor cells are poorly differentiated (high grade), grow in a syncytial pattern, and have an intense associated lymphoplasmacytic infiltrate. These lesions occur more frequently in younger patients and have been associated with mutations of the *BRCA1* gene (although most breast cancers in these patients are *not* medullary).

Mucinous/colloid carcinomas (1%–2%). These tend to be well-circumscribed masses and are characterized microscopically by nests of tumor cells dispersed in large pools of extracellular mucus; the cells tend to have uniform, low-grade nuclei. They are more common in older patients.

Tubular carcinomas. These are characterized by the presence of well formed tubular or glandular structures infiltrating the stroma. The tubules tend to be elongated, many have pointed ends, and the cells composing the tubules often have apical cytoplasmic protrusions or "snouts." They are typically low grade and may be associated with low-grade DCIS.

Metaplastic carcinoma. These are well-circumscribed lesions of mixed epithelial and sarcomatoid components, as well as primary squamous or mixed adenocarcinoma and squamous carcinoma. Whether these tumors have a worse prognosis than ordinary invasive ductal cancers is unclear. Some studies suggest that tumors in which the squamous cell component predominates appear to be more aggressive and are frequently treatment refractory when compared with other infiltrating ductal cancers (195).

Adenoid cystic carcinoma. This lesion has a distinctive histologic pattern that is morphologically identical to adenoid cystic carcinoma found in the salivary glands. Histologic grading based on the percentage of solid areas may have prognostic significance. They can present as painful breast masses.

Primary Nonepithelial Breast Malignancies

The major categories of nonepithelial breast tumors include PTs, sarcomas (primary and treatment-related), and primary breast lymphomas.

Cytosarcoma Phyllodes

PTs are the most common nonepithelial tumors (<0.5% of all breast tumors). They frequently present as a palpable mobile lesion in women in their 40s. Clinical examination may be comparable to that of an FA, but a recent increase in size should raise the suspicion of a PT. Macroscopically, they are described as being large (average size: 3–5 cm), fleshy tumors that may have central areas of necrosis and can be indistinguishable from FAs. Classical microscopic features include a leaf-like architecture consisting of elongated cleft-like spaces that contain papillary projections of epithelial-lined stroma with varying degrees of hyperplasia and atypia. The stromal elements are a key component in the differentiation of PTs from FAs, and in distinguishing a benign from a malignant PT. Histologic assessment categorizes PT into benign, borderline, or malignant lesions based on features such as the degree of stromal cellular atypia, mitotic activity, tumor margins (infiltrative versus circumscribed), and the presence or absence of stromal overgrowth (196). Unfortunately, such features are poor predictors of clinical outcome.

Due to the low incidence of these lesions, current management is guided by small, single-institutional retrospective data. Because all PT have malignant potential, it is recommended that these lesions be excised; however, whether they should be excised by enucleation or with a clear margin (1 cm) is controversial. Available data suggests variable recurrence rates of 10% to 65% (197). Mastectomy is a valid surgical option; however, there is no data to suggest that it will confer any survival benefit. Axillary dissection is usually not needed because axillary lymph node involvement is only rarely reported. Systemic therapy is not indicated and adjuvant RT is generally unnecessary.

Metastatic disease seems to be rare, with a reported rate of less than 5% of all PTs, and survival rates with metastatic disease can vary greatly.

Sarcomas (Primary and Secondary)

A sarcoma of the breast is a rare histologic diagnosis. The causative factor cannot be identified in most primary breast sarcomas, but secondary breast sarcomas are usually associated with prior RT and conditions causing chronic lymphoedema. Lymphangiosarcomas of the upper extremity, breast, and axilla arising in women with chronic lymphedema after breast cancer therapy were initially described by Stewart and Treves, and this syndrome is now designated Stewart-Treves syndrome. The average latency period between prior ionizing radiation and breast sarcoma is approximately 15 years (range: 0–30 years). The latency period is shorter for angiosarcomas, which tend to arise 5 to 7 years' posttreatment. The increased use of breast prostheses has raised the suspicion that they may confer a risk for secondary sarcoma; however, there is no conclusive evidence of this. Genetic abnormalities such as Li-Fraumeni syndrome, Gardner syndrome, or neurofibromatosis type 1 can sometimes predispose to sarcomas, and environmental factors such as alkylating agents, arsenic compounds, vinyl chloride, herbicides, immunosuppressive agents, human immunodeficiency virus (HIV), and human herpes virus type 8 have also been implicated.

Clinically, breast sarcoma often presents as a large, painless, firm mass within the breast, with tumor size ranging from 1.5 cm to 30 cm. Angiosarcomas may be associated with discoloration, an overlying bluish tint to the skin, or erythema. Clinically and mammographically, these tumors may be mistaken for benign lesions such as FAs; however, they exhibit more rapid growth patterns. Breast sarcomas spread by direct local invasion or hematogenously; regional lymph node involvement is rare except in the setting of widespread metastatic disease. Excisional biopsy is often required for definitive diagnosis. In general, fibrosarcomas, angiosarcomas, malignant fibrous histiocytomas (MFH), and liposarcomas comprise the major subtypes.

Prognosis for primary breast sarcomas is highly dependent upon histologic grade and tumor size. Treatment is influenced by histologic grade and tumor size. As long as adequate tumor-free margins can be achieved, wide-local excision over mastectomy is an acceptable approach. Axillary sampling should be performed.

The overall prognosis of secondary sarcoma is poor. (Median survival durations average 2.3 years, and 5-year survival rates average 27%–35%.) Surgery is the only potentially curative modality, but is often difficult in previously irradiated tissue. RT has also been used, but with little success. The benefit from chemotherapy tends to be short-lived however; response rates as high as 45% are reported with doxorubicin-based regimens (198). The prognosis for the angiosarcoma subtype of treatment-related sarcomas is particularly poor, with high rates of local recurrence. The majority are high-grade lesions that metastasize early, most often to the lung and liver.

Primary Lymphomas

Primary lymphoma of the breast accounts for less than 1% of all extranodal lymphomas. The vast majority are non–Hodgkin lymphomas, although Hodgkin disease has been reported.

The most frequent clinical presentation is a unilateral, painless breast mass in an older woman (average age at diagnosis: 55–60 years); 10% can be bilateral (a less-common clinical scenario is that of a woman of childbearing age who presents during or immediately after pregnancy). Ipsilateral axillary lymphadenopathy is present in more than one third of cases and is characteristically firm and rubbery. There are no characteristic imaging findings. The most common histologic subtype is a B-cell lymphoma. T-cell lymphomas are rare and are associated with an aggressing clinical course.

Staging is according to the Ann Arbor staging system. Prognosis and treatment are similar to lymphomas of the same stage and histology in other locations. Surgery may be required for definite diagnosis, but not for treatment as lymphomas are highly sensitive to radiation and chemotherapy.

Paget Disease of the Breast

Paget disease of the breast (PD) accounts for approximately 2% of all breast cancers diagnosed annually in the United States. It typically presents with scaling, eczematous skin on the nipple/areolar complex that may be accompanied by a change in sensation of the nipple, nipple discharge, or a palpable (or mammographic) mass. Diagnosis is confirmed by full-thickness skin biopsy, and the pathologic hallmark is the presence of malignant, intraepithelial adenocarcinoma cells (Paget cells) occurring singly or in small groups within the epidermis of the nipple. Most patients will have an underlying breast cancer (in situ and/or invasive).

The prognosis of PD is based on the underlying breast cancer. Controversy regarding the pathogenesis of PD has led to treatment uncertainty (nipple-areolar resection alone, resection followed by breast irradiation, or biopsy followed by ipsilateral breast irradiation). The European Organization for Research and Treatment of Cancer (EORTC) conducted a prospective study of BCT for PD (199). Of the 61 patients with histologically proven PD, 97% had no associated palpable mass, and 84% had a normal mammogram. Patients underwent nipple-areolar resection with microscopically negative margins, followed by whole-breast irradiation. Associated DCIS was present in 93%, and the remainder had no underlying carcinoma. At a median follow-up of 6.4 years, the local recurrence rate was 6.5% ($n = 4$; 3 invasive, 1 DCIS), concluding that mastectomy and BCT appear to be acceptable options for women with PD. As most underlying lesions in this setting are DCIS, axillary node sampling should be guided by the level of suspicion of the underlying lesion (grade, size, microinvasion, etc.). PD associated with a palpable mass is likely to be more advanced in stage (i.e., larger size, more frequent invasive disease and axillary node positivity, and multifocal underlying disease) than cases without a mass. A recent study assessed the outcome of 104 patients with PD with an associated mass treated by either breast-conserving approaches ($n = 12$) or mastectomy ($n = 92$), and reported comparable local control and survival rates between the two.

The prognosis of PD is dependent upon the underlying cancer and nodal status. Recommendations regarding adjuvant therapy should be based on the characteristics of any associated carcinoma or axillary node metastases.

Staging

The tumor staging system for breast cancer is published by the American Joint Committee on Cancer (AJCC). This was recently modified in 2002. As compared with the previous edition (1997), changes include identifiers to indicate use of innovative technical approaches (e.g., sentinel lymph node dissection and immunohistochemical or molecular techniques); a size-based discrimination between isolated tumor cells and micrometastases; a reclassification of nodal status by the number of involved axillary lymph nodes; and a reclassification of metastasis to IMN and supraclavicular nodes (200). Subsequent analyses have shown that these changes dramatically affect stage-specific survival (201).

Prognostic/Predictive Factors

The clinical relevance of prognostic and predictive factors is under constant evaluation. Current practice supports the clinical relevance of factors such as age, tumor, nodes, metastasis (TNM) staging, histologic tumor type and grade, lymphovascular invasion, mitotic index, and ER/PR/*HER2/neu* status. Literature review reveals more than 100 putative prognostic and predictive factors for breast cancer; however, few appear particularly promising. Available data is often confounded by selection size and bias, and the lack of prospective data. Of those with potential promise, one of the most widely studied is gene expression profiling (GEP).

Gene-expression arrays have the ability to look at the signaling of thousands of genes simultaneously. Investigators have applied this technology in an attempt to identify gene signaling patterns/signatures that are associated with patient outcome and prognoses. Preliminary results, even in small sample sizes, suggest that GEP may provide a powerful tool to determine a prognosis or identify a response to therapy (202,203).

Primary Prevention

Primary prevention involves activities that are aimed at reducing and removing factors that increase risk of breast cancer. The biggest determinants of breast cancer risk are related to endogenous hormone levels and major reproductive events, and therefore do not lend themselves to traditional prevention strategies. Several approaches to reduce the risk of breast cancer have been proposed, including risk-reducing surgery, modulation of risk factors, and chemoprevention. For some women, surgical intervention seems somewhat radical, and it is unlikely that prospective randomized trials evaluating its efficacy will ever be conducted. Risk-factor modulation is associated with poor compliance and is difficult to control; chemoprevention has been the primary focus over the last decade.

Prophylactic Risk-Reducing Mastectomy

Although no randomized prospective studies comparing different techniques of prophylactic mastectomy (PM) or comparing PM with other modalities of breast cancer risk reduction have been conducted, nonrandomized studies have reported a 90% reduction in breast cancer risk after PM (204). However, its efficacy must be considered in terms of surgical complications and psychosocial impact, and patients must be carefully selected for consideration of PM, as only high-risk women are most likely to benefit from the procedure. The two obvious categories of high-risk patients that might potentially benefit from PM are women with a known or suspected genetic predisposition for breast cancer, and patients with a unilateral breast cancer. The recently published Prevention and Observation of Surgical Endpoints (PROSE) study that prospectively followed 483 BRCA mutation carriers who elected for either bilateral PM ($n = 105$) or not ($n = 378$) reported with a (mean follow-up of 6.4 years) that bilateral PM reduced the risk of breast cancer by approximately 95% in women with prior or concurrent bilateral prophylactic oophorectomy (PO), and by approximately 90% in women with intact ovaries (205).

A personal history of breast cancer is a well-established risk factor for development of a new primary breast neoplasm, with an incidence of approximately 0.8% per year in the non-BRCA population, and as high as 5.6% per year for women with known mutations in BRCA1 or BRCA2 (206). Clinical features such as family history, young age at diagnosis, and a history of radiation therapy for the first breast cancer, and pathologic features such as LCIS, invasive lobular cancer, and multicentric cancer, have been reported to suggest an increased risk of developing a bilateral breast cancer. As well as risk reduction, contralateral PM has several other potential benefits (cosmetic, psychological, etc.). Furthermore, there is a small but significant risk that contralateral

PM specimens may be positive for either high-risk lesions or cancer, and patients need to be counseled as such.

Overall, whether or not contralateral PM has any survival benefit remains undetermined as the general consensus is that survival for a breast cancer patient is generally dictated by the first cancer. Patients with one breast cancer are likely to be observed more closely so that a second tumor will be detected at an early stage and likely be treatable with a breast-preserving operation. Ultimately, the decision to undergo PM is highly personal and must be preceded by an in-depth assessment of the woman's risk of breast cancer, and a thorough discussion of the alternative options (close surveillance, chemoprevention, and PO), benefits of the procedure weighed against its potential surgical risks, and psychological impact. Large studies have shown that more than 95% of patients were pleased with the outcome of PM (207).

Prophylactic Risk-Reducing Salpingo-Oophorectomy

Prophylactic risk-reducing salpingo-oophorectomy (PRRSO) has also been evaluated in nonrandomized studies and consistently results in a 50% (or greater) reduction in breast cancer risk (84,106). Not only are BRCA1/BRCA2 mutation carriers at risk of developing a breast cancer, but they are also at risk of developing ovarian cancer. Beyond the childbearing years, PO should be strongly considered by all individuals with hereditary susceptibility to breast cancer (208) as PO can reduce their risk of developing ovarian cancer by 50% to 98%. However, it is important to keep in mind that "prophylactic" procedures are not completely protective and that primary peritoneal cancer poses a small but real risk after PO ($\sim$2%).

Chemoprevention

Several classes of agents are under investigation for chemoprevention. Of these, SERM and AI hold most clinical relevance. Other promising agents include anti-inflammatory agents [aspirin/nonsteroidal anti-inflammatory drugs (NSAIDs)/cyclo-oxygenase 2 (COX-2) inhibitors] (209–211), retinoids (212), and HMG-CoA reductase inhibitors (213).

Four major randomized, prospective, placebo-controlled trials have evaluated the role of tamoxifen in breast cancer chemoprevention (102,214,215). Sample selection and size varied between these trials, and this was reflected in their varied results. A recently published meta-analysis of these four trials concluded that tamoxifen reduced that incidence of breast cancer by 38% (p <0.0001) (216). Of note, this trial also validated previous findings that tamoxifen reduces the incidence of ER-positive tumors, but has no effect on the incidence of ER-negative tumors. Unfortunately, tamoxifen has a number of side effects, some of which may have significant risk, including increased incidence of thromboembolic events and endometrial cancer. Whether or not such side effects increase overall mortality remains to be seen. Overall, it is clear for women at high risk of developing a breast cancer that the benefits of taking tamoxifen outweigh the risks.

Raloxifene is a second-generation SERM that is similar to tamoxifen in terms of its antiestrogenic effects on the breast. However, it differs from tamoxifen as it does not appear to have a proestrogenic effect on the endometrium. Initially investigated for its beneficial effect on bone in postmenopausal women [Multiple Outcomes for Raloxifene Evaluation (MORE) trial] (217), raloxifene was found to reduce the incidence of breast cancer in this population. This motivated a large, randomized double-blind comparing tamoxifen to raloxifene for the prevention of breast cancer [Study of Tamoxifen and Raloxifene (STAR) trial]. Its initial results have concluded that raloxifene is as effective as tamoxifen in reducing the risk of invasive breast cancer, has a lower risk of thromboembolic events and cataracts, but has a non-statistically significant higher risk of noninvasive breast cancer (however, we await the delineation of DCIS versus LCIS). The risk of other cancers, fractures, ischemic heart disease, and stroke was also similar for both drugs.

As discussed previously, in postmenopausal women the ovaries are no longer the primary sources of estrogen. The adrenal glands take over, and the adipose and breast tissue become the principal sites of aromatization. AIs exemethasane, anastrazole, and letrozole are 3 FDA-approved AIs that have been shown to have comparable efficacy to SERMs (as well as a different side effect profile) in the adjuvant treatment of breast cancer (218–220). Three trials [Arimidex, Tamoxifen Alone or in Combination (ATAC), National Cancer Institute of Canada (NCIC) MA-17, and Intergroup Exemestane Study (IES)] that compared the use of AIs in sequence with, or in lieu of, tamoxifen in the adjuvant setting have reported reductions in the risk of contralateral cancer with AIs, thereby suggesting that AIs may be efficacious primary chemopreventative agents. Clinical trials evaluating their potential are ongoing.

Management

Surgery

From risk-reducing procedures to diagnosis, staging, treatment, reconstruction, palliation and posttreatment follow-up, the role of the surgeon in breast cancer management is vast.

Diagnosis

Although the introduction of sterotactic core biopsy of nonpalpable lesions has facilitated a less-invasive approach to diagnosis, not all lesions are suitable for small congenital nevi (SCN), and both discordance and underestimation are a reality; as a result, excisional biopsy is often required. Nonpalpable lesions not amenable to percutaneous biopsy techniques require image-guided localization and surgical excision, and the primary goal of a surgical biopsy is to achieve a tissue diagnosis. Needle localization can be challenging for the radiologist; different imaging modalities and multiple wires may be required. Success is dependent on good communication between the radiologist and surgeon.

The incision should be made over the lesion within the boundaries of potential incisions for further definitive therapy. The amount of tissue excised will depend on the level of suspicion and the size of the mass. In general, extensive dissection is not recommended as the procedure is diagnostic and tumor-free margins might be difficult to achieve. Once the lesion has been excised, careful palpation of the lesion and the cavity walls is important to ensure that the tumor has not been breached and has been excised within a capsule of macroscopically normal breast tissue. All specimens should be orientated and sent to pathology, where the margins should be inked and formal histopathologic assessment performed.

Staging

Axillary node status is the single most important prognostic variable in breast cancer, and systemic therapy is based on the presence of nodal disease. Traditionally, axillary dissection (ALND) was required to assess the nodal status of patients, but sentinel lymph node biopsy (SLNB) can spare patients axillary dissection by accurately sampling the axilla (4). SNLB is a diagnostic staging procedure based on the hypothesis that the breast drains as single unit to a few common nodes in the axilla, thereby disseminating tumor cells that colonize one or a few lymph nodes before involving others. This hypothesis has been validated by prospective trials that have consistently reported sensitivity of SLNB in the range of 90% to 98%, and false-negative rates of 2% to 4%. Lymphatic mapping is an essential element of SLNB, demonstrating nonaxillary sites of drainage in 19% to 49% (221). The clinical relevance of nonaxillary SLNB involvement in early stage breast cancer remains uncertain. Clinical examination of the axilla is unreliable for evaluating nodal status in breast cancer patients. Even intraoperative examination is challenging as malignant nodes may appear completely normal, and reactive adenopathy may be indistinguishable from gross metastasis. The high false-positive rate associated with clinical examination means that clinically positive nodes alone are not a clear justification for full lymph node dissection, suggesting a wider role for SLNB (18,19).

Although the morbidity of SLNB is less than that of ALND, SLNB is not completely without morbidity. Assessing the histopathologic features of the tumor remains a useful goal to eliminate the morbidity of ALND or SLNB; however, to date, no predictive models have exceeded the high level of accuracy associated with SLNB. Importantly, despite relatively short follow-up, current data suggests that axillary local recurrence after a negative SLNB is extremely rare and comparable to that of ALND (222).

In all, despite wide variations in technique, the results of SLNB appear to be constant. SLNB is suitable for virtually all patients with clinical stage T1-2N0 invasive breast cancer (223) and may also have a role in DCIS (183), multicentric disease (224), PM (225), following neoadjuvant chemotherapy (226), and in ipsilateral breast tumor recurrence (IBTR) after breast conservation (227).

Treatment

From radical mastectomy to BCT, the last 35 years have witnessed an interesting evolution in the role of the surgeon in the treatment of breast cancer. The focus of clinical trials has been on curable disease (stage 0–III); only recently has it been on locally advanced stage III cancer.

DCIS

For decades, mastectomy was considered the treatment of choice for DCIS. Several studies evaluated the outcome of patients treated with lumpectomy alone and reported local recurrence rates of 10% to 15% (228), and (although criticized for selection bias, lack of margin status, and short follow-up), these studies showed that most recurrences occur at the site of the original excision. There has been no randomized prospective trial comparing mastectomy versus wide-local excision alone for DCIS. Randomized trials have shown that the addition of RT to surgical excision alone reduces the rate of ipsilateral breast recurrence in patients with DCIS (229). Furthermore, the addition of tamoxifen to surgical excision plus RT provides a modest additional reduction in ipsilateral breast recurrences and new contralateral primary cancers. Of note, none of these trials demonstrate a survival difference among treatment arms. Clearly there exists a subgroup of patients who can safely be treated with surgical excision alone; however, such a low-risk population remains undefined. Most surgeons now would favor breast conservation over mastectomy. However, patient selection remains a significant clinical challenge. Examination of re-excision specimens in patients with DCIS shows that the likelihood of further disease is related to the resection margin and, although there is a very low risk of death associated with DCIS, there is good evidence that surgical resection margins free of DCIS should be obtained (230).

Invasive disease (stage I–III)

From extended and super-radical mastectomy to BCT, over the last century, there has been a fascinating, evidence-based evolution in the surgical management of early breast cancer (Fig. 13.10).

Decades of clinical trials have consistently shown that early-stage breast cancer can be successfully managed by BCT (lumpectomy followed by radiation) or mastectomy (Table 13.5), and the current standard of care is that the primary treatment of localized breast cancer is either breast-conserving surgery and radiation therapy, or mastectomy (with or without breast reconstruction).

Patients suitable for BCT (table of contraindications, Table 13.6) (231) should be counseled about margin re-excision, postoperative radiation, surveillance, and the risk of local recurrence. Adequate margins are an essential component of BCT; numerous studies have correlated lumpectomy margin status with risk of local recurrence (232). Direct inspection and palpation of the specimen and the cavity may reveal residual areas of disease. Re-excision is sometimes required and is best done at the time of first operation. Orientation of re-excision specimens is fundamental. One of the major controversies surrounding

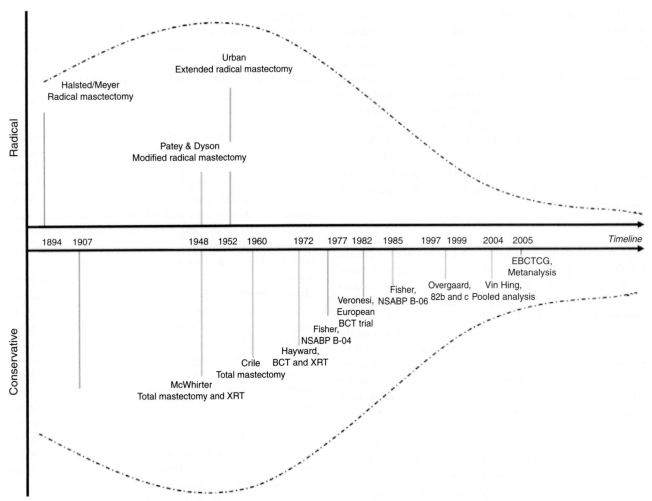

FIGURE 13.10 The evolution of the ideal treatment approach to early-stage invasive breast cancers. The horizontal line illustrates the "ideal treatment." Treatments above this line are associated with increased patient morbidity, and treatments below the line are associated with increased patient risk. EBCTCG, Early Breast Cancer Trialists Collaborative Group; NSABP, National Surgical Adjuvant Breast and Bowel Project; BCT, breast-conservation therapy; XRT, radiotherapy.

BCT is the fact that there is neither a universally accepted method of assessing margin status nor a way of defining the optimal tumor-free margin.

Centered in the midst of this BCT evolution has been the issue of "local control, does it matter?" All modern clinical trials of breast conservation have consistently shown that negative margins and postoperative RT decrease the rate of local recurrence, but have failed to demonstrate a survival benefit from improved locoregional control. Many investigators have refused to accept this finding, citing statistical limitations of the available studies, and despite progressive attempts to refine the surgical component of BCT (lumpectomy, segmentectomy, or quadrantectomy), neither the extent of local breast surgery nor the management of the axillary nodal basin have been shown to impact survival (233). However, the recently published landmark meta-analysis from the Early Breast Cancer Trialists Collaborative Group (EBCTCG) has provided us with comprehensive evidence that optimal local control does matter (234).

An estimated 25% of patients with invasive disease will either be unsuitable for BCT or will choose mastectomy. In addition, of the 75% of women with invasive disease who are suitable for BCT, between 10% and 20% will ultimately require a mastectomy for residual disease (persistent positive margins). For those patients who choose mastectomy, reconstruction should be offered. Total mastectomy (removal of the breast and underlying pectoralis major fascia) and SLNB, or modified radical mastectomy (complete removal of the breast, the underlying pectoralis major fascia, and an ALND) is a reasonable option. In selected patients, skin-sparing mastectomy (SSM) with SLNB/ALND can facilitate immediate breast reconstruction. Suitable candidates for SSM include those undergoing PM, patients with DCIS, or those with small primary tumors without lymphovascular invasion. SSM is contraindicated in those with inflammatory cancer. Using such selection criteria should result in a local recurrence rate comparable to that of traditional mastectomy. The true SSM removes the nipple-areolar complex. There is evidence to

TABLE 13.5

Prospective Randomized Trials Comparing Mastectomy and Axillary Dissection to Breast-Conservation Therapy

Clinical Trial	Dates	n	TNM	Margin Status	XRT Boost	Follow-up (yr)	Local Recurrence (%)		Overall Survival (%)	
							Mx	BCT and XRT	Mx	BCT and XRT
Institute Gustave Roussy (France)	1972–1979	179	≤2 cm N0N1 M0	2 cm	Yes	14.5	11	11.4	6, 5	72
National Tumour Institute (Milan)	1973–1980	701	≤2 cm N0N1 M0	Wide free	Yes	20	2.3	8.8	41.2	41.7
NSABP B06	1976–1984	1,217	≤4 cm N0N1 M0	Tumor free	Yes	20	10.2	14.3	47.2	46.2
National Cancer Institute, U.S.	1979–1987	247	≤5 cm N0N1 M0	Grossly free	Yes	10	10	18	7, 5	77
EORTC	1980–1986	874	≤5 cm N0N1 M0	1 cm	Yes	8	10	15	64	66
Danish Breast Cancer Group	1983–1987	859	Any size N0N1 M0	Grossly free	Yes	6	4	3	82	79

TNM, tumor, nodes, metastasis; N0, node negative; N1, node positive; M0, no distant metastasis; XRT, radiotherapy; Mx, mastectomy; BCT, breast-conservation therapy; XRT, radiotherapy; EORTC, European Organization for Research and Treatment of Cancer.

suggest that in selected patients, SSM with nipple-areolar preservation may be a viable option (235); however, such data awaits further validation.

Between 10% and 40% of those with a positive SLNB will have metastatic disease in the remaining axillary nodes. Pathologic size, lymphovascular invasion, method of detection, number of positive sentinel lymph nodes (SLNs), and number of negative SLNs, appear to be associated with the likelihood of additional, non-SLN metastases (236). Owing to the close proximity of the axillary nodes to the nerves and vessels of the axilla, residual nodal disease can

TABLE 13.6

ᵃContraindications to Breast-Conservation Therapy (BCT)

Absolute	Multicentric disease; previous irradiation to that area; multiple, persistent positive margins; pregnancy (first or second trimester); collagen vascular disease.
Relative	Tumor size; breast size; pregnancy (third trimester).

ᵃReprinted with permission from Borgen PI, Moore MO, Heerdt AS, et al. Breast-conservation therapy for invasive carcinoma of the breast. *Curr Probl Surg* 1995;32:190–247.

lead to obvious morbidity, but whether residual disease affects overall survival is more controversial (237). In all, there is compelling evidence to suggest that untreated axillary disease can affect survival by acting as the source of disseminating cells. The current standard of care is to offer completion ALND to optimize local control, and we await the results of the American College of Surgeons Oncology Group (ACSOG) Z11 trial for definite proof as to whether more surgery, radiation, or both, will contribute to overall survival.

Locally advanced breast cancer

Locally advanced breast cancer (LABC) encompasses a group of clinical entities (stage IIIA or B breast carcinoma, inflammatory disease and locally recurrent/persistent disease) that present in the absence of distant disease. Although there are some randomized, controlled trials evaluating various treatment modalities for LABC, most of the data comes from retrospective reviews and Phase II studies. Traditionally, if tumors showed any of the characteristic "grave signs," (chest-wall fixation, skin edema, ulceration, the presence of satellite nodules, inflammation, matted or fixed axillary nodes, supraclavicular node involvement, or ipsilateral arm edema), they were felt to be inoperable and were associated with a 20% 5-year survival rate (238). The current approaches with AC or neoadjuvant chemotherapy, followed by surgery and RT, are associated with significantly improved survival rates (239,240). In addition, neoadjuvant chemotherapy can decrease the size of the primary tumor, thereby allowing for breast-conserving surgery in women who might not otherwise qualify. Trials that compared neoadjuvant to adjuvant appear comparable, but neoadjuvant has the added advantage of assessing response to treatment and the increased likelihood of successful breast preservation in women with large tumors.

For patients undergoing neoadjuvant therapy, the timing of SLNB (i.e., before or after systemic therapy) has been cause for much debate. Neoadjuvant chemotherapy can convert clinically apparent axillary nodes to pathologically negative status. A concern with inflammatory breast cancer is that the false-negative rate for SLNB will be high because of the presence of partially obstructed, functionally-abnormal subdermal lymphatics. Guidelines from ASCO do not recommend the routine use of SLNB for patients with tumor sizes greater than 5 cm, T4 primaries (i.e., skin and/or chest wall invasion), or inflammatory breast cancer; however, there is no consensus as to the best approach (241).

Reconstruction

Breast reconstruction is a significant contributor to the restoration of a woman's psychological and physical well-being, which is an important component of breast cancer management. Immediate reconstruction is an oncologically safe procedure. It offers better cosmetic outcome, reduced risk of anesthesia-related complications, and psychological benefits for the patient, and is the approach of choice for most women. Reconstruction options include reconstruction with implants or autologous tissue (pedicle or free myocutaneous flaps).

Breast reconstruction is complex, and careful patient counseling and selection are essential for successful outcome. Several factors will determine a patient's suitability (disease stage, comorbidities, adjuvant RT, or chemotherapy, preexisting implants) and optimal procedure (body habitus, mastectomy/partial mastectomy/lumpectomy, patient expectation).

Surgical Palliation

The National Cancer Center Consortium Network (NCCN) recommends that the main goals in the treatment of metastatic breast cancer should be to control the disease, improve quality-of-life, and prolong survival (242). As such, current therapy for stage IV breast cancer is "metastasis-directed" and primarily employs systemic therapy. Conventional wisdom holds that treatment of local disease is indicated only in the presence of symptoms.

The development of more sophisticated imaging technology has improved the detection of small foci of distant disease, potentially upgrading women to stage IV at an earlier time point in the natural history of their disease. This diagnostic stage-shift has been associated with a clear "within stage" (167) decrease in tumor burden, which suggests that the current stage IV population is very different from that of 15 years ago. Clinical studies are continually updating and

clarifying the roles of chemotherapy, hormonal therapy, and biological therapy in stage IV disease, and such advances in systemic therapies have improved survival times for selected patients (243). In addition, a surgical approach to metastatic disease has provided some evidence that an aggressive multimodal approach to patients with limited metastatic disease may provide a survival benefit (244,245). Three recently published retrospective reviews of population-based cancer registries have suggested a potential survival benefit from complete excision of the primary tumor in patients with stage IV disease (246–249), but caution is warranted in interpreting the results of comparative studies due to the selection bias that is inherent in such reports. There are no randomized trials showing that resection of any metastatic site prolongs survival compared with systemic treatment alone; therefore whether surgery prolongs survival in the setting of metastatic disease has not been conclusively proved.

Radiotherapy

RT plays an important role in the management of breast cancer at every stage of the disease. The choice of radiation therapy techniques varies greatly between centers, and promising new approaches such as intraoperative radiation therapy (IORT) are being developed in specialized centers.

Successful treatment of DCIS begins with wide-local excision or mastectomy. Two prospective, randomized trials (NSABP B17 and EORTC 10853) (102,229) have assessed the value of postlumpectomy radiation for patients with DCIS. Analyzing more than 1,800 patients at a median follow-up of 8 and 4 years, respectively, these studies reported a significantly decreased risk of ipsilateral breast cancer recurrence (12.1% versus 26.8% overall; 3.9% versus 13.4% invasive recurrence) and improved local relapse-free survival rates (91% versus 84%). However, other investigators advocate the treatment of DCIS with radiation alone (250–252).

In contrast to DCIS, numerous prospective randomized trials have established the role of RT in the management of invasive disease postlumpectomy (all patients) and postmastectomy (select patients). Such studies have consistently shown that optimal local control with adequate surgery and postoperative radiation decreases the risk of local recurrence. Although it seemed intuitive that optimizing local control would infer a survival advantage, for many reasons (sample size, short follow-up, etc.), these studies failed to reliably prove any overall survival benefit. Considering only unconfounded prospective randomized clinical trials (i.e., no difference in the treatment groups in terms of chemotherapy), the EBCTCG performed a meta-analysis combining all individual patient data (including initial characteristics, surgical procedures, RT regimens, local recurrence definitions, and causes of death) for 42,080 women who collectively took part in 78 treatment comparisons (RT versus none, more versus less surgery, and more surgery versus RT). They found that in the hypothetical absence of any other cause of death, postoperative RT for patients with a high risk of local recurrence confers a 20% absolute reduction in the risk of local recurrence at 5 years, and may lead to a 5% absolute reduction in the risk of breast cancer-specific mortality at 15 years.

Downstaging patients with large primary tumors and/or extensive nodal disease with neoadjuvant chemotherapy and RT may open the doors to BCT (253,254). The treatment of inflammatory carcinoma can be more challenging. A recent report suggests that a combined-modality approach (neoadjuvant chemotherapy followed by mastectomy, and AC with accelerated hyperfractionated radiation) has transformed what was once a disease with local control rates less than 50% to one with local control rates in the order of 70% to 80% (255).

Radiation therapy also plays a role in the management of occult disease. A standard approach to a patient who presents with axillary disease without an identifiable primary is to give up to eight cycles of neoadjuvant therapy, followed by local excision of all gross disease, followed by radiation to the breast and the axilla. Such an approach has been reported to be associated with high rates of locoregional control. RT can also be an effective tool in the management of patients with stage IV disease with a symptomatic primary or metastatic lesion (256).

Ultimately, although there are survival (disease-free and overall) benefits associated with RT, we caution that radiation is not without risks. It is not unreasonable to suggest that for some women, the absolute benefit of RT would be negligible, thereby making omission reasonable. For others, the absolute benefit in terms of breast cancer risk may be real, but may be comparable to the potential risks involved; approaches such as partial radiation or IORT may be more appropriate. Finally, it is worth mentioning that concern has been raised that cells that carry a BRCA1/BRCA2 mutation may be exquisitely sensitive to radiation; therefore BRCA1/BRCA2 mutation carriers may show greater radiation–related toxicity that those without mutations. To date, this data is inconclusive (257,258).

Chemotherapy

The last 30 years have witnessed an explosion of cytotoxic agents to treat micrometastatic disease. Numerous trials support the role of chemotherapy in the neoadjuvant, adjuvant, and metastatic settings in terms of disease-free and overall survival, and have sought to optimize outcome in terms of agent, dose delivery, sequence, and single versus combined modality therapy. A thorough discussion is beyond the scope of this chapter.

In June 2005, the EBCTCG combined the results of 194 unconfounded randomized trials of systemic adjuvant treatment [cyclophosphamide, methotrexate, fluorouracil (CMF)/anthracycline-based combinations such as fluorouracil, doxorubicin, cyclophosphamide (FAC)/or fluorouracil, epirubicin, cyclophosphamide (FEC) and tamoxifen, or ovarian suppression] for early breast cancer in

approximately 150,000 women, many with long-term follow-up, in an incredibly comprehensive meta-analysis. Although none of the included trials included modern agents such as taxanes, trastuzumab, or modern AIs, the group concluded that in the adjuvant setting for patients with early-stage disease, the use of these more traditional agents was associated with a substantial reduction in both 5-year recurrence and 15-year mortality (243).

However, the heterogeneity of breast cancer is reflected in its varied response to chemotherapy. For instance, without chemotherapy, the 10-year survival rate can approach 98% for some tumors, whereas up to 30% of patients with potentially curable disease (stage 0–III) will develop distant metastases. Although some pathologic parameters (ER/PR/HER2/neu status, size of tumor) can help predict outcome with chemotherapy, their contribution is somewhat limited. Molecular signatures that predict outcome to chemotherapy have been developed (259) and validated (oncotype DX/NSABP B14). As with all forms of treatment, several factors (absolute risk of recurrence/relapse, potential toxicity, patient's needs, objectives and understanding) should be taken into account when considering AC. Controversy exists as to the entry criteria for chemotherapy and is the subject of much debate. For example, in the United States, the NCCN recommends adjuvant therapy as a routine treatment for all patients with 1-cm tumors, regardless of nodal status. In contrast, these patients would not be treated according to standards in Europe. In the current era of efficacious hormonal and molecular therapies, it is likely that many women might safely forego chemotherapy; however, an accurate method of identifying such patients remains undefined.

Chemotherapy plays an important role in the management of locally advanced disease. Patients with operable disease may be candidates for neoadjuvant chemotherapy, which may downstage the primary tumor, permitting less-extensive surgery (breast conservation). Those with inoperable disease are offered chemotherapy as a first line. Current regimes include a taxane (paclitaxel or docetaxel). Not all patients will respond to neoadjuvant therapy.

As most breast cancer death is related to metastatic disease, current therapy for stage IV breast cancer is "metastasis-directed." Chemotherapy, along with hormone and molecular therapies, are the mainstay of treatment. The decision whether to treat with chemotherapy or hormonal therapy as a first-line agent depends on factors such as ER/PR status, age of the patient and disease-free interval. The duration of treatment can be intermittent or continuous, and the patients' previous therapies, comorbidities, and HER2/neu status will determine which agent is used. This technique remains investigational, however. In all, an anthracycline-based regimen is the most frequent first-line agent. Paclitaxel is used as a first-line agent for patients previously treated with anthracyclines, or patients deemed unsuitable for doxorubicin-based agents.

Hormonal Therapy

Endocrine therapy is the most important systemic treatment for women with hormone receptor–positive breast cancer. Although the addition of AC to hormonal therapy can further reduce the risk of disease recurrence (260), the benefits of chemotherapy are generally greater in women with hormone receptor–negative disease than hormone receptor–positive disease, particularly when women with receptor-positive disease receive adjuvant endocrine therapy (261).

For the last three decades, tamoxifen, which works by competitively antagonizing hormonal receptors in breast cancer cells, has been the standard of care for adjuvant therapy for any woman with hormone receptor–positive early breast cancer (including DCIS), regardless of menopausal status, nodal status, or stage of disease. Comprehensive meta-analyses have proved its role in the adjuvant setting in improving both disease-free and overall survival.

Ovarian ablation as an adjuvant treatment has been reported to result in an 18% proportional reduction in the risk of breast cancer–related death in women younger than 50 (243). In the premenopausal setting, the addition of goserelin (gonadotropin hormone-releasing hormone) to tamoxifen seems to improve survival in women with estrogen receptor–positive disease. This method has already been proved as effective as chemotherapy in preventing recurrence, and ongoing trials are aiming to better define its role in the adjuvant setting and, in particular, the optimal duration of ovarian suppression.

In the postmenopausal setting, AIs have revolutionized the adjuvant treatment of hormone-responsive cancers of all stages. The current standard of care has come to include AIs, as an alternative, in sequence, after 5 years of tamoxifen. However, whether 5 years of an AI alone or 5 years of sequential therapy is the more beneficial treatment approach awaits longer follow-up of the disease-free and overall survival rates in the respective studies. Finally, although the indication for the use of extended adjuvant therapy with 5 years of letrozole after 5 years of tamoxifen, or the use of letrozole monotherapy for 5 years, was recently approved, wide application is pending FDA approval.

Hormone-therapy resistance is an unfortunate reality and is the focus of extensive research. The mechanisms remain undefined.

Molecular Therapy

Molecular targeting compounds that are directed against the known molecular pathways involved in breast cancer [type I growth factors (*HER-2/neu*; EGFR), angiogenesis, cyclooxigenase-2, tyrosine kinase pathway, etc.] have been the subject of intense research over the last two decades. Currently, trastuzumab is the first agent approved for therapy of *HER-2/neu* overexpressing tumors; however, several other compounds directed against different targets have entered clinical evaluation.

Gene Therapy

The delineation of the molecular basis of neoplasia provides the possibility of specific intervention by gene therapy through the introduction of genetic material for therapeutic purposes. In this regard, several gene therapy approaches have been developed for the treatment of cancer:

- Mutation compensation (e.g., TSG replacement) (262)
- Molecular chemotherapy (renders cells more chemosensitive) (263)
- Genetic immunopotentiation (264)
- Proapoptotic gene therapy (265)
- Antiangiogenic gene therapy (266)
- Genetic modulation of resistance/sensitivity (267)

Clinical trials have been initiated to evaluate the safety, toxicity, and efficacy of each of these approaches, and combined modality therapy with gene therapy and chemotherapy or radiation therapy has shown promising results.

Special Considerations

Male Breast Cancer

Male breast cancer is a rare disease; less than 1% of all breast cancer patients are male. [Rates vary widely and can be as high as 15% in countries such as Uganda and Zambia, where parasitic liver disease is endemic. Suggested risk factors for male breast cancer include genetic abnormalities (BRCA2, Kleinfelter syndrome 47XXY), previous exposure to ionizing radiation, liver disease, testicular damage, obesity, excess alcohol intake, and occupation.] However, most male breast cancer patients have no identifiable risks. Most significantly, up to 20% of men with breast cancer have a first-degree relative with the disease; between 4% and 40% of male breast cancers are thought to result from a BRCA1/BRCA2 mutation (BRCA2 > BRCA1) (268).

The most common presenting symptom is a painless lump. There is no convincing data to suggest that gynecomastia increases the risk of male breast cancer. MG is an effective diagnostic modality with sensitivity and specificity of more than 90%. Similar to female breast cancer, the most common histologic subtype is invasive ductal carcinoma, and most tumors are ER/PR-positive. Management is similar to female breast cancer with similar focus on optimal local control and nodal status. Tamoxifen is frequently recommended as an adjuvant hormonal therapy, and retrospective studies report improved disease-free survival (269). The use of AI has not been evaluated; however, available data on AC suggests a survival benefit is limited (270). Hormonal therapy is the primary modality used to treat advanced disease. Endocrine ablation (surgical or medical) is associated with substantial response rates (271).

Male breast cancer typically presents with more extensive disease than female breast cancer and, as such, carries a worse prognosis. Age, nodal status, and ER/PR status are important prognostic and predictive factors.

REFERENCES

1. Romrell LJ, Bland K. Anatomy of the breast, axilla, chest wall and related metastatic sites. In: Bland K, Copeland EM III, eds. *The Breast, comprehensive management of benign and malignant disorders*, 3rd ed. Philadelphia: WB Saunders, 2004.

2. Osborne MJ. Anatomy of the breast. In: Harris JR, Lippmann ME, Morrow M, et al. eds. *Diseases of the breast*, 3rd ed. Lippincott Williams & Wilkins, 2004.

3. Klauber-DeMore N, Bevilacqua JL, Van Zee KJ, et al. Comprehensive review of the management of internal mammary lymph node metastases in breast cancer. *J Am Coll Surg* 2001;193(5):547–555.

4. Cody HS. Sentinel lymph node biopsy for breast cancer: does anybody not need one? *Ann Surg Oncol* 2003;10(10):1131–1132.

5. Krag D, Weaver D, Ashikaga T, et al. The sentinel node in breast cancer. *N Engl J Med* 1998;339:941–946.

6. Morrow M. Therapeutic value of axillary lymph node dissection. In: Bland K, Copeland EM III, eds. *The breast*, 3rd ed. Philadelphia: WB Saunders, 2004.

7. Rampaul RS, Mullinger K, Macmillan RD, et al. Incidence of clinically significant lymphoedema as a complication following surgery for primary operable breast cancer. *Eur J Cancer* 2003;39(15):2165–2167.

8. Sakakura T. Mammary embryogenesis. In: Neville MC, Daniel CW, eds. *The mammary gland: development regulation and function*, New York: Plenum Publishing, 1987:37–66.

9. Howard BA, Gusterson BA. Human breast development. *J Mammary Gland Biol Neoplasia* 2000;5(2):119–137.

10. Russo J, Russo IH. Development of the humanmammary gland. In: Neville MC, Daniel CW, eds. *The mammary gland: development regulation and function*. New York: Plenum Publishing, 1987:67–93.

11. Potten CS, Watson RJ, Williams GT, et al. The effect of age and menstrual cycle upon proliferative activity of the normal human breast. *Br J Cancer* 1988;58(2):163–170.

12. Hussain Z, Roberts N, Whitehouse GH, et al. Estimation of breast volume and its variation during the menstrual cycle using MRI and stereology. *Br J Radiol* 1999;72(855):236–245.

13. Houssami N, Cheung MN, Dixon JM. Fibroadenoma of the breast. *Med J Aust* 2001;174(4):185–188.

14. Berry DA, Cronin KA, Plevritis SK, et al. Cancer Intervention and Surveillance Modeling Network (CISNET) Collaborators. Effect of screening and adjuvant therapy on mortality from breast cancer. *N Engl J Med* 2005;353:1784.

15. Lau S, Kuchenmeister I, Stachs A, et al. Pathologic nipple discharge: surgery is imperative in postmenopausal women. *Ann Surg Oncol* 2005;12(7):546–551.

16. Simmons R, Adamovich T, Brennan M, et al. Nonsurgical evaluation of pathologic nipple discharge. *Ann Surg Oncol* 2003;10(2):113–116.

17. Van Zee KJ, Ortega Perez G, Minnard E, et al. Preoperative galactography increases the diagnostic yield of major duct excision for nipple discharge. *Cancer* 1998;82(10):1874–1880.

18. Fisher B, Wolmark N, Bauer M, et al. The accuracy of clinical nodal staging and of limited axillary dissection as a determinant of histologic nodal status in carcinoma of the breast. *Gynecol Obstetynecol Obstet* 1981;152:765–772.

19. Specht MC, Fey JV, Borgen PI, et al. Is the clinically positive axilla in breast cancer really a contraindication to sentinel lymph node biopsy? *J Am Coll Surg* 2005;200(1):10–14.

20. Pisano ED, Gatsonis C, Hendrick E, et al. Digital Mammographic Imaging Screening Trial (DMIST) Investigators Group. Diagnostic performance of digital versus film mammography for breast-cancer screening. *N Engl J Med* 2005;353(17):1773–1783.

21. Liberman L, Menell JH. Breast imaging reporting and data system (BI-RADS). *Radiol Clin North Am* 2002;40(3):409–430.

22. Boyd NF, Dite GS, Stone J, et al. Heritability of mammographis density, a risk factor for breast cancer. *N Engl J Med* 2002;347:886–894.

23. Moy L, Slanetz PJ, Moore R, et al. Specificity of mammography and US in the evaluation of a palpable abnormality: retrospective review. *Radiology* 2002;225:176.

24. Morris EA. Review of breast MRI: indications and limitations. *Semin Roentgenol* 2001;36(3):226–237.

25. Liberman L. Breast cancer screening with MRI–what are the data for patients at high risk? *N Engl J Med* 2004;351(5):497–500.

26. Buchanan CL, Morris EA, Dorn PL, et al. Utility of breast magnetic resonance imaging in patients with occult primary breast cancer. *Ann Surg Oncol* 2005;12(12):1045–1053.

27. Julius T, Kemp SE, Kneeshaw PJ, et al. MRI and conservative treatment of locally advanced breast cancer. *Eur J Surg Oncol* 2005;31(10):1129–1134.

28. Bartella L, Morris EA, Dershaw DD, et al. Proton MR spectroscopy with choline peak as malignancy marker improves positive predictive value for breast cancer diagnosis: preliminary study. *Radiology* 2006;239(3):686–692.

29. Wahl RL, Siegel BA, Coleman RE, et al. PET Study Group. Prospective multicenter study of axillary nodal staging by positron emission tomography in breast cancer: a report of the staging breast cancer with PET Study Group. *J Clin Oncol* 2004;22:277–285.

30. Port ER, Yeung H, Gonen M, et al. 18F-2-fluoro-2-deoxy-D-glucose positron emission tomography scanning affects surgical management in selected patients with high-risk, operable breast carcinoma. *Ann Surg Oncol* 2006;13(5):677–684.

31. Lumachi F, Tregnaghi A, Ferretti G, et al. Accuracy of ultrasonography and (99m)Tc-sestamibi scintimammography for assessing axillary lymph node status in breast cancer patients. A prospective study. *Eur J Surg Oncol* 2006;32:933–936. [Epub ahead of print].

32. Lumachi F, Ermani M, Marzola MC, et al. Relationship between prognostic factors of breast cancer and 99mTc-sestamibi uptake in patients who underwent scintimammography: multivariate analysis of causes of false-negative results. *Breast* 2006;15(1):130–134.

33. Liu Z, Stevenson GD, Barrett HH, et al. Imaging recognition of inhibition of multidrug resistance in human breast cancer xenografts using 99mTc-labeled sestamibi and tetrofosmin. *Nucl Med Biol* 2005;32(6):573–583.

34. Liberman L, Tornos C, Huzjan R, et al. Is surgical excision warranted after benign, concordant diagnosis of papilloma at percutaneous breast biopsy? *AJR Am J Roentgenol* 2006;186(5):1328–1334.

35. Rohan TE, Miller AB. Hormone replacement therapy and risk of benign proliferative epithelial disorders of the breast. *Eur J Cancer Prev* 1999;8(2):123–130.

36. Tan-Chiu E, Wang J, Costantino JP, et al. Effects of tamoxifen on benign breast disease in women at high risk for breast cancer. *J Natl Cancer Inst* 2003;95(4):302–307.

37. Dupont WD, Page DL. Risk factors for breast cancer in women with proliferative breast disease. *N Engl J Med* 1985; 312(3):146–151.

38. Hartmann LC, Sellers TA, Frost MH, et al. Benign breast disease and the risk of breast cancer. *N Engl J Med* 2005;353(3):229–237.

39. Haagenson CD. *Diseases of the breast*, 3rd edn. Philadelphia: WB Saunders, 1986.

40. Jackman RJ, Nowels KW, Shepard MJ, et al. Stereotaxic large-core needle biopsy of 450 nonpalpable breast lesions with surgical correlation in lesions with cancer or atypical hyperplasia. *Radiology* 1994;193(1):91–95.

41. Fearon ER, Vogelstein B. A genetic model for colorectal tumorigenesis. *Cell* 1990;61:759.

42. Lakhani SR. In-situ lobular neoplasia: time for an awakening. *Lancet* 2003;361:96.

43. Simpson PT, Reis-Filho JS, Gale T, et al. Molecular evolution of breast cancer. *J Pathol* 2005;205:248–254.

44. Mommers EC, Leonhart AM, Falix F. et al Similarity in expression of cell cycle proteins between *in situ* and invasive ductal breast lesions of same differentiation grade. *J Pathol* 2001;194(3):327–333.

45. Singletary SE. A working model for the time sequence of genetic changes in breast tumorigenesis. *J Am Coll Surg* 2002;194(2):202–216.

46. Cifone MA, Fidler IJ. Increasing metastatic potential is associated with increasing genetic instability of clones isolated from murine neoplasms. *Proc Natl Acad Sci USA* 1981;78(11):6949–6952.

47. Lakhani SR, Chaggar R, Davies S, et al. Genetic alterations in "normal" luminal and myoepithelial cells of the breast. *J Pathol* 1999;189:496–503.

48. Allred DC, Mohsin SK. Biological features of premalignant disease in the human breast. *J Mammary Gland Biol Neoplasia* 2000;5:351–364.

49. Ellsworth DL, Ellsworth RE, Liebman MN, et al. Genomic instability in histologically normal breast tissues: implications for carcinogenesis. *Lancet Oncol* 2004;5(12):753–758.

50. Oved S, Yarden Y. Signal transduction: molecular ticket to enter cells. *Nature* 2002;416:133–136.

51. Schechter AL, Stern DF, Vaidyanathan L, et al. The neu oncogene: an erb-B-related gene encoding a 185,000-Mr tumour antigen. *Nature* 1984;312(5994):513–516.

52. Yamamoto T, Ikawa S, Akiyama T, et al. Similarity of protein encoded by the human c-erb-B-2 gene to epidermal growth factor receptor. *Nature* 1986;319(6050):230–234.

53. Kwong KY, Hung MC. A novel splice variant of HER2 with increased transformation activity. *Mol Carcinog* 1998;23(2):62–68.

54. Graus-Porta D, Beerli RR, Daly JM, et al. ErbB-2, the preferred heterodimerization partner of all ErbB receptors, is a mediator of lateral signaling. *EMBO J* 1997;16(7):1647–1655.

55. Cohen BD, Kiener PA, Green JM, et al. The relationship between human epidermal growth-like factor receptor expression and cellular transformation in NIH3T3 cells. *J Biol Chem* 1996;271(48):30897–30903.

56. Slamon DJ, Clark GM, Wong SG, et al. Human breast cancer: correlation of relapse and survival with amplification of the HER-2/neu oncogene. *Science* 1987;235(4785):177–182.

57. Bast RC Jr, Ravdin P, Hayes DF, et al. American Society of Clinical Oncology Tumor Markers Expert Panel. 2000 update of recommendations for the use of tumor markers in breast and colorectal cancer: clinical practice guidelines of the American society of clinical oncology, *J Clin Oncol* 2001;19:1865–1878.

58. Van de Vijver MJ, Peterse JL, Mooi WJ, et al. Neu-protein overexpression in breast cancer. Association with comedo-type ductal carcinoma *in situ* and limited prognostic value in stage II breast cancer. *N Engl J Med* 1988;319(19):1239–1245.

59. Gusterson BA, Machin LG, Gullick WJ, et al. Immunohistochemical distribution of c-erbB-2 in infiltrating and *in situ* breast cancer. *Int J Cancer* 1988;42(6):842–845.

60. Carlomagno C, Perrone F, Gallo C, et al. c-erb B2 overexpression decreases the benefit of adjuvant tamoxifen in early-stage breast cancer without axillary lymph node metastases. *J Clin Oncol* 1996;14(10):2702–2708.

61. Cobleigh MA, Vogel CL, Tripathy D, et al. Multinational study of the efficacy and safety of humanized anti-HER2 monoclonal antibody in women who have HER2-overexpressing metastatic breast cancer that has progressed after chemotherapy for metastatic disease. *J Clin Oncol* 1999;17(9):2639–2648.

62. Slamon DJ, Leyland-Jones B, Shak S, et al. Use of chemotherapy plus a monoclonal antibody against HER2 for metastatic breast cancer that overexpresses HER2. *N Engl J Med* 2001;344(11):783–792.

63. Niehans GA, Singleton TP, Dykoski D, et al. Stability of HER-2/neu expression over time and at multiple metastatic sites. *J Natl Cancer Inst* 1993;85:1230–1235.

64. Nahta R, Esteva FJ. HER-2-targeted therapy: lessons learned and future directions. *Clin Cancer Res* 2003;9:5078–5084.

65. Cardoso F, Durbecq V, Larsimont D, et al. Correlation between complete response to anthracycline-based chemotherapy and topoisomerase II-alpha gene amplification and protein overexpression in locally advanced/metastatic breast cancer. *Int J Oncol* 2004;24(1):201–209.

66. Kinzler KW, Vogelstein B. Cancer-susceptibility genes. Gatekeepers and caretakers. *Nature* 1997;386(6627):761, 763.

67. Knudson AG. Hereditary cancer: two hits revisited. *J Cancer Res Clin Oncol* 1996;122(3):135–140.

68. Lacroix M, Leclercq G. The "portrait" of hereditary breast cancer. *Breast Cancer Res Treat* 2005;89(3):297–304.

69. DeMarco TA, Loffredo CA, Sampilo ML, et al. On using a cancer center cancer registry to identify newly affected women eligible for hereditary breast cancer syndrome testing: practical considerations. *J Genet Couns* 2006;15(2):129–136.

70. Szabo CI, King MC. Population genetics of BRCA1 and BRCA2. *Am J Hum Genet* 1997;60:1013–1020.

71. Martin AM, Blackwood MA, Antin-Ozerkis D, et al. Germline mutations in BRCA1 and BRCA2 in breast-ovarian families from a breast cancer risk evaluation clinic. *J Clin Oncol* 2001;19:2247–2253.

72. Newman B, Mu H, Butler LM, et al. Frequency of breast cancer attributable to BRCA1 in a population-based series of American women. *JAMA* 1998;279(12):915–921.

73. Kim SW, Lee CS, Fey JV, et al. Prevalence of BRCA2 mutations in a hospital based series of unselected breast cancer cases. *J Med Genet* 2005;42(1):e5.

74. Struewing JP, Hartge P, Wacholder S, et al. The risk of cancer associated with specific mutations of BRCA1 and BRCA2 among Ashkenazi Jews. *N Engl J Med* 1997;336(20):1401–1408.

75. Hall JM, Lee MK, Newman B, et al. Linkage of early-onset familial breast cancer to chromosome 17q21. *Science* 1990;250(4988):1684–1689.

76. Wooster R, Neuhausen SL, Mangion J, et al. Localization of a breast cancer susceptibility gene, BRCA2, to chromosome 13q12-13. *Science* 1994;265(5181):2088–2090.

77. King MC, Marks JH, Mandell JB, New York Breast Cancer Study Group. Breast and ovarian cancer risks due to inherited mutations in BRCA1 and BRCA2. *Science* 2003;302:643.

78. Narod SA. Modifiers of risk of hereditary breast and ovarian cancer. *Nat Rev Cancer* 2002;2:113.

79. Kramer JL, Velazquez IA, Chen BE, et al. Prophylactic oophorectomy reduces breast cancer penetrance during prospective, long-term follow-up of BRCA1 mutation carriers. *J Clin Oncol* 2005;23:8629.

80. Hashizume R, Fukuda M, Maeda I, et al. The RING heterodimer BRCA1-BARD1 is a ubiquitin ligase inactivated by a breast cancer-derived mutation. *J Biol Chem* 2001;276(18):14537–14540.

81. Wooster R, Bignell G, Lancaster J, et al. Identification of the breast cancer susceptibility gene BRCA2. *Nature* 1995;378:789–792.

82. Antoniou A, Pharoah PD, Narod S, et al. Average risks of breast and ovarian cancer associated with BRCA1 or BRCA2 mutations detected in case series un selected for family history: a combined analysis of 22 studies. *Am J Hum Genet* 2003;72:1117–1130.

83. Kauff ND, Satagopan JM, Robson ME, et al. Risk-reducing salphingo-oophorectomy in women with a BRCA1 or BRCA2 mutation. *N Engl J Med* 2002;346:1609–1615 (2006 update).

84. Hartge P, Chatterjee N, Wacholder S, et al. Breast cancer risk in Ashkenazi BRCA1/2 mutation carriers effects of reproductive history. *Epidemiology* 2002;13:255–261.

85. Jernstrom H, Lerman C, Ghadirian P, et al. 1999 Pregnancy and risk of early breast cancers in carriers of BRCA1 and BRCA2. *Lancet* 1999;354:1846–1850.

86. Jernstrom H, Lubinski J, Lynch HT, et al. Breast-feeding and the risk of breast cancer in BRCA1 and BRCA2 mutation carriers. *J Natl Cancer Inst* 2004;96(14):1094–1098.

87. Cullinane CA, Lubinski J, Neuhausen SL, et al. Effect of pregnancy as a risk factor for breast cancer in BRCA1/BRCA2 mutation carriers. *Int J Cancer* 2005;117(6):988–991.

88. Narod SA, Dube MP, Klijn J, et al. Oral contraceptive and the risk of breast cancer in BRCA1 and BRCA2 mutation carriers. *J Natl Cancer Inst* 2002;94(23):1773–1779.

89. King TA, Gemignani ML, Li W, et al. Increased progesterone receptor expression in benign epithelium of BRCA1 related breast cancer. *Cancer Res* 2004;64:5051–5053.

90. Ferro P, Catalano MG, Dell'Eva R, et al. The androgen receptor CAG repeat: a modifier of carcinogenesis? *Mol Cell Endocrinol* 2002;193(1–2):109–120.

91. Irvine RA, Ma H, Yu MC, et al. Inhibition of p160-mediated coactivation with increasing androgen receptor polyglutamine length. *Hum Mol Genet* 2000;9:267–274.

92. Rebbeck TR. Inherited predisposition and breast cancer: modifiers of BRCA1/2-associated breast cancer risk. *Environ Mol Mutagen* 2002;39(2–3):228–234.

93. Gayther SA, Warren W, Mazoyer S, et al. Germline mutations of the *BRCA1* gene in breast and ovarian cancer families provide evidence for a genotype-phenotype correlation. *Nat Genet* 1995;11:428–433.

94. Thompson D, Easton D. Breast Cancer Linkage Consortium. Variation of *BRCA1* cancer risks by mutation position. *Cancer Epidemiol Biomarkers Prev* 2002;11(4):329–336.

95. Grade K, Hoffken K, Kath R, et al. *BRCA1* mutations and phenotype. *J Cancer Res Clin Oncol* 1997;123:69–70.

96. Amirimani B. Polymorphisms in XRCC1 and XPD as breast cancer risk modifiers in *BRCA1* mutation carriers. *Am J Hum Genet* 2001;69(Suppl 4):206.

97. Scully R, Chen J, Ochs RL, et al. Dynamic changes of BRCA1 subnuclear location and phosphorylation state are initiated by DNA damage. *Cell* 1997;90(3):425–435.

98. Sharan SK, Morimatsu M, Albrecht U, et al. Embryonic lethality and radiation hypersensitivity mediated by Rad51 in mice lacking Brca2. *Nature* 1997;386(6627):804–810.

99. Pierce LJ, Levin AM, Rebbeck TR, et al. Ten-year multi-institutional results of breast-conserving surgery and radiotherapy in BRCA1/2-associated stage I/II breast cancer. *J Clin Oncol* 2006;24(16):2437–2443, Epub 2006 Apr 24.

100. Brekelmans CT, Seynaeve C, Bartels CC, et al. Rotterdam Committee for Medical and Genetic Counseling. Effectiveness of breast cancer surveillance in BRCA1/2 gene mutation carriers and women with high familial risk. *J Clin Oncol* 2001;19(4):924–930.

101. Warner E, Plewes DB, Hill KA, et al. Surveillance of BRCA1 and BRCA2 mutation carriers with magnetic resonance imaging, ultrasound, mammography, and clinical breast examination. *JAMA* 2004;292(11):1317–1325.

102. Fisher B, Costantino JP, Wickerham DL, et al. Tamoxifen for prevention of breast cancer: report of the national surgical adjuvant breast and bowel project P-1 study. *J Natl Cancer Inst* 1998;90(18):1371–1388.

103. Powles TJ. Status of antiestrogen breast cancer prevention trials. *Oncology* (Williston Park). 1998;12(3, Suppl 5):28–31.

104. Narod SA, Risch H, Moslehi R, et al. Hereditary Ovarian Cancer Clinical Study Group. Oral contraceptives and the risk of hereditary ovarian cancer. *N Engl J Med* 1998;339(7):424–428.

105. Rosen PP, Groshen S, Kinne DW. Prognosis in T2N0M0 stage I breast carcinoma: a 20-year follow-up study. *J Clin Oncol* 1991;9(9):1650–1661.

106. Rebbeck TR, Levin AM, Eisen A, et al. Breast cancer risk after bilateral prophylactic oophorectomy in BRCA1 mutation carriers. *J Natl Cancer Inst* 1999;91:1475–1479.

107. Rebbeck TR, Lynch HT, Neuhausen SL, et al. Prevention and Observation of Surgical End Points Study Group. Prophylactic oophorectomy in carriers of BRCA1 or BRCA2 mutations. *N Engl J Med* 2002;346:1616–1622.

108. Struewing JP, Watson P, Easton DF, et al. Prophylactic oophorectomy in inherited breast/ovarian cancer families. *J Natl Cancer Inst Monogr* 1995;17:33–35.

109. Hollstein M, Sidransky D, Vogelstein B, et al. p53 mutations in human cancers. *Science* 1991;253(5015):49–53.

110. Silvestrini R, Benini E, Daidone MG, et al. p53 as an independent prognostic marker in lymph node-negative breast cancer patients. *J Natl Cancer Inst* 1993;85(12):965–970.

111. Allred DC, Clark GM, Elledge R, et al. Association of p53 protein expression with tumor cell proliferation rate and clinical outcome in node-negative breast cancer. *J Natl Cancer Inst* 1993;85(3):200–206.

112. Isola J, Visakorpi T, Holli K, et al. Association of overexpression of tumor suppressor protein p53 with rapid cell proliferation and poor prognosis in node-negative breast cancer patients. *J Natl Cancer Inst* 1992;84(14):1109–1114.

113. Malkin D, Li FP, Strong LC, et al. Germ line p53 mutations in a familial syndrome of breast cancer, sarcomas, and other neoplasms. *Science* 1990;250(4985):1233–1238.

114. Eng C. Genetics of Cowden syndrome: through the looking glass of oncology. *Int J Oncol* 1998;12(3):701–710.

115. Giardiello FM, Brensinger JD, Tersmette AC, et al. Very high risk of cancer in familial Peutz-Jeghers syndrome. *Gastroenterology* 2000;119(6):1447–1453.

116. Thomas HV, Reeves GK, Key TJ. Endogenous estrogen and postmenopausal breast cancer: a quantitative review. *Cancer Causes Control* 1997;8(6):922–928. Review; 8(6):922–928.

117. Hankinson SE, Willett WC, Manson JE, et al. Plasma sex steroid hormone levels and risk of breast cancer in postmenopausal women. *J Natl Cancer Inst* 1998;90(17):1292–1299.

118. Feigelson HS, Ross RK, Yu MC, et al. Genetic susceptibility to cancer from exogenous and endogenous exposures (Review). *J Cell Biochem Suppl* 1996;25:15–22.

119. Feigelson HS, Shames LS, Pike MC, et al. Cytochrome P450c17alpha gene (CYP17) polymorphism is associated with serum estrogen and progesterone concentrations. *Cancer Res* 1998;58(4):585–587.

120. Feigelson HS, McKean-Cowdin R, Pike MC, et al. Cytochrome P450c17alpha gene (CYP17) polymorphism predicts use of hormone replacement therapy. *Cancer Res* 1999;59(16):3908–3910.

121. Jernstrom H, Vesprini D, Bradlow HL, et al. Re: CYP17 promoter polymorphism and breast cancer in Australian women under age forty years. *J Natl Cancer Inst* 2001;93(7):554–555.

122. Feigelson HS, Coetzee GA, Kolonel LN, et al. A polymorphism in the CYP17 gene increases the risk of breast cancer. *Cancer Res* 1997;57(6):1063–1065.

123. Lavigne JA, Helzlsouer KJ, Huang HY, et al. An association between the allele coding for a low activity variant of catechol-O-methyltransferase and the risk for breast cancer. *Cancer Res* 1997;57(24):5493–5497.

124. Millikan RC, Pittman GS, Tse CK, et al. Catechol-O-methyltransferase and breast cancer risk. *Carcinogenesis* 1998;19(11):1943–1947.

125. Sorlie T, Tibshirani R, Parker J, et al. Repeated observation of breast tumor subtypes in independent gene expression data sets. *Proc Natl Acad Sci USA* 2003;100(14):8418–8423. Epub 2003 Jun 26.

126. Farmer P, Bonnefoi H, Becette V, et al. Identification of molecular apocrine breast tumors by microarray analysis. *Oncogene* 2005;24(29):4660–4671.

127. Moe RE, Anderson DO. Distinctive biology of pleomorphic lobular carcinoma of the breast. *J Surg Oncol* 2005;90(2):47–50.

128. De Vivo I, Hankinson SE, Colditz GA, et al. A functional polymorphism in the progesterone receptor gene is associated with an increase in breast cancer risk. *Cancer Res* 2003;63(17):5236–5238.

129. Early Breast Cancer Trialists' Collaborative Group. Tamoxifen for early breast cancer: an overview of the randomised trials. *Lancet*. 1998;351(9114):1451–1467.

130. Harvey JM, Clark GM, Osborne CK, et al. Estrogen receptor status by immunohistochemistry is superior to the ligand-binding assay for predicting response to adjuvant endocrine therapy in breast cancer. *J Clin Oncol* 1999;17(5):1474–1481.

131. Cui X, Schiff R, Arpino G, et al. Biology of progesterone receptor loss in breast cancer and its implications for endocrine therapy. *J Clin Oncol* 2005;23(30):7721–7735.

132. Steroid receptors in breast cancer: an NIH concensus development conference, Bethesda, Maryland, June 27–29, 1979. *Cancer* 1980;46(Suppl 12):2759.

133. Talley LI, Grizzle WE, Waterbor JW, et al. Hormone receptors and proliferation in breast carcinomas of equivalent histologic grades in pre- and postmenopausal women. *Int J Cancer* 2002;98(1):118–127.

134. Shaaban AM, Sloane JP, West CR, et al. Breast cancer risk in usual ductal hyperplasia is defined by estrogen receptor-alpha and Ki-67 expression. *Am J Pathol* 2002;160(2):597–604.

135. Bissell MJ, Rizki A, Mian IS. Tissue architecture: the ultimate regulator of breast epithelial function. *Curr Opin Cell Biol* 2003;15(6):753–762.

136. Paget S. The distribution of secondary growths in cancer of the breast. *Lancet* 1889;1:571–573.

137. Fidler IJ. The pathogenesis of cancer metastasis: the 'seed and soil' hypothesis revisited. *Nat Rev Cancer* 2003;3(6):453–458.

138. Fidler IJ. Selection of successive tumour lines for metastasis. *Nat New Biol* 1973;242(118):148–149.

139. Muller A, Homey B, Soto H, et al. Involvement of chemokine receptors in breast cancer metastasis. *Nature* 2001;410(6824):50–56.

140. Minn AJ, Gupta GP, Siegel PM, et al. Genes that mediate breast cancer metastasis to lung. *Nature* 2005;436(7050):518–524.

141. Karrison TG, Ferguson DJ, Meier P. Dormancy of mammary carcinoma after mastectomy. *J Natl Cancer Inst* 1999;91:80–85.

142. Klauber-DeMore N, Van Zee KJ, Linkov I, et al. Biological behavior of human breast cancer micrometastases. *Clin Cancer Res* 2001;7(8):2434–2439.

143. Demicheli R, Retsky MW, Swartzendruber DE, et al. Proposal for a new model of breast cancer metastatic development. *Ann Oncol* 1997;8:1075–1080.

144. Guidi AJ, Fischer L, Harris JR, et al. Microvessel density and distribution in ductal carcinoma *in situ* of the breast. *J Natl Cancer Inst* 1994;86(8):614–619.

145. Weidner N, Folkman J, Pozza F, et al. Tumor angiogenesis: a new significant and independent prognostic indicator in early-stage breast carcinoma. *J Natl Cancer Inst* 1992;84(24):1875–1887.

146. Weidner N, Semple JP, Welch WR, et al. Tumor angiogenesis and metastasis–correlation in invasive breast carcinoma. *N Engl J Med* 1991;324(1):1–8.

147. Miller, KD. E2100: a randomized phase III trial of paclitaxel versus paclitaxel plus bevacizumab as first-line therapy for locally recurrent or metastatic breast cancer. Data presented at the 41st *Annual Meeting of the American Society of Clinical Oncology*, Orlando, May 16, 2005.

148. Spratt JS, Meyer JS, Spratt JA. Rates of growth of human neoplasms: Part II. *J Surg Oncol* 1996;61(1):68–83.

149. Norton L. Conceptual and practical implications of breast tissue geometry: toward a more effective, less toxic therapy. *Oncologist* 2005;10(6):370–381.

150. Milde-Langosch K, Bamberger AM, Rieck G, et al. Overexpression of the p16 cell cycle inhibitor in breast cancer is associated with a more malignant phenotype. *Breast Cancer Res Treat* 2001;67(1):61–70.

151. Emig R, Magener A, Ehemann V, et al. Aberrant cytoplasmic expression of the p16 protein in breast cancer is associated with accelerated tumor proliferation. *Br J Cancer* 1998;78(12):1661–1668.

152. Roy PG, Thompson AM. Cyclin D1 and breast cancer. *Breast* 2006;15(6):718–727.

153. Husdal A, Bukholm G, Bukholm IR. The prognostic value and overexpression of cyclin A is correlated with gene amplification

154. Berglund P, Landberg G. Cyclin e overexpression reduces infiltrative growth in breast cancer: yet another link between proliferation control and tumor invasion. *Cell Cycle* 2006;5(6):606–609. Epub 2006 Mar 15.

155. Tan AR, Swain SM. Review of flavopiridol, a cyclin-dependent kinase inhibitor, as breast cancer therapy. *Semin Oncol* 2002;29(3, Suppl 11):77–85.

156. Trigo Perez JM, Gil M, Miles D, et al. A multicenter phase II study of the cell cycle inhibitor Ro 31–7453 in patients with metastatic breast cancer who have failed chemotherapy with an anthracycline and a taxane. *Proc Am Soc Clin Oncol* 2003;22:16.

157. Adair F, Berg J, Joubert L, et al. Long-term followup of breast cancer patients: the 30-year report. *Cancer* 1974;33(4):1145–1150.

158. Walter SD, Day NE. Estimation of the duration of a pre-clinical disease state using screening data. *Am J Epidemiol* 1983;118(6):865–886.

159. Andersson I. What can we learn from interval carcinomas. Recent results. *Cancer Res* 1984;90:161–163.

160. Tabar L, Fagerberg CJ, Gad A, et al. Reduction in mortality from breast cancer after mass screening with mammography. Randomised trial from the Breast Cancer Screening Working Group of the Swedish National Board of Health and Welfare. *Lancet* 1985;1(8433):829–832.

161. Shapiro S, Venet W, Strax P, et al. Ten to fourteen-year effect of screening on breast cancer mortality. *J Natl Cancer Inst* 1982;69(2):349–355.

162. Saphner T, Tormey DC, Gray R. Annual hazard rates of recurrence for breast cancer after primary therapy. *J Clin Oncol* 1996;14:2738–2746.

163. O'Shaughnessy J. Extending survival with chemotherapy in metastatic breast cancer. *Oncologist* 2005;10(Suppl 3):20–29.

164. Lynch MD, Cariati M, Purushotham AD. Breast cancer, stem cells and prospects for therapy. *Breast Cancer Res* 2006;8(3):211.

165. Hortobagyi GN, De la Garza Salazar J, Pritchard K, et al. The global breast cancer burden: variations in epidemiology and survival. *Clin Breast Cancer* 2005;6(5):391–401.

166. American Cancer Society. *Breast cancer facts & figures, 1999–2000.* Atlanta: American Cancer Society, 1999.

167. Elkin EB, Hudis C, Begg CB, et al. The effect of changes in tumor size on breast carcinoma survival in the U.S.: 1975–1999. *Cancer* 2005;104(6):1149–1157.

168. Li CI, Daling JR, Malone KE. Incidence of invasive breast cancer by hormone receptor status from 1992 to 1998. *J Clin Oncol* 2003;21:28.

169. Smigal C, Jemal A, Ward E, et al. Trends in breast cancer by race and ethnicity: update 2006. *CA Cancer J Clin* 2006;56(3):168–183.

170. Polite BN, Olapade OI. Breast cancer and race: a rising tide does not lift all boats equally. *Perspect Biol Med* 2005;48(Suppl 1):S166–S175.

171. Vogel VG. Breast cancer risk factors and preventative approaches to breast cancer. In: Kavanagh J, Singletary SE, Einhorn N, et al. eds. *Cancer in women.* Cambridge: Blackwell Science, 1998.

172. withseer.cancer.gov/csr/1975_2000/results_merged/topic_lifetime_risk.pdf.

173. American Cancer Society. *Surveillance research.* American Cancer Society, 1999.

174. Collaborative Group on Hormonal Factors and Breast Cancer. Familial breast cancer: collaborative reanalysis of individual data from 52 epidemiological studies including 58,209 women with breast cancer and 101,986 women without the disease. *Lancet* 2001;358:1389.

175. Maztracci CL, Tjan S, Bane AL, et al. E-cadherin alterations in atypical lobular hyperplasia and lobular carcinoma *in situ* of the breast. *Mod Pathol* 2005;18(6):741–751.

176. Lagios MD, Margolin FR, Westdahl PR, et al. Mammographically detected duct carcinoma *in situ.* Frequency of local recurrence

following tylectomy and prognostic effect of nuclear grade on local recurrence. *Cancer* 1989;63(4):618–624.

177. Solin LJ, Yeh IT, Kurtz J, et al. Ductal carcinoma *in situ* (intraductal carcinoma) of the breast treated with breast-conserving surgery and definitive irradiation. Correlation of pathologic parameters with outcome of treatment. *Cancer* 1993;71(8):2532–2542.

178. Silverstein MJ, Poller DN, Weisman JR, et al. Prognostic classification of breast ductal carcinoma-in-situ. *Lancet* 1995;345(8958):1154–1157.

179. Bellamy CO, McDonald C, Salter DM, et al. Noninvasive ductal carcinoma of the breast: the relevance of histologic categorization. *Hum Pathol* 1993;24(1):16–23.

180. O'Malley FP, Page DL, Dupont EH, et al. Ductal carcinoma *in situ* of the breast with apocrine cytology: definition of a borderline category. *Hum Pathol* 1994;25(2):164–168.

181. Ashworth MT, Haggani MT. Endocrine variant of ductal carcinoma *in situ* of breast: ultrastructural and light microscopical study. *J Clin Pathol* 1986;39(12):1355–1359.

182. Warnberg F, Nordgren H, Bergh J, et al. Ductal carcinoma *in situ* of the breast from a population-defined cohort: an evaluation of new histopathological classification systems. *Eur J Cancer* 1999;35(5):714–720.

183. Klauber-Demore N, Tan K, Liberman L, et al. Sentinel lymph node biopsy: is it indicated in patients with high-risk ductal carcinoma-in-situ and ductal carcinoma-in-situ with microinvasion? *Ann Surg Oncol* 2000;7(9):636–642.

184. Foote FW, Stewart FW. Lobular carcinoma *in situ*. *Am J Pathol* 1941;17:491–495.

185. Urban J. Bilaterality of cancer of the breast: Biopsy of the opposite breast. *Cancer* 1967;20:1867–1870.

186. Rosen PP, Koslof C, Lieberman PH, et al. Lobular carcinoma *in situ* of the breast. Detailed analysis of 99 patients with average follow-up of 24 years. *Am J Surg Pathol* 1978;2(3):225–251.

187. Rosen PP, Senie R, Schottenfeld D, et al. Noninvasive breastcarcinoma: frequency of unsuspected invasion and implications for treatment. *Ann Surg* 1979;189(3):377–382.

188. Haagenson CD, Lane N, Lattis R, et al. Lobular neoplasia (so-called lobular carcinoma *in situ*) of the breast. *Cancer* 1978;42(2):737–769.

189. Page DL, Dupont WD, Rodgers LW, et al. Atypical hyperplastic lesions of the female breast. A long-term follow-up study. *Cancer* 1985;55(11):2698–2708.

190. Page DL, Schuyler PA, Dupont WD, et al. A typical lobular hyperplasia as a unilateral predictor of breast cancer risk: a retrospective cohort study. *Lancet* 2003;361(9352):125–129.

191. Lakhani SR. In-situ lobular neoplasia: time for an awakening. *Lancet* 2003;361(9352):96.

192. Lakhani SR, Audresch W, Cleton-Jenson JM, et al. The management of lobular carcinoma *in situ* (LCIS). Is LCIS the same as ductal carcinoma *in situ* (DCIS)?. *Eur J Cancer* 2006;42(14):2205–2211.

193. Li CI, Moe RE, Daling JR. Risk of mortality by histologic type of breast cancer among women aged 50 to 79 years. *Arch Intern Med* 2003;163(18):2149–2153.

194. Ferlicot S, Vincent-Salamon J, Melioni J, et al. Wide metastatic spreading in infiltrating lobular carcinoma of the breast. *Eur J Cancer* 2004;40(3):336–341.

195. Hennessy BT, Khrishnamurty S, Giordiano S, et al. Squamous cell carcinoma of the breast. *J Clin Oncol* 2005;23(31):7827–7835.

196. Anderson BO. Phyllodes Tumors. In: Harris JR, Lippman ME, Morrow M, et al. eds. *Diseases of the breast*, 3rd ed. Philadelphia: Lippincott Williams & Wilkins, 2004:669.

197. Chen WH, Cheng SP, Tzen CY, et al. Surgical treatment of phyllodes tumors of the breast: retrospective review of 172 cases. *J Surg Oncol* 2005;91(3):185–194.

198. Des Guetz G. Postirradiation sarcoma: clinicopathologic features and results of chemotherapy (abstract). *Proc Am Soc Clin Oncol* 2002;21:404a.

199. Bijker N, Rutgers EJ, Duchateau JL, et al. Breast-conserving therapy for Paget disease of the nipple. A prospective European Organization for Research and Treatment of Cancer study of 61 patients. *Cancer* 2001;91:472.

200. AJCC (American Joint Committee on Cancer). In: Greene FL, Page DL, Fleming ID, et al. eds. *Cancer staging manual*, 6th ed. New York: Springer-Verlag, 2002:223–240.

201. Woodward WA, Strom EA, Tucker SL, et al. Changes in the 2003 American joint committee on cancer staging for breast cancer dramatically affect stage-specific survival. *J Clin Oncol* 2003;21(17):3244–3248.

202. Van de Vijver MJ, HE YV, Van't Veer LJ, et al. A gene-expression signature as a predictor of survival in breast cancer. *N Engl J Med* 2002;347:1999–2009.

203. Van't Veer LJ, Paik F, Hayes DF. Gene expression profiling of breast cancer: a new tumor marker. *J Clin Oncol* 2005;23(8):1631–1635.

204. Hartmann LC, Schaid DJ, Woodes JE, et al. Efficacy of bilateral prophylactic mastectomy in women with a family history of breast cancer. *N Engl J Med* 1999;340:7–84.

205. Rebbeck TR, Freibel T, Lynch HT, et al. Bilateral prophylactic mastectomy reduces breast cancer risk in BRCA1 and BRCA2 mutation carriers: the PROSE Study Group. *J Clin Oncol* 2004;22(6):1055–1062. Epub 2004 Feb 23.

206. Frank TS, Manley SA, Olapade OI, et al. Sequence analysis of BRCA1 and BRCA2: correlation of mutations with family history and ovarian cancer risk. *J Clin Oncol* 1998;16:2417–2425.

207. Borgen PI, Hill ADK, Tran KN, et al. Patient regrets after bilateral prophylactic mastectomy. *Ann Surg Oncol* 1998;5(7):603–606.

208. Schrag D, Kuntz JM, Garber JE, et al. Life expectancy gains from cancer prevention strategies for women with breast cancer and BRCA1 or BRCA2 mutations. *JAMA* 2000;283:617–624.

209. DuBois RN. Aspirin and breast cancer prevention: the estrogen connection. *JAMA* 2004;291:2488–2489.

210. Arun B, Gros P. The role of COX-2 inhibition in breast cancer treatment and prevention. *Semin Oncol* 2004;31:22–29.

211. Terry MB, Gammon MD, Zhang FF, et al. Association of frequency and duration of aspirin use and hormone receptor status with breast cancer risk. *JAMA* 2004;291:2433–2440.

212. Singletary SE, Atkinson EN, Hoque A, et al. Phase II clinical trial of N-(4-hydroxyphenyl)retinamide and tamoxifen administration before definitive surgery for breast neoplasia. *Clin Cancer Res* 2002;8:2835–2842.

213. Denoyelle C, Vasse M, Korner M, et al. Cerivastatin, an inhibitor of HMG-CoA reductase, inhibits the signaling pathways involved in the invasiveness and metastatic properties of highly invasive breast cancer cell lines: an *in vitro* study. *Carcinogenesis* 2001;22:1139–1148.

214. Cuzick J, Forbes J, Edwards R, et al. First results from the International Breast Cancer Intervention Study (IBIS-I): a randomised prevention trial. *Lancet* 2002;360:817–824.

215. Veronesi U, Mainsonneuve P, Costa A, et al. Prevention of breast cancer with tamoxifen: preliminary findings from the Italian randomised trial among hysterectomized women. *Lancet* 1998;352:93–97.

216. Cuzick J, Powles L, Veronesi U, et al. Overview of the main outcomes in breast-cancer prevention trials. *Lancet* 2003;361:296–300.

217. Cummings SR, Eckert S, Kruger KE, et al. The effect of raloxifene on risk of breast cancer in postmenopausal women: results from the MORE randomized trial. Multiple outcomes of raloxifene evaluation. *JAMA* 1999;281:2189–2197.

218. Goss PE, Inge J, Martino S, et al. A randomized trial of letrozole in postmenopausal women after 5 years of tamoxifen therapy for early-stage breast cancer. *N Engl J Med* 2003;349:1793–1802.

219. Coombes RC, Hall E, Gibson LJ, et al. A randomized trial of exemestane after two to three years of tamoxifen therapy in postmenopausal women with primary breast cancer. *N Engl J Med* 2004;350:1081–1092.

220. Baum M, Buzdar A, Cusick J, et al. Anastrozole alone or in combination with tamoxifen versus tamoxifen one for adjuvant treatment of postmenopausal women with early-stage breast cancer: results of the ATAC(Arimidex, Tamoxifen Alone or in Combination) trial efficacy and safety update analyses. *Cancer* 2003;98:1802–1810.

221. Jansen L, Doting MH, Rutgers EJ, et al. Clinical relevance of sentinel lymph nodes outside the axilla in patients with breast cancer. *Br J Surg* 2000;87:920–925.

222. Naik AM, Fey J, Gemignani M, et al. The risk of axillary relapse after sentinel lymph node biopsy for breast cancer is comparable with that of axillary lymph node dissection: a follow-up study of 4008 procedures. *Ann Surg* 2004;240:462–468.

223. Bedrosian I, Reynolds C, Mick R, et al. Accuracy of sentinel lymph node biopsy in patients with large primary breast tumors. *Cancer* 2000;88:2540–2545.

224. Schrenk P, Wayand W. Sentinel-node biopsy in axillary lymph-node staging for patients with multicentric breast cancer. *Lancet* 2001;357:122.

225. Dupont EL, Khun MA, McCann C, et al. The role of sentinel lymph node biopsy in women undergoing prophylactic mastectomy. *Eur J Nucl Med* 1999;26(Suppl):S72.

226. Breslin TM, Cohen L, Sahin A, et al. Sentinel lymph node biopsy is accurate after neoadjuvant chemotherapy for breast cancer. *J Clin Oncol* 2000;18:3480–3486.

227. Port ER, Fey J, Gemignani M, et al. Reoperative sentinel lymph node biopsy: a new option for patients with primary or locally recurrent breast carcinoma. *J Am Coll Surg* 2002;195:167–172.

228. Swallow CJ, Van Zee KJ, Sacchini V, et al. Ductal carcinoma *in situ* of the breast: progress and controversy. *Curr Probl Surg* 1996;33(7):553–600.

229. Julien JP. Radiotherapy in breast-conserving treatment for ductal carcinoma *in situ*: first results of the EORTC randomized phase III trial 10853. *Lancet* 2000;355:528–533.

230. Kell MR, Morrow M. An adequate margin of excision in ductal carcinoma *in situ*. *Br Med J* 2005;331(7520):789–790.

231. Borgen PI, Moore MO, Heerdt AS, et al. Breast-conservation therapy for invasive carcinoma of the breast. *Curr Probl Surg* 1995;32:190–247.

232. Singletary SE. Surgical margins in patients with early-stage breast cancer treated with breast conservation therapy. *Am J Surg* 2002;184:383–393.

233. Veronesi U, Banfi A, Del Vecchio M, et al. Comparison of Halsted mastectomy with quadrantectomy, axillary dissection, and radiotherapy in early breast cancer: long-term results. *Eur J Cancer Clin Oncol* 1986;22(9):1085–1089.

234. Clarke M, Collins R, Darbv S, et al. EBCTCG effects of radiotherapy and of differences in the extent of surgery for early breast cancer on local recurrence and 15-year survival: an overview of the randomised trials. *Lancet* 2005;366(9503):2087–2106.

235. Gerber B, Krause A, Remer T, et al. Skin-sparing mastectomy with conservation of the nipple-areola complex and autologous reconstruction is an oncologically safe procedure. *Ann Surg* 2003;238(1):120–127.

236. Van Zee KJ, Mannaseh DM, Bevilaqua JL, et al. A nomogram for predicting the likelihood of additional nodal metastases in breast cancer patients with a positive sentinel node biopsy. *Ann Surg Oncol* 2003;10(10):1140–1151.

237. Fisher B, Redmon C, Fisher ER, et al. Ten-year results of a randomized clinical trial comparing radical mastectomy and total mastectomy with or without radiation. *N Engl J Med* 1985;312:674–681.

238. Haagenson CD. Criteria of inoperability. *Am Surg* 1943;118:859.

239. National Comprehensive Cancer Network (NCCN) guidelines for treatment of breast cancer. Available at www.nccn.org /professionals/physician_gls/default.asp (Accessed March 7, 2005).

240. Schwartz GF, Hortobagyi HN. Proceedings of the consensus conference on neoadjuvant chemotherapy in carcinoma of the breast, April 26–28, 2003, Philadelphia, Pennsylvania. *Cancer* 2004;100(12):2512–2532.

241. Lyman GH, Giuliano AE, Somerfeld ME, et al. American Society of Clinical Oncology guideline recommendations for sentinel lymph node biopsy in early-stage breast cancer. *J Clin Oncol* 2005;23(30):7703–7720. Epub 2005 Sep 12.

242. National Comprehensive Cancer Network. Clinical practice guidelines in oncology *Breast Cancer* 2003, Version 3.

243. Early Breast Cancer Trialists' Collaborative Group (EBCTCG). Effects of chemotherapy and hormonal therapy for early breast cancer on recurrence and 15-year survival: an overview of the randomized trials. *Lancet* 2005;365(9472):1687–1717.

244. Vlastos G, Smith DA, Singletart SE, et al. Long-term survival after an aggressive surgical approach in patients with breast cancer metastasis. *Ann Surg Oncol* 2004;11(9):869–874.

245. Pocard M, Poulliart P, Asselain B, et al. Hepatic resection for metastatic breast cancer metastases: results and prognosis (65 cases). *Ann Chir* 2001;126:413–420.

246. Khan SA, Stewart AK, Morrow M. Does aggressive local therapy improve survival in metastatic breast cancer? *Surgery* 2002;132(4):620–626; discussion 626–627.

247. Carmichael AR, Anderson DE, Chetty U, et al. Does local surgery have a role in the management of stage IV breast cancer? *Eur J Surg Oncol* 2003;29:17–19.

248. Babiera G, Rau R, Feng L, et al. Effect of primary tumor extirpation in breast cancer patients who present with stage IV disease and an intact primary tumor. *Ann Surg Oncol* 2006;13(6):776–782. Epub 2006 Apr 17.

249. Rapiti E, Verkooijen HM, Vlastos G, et al. Complete excision of primary breast tumor improves survival of patients with metastatic breast cancer at diagnosis. *J Clin Oncol* 2006;24(18):2743–2749. Epub 2006 May 15.

250. Kestin LL, Goldstein MS, Martinez AA, et al. Mammographically detected ductal carcinoma *in situ* treated with conservative surgery with or without radiation therapy: patterns of failure and 10-year results. *Ann Surg* 2000;231:235–245.

251. Silverstein MJ, Barth A, Poller DN, et al. Ten-year results comparing mastectomy to excision and radiation therapy for ductal carcinoma *in situ* of the breast. *Eur J Cancer* 1995;31A(9):1425–1427.

252. Page DL, Silverstein MJ. Ductal carcinoma *in situ*. The success of breast conservation therapy: a shared experience of two single institutional nonrandomized prospective studies. *Surg Oncol Clin N Am* 1997;6(2):385–389.

253. Sadeski S, Oberman B, Zipple D, et al. Breast conservation after neoadjuvant chemotherapy. *Ann Surg Oncol* 2005;12(6):480–487. Epub 2005 Apr 19.

254. Hortobagyi GN, Ames FC, Buzdar AU, et al. Management of stage III primary breast cancer with primary chemotherapy, surgery, and radiation therapy. *Cancer* 1988;62:2507–2516.

255. Bristol IJ, Buchholz TA. Inflammatory breast cancer: current concepts in local management. *Breast Dis* 2005–2006;22:75–83.

256. Maher EJ. The use of palliative radiotherapy in the management of breast cancer. *Eur J Cancer* 1992;28(2–3):706–710.

257. Andrieu N, Easton DF, Chang-Claude J, et al. Effect of chest X-rays on the risk of breast cancer among BRCA1/2 mutation carriers in the international BRCA1/2 carrier cohort study: a report from the EMBRACE, GENEPSO, GEO-HEBON, and IBCCS Collaborators' Group. *J Clin Oncol* 2006;24(21):3361–3366. Epub 2006 Jun 26.

258. Pierce LJ, Strawdemann M, Narod SA, et al. Effect of radiotherapy after breast-conserving treatment in women with breast cancer and germline BRCA1/2 mutations. *J Clin Oncol* 2000;18(19):3360–3369.

259. Kattan MW, Giri D, Panageas DA, et al. A tool for predicting breast carcinoma mortality in women who do not receive adjuvant therapy. *Cancer* 2004;101(11):2509–2515.

260. Fisher B, Dignam M, Wolmark N, et al. Tamoxifen and chemotherapy for lymph node-negative, estrogen receptor-positive breast cancer. *J Natl Cancer Inst* 1997;89:1673–1682.

261. Berry DA. Effects of improvements in chemotherapy on disease-free and overall survival of estrogen-receptor negative, node-positive breast cancer: 20-year experience of the CALGB and U.S. Breast Intergroup. *Breast Cancer Res Treat* 2004;88(Abstr 29, Suppl 1):S17.

262. Nielsen LL, Dell J, Maxwell E, et al. Efficacy of p53 adenovirus-mediated gene therapy against human breast cancer xenografts. *Cancer Gene Ther* 1997;4:129–138.

263. Majumdar AS, Zolotorev A, Samuel S, et al. Efficacy of herpes simplex virus thymidine kinase in combination with cytokine gene therapy in an experimental metastatic breast cancer model. *Cancer Gene Ther* 2000;7:1086–1099.

264. Strong TV. Gene therapy for carcinoma of the breast genetic immunotherapy. *Breast Cancer Res* 2000;2:15–21.

265. Griffith TS, Anderson RD, Davidson BL, et al. Adenoviral-mediated transfer of the TNF-related apoptosis-inducing ligand/Apo-2 ligand gene induces tumor cell apoptosis. *J Immunol* 2000;165:2886–2894.

266. Oga M, Takenaga A, Sato Y, et al. Inhibition of metastatic brain tumor growth by intramuscular administration of the endostatin gene. *Int J Oncol* 2003;23:73–79.

267. Lebedeva S, Bagdosorova S, Tyler T, et al. Tumor suppression and therapy sensitization of localized and metastatic breast cancer by adenovirus p53. *Hum Gene Ther* 2001;12:763–772.

268. Thorlacius S, Sigurssdon S, Bjarnatdottir H, et al. Study of a single *BRCA2* mutation with high carrier frequency in a small population. *Am J Hum Genet* 1997;60:1079–1084.

269. Goss PE, Reid C, Pintilie M, et al. Male breast carcinoma: a review of 229 patients who presented to the Princess Margaret Hospital during 40 years: 1955–1996. *Cancer* 1999;85:629–639.

270. Giordano SH. Adjuvant systemic therapy for male breast cancer. *Cancer* 2005;104:235–264.

271. Kantarjian H, Yap HY, Hortobagni HN. Hormonal therapy for metastatic male breast cancer. *Arch Intern Med* 1983;143:237–240.

CHAPTER 14

The Endocrine System

Mark S. Cohen and L. Michael Brunt

This chapter is a review of the anatomy and physiology of the endocrine system, using an organ-system approach and including discussion of functional endocrine disorders of importance in surgical practice. Every attempt has been made to integrate the pathophysiologic basis of these functional disorders with their clinical presentation and management.

THE THYROID

Anatomy and Development

The anlage of the thyroid gland first appears embryologically at 3 to 4 weeks of development as a thickening of epithelium in the floor of the pharyngeal gut. The thyroid primordium subsequently migrates caudally, remaining connected with the floor of the pharynx by the thyroglossal duct. This duct normally obliterates and disappears by the end of the second month, marking its origin from the junction of the middle and posterior thirds of the tongue by a small dimple, the foramen cecum. Follicles containing colloid are visible by the end of the third month, at which time concentration of iodide and synthesis of T_4 are apparent. During its descent, the thyroid acquires from the ultimobranchial body parafollicular cells that secrete calcitonin.

Several clinically important developmental abnormalities of the thyroid gland may occur. Complete failure of the thyroid anlage to develop results in absence of the thyroid gland (athyreosis), a rare cause of neonatal hypothyroidism and cretinism. Thyroid dysgenesis due to abnormal morphogensis of thyroid follicular cells is the most common cause of congenital hypothyroidism with an incidence of 1 in 3,500 newborns (1). Thyroid tissue also may develop at ectopic sites along the pathway of normal descent of the thyroid gland. Differentiation of thyroid tissue may occur in the setting of a complete arrest in migration (lingual thyroid) or may occur in ectopic suprathyroid or infrathyroid sites and the mediastinum. Lingual thyroid occurs in approximately 1 in 3,000 cases of thyroid disease and is the most common site for functioning ectopic thyroid tissue. In

approximately 70% of cases, it is the patient's only thyroid tissue. Thyroglossal duct cyst is the most common clinically important thyroid developmental abnormality. Thyroglossal cysts arise from persistence of a portion of the thyroglossal duct as a sinus tract or cyst and usually present as midline neck masses that first appear during childhood or adolescence.

The thyroid gland in the adult weighs approximately 20 g, making it the largest of the endocrine organs. It consists of two lateral lobes connected by a narrow isthmus. A pyramidal lobe formed by differentiation of cells of the lower thyroglossal duct into thyroid tissue may sometimes be found at the superior aspect of the isthmus (Fig. 14.1). The isthmus of the gland crosses the trachea just below the cricoid cartilage, and the lateral lobes cover the lower halves of the thyroid cartilages. The right lobe is often slightly larger than the left and tends to enlarge to a greater degree in patients with diffuse goiters. The gland lies deep to the superficial strap muscles of the neck (sternothyroid and sternothyroid muscles) and is related laterally to the sternocleidomastoid muscle and the carotid sheath. It attaches to the cricoid cartilage and tracheal rings by bands of connective tissue termed *Berry's ligament*.

Histologically, the thyroid is organized into varying sized follicles which are the site of synthesis and secretion of thyroid hormone. The follicles are comprised of a single layer of cuboidal cells, which surround a central space that is filled with colloid containing thyroglobulin. The thyroid cell is polarized such that uptake of iodide occurs at the basal pole and iodination of thyroglobulin (Tg) takes place at the apical pole. The thyroid also contains the C cells or parafollicular cells which produce calcitonin. In the normal thyroid, the C cells are difficult to see with routine histologic stains but can be identified easily by immunohistochemic staining for calcitonin.

The blood supply to the thyroid (Fig. 14.2) is derived from two main sources: the superior thyroid artery, a branch of the external carotid artery, and the inferior thyroid artery, a branch of the thyrocervical trunk of the subclavian artery. The superior thyroid artery enters the gland at the superior

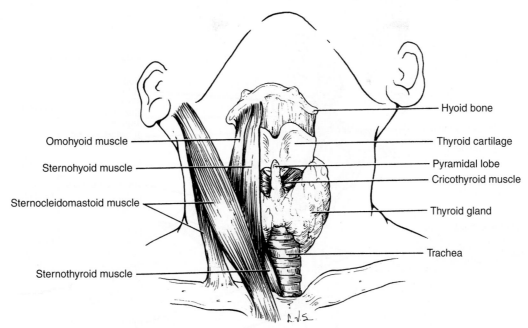

FIGURE 14.1 Gross anatomy of the human thyroid. (From Greenspan FS, Rapoport B. Thyroid gland. In: Greenspan FS, ed. *Basic and clinical endocrinology*, 3rd ed. Norwalk: Appleton & Lange, 1991:189. Reprinted by permission.)

pole, whereas the inferior artery enters the lateral aspect of each lobe. The inferior artery also provides a majority of the blood supply to the parathyroid glands, which can be important to consider during thyroidectomy. The thyroid ima artery is a variably sized vessel that may originate from the innominate artery, the aortic arch, or the lower end of the common carotid artery. It passes upward anterior to the

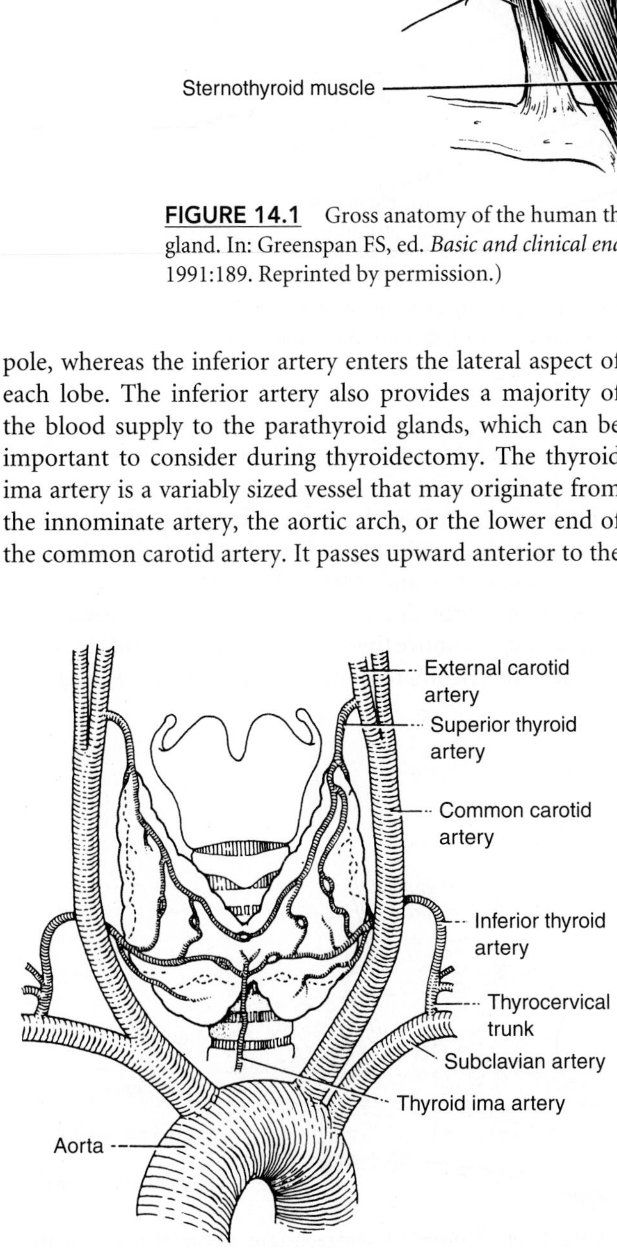

FIGURE 14.2 Arterial supply to the thyroid gland. The thyroid ima artery is frequently absent. (From Tzinas S, Droulias C, Harlaftis N, et al. Vascular patterns of the thyroid gland. *Am Surg* 1976;42:640. Reprinted by permission.)

trachea to enter the posterior aspect of the inferior border of the thyroid. Although usually small, it may be a sizable vessel and, if unrecognized, a source of troublesome bleeding during thyroidectomy. This rich vascular network provides the thyroid with a blood flow of 4 to 6 mL/g/min, more than the kidney and 50 times as much as the body as a whole (2). In diffuse thyrotoxic states, thyroid blood flow may reach greater than 1 L/min, and this increased flow may be identifiable as a thrill or bruit over the gland.

Blood exits the thyroid through the superior, middle, and inferior thyroid veins. The superior thyroid vein runs parallel with the superior thyroid artery and empties into the internal jugular vein. The middle thyroid vein also drains into the internal jugular vein, but no artery accompanies it. The inferior thyroid veins are the largest and most variable of the thyroid veins. They descend from the inferior poles of the gland to empty into the right and left innominate veins.

The lymph nodes that drain the thyroid (Fig. 14.3) can be categorized according to superior, inferior, and lateral drainage patterns (3). The superior aspect of the isthmus and median aspects of the lateral lobes drain upward into the prelaryngeal (delphian) nodes just above the isthmus and beyond to the digastric node group (level 2). The inferior lymph vessels follow the inferior thyroid veins to drain into the pretracheal and innominate node (level 6). Lymphatics that drain the lateral lobes course with the vascular supply to drain into the internal jugular, recurrent laryngeal, paratracheal, and paraesophageal lymph node chains (levels 3, 4 and 5). Each of these lymph node groups are common sites of metastatic spread in patients with thyroid carcinoma. Submandibular (level 1) and mediastinal lymph nodes (level 7), however, are rarely involved.

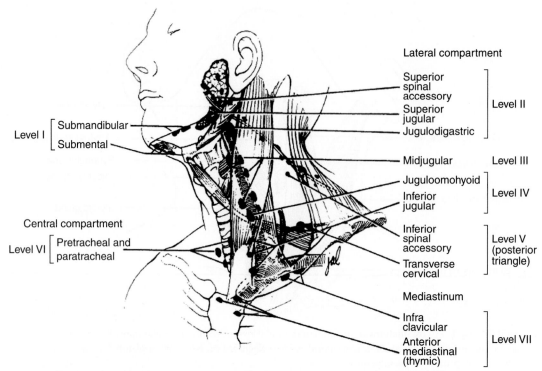

FIGURE 14.3 Diagramatic representation of nodal groupings of lymphatic drainage in the neck. (From Musholt TJ, Moley JF. Management of persistent or recurrent medullary thyroid carcinoma. *Prob Gen Surg* 1997;14:89–110. Reprinted with permission.)

The precise anatomic relation of the thyroid to the laryngeal nerves must be understood for thyroid surgery to be performed safely. The recurrent laryngeal nerve is a branch of the vagus nerve. On the right side, the recurrent nerve arises from the vagus at the level of the subclavian artery. It then loops from anterior to posterior around the right subclavian artery and passes upward in the tracheoesophageal groove. The left recurrent nerve arises from the vagus at the level of the aortic arch where it loops beneath the ligamentum arteriosum before ascending in a manner similar to the right. The recurrent laryngeal nerve is usually found in the tracheoesophageal groove along the posterior aspect of the thyroid gland (Fig. 14.4). It crosses the inferior thyroid artery at the middle third of the gland and may run behind the artery, between its branches, or in front of it. The nerve often has more than one trunk, each of which must be preserved. In approximately 1% of cases, the right nerve is nonrecurrent and enters the larynx directly. A nonrecurrent left nerve is even less common and is usually associated with a right-sided aortic arch. The recurrent nerves penetrate the cricothyroid membrane to form the nerve's terminal branch, the inferior laryngeal nerve. The inferior laryngeal nerve innervates all of the muscles of the larynx except the cricothyroid and supplies sensation to the trachea and subglottic region of the larynx. Unilateral paralysis of the inferior laryngeal nerve from recurrent nerve injury results in paralysis of the vocal cord on that side. The vocal cord becomes bowed outward and can be neither abducted nor adducted. The lack of apposition of the vocal cords produces hoarseness. With time, however, the paralyzed cord may move toward the midline and the voice may improve or even become normal.

The superior laryngeal nerve is a branch of the inferior (nodose) ganglion of the vagus. At the level of the hyoid bone, it splits into internal and external branches (Fig. 14.5). The internal branch provides sensation to the pyriform fossa and laryngeal mucosa above the vocal cords. The external branch innervates the cricothyroid muscle and is of greater surgical

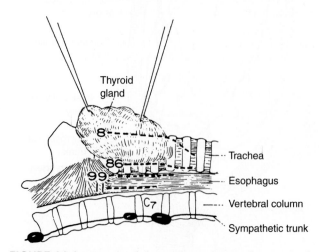

FIGURE 14.4 Course of the recurrent laryngeal nerve in the normal adult. Lateral view of the course of the recurrent laryngeal nerve at the level of the thyroid gland in 102 cadavers. (From Skandalakis JD, Droulias C, Harlaftis N, et al. The recurrent laryngeal nerve. *Am Surg* 1976;42:631. Reprinted by permission.)

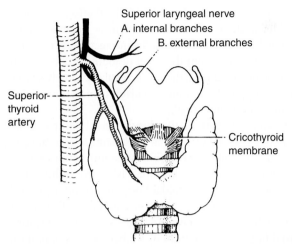

FIGURE 14.5 Relationship of the internal and external branches of the superior laryngeal nerve, the superior thyroid artery, and the upper pole of the thyroid. (From Droulias C, Tzinas S, Harlaftis N, et al. The superior laryngeal nerve. *Am Surg* 1976;42:636. Reprinted by permission.)

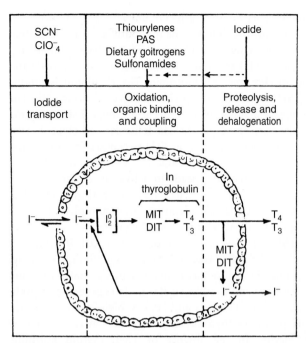

FIGURE 14.6 Pathway of biosynthesis of thyroid hormone. Shown at the top are inhibitors of the various steps in hormone synthesis. SCN, PAS, MIT, monoiodotyrosine; DIT, diiodotyrosine. (From Ingbar SH. The thyroid. In: Wilson JD, Foster DW, eds. *Textbook of endocrinology*, 7th ed. Philadelphia: WB Saunders, 1985:686. Reprinted by permission.)

importance. It travels with the superior thyroid artery and turns medially to enter the cricothyroid above where the superior thyroid artery branches at the superior pole of the thyroid gland. If the external branch of the superior laryngeal nerve is injured during thyroidectomy, the cricothyroid is paralyzed and the vocal cords cannot be tensed. This results in a loss of timbre and volume in the voice, causing the voice to tire easily and making singing and shouting difficult.

Physiology

The thyroid gland produces two biologically active hormones, L-3,5,3′5′-tetra iodothyronine (thyroxine or T_4) and L-3,5,3′-triiodothyronine (T_3), which are essential for normal growth and development and for regulation of cellular metabolism. Figure 14.6 shows the sequential steps in the biosynthetic pathway for thyroid hormone. Thyroxine accounts for approximately 90% of thyroid hormone secreted by the gland whereas T_3 accounts for 9% and reverse T_3, which is not biologically active, accounts for the remaining 1%. Synthesis of thyroid hormone depends on a supply of iodine that comes from dietary sources. In the United States, the average daily intake of iodine ranges from 200 to 500 μg (4). After absorption, iodine is taken up by the thyroid follicular cells by an active transport process, called the *iodide trap*, which transports inorganic iodide [I^-] intracellularly against its electrical and concentration gradients. The iodide-trapping mechanism allows the thyroid to store large quantities of iodine (8,000 μg and 90% of total body iodine), most of which has been organified. The effectiveness of iodide trapping is sometimes assessed by the thyroid/serum (T/S) ratio, which is usually measured with radioactive iodide. A normal T/S ratio in a euthyroid person is usually approximately 30, indicating the follicular iodide concentration is 30 times that of the serum. Both thyroid-stimulating hormone (TSH) and organic iodine regulate this process.

TSH stimulates iodine uptake, and excess iodide, once it has become organified, inhibits it. The monovalent anions perchlorate and pertechnetate are competitive inhibitors of iodide trapping.

Upon entering the follicular cell, iodine is oxidized by hydrogen peroxide and then organified by a process that results in iodination of tyrosine residues on the Tg molecule to form monoiodotyrosine (MIT) and diiodotyrosine (DIT). This process is catalyzed by the enzyme thyroid peroxidase (TPO), which is a membrane-bound glycoprotein of molecular weight (MW) 102,000. The formation of the biologically active iodothyronines T_3 and T_4 then proceeds by a coupling reaction, also catalyzed by TPO, involving MIT and DIT. MIT combines with DIT to yield T_3, and two molecules of DIT are coupled to form T_4. TSH positively regulates the organic iodination and coupling process, whereas antithyroid drugs and high concentrations of iodide (Wolff-Chaikoff effect) inhibit it. Once organified, iodine is no longer a part of the intracellular pool of iodide and cannot be affected by competitive inhibitors of iodide transport. Two mechanisms regulate secretion of thyroid hormones: (i) a classic feedback loop that involves the pituitary and hypothalamus, and (ii) an intrinsic thyroid autoregulatory process mediated by glandular content of iodine.

TSH or *thyrotropin* is a 28,000 MW glycoprotein produced by cells of the anterior pituitary and is the principal agent that modulates thyroid function and thyroid cell growth. TSH exists as a heterodimer that is comprised of both α and β subunits. The α subunit is identical to that of two other pituitary glycoprotein hormones [luteinizing hormone (LH) and follicle stimulating hormone (FSH)] and human chorionic gonadotropin. The β subunit is unique to TSH and confers its specificity and biologic activity. The biological actions of TSH occur through TSH receptors on the surface of the thyroid follicular cell (type 1 TSH receptors) and on type 2 TSH receptors in adipocytes, lymphocytes, fibroblasts, and the gonads. Activation of TSH type 1 receptors leads to activation of the guanine-nucleotide–binding protein ($G_s\alpha$) that activates adenylate cyclase and the cyclic adenosine monophosphate (cAMP) and phospholipase C (PLC) signaling systems.

TSH has many effects on the thyroid cell. It stimulates all phases of iodide metabolism, including iodine trapping, organification of iodide, iodination of Tg, and promoting release of T_3 and T_4 from Tg. It stimulates gene transcription and synthesis of both Tg and TPO. At higher concentrations, TSH promotes thyroid cell growth and increases thyroid vascularity. In the absence of TSH, thyroid hormone production decreases and atrophy of the gland occurs.

TSH secretion is stimulated by thyrotropin-releasing hormone (TRH) and is inhibited by thyroid hormone. TRH is produced in the supraoptic and paraventricular nuclei of the hypothalamus and is released into the hypophyseal-portal system, through which it is transported to the cells of the anterior pituitary. TRH stimulates both secretion and synthesis of TSH but is not itself affected by the level of thyroid hormones. Inhibition of TSH secretion by thyroid hormones is a function of the rate of secretion of T_4 by the thyroid, serum levels of T_3, and the rate of intrapituitary conversion of T_4 to T_3 (4).

Thyroid hormonogenesis is also regulated in a TSH-independent manner by the availability and glandular content of iodide. Iodide depletion enhances iodide transport and stimulates hormone synthesis. In the presence of excess iodide, however, both iodide transport and hormone synthesis are suppressed (Wolff-Chaikoff effect). In normal individuals, these effects are transient as decreased iodide trapping leads to a decrease in the intraglandular content of iodine and escape from the effect of iodine occurs. Thyroid hormone production is, therefore, regulated closely so that a constant supply of hormone is available to meet the metabolic demands of the individual.

A unique feature of the thyroid gland compared with other endocrine organs is that it contains a large hormone store but has a slow overall hormone utilization rate. This large reserve of thyroid hormone is stored within the Tg molecule. Most intrathyroidal hormone within Tg is in the form of T_4 that may exceed the concentration of T_3 by 10-fold or more. In addition, there are large extrathyroidal stores of thyroid hormone (one third of the body's T_4 supply) in the liver and kidney. The pool of T_4 in these organs is much greater than that of T_3; however, T_4 turnover is much slower than that of T_3. At a T_4 production rate of 80 μg/d, the thyroid has enough reserve to maintain normal hormone levels for 2 to 3 weeks in the event of a block in synthesis. Considering the critical role of thyroid hormone in metabolism and calorigenesis, this provides the organism with an important protective mechanism against hormone depletion.

Tg is a 660,000 MW glycoprotein that is virtually the sole constituent of the follicular colloid. As noted previously, the Tg molecule contains the tyrosine residues, where MIT, DIT, T_3, and T_4 are formed and stored. TSH stimulates endocytosis of Tg colloid droplets into the follicular cell. Pseudopodia on the follicular cell engulf the Tg droplet forming a membrane-bound droplet inside the cell which fuses with a lysosome to form a phagosome where the Tg is hydrolyzed to T_3, T_4, rT_3, MIT, and DIT. Thyroid deiodinase, which is specific for iodotyrosines (MIT and DIT) but not iodothyronines (T_3 and T_4), releases iodine from the iodotyrosines to be reused in the iodination of new Tg. The iodothyronines are then released out of the cell into the blood stream (Fig. 14.7) (5) This process of endocytosis, proteolysis, and release is stimulated by TSH and inhibited by excess iodine

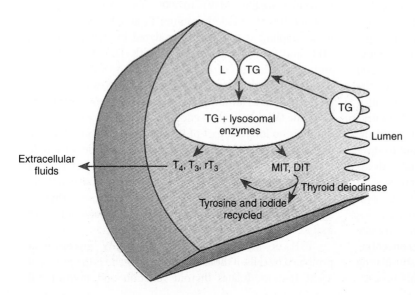

FIGURE 14.7   Schematic pathway of thyroid hormone secretion. Thyroglobulin (Tg) is endocytosed and fused with a lysosome (L) that contains proteolytic enzymes which hydrolyze Tg, releasing the thyroid hormones. Iodinated tyrosines [monoiodotyrosine (MIT) and diiodotyrosine (DIT)] are deiodinated by thyroid deiodinase. Porterfield SP. Thyroid Gland. In: *Endocrine Physiology*, 2nd ed. St. Louis: Mosby, 2001:59–84.

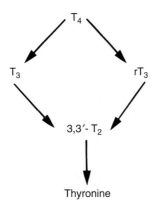

FIGURE 14.8 Pathway of sequential deiodination of thyroxine to its metabolites. Approximately 90% of the T_4 secreted daily by the thyroid is metabolized through this pathway. Kinetic analysis indicates that approximately 35% of T_4 is converted to T_3 and 40% to rT_3. Reverse T_3 and $3,3'$-T_2 are biologically inactive.

and by lithium. Iodine mediates its effect in part by inhibition of TSH-induced stimulation of thyroid adenylate cyclase and by increasing the resistance of Tg to proteolysis. Despite the efficient storage mechanism of the thyroid, Tg is detectable in small quantities in the serum of normal individuals. Elevated serum levels of Tg may be seen in patients with benign or differentiated thyroid tumors. After complete removal of the tumor, Tg levels return to normal. In patients with differentiated thyroid cancer, Tg may be useful as a tumor marker to follow patients postoperatively for development of metastatic tumor. Large amounts of Tg may also be released into the circulation after thyroid surgery and in patients with radiation-induced or subacute thyroiditis.

The pathway for metabolism of thyroid hormone is shown in Figure 14.8 (4). All of circulating T_4 and approximately 20% of T_3 result from direct secretion by the thyroid. The remainder of T_3 comes from peripheral conversion of T_4 to T_3. Approximately 80% of circulating T_4 undergoes extrathyroidal deiodination to T_3 or reverse T_3 (rT_3). Reverse T_3 derives exclusively from T_4 and has little biologic activity. T_3 and rT_3 metabolize to $3,3'$-diiodothyronine ($3,3'$-T_2), which undergoes further deiodination and is excreted in the urine as thyronine.

T_3 has approximately three times the biologic activity of T_4. The half-life for T_3 is 3 days and for T_4 is 7 to 10 days. Consequently, patients undergoing thyroidectomy for hyperthyroidism should continue treatment with β-blockade for 2 weeks postoperatively to avoid the untoward effects of residual circulating hormone.

Most circulating thyroid hormone is reversibly bound to three plasma proteins: thyronine-binding globulin (TBG), thyroxine-binding prealbumin (TBPA) also called *transthyretin* (TTR), and *albumin*. The extent to which thyroid hormone is bound to these carrier proteins (Table 14.1) is a function of their concentration, binding capacity, and affinity for T_3 and T_4. The high affinity of TBG for T_3 and T_4 makes it the major thyroid hormone binding protein. Virtually no T_3 is bound to TBPA because of the low affinity of interaction between the two. Because protein-bound T_3 and T_4 are biologically inactive, the metabolic state of the patient is determined by the level of free hormone. As most thyroid hormone is protein bound, changes in the plasma concentrations of TBG may affect the total T_4 concentration without altering the serum level of free T_4. In conditions associated with alterations in TBG levels (pregnancy and oral contraceptive use), therefore, free T_4 levels are normal and the patient is clinically euthyroid.

The thyroid hormones exert their metabolic effects at the cellular level after uptake and binding to specific receptors for T_3 in the cell nucleus. There are two T_3 receptor genes (α on chromosome 17 and β on chromosome 3), and the T_3 receptors are themselves members of a family of hormones responsive to nuclear transcription factors (6). These T_3 receptors bind to regulatory regions of genes, termed *thyroid hormone–response elements*, and modify their expression (by regulating gene transcription of certain messenger ribonucleic acids (mRNAs) in various tissues in response to stimulation with T_3. Recent discoveries of coregulatory proteins (thyroid receptor interacting proteins; *Trips*) for nuclear receptors clearly indicate that thyroid hormone receptors do not mediate the hormone signal alone, but require extensive cooperation and complex interplay with many cellular proteins (6).

The numerous effects of thyroid hormones on body metabolism are listed in Table 14.2. Thyroid hormone

TABLE 14.1

Characteristics of Serum Thyroid Hormone–Binding Proteins

Protein	MW	Plasma Concentration	Capacity for T_4	Affinity T_4	(M^{-1}) T_3
Thyronine-binding globulin	60,000	2 mg/dL	20 μg/dL	2×10^{10}	2×10^9
Thyronine-binding prealbumin	50,000	25 mg/dL	250 μg/dL	1.5×10^8	2.5×10^5
Albumin	69,000	4 g/dL	High	1.5×10^6	1×10^7

MW, molecular weight; T_4, tetraiodothyronine; T_3, 3, 5, 3′, triiodothyronine.
From Gavin LA. Thyroid physiology and testing and thyroid function. In: Clark O, ed. *Endocrine surgery of the thyroid and parathyroid glands.* St. Louis: C.V. Mosby Co., 1985;7. Reprinted with permission.

TABLE 14.2

Actions of Thyroid Hormones

Parameter/Organ System	Action
Developmental	Essential for normal neural and skeletal development
Calorigenesis	O_2 consumption[a]
	Basal metabolic rate
Intermediary metabolism	Protein synthesis
	Synthesis/degradation of cholesterol
	Lipolysis
	Glycogenolysis and gluconeogenesis
Cardiovascular	Heart rate and myocardial contractility
Sympathetic nervous system	Sensitivity to catecholamines
	Catecholamine receptors in cardiac muscle
	Possible Amplification of catecholamine effects at post receptor site
Endocrine	Steroid hormone release
Hematopoietic	Erythropoiesis
	2,3 DPG production
	Maintain hypoxic and hypercapnic drives
Musculoskeletal	Bone turnover
	Urinary hydroxyproline excretion
	↑ Rate of muscle relaxation

2,3 DPG, 2,3-diphosphoglycerate.
[a]Occurs in all tissues except brain, spleen, and testis.

regulates calorigenesis by increasing oxygen consumption and elevating the basal metabolic rate (BMR). It affects protein, carbohydrate, and lipid metabolism and is necessary for normal growth and development. It also increases the sensitivity of the sympathetic nervous system to the effects of catecholamines, which accounts for many clinical features seen in patients with hyperthyroidism.

Inhibitors of Thyroid Hormone Synthesis and Secretion

Thionamides

Propylthiouracil (PTU) and methimazole (Tapazole) are members of the thionamide class of antithyroid drugs commonly used in the treatment of hyperthyroidism. These agents may be used either as primary therapy for Graves disease or in preparation for radioiodine therapy or surgery. The thionamides act principally by interfering with TPO-mediated iodination of tyrosine residues in Tg, which is a critical step in synthesis of thyroxine and T3 (7). PTU has the additional effect of inhibiting the enzyme 5'-monodeiodinase which regulates peripheral conversion of T_4 to T_3. This latter action may be a consideration when a rapid effect is needed in patients with severe thyrotoxicosis. Some immunosuppressive effect of these drugs may also occur such as a reduction in anti-TSH receptor antibodies and induction of apoptosis in intrathyroidal lymphocytes (8). In up to 40% to 50% of

adults with Graves disease, long-term remissions may occur after withdrawal of antithyroid medications. PTU is usually administered in a dose of 100 to 300 mg given every 8 hours. Methimazole has the advantage of a single daily dose. Methimazole also crosses the placenta more readily than PTU and has been associated with an increased risk of congenital anomalies and therefore, in North America, PTU is preferred in thyrotixic pregnant patients. The most serious potential side effect associated with thionamide therapy is agranulocytosis that develops in approximately 0.35% of cases and is usually reversible on cessation of the offending agent.

Iodine

Iodine acts by inhibiting release of thyroid hormone and the organic binding process. This latter action (acute Wolff-Chaikoff effect) is transient, and escape occurs after a few days of therapy. Pharmacologic doses of iodine (>6 mg/d) are required for the antithyroid effect to occur.

Other Agents

Glucocorticoids suppress the hypothalamic-pituitary-thyroid axis and, in pharmacologic doses, lower serum TSH and T_4 levels. They also lower serum T_3 levels by inhibiting peripheral T_4 to T_3 conversion. Pituitary secretion of TSH is also inhibited by dopamine. Lithium inhibits release of thyroid hormone and may induce goitrous hypothyroidism in susceptible individuals.

Adrenergic antagonists (β blockers) do not inhibit thyroid hormone synthesis, but they are extremely valuable in controlling the peripheral manifestations of increased catecholamine sensitivity in patients with thyrotoxicosis. Propranolol (Inderal) has the added benefit of blocking peripheral conversion of T_4 to T_3.

Tests of Thyroid Function

The initial screening for suspected thyroid disorders should consist of measurement of serum TSH. Current generation TSH assays, which have a sensitivity level of 0.02 μU/mL, reliably distinguish euthyroid subjects from patients with hyper- or hypothyroidism. TSH levels are low or suppressed in hyperthyroidism and are elevated in hypothyroidism (9,10). An abnormal TSH should be further investigated by measurement of thyroid hormone levels.

Tests available for determination of thyroid hormone levels include total T_4, free T_4, and total and free T_3. Serum total T_4 assays measure both free and protein-bound hormone. Because changes in total T_4 can result from alterations in either hormone production or hormone binding to serum proteins, an accurate diagnosis of thyroid dysfunction requires measurement of free T_4. Free T_4 is measured either by an indirect technique or by equilibrium dialysis (10). Measurement of serum total and free T_3 concentrations are not routinely employed in screening but are reserved mainly for the diagnosis of T_3 toxicosis, which accounts for 5% or less of cases of hyperthyroidism.

Estrogens have the ability to nonspecifically stimulate the synthesis of TBG. In pregnancy, the levels of TBG may rise to a level where total T_4 is twice that of the nonpregnant state (11). Free T_4 levels, however, will remain in the normal range. It is, therefore, important to consider this effect of estrogens on TBG and T_4 levels to avoid misdiagnosing hyperthyroidism in this scenario.

Radioactive Iodine Uptake

The radioactive iodine uptake (RAIU) test measures the thyroid content of radioactive iodine after an orally administered dose of iodine 123 (^{123}I) (100 μCi). In healthy subjects, the percent uptake at 24 hours should be 15% to 30%. ^{123}I is the radioisotope commonly employed because of the shorter half-life and minimal radiation exposure compared with iodine 131 (^{131}I). The RAIU is no longer widely used because of the availability of more precise biochemical tests and the decrease in normal values for RAIU that have occurred because of dietary iodine supplementation. Current use of the RAIU test in the diagnosis of hyperthyroidism is subsequently discussed.

Calcitonin

Calcitonin is a 32-amino acid peptide secreted by the parafollicular, or C cells, of the thyroid. Calcitonin radioimmunoassay has been useful for identifying patients with medullary thyroid carcinoma (MTC), a C cell neoplasm of the thyroid. In most patients with MTC, the diagnosis can be established by demonstration of elevated basal plasma calcitonin levels. Patients with MTC, but not normal individuals, also exhibit an increase in plasma calcitonin after intravenous administration of calcium and pentagastrin. In cases of familial MTC and the multiple endocrine neoplasia type 2 (MEN 2) syndrome, monitoring with the sensitive calcitonin assay and in some cases using provocative testing with calcium-pentagastrin is a valuable biochemical method for screening patients at risk for the disease and monitoring patients for disease recurrence after thyroidectomy.

Tests for Autoimmune Thyroid Disease

Detection of autoantibodies to thyroid antigens may be useful diagnostically in the evaluation of patients with autoimmune thyroid disorders such as Graves disease and Hashimoto thyroiditis. *Antithyroid peroxidase* antibodies are present in high titer in 95% of patients with Hashimoto thyroiditis and 80% with Graves disease. In these conditions, antithyroglobulin antibodies are also detectable but in a lower percentage of cases. Graves disease is caused by circulating antibodies that bind to and stimulate the TSH receptor on thyroid follicular cells.

Thyroid Scintigraphy

Imaging of the thyroid with radionuclide agents is useful in identification of hyperfunctioning nodules and in following patients with differentiated thyroid cancers after thyroidectomy. Formerly, thyroid scintigraphy was used to screen patients for hypofunctioning or cold thyroid nodules. However, because cold nodules are only associated with a 10% to 15% incidence of malignancy, this test is not very specific for

assessing cancer risk and has been supplanted in this role by ultrasonography and fine-needle aspiration (FNA) biopsy. The two agents most commonly used in thyroid imaging are radioactive iodine and ^{99m}Tc pertechnetate. Technetium is trapped by the thyroid but not organified and, consequently, has a short half-life (6 hours) and a low associated radiation dose (10 mrad). Unlike radioactive iodine, technetium is not affected by drugs that inhibit organification (PTU and methimazole). Because of the short half-life and the requirement for earlier imaging, technetium radioactivity may appear in the salivary glands or major vascular structures. Patients with suspected lingual thyroid, ectopic thyroid, or substernal goiter, therefore, may need to undergo scanning with ^{123}I. Both the ^{123}I and ^{131}I radioisotopes are used clinically. ^{123}I has the advantage of a low dose of radiation (30 mrad) and short half-life (12 hours) compared with ^{131}I (500 mrad and a half-life of 8 days).

Patients with differentiated thyroid carcinoma in whom screening is done to search for distant metastases should be screened with ^{131}I. Well-differentiated thyroid cancer is generally well visualized on ^{131}I imaging, but may be poorly seen on fluoro-deoxy-glucose (FDG) positron emission tomography (PET) imaging due to the relatively low metabolic activity of the lesions. In contrast, poorly differentiated thyroid carcinoma is seen well on FDG imaging, but less well visualized on ^{131}I imaging. PET imaging may be useful if the tumor burden is suspected to be greater than that seen on ^{131}I scans (12,13).

Hyperthyroidism

Thyrotoxicosis is the clinical state produced by excess circulating thyroid hormone. Table 14.3 demonstrates the frequency of signs and symptoms in affected organ systems.

TABLE 14.3

Symptoms and Signs in 243 Patients with Thyrotoxicosis

Symptom	Percentage	Sign	Percentage
Nervousness	99	Tachycardia[a]	100
Increased sweating	91	Goiter[a]	100
Heat intolerance	89	Skin changes	97
Palpitations	89	Tremor	97
Fatigue	88	Thyroid bruit	77
Weight loss	85	Eye signs	71
Tachycardia	82	Atrial fibrillation	10
Dyspnea	75		
Weakness	70		
Increased appetite	65		
Eye complaints	54		
Diarrhea	23		

[a]Patients with normal pulse rate or absence of a goiter have been observed in some series.

From Williams RH. Thiouracil treatment of thyrotoxicosis; results of prolonged treatment. *J Clin Endocrinol* 1946;6:3–4. Reprinted with permission.

Elevation of the BMR, increased appetite, heat intolerance, and a slight elevation in body temperature are all manifestations of the accelerated rate of energy metabolism and heat production. The increased rate of protein synthesis and degradation causes increased protein turnover, negative nitrogen balance, weight loss, muscle wasting, and hypoalbuminemia.

Some of the most pronounced features of thyrotoxicosis are seen in the cardiovascular system. Tachycardia is invariably present, and approximately 10% of patients develop atrial fibrillation that may be refractory to medical therapy until control of the thyrotoxicosis is achieved. High output congestive heart failure is sometimes seen, but this occurs primarily in patients with preexisting cardiac disease. Excess thyroid hormone mediates its cardiac effects in part by a cardiac stimulatory action resulting in increased heart rate, contractility, and cardiac output. Thyroid hormones have direct actions on the myocardium, increasing myosin, actin, and membrane Na-K ATPase contents as well as myosin ATPase activity. In addition hyperthyroidism increases myocardial sensitivity to the effects of circulating catecholamines by increasing the number of adrenergic receptors in the heart. The latter explains some of the beneficial actions of β-blockade in patients with thyrotoxicosis-related cardiac symptoms.

Table 14.4 lists the various causes of thyrotoxicosis. The most common cause of hyperthyroidism in Western countries is Graves disease, also known as *diffuse toxic goiter* (5,14). An autoimmune basis for the development of Graves disease is well established. The pathogenesis involves the production of autoantibodies (IgGs) to the TSH receptor.

These thyroid-stimulating antibodies (TSAb) are directed against various sites within the follicular cell membrane, some being cytotoxic, while others activate adenylate cyclase and cAMP, which in turn stimulates increased thyroid vascularity, growth, and hormone release, often leading to goiter formation. The mechanism of autoantibody formation is unknown but probably results from regulatory abnormalities in both B- and T-lymphocyte immune responses. Genetic factors also appear to play a role in disease development because an increased incidence exists in relatives of affected individuals. An increase in frequency of human leukocyte antigen (HLA)-B8 and HLA-DR3 haplotypes in Caucasians, HLA-BW46 in Chinese individuals, and HLA-BW35 in those of Japanese descent, has also been observed in patients with Graves disease (5). There is a notable familial predisposition for this disorder with a strong female predominance (up to 10-fold that of males).

Toxic multinodular goiter (Plummer disease) is a less common cause of hyperthyroidism; it usually develops slowly over a prolonged period in patients with a longstanding goiter. This disease is characterized by multiple heterogeneous autonomously functioning nodules. The role of iodine in the development of this disorder is unclear, but in areas of iodine deficiency and endemic goiter, the administration of iodine may cause hyperthyroidism (Jod-Basedow phenomenon). Toxic adenoma is a less common cause of hyperthyroidism in North America and is more likely to be seen in areas of iodine deficiency than if there is sufficient iodine in the diet. Toxic adenomas are follicular adenomas whose function is not TSH dependent. The pathogenesis is unknown but recently mutations in $G_s\alpha$ resulting in chronic activation of the adenylate cyclase-cAMP cascade have been identified in some patients with autonomously functioning thyroid adenomas. TSH-secreting tumors of the anterior pituitary are a rare cause of hyperthyroidism. Trophoblastic tumors (hydatidiform mole, choriocarcinoma, and metastatic embryonal carcinoma) induce hyperthyroidism through production of a thyroid stimulator similar to TSH.

Thyrotoxicosis may also occur in the absence of hyperthyroidism from either an increased rate of release of stored hormone (thyroiditis) or from extrathyroidal sources of thyroid hormone. Factitious thyrotoxicosis from the exogenous administration of excess amounts of thyroid hormone usually occurs in patients with psychiatric disorders or medical–paramedical backgrounds. Struma ovarii is an uncommon cause of thyrotoxicosis, which results from excess thyroid hormone production by an ovarian teratoma. Rarely, functioning metastases from thyroid carcinoma may produce enough hormone to cause thyrotoxicosis. Each of these conditions can be differentiated from primary thyroid sources of thyrotoxicosis by the RAIU test.

The concentration of serum free T_4 is increased in most (95%) patients with hyperthyroidism. The ultrasensitive TSH assay has greatly facilitated confirmation of the diagnosis because it reliably distinguishes TSH levels in normal individuals (0.3–0.5 μU/L) from the suppressed levels

---

TABLE 14.4

Causes of Thyrotoxicosis

Increased Hormone Production by the Thyroid[a]
Graves disease
Toxic multinodular goiter
Toxic adenoma
TSH-secreting pituitary tumor
Trophoblastic tumor
Iodine induced (Jod Basedow)

Not Associated with Increased Hormone Production by the Thyroid[b]
Factitious thyrotoxicosis
Subacute thyroiditis
Chronic thyroiditis with transient thyrotoxicosis
Ectopic thyroid tissue (struma ovarii, functioning metastatic thyroid carcinoma)

[a]Associated with increased values of RAIU except for iodine induced hyperthyroidism.
[b]Associated with decreased RAIU values.
TSH, thyroid-stimulating hormone; RAIU, radioactive iodine uptake.
Modified from Ingbar S.H. The thyroid. In: Williams RH ed. *Textbook of endocrinology*, 7th ed. Philadelphia: WS Saunders, 1985;743. Reprinted with permission.

(<0.1 μU/L) of hyperthyroid patients. The presence of an elevated serum-free T_4 level together with a suppressed serum TSH level establishes the diagnosis. If the serum-free T_4 level is normal and the TSH level is low, the patient may have T_3 toxicosis as evidenced by an elevated serum free T_3 level. In patients with TSH-secreting pituitary tumors, serum T_4 and T_3 levels are elevated and serum TSH is normal or increased. Caution must be exercised in evaluating patients who are pregnant or taking oral contraceptives, as the serum total T_4 and T_3 may be elevated because of an increase in the concentration of thyroxine-binding globulin. In the absence of thyroid disease, the serum TSH concentration in such individuals is normal.

Once the diagnosis of hyperthyroidism is established biochemically, the etiology must then be determined. If the patient has a diffusely enlarged goiter and exophthalmos, the diagnosis is Gravesdisease and no further tests are necessary. Patients with a nodular thyroid gland should have a radioactive iodine scan. Concentration of iodine in one or more nodules with suppressed uptake in the rest of the gland suggests a toxic adenoma or toxic multinodular goiter. If one of these etiologies is not confirmed, the patient should have a RAIU test. If the uptake is increased, the most likely diagnosis is Graves disease. If the RAIU is low, the thyrotoxicosis may be the result of thyroiditis or an ectopic or exogenous source of thyroid hormone.

Thyroid Storm

Thyroid storm is a life-threatening complication of severe thyrotoxicosis that requires emergent medical intervention (15). Fortunately, with improved medical treatment of thyrotoxicosis and better preparation of patients undergoing thyroidectomy, thyroid storm is rarely seen. However, the mortality from this condition, if untreated, remains between 20% and 30% (16). Infection, trauma, and surgery are the usual precipitating events. The clinical manifestations of thyroid storm are those of profound hypermetabolism: fever (which may be extreme), profuse sweating, and marked tachycardia. Congestive heart failure and pulmonary edema may develop. Nausea, vomiting, and abdominal pain are commonly present. The patient appears restless and tremulous and may become delirious and psychotic. If this complication is not recognized and treated, progression to stupor and coma occurs and death inevitably results. Treatment is directed at correction of the thyrotoxicosis and the precipitating event. Both PTU at a dose of 200 to 250 mg every 6 hours (or methimazole 20 mg every 4 hours) and inorganic iodide should be administered to block synthesis and to slow the release of thyroid hormone, unless the thyroid storm has occurred after thyroidectomy. Patients with allergies to thionamides should take lithium carbonate (300 mg every 6 hours). Propranolol is given to block adrenergic effects (80–120 mg orally every 6 hours or 1–3 mg IV every 4–6 hours) and dexamethasone may aid in inhibiting peripheral conversion of T_4 to T_3. General supportive measures include fever reduction and administration of glucose-containing fluids.

Hypothyroidism

The causes of hypothyroidism include primary thyroid gland failure, pituitary insufficiency, resistance to thyroid hormone, and prior ablative procedures (surgery or radioactive iodine administration). The clinical manifestations of hypothyroidism depend more on severity of the hormone insufficiency and age of onset than on the etiology of the disorder. Thyroid hormone is essential for central nervous system development and for skeletal growth and maturation. In infants, untreated hypothyroidism can cause permanent mental and growth retardation (cretinism). Childhood hypothyroidism is characterized by delayed growth and poor intellectual development. Common signs and symptoms of hypothyroidism in adults are listed in Table 14.5. Treatment, consisting of replacement therapy with exogenous thyroid hormone, is highly successful, but it may take several weeks to months for the physical manifestations to disappear.

Measurement of serum TSH and T_4 should be the initial screening test in the evaluation of patients with clinically suspected hypothyroidism. The presence of a low serum-free T_4 level and elevated TSH establishes the diagnosis. Hypothyroidism secondary to pituitary failure is characterized by both decreased serum T_4 and TSH levels and is much less common than primary gland failure. The diagnosis of hypothyroidism in sick patients may be more difficult because of changes in thyroid hormone secretion and alterations in plasma-binding proteins that occur in severe illness. Serum total T_4 and the free T_4 index are frequently depressed in the critically ill, whereas TSH levels should be elevated in hypothyroid sick patients. However, one must be cautious in interpreting TSH results in patients on dopamine or pharmacologic doses of steroids because, in hypothyroid subjects, these agents may suppress TSH levels into the normal range.

TABLE 14.5

Signs and Common Symptoms of Adult Patients with Hypothyroidism

Loss of energy/fatigue	Myxedema of the skin
Cold intolerance	Delayed deep tendon reflex responses
Decreased appetite	Bradycardia
Weight gain	Low voltage electrocardiogram (ECG)
Decreased BMR	Thin, brittle hair
Constipation	Dry, cold skin
Muscle aches and stiffness	Goiter
Intellectual lethargy	Thick tongue
Slowed speech	Somnolence
Congestive heart failure	Hoarseness
Sexual dysfunction (decreased libido, irregular and heavy menses)	

BMR, basal metabolic rate.

THE PARATHYROIDS

Anatomy and Development

The parathyroid glands first appear embryologically during the sixth week of gestation. The superior parathyroids arise from the fourth branchial pouch, as does the ultimobranchial body. This latter structure eventually separates from the parathyroid as it joins the thyroid gland to form the C cells. The inferior parathyroids along with the thymus are derived from the third branchial pouches.

Variability in the extent and direction of migration of the parathyroids during development can lead to considerable variation in their anatomic location in the adult (Fig. 14.9) (17). The superior parathyroids are usually embedded in fat along the posterior surface of the middle or upper portions of the thyroid lobes posterolateral to the recurrent laryngeal nerve and approximately 1 cm above the junction of the nerve and the inferior thyroid artery. Occasionally, a superior parathyroid may be found within the substance of the thyroid gland. Other aberrant sites for the superior parathyroids include the tracheoesophageal groove, retroesophageal space, and posterior mediastinum. The inferior parathyroids are located more ventrally than the superior glands, anteromedial to the recurrent laryngeal nerve, and near the lower pole of the thyroid or in the thyrothymic ligament. Because of its embryologic association with the thymus, an inferior parathyroid gland may be found embedded in the thymic tissue in the lower neck. In approximately 2% of cases, an inferior gland will be located deep within the thymus in the anterior mediastinum. Other aberrant sites for the inferior parathyroids are lateral to the trachea at the level of the lower pole of the thyroid, the carotid sheath, and rarely, the pharyngeal mucosa. Regardless of location, the position of the glands is symmetrical in a high percentage of cases.

Four parathyroid glands are present in most individuals. Studies in which serial embryologic sections have been examined have demonstrated at least four parathyroid glands in every case (18). In an autopsy study of 503 cadavers, Akerstrom et al. (17) found four or more parathyroids in 97% of cases. Supernumerary, or fifth, parathyroid glands, which have been reported in 6% to 13% of cases, may arise from division of one or more of the four main parathyroids during development. Such supernumerary glands are commonly located within the thymus.

The primary blood supply to the parathyroids comes from the inferior thyroid artery, an important consideration during thyroidectomy, but contributions may also be received from the superior thyroid artery or the thyroidea ima artery. The venous drainage is through the superior, inferior, and middle thyroid veins.

Grossly, the parathyroids are oval shaped and each weighs approximately 40 to 60 mg. Typically, the lower glands are slightly heavier than the upper glands. The parathyroids are

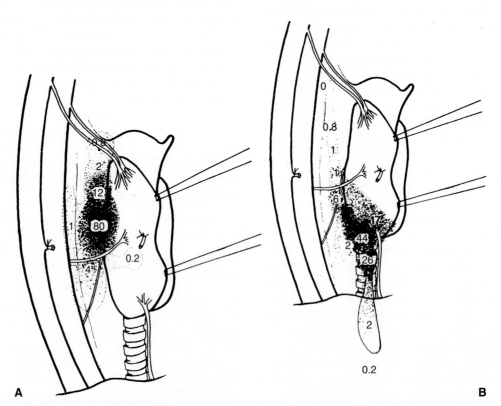

FIGURE 14.9   Locations of the superior (**A**) and inferior (**B**) parathyroid glands. The more common locations are indicated by the darker shading. The numbers represent the percentages of glands found at the different locations. (From Akerstrom G, Malmaeus S, Bergstrom R. Surgical anatomy of human parathyroid glands. *Surgery* 1984;95:17. Reprinted by permission.)

distinguished from adjacent fat and lymph nodes by their red-brown or tan color. Architecturally, the parathyroid glands are composed of cords and sheets of cells arranged within a fatty stroma. The chief cell is the primary cell in the parathyroid that synthesizes and secretes parathyroid hormone (PTH), an 84-amino acid protein. Oxyphil cells are slightly larger cells than the chief cells and are characterized by a central pyknotic nucleus, eosinophilic cytoplasm, and abundant mitochondria. Oxyphil cells first appear at puberty and increase in number with advancing age, but they rarely make up more than 5% of the total cells in the gland. Water-clear cells are glycogen-laden cells that have a clear cytoplasm. Water-clear cell hyperplasia is a rare cause of hyperparathyroidism (HPT).

Physiology

Mineral Metabolism

The principal function of the parathyroid glands and PTH is regulation of bone mineralization and maintenance of calcium and phosphate homeostasis. Most calcium and phosphate within the body is found in an insoluble form within the skeleton. Calcium, phosphate, and magnesium are also essential for a variety of normal cellular and metabolic processes. The need for precise homeostatic control of these minerals is illustrated by the serious clinical consequences of acute derangements in plasma levels of these ions.

The distribution and body content of calcium, phosphate, and magnesium in the tissues and blood is shown in Table 14.6 (14,15). The average daily intake of calcium is 500 to 1,000 mg, most of which is absorbed in the upper small intestine by a process dependent on the active vitamin D_3 metabolite calcitriol (1,25-dihydroxycholecalciferol). Normal plasma levels of calcium vary slightly among laboratories but generally range from 8.5 to 10.2 mg/dL (2.2–2.5 mmol/L). Plasma calcium is evenly distributed between ionized (46%) and protein-bound (46%) phases, with a smaller percentage (8%) that is complexed with organic anions such as citrate. Approximately 80% of protein-bound calcium is complexed with albumin. Protein-bound calcium is not biologically active, and changes in serum protein have little effect on the concentration of

the ionized physiologically active fraction. The percentage of total plasma calcium that is protein bound is, however, affected by changes in plasma pH, as hydrogen ion competes with calcium for the same binding site on plasma proteins. This results in an increase in the percentage of ionized calcium in acidosis, whereas in alkalosis, the proportion of ionized calcium ion is decreased.

Extracellular calcium is necessary for the normal activity of a number of physiologic processes, including bone formation, coagulation, and neuromuscular function. Calcium also plays a critical role in a number of intracellular regulatory systems and second messenger pathways, including the cAMP second messenger system. Calcium is excreted through the urine (100 to 200 mg/d), feces (600 mg/d), and sweat (<100 mg/d). Normally, the kidney reabsorbs 98% to 99% of the filtered calcium load. Consequently, urinary calcium excretion rates of greater than 500 mg/d are unusual, even in patients with marked hypercalcemia.

Inorganic phosphate deposited in the mineral phase of bone accounts for approximately 85% of total body phosphate. Unlike calcium, phosphate is also distributed widely in nonosseous tissues in both an inorganic form and as a component of cellular macromolecules. These macromolecules include phospholipids and phosphoproteins that are integral components of cellular membranes, nucleic acids, glycogen, and other intermediates of carbohydrate metabolism. Phosphates also serve as substrates for the enzymes of glycolysis, respiration, and the formation of high-energy phosphate bonds [adenosine triphosphate (ATP)]. They are critical for normal muscular contraction and transmission of nerve impulses. Severely hypophosphatemic patients will have decreased nerve conductance, which may manifest as weakness or in ventilator-dependant patients, may impair spontaneous respiratory mechanics. Approximately 70% of the phosphate ingested daily is absorbed, primarily in the small intestine. Unlike calcium, plasma proteins bind 15% of circulating phosphate, with the remaining 85% circulating as free ion or complexed with other cations. Normal serum phosphate levels range from 2.5 to 4.5 mg/dL in the adult and from 5 to 6 mg/dL in children. Serum phosphate levels may vary daily

TABLE 14.6

Body Content and Distribution of Calcium, Phosphate, and Magnesium

	Calcium	Phosphate	Magnesium
Specific tissue distribution			
Skeleton	99%	86%	53%
Extracellular fluid	0.1%	0.03%	1%
Cells	1%	14%	46%
Total body content[a]	20–25 g/kg	11–14 g/kg	25 g

[a]g/kg fat-free tissue.
From Tietgens ST, Leinung MC. Thyroid storm. *Med Clin North Am* 1995;79:169–184.
Modified from Aurbach GD, Marx SJ, Spiegel AM. Parathyroid hormone, calcitonin, and the calciferols. In: Wilson JD, Foster DW, eds. *Textbook of endocrinology*, 7th ed. Philadelphia: WB Saunders, 1985; Reprinted with permission.

by up to 1.5 mg/dL and are influenced by several factors, including diet, age, and secretion of PTH and other hormones. Inorganic phosphate is freely filtered by the kidney where approximately 90% is reabsorbed, mostly in the proximal tubule.

Magnesium is the most common divalent intracellular cation and functions in the activation of enzyme systems, cellular metabolism, and neuromuscular electrical activity. Total body magnesium content is 25 g, half of which is in bone and only 1% of which is in the extracellular fluid. Because only 20% of magnesium is protein bound, serum levels (normal range 1.5–2.2 mg/dL) are not influenced greatly by changes in serum proteins. The average dietary intake of magnesium is about 300 mg (25 mEq), 50% of which is absorbed. Magnesium is cleared by the kidney in a manner similar to calcium.

Parathyroid Hormone, Calcitonin, and Vitamin D
Parathyroid Hormone
PTH is an 84-amino acid peptide (9,400 Da) secreted by the parathyroid glands. Serum calcium is the major regulator of PTH secretion. Increased serum calcium levels inhibit PTH secretion whereas decreased calcium levels stimulate release. The effects of calcium on PTH secretion are mediated through the calcium sensing receptor on the parathyroid cell surface. Stimulation of the calcium-sensing receptor by low or falling serum calcium levels results in PTH secretion within seconds. The calcium set point at which PTH secretion is 50% of maximal occurs at a serum ionized calcium of 4 mg/dL (1 mmol/L). Hypocalcemia also stimulates parathyroid cell growth whereas metabolites of vitamin D have an inhibitory effect. Magnesium also affects PTH secretion in a manner qualitatively similar to calcium, although it is much less potent. Severe hypomagnesemia paradoxically inhibits PTH secretion, probably by interfering with intracellular secretory mechanisms. As a result, hypocalcemia associated with profound hypomagnesemia will not respond to calcium administration until the hypomagnesemia has been corrected. Secretion of PTH is unaffected by serum phosphate levels. After secretion, the PTH molecule is degraded within minutes into biologically inactive peptides. Full biologic activity resides within the first 34 N-terminus amino acids. Bioactive N-terminus PTH fragments are cleared rapidly from the circulation, whereas biologically inactive C-terminus fragments persist longer in the circulation, especially in the setting of chronic renal insufficiency.

PTH regulates the level of calcium in the extracellular fluid by direct effects on the kidney and bone and, indirectly, through the gastrointestinal (GI) tract. In the kidney, PTH increases calcium reabsorption in the proximal convoluted tubule. This effect on calcium clearance is rapid and is associated with increased urinary secretion of sodium, potassium, and bicarbonate. In the skeleton, PTH increases mobilization of calcium from bone to blood in two phases: (i) a rapid phase that results from mobilization of bone in equilibrium with the extracellular fluid, and (ii) a slow phase that depends on activation of enzymes that promote bone resorption. PTH also indirectly increases the rate of calcium absorption from the intestinal tract through its effects on vitamin D. It also regulates phosphate metabolism by increasing renal clearance of phosphate and increasing release of phosphate from bone. The effects of PTH are mediated through type 1 PTH (PTH-1) receptors in bone, kidney, and intestines. The PTH-1 receptor in these cells is coupled to the heterotrimeric guanine nucleotide-binding (G) protein containing the stimulatory alpha subunit (Gαs), which stimulates the formation of cAMP and the activation of the protein kinase A (PKA)-signaling cascade. The PTH-1 receptor can also activate the phospholipase C/protein kinase C (PLC/PKC) signaling pathway, most likely through the Gαq-containing G protein heterotrimer, although this signaling response to PTH is generally not as sensitive or as robust as the cAMP/PKA pathway. The end result of PTH-1 receptor activation in these target cells is the release of calcium from bone, the stimulation of calcitriol (1,25-dihydroxyvitamin D_3) production, and the retention of calcium from the glomerular filtrate. A second type of PTH receptor (type 2 PTH receptor) is found in the brain and intestines; the principal ligand for this receptor differs from PTH and its biological function is unknown (19).

Calcitonin
Calcitonin is a polypeptide of 32 amino acids and is produced in the parafollicular C-cells of the thyroid gland. The principal action of calcitonin is to lower serum calcium and phosphate levels by acutely inhibiting osteoclastic bone resorption. Calcitonin also has a phosphaturic effect on the kidneys, which is independent of PTH. Calcitonin secretion is stimulated by increased serum calcium levels, gastrin, secretin, and cholecystokinin (CCK) and is inhibited by low calcium concentrations. Clinically, calcitonin has been used in pharmacologic doses to lower serum calcium levels acutely in patients with severe hypercalcemia and to treat Paget disease. However, neither patients with elevated calcitonin levels (MTC) nor patients with calcitonin deficiency (thyroidectomy) have significant alterations in calcium homeostasis. The precise physiologic role of calcitonin in human bone and mineral metabolism is unclear. It may be more important in protecting the skeleton during periods of calcium stress than in maintaining plasma calcium homeostasis. Calcitonin has a short half-life (~10 minutes) and is degraded primarily in the kidneys (20).

Vitamin D
The D vitamins (calciferols) are a group of fat-soluble vitamins found in virtually all living plants and animals. Only a few foods (fish liver oils, egg yolk, and liver) contain vitamin D. The principal nutritional source of vitamin D comes from exposure to sunlight. In humans, the precursor for vitamin D_3 (7-dehydrocholesterol) is found in the skin and epidermis. After exposure to ultraviolet radiation, this precursor is converted to vitamin D_3 (cholecalciferol). Vitamin D_3 then undergoes hydroxylation in the liver to form 25-hydroxycholecalciferol (25-OH-D_3) (Fig. 14.10).

Site	Vitamin D metabolite
Skin	7–Dehydrocholesterol
	↓ Ultraviolet radiation
	Cholecalciferol (vitamin D$_3$)
Liver	↓ 25–Hydroxylase
	25– (OH) –vitamin D$_3$
Kidney	↓ 1α–Hydroxylase
	1, 25– (OH)$_2$–vitamin D$_3$

FIGURE 14.10 Metabolic pathway for vitamin D. 1α-Hydroxylase activity in the kidney is regulated positively by parathyroid hormone (PTH) and is the rate-limiting step in the vitamin D metabolism pathway.

Approximately 5% to 30% of 25-OH-vitamin D$_3$ is excreted into the bile and enters the enterohepatic circulation. Further hydroxylation by 1α-hydoxylase in the kidney leads to the formation of 1,25-dihydroxycholecalciferol (1,25(OH)$_2$-D$_3$; calcitriol), the most potent, active natural metabolite of vitamin D. Both PTH and serum phosphate levels directly regulate 1α-hydoxylase activity. Vitamin D acts on the intestine to increase absorption of calcium by stimulating synthesis of a calcium-binding protein that promotes calcium transport across the intestinal cell. Vitamin D also increases, to a lesser extent, intestinal absorption of phosphate and magnesium. It has an antirachitic effect on bone and increases mobilization of calcium and phosphate from bone to blood. Clinically, low circulating calcitriol levels are seen in hypoparathyroidism, neonatal hypocalcemia, secondary HPT, rickets, and osteomalacia.

Tests of Parathyroid Function

Biochemical Tests

Measurement of total serum calcium is the most useful screening test for identifying patients with disorders of the parathyroid glands. In most laboratories, the upper limit of normal for serum calcium ranges from 10.2 to 10.4 mg/dL. Patients with hypercalcemia should undergo further diagnostic evaluation for HPT. Because approximately 50% of serum calcium is protein bound, changes in serum proteins (albumin) and other anions may significantly affect the total serum calcium level in the blood. Ionized calcium more accurately reflects the physiologic state of calcium homeostasis and its measurement should be carried out in equivocal cases.

Other biochemical abnormalities commonly seen in patients with HPT include hypophosphatemia from the phosphaturic actions of PTH and hyperchloremic metabolic acidosis from increased urinary excretion of bicarbonate. Elevation of the chloride:phosphate ratio to greater than 33 is seen in many patients with HPT. Patients with bone disease from HPT often have an increase in serum alkaline phosphatase. Hypomagnesemia is present in approximately 5% to 10% of patients with primary HPT. If hypocalcemia develops after parathyroidectomy and associated hypomagnesemia exists, the hypocalcemia will be refractory to calcium administration until the serum magnesium level has been normalized.

Parathyroid Hormone Assay

Demonstration of an elevated serum PTH level in conjunction with hypercalcemia is diagnostic of HPT. Total and ionized serum calcium levels should be measured at the same time as serum PTH in order to properly interpret the results. Various types of PTH immunoassays have been used based on the region of the PTH molecule that is recognized (21). The assay of choice is one that measures the intact PTH molecule, which eliminates the problem of detection of inactive fragments of PTH in the circulation associated with region specific PTH assays. The intact PTH assay employs a two-site double antibody technique in which one antibody reacts with the N-terminus of the molecule and the second antibody recognizes the C-terminus region. These two antibodies are bound simultaneously by intact PTH molecules, and the bound antibodies are then detected with either radioactive or chemiluminescent tags. The sensitivity of the intact PTH assay in the detection of patients with primary HPT ranges from 90% to 97%, and the specificity of the assay nears 100%. The intact PTH assay also reliably differentiates patients with HPT from those with hypercalcemia of malignancy. parathyroid hormone–related protein (PTHrP), a hypercalcemia-causing factor released by many tumors, is not detected by the intact PTH assay. Recently, PTHrP has been shown to have an important role in normal skeletal development as shown by the neonatal lethal phenotype of mice having the *PTHrP* gene deleted (22–24). PTHrP binds to the same PTH-1 receptor as PTH, and induces the same second messenger signaling responses.

Nephrogenous cAMP determination is currently most useful in evaluating patients with hypoparathyroidism and in identifying states of PTH resistance.

Hyperparathyroidism

Primary Hyperparathyroidism

Primary HPT is the result of excessive secretion of PTH by one or more parathyroid glands. While PTH hypersecretion can occur physiologically in response to calcemic stress, primary HPT is characterized by high concentrations of PTH in association with elevated plasma calcium concentrations. The etiology of HPT in most cases is unknown and while there do not appear to be any well-established predisposing factors, a history of childhood irradiation to the face and neck is obtained in as many as 15% to 25% of patients. An altered set point in the level of ionized calcium at which PTH secretion is suppressed has also been demonstrated in patients with HPT, but the role of this physiologic abnormality in initiating the development of HPT is uncertain.

Approximately 80% to 85% of cases of primary HPT are the result of a single parathyroid adenoma, whereas the remaining 15% to 20% can be attributed to multigland disease. Parathyroid adenomas may be monoclonal or oligoclonal in nature. In most cases, the genetic basis for the development of parathyroid adenomas or hyperplasia is unknown. Recent molecular studies have begun to identify genetic factors associated with the development of parathyroid gland neoplasms in some groups of patients (22,24–26). Two specific genes have been implicated in the pathogenesis of parathyroid adenomas: the *cyclin D1/PRAD1* oncogene and the *MEN 1* tumor suppressor gene. Cyclin D1 (also known as *PRAD-1*) is an integral component of the cell-cycle regulatory machinery, acting with cyclin dependent kinases to drive progression through the G1/S checkpoint. The *cyclin D1* oncogene is activated in a subset of parathyroid adenomas, in which a chromosome 11 inversion brings the *cyclin D1* gene under the influence of the 5'-regulatory region of the *PTH* gene, leading to cyclin D1 overexpression (Fig. 14.11) (23). Cyclin D1 overexpression is found in 20% to 40% of parathyroid adenomas. Genetic defects have also been identified in patients with MEN types 1 and 2A, each of which have associated parathyroid hyperplasia and an autosomal dominant inheritance pattern (see "Multiple Endocrine Neoplasia Syndromes"). Mutations in the *MEN 1* gene have been identified in approximately 20% of parathyroid adenomas. The hyperparathyroidism-jaw-tumor syndrome is characterized by HPT, ossifying tumors of the jaw, Wilms tumors, renal cysts, and renal hamaratomas. It is inherited as an autosomal dominant trait and caused by a mutation on chromosome 1q24. The syndromes of familial hypocalciuric hypercalcemia (FHH) and neonatal severe HPT occur as a result of mutations in the calcium-sensing receptor gene on chromosome 3 (27). Abnormal expression of the tumor suppressor gene p53 and inactivation of the retinoblastoma gene have also been described in some patients with parathyroid carcinoma. Mutations in the *HRPT2* tumor suppressor gene have also been identified in sporadic parathyroid carcinomas (28).

Patients with primary HPT lack the adaptive mechanisms that normally protect the individual against hypercalcemia. Excessive secretion of PTH with its direct effects on the kidney and indirect actions on the intestine through vitamin D prevents a compensatory increase in urinary and intestinal losses of calcium from occurring. With mild states of hypercalcemia (<11.5 mg/dL), calcium is reabsorbed efficiently by the kidney, and urinary calcium levels may remain normal. With more severe hypercalcemia, however, the renal tubular mechanism is overwhelmed and hypercalciuria results. Decreased renal tubular reabsorption of phosphate leads to increased urinary phosphate excretion and hypophosphatemia. Excess PTH also causes decreased urinary excretion of hydrogen ion and increased excretion of bicarbonate. The hyperchloremic acidosis that results further aggravates the effects of hypercalcemia by increasing the fraction of ionized calcium in the circulation.

Conditions that must be distinguished from HPT in the differential diagnosis of hypercalcemia are shown in Table 14.7. The majority of these disorders can be excluded by a careful history and physical examination, family history, and review of medications (vitamin D, thiazides, alkali, and lithium, and measurement of intact PTH. Hypercalcemia of malignancy is generally characterized by low PTH levels. Patients who present with marked hypercalcemia (calcium >12.5 mg/dL) or the combination of hypercalcemia and weight loss, anemia, or an elevated erythrocyte sedimentation rate should undergo a careful search for an occult malignancy. The mechanisms of development of hypercalcemia in malignancy are discussed under "Endocrine Manifestations of Nonendocrine Malignancies," in the subsequent text.

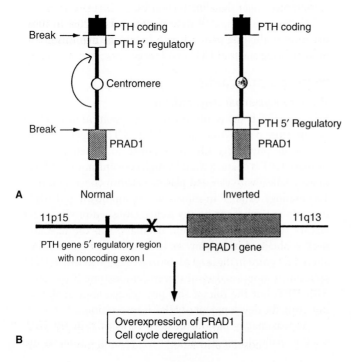

FIGURE 14.11 Schematic illustration of the mechanism of gene rearrangement and overexpression of the protooncogene PRAD1 in a subset of parathyroid adenomas.
A: Pericentromeric inversion of chromosome 11 results in juxtaposition of the *PTH* gene and the *PRAD1* gene.
B: Molecular structure of the rearranged PTH/PRAD gene complex. The X marks the chromosomal breakpoint between the *PTH* gene regulatory region from 11p15 and the *PRAD1* gene from 11q13. (From Habener JF, Arnold A, Potts JT Jr. Hyperparathyroidism. In Degroot LJ, ed. *Endocrinology.* Philadelphia: WB Saunders, 1995;1044–1057. Reprinted with permission.)

TABLE 14.7

Differential Diagnosis of Hypercalcemia

Due to increased serum PTH

Primary hyperparathyroidism (HPT)
Tertiary HPT
Familial HPT (MEN 1, MEN 2A, HPT-jaw tumor syndrome)
Parathyroid carcinoma

Not due to increased serum PTH

Drug-induced hypercalcemia (thiazides, furosemide,
   vitamin D, calcium, vitamin A, lithium)
Granulomatous diseases (sarcoidosis, tuberculosis,
   berylliosis)
Genetic diseases (familial hypocalciuric hypercalcemia)
Immobilization
"Idiopathic" hypercalcemia
Malignancy (PTHrP related, skeletal metastases, some
   hematologic malignancies)
Nonparathyroid endocrine diseases (Addison disease, hyper-
   and hypothyroidism)

PTH, parathyroid hormone; MEN, multiple endocrine neoplasia;
PTHrP, parathyroid hormone-related protein.

TABLE 14.8

Clinical Manifestations of Hyperparathyroidism

Organ System	Clinical Manifestations
Renal	Polyuria, nocturia, nephrolithiasis, nephrocalcinosis
Musculoskeletal	Proximal muscle weakness, calcific tendinitis, chondrocalcinosis, pseudogout, osteitis fibrosa cystica
Central nervous system	Impaired mentation, loss of recent memory, lethargy, insomnia, emotional lability, depression, somnolence, coma
Gastrointestinal	Anorexia, nausea, vomiting, dyspepsia, constipation
Skin	Pruritus
Ophthalmologic	Band keratopathy
Cardiovascular	Hypertension, heart block

FHH, or familial benign hypercalcemia, is a rare condition characterized by asymptomatic or mildly symptomatic hypercalcemia, hypocalciuria, hypermagnesemia, and normal or low PTH levels. This disorder is inherited as an autosomal dominant trait with the phenotype diagnosed soon after birth, and the parathyroid glands are usually either normal in size or slightly enlarged. While the penetrance of FHH approaches 100%, affected individuals exhibit virtually none of the morbidity generally associated with hypercalcemia. Physiologic and biochemical studies on individuals with FHH demonstrate abnormal responses of both the kidney and the parathyroid glands to calcium. Although the precise genetic defect is unknown, linkage analyses have demonstrated that the disease locus in most FHH families is located on the long arm of chromosome 3 and in one family, an FHH locus maps to chromosome 19p32.

The basis for the development of FHH appears to be mutations in the calcium-sensing receptor gene on chromosome 3 that regulates the parathyroid gland set point and modulates the extracellular calcium concentration (27). Patients with FHH are usually asymptomatic and are not rendered eucalcemic by parathyroidectomy. FHH can be distinguished from primary HPT by demonstrating a low 24-hour urinary calcium excretion. Neonatal severe HPT is a rare life-threatening disorder characterized by very high serum calcium concentrations (>15 mg/dL). Genetic analyses of FHH families with neonatal severe HPT demonstrate that this disorder can be transmitted as an autosomal recessive trait tightly linked to the FHH locus (odds >350,000:1) on chromosome 3q2 (29). Individuals with severe neonatal HPT are homozygous for the FHH mutation; heterozygous mutations are associated with a milder form of disease.

The clinical features of primary HPT are shown in Table 14.8. With the widespread use of biochemical screening tests, most patients with primary HPT are asymptomatic or have mild, nonspecific symptoms (muscle weakness and fatigue) at the time of diagnosis. The classic findings of osteitis fibrosis cystica with bone cysts and fractures are rarely seen. The principal radiographic sign of osteitis fibrosis cystica is subperiosteal bone resorption, which is best seen in the distal phalanx of the index finger. Other sites for development of subperiosteal erosions include the proximal tibia and femur, distal clavicles, and skull. The classic findings of parathyroid bone disease are rarely seen now in patients with primary HPT. However, osteopenia develops in 25% of patients, which may increase the subsequent long-term risk of osteoporosis and vertebral and other fractures. Successful parathyroidectomy is accompanied by an increase in bone mass in these patients. Nephrolithiasis occurs in 20% to 30% of patients. Extraskeletal calcification from deposition of calcium-phosphate crystals in the soft tissues may occur if the calcium-phosphate solubility product exceeds 70. Calcific tendinitis and chondrocalcinosis with joint pain and nephrocalcinosis with impairment of renal function may result.

Secondary Hyperparathyroidism

Secondary HPT represents an adaptive response to a disruption in maintenance of normal calcium and phosphorus homeostasis which occurs most commonly due to chronic renal failure (30). Vitamin D deficiency can also lead to secondary elevation in PTH. The pathophysiologic basis for the development of secondary HPT is outlined in Figure 14.12. As renal function declines, phosphate excretion decreases and the serum phosphate concentration increases. This leads to a transient decrease in serum calcium concentration, which in turn stimulates secretion of PTH by the parathyroid glands. Serum calcium and phosphate levels return to normal as a result of the phosphaturic actions of PTH and mobilization

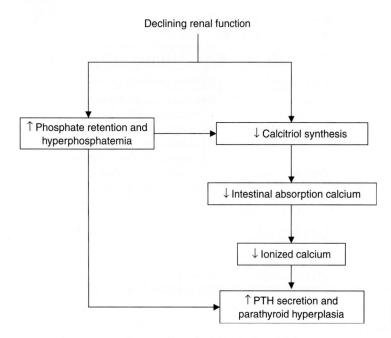

FIGURE 14.12 Pathogenesis of secondary hyperparathyroidism.

of skeletal calcium. With a decrease in glomerular filtration to less than 20 to 25 mL/min, PTH secretion cannot increase phosphate excretion further and hyperphosphatemia occurs. Chronic hyperphosphatemia results in increased PTH secretion and parathyroid cell proliferation. As this cycle is progressively repeated, parathyroid hyperplasia and secondary HPT gradually develop. Abnomalities in vitamin D metabolism also contribute to the pathophysiology of secondary HPT. Both the hyperphosphatemia and the loss of nephron function result in reduced conversion of decreased production of $1,25(OH)_2$-D_3 or calcitriol, which in turn leads to reduced intestinal absorption of calcium and exacerbation of the hypocalcemia. Calcitriol also has a direct inhibitory effect on PTH secretion, which is diminished as a result of its reduced synthesis.

The combined effects of increased PTH and reduced vitamin D levels in patients with chronic renal failure produce a complex array of skeletal abnormalities termed *renal osteodystrophy* (31). Characteristically, renal osteodystrophy consists of varying degrees of osteitis fibrosa cystica, generalized osteoporosis, osteomalacia, osteosclerosis, and growth retardation. The typical lesions of osteitis fibrosa cystica include subperiosteal bone resorption and the formation of bone cysts and cyst-like areas within the bone (brown tumors). Osteosclerosis occurs as a result of an increase in the thickness and number of trabeculae in spongy bone and is responsible for the "rugger jersey" appearance of the spine on plain radiographs. The combined effects of osteitis fibrosa cystica and osteosclerosis may give the skull a mottled, granular (salt and pepper) radiographic appearance. Bone pain with fractures, soft tissue calcification, and pruritus are the predominate clinical manifestations of secondary HPT. Treatment consists of dietary restriction of phosphate (including phosphate-binding antacids), calcium supplementation, and vitamin D therapy. Surgical parathyroidectomy is reserved for patients

who develop progressive symptoms or complications on medical therapy such as bone pain or fracture, pruritus or calciphylaxis.

Tertiary Hyperparathyroidism
Tertiary HPT is a condition that presents secondary to long-standing secondary HPT and is characterized by the development of autonomous hypersecretion of PTH causing hypercalcemia. While the etiology is largely unknown, changes occur in the set point of the calcium-sensing mechanism to hypercalcemic levels. This condition is most commonly observed in patients with chronic secondary HPT and often after renal transplantation. The hypertrophied parathyroid glands fail to return to normal and continue to oversecrete PTH, despite serum calcium levels that are often within the reference range or mildly elevated. Hypertrophied glands secrete PTH autonomously and cause hypercalcemia, even after withdrawal of calcium and calcitriol therapy. With high phosphate levels and high calcium-phosphate products, calcinosis may occur. Treatment involves total parathyroidectomy with autotransplantation or $3\frac{1}{2}$ gland subtotal parathyroidectomy.

Hypoparathyroidism
Parathyroid Hormone–Deficient Hypoparathyroidism
Hypoparathyroidism may develop either as a result of a deficiency in secretion of PTH or end organ resistance to PTH (pseudohypoparathyroidism) (32). The causes of PTH-deficient hypoparathyroidism are shown in Table 14.9. Injury to the parathyroid glands during surgery accounts for most of these cases and is most commonly seen in patients undergoing extensive thyroidectomy for cancer, reoperative parathyroidectomy, or from failed autograft function after total parathyroidectomy. The pathophysiologic consequences of PTH deficiency are (i) decreased bone resorption,

TABLE 14.9

Causes of Parathyroid Hormone (PTH)–Deficient Hypoparathyroidism

Etiology	Basis for PTH Deficiency
Postsurgical	Loss of all functional parathyroid tissue
Congenital	Congenital absence of parathyroids and thymus (DiGeorge syndrome)
Idiopathic[a]	Unknown (? circulating parathyroid autoantibodies)
Functional	Chronic hypomagnesemia

[a]Idiopathic hypoparathyroidism has been categorized into early- and late-onset forms. The early-onset form of hypoparathyroidism, also termed the *multiple endocrine deficiency-autoimmune-candidiasis syndrome*, has a genetic origin and is often associated with circulating parathyroid and adrenal autoantibodies. The late-onset form does not have associated autoantibodies, occurs sporadically, and has an unknown pathogenesis.

From Arnaud CD, Kolb FO. The calciotropic hormones and metabolic bone disease. In Greenspan FS, ed. *Basic and clinical endocrinology*, 3rd ed. Norwalk: Appleton & Lange, 1991;249–322.

(ii) increased renal clearance of calcium, (iii) decreased renal phosphate excretion, and (iv) decreased renal production of $1,25(OH)_2\text{-}D_3$, which results in decreased intestinal absorption of calcium. Biochemically, these patients are hypocalcemic, are hyperphosphatemic, and have low to absent circulating levels of PTH.

Hypoparathyroidism is characterized clinically by increased neuromuscular excitability, which first manifests itself acutely as paresthesias around the mouth, fingertips, and feet. Progressive hypocalcemia may cause tetany with carpopedal spasms, hyperventilation, and ultimately, convulsions. The alkalosis that results from hyperventilation may worsen the hypocalcemia by increasing the fraction of ionized calcium bound to plasma proteins. Other consequences of long-standing hypoparathyroidism include extrapyramidal neurologic disorders (parkinsonism), cataracts, prolonged QT interval on electrocardiogram (ECG), heart block, dental abnormalities, and intestinal malabsorption. Treatment consists of replacement therapy with oral calcium and vitamin D. Acute hypocalcemia and tetany require emergency treatment with intravenous calcium.

Pseudohypoparathyroidism and Pseudopseudohypoparathyroidism

Pseudohypoparathyroidism (PHP) is a rare familial disorder characterized by target tissue resistance to PTH, hypocalcemia, hyperphosphatemia, and congenital defects in growth and skeletal development. The molecular defects in the gene (GNAS1) encoding the α subunit of the stimulatory G protein ($G_s\alpha$) contribute to at least three different forms of the disease: PHP type 1a, PHP type 1b, and pseudopseudohypoparathyroidism (pseudo-PHP). PHP type 1a is inherited in an autosomal dominant pattern and all patients are heterozygous, having one normal $G_s\alpha$ allele and one mutant allele (33). It is caused by loss of function mutations in $G_s\alpha$ such that PTH does not stimulate activation of the c AMP

cascade. Parathyroid function is normal in these individuals and circulating PTH levels are increased appropriately for the degree of hypocalcemia. The biochemical abnormalities are similar to those seen in patients with surgical hypoparathyroidism, except for the elevated PTH levels. This disorder can also be distinguished from other causes of hypoparathyroidism by the failure of these patients to increase nephrogenous cAMP levels in response to exogenously administered PTH. The treatment is the same as for patients with PTH-deficient hypoparathyroidism.

Patients with PHP type 1b are biochemically and genetically distinct from type 1a patients in that they have normal expression of Gsa protein in accessible tissues, and manifest hormonal resistance limited to PTH target tissues. PTH resistance may be limited to the kidney, with PTH responsiveness preserved in the bone, as evidenced by the hyperparathyroid skeletal lesions observed in these patients. The severity of PHP type 1b can vary considerably even within a single kindred. Current data suggest that a molecular defect in the GNAS1 gene may also be responsible for at least some forms of PHP type 1b. A mutant promoter or enhancer region of the GNAS1 gene that has lost the ability to support expression of Gsa in the kidney but not in other tissues may be responsible for the renal resistance to PTH.

Pseudo-PHP is characterized by the same skeletal developmental defects as PHP, but it is distinguished by a lack of associated biochemical abnormalities. Serum calcium and phosphate levels are normal and no treatment is necessary.

THE PITUITARY

Anatomy and Development

The pituitary gland lies within the bony sella turcica (Turkish saddle), which is formed as a recess within the sphenoid bone in the anterior cranial fossa. The pituitary is surrounded by dura. The roof of the sella is formed by a reflection of dura attached to the clinoid processes (the diaphragma sella) (Fig. 14.13). In 10% of patients, the diaphragma sella is very thin, and in 40%, a 5-mm opening is present that may allow pituitary tumors to enlarge into the suprasellar region (34). The floor of the sella is formed by the roof of the sphenoid sinus that provides surgical access to the pituitary. Laterally, the pituitary is bounded by the cavernous sinus and the carotid artery; cranial nerves III, IV, and VI cross this sinus just lateral to the sella. The optic chiasm is located 5 to 10 mm above the diaphragma sella and is anterior to the pituitary stalk. The proximity of these structures to the pituitary can cause cranial nerve palsies and visual field defects in patients with pituitary tumors. The pituitary gland normally weighs 500 to 900 mg and measures $15 \times 10 \times 6$ mm. The size of the gland may increase twofold in pregnancy.

The pituitary is divided anatomically and functionally into two parts: the adenohypophysis and the neurohypophysis (Fig. 14.13). The adenohypophysis, derived embryologically from Rathke pouch, is divided anatomically into the

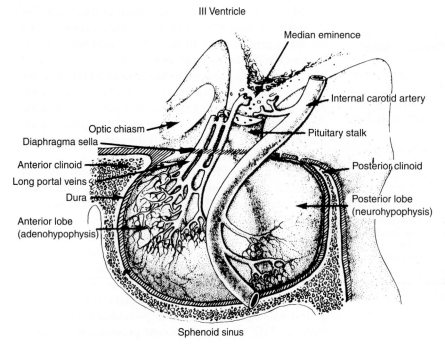

FIGURE 14.13 Anatomic relationships and blood supply of the pituitary gland. (From Frohman LA. Diseases of the anterior pituitary. In: Felig P, Baxter JD, Broadus AE, et al. eds. *Endocrinology and metabolism.* New York: McGraw-Hill, 1981:152. Reprinted by permission of McGraw-Hill, Inc.)

anterior lobe (pars distalis), pars intermedia, and pars tuberalis. In humans, the pars intermedia is indistinct and the anterior lobe, or par distalis, is the main source of pituitary hormone secretion. The neurohypophysis is an anatomic extension of the central nervous system derived from the neural primordia. It consists of the median eminence (infundibulum), the pituitary stalk (infundibular stem), and the posterior lobe (infundibular process).

Pituitary blood flow, which ranges from 0.5 to 0.8 mL/g/min, is the richest blood flow of any organ in the body. The adenohypophysis has no direct arterial supply but is supplied by venous blood from long portal veins connecting the median eminence of the hypothalamus and the anterior pituitary. Short portal venous channels from the posterior pituitary also contribute to the blood supply to the anterior lobe. The posterior pituitary receives arterial blood directly from the internal carotid artery through the middle and inferior hypophyseal arteries, which also supply the median eminence of the hypothalamus. Consequently, blood entering the posterior pituitary is outside of the blood–brain barrier. Blood exits the pituitary through the cavernous sinus, which drains into the superior and inferior petrosal sinuses and then into the jugular bulb and vein. Sampling of inferior petrosal sinus blood for pituitary hormones can be a useful technique for the diagnosis and localization of pituitary tumors, especially in patients with Cushing syndrome (35).

Physiology

Posterior Pituitary

The posterior pituitary or neurohypophysis secretes two nonapeptides (9 amino acids): oxytocin and vasopressin or antidiuretic hormone (ADH) differing only by 2 amino acids. These hormones are each synthesized as preprohormones in axonal cell bodies of the supraoptic and paraventricular nuclei of the hypothalamus. Also synthesized by those hypothalamic neurons are carrier proteins called neurophysins, which bind specifically to the neurohypophyseal hormones. This hormone–neurophysin complex is then transported by the hypothalamic neurons to their termination point on capillaries in the posterior lobe of the pituitary where the active peptide and neurophysin are cleaved and released into the systemic circulation.

The principal action of vasopressin is to increase the permeability of the distal nephron to water, promoting water absorption in the collecting ducts of the kidney. Increased secretion of vasopressin causes concentration of the urine (maximum 1,200 mOsm/kg water) and a decline in urine output (to as little as 0.5 mL/min). In the absence of vasopressin, such as occurs in patients with diabetes insipidus, urine osmolality may fall to as low as 30 mOsm/kg water and urine flow may increase to 15 to 20 mL/min. Vasopressin also exerts a constrictive effect on peripheral arterioles elevating blood pressure. Release of vasopressin occurs in response to an increase in plasma osmolality (>285 mOsm) or decrease in plasma volume of 5% or more.

Oxytocin acts on uterine smooth muscle cells to increase the frequency and strength of contractions and stimulates the myoepithelial cells of the breast surrounding the mammary gland alveoli to induce milk ejection. Estrogens increase the uterine response to oxytocin whereas progesterones decrease the response. Oxytocin carries a short half-life (3–5 minutes) and is degraded in the liver and kidney primarily but also in the uterus and mammary glands.

Anterior Pituitary

The anterior pituitary secretes six major hormones: growth hormone (GH), adrenocorticotropic hormone (ACTH), prolactin (PRL), TSH, FSH, and LH. Secretion of these hormones is controlled primarily by hypothalamic hormones synthesized in the arcuate and other hypothalamic nuclei. These hypophyseal hormones are secreted into portal hypophyseal vessels, which connect the median eminence of the hypothalamus with capillary networks that bathe the cells of the adenohypophysis.

Growth Hormone

GH is a 191-amino acid peptide whose primary function is promotion of linear growth of bone, muscle, and the visceral organs. Thirty percent to 40% of GH in serum is bound to the N-terminal (extracellular) domain of its receptor (GH-binding protein). The GH receptor is a member of the cytokine/GH/PRL/erythropoietin receptor family associated with cytosolic tyrosine kinase proteins. The growth-promoting action of GH is mediated by the somatomedins, a group of polypeptide insulin-like growth factors synthesized in the liver. GH acts through the somatomedins to increase amino acid uptake, increase protein synthesis, and decrease protein catabolism by promoting mobilization of fat as a fuel source. GH also interferes with glucose uptake and carbohydrate use by cells. This causes an increase in glucose levels and stimulation of insulin release. Hypothalamic control of GH secretion is mediated by growth hormone-releasing hormone (GHRH) and somatostatin (SST) (GH-inhibitory hormone). A variety of neural, physiologic, metabolic, and hormonal factors affect the rate of GH secretion and these are listed in Table 14.10. Secretion follows diurnal rhythms and is episodic with peak secretory episodes occurring during the early morning before wakening [deep slow-wave stages (III and IV) of sleep]. GH deficiency before puberty is known as *dwarfism*, whereas excess during this time is known as *gigantism*. Acromegaly is a condition of GH excess following puberty and closure of the epiphyses leading to appositional bone growth as well as soft tissue growth and visceral enlargement (36).

Prolactin

PRL is a 199-amino acid single-chain peptide whose primary action is stimulation of postpartum lactation. Stimulating factors of PRL secretion include pregnancy, lactation or breast manipulation, stress, sleep, vasoactive intestinal peptide (VIP), TRH, gastroinhibitory peptide (GIP), secretin, glucagon, and dopamine antagonists. Although physiologic levels of PRL do not affect gonadal function, hyperprolactinemia from PRL-secreting pituitary tumors causes hypogonadism in both men and women. PRL-secreting tumors account for 30% to 50% of all pituitary tumors (37). Unlike other anterior pituitary hormones, hypothalamic control of PRL secretion is primarily inhibitory. Dopamine appears to be the principal PRL inhibitory factor secreted by the hypothalamus and its inhibitory effects predominate over stimulatory factors.

Adrenocorticotropic Hormone

ACTH is synthesized by the corticotroph cells of the pituitary as part of a large precursor molecule pro-opiomelanocortin (MW 28,500). This precursor molecule is processed into several smaller, biologically active amino acid fragments that include ACTH (amino acids 1–39), β-lipotropin (amino acids 1–91), and β-endorphin (amino acids 61–91). The principal action of ACTH is to stimulate secretion of glucocorticoids, mineralocorticoids, and androgenic steroids from the adrenal cortex. The most important mediator of ACTH secretion is corticotropin-releasing factor (CRF), produced by the hypothalamus. CRF stimulates ACTH secretion in a pulsatile manner, peaking in the early morning and progressively declining to a nadir in the late afternoon or evening. ACTH secretion is also stimulated physiologically by many types of stressors including pain, trauma, infection, hypoxia, cold exposure, and acute hypoglycemia. Negative feedback control of ACTH release is maintained by cortisol and synthetic glucocorticoids at the level of the hypothalamus and pituitary. Extra-adrenal actions of ACTH include skin darkening and stimulation of lipolysis. In the circulation, ACTH has a short half-life of 7 to 12 minutes.

Thyroid-Stimulating Hormone

TSH is a large glycoprotein synthesized by the pituitary thyrotrophs. The primary action of TSH is to regulate growth and metabolism of the thyroid gland. TSH binds to specific receptors in the thyroid where it stimulates uptake of iodide and synthesis and release of thyroid hormone. TSH secretion is regulated by both stimulatory (TRH) and inhibitory (SST) factors produced by the hypothalamus and by negative feedback inhibition of the hypothalamic-pituitary axis by thyroid hormone.

TABLE 14.10

Regulating Factors of Growth Hormone Secretion

Factors Inhibiting GH Secretion	Factors Stimulating GH Secretion
Hormonal	*Hormonal*
IGF, hypothyroidism, somatostatin	TRH, ADH, glucagon, GRH, Dopamine, uncontrolled DM
Metabolic	*Metabolic*
Hyperglycemia	Decreased blood glucose, high levels of leucine and arginine
Physiologic	*Physiologic*
Aging process, childhood emotional deprivation	Stress, puberty, exercise, deep slow-wave sleep
Drugs	*Drugs*
Dopamine antagonists	Dopamine agonists

GH, growth hormone; IGF, insulin-like growth factor; TRH, thyrotropin releasing hormone; ADH, antidiuretic hormone; GRH, growth hormone releasing hormone; DM, diabetes mellitus.

Gonadotropins

FSH and LH are glycoproteins, each of which is composed of an α subunit and a β subunit. The α subunits are identical, and specific biologic activity resides in the β subunit. The gonadotropins bind specific receptors in the ovaries and testes, where they stimulate production of sex steroids and promote gametogenesis. In males, LH stimulates production of testosterone by the interstitial cells (Sertoli cells) of the testis, and FSH stimulates testicular growth. FSH also stimulates the Sertoli cells to produce an androgen-binding protein, which is essential for the development of the high local concentrations of testosterone required for normal spermatogenesis. Both gonadotropins are required for the process of sperm maturation. In females, LH stimulates estrogen and progesterone production by the ovary. The midcycle surge of LH causes ovulation, and continued LH secretion stimulates the corpus luteum to make progesterone. FSH controls maturation of the ovarian follicle, which secretes estrogen under the influence of both FSH and LH.

Both LH and FSH are secreted from the gonadotrope cell in the anterior pituitary. This secretion is regulated by the hypothalamic hormone gonadotropin-releasing hormone (GnRH) and by positive and negative feedback mechanisms involving the sex steroid hormones. GnRH is a decapeptide, formed in the preoptic and arcuate areas of the hypothalamus, which maintains basal gonadotropin secretion, generates the midcycle surge in gonadotropins necessary for ovulation, and regulates the onset of puberty. Secretion of GnRH is pulsatile, with hourly secretory bursts that cause a similar pattern of release of both FSH and LH. Pituitary sensitivity to the effects of GnRH is also increased by estrogen, and rising estrogen levels during the menstrual cycle provide the stimulus for the ovulatory surge in FSH and LH (positive feedback). Secretion of gonadotropins also occurs in response to stress, sexual stimuli, and castration. Stimulation of FSH and LH production are also seen in response to decreased circulating levels of sex hormones in patients with primary gonadal failure (negative feedback).

THE ADRENAL

Anatomy and Development

The adrenal gland is composed of a cortex and medulla, which have separate embryologic origins. The adrenal cortex arises from the coelomic mesoderm between the fourth and sixth weeks of gestation. The adrenal medulla is derived from cells of the neural crest that also form the sympathetic nervous system and the sympathetic ganglia. Some of these neural crest cells migrate into the adrenal cortex to form the adrenal medulla, but chromaffin tissue may also develop in extra adrenal sites in the para-aortic and paravertebral regions (Fig. 14.14). The most common site for extra-adrenal chromaffin tissue is the organ of Zuckerkandl, located adjacent to the aorta near the origin of the inferior mesenteric artery.

The adrenal glands each weigh approximately 4 g and are located in the retroperitoneum along the superior-medial

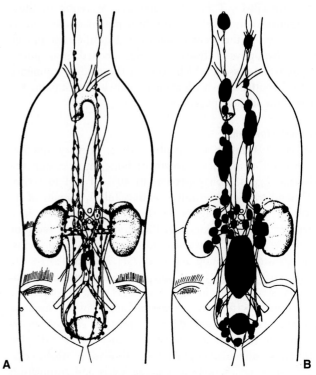

FIGURE 14.14 Distribution of chromaffin tissue in the newborn compared with distribution of extra adrenal pheochromocytomas. Extra-adrenal pheochromocytomas (**A**) occur in and around the sympathetic ganglia in an anatomic distribution that parallels that of extra-adrenal chromaffin tissue in the newborn (**B**). (From Landsberg L, Young JB. Catecholamines and the adrenal medulla. In: Wilson RH, Foster DW, eds. *Textbook of endocrinology*, 7th ed. Philadelphia: WB Saunders, 1985:935. Reprinted by permission.)

aspect of the kidneys (Fig. 14.15). A fibrous capsule surrounds the glands, which have a golden-yellow appearance because of their high lipid content. The adrenal glands measure 3 to 5 cm in length and width and 4 to 6 mm in thickness. The left gland is slightly larger and thicker than the right. The adrenal glands are highly vascularized and receive arterial blood from branches of the inferior phrenic artery, aorta, and renal arteries. Within the gland, a sinusoidal plexus is formed, which drains into a single, central vein. The right adrenal vein is short and wide and exits the gland medially to enter the posterior aspect of the inferior vena cava. The left adrenal vein exits anteriorly and usually drains into the left renal vein, although it may occasionally enter the inferior vena cava directly. As a result, adrenal venous catheterization is accomplished more easily on the left than on the right.

The adrenal cortex accounts for 80% to 90% of total gland weight and is composed of three zones histologically. The outer zona glomerulosa is the exclusive site for mineralocorticoid synthesis, whereas the large central zona fasciculata and inner zona reticularis produce both cortisol and androgens. The cells of the adrenal medulla account for approximately 10% to 20% of the gland, are polyhedral in shape, and are arranged in clumps and cords around blood

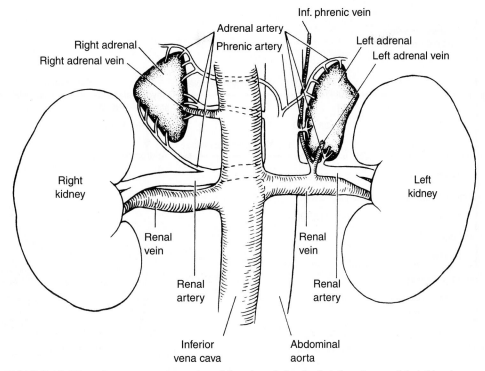

FIGURE 14.15   Schematic representation of the adrenal glands, their location, and their blood supply. (From Baxter JD. The adrenal cortex. In: Felig P, Baxter JD, Broadus AE, et al. eds. *Endocrinology and metabolism*, 2nd ed. New York: McGraw-Hill, 1987:513. Reprinted by permission of McGraw-Hill, Inc.)

vessels. Most of the blood supply to the medulla comes from venous blood draining through the cortex. This provides the adrenal chromaffin cells with a high local concentration of cortisol, which induces the enzyme phenyl ethanolamine-*N*-methyltransferase (PNMT) required for conversion of norepinephrine to epinephrine. A direct arterial supply to the adrenal medulla is also present, primarily to cells that predominately secrete norepinephrine. The adrenal medulla is innervated by preganglionic fibers of the sympathetic nervous system.

The Adrenal Cortex

Physiology

The adrenal cortex secretes three major hormones: cortisol, androgens, and aldosterone. The biosynthetic pathway for these hormones and their intermediates is shown in Figure 14.16. Because of the differences in enzymatic activity between the zona glomerulosa and the zona fasciculata and reticularis, the adrenal cortex functions as two separate entities. The zona glomerulosa is the exclusive site of production of aldosterone because it lacks the 17α-hydroxylase enzyme necessary for synthesis of 17α-hydroxyprogesterone and 17α-hydroxypregnenolone, which are the precursors for synthesis of cortisol and the adrenal androgens. The zona fasciculata and reticularis function as a unit to produce cortisol, androgens, and small amounts of estrogen, but they lack the enzymes necessary for conversion of 18-hydroxycorticosterone to aldosterone.

Cholesterol is the precursor from which all adrenal steroids are synthesized. Conversion of cholesterol to pregnenolone is the rate-limiting step in adrenal steroidogenesis and is the major site of action of ACTH.

Glucocorticoids

Secretion of cortisol is regulated by the hypothalamus and pituitary through secretion of CRF and ACTH. Neuroendocrine control of this process is maintained by three mechanisms: (i) episodic secretion and the circadian rhythm of ACTH; (ii) stress responsiveness of the hypothalamic-pituitary-adrenal axis; and (iii) feedback inhibition of corticotropin-releasing hormone (CRH) and ACTH secretion by cortisol. Cortisol, like ACTH, is secreted in a pulsatile manner, and plasma levels closely parallel those of ACTH (Fig. 14.17). Superimposed on this episodic secretory pattern is a circadian rhythm that results in peak cortisol levels in the early morning and a nadir in the late evening. Physical and emotional stress (trauma, surgery, and hypoglycemia) increase cortisol secretion by stimulating release of CRF and ACTH from the hypothalamus and pituitary, respectively.

Circulating cortisol is more than 90% bound to plasma proteins, 75% that is bound to corticosteroid-binding globulin (CBG) and 15% to albumin. Biologic activity resides in the nonprotein-bound fraction, which has a circulatory half-life of 70 to 120 minutes. Normal daily production of cortisol is 10 to 30 mg. The liver is the major site of metabolism of cortisol where it is inactivated

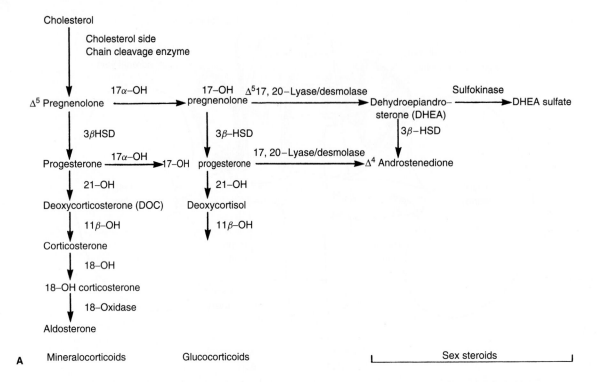

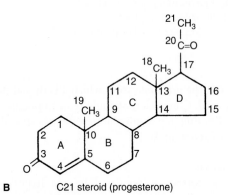

B   C21 steroid (progesterone)

FIGURE 14.16   **A:** Biosynthetic pathway for adrenal steroid synthesis. OH, hydroxylase; *3β*-HSD, *3β*-hydroxy- *δ⁵*-steroid dehydrogenase; *17*-HSO, 17-hydroxysteroid oxireductase. (From Conte FA, Grumbach MM. Pathogenesis, classification, diagnosis, and treatment of anomalies of sex. In: DeGroot LJ, ed. *Endocrinology*, 2nd ed. Philadelphia: WB Saunders, 1989:1825. Reprinted by permission.) **B:** Basic C21 steroid structure of the adrenocortical steroids. The letters in the formula for progesterone identify the *A, B, C,* and *D* rings; the numbers identify the position of each atom within the C21 structure. (From Ganong WF. *Review of medical physiology*. 14th ed. Norwalk, CT: Appleton & Lange, 1989:294.)

as well as conjugated with glucuronide or sulfate for easier excretion by the kidney. Two major metabolites are 17-hydroxycorticosteroids and 17-ketosteroids, which are excreted in the urine.

The glucocorticoids exert their effects through their actions on intermediary metabolism and through interactions with a broad range of cells and tissues. Corticosteroids diffuse into target cells and interact with intracellular cytosolic receptor proteins. The receptor is bound to other proteins including a heat shock protein (HSP). As the hormone binds to the receptor-HSP complex, the HSP is released and the hormone–receptor complex is activated. The activated glucocorticoid–receptor hormone complex then enters the cell

nucleus where it binds to specific hormone-responsive deoxyribonucleic acid (DNA) sequences called *glucocorticoid-response elements* (38). Glucocorticoid-specific genes are then activated, leading to gene transcription and synthesis of proteins that mediate the glucocorticoid response. The types of proteins synthesized and their ability to stimulate or inhibit other biologic activities varies widely as a result of the differential expression of specific genes in the different cell types.

The metabolic effects of the glucocorticoids include stimulation of hepatic gluconeogenesis and glycogen synthesis, inhibition of protein synthesis, increased protein catabolism, and lipolysis of adipose tissue. The increased release of amino acids from muscle protein and release of glycerol and free

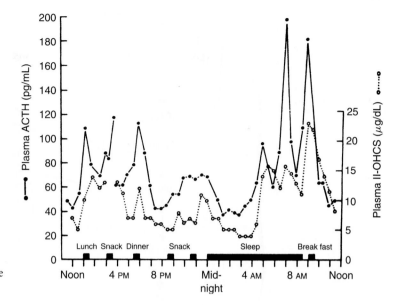

FIGURE 14.17 Fluctuations in plasma adrenocorticotropic hormone (ACTH) and glucocorticoids (11-hydroxy-corticosteroids) throughout the day. Note the greater ACTH and glucocorticoid levels in the morning before awakening. (From Krieger DT, Allen W, Rizzo F, et al. Characterization of the normal temporal pattern of plasma corticosteroid levels. *J Clin Endocrinol Metab* 1971;32:266. Reprinted by permission of The Endocrine Society.)

fatty acids from fat provide the substrates for hepatic gluconeogenesis. In addition, glucocorticoids increase the hepatic response to the gluconeogenic hormones (glucagon and catecholamines) and increase glycogen synthesis. Peripheral uptake of glucose in most tissues (except liver, brain, and red blood cells) is inhibited and may cause hyperglycemia and increased insulin secretion, especially in states of chronic cortisol excess.

Glucocorticoids cause loss of collagen and impair wound healing by inhibition of fibroblast activity. They inhibit bone formation, stimulate bone resorption, reduce intestinal absorption of calcium, and induce negative calcium balance, all of which contribute to the development of steroid-induced osteoporosis. Glucocorticoids also have numerous anti-inflammatory actions, which include inhibition of leukocyte mobilization and function, decreased migration of inflammatory cells to sites of injury, and decreased production of inflammatory mediators (e.g., interleukin-1, leukotrienes, and bradykinins). These properties may account for the increased susceptibility to infection of patients who suffer from chronic steroid excess.

Glucocorticoids are involved in stimulating gastric acid secretion and are necessary for maintaining the integrity and function of the GI tract. Cortisol stimulates erythropoietin and red blood cell production, inhibits vasopressin secretion and action, and psychologically alters mood and behavior causing insomnia and decreasing deep sleep. The glucocorticoids are also essential for cardiovascular stability including the vascular response to catecholamines, as evidenced by the cardiovascular collapse that occurs in patients with acute adrenal insufficiency.

Androgens

The zona reticularis is the primary site for androgen synthesis. Dehydroepiandrosterone (DHEA) is the principal C-19 sex steroid produced by the adrenal and its sulfated derivative DHEA-sulfate and androstenedione are also formed. The adrenal androgens have weak direct biologic activity, but in the periphery they undergo conversion to the active androgens testosterone and dihydrotestosterone. Increased production of adrenal androgens may occur in patients with Cushing syndrome, adrenal carcinoma, and congenital adrenal hyperplasia. In healthy men, adrenal androgens account for less than 5% of total testosterone production, and so the clinical effects of excess adrenal synthesis are minimal. In prepubertal boys, however, increased production of androgen may be manifested by the early development of secondary sexual characteristics and penile enlargement. In women, the adrenal is the major source of androgens and in pubertal females these androgens stimulate pubic and axillary hair development. Excess androgen production in women is manifested by the development of acne, hirsutism, virilization, and amenorrhea. Increased production of estrogen causes gynecomastia in men and precocious breast development and menstrual bleeding in women.

Aldosterone

The principal actions of aldosterone are maintenance of extracellular fluid volume and regulation of sodium and potassium balance. The major physiologic regulator of aldosterone secretion is the renin-angiotensin system (Fig. 14.18). The plasma potassium concentration and, to a lesser extent, plasma sodium and ACTH also influence aldosterone secretion. Renin is an enzyme secreted by the juxtaglomerular cells of the kidney in response to decreased pressure in the renal afferent arterioles. Decreases in plasma sodium concentration sensed by osmoreceptors in the cells of the macula densa promote renin release as well. Renin secretion is also stimulated by hyperkalemia and inhibited by potassium depletion. Renin converts angiotensinogen (a 14-amino acid plasma peptide) into angiotensin I, a decapeptide that is in turn altered in the lung by angiotensin-converting enzyme (ACE) to form angiotensin II (an octapeptide). Angiotensin II is a potent vasoconstrictor that is important in maintaining

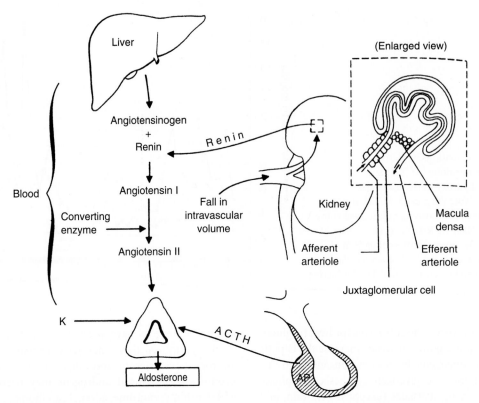

FIGURE 14.18 Regulation of aldosterone secretion. A fall in blood volume, a fall in blood pressure, or vasoconstriction of the renal arteries produces a decrease in pressure in the afferent arteriole leading to a release of renin from the juxtaglomerular cells and stimulation of the renin-angiotensin-aldosterone axis. Adrenocorticotropic hormone (ACTH) and hyperkalemia also stimulate release of aldosterone. (From Bergland RM, Gann DS, De Maria EJ. The pituitary and adrenals. In: Schwartz SI, ed. *Principles of surgery*, 5th ed. New York: McGraw-Hill, 1989:1566. Reprinted by permission of McGraw-Hill, Inc.)

blood pressure in response to hemorrhage and hypovolemia. It also directly stimulates cells of the zona glomerulosa to secrete aldosterone. Aldosterone then stimulates renal tubular reabsorption of sodium in exchange for potassium and hydrogen ion secretion. The net effect is fluid reabsorption and expansion of the intravascular volume.

Pathophysiology

Cushing Syndrome

Signs and Symptoms. Cushing syndrome refers to the constellation of signs and symptoms that result from chronic glucocorticoid excess. The most common source of Cushing syndrome is iatrogenic administration of glucocorticoids. ACTH-secreting tumors of the pituitary are the most common cause of spontaneous Cushing syndrome. Pituitary Cushing from an ectopic ACTH-secreting pituitary tumor, also termed *Cushing disease*, accounts for approximately 70% of all cases of Cushing syndrome. Ectopic ACTH-secreting tumors comprise 15% of cases and are associated most commonly with small cell carcinomas of the lung. Primary adrenal tumors (adenomas and carcinoma) account for 15% to 20% of cases.

The clinical symptoms and signs associated with Cushing syndrome are shown in Table 14.11. Obesity is the most constant feature and is characteristically centrally distributed

TABLE 14.11	
Clinical Features of Cushing Syndrome	
Features	*Percentage*
Obesity	94
Facial plethora	84
Hirsutism	82
Menstrual disorders	76
Hypertension	72
Muscular weakness	58
Back pain	58
Striae	52
Acne	40
Psychologic symptoms	40
Bruising	36
Congestive heart failure	22
Edema	18
Renal calculi	16
Headache	14
Polyuria-polydipsia	10
Hyperpigmentation	6

From Baxter JD, Tyrrel JB. The adrenal cortex. In: Felig P, Baxter J, Braodus A, et al. eds. *Endocrinology and metabolism.* New York: McGraw-Hill, 1981; Reprinted with permission.

around the face, trunk, neck, and abdomen. Skin changes occur frequently and include increased fragility, bruising, and skin striae. Hyperpigmentation is seen most commonly in patients with ectopic ACTH production. Hirsutism from increased secretion of adrenal androgens is frequently present in women, but virilism is uncommon except in patients with adrenal carcinoma. Increased production of adrenal androgens also causes gonadal dysfunction manifested by amenorrhea and infertility. In males, increased production of cortisol may cause decreased libido, reduction in body hair, and testicular atrophy.

The essential steps in the laboratory evaluation of patients with Cushing syndrome are (i) documentation of excess adrenal cortisol production, and (ii) differentiation of ACTH-dependent from independent causes, and localization of the source. An outline of the approach to the diagnostic evaluation of Cushing syndrome is given in Figure 14.19.

Biochemical Screening Tests for the Diagnosis of Cushing Syndrome

Plasma Cortisol. Because of the episodic nature of ACTH and cortisol secretion, plasma cortisol levels vary greatly with the assay method employed and the time of day that the sample is obtained. Cortisol levels obtained at 4 p.m. are usually approximately half those obtained at 8 a.m. Patients with Cushing syndrome lose this diurnal variation in cortisol levels but because of variation in levels, random cortisol determinations are not reliable in making the diagnosis.

Urinary Free Cortisol. The most useful diagnostic test in the initial evaluation of patients with suspected Cushing

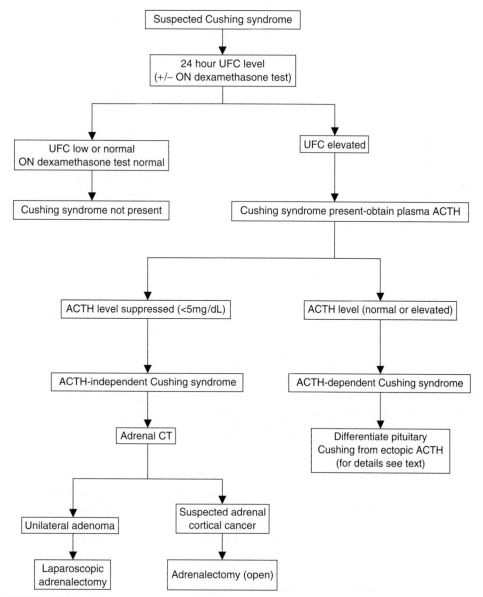

FIGURE 14.19 Schematic algorithm for diagnosis, etiology, and treatment of Cushing syndrome. UFC, uinary free cortisol; ACTH, adrenocorticotropic hormone; CT, computed tomography.

syndrome is measurement of urinary free cortisol. Normally, less than 1% of cortisol is excreted in the urine, but with increased rates of cortisol secretion, corticotropin-binding globulin becomes saturated and free cortisol is excreted. Elevated urinary cortisol levels are present in more than 90% of patients with Cushing syndrome. This test, however, may not detect mild degrees of hypercortisolism and false-positive elevations can occur with other medical and psychiatric illnesses.

Low-Dose Dexamethasone Suppression Test. Dexamethasone is a synthetic glucocorticoid with enhanced biologic activity compared with cortisol because of its higher affinity for the glucocorticoid receptor. Dexamethasone suppresses pituitary secretion of ACTH and adrenal production of corticosteroids through feedback inhibition of the hypothalamic-pituitary-adrenal axis. The single, low-dose dexamethasone suppression test is *a simple and useful screening test for* Cushing syndrome. In the single-dose dexamethasone test, 1 to 3 mg of dexamethasone is given orally at 11 p.m. and plasma cortisol measured at 8 a.m. the next morning. Suppression of plasma cortisol to less than 3 μg/dL excludes the diagnosis of Cushing syndrome. Patients with plasma cortisol levels greater than 10 μg/dL are likely to have Cushing syndrome and require further testing. False-negative results with this test are rare, as greater than 98% of patients with Cushing syndrome have an abnormal response to the overnight dexamethasone test. False-positive results occur in approximately 15% of obese patients and 25% of hospitalized chronically ill patients. In the 2-day low-dose dexamethasone test, 24-hour urine collections for 17-hydroxycorticosteroids are obtained before and during the second day of administration of 0.5 mg dexamethasone every 6 hours. This test is cumbersome and time consuming and requires collection of 24-hour urine specimens. It is associated with both false-positive and false-negative results and is no longer recommended for the biochemical diagnosis of Cushing syndrome.

17-Hydroxycorticosteroids and 17-Ketosteroids. Measurement of urinary metabolites of cortisol are less useful in the diagnosis of Cushing syndrome than urinary free cortisol levels. 17-Ketosteroids are produced from metabolism of both cortisol and androgens. Although they may be elevated in patients with adrenal androgen excess, they are less specific and sensitive than plasma androgen assays. Plasma testosterone levels should be measured in patients with virilizing features.

Tests to Determine the Etiology of Cushing Syndrome

Plasma Adrenocorticotropic Hormone. Plasma ACTH levels are used to differentiate ACTH-dependent (pituitary and ectopic ACTH-secreting tumors) from adrenal causes of Cushing syndrome (Fig. 14.20). In patients with cortisol-secreting primary adrenal neoplasms, ACTH levels are suppressed (<5 pg/mL). Patients with pituitary Cushing

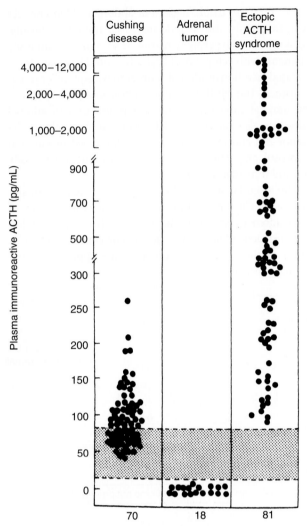

FIGURE 14.20 Basal plasma adrenocorticotropic hormone (ACTH) concentrations in patients with spontaneous Cushing syndrome. (From Scott AP, Bloomfield GA, Lowry PJ, et al. Pituitary adreno-corticotropin and the melanocyte stimulating hormones. In: Parson JA, ed. *Peptide hormones.* Baltimore: University Park Press, 1976:266.)

syndrome should have ACTH levels that are normal or moderately elevated (15–200 pg/mL). Markedly elevated ACTH levels are often seen in patients with ectopic ACTH-secreting tumors, although some overlap exists with levels seen in Cushing disease.

High-Dose Dexamethasone Test. The high-dose dexamethasone test has been used to distinguish pituitary from nonpituitary causes of ACTH-dependent Cushing syndrome. The rationale for this test is that supraphysiologic doses of glucocorticoids will suppress the hypothalamic-pituitary axis, ACTH secretion, and cortisol production in patients with ACTH hypersecretion from a pituitary tumor but will not affect cortisol production in patients with primary adrenal neoplasms or ectopic ACTH-secreting tumors. The single-dose 8 mg dexamethasone test is simpler to perform and more reliable than the 2-day test. A basal level of plasma cortisol is obtained at 8 a.m. on the day before the test. A single 11 p.m. dose of 8 mg dexamethasone is given orally, and plasma cortisol is measured at 8 a.m. the next day. The 2-day high-dose dexamethasone test is performed in a manner identical to the 2-day low-dose test, except dexamethasone is given in a dose of 2 mg every 6 hours and urinary 17-hydroxycorticosteroids are measured. With either test, patients with pituitary Cushing syndrome should have suppression of plasma or urinary corticosteroids to less than 50% of the basal level, whereas cortisol levels in patients with ectopic ACTH production or primary adrenal tumors are usually unchanged. However, 20% to 30% of patients with mildly increased corticotropin secretion and pituitary Cushing syndrome fail to suppress steroid production to less than 50% of baseline, and some patients with ACTH-secreting tumors do suppress plasma and urine steroids to this level. Therefore, the overall diagnostic accuracy of the high dose dexamethasone suppression test is only 70% to 80% (39).

Corticotropin-Releasing Hormone Stimulation. The CRH stimulation test may also be used to differentiate the etiology of Cushing syndrome. A single intravenous dose of ovine CRH is given and serum cortisol and ACTH levels are obtained every 15 minutes for an hour. Patients with a pituitary source (Cushing disease) will demonstrate an increase in ACTH levels in response to CRH. A rise of greater than 35% is considered diagnostic for the disease. Patients with adrenal or extra-adrenal sources of hypercortisolism have little to no change in ACTH levels after CRH administration.

Radiologic Tests. Once the biochemical evaluation of the patient with Cushing syndrome has been completed, radiographic localization of the source of the Cushing syndrome should be carried out. The most common ectopic ACTH-producing tumors are small cell lung carcinomas or bronchial or thymic carcinoids. Most of these tumors can be detected by computed tomography (CT) scanning or by radionuclide imaging with indium 111(^{111}I)–labeled octreotide analogs which detect tumors that express SST receptors. Gadolinium-enhanced magnetic resonance imaging (MRI) of the pituitary will demonstrate an adenoma in more than 60% of patients with pituitary Cushing syndrome. A CT scan of the adrenal glands is the preferred localization modality in patients with suspected adrenal Cushing syndrome, although MRI may be used as well. If the results of these studies are negative and the etiology of the ACTH-dependent Cushing syndrome is still unclear, then bilateral inferior petrosal sinus sampling for ACTH should be carried out because the most likely etiology is an occult pituitary tumor.

Inferior Petrosal Sinus Sampling. The most direct method to differentiate pituitary from nonpituitary causes of ACTH-dependent Cushing syndrome is measurement of inferior petrosal sinus blood for ACTH with and without CRH stimulation. This procedure requires a highly-skilled interventional radiologist who can reliably cannulate both inferior petrosal sinuses. Simultaneous measurements of peripheral and bilateral inferior petrosal sinus and plasma ACTH levels are carried out both before and after administration of 100 μg of CRH intravenously. A basal or stimulated inferior petrosal sinus:peripheral ACTH ratio of greater than 3.0 reliably indicates pituitary Cushing disease, and a gradient less than 1.8 is diagnostic of an ectopic ACTH-secreting tumor (40). This technique may also serve to localize the microadenoma within the pituitary gland if the ACTH gradient lateralizes to only one petrosal sinus. The sensitivity and specificity of this procedure are between 80% to 90% or even higher in experienced hands (40,41).

Disorders of Excess Adrenal Androgen Production. Adrenal causes of excess androgen production include Cushing syndrome, adrenal carcinoma, and congenital adrenal hyperplasia. Congenital adrenal hyperplasia refers to a group of autosomal recessive disorders characterized by defects in the synthesis of cortisol. This impaired production of cortisol stimulates ACTH release, which leads to adrenal hyperplasia and increased production of adrenal androgens and androgen precursors. The most common cause (95% of cases) of congenital adrenal hyperplasia is 21α-hydroxylase deficiency. There are three types of 21α-hydroxylase deficiency: classic salt wasting, classic non–salt wasting, and nonclassic. Classic forms are more severe and present in infancy or early childhood with virilization and adrenal insufficiency, with or without salt wasting. The nonclassic form is milder and exhibits hyperandrogenism without cortisol deficiency. In the classic salt-wasting variety, severe electrolyte and fluid losses may develop in up to 80% of patients with 21α-hydroxylase deficiency because of an associated defect in aldosterone production.

In adults, excess adrenal androgens cause testicular atrophy in males and hirsutism, acne, and irregular or absent menses in women. Virilism in women, from marked excess production of adrenal androgens, is characterized by male pattern baldness, clitoral enlargement, and development of masculine features, including increased muscle bulk and deepening of the voice. The diagnosis of androgen excess is made most accurately by measurement of plasma androgen levels, including DHEA, DHEA sulfate, testosterone, and dihydrotestosterone. Plasma androgens are elevated in approximately 85% of women with hirsutism. Other causes of hirsutism and virilism in women include the polycystic ovary syndrome and androgen-secreting ovarian tumors.

Primary Aldosteronism

Primary hyperaldosteronism due to spontaneous increased production of aldosterone by the adrenal glomerulosa cells results, termed *Conn syndrome*, is characterized by hypertension and hypokalemia in conjunction with suppression of plasma renin activity (PRA) (42). Excess aldosterone leads to sodium retention and expansion of the extracellular fluid volume, which feeds back on the renal juxtaglomerular cells and macula densa to shut off renin production. Both potassium and hydrogen ion are excreted in the urine in exchange for sodium, which results in potassium depletion and alkalosis. Movement of hydrogen ion into the cells to replace intracellular potassium also contributes to the alkalosis. Mild glucose intolerance may accompany significant potassium depletion.

The symptoms and signs of primary aldosteronism are nonspecific and include fatigue, weakness, and nocturia. With severe potassium depletion, patients may develop increased thirst, polyuria, and paresthesias. Hypertension is moderate to severe and may be refractory to standard medical management.

The diagnosis of primary aldosteronism should be suspected in any patient with spontaneous hypokalemia and hypertension. However, up to 60% of patients may not be hypokalemic, because of dietary restriciton in sodium intake, which can ameliorate potassium losses as the amount of sodium available for reabsorption in the distal tubule decreases. Other laboratory features of primary aldosteronism include elevation of serum sodium and bicarbonate levels. Initial screening should consist of measurement of plasma aldosterone concentration (PAC) and PRA. A PAC:PRA ratio of greater than 20 to 30 with a PAC greater than 15 ng/dL and suppressed PRA is suggestive of the diagnosis (43). Patients with an elevated PAC:PRA ratio should have further biochemical confirmation of the diagnosis by measurement of 24-hour urine aldosterone excretion rates while on a high sodium diet or plasma aldosterone after intravenous saline loading.

The principal causes of primary aldosteronism are aldosterone-producing adenomas (60% of cases) and idiopathic hyperaldosteronism (40%) from bilateral adrenal cortical hyperplasia. Adrenal carcinoma is an extremely rare cause of hyperaldosteronism. Differentiation of an aldosterone-producing adenoma from idiopathic hyperaldosteronism is important clinically because adenomas are treated by adrenalectomy whereas idiopathic hyperaldosteronism is managed medically. A diagnostic algorithm for managing primary hyperaldosteronism is outlined in Figure 14.21. Once the diagnosis has been confirmed biochemically, adrenal imaging should be carried out with CT or MRI. Patients with a unilateral macroadenoma (>1 cm) and a normal contralateral adrenal may be considered for unilateral adrenalectomy. However, adrenal vein sampling is recommended in cases of bilateral nodules, unilateral microadenoma (<1 cm) or normal adrenals to determine if there is a lateralizing source of increased aldosterone production. For adrenal vein sampling, aldosterone and cortisol levels are measured from both adrenal veins and the inferior vena cava. An aldosterone to cortisol ratio that is at least four to five times greater on one side compared to the other is considered diagnostic for a unilateral adenoma.

Inherited forms of primary hyperaldosteronism account for 1% of cases and include familial hyperaldosteronism (FH) types I and II. FH-I is inherited in an autosomal dominant manner as a result of meiotic crossover of the 11β-hydroxylase gene and the aldosterone synthase gene. The resulting fusion product stimulates ACTH-dependent aldosterone production as well as production of 17-hydroxylated analogs of 18-hydroxycortisol in the zona fasciculata (43). Adenoma formation is rare in this type. FH type II is also inherited in an autosomal dominant manner; however, its gene locus has not yet been identified. Patients with type-II disease, however, do exhibit a high rate of adenoma formation.

Secondary Hyperaldosteronism

Elevation of plasma aldosterone in response to increased renin production by the kidney is termed *secondary aldosteronism* and may be caused by a variety of conditions, including renovascular hypertension, decreased intravascular volume (congestive heart failure, nephrosis, cirrhosis), Bartter syndrome, and normal pregnancy. Adrenal function is normal and aldosterone secretion increases in response to elevated plasma renin and angiotensin. Treatment should be directed at the underlying disorder.

Adrenal Insufficiency

Adrenal insufficiency occurs most commonly in surgical patients as a result of chronic cortisol administration with suppression of adrenal cortical function. The primary cause of spontaneous adrenal insufficiency in industrialized countries is autoimmune adrenal disease and in the developing world is tuberculosis (44). Other causes of adrenal insufficiency include bilateral adrenal hemorrhage, adrenal metastases, and postsurgical after adrenalectomy. Chronic adrenal insufficiency (Addison disease) is characterized by hyperpigmentation of the skin [which is the result of chronic hypersecretion of melatonin, a product from the ACTH precursor pro-opiomelano-cortin (POMC)], weakness, fatigue, anorexia, weight loss, nausea, vomiting, salt-craving, and hypotension. Many of the symptoms are nonspecific and, therefore, patients may go undiagnosed for a long time. In patients with inadequate adrenal reserve, the stress of surgery, trauma, infection, or dehydration may precipitate an acute adrenal crisis. Acute adrenal insufficiency is characterized by unexplained vascular collapse with hypotension and shock. Abdominal pain, weakness, depressed mentation, and fever are also commonly present. Patients with unexplained cardiovascular collapse in whom the diagnosis is suspected should be treated empirically with replacement corticosteroids to avoid the lethal consequences of this condition.

Biochemical manifestations of adrenal insufficiency include hyponatremia, hyperkalemia, hypoglycemia, and azotemia, with increased blood urea nitrogen and creatinine concentrations. The diagnosis is confirmed by measurement of plasma or urinary cortisol levels. In primary adrenal insufficiency, 8 a.m. plasma cortisol levels are usually low (<3 μg/dL) and plasma ACTH is high (>100 pg/mL). Plasma ACTH levels are low or inappropriately normal if pituitary failure or hypothalamus pathology is the cause (44). In patients with partial adrenal insufficiency, determination of

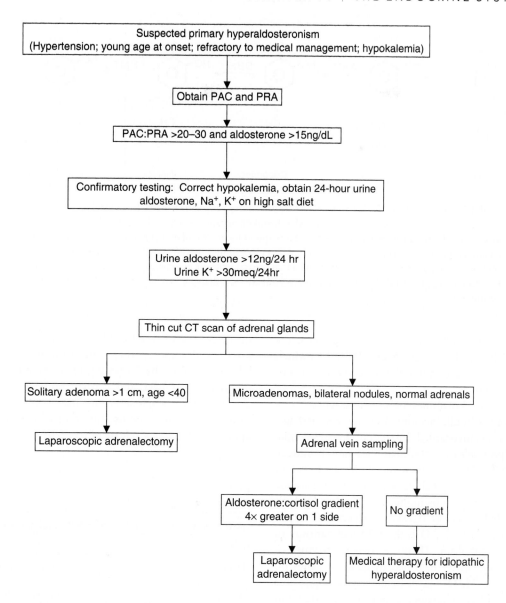

FIGURE 14.21   Schematic algorithm for the diagnosis and treatment of primary hyperaldosteronism. PAC, plasma aldosterone concentration; PRA, plasma renin activity; CT, computed tomography.

adrenocortical reserve with the ACTH stimulation test is necessary to establish the diagnosis. In the acute setting, this condition is often diagnosed when hypotension with vasopressor requirement is corrected by administration of glucocorticorticoids. For the ACTH stimulation test, 250 μg of synthetic ACTH is administered intravenously and plasma cortisol levels are measured at 0, 30, and 60 minutes. A plasma cortisol of greater than 18 μg/dL at either 30- or 60-minute time point is considered a normal response. Pituitary-adrenal reserve in patients with adrenal insufficiency can also be assessed with the metyrapone test. Metyrapone inhibits 11β-hydroxylase activity and thereby blocks conversion of 11-deoxycortisol to cortisol. In patients given metyrapone, 11-deoxycortisol production should increase as ACTH secretion increases in response to the decrease in plasma cortisol levels. An increase in 11-deoxycortisol levels

(>7 μg/dL) in response to metyrapone is indicative of normal pituitary and adrenal function.

Adrenal Medulla

The pathway for catecholamine biosynthesis is shown in Figure 14.22. Hepatic synthesis of tyrosine from phenylalanine and dietary sources provide the substrate for catecholamine synthesis. The enzymes necessary for catecholamine synthesis are found in all chromaffin tissues except for PNMT, which is present only in the adrenal medulla, organ of Zuckerkandl, and select central nervous system neurons. High local concentrations of cortisol (as found in the adrenal medulla) are necessary for induction of PNMT activity. Catecholamines are stored in chromaffin granules within the sympathetic nerve terminals and in the cells of the adrenal medulla. Secretion of catecholamines is

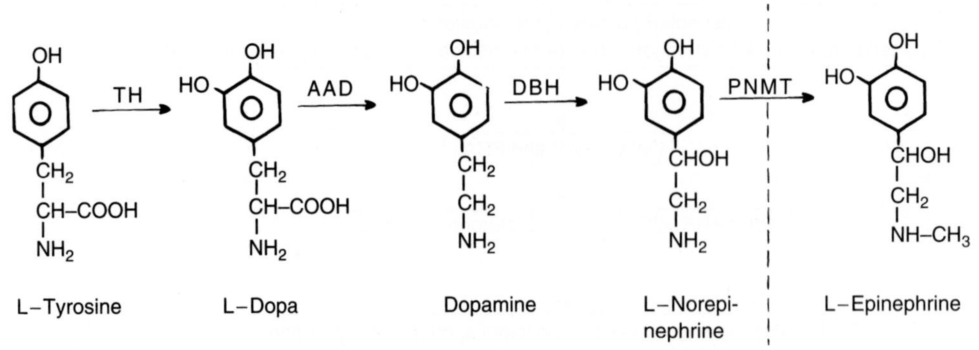

FIGURE 14.22 Biosynthetic pathway for catecholamines. Tyrosine hydroxylase (TH), aromatic-L-amino acid decarboxylase (L-AADC), and dopamine-β-hydroxylase (DBH) catalyze formation of norepinephrine from tyrosine. Subsequent formation of epinephrine, catalyzed by phenyl ethanolamine-N-methyltransferase (PNMT), takes place in the adrenal medulla and in neurons of the central nervous system and peripheral ganglia that use epinephrine as a neurotransmitter. (From Bondy PK, Rosenberg LE. *Metabolic control and disease*, 8th ed. Philadelphia: WB Saunders, 1980;1626, with permission.)

initiated by release of acetylcholine from preganglionic nerve fibers. Acetylcholine then induces cell depolarization, which results in an influx of calcium into the cell and exocytosis of neurosecretory granules.

Secretion of catecholamines occurs in response to a variety of stressful stimuli, including exercise, hemorrhage, surgery, angina or myocardial infarction, hypoglycemia, and anoxia. Upon release, catecholamines rapidly induce their biologic effect and are then metabolized by one of several mechanisms. These include reuptake by sympathetic nerve endings, metabolism by monoamine oxidase (MAO), catechol-O-methyltransferase (COMT), or excretion by the kidney. Deamination by MAO is the principal pathway of catecholamine metabolism. There are two isoenzymes of MAO, MAO-A and MAO-B, coded by adjacent genes on the X chromosome. MAO-A is the main enzyme responsible for deamination of catecholamines. Both epinephrine and norepinephrine are metabolized by the combination of MAO and aldehyde reductase or aldose to the metabolite 3,4-dihydroxyphenylglycol (DHPG). The second primary pathway of catecholamine metabolism involves COMT-catalyzed O-methylation of epinephrine to metanephrine, dopamine to methoxytyramine, and norepinephrine to normetanephrine. COMT is present in two isoenzymes, a membrane-bound form and a soluble form, both encoded by the same gene but differing in a terminal amino acid anchor allowing attachment to the endoplasmic reticular membrane. COMT is the enzyme responsible for metabolism of most circulating catecholamines.

The catecholamines exert their biologic effects by interaction with specific cell-surface receptors. The types of receptors and effects they mediate in the various target tissues are outlined in Table 14.12 (45). The principal physiologic effect of α-receptor stimulation is vasoconstriction. Two types of β-receptors exist. The β_1-receptors mediate inotropic and chronotropic stimulation of cardiac muscle, whereas β_2-receptors induce relaxation of smooth muscle

in noncardiac tissues, including blood vessels, the bronchi, uterus, and adipose tissue. Catecholamines also affect cellular metabolism by increasing O_2 consumption and heat production. In liver and cardiac muscle, they stimulate glycogenolysis, which serves to increase the availability of carbohydrate for tissue use. In adipose tissue, they induce lipolysis and increase release of free fatty acids and glycerol.

TABLE 14.12

Adrenergic Responses of Selected Tissues

Organ Or tissue	Receptor	Effect
Heart (myocardium)	β_1	Increased force and rate of contraction
Blood vessels	α	Vasoconstriction
	β_2	Vasodilatation
Kidney	β	Increased renin release
Gut	α, β	Decreased motility and increased sphincter tone
Pancreas	α	Decreased release of insulin and glucagon
	β	Increased release of insulin and glucagon
Liver	α, β	Increased glycogenolysis
Adipose tissue	β	Increased lipolysis
Most tissues	β	Increased calorigenesis
Skin (apocrine glands)	α	Increased sweating
Bronchioles	β_2	Dilation
Uterus	α	Contraction
	β_2	Relaxation

From Goldfien A. Adrenal medulla. In: Greenspan FS, ed. *Basis and clinical endocrinology*, 3rd ed. Norwalk: Appleton & Lange, 1991;387. Reprinted with permission.

Both norepinephrine and epinephrine inhibit insulin secretion.

Pheochromocytoma

Pheochromocytomas are catecholamine-secreting tumors that arise from chromaffin tissue. Most pheochromocytomas (85%–90%) arise in the adrenal gland, but they may occur in any site where chromaffin tissue is found. Several features of pheochromocytomas are characterized by a 10% frequency of distribution: 10% extra adrenal, 10% bilateral, 10% in children, 10% familial, and 10% malignant. The signs and symptoms of pheochromocytomas are related to the effects of sustained and/or paroxysmal secretion of norepinephrine and epinephrine (46,47). Paroxysmal attacks from pheochromocytomas often begin as a pounding in the chest from forceful cardiac contractions induced by the β_1-receptor–mediated increase in cardiac output. These symptoms may progress to involve the trunk and head and commonly cause headaches. Hands and feet become cool, moist, and pale from α-receptor–induced peripheral vasoconstriction. Blood pressure may become markedly elevated from the combination of intense vasoconstriction and increased cardiac output. Temperature elevation, flushing, and sweating may result from hypermetabolism and from a reduction in heat loss secondary to peripheral vasoconstriction. Marked anxiety and an impending sense of doom are occasionally present. Most attacks are short lived (<15-minute duration) but occur weekly in 75% of patients. They may be precipitated by postural changes, exertion, intake of certain foods or beverages, emotion, urination, direct tumor stimulation, and the use of certain drugs (e.g., histamine, tricyclic antidepressants, phenothiazide, and metoclopramide) or anesthetic agents, or may occur spontaneously. In some cases, paroxysms in catecholamine surges can result in a hypertensive crisis leading to severe headaches, diaphoresis, visual disturbances, palpitations, encephalopathy, acute myocardial infarction, congestive heart failure, or even cerebrovascular accident. Treatment of such hypertensive emergencies involves intravenous administration of esmolol and/or phentolamine or sodium nitroprusside. If tachyarrhythmias are also present, preoperative β-blockade with atenolol or metoprolol is appropriate after α-receptor blockade.

The diagnosis of pheochromocytoma is established either by demonstration of elevated levels of urinary catecholamines and metabolites (metanephrines) or plasma fractionated metanephrines (48–50). Urinary vanillylmandelic acid (VMA) is the least specific test because of false-positive tests from ingestion of related foods and is not routinely employed. Once the diagnosis is established, localization with MRI is preferred as pheochromocytomas typically have a bright appearance on TR- weightedMR sequences. ^{123}I-metaiodobenzylguanidine (MIBG) is an agent that is taken up in chromaffin tissues and has been used for pheochromocytoma localization. Its main value is in patients with suspected extra-adrenal tumors or malignant pheochromocytoma.

Preoperative α-receptor blockade with phenoxybenzamine and expansion of intravascular volume by hydration are essential for intraoperative control of blood pressure during adrenalectomy. Patients with marked tachycardia or arrhythmias may also require β-receptor blockage with metoprolol. β-receptor blockade should never be initiated without first achieving α-blockade because a hypertensive crisis can result from unopposed α-stimulation.

Hereditary Pheochromocytomas

Pheochromocytomas may occur as a part of a number of different inherited endocrine tumor syndromes as shown in Table 14.13. Recently, familial paragangliomas of the neck have also been shown to be associated with mutations in the succinate dehydrogenase subunit B (SDHB) and succinate dehydrogenase subunit D (SDHD) genes. (51,52). These

TABLE 14.13

Hereditary Pheochromocytoma Syndromes

Syndrome	Mutation	Chromosome	Frequency
MEN 2A and 2B	RET protooncogene	10q11	30%–50%
Von Hippel-Lindau	VHL tumor suppressor gene	3p25	15%–20%
Neurofibromatosis	NF-1	17q11	1%–5%
Familial paraganglioma and extra-adrenal pheochromocytoma	SDHS[a]	11q23	
	SDHB	1p35-36	
	SDHC	1q21	

[a]Frequency refers to clinical incidence of tumors within individuals affected by the mutation.
The S, B and C are the designation for the specific mutation within the SDH gene. Patients with SDHD mutations are more likely to develop head and neck paragangliomas whereas SDHB mutations are more likely to be associated with extra-adrenal pheos and malignant tumors.
MEN, multiple endocrine neoplasia; SDH, succinate dehydrogenase, SDHS, succinate dehydrogenase subunit H; SDHB, succinate dehydrogenase subunit B; SDHC, succinate dehydrogenase subunit C.

genes encode mitochondrial enzymes involved in oxidative phosphorylation (53). Familial pheochromocytoma may be more common than previously thought. In one recent study, muutations were found in 66 cases (24%); 30 had mutations of von Hippel-Lindau (VHL), 13 of RET, 11 of SDHD, and 12 of SDHB (54).

ENDOCRINE PANCREAS

Cellular Anatomy

The pancreatic islets are nests of endocrine cells scattered throughout the exocrine pancreatic tissue. Although the islet cells comprise only 1% of the total pancreatic cell mass, they are richly vascularized, receiving 10% of total pancreatic blood flow. Four types of cells—A, B, D, and F—have been identified in normal pancreatic islets (Table 14.14). These cells function as major regulators of nutrient metabolism by secretion of glucagon (A cell), insulin (B cell), SST (D cell), and pancreatic polypeptide (PP) (F cell). The development of these cells within the pancreatic ductal epithelium is controlled by expression of a sequence of transcription factors as illustrated in Figure 14.23A. In addition, several peptide growth factors have their origins and targets in the developing endocrine pancreas as shown in Figure 14.23B.

Physiology

Insulin

Synthesis of insulin begins with production of the precursor molecule preproinsulin (MW 11,500) in the endoplasmic reticulum of the β cell. Preproinsulin is cleaved to form proinsulin (MW 9,000), which consists of the α and β chains of the insulin molecule and a connecting peptide as shown in Figure 14.24. Proinsulin is transported to the Golgi apparatus and packaged into secretory granules. With maturation of the granule, proinsulin is enzymatically cleaved to form the 51-amino acid insulin molecule and 31-amino acid C-peptide, which are cosecreted by the β cell. Small amounts of proinsulin are also released into the circulation and may be detected by most antisera used in standard immunoassays for insulin. Normally, 12% to 20% of immunoreactive insulin in the bloodstream is accounted for by proinsulin.

The insulin molecule (MW 5800) consists of α- and β-peptide chains linked by two disulfide bridges (Fig. 14.24). An intra chain disulfide bond also links positions 6 and 11 in the α chain. Circulating insulin has a half-life of 3 to 5 minutes, and approximately 50% is removed from the circulation by a single pass through the liver.

The normal adult pancreas secretes approximately 40 to 50 units of insulin daily. Basal fasting insulin concentrations in normal subjects average 10 μU/mL but may rise to 100 μU/mL after ingestion of a standard meal. Secretion of insulin by the β cell occurs in response to a variety of physiologic stimuli, including glucose, amino acids, fatty acids, and ketone bodies. The most potent of these stimuli for insulin release is glucose. Within a few minutes of food ingestion, insulin levels rise in response to an increase in glucose levels (Fig. 14.25). Peak insulin levels are reached within 30 to 45 minutes of eating and are accompanied by a rapid decline in blood glucose to near basal levels 90 to 120 minutes postprandially. Several of the GI hormones released in response to meal stimulation (GIP, CCK, secretin, and gastrin) further augment the rate of insulin secretion by potentiating the effects of glucose on the β cell.

Insulin exerts its biologic activity through both paracrine effects on adjacent islet cells and more distant endocrine effects on liver, muscle, and adipose tissue. Locally, insulin inhibits glucagon secretion by the α cells. Glucagon secretion is further inhibited by SST, which is released from the pancreatic delta cells in response to many of the same agents that stimulate insulin secretion. In contrast to the selective stimulation of α and δ cells by glucose, ingested amino acids stimulate release of both insulin and glucagon. Consequently, the type of ingested nutrients influences the pattern and rate of islet cell hormone release in response to a meal. The hyperglycemia that results from a predominately carbohydrate meal stimulates insulin secretion, which blunts glucagon release in response to the ingested amino acids. A protein-rich meal, however, results in a relatively greater

---

TABLE 14.14

Cell Types in the Pancreatic Islets

	Approximate Percentage of Islet Volume		
Cell Types	Dorsally Derived[a] (Anterior Head, Body, Tail)	Ventrally Derived[b] (Posterior Portion of Head)	Secretory Products
A cell (α)	20%	<0.5%	Glucagon
B cell (β)	70%–80%	15%–20%	Insulin, C peptide, proinsulin
D cell (δ)	3%–5%	<1%	Somatostatin
F cell (PP cell)	<2%	80%–85%	Pancreatic polypeptide

[a]Arises from embryonic dorsal bud and receives most of blood supply from celiac artery.
[b]Arises from primordial ventral bud and receives blood from superior mesenteric artery.
From Karen JH, Salber PR, Forsham PH, et al. Pancreatic hormone and diabetes mellitus. In: Greenspan FS ed. *Basic and clinical endocrinology*, 3rd ed. Norwalk: Appleton & Lange, 1991;593. Reprinted with permission.

rate of glucagon secretion because amino acids are potent stimulators of α cells but are less effective in stimulating insulin release in the absence of concurrent hyperglycemia. Therefore, the carbohydrate:protein ratio of an ingested meal is an important determinant of the secretion rates of these two hormones.

The principal function of insulin is to promote storage of ingested nutrients. Secreted insulin first reaches the liver where it exerts both anabolic and anticatabolic effects. Insulin binds to the insulin receptor, a transmembrane tyrosine kinase receptor with two α and two β subunits. The α subunits lie external to the cell membrane and contain the hormone binding sites, whereas the β subunits harbor tyrosine kinase on the cytosolic surface. When insulin binds to its receptor, tyrosine kinase is activated leading to autophosphorylation of the β subunits. In addition, the tyrosine kinase phosphorylates cytoplasmic proteins insulin receptor subtrate (IRS) 1 and 2 (IRS-1 and IRS-2). The IRS proteins act as docking sites for protein-mediating insulin actions such as phosphatidyl 3'-kinase. Insulin receptors are downregulated and internalized when circulating insulin levels are high (55).

Insulin increases the synthesis and storage of glucagon and promotes both glycogen synthesis and storage and inhibits its breakdown. It stimulates hepatic synthesis of proteins, triglycerides, and formation of very low density lipoproteins. It reduces cellular catabolism by inhibiting gluconeogenesis, ketogenesis, and hepatic glycogenolysis. In muscle, insulin stimulates synthesis of protein and glycogen, whereas in adipose tissue, it promotes storage of triglycerides, increases glucose transport into adipocytes, and inhibits lipolysis. These endocrine effects are detailed further in Table 14.15.

Glucagon

Glucagon is a 29-amino acid peptide (MW 3,485) secreted by pancreatic α cells. Glucagon has a circulatory half-life of 3 to 6 minutes and is secreted in response to stimulation by amino acids (arginine and alanine), catecholamines, GI hormones (CCK, gastrin, and GIP), glucocorticoids, and sympathetic nerve stimulation. The major target organ of action of glucagon is the liver, where it stimulates breakdown of stored glycogen and promotes hepatic gluconeogenesis from amino acid precursors and ketogenesis from fatty acid precursors.

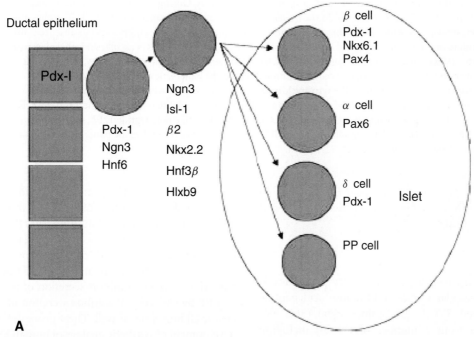

A

FIGURE 14.23   A: Expression of transcription factors in the developing endocrine pancreas from the generation of endocrine cells at the ductal epithelium to their expansion into mature islet cells. Pdx-1, initiates endocrine lineage commitment for cells within the pancreatic ducts, becomes restricted to differentiating β, D and pancreatic polypeptide (PP) cells and is lost from presumptive β cells, and finally becomes restricted to mature β cells where it controls insulin and Glut-2 gene expression. The pre-endocrine cell type derived from ducts has a transcription factor expression signature of Pdx-1, neurogenin 3 (Ngn3), Isl-1, Nkx2.2, β_2 and Pax6. Subsequent differentiation of β cells requires the additional expression Nkx6.1 and Pax4 with a reduction in Ngn3 and β_2. Presumptive endocrine cells also express hepatocyte nuclear factor 6 (Hnf6), Hnf3β and Hlxb9, the latter controlling migration away from the ducts. Hnf3β is a transcriptional regulator of Pdx1, and is itself regulated by Hnf6. Hnf6 also controls expression of neurogenin 3 (Ngn3) which continues to be expressed throughout islet formation until the point of final commitment of the endocrine lineages. (Adapted and modified from Hill D. Development of the endocrine pancreas. *Rev Endocr Metab Disord* 2005;6:229–238.)

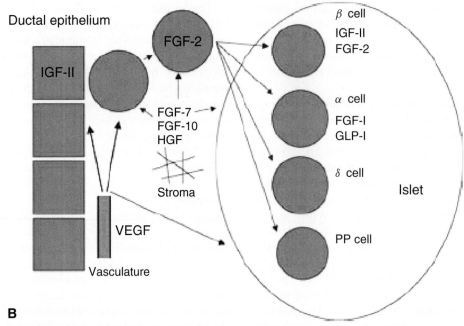

FIGURE 14.23   (*continued*) **B:** Proposed cellular origins of and target tissues of peptide growth factors during the development of the endocrine pancreas. Fibroblast growth factors (FGF) are involved in early pancreatic induction from gut endoderm, and the high affinity FGF receptor, FGFR1, has been localized to ductal epithelial cells and to small developing islets. During development of the endocrine pancreas, FGF-7 is expressed within the mesenchyme adjacent to the pancreatic ducts. FGF-10 has also been shown to be expressed within pancreatic mesenchyme in the mouse embryo and its absence causes a failure of ductal branching and an absence of endocrine progenitor cells. Vascular endothelial growth factor (VEGF) is a potent mitogen for endothelial cells, increases vascular permeability, and acts as a morphogen to induce endocrine cell commitment within the pancreatic ducts. Hepatocyte growth factor (HGF) and its receptor the tyrosine kinase *met*, are also expressed within adjacent epithelial tissues and appear to be involved in regulation of proliferation and differentiation pancreatic epithelial and islet cells. IGF, insulin-like growth factor; GLP-1, glucagon-like polypeptide 1, PP, pancreatic polypeptide. (Adapted and modified from Hill D. Development of the endocrine pancreas. *Rev Endocr Metab Disord* 2005;6:229–238.)

The major physiologic role of glucagon, therefore, is to provide the organism with a fuel source between meals and during periods of fasting.

Somatostatin

SST derives its name from its GH inhibitory properties. It occurs in two molecular forms—a 14-amino acid peptide termed *SST-14* and *SST-28* (28 amino acids) (56). SST has been isolated from a number of tissues, including the hypothalamus, GI tract, and pancreas. It acts through specifc SST receptors that belong to the G protein family of receptors. Five different SST receptor subtypes have been identified, each encoded by distinct genes located on different chromosomes. SST mediates its effects on target tissues through its receptors in a variety of pathways: through inhibition of cAMP, by reduction of calcium fluxes, and by stimulation of tyrosine phosphatase activity (56).

In the central nervous system, SST acts as a neurotransmitter and regulates the release of GH and TSH. In the GI tract, secretion occurs in response to the same stimuli that promote insulin release, including glucose, arginine, and other GI hormones. The principal function of SST in digestion is to slow movement of nutrients from the intestinal tract into the circulation. It accomplishes this purpose by reducing gastric emptying time, decreasing gastric production of gastrin and gastric acid, decreasing pancreatic exocrine secretion, and reducing splanchnic blood flow. SST acts in a paracrine manner to inhibit secretion of insulin, glucagon, and PP by islet cells. It inhibits secretion of other nonpancreatic GI hormones as well. These properties of SST and the development of synthetic analogs of human SST (octreotide, lanreotide) have led to its clinical use in the treatment of patients with fistulas of the GI tract and pancreas and patients with unresectable neuroendocrine tumors as well as reducing splanchnic blood flow in patients with variceal GI bleeding. Amelioration of hormone-related symptoms has been reported in patients with carcinoid tumors, pancreatic endocrine tumors (gastrinomas, VIP tumors), GH-secreting pituitary tumors, and ACTH-secreting tumors. SST receptor scintigraphy using In 111-labeled octreotide has also been used to image neuroendocrine tumors in patients whose tumors are difficult to localize by conventional imaging modalities.

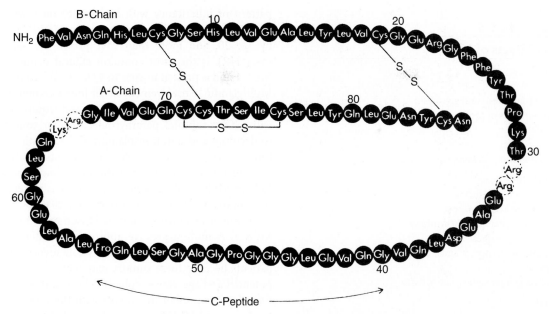

FIGURE 14.24 Structure of human proinsulin. The molecule is cleaved at amino acids 31 to 32 and 64 to 65 to form insulin and C peptide. (From Steiner DF, et al. Structural and immunological studies on human proinsulin. In: Rodriguez RR, Vallance-Owen J, eds. *Proceedings of the seventh congress of the international diabetes federation*, Amsterdam: Excerpta Medica, 1971:281. Reprinted by permission.)

Pancreatic Polypeptide

PP is a 36-amino acid peptide (MW 4,200) secreted by the F cells, which are located principally in the posterior portion of the head of the pancreas. The physiologic action of PP is unknown, but blood levels increase after ingestion of a protein-rich meal, episodes of hypoglycemia, and strenuous exercise. Elevated circulating levels of PP are frequently present in patients with pancreatic endocrine tumors and

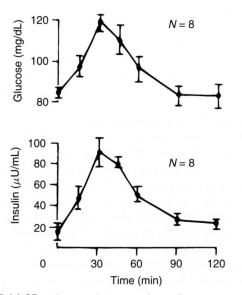

FIGURE 14.25 Plasma glucose and insulin response to a standard 530 kcal breakfast in normal subjects. (From Karam JH, Salber PR, Forsham PH. Pancreatic hormones and diabetes mellitus. In: Greenspan FS, ed. *Basic and clinical endocrinology*, 3rd ed. Norwalk: Appleton & Lange, 1991:593. Reprinted by permission.)

may serve as a biochemical marker for the diagnosis of these neoplasms and their response to therapy.

Pathophysiology

Tumors of the endocrine pancreas may arise from any of the four major cell types normally present in the islets or from neuroendocrine cells of the pancreas that secrete gastrin, VIP, or neurotensin (Table 14.16) The most common pancreatic endocrine tumors are gastrinomas and insulinomas (57,58). The other tumor types occur much less commonly; only a few cases of SST and neurotensin-secreting tumors have been reported. Pancreatic endocrine tumors may occur sporadically or in association with the MEN type 1 syndrome. The clinical and diagnostic features associated with the various tumors are shown in Table 14.16. Benign pancreatic endocrine neoplasms are frequently small and may be difficult to localize. Furthermore, gastrinomas occur three to ten times more commonly in the duodenum than the pancreas (59,60). CT, MRI, and selective mesenteric angiography combined with provocative calcium or secretin infusion to stimulate hormone release have been used to localize these neoplasms. Selective portal venous catheterization with sampling of the venous drainage beds of the pancreas may provide regional localization but is rarely utilized now. SST receptor scintigraphy localizes 90% of hepatic neuroendocrine tumors and 60% to 70% of primary gut neuroendocrine tumors (61). Other modalities to localize PETs include endoscopic ultrasonography and intraoperative ultrasonography. Despite improved methods of preoperative localization, direct palpation of the pancreas and duodenum is often necessary for intraoperative localization.

Multiple Endocrine Neoplasia Syndromes

The MEN syndromes are a group of familial disorders characterized by the development of endocrine neoplasms in multiple sites (62). The various components of the MEN syndromes and the frequency of their occurrence are shown in Table 14.17 (63–65). The MEN syndromes are each inherited in an autosomal dominant manner with complete penetrance but variable expressivity of the *MEN* gene. This means that each individual who inherits the *MEN* gene will exhibit some, but not necessarily all, components of the syndrome. Both sexes are affected with equal frequency, and no racial predilection exists.

The incidence of the various components of the MEN syndromes reflects an average frequency that may vary significantly among different kindreds (Table 14.17). The clinical and biochemical characteristics of these neoplasms are similar to the features that develop in patients with sporadic endocrine neoplasms of the same organs.

Multiple Endocrine Neoplasia 1

The endocrine neoplasms associated with MEN 1 are HPT, pituitary tumors, and pancreatic endocrine tumors. Other tumors that are less frequently associated with MEN 1 include adrenal adenomas or hyperplasia, lipomas, and foregut carcinoid tumors (64). MEN 1 has an autosomal dominant

pattern of inheritance with high penetrance, where more than 50% of patients with mutation in *MEN1* gene present by age 20, and more than 95% present by age 40. Primary HPT is the most common clinical manifestation of MEN 1 and is present in 90% to 97% of affected individuals. Multiglandular involvement of all four parathyroid glands with hyperplasia is generally present and requires treatment with either subtotal parathyroidectomy or total parathyroidectomy and autotransplantation. Pancreatic endocrine tumors occur in 30% to 80% of patients. These tumors may be nonfunctioning, but the most common secretory PET in MEN 1 is a gastrinoma, followed in frequency by insulinoma. Conversely, approximately 20% to 25% of patients who present with Zollinger-Ellison syndrome will have MEN 1. A more aggressive approach to pancreatic tumor localization and surgical resection is now advocated for these patients because these tumors may have a high malignant potential and aggressive biologic behavior. If hypercalcemia from HPT is present in patients with the Zollinger-Ellison syndrome and MEN-I, improved control of gastrin secretion may be achieved by parathyroidectomy. This is probably due to the observation that hypercalcemia promotes gastrin release from these pancreatic tumors. The most common pituitary tumor seen in this syndrome is a prolactinoma. Most symptomatic prolactinomas can be controlled medically with bromocriptine and surgery is not often indicated unless the tumor is enlarging or causing compressive symptoms.

The genetic defect responsible for MEN 1 is in a tumor suppressor gene (*MEN 1* gene) consisting of 10 exons that span a 9 kilobase region on the long arm of chromosome 11 (11q13) (66). The product of the *MEN 1* gene is a 610-amino acid protein termed *menin* (67), a nuclear protein (48) (68) whose precise function has not been fully elucidated; however, menin is known to interact with *JunD*, a common transcription factor in many cells. More than 200 mutations in the *MEN 1* gene have been described including missense, nonsense, frameshift, and mRNA splicing defects distributed throughout the coding exons of this gene. No correlation between specific genetic mutations and phenotype expression has yet been identified.

Multiple Endocrine Neoplasia 2

The MEN 2 syndromes are a group of related disorders that include MEN 2A, MEN 2B, and familial non-MEN MTC. The most constant feature of MEN 2 isMTC, a calcitonin-producing neoplasm of the parafollicular or C cells of the thyroid (see "The Thyroid"). MTC occurs in virtually 100% of patients who inherit the affected gene. MTC in these patients is multifocal and bilateral, and is often preceded by the development of C-cell hyperplasia in affected individuals. As discussed previously, calcitonin is a very sensitive biochemical marker for the development of MTC, and provocative stimulation of calcitonin release into the blood by the administration of intravenous calcium and/or pentagastrin is a reliable method for establishing the presence of disease and for monitoring patients after thyroidectomy (69). MTC cells have been shown to synthesize

TABLE 14.16

Biochemical and Clinical Features of the Major Endocrine Pancreatic Tumors

Tumor	Predominant Peptide	Major Cell Type	Clinical Features	Diagnostic Features
Insulinoma	Insulin	B	Fasting hypoglycemia (glucose <50 mg/dL) signs of neuroglucopenia and adrenergic discharge	Elevated fasting plasma insulin, failure of insulin suppression in fasting hypoglycemia (insulin/glucose ratio >0.3)
Gastrinoma	Gastrin	Islet cells	Virulent peptic ulcer disease, diarrhea (Zollinger-Ellison syndrome)	Elevated gastric acid output, elevated plasma gastrin, increased gastrin response to intravenous secretin
Glucagonoma	Glucagon	A	Dermatitis (necrolytic migratory erythema), glucose intolerance, diabetes mellitus, weight loss, anemia	Elevated fasting plasma glucagon
Somatostatinoma	Somatostatin	D	Dyspepsia, mild diabetes mellitus, gallbladder disease, steatorrhea, hypochlorhydria	Elevated fasting plasma somatostatin, hyperglycemia without ketonemia
PPoma	PP	F	Not identified (clinically silent)	Elevated fasting plasma PP
VIPoma	VIP	Non-β islet cells	Profound secretory diarrhea, hypokalemia, hypochlorhydria, acidosis (WDHA syndrome)	Elevated fasting plasma VIP
Neurotensinoma	Neurotensin	N	Diarrhea, diabetes, weight loss, edema, hypotension (may be indistinguishable from VIPoma)	Elevated fasting plasma neurotensin

PP, pancreatic polypeptide; VIP, vasoactive intestinal polypeptide; WDHA, watery diarrhea, hypokalemia, hypochlorhydria.
Modified from Gower WR, Fabri PJ. Endocrine neoplasms (non-gastrin) of the pancreas. *Semin Surg Oncol* 1990;6:98–109. Reprinted with permission.

a number of other peptides, including calcitonin gene–related peptide, ACTH, melanocyte-stimulating hormone, VIP, serotonin, substance P, and SST. Carcinoembryonic antigen may also be secreted by MTC cells and can be a useful marker for monitoring patients for disease activity.

The RET protooncogene on chromosome 10 (10q11.2) has been identified as the gene responsible for both MEN 2A (70,71) and MEN 2B (72). Mutations in the RET protooncogene have been identified in a subset of patients with Hirschsprung disease as well. Most RET mutations are located in exons 10, 11 and 16, making genetic screening for this syndrome more sensitive. Presymptomatic DNA testing in kindred members who are at risk for developing MEN 2A to be now been carried out at an early age in individuals affected with the RET mutation, even if they have normal stimulated plasma calcitonin levels. These recent landmark reports from Wells et al. (73) and Lips et al. (74) mark the first time that a genetic test has been used as the sole basis for initiating surgical therapy for a disease.

Multiple Endocrine Neoplasia 2A

MTC usually develops within the first three decades of life in patients with MEN 2A. Pheochromocytomas, which occur in 30% to 40% of patients, are frequently bilateral and may be preceded by the development of adrenal medullary hyperplasia. HPT is found in 25% to 35% of patients and is often asymptomatic and characterized by generalized parathyroid hyperplasia. Approximately one third of patients with MEN 2A will also develop cutaneous lichen amyloidosis, a skin disorder manifesting as brownish plaques in the epidermis located between the scapulae. There is an association between MEN 2A and Hirschsprung disease, with several MEN 2A patients developing severe GI manifestations in infancy from aganglionosis of the distal bowel.

Multiple Endocrine Neoplasia 2B

MTC occurs in 100% of patients with MEN 2B and behaves in a biologically more virulent manner than in patients with MEN 2A. The incidence of pheochromocytomas is variable, but overall occurs in approximately 50% of patients (75). The most striking feature of MEN 2B is the multiple mucosal neuromas that affect the lips, tongue, eyelids, and conjunctiva. Hypertrophied corneal nerve fibers may be seen on slit-lamp examination. Ganglioneuromas in the GI tract may cause constipation and cause colonic dilatation and megacolon by an unknown mechanism (76). A Marfanoid body habitus with long, thin extremities and muscle wasting is often present.

Familial Non-Multiple Endocrine Neoplasia Medullary Thyroid Carcinoma

Patients with familial non-MEN MTC develop MTC but do not have any of the other associated endocrinopathies.

TABLE 14.17

Components of the Multiple Endocrine Neoplasia Syndromes

Syndrome	Component	Frequency
MEN 1	Parathyroid hyperplasia	90%
	Pancreatic islet tumors	35%–75%
	Pituitary tumors	65%
	Other tumors[a]	5%–10%
MEN 2A	Medullary thyroid carcinoma	100%
	Pheochromocytoma	30%–40%
	Parathyroid hyperplasia	25%–35%
MEN 2B	Medullary thyroid carcinoma	100%
	Pheochromocytoma	50%
	Multiple mucosal neuromas	100%
	Marfanoid body habitus	65%

[a]Includes carcinoids, bronchial adenomas, thyroid adenomas, lipomas, and adrenocortical adenomas.

Shapiro SE, Cote GC, Lee JE, et al. The role of genetics in the surgical management of familial endocrinopathy syndromes. *J Am Coll Surg* 2003;197:818–831.

Lairmore TC, Moley JF, eds. The multiple endocrine neoplasia syndromes. In: Townsend CM, et al. eds. *Sabiston textbook of surgery*, 17th ed. Philadelphia: Elsevier Science, 2004:1071–1087.

MTC in these patients has its onset later in life (fifth or sixth decade) and behaves in a biologically indolent manner compared to MTC in MEN 2A and 2B.

Carcinoid Tumors and the Carcinoid Syndrome

Carcinoid tumors are neuroendocrine tumors that arise in the enterochromaffin or Kulchitsky cells. These cells are a part of the diffuse neuroendocrine system. Kulchitsky cells are found in many tissues, including the crypts of the GI tract and the bronchial epithelium. Carcinoid tumors may develop anywhere throughout the GI tract and are traditionally classified according to the portion of the embryonic gut from which they are derived (foregut, midgut, or hindgut). The most common sites of occurrence, in order of decreasing frequency, are the small bowel, appendix, and rectum (77). Appendiceal and rectal carcinoids are frequently benign whereas most ileal carcinoids are malignant.

Because of their neuroendocrine origin, carcinoid tumors may synthesize and secrete a variety of biologically active substances, including serotonin (5-hydroxytryptamine). The clinical manifestations that result from the release of these humoral mediators into the circulation have been termed the *carcinoid syndrome*. This syndrome is characterized by flushing, diarrhea, bronchospasm, and endocardial fibrosis of the tricuspid and pulmonic valves. Serotonin is the best-documented mediator of the carcinoid syndrome, but other substances (histamine and substance P) are also likely involved. The mediators of the carcinoid syndrome are inactivated after a single pass through the liver. Consequently, the presence of the carcinoid syndrome implies that mediators are being released directly into the systemic circulation. Most cases of carcinoid syndrome, therefore,

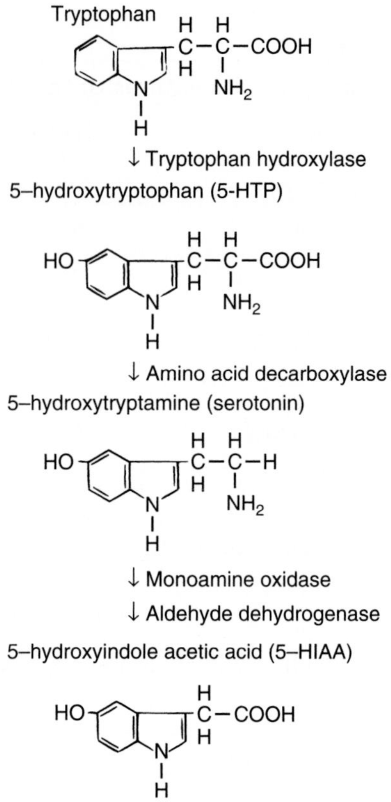

FIGURE 14.26 Pathway of serotonin synthesis and metabolism.

occur in patients with either hepatic metastases from GI tumors or extra-abdominal tumors (bronchial carcinoids) that release their mediators systemically. Overall, less than 1% of GI carcinoids are associated with the development of the carcinoid syndrome.

The pathway for biosynthesis of serotonin is shown in Figure 14.26. The rate-limiting step in this pathway is conversion of tryptophan to 5-hydroxytryptophan by tyrosine hydroxylase (TH). 5-hydroxytryptophan is converted rapidly by amino acid decarboxylase to 5-hydroxytryptamine (serotonin). Foregut carcinoids generally have low levels of amino acid decarboxylase activity and preferentially secrete 5-hydroxytryptophan (Table 14.18). After synthesis, 5-hydroxytryptamine is packaged into neurosecretory granules, which then discharge their contents into the circulation. Most circulating 5-hydroxytryptamine undergoes conversion to 5-hydroxyindole acetic acid (5-HIAA) by the actions of MAO and aldehyde dehydrogenase and is then excreted in the urine. Measurement of urinary 5-HIAA is the most useful diagnostic test in the evaluation of patients with suspected carcinoid tumors or the carcinoid syndrome. The excretion rate of 5-HIAA in healthy subjects is less than 10 mg/24 hr. Chromogranin A is another neuroendocrine tumor marker that is often elevated in patients with carcinoid tumors and has been used to follow patients for tumor recurrence (77). Compared to urinay 5 HIAA levels, chromogranin A is somewhat more likely to be elevated in midgut carcinoids (87% versus 75%) and much more sensitive in the setting

TABLE 14.18

Common Ectopic Hormone Syndromes Caused by Nonendocrine Malignancies

Syndrome	Etiologic Agents	Types of Malignancies
Hypercalcemia	PTH-related protein	Squamous carcinoma (lung, head and neck, renal cell cancer, ovarian cancer, breast cancer)
	Local osteolytic factors[a]	Breast carcinoma, multiple myeloma, lymphomas)
	1, 25 (OH)$_2$ vitamin D	Lymphomas
SIADH	Vasopressin (ADH)	Small cell lung carcinoma
Hypoglycemia	IGF-II	Mesenchymal tumors of trunk (soft tissue sarcomas)
		Gastrointestinal tract malignancies
		Carcinoid tumors
		Adrenocortical carcinoma
Cushing syndrome	ACTH	Bronchial or thymic carcinoid tumors
		Small cell lung carcinoma

[a]Includes cytokines TNF-β, IL-1, IL-6.
PTH, parathyroid hormone; SIADH, syndrome of inappropriate antidiuretic hormone; ADH, antidiuretic hormone; IGF-II, insulin-like growth factor-II; ACTH, adrenocorticotropic hormone; TNF-β, tumor necrosis factor; IL, interleukin.

of foregut (87% versus 31%) or hindgut tumors (100% versus 0%) (78,79). Approximately 90% of carcinoid tumors express type 2 SST receptors (56) and can therefore, often be localized with radioactive labeled octreotide imaging.

ENDOCRINE MANIFESTATIONS OF NONENDOCRINE MALIGNANCIES

Ectopic or inappropriate secretion of peptide hormones is one of the most common paraneoplastic manifestations of nonendocrine malignancies. With the exception of the steroid hormones and thyroid hormone, both of which require specialized enzymatic machinery for synthesis, virtually any hormone can be produced in an ectopic manner. In contrast to hormone secretion by normal endocrine cells, ectopic production of hormones by neuroendocrine tumors is usually not suppressible and may predominantly involve secretion of precursor molecules with reduced biologic activity (see "Hypercalcemia of Malignancy"). Neuroendocrine tumors may also secrete peptides that differ in amino acid sequence from the native hormone but retain their physiologic activity. The identification of ectopic hormone production by a neuroendocrine tumor requires fulfillment of the following criteria: (i) presence of a tumor and association with a clinical hormone syndrome and elevated circulating hormone levels, (ii) resolution of hormonal symptoms with treatment of the tumor, (iii) demonstration of an arteriovenous hormone gradient across the vascular bed of the tumor, (iv) presence of hormone in the tumor tissue, and (v) documentation of synthesis or secretion of hormone by the tumor *in vitro* or by mRNA analysis. The first two criteria are usually sufficient to establish the diagnosis clinically.

The most common clinical syndromes caused by ectopic production of peptide hormones are shown in Table 14.18. In addition, a variety of other hormones may be produced ectopically in patients with neuroendocrine tumors, including human chorionic gonadotropin, GH-releasing hormone, calcitonin, VIP, and erythropoietin.

Hypercalcemia of Malignancy

Malignancy-associated hypercalcemia is the most common endocrine complication of malignancy. It occurs in 3% to 30% of patients with advanced malignancies at sometime during their disease course and is the most common cause of hypercalcemia in hospitalized patients (80). In 98% of cases, the responsible tumor is identifiable at the time of presentation of the hypercalcemia. Common tumor types where hypercalcemia can occur include squamous cell lung cancer, breast cancer, head and neck cancer, renal cancer, and ovarian cancer. While squamous cell lung cancer is the most common cause of hypercalcemia in malignancy, approximately 30% to 40% of patients with breast cancer will manifest some degree of hypercalcemia. Three types of hypercalcemia in malignancy have been categorized: humoral hypercalcemia in malignancy, hypercalcemia with skeletal metastases, and hypercalcemia in hematologic malignancy. In humoral hypercalcemia of malignancy, stimulation of bone resorption by PTHrP is the principal mechanism by which hypercalcemia develops. Elevated serum levels of PTHrP, which has significant N-terminus homology to PTH, are present in up to 80% of hypercalcemic patients with solid tumors (81). PTHrP binds to PTH receptors in kidney and bone and has similar physiologic activity to PTH. It does not cross-react with the PTH antisera used in standard PTH immunoassays. Rarely, ectopic secretion of intact PTH has also been described (80).

Hypercalcemia in patients with breast carcinoma primarily develops in patients with extensive osseous metastases. The administration of estrogen, androgens, or antiestrogen compounds may precipitate the appearance of hypercalcemia. Production of a local osteolytic factor has been implicated as the etiologic agent. The mechanism of hypercalcemia in patients with hematologic malignancies such as multiple myeloma and lymphomas is thought to involve production of hypercalcemia-inducing cytokines responsible for increased bone-rosorption such as tumor necrosis factor β, interleukin-1, and interleukin-6 (82). Some lymphomas have also been reported to secrete the active vitamin D metabolite 1, 25 $(OH)_2$ D, and, therefore, cause hypercalcemia by both increased intestinal absorption of calcium and enhanced osteoclastic bone resorption (80).

Syndrome of Inappropriate Antidiuretic Hormone Secretion

Inappropriate secretion of vasopressin, or ADH, is the second most common endocrine manifestation of malignancy. It occurs in 7% to 8% of patients with small cell lung carcinoma and results in impaired secretion of free water by the kidneys. This results in symptoms of water intoxication and hyponatremia, including weakness, lethargy, somnolence, and confusion. Profound hyponatremia (<110 mEq/L) may cause coma, seizures, and death.

Ectopic Adrenocorticotropic Hormone Syndrome

Many nonendocrine tumors secrete the precursor molecule for ACTH, pro-opiomelanocortin. However, most cases of Cushing syndrome from ectopic ACTH production occur in neuroendocrine cell tumors. In one recent series, bronchial carcinoids and small cell lung cancers were the two most common causes (83). This occurs because only neuroendocrine cells are capable of processing and secreting clinically significant amounts of ACTH from pro-opiomelanocortin. Patients with the ectopic ACTH syndrome do not usually develop the truncal obesity and skin changes typically associated with Cushing syndrome. Instead, weight loss, muscle weakness, wasting, skin pigmentation, and hypokalemia are the usual findings.

Hypoglycemia

A number of nonpancreatic islet cell tumors may cause hypoglycemia. Soft tissue sarcomas of the trunk (chest, abdomen, and retroperitoneum) account for 50% of all cases; another 25% are the result of the other tumors listed in Table 14.18. The presence of hypoglycemia together with suppressed plasma insulin levels suggests the diagnosis. The mechanism of hypoglycemia may involve both increased rates of glucose use by the tumor and secretion of humoral factors (insulin-like growth factor 2) with insulin-like effects.

REFERENCES

1. De Felice M, Di Lauro R. Thyroid development and its disorders: genetics and molecular mechanisms. *Endocr Rev* 2004;25:722–746.
2. Harrison T. The thyroid gland. In: Sabiston, DC, ed. *Textbook of surgery*, Philadelphia: WB Saunders, 1986:579–619.
3. Musholt TJ, Moley JF. Management of persistent or recurrent medullary thyroid carcinoma. *Prob Gen Surg* 1997;14:89–109.
4. Gavin LA. Thyroid physiology and testing of thyroid function. In: Clark, O, ed. *Endocrine surgery of the thyroid and parathyroid glands*, St. Louis: CV Mosby, 1985:1–34.
5. Porterfield SP. Thyroid gland. *Endocrine physiology*. St. Louis: Mosby, 2001:59–84.
6. Cheng SY. Multiple mechanisms for regulation of the transcriptional activity of thyroid hormone receptors. *Rev Endocr Metab Disord* 2000;1:9–18.
7. Cooper D. Antithyroid drugs. *N Engl J Med* 2005;352:905–917.
8. Mitsiades N, Poulaki V, Mitsiades CS, et al. Apoptosis induced by FasL and TRAIL/Apo2L in the pathogenesis of thyroid diseases. *Trends Endocrinol Metab* 2001;12:384–390.
9. Attia J, Margetts P, Guyatt G. Diagnosis of thyroid disease in hospitalized patients: a systematic review. *Arch Intern Med* 1999;159:658–665.
10. Demers L. Thyroid disease: pathophysiology and diagnosis. *Clin Lab Med* 2004;24:19–28.
11. Vaidya B, Anthony S, Bilous M. Detection of thyroid dysfunction in early pregnancy: universal screening or targeted high-risk case finding? *J Clin Endocrinol Metab* 2006;91:1748.
12. Lind P, Kohlfurst S. Respective roles of thyroglobulin, radioiodine imaging, and positron emission tomography in the assessment of thyroid cancer. *Semin Nucl Med* 2006;36:194–205.
13. Choi MY, Chung JK, Lee HY. The clinical impact of 18F-FDG PET in papillary thyroid carcinoma with a negative ^{131}I whole body scan: a single-center study of 108 patients. *Ann Nucl Med* 2006;20:547–552.
14. Schussler-Fiorenza CM, Bruns CM, Chen HT. The surgical management of Graves' disease. *J Surg Res* 2006;133:207–214.
15. Sarlis NJ, Gourgiotis L. Thyroid emergencies. *Rev Endocr Metab Disord* 2003;4:129–136.
16. Tietgens ST, Leinung MC. Thyroid storm. *Med Clin North Am* 1995;79:169–184.
17. Akerstrom G, Malmaeus J, Bergstrom R. Surgical anatomy of the parathyroid glands. *Surgery* 1984;95:14–21.
18. Norris EH. The parathyroid glands and the lateral thyroid in man: their morphogenesis, histogenesis, topographic anatomy, and prenatal growth. *Contrib Embryol* 1937;26:247–294.
19. Gardella TJ, Juppner H. Interaction of PTH and PTHrP with their receptors. *Rev Endocr Metab Disord* 2000;1:317–329.
20. Inzerillo AM, Zaidi M, Huang CL. Calcitonin: physiological actions and clinical applications. *J Pediatr Endocrinol Metab* 2004;17:931–940.
21. Goodman WG. The evolution of assays for parathyroid hormone. *Semin Dial* 2005;18:296–301.
22. Arnold A. Molecular genetics of parathyroid gland neoplasia. *J Clin Endocrinol Metab* 1993;77:1108–1112.
23. Heppner C, Kester MB, Agarwal SK, et al. Somatic mutation of the MEN1 gene in parathyroid tumours. *Nat Genet* 1997;16:375–378.
24. Arnold A. The cyclin D1/PRAD1 oncogene in human neoplasia. *J Investig Med* 1995;43:543–549.
25. Hendy GN. Molecular mechanisms of primary hyperparathyroidism. *Rev Endocr Metab Disord* 2000;1:297–305.
26. Sherr CJ. Cancer cell cycles. *Science* 1996;274:1672–1677.
27. Pollak MR, Brown EM, Wu Chow YH, et al. Mutations in the human Ca2+ sensing receptor gene cause familial hypocalciuric hypercalcemia and neonatal severe hyperparathyroidism. *Cell* 1993;75:1297–1303.

28. Shattuck TM. Somatic and germ-line mutations of the HRPT2 gene in sporadic parathyroid carcinoma. *N Engl J Med* 2003;349:1722–1729.

29. Brown EM. Familial hypocalciuric hypercalcemia and other disorders with resistance to extracellular calcium. *Endocrinol Metab Clin North Am* 2000;29:503–522.

30. Moe SM, Drueke TB. Management of secondary hyperparathyroidism: the importance and challenge of controlling parathyroid hormone levels without elevating calcium, phosphorus, and calcium-phosphorus product. *Am J Nephrol* 2003;23:369–379.

31. Delmez JA, Slatopolsky E. Recent advances in the pathogenesis and therapy of uremic secondary hyperparathyroidism. *J Clin Endocrinol Metab* 1991;72:735–739.

32. Arnaud CD, Kolb FO. The calciotropic hormones and metabolic bone disease. In: Greenspan FS, ed. *Basic and clinical endocrinology*, Norwalk: Appleton & Lange, 1991:247–322.

33. Levin MA. Clinical spectrum and pathogenesis of pseudohypoparathyroidism. *Rev Endocr Metab Disord* 2000;1:265–274.

34. Bergland RM, Gann DS, De Maria EJ. Pituitary and adrenal. In: Schwartz SI, ed. *Principles of surgery*, New York: McGraw-Hill, 1990:1545–1557.

35. Oldfield EH, Doppman JL, Nieman LK, et al. Petrosal sinus sampling with and without corticotropin releasing hormone for the differential diagnosis of Cushing's syndrome. *N Engl J Med* 1991;325:899–905.

36. Melmed S. Acromegaly. *N Engl J Med* 2006;355:2558–2573.

37. Simard MF. Pituitary tumor endocrinopathies and their endocrine evaluation. *Neurosurg Clin N Am* 2003;14:41–54.

38. Rhen T, Cidlowski JA. Antiinflammatory action of glucocorticoids. *N Engl J Med* 2005;353:1711–1723.

39. Findling JW, Doppman JL. Biochemical and radiologic diagnosis of Cushing's syndrome. *Endocrinol Metab Clin North Am* 1994;23:511–537.

40. Invitti C, Giraldi FP, Cavagnini F. Inferior petrosal sinus sampling in patients with Cushing's syndrome and contradicting response to dynamic testing. *Clin Endocrinol* 1999;51:255–257.

41. Findling JW, Raff H. Diagnosis and differential diagnosis of Cushing's syndrome. *Endocrinol Metab Clin North Am* 2001;30:729–747.

42. Ganguly A. Primary aldosteronism. *N Engl J Med* 1998;339:1828–1834.

43. Young WF Jr. Primary aldosteronism: a common and curable form of hypertension. *Cardiol Rev* 1999;7:207–214.

44. Salvatori R. Adrenal insufficiency. *JAMA* 2005;294:2481–2488.

45. Goldfien A. Adrenal medulla. In: Greenspan S, ed. *Basic and clinical endocrinology*, Norwalk: Appleton & Lange, 1991:380–399.

46. Bravo EL, Tagle R. Pheochromocytoma: state-of-the-art and future prospects. *Endocr Rev* 2003;24:539–553.

47. Pacak K, Linehan WM, Eisenhofer G, et al. Recent advances in genetics, diagnosis, localization, and treatment of pheochromocytoma. *Ann Intern Med* 2001;134:315–329.

48. Eisenhofer G, Lenders JW, Linehan WM, et al. Plasma normetanephrine and metanephrine for detecting pheochromocytoma in von Hippel-Lindau disease and multiple endocrine neoplasia type 2. *N Engl J Med* 1999;340:1872–1879.

49. Sawka AM, Jaeschke R, Singh RJ, et al. A comparison of biochemical tests for pheochromocytoma: measurement of fractionated plasma metanephrines compared with the combination of 24-hour urinary metanephrines and catecholamines. *J Clin Endocrinol Metab* 2003;88:553–558.

50. Ilias I, Pacak K. Current approaches and recommended algorithm for the diagnostic localization of pheochromocytoma. *J Clin Endocrinol Metab* 2004;89:479–491.

51. Neumann HP, Pawlu C, Peczkowska M, et al. Distinct clinical features of paraganglioma syndromes associated with SDHB and SDHD gene mutations. *JAMA* 2004;292:943–951.

52. Benn DE, Gimenez-Roqueplo AP, Reilly JR, et al. Clinical presentation and penetrance of pheochromocytoma/paraganglioma syndromes. *J Clin Endocrinol Metab* 2006;91:827–836.

53. Baysal BE, Rerrell RE, Willett-Brozick JE, et al. Mutations in SDHD, a mitochondrial complex II gene, in hereditary paraganglioma. *Science* 2000;287:848–851.

54. Neumann HP, Bausch B, McWhinney SR, et al. Germ-line mutations in nonsyndromic pheochromocytoma. *N Engl J Med* 2002;346:1459–1466.

55. Porterfield SP. Endocrine pancreas. *Endocrine physiology*. St. Louis: Mosby 2001:85–106.

56. de Herder WW, Lamberts SW. Somatostatin and somatostatin analogues: diagnostic and therapeutic uses. *Curr Opin Oncol* 2002;14:53–57.

57. Proye CA. Current concepts in functioning endocrine tumors of the pancreas. *World J Surg* 2004;28:1231–1238.

58. Viola KV, Sosa JA. Current advances in the diagnosis and treatment of pancreatic endocrine tumors. *Curr Opin Oncol* 2004;17:24–27.

59. Norton JA, Fraker DL, Alexander R, et al. Surgery to cure the Zollinger-Ellison syndrome. *N Engl J Med* 1999;341:635–644.

60. Norton JA, Jensen RT. Resolved and unresolved controversies in the surgical management of patients with Zollinger-Ellison syndrome. *Ann Surg* 2004;240:757–773.

61. Modlin IM, Tang LH. Approaches to the diagnosis of gut neuroendocrine tumors. The last word today. *Gastroenterology* 1997;112:583–590.

62. Carney J. Familial multiple endocrine neoplasia: the first 100 years. *Am J Surg Pathol* 2005;29:254–274.

63. Cance WG, Wells SA. Multiple endocrine neoplasia type IIa. *Curr Probl Surg* 1985;22:1–56.

64. Shapiro SE, Cote GC, Lee JE, et al. The role of genetics in the surgical management of familial endocrinopathy syndromes. *J Am Coll Surg* 2003;197:818–831.

65. Lairmore TC, Moley JF, eds. The multiple endocrine neoplasia syndromes. In: Townsend CM Beauchamp D, Evers M, et al. Philadelphia: Elsevier Saunders, 2004:1071–1087.

66. Larrson C, Skogseid B, Oberg K, et al. Multiple endocrine neoplasia type 1 gene maps to chromosome 11 and is lost in insulinoma. *Nature* 1988;332:85–87.

67. Chandrasekharappa SC, Guru SC, Manickamp P, et al. Positional cloning of the gene for multiple endocrine neoplasia type 1. *Science* 1997;276:404–407.

68. Guru SC, Goldsmith PK, Burn AL, et al. Menin, the product of the MEN 1 gene, is a nuclear protein. *Proc Natl Acad Sci USA* 1998;95:1630–1634.

69. Wells SA, Baylin SB, Linehan WM, et al. Provocative agents and the diagnosis of medullary carcinoma of the thyroid gland. *Ann Surg* 1978;188:139–141.

70. Mulligan LM, Kwok JB, Healey CS, et al. Germ-line mutations of the RET proto-oncogene in multiple endocrine neoplasia type 2A. *Nature* 1993;363:458–460.

71. Donis Keller H, Dou S, Chi D, et al. Mutations in the RET proto oncogene are associated with MEN 2A and FMTC. *Hum Mol Genet* 1993;2:851–856.

72. Lairmore TC, Howe JR, Korte JA, et al. Familial medullary thyroid carcinoma and multiple endocrine neoplasia type 2B map to the same region of chromosome 10 as multiple endocrine neoplasia type 2A. *Genomics* 1991;9:181–192.

73. Wells SA, Chi DD, Toshima K, et al. Predictive DNA testing and prophylactic thyroidectomy in patients at risk for multiple endocrine neoplasia type 2A. *Ann Surg* 1994;220:237–250.

74. Lips CJM, Landsvater RM, Hoppener JWM. Clinical screening as compared with DNA analysis in families with multiple endocrine neoplasia type 2A. *N Engl J Med* 1994;331:828–835.

75. Lee NC, Norton JA. Multiple endocrine neoplasia type 2b—genetic basis and clinical expression. *Surg Oncol* 2000;9:111–118.

76. Cohen MS, Phay JE, DeBenedetti MK, et al. Gastrointestinal manifestations of multiple endocrine neoplasia type 2. *Ann Surg* 2002;235:648–655.

77. Sippel RS, Chen H. An update on carcinoid tumors. *Prob Gen Surg* 2003;20:125–133.

78. Oberg K. Carcinoid tumors: molecular genetics, tumor biology and update of diagnosis and treatment. *Curr Opin Oncol* 2002;14:38–45.

79. Bashir S, Gibril F, Ojeaburu JV, et al. Prospective study of the ability of histamine, serotonin, or serum chromogranin levels to identify gastric carcinoids in patients with gastrinomas. *Aliment Pharmacol Ther* 2002;16:1367–1382.

80. Stewart AF. Hypercalcemia associated with cancer. *N Engl J Med* 2005;352:373–379.

81. Strewler GJ. The physiology of parathyroid hormone-related protein. *N Engl J Med* 2000;342:177–184.

82. Grill V, Martin TJ. Hypercalcemia in malignancy. *Rev Endocr Metab Disord* 2000;1:253–263.

83. Isidori AM, Kaltsas GA, Possa C, et al. The ectopic adrenocorticotropin syndrome: clinical features, diagnosis, management, and long-term follow-up. *J Clin Endocrinol Metab* 2006;91:371–377.

SUGGESTED READINGS

Arafah BM, Nasrallah MP. Pituitary tumors: pathophysiology, clinical manifestations and management. *Endocr Relat Cancer* 2001;8:287–305.

Bravo EL, Tagle R. Pheochromocytoma: state-of—the-art and future prospects. *Endocr Rev* 2003;24:539–553.

Carney JA. Familial endocrine neoplasia: the first 100 years. *Am J Surg Pathol* 2005;29:254–274.

Cooper DS. Antithyroid drugs. *N Engl J Med* 2005;352:905–917.

Demers LM. Thyroid disease: pathophysiology and diagnosis. *Clin Lab Med* 2004;24:19–28.

Findling JW, Raff H. Diagnosis and differential diagnosis of Cushing's syndrome. *Endocrinol Metab Clin North Am* 2001;30:729–747.

Ganguly A. Primary aldosteronism. *N Engl J Med* 1998;339:1826–1834.

Lairmore TC. Multiple endocrine neoplasia. In: Norton JA, Bollinger RR, Chang AE, et al. eds. *Surgery: basic science and clinical evidence*, 1st ed. New York: Springer-Verlag, 2001:955–966.

Marx SJ. Hyperparathyroid and hypoparathyroid states. *N Engl J Med* 2000;343:1863–1875.

Pacak K, Linehan WM, Eisenhofer G, et al. Recent advances in genetics, diagnosis, localization, and treatment of pheochromocytoma. *Ann Intern Med* 2001;134:315–329.

Paschke R, Ludgate M. The thyrotropin receptor in thyroid diseases. *N Engl J Med* 1997;337:1675–1681.

Proye CAG, Lokey JS. Current concepts in functioning endocrine tumors of the pancreas. *World J Surg* 2004;28:1231–1238.

Shapiro SE, Cote GC, Lee JE, et al. The role of genetics in the surgical management of familial endocrinopathy syndromes. *J Am Coll Surg* 2003;197:818–831.

Young WF Jr. Primary aldosteronism: a common and curable form of hypertension. *Cardiol Rev* 1999;7:207–214.

CHAPTER 15

The Cardiovascular System

Daniel L. Beckles and Michael A. Wait

Cardiovascular disease is a major cause of morbidity and mortality in modern society and its prevalence is seen in our aging population, with associated risk factors such as obesity and diabetes.

This chapter is designed to be a review of the basic science, anatomy and pathophysiology of the cardiovascular system written for general surgical residents.

Obviously, it is impossible to include every facet of the cardiovascular system in such a review. However, this chapter should allow surgical residents to review the basic scientific principles of the cardiovascular system as it applies to the care of the general surgical patient. This chapter also provides a concise introduction to the pathophysiology of various cardiovascular disorders. A list of selected references follows this chapter, and residents are urged to use these references because they are not only complete but also readable, in-depth sources of information.

BASIC SCIENCE OF THE PERIPHERAL VASCULAR SYSTEM

Arterial Anatomy

The arteries of the body are divided histologically into three layers. The intima is the layer that contains endothelial cells and, in some places, a single layer of subendothelial smooth muscle cells. Beneath the intima, dividing it from the media, is the internal elastic membrane. The media is the major structural component of the artery containing smooth muscle cells, elastin, proteoglycans, and collagen. The media is separated from the third layer, the adventitia, by the external elastic membrane. When a typical endarterectomy is performed, the cleavage plane is superficial to the external elastic membrane. The blood supply for the inner part of the media comes from direct diffusion from the lumen of the blood vessel wall, and the outer part of the media is supplied by smaller penetrating arteries known as *vasovasorum*. The third layer, the adventitia, contains elastic tissue, fibroblasts, and collagen, and provides approximately 60% of the

strength of the blood vessel itself. Large arteries, such as the aorta and first- and second-order branches, have vasa vasorum vessels within the adventitial layer; dilated hypertrophic vasa vasorum on the thoracic and abdominal aorta can be external signs of underlying severe intimal atherosclerosis.

The Role of Endothelium in the Cardiovascular System

The vascular endothelium is a crucial mediator of vascular physiology. Endothelial cells are involved actively in angiogenesis, coagulation, platelet interaction, inflammation, immune response, synthesis of connective tissue components, metabolic functions and, most importantly, the regulation of vascular tone. The endothelium is, of course, normally nonthrombogenic; therefore, platelets do not adhere to an intact, quiescent endothelial lining. Platelets do, however, adhere to inflamed endothelium or to the basal lamina of vessels denuded of their endothelial coverings. Endothelial cells secrete prostacyclin (PGI_2) and nitric oxide [NO, otherwise known as *endothelium-derived relaxing factor* (EDRF)]. Both of these compounds are active mediators of vasodilatation and potent inhibitors of platelet adhesion and aggregation. Endothelial cells also contribute to anticoagulant properties of the intact vessel through the synthesis of thrombomodulin and protein S, both of which activate protein C, a substance synthesized in the liver that suppresses the actions of factor V and VIII of the coagulation cascade. Heparan sulfate, a component of intact endothelial cell membranes, accelerates the inactivation of thrombin and other coagulation factors by plasma antithrombin III. Furthermore, endothelial cells are involved in thrombolysis through the secretion of tissue plasminogen activators.

The vascular endothelium also operates as a critical modulator of vascular tone. EDRFs are synthesized and released in response to a host of exogenous vasoactive substances and to physiologically important neurohumoral mediators. These endothelial dependent vasodilators include platelet-derived products such as adenosine diphosphate (ADP), adenosine triphosphate (ATP), thrombin, and serotonin, as well as local mediators of inflammation, including bradykinin and arachidonic acid derivatives such as prostacyclin (PGI_2). L-arginine serves as a precursor to NO, by action of NO synthase, an endothelial enzyme which can be either constitutive or inducible.

Regulation of vascular tone is not limited to the endothelium. Local mediators, such as adenosine, that control vascular smooth muscle tone independent of the endothelium also play an important role. The inherent differences among vessels and their varying levels of EDRF and responses to endothelial dependant relaxation suggest a highly intricate system in which conduit arteries and resistance arterioles of different organs react to maintain vascular homeostasis and optimal cardiovascular efficiency.

Endothelial dysfunction can either cause or result from hypertension. Atherosclerosis clearly changes the way endothelial cells respond to various stimuli, sometimes causing paradoxical vasoconstriction under conditions that would ordinarily cause vasodilatation. Endothelial injury may occur during surgical procedures in which clamps are placed outside the lumen of the vessel or catheters are placed inside the vessel. Intimal injury can occur during vessel harvest by overdistension of saphenous vein conduit with crystalloid solution. Endothelial dysfunction can also occur in reperfusion of ischemic vascular beds, sometimes with paradoxical responses. In particular, free radicals may inactivate EDRF, allowing counterbalancing vasoconstrictive forces to prevail. Endothelial cell swelling consequent to theischemia/reperfusion (I/R) response can result in a "no-reflow" phenomenon.

The arterial endothelium is an immunologically active surface, tethering and communicating with circulating inflammatory cell in the bloodstream, leading to diapedesis of leukocytes to extravascular sites of tissue injury. Acquired vascular injury and systemic disease states (hyperlipidemia, diabetes, chronic tobacco abuse) have been found to increase endothelial–leukocyte interaction and lead to deleterious inflammation. Chronic inflammation from systemic risk factors can lead to arterial occlusive disease secondary to atherosclerosis, while inflammation after revascularization can produce intimal hyperplasia. Metabolic syndrome, a constellation of type 2 diabetes, central obesity, dyslipidemia, and hypertension is associated with elevated levels of soluble E-selectin, intercellular adhesion molecule 1 (ICAM-1) and vascular cell adhesion molecule 1 (VCAM-1). The presence of these circulating factors is a strong indicator for endothelial activation and subsequent development of arterial occlusive disease secondary to atherosclerosis.

Atherosclerosis

The etiology of atherosclerosis is complex, incompletely understood, and the subject of an enormous amount of research. Basic research centers on the end stage of human atherosclerotic vessels and on the development of atherosclerosis in certain animal models. A great deal of discussion has resulted from large-scale epidemiologic studies. However, no single etiology has been identified. The consensus is that atherosclerosis is the end-stage response of the vessel wall to injury, which includes such diverse insults as physical injury (balloon catheter denuding of endothelium), ischemia, toxins (tobacco and cholesterol), biologic injury (viruses), mechanical stress (hypertension), and immunologic attack (rejection). Four cell types are involved in the response of the vessel wall to injury, including endothelial cells, monocytes, platelets, and smooth muscle cells. Each can release both growth factors and chemoattractants, and induction of endothelial cell adhesion molecule expression exacerbates these inflammatory processes. It seems that one of the earliest events in response to endothelial injury is the tethering of monocytes to the endothelium, and subendothelial deposition. Furthermore, platelets may adhere even to minimally injured endothelial cells. These two cell populations may then stimulate intimal proliferative lesions and, subsequently, smooth muscle proliferation.

The histologic progression of atherosclerosis begins with intimal thickening. Intimal thickening may reflect an adaptive response of the vessel to increased tension on the vessel wall caused by turbulence and alteration in endothelial shear stress. Intimal thickenings have been observed in children and even in infants at or near branch points of vessels and may represent local remodeling of the vessel wall related to growth and the associated redistribution of the tensile stresses. Lipid accumulation is not a prominent feature in this type of intimal thickening, and the lumen generally remains regular and normal in caliber. Intimal thickening is not a clear precursor of lipid-containing atherosclerotic plaques, but both processes do occur in similar locations, and intimal thickening is evident in vessels that are especially susceptible to atherosclerosis.

Fatty streaks are the focal patches of fat infiltrating the intima of vessels. They consist of lipid-laden foam cells, which are probably transformed resident macrophages. Fatty streaks are found with increasing frequency from childhood up into the early adult years. Some seem to resolve at that point, but others may progress to worsening atherosclerotic plaques. There may be a predisposition of the endothelial cells overlying these plaques to disrupt, which would then allow platelet adhesion; this may be the inciting event in the development of a fibrous plaque.

Fibrous plaques are the next stage in the development of typical atherosclerotic lesions. They occur in the immediate subendothelial region and consist of compact and stratified layers of well-organized smooth muscle cells. They are covered with a fibrous cap. A necrotic core often lies in the deeper regions of the plaque and contains a variety of forms of lipid. The most advanced lesions, especially those associated with aneurysmal dilatation, consist of dense fibrous tissue and prominent calcium deposits. Calcifications are often found in advanced plaques, and they may be extensive.

The most common sites for these atherosclerotic lesions to develop are at arterial bifurcations or areas of fixation where turbulent flow is the highest. More specifically, locations that are typical for these focal lesions include all of the aortic branches at their origins, the aortic bifurcation, the iliac bifurcation, the common femoral artery bifurcation, the superficial femoral artery at the Hunter canal (where it is fixed) and the common carotid bifurcation. The consistent finding of arterial occlusive disease at bifurcations likely reflects the concomitant alterations in blood velocity and endothelial shear stress. This concept was described by Zarins et al. in a carotid bulb model that demonstrated that recirculation of blood leads to oscillations in shear stress, and a net reduction in the mean blood velocity. Decreased endothelial shear stress has subsequently been found to be related to increases in ICAM-1 and E-selectin expression and increased leukocyte and platelet residence time. This increased apposition of activated endothelium and inflammatory cells results in the development of atherosclerotic lesions, especially in those with systemic risk factors.

Basic Hemodynamic Principles

Blood flow in the human circulation can be described in terms of strict hemodynamic principles, which are derived from engineering, mathematics, and physiology disciplines. These principles form the theoretic foundation for the understanding and treatment of vascular disease.

There are three pathologic manifestations of arterial disease: obstruction of the lumen, aneurysmal dilatation, and disruption or dissection of the vessel wall. Arterial obstruction may result from atherosclerosis, thrombi, emboli, fibromuscular dysplasia, trauma, or external compression. The significance of an obstructing lesion depends on where it is situated, the degree of the obstruction, its duration, and the compensatory ability of the body to develop collateral pathways around the lesion. Disruption or dissection of the vessel wall with loss of arterial wall integrity can occur with rupture of an existing aneurysm, hemorrhage into and/or rupture of an atherosclerotic plaque (especially in the aorta), dissection of the arterial wall, or as a result of direct trauma.

The foundation for the understanding of these pathologic events involves some basic principles of hemodynamics. Blood flows through the arterial system in response to differences in total fluid energy. Total fluid energy (E) consists of potential energy and kinetic energy (KE). Potential energy is made up of intravascular pressure (IP) and gravitational potential energy (GPE). Kinetic energy represents the ability of blood to do work on the basis of its motion and is proportional to the density (D) of blood and the square of blood velocity (V).

$$E = IP + GPE + KE$$
$$KE = \frac{1}{2}(DV^2)$$

This concept of the energy of the blood having a pressure component, a kinetic component, and a gravitation component is related to why people hang their legs over the side of the bed when they have ischemic rest pain. They are increasing the energy of the blood in their leg by allowing gravity to help pull the blood down to the most ischemic areas. This concept also explains why patients with marginal blood flow experience pain in their toes after they lie flat in bed.

The Bernoulli principle states that when fluid flows from one point to another, total energy along the stream is constant, provided that flow is steady and no frictional energy losses result. In the circulation, this ideal condition is not present, and a portion of the total fluid energy is lost in moving blood through the arterial circulation as heat. As a vessel gets smaller or a stenosis is present within a vessel, potential energy in the form of pressure converts to kinetic energy in the form of velocity. This phenomenon is seen when one's finger is placed over the end of a garden hose, causing the velocity of the water escaping the end to increase greatly.

Energy losses that occur in flowing blood occur either as viscous losses, resulting from friction between adjacent layers of blood, or as inertial losses, related to changes in velocity or direction of flow. Viscosity describes the resistance to flow that occurs because of the intermolecular attraction between fluid layers. The Poiseuille law describes the viscous energy losses that occur. The law states that the pressure gradient along a tube or vessel is directly proportional to the flow (Q), the length of the vessel (L), and the dynamic fluid viscosity (η) and is inversely proportional to the fourth power of the radius (r). Simplifying this equation to "pressure equals flow times resistance" makes it analogous to the Ohm law, which states that pressure is equal to flow times resistance. The predominant factor influencing hemodynamic resistance (R) is the fourth power of the radius.

$$R = \eta 8L/\pi r^4$$

Although the predominant factor in this equation is indeed the radius, the length of the lesion plays an important role as well. As seen in the previous resistance equation, resistance is directly proportional to the length of the lesion. This principle is one reason why a long thin central line has a great deal of resistance compared to a short stubby large bore IV when a patient is given resuscitative fluids or blood rapidly. It also explains why a long tubular stenosis blood vessel is much more clinically important than a short discrete stenosis.

Occlusive Arterial Disease

The degree of arterial narrowing that is required to produce a reduction in blood pressure or in blood flow is called the *critical arterial stenosis*. The pressure or energy drop associated with the stenosis is inversely proportional to the fourth power of the radius. Therefore, an exponential relation exists between energy loss or pressure drop and the reduction of lumen size. Furthermore, the pressure drop across a stenosis varies with the velocity given the same radius of the stenosis. In other words, as blood velocity increases, a stenosis that was not impeding flow may become important and cause decreased flow as well as a pressure drop. This has an important clinical implication. A patient may have a 50% stenosis of an artery and have no symptoms at rest at the cardiac output (CO) necessary for resting nourishment of the muscle bed distal to the stenosis. If the muscle bed requires increased circulation because of increased metabolic demand (exercise), a huge increase in blood flow occurs because of a decrease in the resistance of the distal runoff bed. The CO and, therefore, the velocity of the blood increase to meet these metabolic demands. A previously marginal stenosis may become critical in the sense that pressure will fall across the stenosis; therefore, flow falls as well. The decrease in flow is linearly related to the increase in pressure gradient. Therefore, as a pressure drop across the stenosis increases, flow is similarly decreased across that stenosis. These are the hemodynamic situations that occur in claudication or stable angina.

Generally, significant changes in pressure and flow begin to occur when the arterial lumen has been reduced by 50% of its diameter as reported by arteriography, which correlates with a 75% reduction of cross-sectional area as may be determined intraoperatively, at autopsy studies, or by high-quality duplex scanning. Remember that a stenosis that is not significant at resting flow rates may become significant when flow rates are increased. This fact forms the basis for physiologic testing in the vascular diagnostic laboratory.

There are several other important hemodynamic principles that should be mentioned. As seen from the Poiseuille law, the radius of a stenosis will have a much greater effect on energy losses than its length. Doubling the length of a stenosis will double the energy losses, but reducing the radius by one half increases the energy loss by a factor of 16. As blood traverses a stenosis, the energy losses that occur with contraction and expansion of the blood as it passes into and out of a stenosis are more significant than the viscous energy losses. These inertial losses of contraction and expansion are independent of the length of the stenosis and are especially prominent at the exit of the stenosis rather than at the entrance. Because energy and, therefore, pressure losses are primarily the result of the entrance and exit effects, separate stenoses of equal diameter are more significant than a single stenosis having the same diameter and a length equal to the sum of the other two. Therefore, multiple subcritical stenoses may have the same effect as a single critical stenosis. On the basis of this, several points can be made about stenoses in series. When two stenoses are of similar diameter, removal of one will provide only a modest increase in blood flow. If the stenoses have different diameters, removal of the least severe will have little effect, whereas removal of the most severe will improve blood flow dramatically. It makes no difference whether the most severe stenosis is proximal or distal to the least severe because the hemodynamic result is not affected by the sequence of stenoses. These principles apply only to unbranched arterial segments like the internal carotid artery. Therefore, a patient with tandem lesions, that is, a severe lesion of the internal carotid artery at the bifurcation and a lesser lesion of the carotid siphon, would be expected to be helped considerably if the proximal cervical carotid lesion were treated with carotid endarterectomy.

When complete arterial obstruction occurs, blood must pass through a network of collateral vessels that bypass the occluded segment. The capacity of the collateral circulation varies according to the level and extent of the occlusive lesion. For example, the collateral flow around an occluded superficial femoral artery through the profunda and into the popliteal can compensate to a large extent for an isolated occlusion of the superficial femoral artery. If, however, an iliac stenosis were added above this, flow would be severely limited through the collateral bed. If the iliac stenosis were removed with direct arterial surgery or transluminal angioplasty, although the iliac stenosis was not as severe as the superficial femoral artery occlusion, perfusion to the lower leg would be improved because of increased flow through the collateral system. The unvarying principles that concern collateral vessels are that they are always smaller, longer, and more numerous than the replaced artery and that the collateral resistance would always be greater than that of the original unobstructed artery. Furthermore, the resistance of a collateral system is relatively fixed and cannot change acutely as in the case of a normal artery in which resistance can change to increase or decrease flow.

Aneurysmal Arterial Disease

An arterial aneurysm is defined as an artery that has reached a size two times its normal diameter. Aneurysms occur when the structural components of the arterial wall are weakened. Rupture of an aneurysm occurs when the tangential stress within the arterial wall exceeds its tensile strength. The Laplace law

$$\sigma = Pr/h$$

[σ = wall stress; P = mean pressure; r = vessel radius; h = wall thickness] states that tangential arterial wall tension increases as the IP and the radius of the vessel increases. The relation between tangential stress and blood pressure accounts for the importance of avoiding hypertension in patients with aneurysms. Also, the direct relation between radius and wall tension explains the observed higher incidence of rupture of aneurysms as their size increases. Increases in wall stress can be temporarily offset by increases in vessel wall thickness, such as hypertrophy.

Venous System

The structure of the venous circulation is considerably different from that of the arterial side of the circulation. Most of these differences are related to the differences in the wall of the vein relative to that of the artery. Furthermore, an important characteristic of many veins is the presence of valves, which are essential for their proper function. The distribution and number of valves correspond to those regions in which the effects of gravity are the greatest. Venous valves have a bicuspid structure with a fine connective tissue skeleton covered by endothelium on both surfaces. Their major function is to ensure antegrade flow of blood and prevent the reflux of blood from proximal to distal veins and from deep to superficial veins.

Because of their structure, veins can undergo large changes in volume with little change in transmural pressure. This enlarged volume with minimal pressure change is called *venous capacitance*. Veins are actually stiffer per unit of cross-sectional area than arteries when compared at the same distending pressure. This is because of the paucity of elastic tissue and the prominent venous adventitia, which consists mostly of collagen. In the venous system, a wide range of flow rates can be found. In an upright person, venous pressure at the level of the foot exceeds 100 mm Hg. Obviously, at this high pressure, fluid is forced out of the capillaries into the tissue. Some of this fluid may be picked up by lymphatics; however, the single most important element in preventing the accumulation of interstitial fluid is the calf muscle pump. The calf muscle pump produces important changes in venous volume flow rate and flow direction. It lowers the venous pressure in the dependent leg, reduces venous volume in the exercising muscle, and increases venous return. As stated, in a completely stationary upright individual, the venous pressure is high; however, with a single step, the venous pressure within the foot becomes very low and requires several seconds to return to the resting level. When a normal individual walks, the venous pressure remains at a low level throughout the period of exercise. The calf muscle pump empties the local venous system during contraction of the muscle. With relaxation, the veins expand and the venous pressure is lowered because of the functioning valves. If the valves are incompetent, venous pressure becomes increased as blood refluxes past the valves.

Two common manifestations of abnormal venous function are varicose veins and postthrombotic syndrome. Varicose veins occur when incompetent valves in the saphenous system permit reflux of blood from proximal to distal. Progressive incompetence occurs at each valve as the vein dilates. As valves in the main deep venous trunks dilate, there is a failure of coaptation of the fibrosed valve leaflets, and varicosities occur as a result of the constant increase in pressure transmitted through the standing column of fluid.

Postthrombotic syndrome results in up to 60% of patients after an episode of acute deep venous thrombosis (DVT), with increased risk for chronic deep vein valvular incompetence after each recurrent bout of DVT. Factors that are responsible for the development of the postthrombotic syndrome relate mainly to the status of the deep veins below the knee and the perforating veins that connect the superficial and deep venous circulation. When valvular incompetence occurs in both of these areas, high pressures that can be generated by activation of the calf-pump mechanism cause increased venous hypertension, not only at rest but also during ambulation. This constant venous hypertension may cause transudation of fibrinogen and coagulation factors into the subcutaneous tissue, which produces a significant barrier to the diffusion of oxygen and nutrients to the skin. This resultant brawny discoloration and occasional skin ulceration is known as *venous stasis disease*.

The clinician should recognize the two different clinical syndromes associated with the two main types of venous disease: obstructive venous disease and the venous problems associated with valvular incompetence. Although it would seem that obstructive venous problems would be a more morbid condition, the reverse is actually true. When no direct communication exists between the large and heavy column of blood from the inferior vena cava (IVC) all the way down to the foot, the leg will actually accommodate enlarging alternate routes of outflow. Sudden occlusion of an outflow vein is a fairly morbid event, but the gradual occlusion of these types of veins is not nearly as morbid as was once thought. For example, people tolerated ligation of the vena cava fairly well when it was done for chronic pulmonary embolism. Patients tolerate the removal of the superficial femoral vein for use as a conduit elsewhere with minimal subsequent swelling in the leg. In stark contrast to the relatively mild long-term morbidity of this type of venous problem is the situation in which there are patent veins but no functioning valves between the heart and the ankle. Patients with this anatomic situation generally have morbid venous disease with tensely swollen legs and frequent bouts of venous ulceration on the medial side of their calves and ankles. These patients usually have had prior DVT, which has subsequently recanalized with destruction of the valves. These patients will present with noninvasive studies that show no obstructive lesions but obvious venous disease. Patients with chronic venous insufficiency have to be motivated, with vigilant protection from skin trauma, and treatment of the associated chronic lower extremity pruritis.

The most severe consequence of venous disease is the unhealthy edema associated with it, particularly focal edema. Focal edema occurs in legs in which incompetent perforators allow the direct pressure of the deep venous system to be transmitted to a superficial site. This can cause ulcerations, particularly on the medial side of the leg known as *venous stasis ulcers*. These ulcers can apparently form spontaneously, but they may also be the result of trivial trauma that would heal in any other area but cannot heal in the environment of venous hypertension.

Preventative therapy for chronic venous insufficiency includes the use of elastic support stockings to provide external compression and minimize the amount of edema that occurs during ambulation. Elevation of the legs also helps relieve the symptoms of chronic venous insufficiency by three mechanisms. First, elevation reduces venous pressure by decreasing the effects of gravity. Second, resorption of edema fluid is promoted secondary to decreased hydrostatic pressure. Third, the calf muscle pump will not activate when the limb has been elevated, thereby eliminating ambulatory venous hypertension.

BASIC CARDIAC ANATOMY

This section on cardiac anatomy assumes that the reader has been acquainted with basic cardiac anatomy. The cardiac conduction system, the coronary arteries, and the cardiac valves will be covered in detail in other sections of this chapter.

Endocardium

Although the endocardium seems like a superfluous structure, it is of great importance to the general surgeon. The endocardium serves as a barrier to infectious agents and has proved important in the structural prevention of endocarditis. The endocardium lines all of the cardiac chambers and the cardiac valves. It is continuous with the lining of all vessels within or connecting to the heart. Human beings can tolerate recurrent bacteremias as often as twice a day and not develop bacterial endocarditis. Animal studies have shown that remarkably high doses of intravascular bacteria are well tolerated. However, if the integrity of the endocardium becomes disturbed, the risk of bacterial endocarditis with bacteremia is increased more than 1,000-fold.

Disruption of the endocardium may occur from natural causes, acquired conditions, or from congenital cardiac abnormalities. Deformed cardiac valves will cause repeated abrasion of the valvular endothelium. Extremely narrowed valves or regurgitant valves may also lead to jets aimed at endocardium; such jets have been associated with erosion of the protective lining. Congenital cardiac conditions causing high velocity flow and turbulence, or the jetting of blood, will likewise cause disruption of endocardium.

Iatrogenic interventions that increase the risk of bacterial endocarditis include cardiac catheterization, or the insertion of central venous lines and pulmonary artery (PA) catheters. This phenomenon also explains the markedly increased risk of developing bacterial endocarditis in the early period after cardiac surgery. Endocardial injury should be minimized, and when the patient is at risk, prophylaxis for bacterial endocarditis may be necessary.

Epicardium

The epicardium, or visceral pericardium, covers the entire normal heart. When cardiac injuries require closure, the epicardium holds sutures considerably better than does myocardium. It is now recognized that the visceral epicardium can become involved in the fibrotic process as a consequence of constrictive pericarditis, mandating that the diseased areas of constricting visceral epicardium must be removed at the same time of pericardiectomy, in order to relieve the constrictive/restrictive physiology. Often, that will require intraoperative hemodynamic support on cardiopulmonary bypass (CPB).

Pericardium

The pericardium is not an inert mass of connective tissue. Scanning electron microscopy shows it to be a highly organized tissue with microvilli and cilia for the production and absorption of fluid and the facilitation of movement across the serosal surfaces. The normal amount of pericardial fluid in an adult is approximately 50 mL.

The pericardium may play an important role as a barrier to inflammation from adjacent structures, particularly the lung. Although complete pericardiectomy will not interfere with cardiac function, partial removal of the pericardium in certain locations can leave a situation in which the heart can be subjected to life-threatening herniation. Herniation can be a particular problem after intrapericardial pneumonectomy.

The knowledge of certain features of pericardial anatomy plays an important role in interpreting echocardiograms, preventing complications, and improving the efficiency of emergency open chest resuscitation. Understanding this anatomy also offers alternative routes for exposure in operations around the trachea and great vessels.

Because of the pericardial sac attachment to the diaphragm, attempts at open massage of the ventricles during resuscitation generally will be ineffective unless the pericardium is entered and the hand is placed around the heart within the pericardial sac. Failure to open the pericardium is a common error in emergency resuscitation. In addition, knowledge of the course of the left phrenic nerve along the posterior lateral margin of the pericardium is important because this must be preserved during emergency pericardiotomy. Knowing that the nerve runs in a vertical manner generally means that a vertical incision anterior to the area of the nerve will protect this structure.

Occasionally, traumatic injuries to the PA or pulmonary veins and to the aorta will require emergency opening of the pericardium to obtain control. Knowing that the left and right pulmonary arteries have short courses within the pericardium is helpful. In addition, it is helpful to know that the pulmonary veins have a short free passage within the pericardial space before exiting. These areas can be exposed for control of these structures.

Pericarditis often presents with a characteristic sharp substernal chest pain, a pericardial friction rub, and electrocardiographic changes with widespread ST-segment elevation involving all three standard limb leads and most of the precordial leads. Reciprocal depression is usually found in leads atrioventricular (AV_R) and V_1. Pericarditis without effusion does not directly affect cardiac function. When an effusion does develop, the occurrence of tamponade depends not only on the volume of pericardial fluid but also on its rate of formation. If the effusion has formed slowly, the pericardium may have stretched, and the effect on the heart would be less. When tamponade is present, a paradoxical pulse may develop. This term is actually a misnomer because the pulse amplitude of a normal individual will diminish slightly on inspiration. Therefore, a better term would be an *exaggerated pulse* instead of a *paradoxical pulse*. The normal influence of inspiration on cardiac filling is that the negative intrathoracic pressure draws more blood into the right ventricle, whereas the left ventricle transiently receives less blood because blood stays in the lungs; therefore the left heart ejects less blood. When cardiac tamponade occurs, this normal slight decrease in pressure with inspiration becomes exaggerated. A decline in systolic blood pressure of 15 mm Hg or more with each inspiration is thought to be definite evidence of a pathologic "paradoxical" pulse. Advanced cardiac tamponade produces the Beck triad, which consists of hypotension, distended neck veins, and muffled heart sounds. Clinically, pericardial tamponade is said to exist when a cluster of examination findings exist such as tachycardia, elevated central venous pressure (CVP), diminished pulse pressure, and paradoxical pulse. Confusion not only exists over the definition of a paradoxical pulse, but there are also questions about the usefulness of the term.

Measuring this physical finding accurately is difficult because it requires a quiet room, a cooperative patient, excellent blood pressure taking skills, and a spontaneously breathing patient. Most frustrating, the finding is inconsistent in trauma. The finding of distended neck veins may be absent in the setting of hypovolemia. Positive pressure breathing with high expiratory pressures may cause pulsus paradoxicus, such as in asthma, chronic obstructive pulmonary disease (COPD) with bronchospasm, and in ventilator-assisted patients who demonstrate "auto-PEEP". Therefore, trying to determine whether a paradoxical pulse is present to help make the diagnosis of tamponade is more useful in the chronic setting, such as pericardial effusions which may be seen in uremia or postpericardiotomy syndrome. Similarly, looking for an enlarged heart shadow on a chest radiograph is an unreliable finding; because the pericardium is stiff and inelastic, it may not be enlarged significantly in acute tamponade. The most reliable clinical findings of tamponade will be a relative decrease in CO and blood pressure in the setting of increased venous pressure. Echocardiography has been shown to be the simplest diagnostic test beyond these clinical findings to document a pericardial effusion.

Studies of the influence of tamponade on the heart show that the left ventricle itself is markedly resistant to a reduction in its stroke volume (SV) by direct compression. Most of the effects produced by tamponade actually are associated with impairment of filling of the left and right atria and the right ventricle. Therefore, the overall effect of compression of the other chambers causes impairment of the filling of the left ventricle and subsequent decreased SV and systolic blood pressure. Because the normal SV has been diminished, a compensatory tachycardia then develops. This tachycardia is often insufficient to maintain CO, and a compensatory increase in systemic vascular resistance (SVR) results. The rise in systemic resistance maintains systemic blood pressure at the expense of CO, cardiac oxygen consumption, cardiac work, and tissue perfusion. When intrapericardial pressure continues to rise, systemic vasoconstriction occurs, and CO diminishes until a shock state exists.

As pericardial fluid volume increases, there is little change in pericardial pressure until a point at which the tension in the pericardium reaches near maximum. At this point, a small increase in pericardial volume produces a rapid increase in pressure. Specifically, the slope of the curve becomes steeper as intrapericardial pressure approaches 14 to 15 mm Hg. This phenomenon also explains why, in the emergency treatment of tamponade, the removal of a small amount of fluid may dramatically increase the blood pressure and CO. Removal of as small a volume as 25 mL can allow enough filling of the heart to significantly increase the output. For instance, if the heart is beating 100 times per minute and pumps 10 mL more per stroke, the CO would be improved by 1 L. This small improvement in CO under these dire circumstances

can often mean the difference between the patient surviving until definitive treatment can be rendered and the patient dying of cardiac tamponade.

Because the deleterious effect of tamponade predominantly affects right ventricular filling, giving additional intravascular fluids may cause a temporary improvement. Increased preload for the right ventricle increases the volume filling the right ventricle. This increase improves pulmonary venous return. As the left ventricle filling pressure increases, SV increases, as does systolic pressure.

The fact that a state of tamponade produces systemic vasoconstriction to maintain systemic blood pressure also helps explain the increased potential dangers to a patient in tamponade who undergoes general anesthesia. Peripheral vasodilatation is a common side effect of most anesthetic agents and, under these circumstances, causes a rapid loss of blood pressure. This phenomenon explains the wisdom of prepping a patient's chest before the introduction of general anesthesia if a cardiac tamponade has been suspected. This maneuver then permits the rapid decompression of the pericardial space if needed. Pericardial drainage through a subxyphoid approach under local anesthesia should be strongly considered in patients with tamponade physiology when temporizing measures such as echo-guided pericardiocentesis have failed or are contraindicated. The rapid development of tamponade physiology in the setting of sepsis is a hallmark of purulent pericarditis.

THE CORONARY CIRCULATION

Microcirculation

The coronary perfusion pressure (CPP) is the pressure that drives blood across the coronary microcirculation. Another approximation of this driving force can be determined by subtracting the CVP from the diastolic blood pressure. This is the gradient across which most of the coronary circulation's blood flow is driven. Therefore, as the diastolic blood pressure falls and the CVP (the pressure seen by the coronary sinus) rises, the flow across the coronary microcirculatory bed will lessen. When this driving force is under 25 mm Hg, the patient will usually not survive long unless some intervention is rendered to reverse this situation and to improve the CPP.

The coronary microcirculation is representative of most vascular beds in the body serving muscular tissues. Blood flow through these beds is controlled by a variety of factors. Under conditions of increased oxygen demand or decreased oxygen supply, adenosine is released from most tissues. Adenosine is the nucleoside that results from the breakdown of the high-energy phosphate compounds ATP, ADP, and AMP. It is one of the most potent vasodilators known. Therefore, as adenosine is released into the interstitial fluid, the contiguous arterioles are dilated, resulting in increased flow to the area and, therefore, increased oxygen delivery. Other factors may play a role in the vasodilatation associated with ischemia, including the concentration of oxygen, potassium, prostacyclin, and endothelium-derived relaxing factor. There

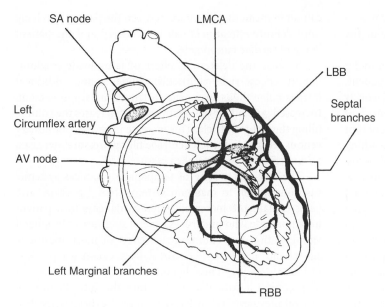

FIGURE 15.1 The left coronary artery distribution and branches along with the main conduction pathways. SA, sinoatrial; LMCA, left main coronary artery; LBB, left bundle bunch; AV, atrioventricular; RBB, right bundle bunch.

is growing evidence that under conditions of profound and prolonged ischemia, these autoregulatory mechanisms are no longer functional, resulting in irreversible vasoconstriction.

In addition to the metabolic factors noted earlier, a number of other agents influence coronary blood flow, including physical and neural factors. The majority (~65%) of coronary blood flow in the left main coronary artery occurs during diastole. In the right coronary artery, coronary blood flow is more evenly distributed between systole and diastole. At higher heart rates (HRs), a lesser percentage of the cardiac cycle occurs during diastole. Therefore, when diastole is shortened by factors such as increased HR, nutrient blood flow diminishes. If the end diastolic pressure (EDP) in the left ventricle is high (as in left ventricular hypertrophy or aortic valve insufficiency) flow through the coronary bed will be less, especially in the subendocardial area. Likewise, if the afterload facing the heart is great [as in severe hypertension or aortic stenosis (AS)], the subendocardium will be deprived of blood flow even further during systole. If the diastolic blood pressure is low and the CVP is high, the CPP can be reduced and coronary blood flow will fall. When sympathetic nerves supplying a nonworking, perfused heart are stimulated, vasoconstriction occurs. However, when sympathetic stimuli exist, the heart works harder and coronary blood flow increases. These changes are influenced primarily by metabolic factors. Cholinergic innervation of the coronary vasculature does not exist. Therefore, it is believed that the sympathetic nervous system does not play an important role in regulating coronary artery blood flow.

Coronary Arteries and Coronary Arterial Disease

The left main and right main coronary arteries provide the primary blood supply to the heart (Figs. 15.1 and 15.2). Normal coronary anatomy consists of three primary coronary arteries supplying the left ventricle. The left anterior descending (LAD) artery supplies the anterior wall and

anterior septum, the circumflex artery supplies the lateral wall, and the right coronary artery supplies the posterior wall and posterior septum. The coronary system is considered right dominant if the right coronary artery supplies the posterior septum. Right coronary dominance is present in approximately 85% to 95% of individuals; patients with bicuspid aortic valve have left coronary dominance approximately 50% of the time.

The most significant pathologic factor involving coronary arteries is atherosclerosis. Atherosclerosis is a process that is thought to occur in response to chronic vessel injury. The injury response includes endothelial dysfunction, infiltration of the vessel wall with blood-borne elements, vascular smooth

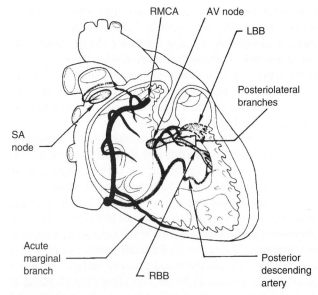

FIGURE 15.2 The right coronary artery distribution and branches along with the main conduction pathways. RMCA, right main coronary artery; AV, atrioventricular; LBB, left bundle bunch; SA, sinoatrial; RBB, right bundle bunch.

muscle cell proliferation, and the accumulation of lipid, resulting in plaque formation. Alterations in endothelial cell function or increased permeability to macromolecules caused by non-denuding vessel injury are thought to be integral to the atherosclerotic process. Eventual calcification is the end result. Although the processes can be slow, occlusion of vessels can occur acutely, particularly if hemorrhage into a plaque occurs. If an acute occlusion of a coronary vessel occurs, then myocardial cells begin to die after 20 minutes of ischemia. After 60 minutes of occlusion, severe myocardial necrosis can exist, but this degree of necrosis has not been a predictable finding. Much depends on the presence of collaterals around the area of stenosis or occlusion. If the stenosis has occurred gradually, then even an acute occlusion may not cause myocardial damage. However, if only a mild stenosis occurs, followed by an acute occlusion secondary to hemorrhage into a plaque, and collaterals have not developed, then extensive myocardial damage often results. The presence or absence of collaterals explains why the results of thrombolytic therapy can be uncertain. If a patient has much in the way of collaterals, then there will often be no significant myocardial damage after clot lysis. However, if there are minimal collaterals, then major damage can occur despite early thrombolytic therapy.

In most patients who develop coronary stenosis, the process develops slowly. These patients usually report stable angina, that is, angina at predictable workloads. The capacity to increase coronary flow with increasing demand is limited; therefore, symptoms develop only during exercise. These patients can frequently be treated medically with β blockers and coronary dilators such as nitroglycerin. Unstable angina, on the other hand, represents a primary decrease in supply in the setting of normal oxygen demand. This is manifest clinically as new-onset angina, crescendo effort angina (increasing angina at diminishing levels of exercise), or rest angina. Rest angina includes stuttering, preinfarction angina. This situation occurs in the setting of plaque instability, usually of nonflow–limiting plaque (<50% diameter reduction); acute or subacute plaque fissuring, platelet clumping, and fibrin scaffold formation develops and resting coronary blood flow is lowered. Coronary arteriography or computed tomographic angiography (CTA) or magnetic resonance angiography (MRA) can delineate areas of acute plaque instability and helps define appropriate therapy, either percutaneous coronary intervention (PCI) or surgical revascularization coronary artery bypass grafting (CABG).

PCI involves balloon dilatation followed almost routinely by the deployment of intracoronary metallic stents. Balloon dilatation causes a controlled dissection of the plaque with expansion and intramural compaction of the residual plaque; it also disrupts the internal elastic lamina, exposing the media to the circulating blood. The "Achilles' heel" of standard balloon angioplasty was elastic recoil, acute thrombosis, and restenosis. Restenosis is caused by migration of myofibroblasts from the media through the disrupted internal elastic lamina, and proliferation of collagen into

plaque, the so-called "fibrous cap." PCI with stents helped solve the problem with elastic recoil, and intensive short-term antiplatelet and antithrombic therapy helped solve the problem with acute thrombosis. Stents are classified as bare metal stents (BMSs) or drug-eluting stents (DESs). A DES typically employs a polymer-based scaffold onto which an antiproliferative drug such as taxol or rapamycin have been secured. Restenosis remains the "Achilles' heel" of BMS, due to in-stent restenosis, which occurs in approximately 34% of patients. DES helped solve the problem of in-stent restenosis, but has not solved the problem of edge stenosis ("candy-wrapper" lesions) and has not been observed to contribute meaningful differences in outcomes when compared to BMS. Also, because DES elute drugs not only inhibit medial myofibroblasts, but also normal coronary endothelial function, patients with DES must have intensive antithrombotic therapy until the time of re-endothelialization of the DES, which requires 6 to 12 months. Interruption of antiplatelet therapy in that time frame risks acute coronary thrombosis, a high percentage of which are fatal. PCI is indicated in patients with either one- or two-vessel or selected three-vessel coronary disease and discrete stenoses. PCI of the left main coronary artery is suitable only for patients who are categorically deemed inoperable. CABG surgery is reserved for patients with symptoms despite maximized medical therapy or when PCI has failed or is contraindicated. Most often, CABG is reserved for patients with severe multivessel coronary arterial disease (CAD), CAD involving the proximal (before the first septal or diagonal branch) left anterior coronary descending (LAD) coronary artery, multivessel disease with severely depressed left ventricular dysfunction, diabetic patients, left main disease, complications of acute myocardial infarction [such as ventricular septal defect (VSD) or acute mitral insufficiency] or concomitant valvular or aortic disease.

Although the techniques of bypass surgery are not germane here, it is important to understand the difference between the various conduits used for CABG. Vein graft options include the greater and lesser saphenous veins. Arterial options include the right and left internal mammary (thoracic) and radial arteries. Vein bypasses provide effective bypass of coronary lesions with a greater than 90% early patency rate. However, vein bypasses may develop a thickened intima with atherosclerotic changes such that vein graft patency rates approximate 50% at 10 to 12 years' follow-up. Although the internal mammary artery (IMA) has a smaller caliber than a vein, it does provide sufficient blood flow, tends to stay free of atherosclerotic occlusion, and has a 10-year patency rate of approximately 95%.

The IMA does have certain features that may contribute to its long-term patency. The blood supply (vasovasorum) of the IMA is confined to the adventitia and does not penetrate the media. The media is nourished entirely from the lumen. Autopsy studies and intravascular ultrasonography (IVUS) show that diseased coronary arteries have intimal thickening, which increases in severity with age. The internal mammary arteries appear to be spared from these changes. Harvested human saphenous veins, which have been subjected to luminal overdistension have shown incomplete endothelial cell coverage in contrast to the internal mammary arteries, which are completely covered. Finally, the internal mammary has a thin-walled media with well-differentiated smooth muscle cells compared with the LAD coronary artery, which exhibits multiple defects in the internal elastic laminae and a thickened intimal layer. Taken together, these studies suggest that important histologic differences exist between the IMA and the coronaries and that these differences may play a role in the IMA's resistance to atherosclerosis. Patients with single left IMA grafts to the LAD have an increased survival when compared to comparable patients with only vein grafts; patients with bilateral IMA grafts have increased graft patency and reoperation-free survival compared to single IMA graft patients.

Small myocardial infarctions have a low mortality. Large myocardial infarctions from occlusion of a large epicardial coronary artery will often cause extensive myocardial damage leading to remodeling, wall thinning, chamber dilation and left ventricular aneurysm formation. Left ventricular (LV) aneurysms expand during systole, removing a portion of the normal SV from left ventricular ejection, leading to congestive heart failure (CHF). Perianeurysmal infarction scar causes unequal myocardial refractory periods, leading to refractory ventricular arrhythmias, the second complication of aneurysm. Mural thrombus within the aneurysm leads to thromboembolism and stroke, a third complication of LV aneurysm. Any complication of LV aneurysm is an indication for surgical repair. Rupture of a true LV aneurysm is extremely uncommon, unlike rupture of an LV pseudoaneurysm, which is much more common; because of that fact, the mere presence of a pseudoaneurysm is sufficient to justify surgical treatment. Massive myocardial infarction can also cause cardiogenic shock if more than 40% of the left ventricle has been lost. Septal myocardial infarctions can cause VSD. This is often associated with a large left-to-right shunt, right-sided overload, pulmonary edema, and often death. Therapy in this case consists of multivessel CABG and closing the defect. Finally, infarction can be associated with rupture of a papillary muscle that supports the mitral valve apparatus. This causes severe mitral regurgitation and heart failure. Therapy requires valve repair or replacement.

Ischemia and Reperfusion Injury

Myocardial dysfunction caused by brief episodes of acute normothermic ischemia (0–20 minutes) is completely reversible with restoration of coronary flow. Prolonged ischemia (6–18 hours) will ultimately progress to irreversible cellular death, even if coronary flow is restored. Chronic, (days to years) sublethal myocardial ischemia can cause dysfunction that is reversed by revascularization; this is referred to as *hibernating myocardium*. However, reperfusion of viable, but prolonged (20 minutes–6 hours), acutely ischemic tissue can exacerbate cellular injury by inducing a complex cascade of pathophysiologic, biochemical, and morphologic changes, leading to prolonged but ultimately reversible myocardial dysfunction referred to as *stunned myocardium*. In fact, reperfusion injury is often far more severe than damage incurred during the ischemic period itself. Reperfusion injury is characterized by cellular edema, intracellular Ca^{2+} overload with subsequent activation of Ca^{2+}-dependent autolytic enzymes, disruption of lipid membranes, and perturbations in mitochondrial structure and function. Restoration of myocardial dysfunction from I/R injury, or stunning, requires many hours to days, to repair oxidized cell membranes, regenerate contractile proteins and high energy phosphate compounds (ATP), and relieve intracellular edema.

Mediators of Reperfusion Injury

Oxygen-Free Radicals

The discovery of the detrimental effects of reintroduction of O_2 to previously ischemic tissues led to the suspicion that highly reactive, unstable oxygen metabolites are important mediators of reperfusion injury. These so-called oxygen-free radicals, which contain one or more unpaired electrons, are derived from molecular O_2 and include the superoxide anion (O_2^-), hydrogen peroxide (H_2O_2), and the extremely potent hydroxyl radical ($\cdot OH$). The rapid generation of these toxic moieties at the onset of reperfusion initiates a series of biochemical processes that causes widespread damage to cellular macromolecules. These pathologic processes include peroxidation of lipid membranes, protein degradation, nucleic acid damage, hemoprotein/cytochrome inactivation, and neutralization of NO. The most damaging effect of oxygen-free radicals is lipid peroxidation, which impairs the normal fluidity and permeability of cell membranes, leading to cellular edema, massive Ca^{2+} and Na^+ overload, and cell lysis.

The sources of reactive oxygen metabolites during reperfusion are multiple. Xanthine oxidase, an enzyme that is activated in ischemic endothelial and parenchymal cells and that uses O_2 and hypoxanthine as substrates, is responsible for most of the superoxide production. Polymorphonuclear cells (PMNs) are also a prolific free radical source, whereas catecholamine oxidation and prostaglandin metabolism are less important mechanisms of reperfusion-associated free radical production. Oxygen-free radical scavengers and antioxidants have been shown both experimentally and clinically to ameliorate reperfusion injury by preventing the production of free radicals or by blocking their pathologic effects after they have been synthesized. Controlled reperfusion with low partial pressure of oxygen (FIO_2 = room air) has been utilized to ameliorate reperfusion pulmonary edema in lung transplantation.

Polymorphonuclear Cells

PMNs are also important mediators of reperfusion injury, but they rely on the priming of reperfused tissues by oxygen-free radicals for their activation and accumulation. For example, free radicals react with endothelial cells to elicit platelet-activating factor (PAF), leukotriene B_4 (LTB_4), and complement 5A (c5A), all of which are chemotactic to neutrophils. In addition, reactive oxygen metabolites induce the expression of the CD11/CD18 complex on the PMN cell surface, the expression of which is a prerequisite to the adherence of PMNs to the microvasculature and their subsequent accumulation in postischemic tissues.

Activated PMNs inflict damage to reperfused endothelial and parenchymal cells in a variety of ways. PMNs release a host of destructive proteolytic enzymes, including elastase, collagenase, gelatinase, lysozyme, and cathepsin G. In addition, as previously mentioned, PMNs are a rich source of oxygen-free radicals by virtue of a superoxide-generating nicotinamide adenine dinucleotide (NAD) oxidase. Finally, activated PMNs produce substantial quantities of hypochlorous acid, a biologically toxic molecule formed by the activity of myeloperoxidase.

The Endothelium in Ischemia and Reperfusion

Our appreciation of the integral role of the endothelium in reperfusion injury continues to evolve. The complexity of the biologic responses mounted by this cell layer is staggering; and it is no longer considered a passive sheet of cells lining the vasculature, but is treated as an organ itself. A host of mediators formed during reperfusion induces endothelial cells to express ICAM-1 and ICAM-2 and endothelial leukocyte adhesion molecule (ELAM). These molecules bind the CD11/CD18 complex on activated neutrophils, thereby facilitating PMN adherence to and migration across the endothelium. In this way, PMNs are able to gain access to the subendothelial parenchymal cells, where they release their destructive enzymes and bioreactive molecules. Endothelial cells also secrete an abundance of soluble factors during reperfusion, including platelet adhesion factors, leukotriene B_4, thromboxane A_2, and endothelin, the latter of which is the most potent vasoconstrictor known. In combination with decreased endothelial secretion of prostacyclin and the inactivation of the endothelial derived vasodilator NO by superoxide, the net deleterious effects of these endothelial factors are vasoconstriction, platelet aggregation, PMN plugging of capillaries, and increased microvascular permeability. The end result is that perfusion of the microcirculation is severely compromised, which manifests as the classic "no-reflow" phenomenon of reperfusion injury. Therefore, limiting ischemic time, preparing and recognizing signs of reperfusion injury and timely supportive treatment remains the cornerstone of management.

CARDIAC VALVULAR DISEASE

There are four cardiac valves in a normal human heart. The semilunar valves (aortic, pulmonic) have a simple passive function: permit the unimpeded, unidirectional flow of blood and prevent regurgitation. The atrioventricular (AV) valves (mitral, tricuspid) have a subvalvar apparatus consisting of papillary muscles and chordae tendinae which participate actively in ventricular ejection (into the aorta and pulmonary artery, respectively) as well as prevent regurgitation into the atria. Cardiac valvular disease can be categorized as congenital or acquired lesions, which disrupt the flow of blood leading to a pressure or volume overloaded state. Cardiac valve prostheses can be classified as mechanical or biological. All U.S Food and Drug Administration (FDA)-approved mechanical valves are constructed of pyrolytic carbon leaflets or solitary discs within a metallic housing and cloth-covered sewing ring. Biologic valves are derived from porcine aortic valves, bovine pericardium, cyropreserved cadaveric human valves, or transplanted autogenous valves (such as the Ross procedure, where the native pulmonic valve is translocated into the aortic position). All mechanical valves mandate antithrombotic treatment with warfarin as a matter of routine; biologic valves routinely do not require such long-term prophylactic treatment. Mechanical valves, properly cared for, have limitless durability, whereas biological valves have a finite survival.

Aortic Stenosis

Most cases of AS are caused by calcification of congenital deformities of the aortic valve, most commonly a bicuspid valve. Other causes include senile calcification or rheumatic valvulitis. AS obstructs outflow from the left ventricle, causing left-ventricular hypertrophy and decreasing left ventricular compliance. The obstruction causes significant left ventricular hypertension while maintaining a normal aortic blood pressure. Diastolic CPP is normal while the intramural tension increases markedly. This decreases coronary blood flow and oxygen supply to the left ventricular myocardium, where the oxygen demand is greatly increased because of increased work. Patients with significant AS are at risk of sudden death. The typical history of AS is a patient with a known cardiac murmur for at least 20 years and the onset of symptoms at the age of 50 or 55. Three classic presenting symptoms of AS include chest pain, syncope, and heart failure. Syncope was formerly thought to result from potentially lethal, self-terminating arrhythmias [ventricular tachycardia (VT) or ventricular fibrillation (VF)], leading to a decreased CO and decreased cerebral blood flow. This is more likely the cause of sudden cardiac death in AS. Syncope is due to an abnormal baroreceptor reflex, where left ventricular intracavitary hypertension leads to a paradoxical decrease in SVR, resulting in transient cerebral hypoperfusion. Chest pain results from subendocardial myocardial ischemia; one third of patients with AS and angina also have significant CAD. CHF is initially the result of diminished left ventricular compliance and diastolic dysfunction; with the onset of afterload mismatch, left ventricular systolic function ultimately fails and the left ventricle dilates. With the onset of any one of the three major symptoms, a patient with AS has a 50% probability of dying within 2 years, and 33% of these patients will have sudden death without the progression of symptoms. An increased risk of death also exists when undergoing noncardiac surgery. AS is suspected from hearing a harsh systolic flow murmur over the precordium and is diagnosed noninvasively with 2-D echocardiography. Hemodynamic assessment of AS and the status of the coronary arteries can be accomplished at cardiac catheterization. Cardiac catheterization is a prerequisite for aortic valve replacement surgery because of the risk of diseased coronary arteries remaining unrevascularized.

When patients with unrelieved AS must undergo noncardiac surgery, every attempt must be made to avoid peripheral hypotension, because this leads to further cardiac ischemia. Therefore, patients with suspected AS should not be treated with vasodilators, especially nitroglycerin. Aortic valve replacement should be reserved for symptomatic patients with significant AS; the only acceptable situation where asymptomatic patients with significant AS should undergo valve replacement are those who are undergoing CABG surgery, as the rate of stenosis progression rises following CABG surgery.

Mitral Stenosis

Approximately 99% of all cases of mitral stenosis result from rheumatic fever and valvulitis. The consequences of a narrowed mitral valve are left atrial hypertension, pulmonary venous hypertension, PA hypertension, and an increased pressure load on the right ventricle. In general, the left ventricle remains normal unless previously injured by rheumatic fever or compromised by coronary artery disease.

Patients with mitral stenosis are at risk of developing atrial fibrillation and peripheral emboli. They are sensitive to volume overload, and the infusion of large amounts of colloid may lead rapidly to pulmonary edema. Anything that increases the pulmonary hypertension of these patients may also lead to tricuspid regurgitation and right heart failure.

The natural history of mitral stenosis is protracted. Frequently, the patient will give a 20- or 25-year history of slowly progressive symptoms consisting first of easy fatigability, progressing to dyspnea on exertion, and finally to severe exercise limitation. Until these patients reach a New York Heart Association Class IV status, they are not at high risk of sudden death, but they are predisposed to all the risks of chronic atrial fibrillation and bacterial endocarditis. All symptomatic patients with significant mitral stenosis should undergo mitral valve reconstruction or replacement.

Pulmonic Stenosis

Pulmonic valvular stenosis is usually the result of congenital heart disease (CHD) and creates a significant pressure overload for the right ventricle. With time, this usually leads to tricuspid regurgitation or decreased compliance of the right ventricle. Although an uncommon condition, surgical intervention has not been recommended unless the systolic pressure within the right ventricle exceeds 50 mm Hg. Treatment currently is balloon valvuloplasty and, in the few unsuccessful cases, open pulmonic valvulotomy or replacement with a cadaveric homograft or a stentless porcine valve.

Tricuspid Stenosis

Tricuspid valvular stenosis is rarely an isolated finding and is most commonly the late result of rheumatic heart disease. Other causes include foregut carcinoid syndrome, especially in the presence of hepatic metastasis; other sympathomimetic states, such as the use of anorexigenic agents (phentermine/fenfluramine), can also cause tricuspid stenosis. Treatment involves repair or replacement, most commonly with bioprosthetic valves. Although the use of a mechanical prosthesis has been reported with success in the tricuspid position, the presence of a mechanical prosthesis virtually excludes the possibility of future transvenous access to the right ventricle for pacemaker lead placement or PA catheter placement.

Aortic Regurgitation

Aortic valvular regurgitation may result from (i) bacterial endocarditis, (ii) traumatic disruption of an aortic leaflet, (iii) rheumatic valvulitis, (iv) congenital valvular disease, (v) ascending aortic dissection, (vi) aortoannular ectasia due to Marfan syndrome or a defect in connective tissue metabolism, or (vii) idiopathic causes. The exact cause in a given case may not be known. The physiologic consequence is volume overload of the left ventricle, which can remain asymptomatic for many years. As a general rule, leaking valves do not cause symptoms or major physiologic consequences until more than 50% of the systolic forward flow returns to the proximal cardiac chamber during diastole. Therefore, aortic regurgitation rarely produces symptoms until the left ventricle constantly ejects more than twice the normal CO. Cardiac compensation occurs through dilatation and hypertrophy. The typical history of aortic regurgitation is that of a cardiac murmur present for 25 to 30 years before the onset of symptoms, often consisting of mild cardiac failure. At that point, the patient generally has a moderately enlarged heart. If the patient is placed on digoxin and diuretics, the symptoms of heart failure will disappear, and the patient may be carried an additional 3 to 10 years before the symptoms recur. Unfortunately, at that point massive cardiac remodeling (eccentric hypertrophy and dilatation) usually occurs, and the patient has a poor long-term prognosis.

The precise timing of valve replacement for aortic insufficiency is important, due to the insidious nature of the disease progression while the patient is still asymptomatic. All symptomatic patients and asymptomatic patients with moderate to severe aortic insufficiency and impaired left ventricular systolic function at rest or with exercise merit valve surgery. These patients are not at great risk of sudden death until they develop angina or persistent heart failure.

Mitral Regurgitation

Mitral regurgitation may be caused by (i) rheumatic valvulitis (rare), (ii) dilated mitral annulus, (iii) stretched or torn chordae tendineae, (iv) ruptured papillary muscle head or papillary muscle, (v) myocardial ischemia, or (vi) bacterial endocarditis. Mitral regurgitation may cause CHF.

Acute mitral regurgitation is most likely to result from ruptured chordae or bacterial endocarditis. Myocardial ischemia may cause mitral valve dysfunction and central regurgitation. Therefore, the etiology must be determined before proceeding to either cardiac or noncardiac treatment of these patients.

Chronic mitral regurgitation is an insidious condition that produces few symptoms until major cardiac enlargement occurs. These patients are at far greater risk of having permanent underlying myocardial damage and limited cardiac reserve.

There are few palliative steps for the management of acute or chronic mitral regurgitation during noncardiac operations. The most important factors are the avoidance of hypertension and prophylactic measures to prevent bacterial endocarditis. The chronic use of afterload reducing agents such as angiotensin-converting enzyme inhibitors (ACE-Is, such as captopril) in an effort to improve symptoms and forestall inevitable surgery is detrimental to the patient, in that it allows the insidious process of progressive LV dysfunction to proceed undetected while the left ventricle continues to undergo deconditioning.

The treatment of significant mitral regurgitation should be mitral repair, which can be accomplished in more than 90% of patients with nonrheumatic mitral regurgitation. Repair usually consists of replacement of ruptured chordae, flail leaflet resection, and downsizing the dilated mitral annulus with a prosthetic ring. Certainly all patients with moderate to severe mitral regurgitation should undergo valve repair or replacement. Of all of the four cardiac valves, a higher percentage of mitral valve patients are asymptomatic at the time of operation, as most of them can experience the benefits of a reliable, durable repair.

Pulmonic Regurgitation

Pulmonic regurgitation most commonly results from severe pulmonary hypertension and should not be surgically addressed until the pulmonary hypertension can be reversed.

Tricuspid Regurgitation

Tricuspid regurgitation usually results from pulmonary hypertension and right ventricular failure, although it may rarely be the result of bacterial endocarditis, especially among illicit drug users. Tricuspid regurgitation can also be associated with long standing mitral regurgitation. Tricuspid regurgitation generally indicates severe right heart failure, and its management is by treatment of right heart failure and pulmonary hypertension if present. Tricuspid annuloplasty can be added to any left-sided heart valve operation without much added operative time or risk.

THE PERIOPERATIVE CARE OF PATIENTS WITH CARDIAC VALVULAR DISEASE

Undergoing Noncardiac Surgery

Aortic Stenosis

AS presents a special problem. In AS, increases in SVR or the development of systemic hypertension can cause increased myocardial oxygen demand, resulting in ischemia and failure. More serious, however, is when hypotension occurs and decreases the coronary artery filling pressures, which may decrease oxygen supply. When patients with AS require noncardiac surgery, the placement of a PA catheter and direct systemic arterial pressure monitoring are indicated to balance these two extremes.

Bacterial Endocarditis

All patients with native cardiac valvular lesions or prosthetic cardiac valves are at an increased risk for the development of bacterial endocarditis. Transient bacteremia from any cause, including surgical or invasive monitoring increases this risk. Bacterial endocarditis has been reported widely with minor trauma and endoscopy and other minor operations. These patients must receive appropriate antibiotic prophylaxis before, during, and for appropriate periods after any surgical or traumatic event. The American Heart Association has published guidelines for antibiotic prophylaxis against bacterial endocarditis. Amoxicillin or ampicillin is given orally 1 hour before the procedure, or clindamycin, azithromycin, or vancomycin for penicillin-class allergic patients. Prophylaxis is given before the invasive procedure, not afterwards, to have an optimal effect.

Anticoagulants

Anticoagulants are used in all patients with mechanical valves and occasionally for patients with bioprosthetic valves to prevent thrombosis of the valve or systemic embolization. As a general rule, patients with homograft valves need not be placed on long-term anticoagulation. Anticoagulation for patients with mechanical valves is maintained with oral anticoagulants (warfarin sodium) to produce a prothrombin time which is approximately 1.5 to 2.0 times normal. A more uniform approach to anticoagulation management is to use the International Normalized Ratio (INR) system. Patients with mechanical valves should have their INR maintained at 2.0 to 2.5 for aortic valves and, 3.0 to 3.5 for mitral valves. The INR range is increased in the setting of atrial fibrillation, prior thromboembolic event, spontaneous echo contrast, or left atrial thrombus.

Managing the anticoagulation of a patient with a mechanical valve around the time of an elective operation is a challenge. Patients who have never had an embolic or thrombotic event, who are in sinus rhythm, and who do not have spontaneous echo contrast by 2-D echo imaging are instructed to discontinue warfarin 4 days before the surgical procedure, and the therapy is reinstated the night of surgery. Oral warfarin should be started soon after the surgery has been completed because it will take several days to reanticoagulate the patient. Patients with a prosthetic valve who are in atrial fibrillation, who have a history of any thromboembolic event, or who have spontaneous echo contrast should stop taking warfarin 4 days before the surgical procedure and administer low molecular weight heparin (enoxapirin, 1 mg/kg subcutaneously twice daily) up to within 12 hours of the time of surgery. Following surgery, in the estimation of the surgeon that perioperative bleeding risk is negligible, low molecular weight heparin and warfarin are restarted until the PT-INR is therapeutic, at which time the heparin is discontinued.

Untreated Cardiac Valvular Lesions and the Postoperative Care of Patients Undergoing Noncardiac Surgery

All patients with untreated cardiac valvular lesions should be considered at high risk of cardiac complications when other operations are being conducted. The problems of bacterial endocarditis and intraoperative management were noted previously. Assume that all of these patients have compromised myocardial function. The early postoperative period will be managed most easily in a critical care area with the use of a PA catheter and direct measurement of systemic arterial pressure. This allows for intermittent measurement of cardiac index (CI) and of SVR index. Maximum cardiac function will be achieved when CI is maintained above 2.5 $L/min/m^2$ and SVR index is maintained below 2,200 $dyne/s/cm^5/m^2$. If this cannot be accomplished by volume replacement, then peripheral vasodilators and inotropic agents should be considered. As previously mentioned, peripheral vasodilators should be avoided in untreated AS. In rare cases, an intra-aortic balloon pump (IABP) should be considered as an adjunct.

CARDIOVASCULAR MONITORING

Cardiovascular monitoring is only one aspect of the appropriate care of ill patients, and all data acquired through the use of electronic or electromechanical devices should be correlated with the visual and physical findings before being accepted as valid.

Although cardiovascular monitoring includes palpation, observation, and a clinical assessment of the adequacy of peripheral perfusion, this section will be limited to a discussion of electrical and electromechanical monitoring of cardiovascular variables.

The direct measurement of cardiovascular variables allows the surgeon to separate three basic components of homeostasis: the state of cardiac function, the adequacy of intravascular volume, and the tone of the peripheral and pulmonary vascular systems. By separating these components, the surgeon can usually make rational decisions concerning the need for and the appropriateness of interventions to correct pathologic states. Under many conditions, the inability to separate the various components of the cardiovascular system will lead to faulty diagnosis and inappropriate and less than optimal treatment.

Application

The application of modern technical cardiovascular monitoring is extensive and should not be applied to all patients. The selection of patients who require monitoring significantly relies on the experience and skill of the surgeon.

Therefore, only general statements will be made here; the details will be discussed with specific diseases. If observation or tests indicate inadequate or inappropriate cardiac function, tissue or organ perfusion, or abnormalities of intravascular volume, then strong consideration should be given to the application of invasive cardiovascular monitoring.

Inadequate or inappropriate cardiac function may be indicated by irregular cardiac rhythm, tachycardia, or bradycardia. Inadequate perfusion of peripheral tissues or individual organs may be indicated by decreased urinary output, signs of peripheral vasoconstriction, or chemical tests suggesting decreased renal or liver function. Adequacy of the intravascular volume can be assessed indirectly by the filling of the venous system, the general state of peripheral perfusion, and by trends in the hematocrit and hemoglobin.

Intravascular Pressure

For more than a century, various methods have been used for the noninvasive measurement of systemic blood pressure. Filling pressure is a surrogate marker of filling volume, which is a more meaningful parameter; pressure is easily measured, but can be altered by changes in volume or chamber/vessel compliance. In ill patients, the measurement of systemic blood pressure by the use of an external pneumatic cuff should always be suspect. Although pressure-measuring systems can be extremely accurate, they are subject to equipment failure and human error in their application. The most accurate measurement of intravascular blood pressure (venous or arterial) is made by the insertion of a fluid-filled tube or a microtransducer directly into a blood vessel. Electromechanical coupling through a transducer converts the mechanical forces of blood pressure to an electrical signal that can be displayed or recorded for monitoring purposes. When fluid-filled monitoring systems are used, small amounts of air within the system or narrowed portions of the catheter system can lead to false readings. A properly positioned and calibrated arterial line is the most accurate form of measuring arterial blood pressure.

The commonly measured IPs include arterial or systemic blood pressure, CVP or right atrial pressure, pulmonary artery pressure (PAP), and PA wedge pressure.

Arterial or Systemic Blood Pressure

Arterial blood pressure is a reflection of cardiac pump function, peripheral vascular compliance, peripheral vascular resistance (PVR), and intravascular blood volume. By itself, neither a high nor a low arterial blood pressure has any diagnostic meaning. In terms of cardiac function, when systolic arterial blood pressure increases, myocardial oxygen consumption increases and the heart requires an increased end-diastolic resting tension of the myocardium. In turn, this requires an increased left ventricular end-diastolic volume, resulting in an increased left atrial pressure (LAP) and pulmonary venous pressure. Because most nutrient blood flow in the coronary arteries occurs during diastole, arterial diastolic pressure is an indirect measurement of the driving force that maintains coronary blood flow and myocardial perfusion. High HRs that reduce the length of diastole or lower arterial diastolic pressures may lead to underperfusion of the myocardium.

Arterial blood pressure is also an indicator of the state of the peripheral vascular system. In elderly patients, when the larger blood vessels are affected by atherosclerosis, rigidity may lead to high peak systolic pressures and low diastolic pressures. However, the behavior of the resistance vessels determines the degree of impedance to flow. If the arterioles are in a high state of tone, impedance may be high and cause an elevation of mean blood pressure.

Central Venous or Right Atrial Pressure

The term *CVP* is used here because of its popularity; however, *right atrial pressure* is a more appropriate term. This measurement determines the right ventricular preload and is a reflection of the adequacy of intravascular volume. In these measurements, it is assumed that the tricuspid valve is normal and, therefore, that the measurement of mean right atrial pressure is a close approximation of the right ventricular end-diastolic pressure.

Pulmonary Artery Pressure

PAP is determined by the state of contractility of the right ventricle, the pulmonary arteriolar tone, and the LAP. As with the left ventricle, increases in pulmonary systolic blood pressure increase oxygen consumption and alter the contractile state of the right ventricle. Pulmonary artery diastolic pressure is an inaccurate reflection of LAP and left ventricular filling pressure. Pulmonary artery diastolic pressure should only be used as a reflection of left ventricular preload when it has been shown to correlate well with PA wedge pressure. This situation does not exist, for example, in PA hypertension.

Pulmonary Artery Wedge Pressure

When assessing the adequacy of filling of the cardiac chambers, the true goal is usually to achieve optimal loading of the left ventricle. Exceptional instances exist in which the right side pressures may be more important. These situations include patients with known pulmonary hypertension or right heart failure. The best measure of left-sided filling would be the left ventricular end-diastolic pressure. The LAP is the best approximation of the left ventricular EDP when the left ventricle is relatively normal. However, these pressures are unobtainable without left heart catheters. Therefore, the ability to measure PA wedge pressure outside of the cardiac catheterization laboratory was a major advance in cardiovascular monitoring. Properly measured, PA wedge pressure is a remarkably accurate measurement of LAP and, assuming a normal mitral valvular apparatus, it is a close approximation of left ventricular end-diastolic pressure. Left ventricular end-diastolic pressure is a reasonable reflection of the end-diastolic resting tension of the myocardium of the left ventricle. The accurate measurement of PA wedge pressure requires the PA wave form to disappear with balloon inflation and be replaced by a properly timed wedge wave form, which is the equivalent of a left atrial wave form. An adequate wedge or left atrial wave form should always include a V wave, which is a positive deflection concomitant with the onset of left ventricular contraction that continues until ventricular relaxation. If a properly timed atrial contraction occurs, an A-wave will be seen during ventricular diastole. Exaggerated V waves may be caused by a noncompliant left ventricle, atrial contraction after closure of the mitral valve (nodal rhythm), mitral regurgitation, or mitral stenosis.

The PA wedge pressure is read most accurately at the "valley" of the ventilatory cycle (end expiration) when the patient is being ventilated. High levels of positive end-expiratory pressure (PEEP) may spuriously raise the PA wedge pressure to some degree. This spurious rise occurs especially when levels of PEEP exceed 10 cm of water. A reasonable rule to factor in the effects of PEEP is to subtract half the PEEP level from the measured wedge; alternatively, the patient can be temporarily disconnected from the ventilator circuit for 10 to 15 seconds while PEEP measurements are taken. In contrast, the pulmonary wedge pressure should be measured at the "peak" of the respiratory cycle (end of inspiration) when the patient is breathing spontaneously.

Substantial risks exist whenever PA wedge pressures are monitored. Complications of PA catheterization include the possibility of thrombosis of the catheter, valve damage, endocarditis, PA rupture, mechanical problems with the catheter such as knots, cardiac arrhythmias, and rupture of the balloon itself. Pulmonary artery rupture usually occurs in the setting of pulmonary hypertension and small branch pulmonary arteries. Complete heart block can occur if the patient already has a left bundle branch block because the catheter can cause right bundle branch block. Therefore, a catheter capable of pacing should be used in this setting. Several techniques exist for the safe placement of PA balloon catheters; however, there is no substitute for caution in the subsequent measurement of wedge pressure. When patients with PA balloon catheters are moved intraoperatively or in the postoperative period, the position of the catheter tip repeatedly shifts. If the catheter advances farther into the PA than its original placement, subsequent inflation of the balloon can lead to rupture of the PA and death. Retraction of the catheter back toward the main PA may place it in a position where inflation of the balloon fails to achieve a wedged condition and will require readjustment. A good general rule is that the PA catheter should not be advanced past the right heart border on the chest radiograph.

The indication for the use of a PA catheter is the need to have precise fluid management of the patient. It is now well known that the ability of even astute clinicians to accurately determine the volume assessment of the patient from the bedside is poor. Therefore, if precise fluid management is mandatory, PA catheter will probably be required. The routine use of PA catheters, even in the setting of acute lung injury, is not supported by evidence-based medicine. The Fluid And Catheter Treatment Trial (FACTT) of The National Heart, Lung, and Blood Institute study randomized

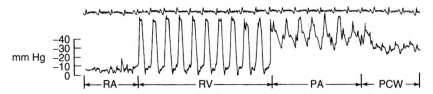

FIGURE 15.3 Pressure waveforms recorded as pulmonary artery catheter is advanced through right atrium (RA) and right ventricle (RV) into pulmonary artery (PA) and to pulmonary capillary wedge (PCW) position.

1,001 patients with acute lung injury to management with and without PA catheters. There was no change in mortality, intensive care unit (ICU) days, or ventilator-free days, but there was a twofold increase in complications, primarily arrhythmias, in the routine PA catheter group.

When the catheter is being placed, the tracings that one will see first will be the minor irregular deflections reflective of the superior vena cava and the slightly greater deflections seen when the catheter is in the right atrium. The right ventricle tracing will show wide deflections with a very low diastolic pressure and a high systolic pressure. Once the catheter has been advanced into the pulmonary artery, the systolic pressures are the same, whereas the diastolic pressures are higher. The wedge pressure tracing will resemble the right atrial pressure tracing and will be characterized by low systolic pressure with a diastolic similar to the PA diastolic. One should never pull the PA catheter back when the balloon is inflated because valvular disruption can occur (Fig.15.3).

Several abnormal waves include the so-called "pseudo wedge" pressure tracing, which is caused by overwedging. This is illustrated in Figure 15.4. An example of a V wave, which results from mitral regurgitation, is illustrated in Figure 15.5.

Blood Flow

Blood flow can be measured directly by electromagnetic flow probes, fast-Fourier arterial waveform analysis, or estimated by 2-D echo (Doppler velocity times cross-sectional area). Two basic catheter techniques are available for the measurement of CO: the Fick principle and the thermodilution method. Neither technique has an accuracy better than ±10% even under ideal circumstances, and under most clinical conditions the accuracy is probably little better than approximately 15% or 20%. The measurement of CO is equal to the HR times the SV and is represented

conventionally as liters per minute. The CI is the CO divided by the body surface area (BSA, m^2).

$$CO = HR \times SV$$
$$CI = CO/BSA$$

The Fick Principle

The Fick principle can be used to determine blood flow. This principle is based on the use of an indicator to measure the blood flow indirectly. To use this approach, the physician must be able to sample blood going into and out of the system. The blood must also carry an indicator. The indicator could be normal substances like oxygen or other indicators such as dyes, carbon monoxide, or cold crystalloid solutions. It is important to know, or be able to estimate accurately, the total exchange of the indicator (I). The most common direct application of the Fick principle is when the blood flow through the lungs is measured. Therefore, when pulmonary blood flow is known, it is assumed to be equal to CO.

The general Fick equation is:

$$\text{Blood flow} = \frac{\text{total exchange of indicator}}{\begin{array}{c}(\text{concentration of indicator entering system} \\ - \text{ concentration of I leaving system})\end{array}}$$

When the Fick principle is applied to the lungs, the equation becomes:

$$\text{Cardiac output} = \frac{\text{oxygen consumption}}{\begin{array}{c}\text{arterial O}_2 \text{ content} \\ - \text{ mixed venous O}_2 \text{ content}\end{array}}$$

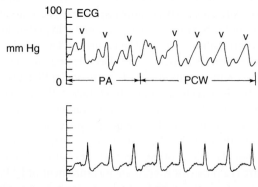

FIGURE 15.5 V waves in acute mitral regurgitation. V wave can be seen immediately following systolic pulmonary artery (PA) waveform, but is more prominent on pulmonary capillary wedge (PCW) waveform. The second wave in PA tracing can be identified as V wave, it peaks at same time following R wave of electrocardiogram (ECG) (0.4 second) as V wave on wedge tracing. Mean wedge pressure is higher than pulmonary artery (PA) diastolic pressure.

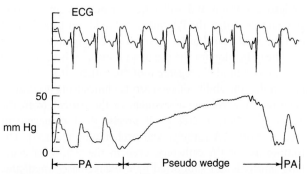

FIGURE 15.4 Pseudo wedge pressure tracing recorded with inflation. ECG, electrocardiogram; PA, pulmonary artery.

Therefore, CO measurement based on the Fick principle ideally requires measurement of the oxygen consumption, arterial oxygen content, and mixed venous oxygen content. It assumes a stable and normal metabolic state. In clinical application, this method may be compromised by several factors. Unless measured directly by a Douglas bag or metabolic cart, the oxygen consumption is assumed based on tables derived from large numbers of normal individuals and may not reflect the condition of the individual patient. Likewise, the metabolic state is assumed to be normal, which is often not the case. Arterial and venous oxygen content are derived indirectly, either from the partial pressure of oxygen (P_{O_2}) or the colorimetrically determined oxygen content O_2 (saturation), and both methods may introduce sizable errors. When the Fick method is used clinically, the number of assumptions and the potential inaccuracies must be taken into account.

Indicator Dilution Technique

In the indicator dilution technique, a marker of known volume is injected into flowing blood and its concentration measured downstream to determine the volume of blood flowing during a specified time period. The method was first developed using various dyes, the concentration of which could be measured colorimetrically. When dyes were used, it was necessary to withdraw enough blood for measurement in a colorimeter. Because the dyes required several hours to dissipate, they accumulated within the bloodstream, thereby limiting the number of determinations that could be made. Furthermore, as the dyes recirculated, the complexity of the analysis of the indicator concentration increased. Present techniques are based on thermodilution, in which a precisely measured quantity of fluid, the temperature of which is known and is lower than that of the circulating blood (usually room temperature), is injected rapidly into the central venous system, and the variation of the temperature of the blood reaching the PA is measured continuously. The greater the magnitude of the temperature drop in the PA per unit time, the lower the rate of blood flow, and vice versa. This is the most popular and probably the most accurate technique available clinically, although its accuracy is seldom better than approximately 15%. However, technical errors that decrease accuracy include the slow or erratic injection of the indicator, inaccurate measurement of the volume of the indicator, inaccurate measurement of the temperature of the indicator, and improper placement of the PA catheter, and tricuspid insufficiency.

Calculated Hemodynamic Variables

Understanding the conversion of cardiovascular measurements to indices and knowing the range of normal indices is important. The importance of indexing certain hemodynamic variables is obvious when the difference in the CO needed for normal function of a 20-kg child as opposed to a 100-kg wrestler is considered. When normal values are reduced to indices, a relatively narrow range of normal values is found. Indexing is conventionally based on BSA employing standard nomograms. CO is reported in liters per minute,

whereas CI is reported in liters per minute per square meter. When the evaluation of systemic flow is reduced to a CI, the ranges for normal output and changes produced by similar aberrations are fairly close for the small child and large adult.

When measurement of CO became possible, these values could be combined with systemic or pulmonary arterial pressures to determine vascular resistance. The calculation of vascular resistance provides an approximation of the state of vascular tone and has become a critical measurement for the appropriate management of critically ill patients. Vascular resistance is calculated by dividing the pressure difference across a vascular bed by the minute blood flow through that bed. These calculations are, as in the case of peripheral vascular hemodynamics, analogous to Ohm law. For the pulmonary vascular bed, this resistance (PVR) is the difference between mean PAP and mean LAP (clinically defined as wedge pressure) divided by CO.

$$PVR = [(\text{mean } PAP - \text{mean } LAP)/CO] \times 80,$$
$$\text{in dyne} \times \text{s/cm}^5$$

PVR may be expressed in terms of "Woods units." Woods units are determined by subtracting the wedge pressure from the mean PAP and dividing by the CO. The two clinical situations in which this terminology is used is in discussing the degree of pulmonary hypertension of patients before repair of congenital defects which result in right-to-left shunting, and when considering heart transplantation. The reason for making this determination is that even a new heart cannot sustain an adequate output in the face of a pulmonary resistance greater than 6 to 8 Woods units. Transplant recipients with irreversible pulmonary hypertension unresponsive to pulmonary vasodilators such as inhaled NO, sodium nitroprusside, high F_{IO_2}, or adenosine would require heart–lung transplantation to have a reasonable chance of survival.

SVR is calculated by determining the difference between the mean arterial pressure (MAP) and the CVP divided by the CO.

$$SVR = [(MAP - \text{mean } CVP)/CO] \times 80,$$
$$\text{in dyne} \times \text{s/cm}^5$$

Although the normal mean pressure ranges vary little from individual to individual, or even between children and adults, CO, as mentioned previously, varies greatly according to the size of the individual. For this reason, resistance index to the total body surface area (TBSA) should be used when monitoring patients. Resistance indices (RI) are calculated by substituting the CI for the CO.

$$PVRI = \frac{([(\text{mean } PAP - \text{mean } LAP)/CO] \times 80)}{TBSA},$$
$$\text{in dyne} \times \text{s/cm}^5$$
$$SVRI = \frac{([(MAP - \text{mean } CVP)/CO] \times 80)}{TBSA},$$
$$\text{in dyne} \times \text{s/cm}^5$$

CARDIAC RHYTHM AND ARRHYTHMIAS

Normal conduction begins with the sinoatrial (SA) node (Figs. 15.1 and 15.2), which conducts electrical activity through atrial tissue to the AV node, down the His bundle, through the Purkinje fibers, finally reaching the ventricles through the left and right bundle branches and causing contraction. When arrhythmias occur, they are caused by either problems with impulse conduction or disorders of impulse formation, that is, automaticity. Impulse conduction problems are the most common cause of arrhythmias. The mechanism is unidirectional block and reentry. Reentry occurs when an electrical impulse comes to a branch point in the conduction system and is transmitted unequally down two parallel pathways. When antegrade conduction is blocked in one path, the area beyond the block remains temporally inactivated. Coming down the other path, the unblocked impulse bypasses the blocked region and then, in retrograde manner, activates the tissue. This can produce a continuous loop of activation. During normal conduction without an antegrade block, the impulses tend to block each other, preventing loop formation. Examples of arrhythmias caused by the reentry mechanism are VT, Wolff-Parkinson-White syndrome, and atrial flutter.

Supraventricular Arrhythmias

Most supraventricular arrhythmias are responsive to treatment. For example, a patient whose symptom at initial examination is a sinus bradycardia can be treated with a vagolytic anticholinergic agent, such as atropine, to speed up the heart rhythm. Sinus tachycardias can be treated with carotid sinus massage to increase vagal tone and to decrease the speed of the rhythm. However, carotid massage should never be used in persons with atherosclerotic disease because cerebral atheroembolism may occur with carotid manipulation. β Blockers, such as propranolol, can also be used in these circumstances. Atrial fibrillation is a common rhythm seen after many kinds of surgery. Approximately a third of all the patients who undergo cardiac surgery will have atrial fibrillation some time in their postoperative period. The mechanism of production remains unclear, but atrial fibrillation is often associated with atrial dilatation, hypoxemia, increased catecholamines, and some element of pulmonary disease. Regardless of the cause, the goal of treatment is to slow conduction through the AV node and control the ventricular rate response with β-blockade, calcium channel antagonists, adenosine, or infrequently digoxin. Atrial fibrillation of greater than 48-hour duration should be anticoagulated to an INR of 1.5 to 2.0, as routine restoration of sinus rhythm following this period can otherwise lead to systemic embolization. Alternatively, transesophageal echocardiography (TEE) can determine accurately the presence or absence of intracavitary thrombus in atrial fibrillation, allowing cardioversion at any time in the absence of clot. Restoration and maintenance of sinus rhythm can be expedited by use of a membrane- stabilizing agent, after ventricular rate has been controlled. The preferred agents are amiodarone, sotalol, procainaminde, or ibutilide. Catheter-based pulmonary vein isolation techniques enjoy a modest success rate (50%–60%) in the treatment of persistent atrial fibrillation. Surgical techniques (biatrial Maze procedure) are associated with up to 90% success rate in permanently ablating atrial fibrillation.

Surgical therapy is possible for certain kinds of supraventricular arrhythmias. Wolff-Parkinson-White syndrome is an arrhythmia that causes tachycardia. The mechanism involves macro reentry, that is, a specific pathway (the Kent bundle) exists separate from, and bypasses, the normal conduction system. These pathways do not have any conduction delay in them analogous to the AV node. Therefore, impulses from the atria reach the ventricles before the normally conducted impulse, which includes the AV node delay. Evidence for this preexcitation can be found in the electrocardiograms (ECGs) of these patients, in slurring of the initial deflection of the QRS occurs, called a *Delta* (δ) *wave*. These pathways can be mapped precisely using electrophysiologic techniques. The impulses usually travel in a retrograde manner during tachycardic episodes. Normal impulses travel through the AV node and are then transmitted rapidly retrograde through these abnormal pathways, resulting in tachycardia. The pathways can be mapped and treated either surgically or with catheter radiofrequency (RF) ablation techniques in the electrophysiology laboratory. When the pathway is ablated, the δ wave should disappear.

Automatic supraventricular tachycardias can also occur; these are arrhythmias that are continuous and related to the firing of a specialized area, usually in the atrium. Often, these constant tachycardias will ultimately cause ventricular dilation and heart failure. They too can be treated surgically by direct ablative techniques or by catheter ablation techniques.

Ventricular Arrhythmias

Ventricular arrhythmias are divided into two basic groups. The first group is VF, which includes polymorphic VT. Polymorphic VT is an irregular-looking rhythm by ECG that is a form of coarse VF. The mechanism for the VF depends on the clinical situation. VF is a disorganized arrhythmia of the ventricle and most often occurs on the basis of a metabolic derangement. Less often it is the result of reentry. This derangement can also be caused by ischemia, most notably associated with an acute myocardial infarction. Automaticity in such a case would be related to dying Purkinje fibers or to metabolic changes in the myocardium. Treatment for these kinds of arrhythmias is related to correction of the metabolic abnormality and pharmacologic agents that decrease the sensitization to abnormal impulses, and make repolarization more uniform. Amiodarone is the preferred agent for VT or fibrillation. Other common drugs used to treat the rate of depolarization are lidocaine derivatives (such as flecainide), moricizine, and procainamide. β Blockers may also be useful in treating ventricular ectopy.

Monomorphic VT is an entirely different arrhythmia. This is a uniform kind of VT that is often associated with ischemic cardiovascular collapse. This arrhythmia often occurs in the first 48 hours after acute myocardial infarction.

In this circumstance, it is the result of automaticity. This arrhythmia more commonly occurs later after myocardial infarct and is caused by a reentry mechanism. When the myocardial infarction occurs, some of the tissue is clearly dead and some absolutely normal. Neither of these kinds of tissue causes arrhythmias. Rather, the injured border zone tissue between the normal and dead tissue provides a substrate for micro reentry. Many unidirectional blocks exist, and as a result, there is an anatomic focus for this arrhythmia. With an anatomic focus, the arrhythmia is less likely to be sensitive to drugs. Frequently, this arrhythmia needs to be treated by electrophysiologic ablation using RF current. Alternatively monomorphic VT can be treated surgically by endocardial resection of the border zone tissue between the normal and nonviable endocardium.

The most common clinical arrhythmia is premature ventricular complexes (PVCs). In the face of an acute myocardial infarction or a metabolic derangement, PVCs can lead to VF. As such, the metabolic derangement needs to be corrected, and PVCs may be suppressed by using lidocaine. However, in the absence of cardiac ischemia, PVCs are a benign arrhythmia. In fact, suppression with drugs often leads to a more malignant form of arrhythmia, VT, or VF. Although the frequency of the PVCs are often suppressed by treatment, the first PVC seen may lead to the malignant arrhythmia. Therefore, the goal of treating a patient with PVCs is to elucidate and treat the cause.

Electrophysiologic Testing

When a persistent ventricular arrhythmia is present, it should be tested to see if it is inducible or if the arrhythmia occurs in the absence of other precipitating factors. Electrophysiologic testing is performed in the laboratory, using catheters in the ventricle to stimulate the heart. If the arrhythmia can be stimulated using multiple PVCs, then the arrhythmia is certainly of the reentry mechanism, and appropriate therapy can be instituted. In addition, electrophysiologic testing allows for serial drug testing to determine if the arrhythmia can be treated pharmacologically, without taking a chance on empiric drug choices. Other treatments for ventricular arrhythmias include endoventricular ablative techniques, which usually involves surgical resection of scar or the use of automatic implantable cardioverter defibrillators.

CARDIAC FUNCTION

The epidemic of CHF is increasing and is most directly related to increasing age, with an incidence of 5% to 7% in patients 50 to 64 years of age and increases 10% to 12% in patients 65 to 75 years old. The underlying etiology of heart failure and prognosis should be factors influencing preoperative risks and benefits of elective general surgery procedures. Life-threatening emergencies will negate this risk/benefit ratio and the intraoperative and postoperative care will determine the patient's outcome.

Determinants of Function and Therapeutic Manipulation of Performance

To treat patients with reduced cardiac function appropriately, it is necessary to have an understanding of the physiologic determinants of cardiac function. Complicating this clinical disease is the preservation of systolic function in 50% of patients with CHF, a 50% prevalence of diastolic dysfunction along with cardiac depressant effects of certain drugs and illnesses. Such an understanding will allow the appropriate surgical care of acutely ill and chronically debilitated patients undergoing elective and high-risk surgical procedures.

There are five basic factors that interact to determine the ability of the heart to function as an effective pump. These factors are also interdependent, and manipulations in one may produce changes in another. They are preload, afterload, electrical state of the heart (rate-chronotropism, rhythm, and conduction-dromotropism), contractility-inotropism, and compliance-lusitropism.

Preload

Preload is the degree of tension on a muscle when it begins to contract. Therefore, the initial filling volume, or pressure, of the left ventricle before contraction determines the sarcomere length and, hence, the muscle performance of the individual fibers. True preload is the end diastolic volume (EDV) of the left ventricle. Ignoring compliance of the heart, EDP of the left ventricle is usually considered a surrogate marker for preload. The physiologic correlate of the sarcomere length-tension relation is the Frank-Starling curve. This curve shows that progressive increases in left ventricular filling volume cause progressive increases in left ventricular developed pressure until a peak level of function is reached. Additional increases in volume beyond this maximum level do not produce improvements in performance. The greater the heart muscle is stretched during filling, the greater the force of contraction and quantity of blood will be pumped into the aorta. This physiologic phenomenon is due to the overlap of actin and myosin filaments that allows the maximum number of cross-bridges between these elements to be formed. This produces the maximum degree of force generation by each cell. Because of the elastic properties of myocardial cells, it is extremely difficult to stretch sarcomeres significantly beyond the peak of the Frank-Starling curve. In fact, any elongation of sarcomeres beyond the peak of the Frank-Starling curve would reduce the overlap of actin and myosin filaments, thereby reducing performance. Therefore, the anatomic correlate of the Frank-Starling curve is the ability of the muscle cell to increase force generation as sarcomere length and ventricular filling volumes increase. Increases in volume beyond that which causes optimum sarcomere length will not improve ventricular performance and may be detrimental. Therefore, the preload, filling volume, or pressure in the left ventricle determines the position of the ventricle on the Frank-Starling curve and predicts cardiac performance. Clinically, a normal left ventricular EDP is 8 to 12 mm Hg; whereas, patients with poor LV function may need higher filling pressures to achieve an adequate CO. However, acutely a left ventricular EDP of greater than 20 to 25 mm Hg is associated with pulmonary congestion and edema.

Preload also depends on the capacitance of the vascular system and the blood volume. Preload can be influenced by volume expansion or contraction and by changes in the capacitance of the venous or arterial circulations. Factors that may reduce venous return to the heart, such as gravitational effects, venodilators, positive pressure ventilation, and PEEP ventilation, may change preload and, therefore, myocardial performance. Therefore, central venous catheters for hemodynamic monitoring may be needed in selected patients with cardiac disease.

Afterload

Afterload is impedance to left ventricular ejection, and is measured indirectly as the pressure in the arterial system distal from the ventricle. We think of afterload as the arterial resistance against which the heart must overcome to eject blood into the total (systemic and pulmonary) circulation. Afterload is defined here as the SVR. The capacitance of the arterial system and the volume of blood contained within the system are the components contributing to the SVR. Therefore, change in either arterial capacitance or blood volume will affect afterload. As myocardial functional reserve is reduced by disease, manipulation of afterload may be an important method of improving ventricular performance.

$$SVR = [(MAP - \text{mean } CVP)/CO] \times 80,$$

$$\text{in dyne} \times \text{s/cm}^5$$

where SVR = systemic vascular resistance, MAP = mean arterial pressure, RA = mean right atrial pressure, and CO = cardiac output.

Because this resistance is the force against which the heart must eject to create forward flow, when the resistance is lowered, the CO should increase.

Two special cases of mechanical afterload manipulation deserve mention: IABPs and military antishock trousers (MAST). The former mechanically decreases afterload while preserving diastolic CPP by deflating just before systolic cardiac ejection and inflating when the aortic valve has closed. This device is useful for unstable patients in cardiogenic shock. The latter, MAST suits, elevate central blood pressure primarily by increasing afterload. Unfortunately, the afterload increase is often peripheral to a large leaking arterial defect in the setting of central penetrating trauma or ruptured aneurysms. This peripheral increase in afterload is the physiologic equivalent of cross clamping the aorta at the level of its bifurcation. Therefore, one must be aware of the effects of this increased afterload on the heart and the aorta or its major branches above this "clamp."

Contractility

The inherent ability of the myocardium to generate force independent of loading conditions is characterized by its inotropic state or contractility. The inotropic state of the myocardium is mostly influenced by the autonomic nervous system (endogenous) and exogenous catecholamines. An assessment of contractility forces can be obtained by measuring the maximum rate of rise of ventricular pressure over time (dp/dt_{max}). This measurement is a basic reflection of contractility as long as preload conditions are held constant and is clinically referred to as the *ejection fraction* (EF).

EF is the ratio of the SV, defined as the volume ejected by the ventricle in systole, to the EDV.

$$EF = SV/EDV = (LVEDV - LVESV)/LVEDV$$

EF is a useful indicator of ventricular function. Normal EF is greater than 65%. Although it depends on preload and afterload conditions, EF can be used to evaluate and compare contractility at baseline.

Compliance

Left ventricular compliance (C), or the relation between the filling pressure (P) and chamber volume (V), is an indicator of the ease of ventricular distensibility.

$$C = \Delta V/\Delta P$$

The physical composition of the myocardium as determined by the underlying disease process influences compliance. Myocardial ischemia, myocardial edema, hypertrophy, amyloidosis, restrictive cardiomyopathies, pericardial disease, and pericardial tamponade decrease ventricular compliance. As compliance decreases, the ventricle becomes stiffer and less distensible. This may produce less diastolic filling (smaller EDV), an increase in left ventricular EDP and decreased cardiac performance.

Electrical State of the Heart

Considering the effect of cardiac rhythm on ventricular performance is also important. Sinus rhythm itself, with the coordinated initial depolarization of the atrium followed by depolarization of the ventricle, has an important influence on myocardial performance. In fact, as ventricular compliance decreases, the "atrial kick" provided in normal sinus rhythm has an even more important contribution to CO, approaching a 25% increase. Therefore, not only is HR a determinant of cardiac performance, but the coordinated depolarization of the cardiac chambers achieved in sinus rhythm also produces a substantial contribution.

CO is defined by the following equation:

$$CO = HR \times SV$$

HR = heart rate; SV = stroke volume. Therefore, increases in HR are directly related to increases in CO. However, as HR increases beyond 90 beats/min, the total CO may actually begin to decrease. SV decreases at faster HRs because the heart cannot fill as completely. Therefore, as HR increases beyond 90 beats/min, the total CO may actually decrease as SV begins to decrease at a faster rate than HR increases. Therefore, tachycardia occurs at the expense of diastole robbing the heart of the time it needs to refill the ventricle. This highlights the importance of rate control therapy in patients with atrial fibrillation.

Measurement of Cardiac Performance

CI is the most frequently used parameter of myocardial performance in surgical patients. Normal CI ranges between 2.5 and 4.5 L/min/m^2. Two clinically applicable methods of determining CO are based on principals of metabolite transport and indicator dilution.

Clinically one can grossly evaluate the adequacy of the CO in relation to end-organ perfusion by several readily available noninvasive parameters such as blood pressure, urine output, extremity perfusion, and level of consciousness. Blood pressure itself is not always a good indicator of CO because there are many compensatory mechanisms that work to actively maintain blood pressure (recall that blood pressure changes occur during the third stage of hypovolemic shock). Because blood pressure is directly related to the product of CO and SVR (BP = CO × SVR), blood pressure may be maintained in the face of a low CO by a high SVR. Urine output is usually a reliable parameter in the absence of diuretic use and an abnormal glomerular filtration rate (GFR), a urine output in adults of greater than 0.5 mL/kg/h implies an adequate output by virtue of adequately perfused kidneys. Extremity perfusion is very worthwhile to evaluate because warm extremities indicate an adequate CO. However, extremity assessment is confounded in patients with peripheral vascular disease who will have cool extremities even with an adequate CO and in septic patients that are febrile. Finally, level of consciousness is useful information. A patient who is alert and awake is obviously receiving adequate brain perfusion and likely has an adequate CO; therefore, an altered mental status is of great concern.

Pharmacologic Interventions

Sympathomimetic Amines

The primary cardiac effects of the sympathomimetic amines (catecholamines) are mediated by way of β-adrenergic receptors. These agents produce an increase in myocardial contractility [by increasing intracellular cyclic adenosine monophosphate (cAMP), which increases calcium release from the sarcoplasmic reticulum], an increase in the frequency of pacemaker discharge in the SA and AV nodes, and an increase in AV node conduction velocity. These agents also produce effects on the vascular system through α- and β-adrenergic receptors. The vasoconstrictor response is mediated by α-adrenergic receptors, and the vasodilator response is mediated by β-adrenergic receptors. The β_{-1} receptors are primarily on the heart, and stimulation leads to an increase in HR and contractility. β_{-2}-Receptors are predominantly on the smooth muscles of blood vessels and bronchi. Stimulation of the β_{-2} receptors leads to vasodilation and bronchodilation. The relative potencies of the various sympathomimetic amines on adrenergic receptors are shown in Table 15.1.

The β-receptor activity of dobutamine is much more important than its α-adrenergic effects. At infusion rates of 5 μg/kg/min, dobutamine acts primarily as a positive inotropic agent by increasing myocardial contractility.

TABLE 15.1

The Relative Potencies and Sites of Influence of the Sympathomimetic Amines

Sympathomimetic Amines Agent	Vascular		Cardiac
	α	β	β
Dobutamine	—	++	++
Dopamine[a]	++	++	++
Epinephrine	++	++	++++
Norepinephrine	+++	—	+++
Isoproterenol	—	++	+++

[a]Dopamine produces mesenteric and renal vascular dilatation by activating dopaminergic receptors. It also acts on α- and β-receptors directly and can cause the release of endogenous norepinephrine.

Dobutamine has more of a chronotropic effect than dopamine and is often limited by tachycardia. Dobutamine also reduces PVR by stimulating the β receptors in the peripheral vasculature. After beginning dobutamine at an initial low dose, increases in dosage are titrated to hemodynamic and clinical improvement.

The effects of dopamine are mediated by three different receptors at low, intermediate, and high dose levels of drug treatment. Therefore, a dose-dependent action of this drug occurs on the renal vasculature, heart, and peripheral vasculature. At low "renal" doses (1–5 μg/kg/min), dopamine has a primary effect on stimulating dopaminergic (DA$_1$) receptors in the renal and mesenteric vasculature. This effect is predominantly vasodilation, resulting in augmentation of renal blood flow.

As intermediate "cardiac" levels of dopamine dosage are achieved in the range of 5 to 10 μg/kg/min, the effect is primarily on increasing cardiac contractility and HR through the β_1 receptors.

As high "pressor" levels of dopamine infusion are reached (10 μg/kg/min), a significant degree of peripheral vasoconstriction results as α-adrenergic receptors are activated. This activation causes a significant elevation of SVR. Maintenance of renal vasodilation is lost at these high infusion rates. This drug also has an arrhythmogenic effect, especially at these high doses.

Epinephrine is a potent α- and β-adrenergic agent with a significant inotropic effect on myocardial contractility. It is also associated with significant α-agonist activity and can increase peripheral arterial vascular tone with all of the potentially negative effects seen with decreased peripheral perfusion. Epinephrine is started at a dose of 0.01 μg/kg/min and can be increased as high as 0.3 μg/kg/min, although at this high sustained dose, renal failure and cutaneous gangrene are at risk of occurring.

Norepinephrine is an extremely potent α-agonist and can be used as a potent pressor agent. Dosage frequently begins in the range of 1 μg/min and can be titrated to increase systemic blood pressure. This agent causes increased activity of all α-receptors with significant elevations in SVR. It may produce marked decreases in coronary, renal, and peripheral perfusion. Peripheral vasoconstriction usually overshadows positive inotropism. However, norepinephrine is specifically indicated in patients with hypotension due to a low SVR and preserved CO such as seen with sepsis, neurogenic shock and post-CPB low SVR states.

Vasopressin is a potent vasoconstrictor agent, directly stimulating smooth muscle V_1 receptors. It is an acceptable substitute for epinephrine in the advanced cardiac life support (ACLS) protocol for resuscitation of VF or pulseless VT, given as 40 units as an IV bolus. The bolus dose for vasoplegic shock is 1U IV and maintenance drip at 0.02 to 1 U/min. A typical dose for diabetes insipidus is 0.5 to 4 units/h.

Isoproterenol has a pure β-adrenergic effect. Its clinical use is usually restricted to situations such as bradyarrhythmias for which enhancement of HR and conditions are desirable such as the denervated heart after transplantation. It is also a potent pulmonary vasodilator.

Levosimendan is one example of a new class of inotropic agents that is currently under investigation and has not been FDA approved. Recall that the typical β-adrenergic agonist class of inotropes exerts their effect by increasing cAMP, which in turn increases sarcoplasmic reticulum release of calcium. Levosimendan works in a cAMP-independent pathway, increasing myofilament (troponin C, actin-myosin cross bridge) sensitivity to available calcium, and is nonarrhythmogenic. It is unique in that it can increase CO without increasing myocardial oxygen demand.

Digitalis Glycosides

Digoxin is the most widely used clinical cardiac glycoside. It has a modest positive inotropic effect on myocardial performance. The effects of digoxin are related to its ability to increase the intracellular calcium available to the myocardial contractile apparatus. This effect is achieved by binding with sarcolemmal sodium potassium ATPase and thereby blocking the active transport of sodium in exchange for potassium. The increased accumulation of sodium within the cell leads to an increased concentration of calcium through the sodium–calcium ion-exchange mechanism. Digitalis-containing compounds also slow conduction through the AV node and can be of therapeutic value in treating supraventricular tachycardias, but have no effect on blunting exercise induced increases in HR.

Digoxin has significant interactions with quinidine, verapamil, and amiodarone, which cause its concentration in the blood to be increased. Remember that the pharmacokinetics of digoxin is such that the equilibration is not achieved until 6 to 8 hours after an oral or intravenous dose. Therefore, serum levels should be measured after equilibration has occurred.

Digitalis preparations can cause toxicity. The most important effects are ventricular arrhythmias. The most typical digitalis-induced rhythm is junctional tachycardia. This rhythm is a wide complex rhythm originating high in the conduction system (near the "junction" of the AV node and the His bundle). Ordinarily, a rhythm originating at this level would have a rate of approximately 40 beats/min. In digitalis toxicity, this rate is usually 80 to 120 beats/min. Digitalis toxicity can also be manifested by systemic signs and symptoms, such as gastrointestinal distress and visual changes such as seeing greens and yellows. Digitalis toxicity is more likely to be seen with hypokalemic and hypomagnesium states. Studies of patients with CHF [Digitalis Investigation Group (DIG) trial] have determined that the efficacy of digoxin is limited to patients with dilated myopathic ventricles (i.e., CHF limited to isolated systolic dysfunction), not to patients with heart failure due to diastolic dysfunction. Digoxin is not a first-line inotrope.

Vasodilators

Nitroprusside is a pure smooth muscle vasodilator that affects all vascular beds, including the arterial, venous, and coronary circulations. Nitroprusside stimulates cyclic guanosine monophosphate (cGMP), which acts as an intracellular second messenger. Treatment is usually initiated at a dose of 0.5 μg/kg/min and is titrated upward for an appropriate response in arterial pressure. Nitroprusside is an extremely effective agent when afterload reduction is required. Its effects are transient and can be reversed rapidly by reducing the dosage or stopping the drug.

Despite its apparent beneficial effect, some evidence suggests that nitroprusside infusion in patients with significant myocardial ischemia can produce a *steal* phenomenon in which coronary blood flow is directed away from the areas of ischemia. Therefore, this agent may not be desirable in such patients.

Nitroprusside is metabolized to cyanide. The cyanide can be metabolized into thiocyanate by the liver and excreted by the kidneys. With normal kidneys, its $t_{1/2}$ is 4 days. However, patients with renal failure may develop thiocyanate toxicity, manifested by tremors, hypoxia, nausea, disorientation, and hypothyroidism. This complication rarely occurs when the drug is used for less than 48 hours. The toxicity can be reversed by infusion of hydroxocobalamin, which converts thiocyanate into cyanocobalamin (vitamin B_{12}).

Nitroglycerin is also a smooth muscle vasodilator, with effects on the coronary and peripheral circulation. Nitroglycerin has a dose-dependent differential action. It acts primarily on veins at low to moderate dosages. At higher dosages, dilatation of the systemic arterial vasculature occurs.

The therapeutic usefulness of nitroglycerin in patients with ischemic coronary artery disease occurs as a result of coronary arterial vasodilation. In addition, a reduction in preload occurs, which produces a decrease in myocardial oxygen consumption. Nitroglycerin is given intravenously with a dose beginning at 50 μg/min and can be titrated upward as required. Oral, sublingual, and dermal forms of this medication are available. Tachyphylaxis to nitroglycerin may develop over time. Options for reestablishing vascular effects include terminating use of the drug for a period of time and treatment with *N*-acetylcysteine.

Hydralazine is an excellent arterial vasodilator, which can be given in bolus doses such as 10 to 50 mg IV every 6 hours.

It is very potent and doses should be started low. Oftentimes it is used as an adjunctive drug to transition patients off the infusion vasodilators, like nitroprusside, over to oral agents for hypertension management.

Amrinone and milrinone are phosphodiesterase inhibitors. They appear to inhibit myocardial cAMP phosphodiesterase activity, producing an increase in the cellular concentrations of cAMP. Amrinone and milrinone therefore have positive inotropic effects: they increase ventricular performance and also appear to act on vascular smooth muscle to produce vasodilation. Both amrinone and milrinone increase CO and decrease systemic and pulmonary vascular resistance. Therefore, they are appropriately considered as inodilators, and have a synergistic effect with β-adrenergic agonists to increase intracellular cAMP. This lowering of pulmonary vascular resistance in patients with pulmonary hypertension gives these drugs unique value in treating right heart failure. Thrombocytopenia has been a problem with amrinone, but not milrinone.

The calcium channel blockers can be used for the treatment of angina pectoris, supraventricular tachycardia, and hypertension. By inhibiting the flux of calcium through myocardial channels, they produce a negative inotropic effect. Furthermore, calcium-dependent activity at the pacemaker cells of the sinus and AV nodes is reduced and causes sinus bradycardia and prolonged AV conduction. These agents produce a vasodilatory action on the coronary and peripheral arterial vasculature by directly interfering with calcium-induced smooth muscle contraction. They also appear to have an antivasospastic activity on the coronary vasculature, as well as muscular CABG conduits such as the radial artery. Many calcium channel blockers are currently available, and they vary in the relative degree of cardiac effect and peripheral vascular effect. Commonly used calcium channel antagonists include nicardipine for vasodilation, and diltiazem for AV nodal conduction control of supraventricular arrhythmias.

Angiotensin-converting enzyme (ACE) inhibitors interfere with the pulmonary conversion of angiotensin I to angiotensin II. Angiotensin II is an extremely potent vasoconstrictor and also promotes adrenal gland release of aldosterone. Aldosterone, in turn, produces systemic vasculature volume expansion through increased renal reabsorption of sodium. The ACE inhibitors have an important role in modifying the renin-angiotensin-aldosterone system. ACE inhibitors produce a significant reduction in systemic vasculature resistance by producing vasodilation and diminishing plasma volume. Treatment with these agents may produce hyponatremia and hyperkalemia (low aldosterone effect).

Adverse effects associated with ACE inhibitors include neutropenia, agranulocytosis, rise in serum creatinine, metallic taste, skin rash, proteinuria, angioedema, a persistent cough, and dysgeusia. An increase in creatinine may suggest underlying renal disease.

Mechanical Assist Devices

Although the vast majority of patients requiring supportive measures for decreased ventricular function respond to conservative medical pharmacologic measures, a small percentage of patients do require more aggressive treatment for survival. A number of mechanical devices are now available for use in such patients. The IABP was the first widely used device for support of the failing heart and is still a mainstay of mechanical ventricular support. Currently, approximately 30 different mechanical circulatory devices are either in use or are in the preclinical phase and two total artificial heart devices are being implanted in humans.

The IABP supports the circulation by implementing the concept of counterpulsation. This theory suggests that the rapid expansion of vascular volume during diastole and the rapid reduction of vascular volume during systole can augment ventricular function significantly. This mechanism provides increased diastolic blood pressure, which causes improved coronary flow and myocardial oxygen supply as well as peripheral perfusion during diastole. It also decreases afterload during systole, which causes improved cardiac performance and reduced myocardial work and oxygen demand. The initial attempts at implementing this theory were unsuccessful because of technical difficulties with the rapid infusion and removal of blood. However, the idea of an intravascular balloon that inflates during diastole and deflates during systole was found to be technically easier to implement than blood manipulation. The IABP works by two actions. First, the rapid inflation of a balloon in the descending aorta early in diastole (firing on the T wave) causes improved diastolic pressure and increased coronary and peripheral perfusion. This mechanism depends on a competent aortic valve, which makes aortic insufficiency an obvious contraindication to its insertion. Second, just before systole (deflating on the R wave), the IABP rapidly deflates and lowers afterload, thereby producing improved myocardial performance by reducing peripheral resistance. Basically, the IABP provides systolic unloading and diastolic augmentation allowing the heart to increase performance at a lower energy demand.

Although the IABP is an effective means of mechanically augmenting ventricular performance, it depends on at least some remaining left ventricular function. In end-stage left ventricular failure, the IABP is of little value. Currently, there are three main conceptual indications for mechanical assist devices: bridge to recovery, bridge to transplant, and destination therapy. The criteria for left ventricular assist device (LVAD) placement are blood pressure less than 90 mm Hg (systolic) and CI less than 1.8 L/min/m^2 despite LAP of 25 mm Hg on maximal inotropic and intra-aortic balloon pump support.

The LVAD is capable of supporting the entire systemic and/or pulmonary circulation when ventricular performance is severely compromised. A variety of devices have been developed as LVAD pumps. These include roller pumps, centrifugal (vortex) pumps, impeller turbines, and pneumatic pulsatile pumps. Each system has its inherent advantages and disadvantages and represents the development of newer technologies.

CONGENITAL HEART DISEASE

CHD remains an important public health problem in the United States, with an incidence of 8/1,000 live births. This commonly quoted percentage is an underestimation because it does not include common asymptomatic childhood problems which may present in adulthood such as patent ductus arteriosus (PDA), coronary artery anomalies, bicuspid aorta with aortic valve stenosis, mitral valve prolapse and atrial septal defects (ASDs). The diagnosis of CHD is usually made by 1 week of age in 40% to 50% of cases and 50% to 60% of all cases are diagnosed by the first month of life after birth. Currently, there are an estimated 1 million people in the United States older than age 20 with CHD and more than 85% of infants with CHD are expected to reach adulthood. Therefore, it is probable that every general surgeon will encounter patients who have treated or untreated CHD. The diagnosis and clinical management requires multidisciplinary collaborations for optimal care, prevention of complications and long-term follow-up.

Classification of Congenital Heart Disease

There are more than 100 anatomic diagnoses for CHD, and most patients have 2 or 3 diagnoses combined. Traditionally, CHD can be categorized into either acyanotic or cyanotic lesions. There are only four major categories into which the diseases are classified, and by understanding these basic classifications, it is relatively easy to understand the pathophysiology of the underlying congenital lesions.

Cyanotic Conditions

Cyanotic lesions are caused by the presence of desaturated blood in the systemic circulation, which may be due to diminished pulmonary blood flow with obligatory right-to-left shunts or chronically increased pulmonary blood flow ultimately resulting in increased pulmonary vascular resistance with late onset right-to-left shunt (tardive cyanosis). Most patients with cyanotic heart disease do not survive to adulthood without surgical intervention and the most common causes of cyanotic CHD in the adult are tetralogy of Fallot (TOF) and Eisenmenger syndrome. The most common causes of cyanotic CHD in pediatric populations are transposition of great vessels (TGV), TOF, total anomalous pulmonary venous return (TAPVR), tricuspid atresia-pulmonary atresia, hypoplastic left heart syndrome (HLHS) and truncus arteriosus.

TOF, the most common cyanotic CHD after infancy is characterized by the presence of (i) a large VSD, (ii) an aorta that overrides the left and right ventricles, (iii) pulmonary stenosis and (iv) infundibular right ventricular hypertrophy. Patients with TOF who have received no medical treatment are always at major risk of the sudden onset of a significant increase in right ventricular outflow tract obstruction, resulting in extreme right-to-left shunting and consequent severe myocardial and cerebral hypoxia. This may be precipitated by endogenous catecholamines, any activity that increases pulmonary resistance (crying and Valsalva maneuver), or the administration of any pharmacologic agents that either increase myocardial contractility (catecholamines, calcium) or decrease peripheral resistance (systemic vasodilators and phlebotomy). The only known effective, nonoperative treatment of cyanotic TOF is the administration of pharmacologic agents that decrease myocardial contractility (β blockers or calcium channel blockers). Although patients with TOF are not usually cyanotic at birth; cyanosis often develops later in life.

Eisenmenger syndrome is seen in patients with a large left-to-right shunt (e.g., ASD, VSD, PDA) that chronically causes pulmonary vascular occlusive disease and pulmonary hypertension with eventual reversal of the direction of shunting. Treatment options for Eisenmenger syndrome are lung transplantation with repair of the shunt lesion, or combined heart–lung transplant if the cardiac shunt lesion is irreparable or if the right ventricle is felt to be dysfunctional beyond hope of recovery.

A natural response to arterial desaturation is the development of secondary polycythemia, which in and of itself may lead to intermittent diffuse intravascular coagulation and its consequences. In preparation for noncardiac surgery, prophylactic phlebotomy is recommended for patients with a hematocrit above 65%. Meticulous management of anesthesia, avoidance of volume depletion and prevention of iatrogenic paradoxical embolization are essential. A specific diagnosis is extremely important if it becomes necessary to operate electively on a cyanotic patient with CHD. When the anatomy is understood, the development of a rational plan for management is possible.

Acyanotic Conditions

Acyanotic lesions include those with simple left-to-right shunt physiology and obstructive outflow or regurgitant valvular lesions. The more common lesions are ASDs, VSDs, PDA, biscuspid aortic valve (BAV), coarctation of the aorta, and pulmonary stenosis.

Immediately after birth, the normally high fetal pulmonary vascular resistance falls below the SVR. Therefore, any communication between the systemic and pulmonic circuits will cause left-to-right shunting and recirculation of blood. These abnormal communications can occur at the great vessel level (PDA and truncus arteriosus), at the ventricular level (VSD), at the atrial level (ASD), or at both atrial and ventricular levels (AV canal). The consequence of this type of shunt is enlargement either of the blood vessels or the cardiac chambers that must carry the increased volume and flow of blood. The size of the shunt and compliance of the myocardium determines the timing of surgical intervention and outcomes. Heart failure, severe pulmonary vascular disease, and pulmonary hypertension with reversal of the direction of shunting can result.

A permanently narrowed valve or blood vessel causes increased resistance to blood flow and requires an increased proximal pressure to maintain the required level of flow. Beginning on the left side of the heart and working backward, it is possible to outline the various causes of obstructing lesions: the obstruction may occur in the aorta (coarctation, hypoplastic aortic arch); at the aortic valve (valvular stenosis, BAV); or as a consequence of an abnormal left ventricle [hypoplastic left ventricle; idiopathic hypertrophic subaortic stenosis (IHSS); and mitral valvular atresia]. Obstruction may occur within the pulmonary vascular circuit (pulmonary venous stenosis, hypoplastic pulmonary arteries, and pulmonary valvular stenosis). Right ventricular causes include hypoplastic right ventricle and tricuspid atresia. If no intravascular or intracardiac shunts exist, the consequence of valvular or vascular obstruction is the increased stress on the cardiac chamber, which must sustain the increased pressure and without surgical intervention will lead to heart failure.

Pulmonary Complications in Congenital Heart Disease

Pulmonary Artery Hypertension

Pulmonary artery hypertension, in its simplest terms, indicates high blood pressure within the PA and by definition exists when the mean PA blood pressure exceeds 30 mm Hg. The cause may be increased pulmonary vascular resistance, increased pulmonary blood flow, or pulmonary venous obstruction.

Increased Pulmonary Vascular Resistance

Determining whether the increased pulmonary vascular resistance is fixed or dynamic is important. Dynamic increases in pulmonary vascular resistance can be controlled by pulmonary vasodilators (such as nitroglycerin, NO, adenosine, high FIO_2, isoproterenol, nitroprusside, etc.) and imply that correction of the congenital cardiac condition may allow pulmonary hypertension to resolve.

Increased Pulmonary Blood Flow

When pulmonary hypertension is the result of high pulmonary flow, as occurs with large VSD, pulmonary vascular resistance initially may be normal or only slightly elevated. The use of pulmonary vasodilators may lead to overt, high-output cardiac failure. The consequence of untreated long term excessive pulmonary blood flow is medial smooth muscle hypertrophy, intimal thickening, plexiform changes and ultimately thrombosis; this ultimately leads to irreversible pulmonary hypertension with consequent right-to-left shunting and tardive (late onset) cyanosis if intracardiac shunt persists. This is called *Eisenmenger syndrome*.

Pulmonary Venous Obstruction

Total or partial anomalous pulmonary venous return occurs when the pulmonary veins drain into a vessel or chamber other than the left atrium. This includes supracardiac, retrocardiac, and infracardiac subtypes. Supracardiac TAPVR involves pulmonary venous drainage into a branch of the innominate vein or persistent left superior vena cava, and drain into the right superior vena cava or right atrium. Intra-, or retrocardiac TAPVR drains into a common vertical vein or chamber (cor triatrium sinister) posterior to the left atrium,

which typically communicates to the left atrium through a restrictive foramen. Infracardiac TAPVR drains pulmonary venous blood into a vertical vein that communicates with the IVC or hepatic veins below the diaphragm. Common to each of the subtypes is the classification of "obstructed" TAPVR, in which the communication to the left atrium is restrictive and causes pulmonary venous hypertension, which in turn causes pulmonary arterial hypertension. This presents in the neonatal period and requires emergent surgical repair. Finally, repair of TAPVR can be complicated by branch pulmonary vein obstruction by stenosis of the orifice of the pulmonary vein, which can result in recurrent pulmonary hypertension.

Natural History and Variability

The natural history of CHD varies greatly. This relates not only to the dynamic character of certain conditions but also to the natural progression of diseases. Of all of the infants born with VSD, it is thought that 25% to 40% of the defects will close at 2 years of age; 90% of those that eventually close do so by 10 years of age. However, of all the children born with TGV, less than 10% will survive to the age of 1 year without surgical intervention. However, coarctation of the aorta may not become evident or be diagnosed until the age of 4 or 5. Remarkably, TOF may remain asymptomatic in 33% of children to the age of 1 year.

Significance for Noncardiac Surgery

Emboli

Any patient with an intracardiac or great vessel shunt has a major risk of either pulmonary or systemic emboli. The meticulous management of all peripheral and central lines is critical. A small bolus of air lodged in the coronary or cerebral vessel can have lethal consequences. The disruption of a clot from the tips of central catheters can likewise be catastrophic. For these reasons, PA catheters placed for hemodynamic monitoring are removed early in the postoperative course.

Arterial Desaturation

Even small right-to-left intracardiac shunts will cause major decreases in arterial PO_2. This cannot be corrected by increasing FIO_2. If the desaturation is a consequence of dynamic right ventricular outflow obstruction, that is, TOF, then the judicious application of β blockers may be helpful. If the magnitude of an intracardiac shunt is the result of increased pulmonary vascular resistance from alveolar hypoxia or atelectasis, appropriate alterations in ventilation may be indicated. Most important, the surgeon must have an appreciation of the cause of arterial desaturation, baseline arterial blood gases and the specific anatomy before developing a rational management plan.

Bacterial Endocarditis

There have been major changes in the epidemiology of infective endocarditis and considerations for prophylaxis in adult CHD are reviewed by the American Heart Association. The increased survival of CHD patients and the use of cardiovascular prosthetic devices along with emerging drug resistant organisms with mortality as high as 30% emphasizes primary prevention. In general, all patients with uncorrected CHD should receive prophylactic antibiotics with few exceptions when undergoing noncardiac operations of any type. All patients withVSDs should receive antibiotic prophylaxis whereas patients with ASDs do not need antibiotics unless there are associated valvular lesions. Patients with CHD should also be considered at risk when they have sustained major trauma or when the placement of temporary central lines becomes necessary.

Venous Anomalies

Cardiac venous anomalies are remarkably common, but few have physiologic consequences. The most important is anomalous pulmonary venous return in which some or all of the pulmonary veins fail to attach to the left atrium and, instead, return oxygenated blood to the right side of the heart. This generally causes a left-to-right shunt, but in its mild forms can be asymptomatic. Another venous anomaly is persistence of the embryologic left superior vena cava. The left superior vena cava usually drains into the coronary sinus. Knowledge of this fact can be important when placing central venous lines, PA catheters, and coronary sinus cardioplegic catheters.

The Systemic Response to Cardiopulmonary Bypass

Since the inception of the use of CPB for open heart surgery in 1953, insight into the complex physiologic and patho-physiologic consequences of extracorporeal circulation has made CPB a relatively safe procedure currently. CPB is used most commonly to maintain a bloodless, quiescent field for cardiac surgery procedures. A venous cannula siphons blood through gravity from the right atrium or superior and IVC into a venous reservoir. Blood then enters a membrane or bubble oxygenator, which provides oxygen and eliminates CO_2. A heat exchanger serves to control the blood temperature for systemic cooling and subsequent rewarming. Finally, a roller or centrifugal pump returns arterial blood to the systemic circulation by way of an arterial cannula in the ascending aorta or femoral artery. Intense anticoagulation with heparin sodium is required before the institution of CPB to prevent clotting of the patient's blood after exposure to the foreign surfaces of the circuit.

Physiologic Effects

CPB is associated with disruption in baseline homeostasis and a well-orchestrated team of professionals including perfusionist, surgeon, anesthesia and operating room support is essential for each step throughout the surgery. The patient's overall medical conditions along with the underlying cardiac abnormalities create a challenge in predicting the compensatory abilities of each patient. Hence, monitoring of the patient is of utmost importance and includes the use of a PA (Swan-Ganz) catheter, arterial lines, urinary catheter and temperature probe. Further input is communicated as a constant gross assessment of the heart and great vessels for volume, perfusion status and arrhythmias in the operating field. Electrolytes, pH, and coagulation profiles are also monitored and appropriately controlled during the duration of CPB.

Perfusion flow rates on CPB generally are maintained at approximately 2 L/min/m^2, yielding mean perfusion pressures in the range of 50 to 70 mm Hg. Continuous flow rates are believed to adequately perfuse the microcirculation, as evidenced by appropriate mixed venous O_2 levels; therefore, most pumps in clinical use now generate nonpulsatile flow.

The hematocrit is normally diluted to approximately 30% during CPB as a result of the use of asanguinous crystalloid and colloid circuit prime. Serial hematocrit levels are drawn during CPB and corrected as indicated. Many studies have shown an increase in morbidity as a direct correlate to the number of blood products transfused.

Most surgeons employ varying degrees of systemic hypothermia during CPB to enhance myocardial and cerebral protection. In general, moderate hypothermia (28°C–32°C) is considered adequate for coronary artery bypass and valve procedures. However, deep hypothermia to 15°C is required for complex congenital repairs or replacement of the ascending and arch aorta, procedures which mandate the use of low-flow perfusion or circulatory arrest to establish a completely bloodless field. Most patients tolerate even deep hypothermia without any apparent adverse sequelae, as long as rewarming to normothermia is complete before the cessation of CPB. However, rapid fluctuations in SVR are not unusual during the rewarming phase, often necessitating pharmacologic intervention to maintain perfusion pressures within the desired range.

Immediately after the institution of CPB, an abrupt increase occurs in blood levels of renin, angiotensin, aldosterone, antidiuretic hormone, and catecholamines. These levels remain elevated for the duration of CPB. Cortisol decreases initially but reaches supraphysiologic levels by the end of bypass. T_3 and T_4 are decreased significantly throughout the period of CPB and may remain so for several days postoperatively. The mechanisms whereby these endocrine alterations occur are unclear, but nonpulsatile flow has been implicated in some instances.

Pathophysiologic Effects

Most patients tolerate a period of CPB without any apparent untoward effects. However, CPB may incite an unpredictable, adverse systemic response which can culminate in multiple organ dysfunction and thereby contribute substantially to cardiac surgical morbidity and mortality (Table 15.2). Although many of the mechanisms underlying these complex pathologic responses remain to be elucidated, there is compelling evidence that the inflammatory response to CPB with the production of cytokines has a major role. Also, nonphysiologic blood flow patterns, shear stresses, exposure of blood to nonendothelial surfaces and patients' preexisting organ dysfunction are

TABLE 15.2

Organ Dysfunction Associated with Cardiopulmonary Bypass

Systemic	Adverse Effect	Presumed Etiology
CNS	Cerebrovascular accident	Macroembolization (calcium, air, atherosclerotic debris)
		Microembolization (fat, cellular/fibrin aggregates)
		Inadequate cerebral perfusion (watershed)
	Neuropsychiatric changes ("postpump delirium")	Inflammatory mediators
		Inadequate cerebral perfusion
	Depressed consciousness	Inflammatory mediators
		Inadequate cerebral perfusion
	Seizure activity	Any of the above
Pulmonary	Acute lung injury	Reperfusion injury
		Leukosequestration
		Inflammatory mediators
	Pulmonary edema	Increased interstitial fluid
		Increased capillary permeability
Gastrointestinal	Pancreatitis	Nonpulsatile flow, hypoperfusion
	Acalculous cholecystitis	Hypoperfusion
Renal	Acute renal failure	Inflammatory mediators
		Hypoperfusion
Hematologic	Excessive bleeding	Platelet dysfunction, or thrombocytopenia
		Hyperfibrinolysis
		Inadequate heparin reversal with protamine sulfate
		Hypofibrinogenemia or dysfibrinogenemia

CNS, central nervous system.

involved. There seems to be a direct correlation between the duration of CPB and the risk of development of the "post-CPB syndrome."

Because most CPB pumps do not provide pulsatile blood flow, the body's visceral capillary beds may depend on pulsatility for optimal perfusion and autoregulation of nutrient flow. This premise has led to the conclusion that nonpulsatile arterial flow is partly responsible for organ dysfunction after CPB. This argument is especially cogent with regard to "postpump" pancreatitis.

Shear stress is inherent in CPB due to the pumping/rolling mechanism involved to move blood through the circuit. Suction lines and turbulence at the end of the arterial cannula may create deleterious shear stresses to which the cellular elements of the blood are particularly sensitive. Red blood cells may be hemolyzed and/or their life spans considerably shortened. In addition, T-cell function may remain depressed for several days postoperatively.

Contact of blood with the artificial surfaces of the CPB circuit may activate a systemic inflammatory cascade, which includes the complement system, coagulation, fibrinolysis, and the kallikrein system. Leukocyte activation and platelet dysfunction also occur. This nonspecific inflammatory response is the most important pathophysiologic stimulus for the "post-CPB syndrome," the hallmarks of which are increased microvascular permeability, leukocytosis, diffuse interstitial edema, and multiple organ dysfunction.

During CPB, contact of the complement proteins with nonendothelial surfaces activates the alternative pathway, yielding dramatically increased levels of the anaphylatoxins, C3a and C5a. Both of these mediators cause vasoconstriction and increased capillary permeability. In addition, C5a can activate monocytes and neutrophils and induces binding of the latter to the vascular endothelium, resulting in organ dysfunction. A prospective trial [pexelizumab for the reduction of infarction and mortality (PRIMO-CABG)] of an antibody to C5a (pexelizumab) resulted in a modest decrease in nonfatal perioperative myocardial infarction but had no effect on stroke or death. The nonendothelial surfaces of the CPB circuit and exposed collagen from tissue injury cause factor XII activation, which can lead to microthrombi formation, consumption of clotting factors, and subsequent end-organ dysfunction. Furthermore, factor XIIa can activate the kallikrein system, resulting in the eventual elaboration of bradykinin. The effects of bradykinin include increased vascular permeability and vasodilation.

Fibrinolysis is increased during and after CPB, due to contact activation of Hageman factor (activated factor XII).

Fibrin degradation products may impair fibrin polymerization and platelet function, and are also capable of injuring the vascular endothelium. Microcirculatory occlusion from fibrin polymers results in end-organ dysfunction. In addition, fibrinogen adsorbed to the pump circuit activates platelets and can induce platelet thrombi formation. Despite the use of therapeutic heparinization, total thrombin inhibition is never complete and pathologic microvascular thrombin formation and excessive bleeding can result from CPB. Pathologic, coagulopathic bleeding following CPB is treated with heparin reversal with protamine, and blood component replacement therapy when appropriate. For life-threatening bleeding despite administration of plasma, platelets, and cryoprecipitate, administration of activated recombinant factor VII (NovaSeven) can often control coagulopathic microvascular bleeding.

The total leukocyte count falls immediately after the onset of CPB due to hemodilution, but as bypass progresses, demargination produces a leukocytosis. Complement-activated neutrophils may cause tissue destruction by releasing proteases such as elastase, as well as toxic oxygen-derived free radicals. Intrapulmonary leukosequestration of activated neutrophils after cessation of CPB has been implicated in lung reperfusion injury. Additionally, monocytes activated during CPB liberate the inflammatory cytokines: tumor necrosis factor, interleukin-1, and interleukin-6, which may be associated with fever, hypotension, and organ dysfunction after cardiac surgery (cytokine release syndrome, or "cytokine storm"). Leukoreduction by filter removal of white blood cellS (WBCs) out of the CPB blood reservoir has been shown to be efficacious but demonstrably reliable benefit has been inconsistent. Aprotinin is a serine protease inhibitor that inhibits plasminogen activity as well as kallikrein activity, and is used as an anticoagulation adjunct during CPB as an antifibrinolytic agent. It preserves platelet function and limits bleeding complications consequent to CPB, as well as demonstrating anti-inflammatory effects in terms of limiting cerebral edema.

Various forms of particulate material have been implicated as emboli during CPB. These include atherosclerotic material, calcific plaques, and lipid globules generated from the subcutaneous fat and sternal marrow. Various groups have shown the presence of lipid microemboli in postmortem brain studies of patients who have undergone CPB. Cannula-based distal embolization filters have demonstrated the ability to remove macroparticulate material, but the impact on neurocognitive outcomes have not been uniformly favorable. Neurocognitive deficits among patients who have undergone CPB have been a subject of intense investigation. Multicenter registry data on CABG patients have shown an incidence of new, focal neurologic deficits or stupor of approximately 3%, and global cognitive dysfunction in an additional 3%; the in-hospital mortality rate of this subset of patients was seven fold higher than the neuron-intact patient group. Various studies are currently looking at means of reducing postoperative neurocognitive deficits by careful monitoring and treatment of these patients.

GLOSSARY

Total fluid energy

$$E = IP + GPE + KE$$

Total fluid energy (E) consists of potential energy and kinetic energy (KE). Potential energy is made up of intravascular pressure (IP) and gravitational potential energy (GPE).

Kinetic energy

$$KE = \frac{1}{2}(DV^2)$$

Kinetic energy (KE) represents the ability of blood to do work on the basis of its motion and is proportional to the density (D) of blood and the square of blood velocity (V).

Bernoulli principle states that when blood flows from one point to another, total energy along the stream is constant, provided that flow is steady and there are no frictional energy losses. Therefore, if the stream narrows, the velocity of the stream must increase to keep the total energy of the stream constant at that point. This principle allows Doppler scans to detect arterial stenoses.

Poiseuille law

$$\text{Flow } (Q) = \frac{\pi r^4 (P)}{8\eta L}$$

$$\text{Resistance } (R) = \frac{8\eta L}{\pi r^4}$$

This law describes the viscous energy losses that occur in a system of moving fluids. The pressure gradient along a tube or vessel is directly proportional to the flow (Q) and the length of the vessel (L) as well as the fluid viscosity (η), and is inversely proportional to the fourth power of the radius (r). This relation is analogous to Ohm law, which states that pressure is equal to flow times resistance (R).

Laplace law $\sigma = Pr/h$ (σ, wall stress; P, mean pressure; r, vessel radius; h, wall thickness) Laplace law defines the tension on the wall of a vessel (σ) as being directly proportional to the pressure (P) and the radius (r) of the vessel, divided by the wall thickness.

Coronary perfusion pressure

$$CPP = DBP - RA$$

Coronary perfusion pressure (CPP) is defined as the pressure that drives the blood across the microcirculation of the coronary circulation. Because most nutrient blood flow occurs during diastole, the driving pressure is the diastolic blood pressure (DBP). The gradient is determined by subtracting from the DBP the right atrial pressure (RA), which reflects the back pressure on the coronary sinus. The units are mm Hg.

Cardiac output

$$CO = HR \times SV$$

Cardiac output (CO) is defined as the amount of blood pumped per minute. This is determined by the heart rate (HR) and the stroke volume (SV). The units are L/min.

The cardiac index

$$CI = CO/BSA$$

The cardiac index (CI) is the cardiac output divided by the body surface area (BSA). The units are L/min/m^2.

Pulmonary vascular resistance

$$[(\text{mean } PAP - \text{mean } LAP)/CO] \times 80,$$

$$\text{in dyne} \times \text{s/cm}^5$$

The pulmonary vascular resistance (PVR) is the difference between the mean pulmonary artery pressure (PAP) and the mean left atrial pressure (LAP) (pulmonary wedge pressure) divided by cardiac output (CO). The units are dyne $\times$ s/cm^5. Woods units are obtained by dividing PVR by 80.

Systemic vascular resistance

$$SVR = [(MAP-\text{mean } CVP)/CO] \times 80,$$

$$\text{in dyne} \times \text{s/cm}^5$$

Systemic vascular resistance (SVR) is the difference between the mean arterial pressure (MAP) and the central venous pressure (CVP) divided by the cardiac output. The units are dyne $\times$ s/cm^5.

Ejection fraction   (EF) is the ratio of the stroke volume (SV) to the end diastolic volume (EDV) which reflects the amount of blood ejected by the ventricle during systole. This is calculated easiest using echocardiography, nuclear medicine studies, or a ventriculogram done at cardiac cath.

$$EF = SV/EDV$$

Fick equation   is used to determine total blood flow and is determined by the exchange of an indicator divided by the concentration of this indicator entering the system and the concentration of the indicator leaving the system. When the Fick principles are applied to the lungs, the equation uses oxygen consumption and content.

Cardiac Output (Fick)

$$CO = VO_2/(CaO_2 - CVO_2)$$

Oxygen consumption divided by arterial O_2 content minus mixed venous O_2 content (generally the oxygen consumption is approximated from tables of normal values for the type of patient being studied).

SUGGESTED READINGS

Rutherford RB, ed. *Vascular surgery*. Philadelphia: WB Saunders, 1989.

Burton AC. *Physiology and biophysics of the circulation*, 2nd ed. Chicago: Year Book Medical, 1972.

Bergan JJ, Yao JST, eds. *Venous disorders*. Philadelphia: WB Saunders, 1991.

Hurst JW, Logue RB, Schlant RC, eds. *The heart: arteries and veins*, 4th ed. New York: McGraw-Hill, 1978.

Berne RM, Levy MN. *Cardiovascular physiology*, 5th ed. St. Louis: CV Mosby, 1986.

Kirklin JW, Barratt-Boyes BG. *Cardiac surgery: morphology, diagnosis criteria, natural history, techniques, results, and indications*. New York: Wiley-Liss, 1986.

Tribble CG, Nolan SP. Current prosthetic cardia valves: a review. *New Dev Med* 1988;3(2): 47–53.

Fozzard HA, Haber E, Jennings RB, et al. eds. *The heart and cardiovascular system: scientific foundations*. New York: Raven Press, 1986.

Ross R. The pathogenesis of atherosclerosis: a perspective for the 1990's. *Nature* 1993;362: 801–809.

Ferri C, Deseridi G, Valenti M, et al. Early upregulation of endothelial adhesion molecules in obese hypertensive men. *Hypertension* 1999;34: 568–573.

Zarins CK, Zatine MA, Giddens DP, et al. Shear stress regulation of artery lumen diameter in experimental atherosclerosis. *J Vasc Surg* 1987;5: 413–420.

Ku DN, Giddens DP, Zarine CK, et al. Pulsatile flow and atherosclerosis in the human carotid bifurcation: positive correlation between plaque location and low and oscillating shear stress. *Arteriosclerosis* 1985;5: 293–302.

Kaza AK, Kern JA. Management of the post surgical valve disease patient. In: Crawford MH, DiMarco JP, eds. *Cardiology*, 1st ed. London: Mosby, 2001: 16.1–16.8.

ECC Committee, Subcommittees, and Task Forces of the American Heart Association. American Heart Association Guidelines for cardiopulmonary resuscitation and emergency cardiovascular care. *Circulation* 2005;112(24, Suppl iv): 1–203.

Bashore T, Cabell C, Rowler V. Update on infective endocarditis. *Curr Prob Cardiol* 2006;31(4): 274–352.

Roach GW, Kanchuger M, Mora Margaro C, et al. Adverse cerebral outcomes after coronary artery bypass surgery. Multicenter study of perioperative research group and the Ischemia Research and Education Foundation investigation. *N Engl J Med* 1996;335: 1857–1863.

CHAPTER 16

The Respiratory System

Herman A. Heck, Jr. and Michael G. Levitzky

The human body is an aerobic organism; its tissues require oxygen for energy production. Carbon dioxide is a by-product of this aerobic metabolism and it and its volatile acid, carbonic acid, are detrimental to subcellular function. The lungs are the main organs of the respiratory system. Their primary function is the attainment of oxygen from the environment, its transport to the circulatory system for subsequent distribution to the cells of various tissues of the body, and the removal from the body of carbon dioxide produced by these same cells. Secondary important functions of the respiratory system include acid–base balance, phonation, olfaction, modification of the inspired air, and pulmonary defense and metabolism. An understanding of the morphology of the respiratory system and of the physiologic determinants of these basic functions is important to the surgeon in his or her care of the patient with respiratory pathology, as well as for the management of ventilated patients or patients undergoing general anesthesia.

This section is not intended as a treatise of the anatomy or pathology of the respiratory system, but rather as a concise review of the salient features of structure and function of the normal respiratory system and how this function is altered with various pathologic states. In presenting the subject in this way it is hoped that one will gain a better understanding of the basis for treatment of various respiratory problems encountered in surgical practice. Commonly used formulas for ventilation and respiration are included in Appendix A.

STRUCTURE AND FUNCTION

Airways

Nasopharynx

Every day approximately 10,000 L of air containing microorganisms, potentially toxic particles or gases, and other irritants are inspired into the airways. With nasal breathing, one role of the nasopharynx is to filter and condition air entering the more delicate tissues of the lower respiratory tract. Initially, nasal vibrissae remove larger particles of greater than 10 to 15 μ in size. As air passes over the nasal turbinates, which provide a surface area of approximately 160 cm^2, it is humidified and thermally regulated, and intermediate-sized particles are removed by the mucous lining and by the posterior pharynx and palate as a result of the abrupt change in direction of bulk airflow. Abrupt, limited inspiration—*sniffing*—allows olfactory detection of potentially hazardous aerosols before they may be transported by bulk airflow to the lower respiratory tract. Efficient airflow through the upper airway also depends on an unobstructed pharynx, the patency of which is regulated by reflex neuromuscular mechanisms involving the pharyngeal dilators.

Tracheobronchial Tree

After passing the nasopharynx, air enters the tracheo-bronchial tree through the larynx. This organ, by virtue of the epiglottis and true vocal chords, offers protection from aspiration of matter from the gastrointestinal tract with which the trachea has a common orifice. The trachea then bifurcates into left and right bronchi with subsequent progressive, dichotomous branching into as many as 23 generations of smaller airways in the adult to form three pulmonary lobes on the right and two on the left, constituting 18 *anatomic* bronchopulmonary segments—8 on the left and 10 on the right (Fig. 16.1). The first 16 generations of airways (the conducting zone) are incapable of gas exchange (Fig. 16.2). These, along with the nasopharynx, larynx, and trachea constitute the *anatomic dead space*, and they offer most of the remaining resistance to respiratory airflow. Gas exchange occurs in the last seven generations of airways (the transitional and respiratory zones), which are composed of the basic functional respiratory unit, the *acinus*. These airways would ordinarily be expected to contribute extensively to the total airway resistance because of their larger numbers and smaller diameters. In fact, because they are in parallel, their individual resistances are added reciprocally and, therefore, contribute very little to the total airway resistance.

The airways can be divided into three major groups based on location and histology. The trachea, major lobar

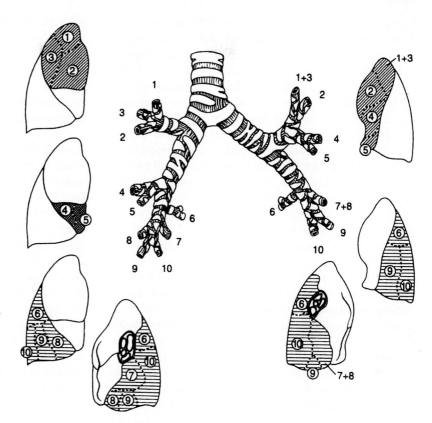

FIGURE 16.1 Anatomy and nomenclature of the bronchopulmonary segments. (From Rice TW. Chapter 20: anatomy of the lung. In: Pearson PG, Cooper JD, Deslauriers J, et al. eds. *Thoracic surgery*, 2nd ed. Philadelphia: Churchill Livingston, 2002:428–441. (Reproduced with permission.)

	Generation		Diameter (cm)	Length (cm)	Number	Total cross sectional area (cm²)
Conducting zone	Trachea	0	1.80	12.0	1	2.54
	Bronchi	1	1.22	4.8	2	2.33
		2	0.83	1.9	4	2.13
		3	0.56	0.8	8	2.00
	Bronchioles	4	0.45	1.3	16	2.48
		5	0.35	1.07	32	3.11
	Terminal bronchioles	16	0.06	0.17	6×10^4	180.0
Transitional and respiratory zones	Respiratory bronchioles	17				
		18				
		19	0.05	0.10	5×10^5	10^3
	Alveolar ducts	T_3 20				
		T_2 21				
		T_1 22				
	Alveolar sacs	T 23	0.04	0.05	8×10^6	10^4

FIGURE 16.2 Schematic diagram of segmental airway branching with corresponding numbers and dimensions. (Figure after Weibel ER. *Morphometry of the human lung*. Berlin: Springer-Verlag, 1963; data from Bouhuys SA. *The physiology of breathing*. New York: Grune & Stratton, 1977:26–42; with permission.)

bronchi, and segmental bronchi constitute the first group. They have cartilaginous walls with little smooth muscle and are lined with ciliated, pseudostratified, columnar epithelium interspersed with mucus secreting *goblet* cells and specialized submucosal glandular cells. The mucus secreted by these cells covers the cilia, which beat in a cephalad direction at frequencies of 600 to 900 cycles per minute, transporting mucus at increasing linear velocities of between 5 and 20 mm/min as it progresses more proximally in the tracheobronchial tree. This *mucociliary escalator* is a major defense mechanism of the tracheobronchial tree and is responsible for removal of particulate matter in the size range of 2 to 10 μ that has settled or impacted on the proximal airways. Submucosal glandular cells also secrete lactoferrin, which is an important bacteriostatic agent in pulmonary defense.

The second group of airways consists of membranous and terminal bronchioles that, by definition, do not contain cartilage and have a relatively large amount of circumferential smooth muscle and elastic fibers. Interspersed within these more distal bronchioles are neuroendocrine *amine precursor uptake and decarboxylase* (APUD) cells—also known as *Kulchitsky* cells and *mast cells*. The former are embryologically derived from the neural crest ectoderm and are rich in amine and peptide hormones such as serotonin, vasopressin, norepinephrine, and vasoactive intestinal peptide, among many others. These cells may be involved in neurohormonal regulation of pulmonary vascular or bronchial responses, especially hypoxia-sensitive chemoreceptor mediated responses (1) Normal embryologic developmental branching of the fetal lung seems to be dependent on one of its peptides—bombesin (2). Other peptides seem to be responsible for the manifestations of various paraneoplastic syndromes caused by their pathologic overexpression with the development of various neuroendocrine tumors of the lung, especially small cell carcinoma (3).

Mast cells are capable of secreting histamine, lysosomal enzymes, leukotrienes, platelet-activating factor, neutrophil and eosinophil chemotactic factors, and serotonin, and are implicated in bronchoconstriction, anaphylactic reactions, immune or inflammatory responses of the lung, and in the initiation of certain cardiopulmonary reflexes (4). These terminal bronchioles are innervated by the autonomic nervous system: cholinergic, parasympathetic, postganglionic efferent fibers, supplied through the vagus nerve, cause bronchoconstriction and enhance glandular secretion; adrenergic, sympathetic fibers cause bronchodilation and inhibit glandular secretion. α and β_2 Receptors, which are responsible for topically or humorally mediated bronchoconstriction and bronchodilation, respectively, are also present. The bronchial smooth muscle is predominantly under parasympathetic tone and a normal circadian rhythm exists with morning bronchoconstriction and evening bronchodilation, which may explain why patients with airway diseases develop respiratory distress more frequently in the morning. Other factors may also cause generalized reflex bronchoconstriction, including inhalation of chemical and particulate irritants,

production of thromboxane by platelets, production of histamine by mast cells, certain leukotrienes, cool temperatures, and stimulation of arterial chemoreceptors. Decreased CO_2 in the conducting bronchioles causes local bronchoconstriction, whereas increased CO_2 and hypoxia cause local bronchodilation. These local responses are likely important in optimizing ventilation-perfusion ($\dot{V}/\dot{Q}$) matching.

The last seven generations of respiratory bronchioles, alveolar ducts, and alveolar air sacs constitute the third group of airways consisting of approximately 130,000 *acini*, with 2,300 alveoli per acinus, or approximately 300 million alveoli. These alveoli are partitioned and interconnected by alveolar septae and are perforated with interalveolar communications, called *pores of Kohn*, which are portals for collateral ventilation and macrophage transit. They are enveloped in up to 280 billion pulmonary capillaries forming *alveolar-capillary units* affording between 50 to 100 m^2 of surface area through which gas exchange by diffusion may occur. The columnar epithelium lining characteristic of the more proximal airways becomes cuboidal at this level and a more specialized secretory cell, the *Clara cell* in the terminal and respiratory bronchioles, progressively replaces submucosal glandular cells and goblet cells. The primary function of Clara cells is to synthesize, store and secrete specialized lipids, proteins and glycoproteins used in certain metabolic functions, and in defense of the lung (5). Among these are surfactant-associated proteins (SP-A, B, C, and D) which promote the transformation of the intracellular lamellae of *type II pneumocytes* into the tubular myelin of surfactant, enhance adsorption of surfactant to the liquid phase of the air–fluid interface within the alveolus, stimulate the endocytic reuptake and recycling of previously secreted phospholipids, and assist in phagocytosis of bacteria by alveolar macrophages.

Ninety percent to 95% of the alveolar surface is composed of a single thin layer of squamous epithelial cells, the *type I pneumocytes*, that constitute the primary diffusion surface of the alveolar-capillary unit. Interspersed among these are more numerous cuboidal type II pneumocytes that serve the dual function of production of pulmonary surfactant and surfactant-related proteins, and the regeneration of type I pneumocytes. *Pulmonary surfactant* is primarily (90%) phospholipid that is secreted as tubular myelin originating from lamellae of the type II pneumocyte and forms a monomolecular film between the air–liquid interface of the inflated alveolus (6). Its purpose is twofold. First, it reduces surface tension, proportionately counteracting the inward elastic recoil of alveoli of varying sizes, tending to equalize individual pressures within alveoli thereby stabilizing their inflation. Second, surfactant helps counterbalance the hydrostatic force of capillary blood, which would otherwise tend to facilitate the development of pulmonary edema. Its salutary effects are impaired by, among other things, smoking and hyperoxia.

A third type of alveolar cell is the amoeboid scavenger cell, the *alveolar macrophage*. This versatile cell is highly mobile and is immunologically responsive to foreign body or antigen intrusion. It is responsible for phagocytosis of particles, viruses and bacteria less than 2 μ, for their destruction by means of reactive oxygen metabolites, interferon, and proteolytic enzymes, and for the secretion of cytokines, leukotrienes, and immunoregulatory mediators that are responsible for the humoral and cellular immune and inflammatory responses of the lung (7).

Chest Wall

Expansion of the lungs is a passive phenomenon and is reliant on an intact chest wall and its associated muscles of respiration. The chest wall is composed of 12 pairs of ribs, the vertebrae, and the sternum (which form the bony thoracic cage), the external, parasternal, and internal intercostal muscles, the scalene muscles, the diaphragm, and the visceral and parietal pleurae. Accessory muscles of respiration are those that may be recruited during deep inspirations, active expirations, situations of physical stress, or in certain pathologic situations. They include the abdominal muscles (the rectus abdominus, in particular), and the sternocleidomastoid, sternohyoid, and sternothyroid muscles. The thorax serves as a rigid protective cage for the lungs and other intrathoracic organs, and maintains an intrathoracic space in which a negative pressure is created by the intrinsic outward elastic recoil of the curved ribs and cartilages. Changes in the configuration of the thoracic cavity serve as the respiratory pump.

Pleura

The lung and the inner thorax are covered with the visceral and parietal pleura, respectively. These are single layers of mesothelial cells 30 to 40 μm in thickness and composed of two layers, an outer mesothelial layer and an underlying connective tissue/fibroelastic layer that contain blood vessels, lymphatics, and neural elements. The pleural space lies between these two layers and extends from the apex of the thorax, above the first rib, to lay reflected deep within the costophrenic and costomediastinal spaces to allow for increased volume with maximal inspiration. The parietal pleura contains corpuscular sensory endings and free somatic nerve endings which are sensitive to pain. The visceral pleura is supplied by vagal and sympathetic nerves. The primary function of the visceral pleura is lubrication by virtue of an abundance of microvilli that produce a hyaluronic acid glycoprotein, which allows easy slippage of the pleural surfaces with normal respiratory motions (8). The main role of the parietal pleura is absorption, mostly through its lymphatics. The usual volume of pleural fluid is only 5 to 15 mL, with a daily turnover rate of approximately 250 to 300 mL (9). This fluid is usually produced by the more cephalad parietal pleura in accordance with Starling forces (intrapleural pressure is more negative), and flows along a vertical pressure gradient to the more dependent costophrenic and lobar regions to be reabsorbed, again, by the parietal pleura through pores in the mesothelium called *stomata*. These stomata vary in size between 2 to 10 μm with respiration, and empty to submesothelial lymphatic lacunae

that coalesce to form valved lymphatic drainage channels with a clearance capacity approximating 30 times the normal capability of fluid production.

Muscles of Respiration

The muscles of respiration are striated skeletal muscles that perform the "work of breathing" and generally require 1% to 2% of total body oxygen consumption under conditions of normal quiet breathing. They are stimulated by anterior horn neurons of the spinal cord and transmit impulses for depolarization through cholinergic motor end plates. Their force of contraction is dependent on the number of fibers stimulated, the frequency of stimulation, and the lengths of the muscle fibers stimulated (10). Ninety percent of the maximal force of contraction is achieved at stimulation rates of 35 Hz (impulses per second). Under usual conditions, inspiratory muscles are capable of generating maximal inspiratory pressures (P_{Imax}) of up to −100 cm H_2O and expiratory muscles are capable of generating maximal expiratory pressures (P_{Emax}) of up to +150 cm H_2O. However, with normal, quiet breathing, inspiratory pressures are generally in the range of −5 to −10 cm H_2O at neural stimulation rates of 10 to 20 Hz.

Respiratory muscle fatigue may occur at low stimulating frequencies against high resistances as a result of primary muscle injury, usually from oxygen-free radical generation, or at high frequencies in excess of 50 Hz as a result of persistent electrolyte shifts due to membrane depolarization. Hypoxia reduces inspiratory muscle endurance for sustaining a contractile effort whereas hypercapnia reduces both the strength of contraction as well as endurance. Resting length–tension properties of muscles of inspiration, especially the diaphragm, may affect their force of contraction under acute or subacute circumstances. Hyperinflation, as occurs with conditions of air trapping, increases the radius of curvature of the diaphragm and shortens its normal resting length, thereby diminishing its contractile force in accordance with the law of Laplace and the length–tension properties of skeletal muscle. Abdominal distension or recumbency in the obese patient overstretches the diaphragm beyond its optimal length–tension properties, which also diminishes contractile force. Under chronic conditions such as chronic obstructive pulmonary disease (COPD) or ascites, adaptation of the muscle's length–tension properties may eventually occur such that contractile force may partially recover. Pathologic states affecting muscles of respiration fall, generally, into four categories: (i) motor neuronal disease, such as Guillain-Barré syndrome, (ii) demyelinating polyneuropathy, as with vasculitis, drugs, or toxins (lead, organophosphates, etc.), (iii) neuromuscular end plate disease, such as myasthenia gravis, Eaton-Lambert syndrome, botulism or envenomation, etc., and (iv) myopathy, such as with hypothyroidism, electrolyte disturbances, dystrophies and poliomyelitis, and so on (11).

The diaphragm is the primary muscle of inspiration and is composed of approximately 50% type I (slow-twitch, high endurance) skeletal muscle fibers and 50%

type II (fast-twitch, increased force) fibers, which allows it to function at up to 50% of its maximal force or velocity thresholds for long periods of time without fatigue. Efficiency is governed by the two basic principles of skeletal muscle function: (i) shorter and excessively long resting lengths decrease force-generating capacity for a given stimulus, and (ii) velocity of contraction is inversely proportional to the force-generating capacity (12). This becomes important with hyperinflation disease states where the generation of adequate force required for thoracic expansion requires both increased motor-neuronal recruitment and increased rate of firing. This may lead to early muscle fatigue and dyspnea, and subsequent respiratory failure. The diaphragm is innervated by the phrenic nerves, which leave the spinal cord at the third through fifth cervical segments. With a person in the supine position, the diaphragm is responsible for approximately two thirds of the air that enters the lung with normal quiet respiration (*eupnea*); in the upright position, it is responsible for approximately one third to one half of the tidal volume (V_T). Peripherally, the diaphragm inserts on the sternum, the lower six ribs, and on the vertebral column by means of its crurae. Centrally, it inserts on the central tendon of the diaphragm, which is confluent with the pericardium. Diaphragmatic excursion during eupneic breathing is 1 to 2 cm, elongating the thoracic cavity and increasing its volume. With deep inspiration, the diaphragm may descend as much as 10 cm at which point it reaches the limits of compliance of the abdominal wall and the intra-abdominal viscera. At this point, further increase in thoracic volume occurs with elevation of the lower ribs, increasing the anterior-posterior and lateral diameters as it contracts against the fixed central tendon.

The external intercostals (innervated by intercostal nerves from thoracic spinal segments 1 through 11), the scalene muscles, and the parasternal muscles, when required for greater inspiratory effort, contract simultaneously with the diaphragm to increase the anterior-posterior dimensions of the thoracic cage and the distance between individual ribs. As the ribs rotate upward about their axes, the intrathoracic volume is further increased. With heavy exercise, the inspiratory phases of coughing and sneezing, and with certain pathologic states such as asthma or emphysema, the accessory inspiratory muscles, such as the sternocleidomastoid muscle, can further increase the anterior-posterior dimensions of the chest wall by elevating the sternum.

Expiration is largely a passive phenomenon due to the unopposed inward elastic recoil of the lung. However, during exercise, speech, singing, the expiratory phases of coughing and sneezing, and certain pathologic states such as chronic bronchitis, active expiration is required. The muscles of expiration are the abdominal wall muscles and the internal intercostal muscles. Contraction of the abdominal muscles increases intra-abdominal pressure and pushes the relaxed diaphragm upward into the thorax. Contraction of the internal intercostal muscles pulls the ribs downward about their axes, decreasing the anterior-posterior dimensions of the thorax. Positive intrapleural pressure (PIP)

is usually generated during such active expiration, the degree dependent upon the strenuousness of the forced expiration and the resistive attributes of the thorax, lung and airways.

The Pulmonary Vasculature

Pulmonary Circulation

The lungs receive the entire cardiac output from the right ventricle consisting of mixed venous blood returning from metabolically active tissues of the body. The right ventricle pumps this blood into a progressively less muscular, thin-walled, distensible and compressible, low-pressure vascular system, which is highly subject to the influence of intrapleural and intra-alveolar pressures. What little smooth muscle these pulmonary arteries have is innervated by the autonomic nervous system to vessels of 30 μ or larger. Sympathetic stimulation increases vessel tone causing vessels to become less distensible; parasympathetic stimulation causes vasodilatation. These pulmonary arteries progressively branch, roughly following the airways, into a network of capillaries that richly encompass the alveoli, forming alveolar-capillary units where gas exchange occurs. These capillaries have an average diameter of 6 μ and are separated from the alveoli by an alveolar-capillary diffusion barrier of approximately 0.2 to 0.5 μ in thickness. This barrier consists of a thin layer of surfactant, the alveolar epithelium and basement membrane, the interstitium, and the capillary endothelium and basement membrane. The pulmonary venules and veins join progressively, frequently in the loose connective tissue septae and interlobar spaces that do not follow the bronchial anatomy as closely as the pulmonary arterial distribution. They normally empty into the left atrium for subsequent distribution of oxygenated blood to the body. The pulmonary circulation is a high-flow, low-pressure system (mean pulmonary arterial pressure of approximately 15 mm Hg) with a transpulmonary vascular gradient between the pulmonary artery and pulmonary vein of approximately 8 mm Hg. Under normal circumstances, the lungs contain 250 to 300 mL of blood/m^2 of body surface area, 60 to 70 mL/m^2 being located in the pulmonary capillaries. The velocity of flow through the pulmonary circulation, and in particular the capillary bed, depends on cardiac output. Under usual resting circumstances, a red cell traverses the alveolar-capillary gas exchange area in 0.75 to 1.2 seconds and traverses the pulmonary circulation in 4 to 5 seconds.

Because the pulmonary and systemic circulations are in series, the outputs of each must be equal in order to prevent overfilling of one or the other. Yet the ratios of the pressure differentials across the respective circuits are of a magnitude of ten, with the pulmonary pressure differential being the lower. Therefore, the pulmonary vascular resistance must be one tenth of the systemic vascular resistance. This is possible because of the morphologic features alluded to previously and because of the relatively minimal hydrostatic (gravitational) forces which the pulmonary circulation must overcome. Furthermore, the uniformity of the metabolic and perfusion demands of its vascular bed, in contradistinction to that of the systemic circulation, also makes this feasible. This resistance is fairly equally distributed among the pulmonary arteries, the pulmonary capillary bed, and the pulmonary veins (in contrast to the systemic circulation, in which approximately 70% of the total vascular resistance resides in the arteries), and is largely determined by passive, extravascular forces such as gravity, lung volume, alveolar and pleural pressures, and right ventricular output, as opposed to alterations in pulmonary vascular tone. These forces create a transpulmonary vascular pressure gradient (a pressure differential between inside and outside of the pulmonary vessel) which, as it becomes greater, increases the vessel diameter and decreases the pulmonary vascular resistance proportional to the radius to the fourth power (see *Poiseuille Law*, Glossary). As it becomes less, the opposite effect occurs such that a negative transpulmonary vascular pressure gradient could result in vessel collapse.

With normal negative–pressure inspiration, lung volumes increase and intrapleural pressure becomes more negative. As the alveoli expand, the pulmonary capillaries between them elongate, thereby decreasing their radii and increasing resistance. On the other hand, the diameters of extra-alveolar capillaries at the juncture of alveolar septae are increased by radial traction, thereby expanding their radii, increasing the transpulmonary vascular pressure gradient, and lowering their resistances. Larger extra-alveolar vessels subject to negative intrapleural pressures have their transpulmonary vascular pressure gradients increased, distending them and, likewise, decreasing their resistance. However, the overall increase in resistance of the capillaries generally exceeds the concomitant decrease in resistance of the larger vessels. Because alveolar and extra-alveolar vessels may be considered two groups of resistances in series, their resistances are additive at any given lung volume and, therefore, total pulmonary vascular resistance increases with inspiration. With forced expiration, compression of the larger extra-alveolar vessels exceeds the decrease in resistance within the capillaries. Therefore, the effect of lung volume on pulmonary vascular resistance is such that total pulmonary vascular resistance is lowest near the functional residual capacity (FRC) at the end of normal expiration, and increases with higher or lower lung volumes. With the special situation of positive pressure ventilation, intrapleural pressure is positive, increasing the resistance to blood flow in both the capillaries and the extravascular vessels. If high enough, this PIP may also compress the intrathoracic vena cavae, decreasing venous return to the heart, such that impaired right and left heart diastolic filling could significantly impair cardiac output under these circumstances (13).

During exercise, cardiac output can increase several fold with only a minimal increase in pulmonary artery pressure, indicating that pulmonary vascular resistance has decreased accordingly. As stated previously, this is the result of passive forces that initiate two distinct passive mechanisms—*distension* and *recruitment*. Distension occurs by virtue of the vessel's increased capacitance with greater volumes because of its morphologic uniqueness as discussed previously. Recruitment refers to the opening of new, previously closed capillaries by virtue of slight increases in perfusion pressure that overcome their critical opening pressures. Opening pressures are determined by increased vascular tone, hydrostatic forces, and/or intra-alveolar pressure. In situations of decreased right ventricular output (volume depletion), pulmonary vascular resistance increases as vessels are less distended and fewer are perfused. Vascular tone may also be humorally modulated. Histamine, thromboxane, endothelin, hypoxia, hypercapnia and certain prostaglandins (F and E) cause vasoconstriction, whereas β-adrenergic agonists such as isoproterenol, acetylcholine, prostaglandins (PGE$_1$) and prostacyclin (PGI$_2$) cause vasodilatation.

Bronchial Circulation

Bronchial arteries arise from the aorta and intercostal arteries and supply oxygenated arterial blood at systemic pressures to, among other thoracic organs, the tracheobronchial tree down to the level of the terminal bronchioles, and to the lymph nodes of the lung. Usually inconsequential connections also exist between the bronchial and pulmonary capillary circulation, which during certain pathophysiologic states become functional (i.e., with pulmonary embolism or congenital absence of portions of the pulmonary arterial tree). The bronchial arterial system has dual venous drainage consisting of unsaturated blood draining to both the azygous/hemiazygous systemic venous system, and to the oxygenated venous blood of the pulmonary venous system. This latter bypassing of the pulmonary capillary bed, along with unsaturated blood returning directly to the left ventricle from Thebesian veins of the heart, constitutes an *anatomic right-to-left shunt*. This is usually 2% to 5% of the normal cardiac output and partly accounts for the systemic arterial saturation generally being less than 100%.

Capillary-Interstitium/Lymphatic Dynamics

Lung capillaries are continuous membrane capillaries, meaning that a dense, continuous basement membrane supports adjacent vascular endothelial cells that are separated by narrow intercellular clefts. Together, these form the vascular-side boundary of the interstitium. The clefts are permeable to smaller solutes such as electrolytes and glucose. The endothelial cells themselves contain transendothelial channels, or "pores," that are highly selective to larger molecules such as albumin and lipoprotein, thereby limiting their escape to the interstitium under ordinary circumstances. The interstitium is a highly compliant space between the basement membranes of the capillaries and the alveoli. It is composed primarily of a loose aggregation of collagen, transudated fluid and its contained solutes, immunologic cellular constituents, and hyaluronate, a proteoglycan that is the major component determining the oncotic pressure of the interstitium. Lymphatic capillaries drain the interstitium to larger lymphatic vessels containing valves and smooth muscle, which in conjunction with tissue motion act as lymphatic pumps. These larger capillaries direct excess interstitial fluid toward the intrathoracic venous system, specifically the subclavian veins, by way of lymphatic ducts. There is essentially no reabsorption of filtered interstitial fluid toward the venous end of the pulmonary capillary bed. There is, however, continuous movement of fluid from the vascular space into the interstitium and back to the vascular space by way of the lymphatics, the net effect being the maintenance of an almost constant and small interstitial fluid volume with an interstitial hydrostatic pressure of approximately −5 to −7 mm Hg. This dynamic interstitial fluid flux is governed by the modified Starling equation for capillary fluid exchange:

$$Q_f = K_f[(P_c - P_{is}) - \delta(\pi_{pl} - \pi_{is})]$$

In essence, this states that the net flow of fluid (Q_f) is determined by the *capillary filtration pressure* ($P_c - P_{is}$) minus the *capillary absorptive force* [$\delta(\pi_{pl} - \pi_{is})$], as modified by a filtration coefficient (K_f) that is determined by the permeability of the capillary endothelium to fluid, and the capillary surface area. The capillary absorptive force is essentially the osmotic pressure differential across the capillary membrane caused by the differences in protein oncotic pressure within the capillaries and interstitial tissue. It is also modified by an *osmotic reflection coefficient* (δ), which describes the permeability of the capillary wall to a particular protein molecule—albumin being the predominant protein of concern in this case. The coefficient is 1.0 when the capillary wall is impermeable to a protein and zero when a protein is able to move out of the capillary unrestricted. The overall coefficient of the lung is approximately 0.75 and is relatively low compared with most other organs of the body. As such, it allows for relatively more efficient protein and lipid flux, a characteristic particularly propitious considering the necessity for surfactant production and recycling.

Certain safety mechanisms concerning pulmonary tissue edema exist as a function of the unique properties of the interstitium and the Starling phenomenon. First, although ultimately rather compliant, the initial portion of the compliance curve for the interstitium is flat. This suggests that for initial increases in capillary hydrostatic pressure, only a relatively small amount of fluid is leaked into the interstitium that generates, in turn, a proportionately higher interstitial pressure. This tends to oppose the capillary hydrostatic pressure and contain the fluid leak. As more fluid enters the interstitium, the compliance increases and results in only moderate increases in interstitial pressure for correspondingly larger amounts of fluid flux. This increase in capacitance tends to maximize lymphatic flow away from the interstitium while steadily limiting interstitial hydrostatic forces, which might exceed critical pressures that would cause alveolar flooding. Furthermore, dilution of the interstitium and high lymphatic flow decreases the interstitial protein concentration, which would tend to increase the capillary absorptive force and favor retention of fluid within the vascular space. These safety factors normally allow the capillary hydrostatic pressure to reach between 25 to 30 mm Hg before alveolar flooding occurs. Ultimately, however, as more volume accumulates and the capacity of the lymphatic sump is reached, the interstitium approaches

the limits of its compliance and interstitial hydrostatic forces exceed the resistive forces of the alveoli resulting in pulmonary edema.

Respiratory Control

The Medullary Respiratory Center

Breathing is spontaneously initiated in the central nervous system, specifically in the reticular formation of the medulla beneath the fourth ventricle, which modulates respiration by way of the phrenic nerves and through a final common pathway consisting of the spinal cord and its segmental intercostal nerves. This spontaneously generated, rhythmic cycle of inspiration and expiration is involuntary in the eupneic state, although it can be voluntarily modified, altered, or suppressed by several mechanisms in order to accommodate various circumstances—as with the increased respiratory demands of exercise or while speaking. These mechanisms include reflexes arising in the lungs, airways, and cardiovascular system, receptors in contact with the cerebrospinal fluid, and commands from higher centers of the brain. Spontaneous alveolar ventilation is involuntary. It is determined by the interval between successive discharges of respiratory neurons [dictating the respiratory rate (RR)] and the frequency and duration of discharges transmitted by individual nerve fibers to their respective motor units as well as the number of motor units activated with each inspiration or expiration (dictating the depth or V_T). Additional voluntary pathways from the cerebral cortex can bypass the medullary respiratory center to directly influence α-motor neurons of the spinal cord that are involved in respiratory muscle control, particularly the accessory muscles of respiration.

Two groups of respiratory neurons in the medullary respiratory center, the dorsal respiratory group and the ventral respiratory group, are the primary organelles of inspiratory and expiratory control, respectively, and influence the rhythm of breathing. The dorsal respiratory group consists primarily of inspiratory neurons and is the principal initiator of phrenic nerve activity. The *nucleus tractus solitarius* within this group receives visceral afferent fibers through the ninth (glossopharyngeal) and 10th (vagus) cranial nerves, which carry information about arterial P_{O_2}, P_{CO_2}, and pH from the chemoreceptors of the aortic and carotid bodies and information concerning systemic arterial blood pressure from the arotic and carotid baroreceptors. It also receives vagal afferent input from pulmonary stretch receptors. Therefore, this area would also appear to be the site of integration of various inputs that are involved in the *reflex* alteration of the otherwise spontaneous pattern of respiration.

Several groups of nuclei comprise the ventral respiratory group, which consists of both inspiratory and expiratory motor neurons. One group consists of primarily ipsilateral vagal motor neurons that innervate the accessory muscles of the larynx, pharynx and tongue, and are involved in maintaining patency of the proximal upper airway. A second group of inspiratory neurons projects predominantly to the contralateral external intercostal muscles and the diaphragm and thereby coordinates inspiration initiated by these muscles. A third group of mostly expiratory motor neurons projects to the internal intercostal muscles and the abdominal muscles used in active expiration.

The Pontine Respiratory Center

The pontine respiratory center includes the apneustic center and the pontine respiratory groups of nuclei—the pneumotaxic center. The apneustic center, located in the brain stem between the more cephalad pontine respiratory nuclei and the more caudal dorsal and ventral respiratory groups, is the site of the inspiratory "cutoff switch." It is where integrated information from afferent visceral fibers is projected and subsequently used to modulate respiration by terminating the otherwise sustained inspiration initiated in the dorsal respiratory group in cyclic manner. The pontine respiratory groups of nuclei modulate the apneustic center, further fine-tuning and synchronizing this cyclic breathing pattern. It does so by serving as the integration site of various reflex afferents located in the lungs, the cardiovascular system, and various other areas of the body that may have an impact on respiration.

Spinal Pathways and Reflex Mechanisms

Axons projecting from the dorsal and ventral respiratory groups, the cortex, and other supraspinal sites descend in the spinal white matter to influence the muscles of respiration through the segmental intercostal nerves. At the level of the spinal anterior horn respiratory motor neurons, there is integration of descending influences as well as local spinal reflexes, such as inhibitory spinal motor interneurons that may inhibit inspiratory afferent pathways when expiratory activity excites the appropriate motor neurons. Ascending pathways in the spinal cord also carry information from pain, touch, temperature, and proprioception that can also influence respiration.

Local reflexes that modulate respiration originate from many parts of the body and include stretch receptors in the lung, receptors in the upper airways and passages, cardiovascular and pulmonary vascular receptors, and receptors arising in muscles, tendons and skin. One such group of local reflexes is the *Hering-Breuer* inflation reflex and the Hering-Breuer deflation reflex, which are elicited primarily by stimulation of stretch receptors within the lung. The Hering-Breuer inflation reflex is initiated by vagally innervated stretch receptors within the smooth muscle of the airways when a maintained distension of the lung occurs. This acts to minimize the work of breathing by limiting large V_{TS} and preventing overdistension of alveoli. Transient reflex apnea or slowing of the respiration, bronchodilation, tachycardia and systemic vascular constriction occurs with moderate inflations. Decreases in heart rate and systemic vascular resistance may occur with larger inflations. At a more physiologic level, this reflex may play a role in influencing normal cyclic respirations through afferent feedback to the pneumotaxic center, essentially determining the length of the expiratory phase of respiration. The Hering-Breuer deflation reflex increases the rate and depth of ventilation with sudden deflation of the lung, as might occur with a pneumothorax. It may also be instrumental in the "sigh" mechanism, which is important in the prevention of atelectasis.

Various vascular reflexes within the pulmonary and systemic circulations are also capable of influencing respiration. *Juxtapulmonary-capillary receptors (J-receptors)* located in the walls of terminal arterioles associated with various pulmonary capillary beds respond to extremes of pressure change. They may cause tachypnea and/or a feeling of dyspnea with high capillary pressures, as may occur with pulmonary vascular congestion. With very low capillary pressures, as may occur with sudden pulmonary embolism, a decrease in ventilation is mediated through this reflex.

Systemic arterial *baroreceptors* are stretch receptors that are located within the carotid sinus at the bifurcation of the common carotid artery, and in the arch of the aorta. The afferent pathway from the carotid baroreceptor is a branch of the glossopharyngeal nerve (Hering nerve), and that from the aortic baroreceptors is the vagus nerve. Their stimulation by arterial hypertension causes brief reflex apnea and bronchodilation, as well as bradycardia and vasodilatation.

Still other respiratory reflexes are mediated through receptors whose afferent pathways follow the segmental intercostal nerves of the muscles, tendons, and joints of the thoracic cage and ascend through the spinal cord to the pontine respiratory center. Their stimulation generally increases ventilation and, therefore, may play a role in adjusting ventilatory effort to the elevated workloads of exercise thereby optimizing the work of breathing. Afferent input from proprioceptors and muscle spindle cells located in the joints, muscles, and tendons of exercising limbs plays an important role in initiating the immediate increase in minute ventilation (V_E) in response to heavy exercise until such time as other chemoreceptor, reflex, and humoral control mechanisms can take over. This response is coordinated in the hypothalamus, along with a similarly appropriate cardiovascular response, influenced to some degree by conditioned reflex cortical input. Somatic pain causes reflex hyperpnea; visceral pain causes apnea or hypoventilation.

Peripheral systemic arterial chemoreceptors are located bilaterally in the carotid bodies at the bifurcation of the common carotid arteries and in the aortic bodies in the arch of the aorta. They have similar afferent pathways as the baroreceptors. They respond to, among other things, local changes such as hypercapnia and low pH and act in a negative feedback loop to supply the central respiratory controller with the afferent information necessary to make proper adjustments in V_E in order to keep the overall acid–base milieu of the body normal. Additionally, peripheral chemoreceptor stimulation specifically involving the carotid bodies is also responsible for initiating reflex responses to sustained hypoxemia. The additional effects of stimulation of these receptors under this condition are bradycardia, hyperpnea, bronchoconstriction, dilation of the upper airways, and increased blood pressure.

Central chemoreceptors are located bilaterally near the ventrolateral surface of the medulla in the brain stem and are not in contact with arterial blood, but rather with cerebrospinal fluid. They are, therefore, on the brain side of the blood–brain barrier. As with the peripheral arterial chemoreceptors, they respond to local increases in P_{CO_2} and hydrogen ion concentration. They do not respond to hypoxemia.

Arterial and cerebrospinal fluid partial pressures of carbon dioxide are normally the most important factors affecting the ventilatory control system in establishing V_T and V_E. Over a range of 20 to 60 mm Hg the stimulation rate of these chemoreceptors changes linearly with changes in arterial P_{CO_2} and/or hydrogen ion concentration. Hypoxemia affecting peripheral arterial chemoreceptors also increases this ventilatory response; therefore, for any given level of P_{CO_2}, the ventilatory response is greater at a lower arterial P_{O_2}. Metabolic acidosis also shifts this response curve to the left. There are other influences that induce respiratory depression by shifting this curve to the right. Among these are narcotics, anesthesia, endogenous endorphin production, chronic obstructive lung disease, and sleep.

The blood–brain barrier allows only carbon dioxide to rapidly diffuse through it and is relatively impervious to plasma bicarbonate and hydrogen ions. Furthermore, cerebrospinal fluid has a lower protein buffering capacity than plasma and lacks the additional buffering capacity of hemoglobin, and therefore has an intrinsically lower pH than arterial blood. The primary buffer in the cerebrospinal fluid is bicarbonate, formed mainly through the enzymatic action of carbonic anhydrase within the choroid plexus. As a result of these unique differences, arterial hypercapnia will lead to greater changes in cerebrospinal fluid hydrogen ion concentration than it will in arterial blood. This phenomenon allows the central medullary chemoreceptors to function as the major regulator of ventilation with respect to small, chronic, steady state fluxes in P_{CO_2} and pH. The peripheral arterial chemoreceptors serve as rapid-response, short-term regulators to more extreme changes in P_{CO_2} and pH. Peripheral chemoreceptors, being affected by progressive hypoxemia, are also responsible for offsetting the direct depressant effect of hypoxemia on the central respiratory controller.

Cheyne-Stokes respiration is an abnormal respiratory pattern consisting of periods of hyperpnea alternating with periods of apnea, which derives from relative hypersensitivity of the peripheral respiratory controllers to CO_2 under certain unusual circumstances. It may occur with subacute hypoxemia and markedly slowed circulatory transit times (i.e., congestive heart failure) when, as a result of elimination of the damping effect of oxygen on carotid body sensitivity to CO_2 and with the delay in transit time of CO_2 elimination, extremes of partial pressure changes in the peripheral circulation reaching the carotid body lead to exacerbated swings of the normal respiratory cycle (14). Under certain circumstances, physiologic states of deep rapid eye movement (REM) sleep and certain levels of anesthesia may occasionally

cause bradycardia, hypoventilation and hypoxemia, with similar effects.

NORMAL VENTILATION

Mechanics of Breathing

The bony thorax, primarily because of curvature of the ribs, has a resting *outward* elastic recoil force. The lung, with its fibroelastic tissue, as well as the surface tension of the distended alveoli that are prone to collapse, has a resting *inward* elastic recoil force. The balance between these opposing forces, the outwardly expanding chest wall tending to hold the alveoli open in opposition to their inward elastic recoil, is the basis for normal ventilation mechanics. Alveoli expand only in a passive manner in response to a transmural pressure gradient across alveolar walls that tend to distend them. This is accomplished during negative-pressure breathing by increasing intrathoracic volume, thereby making the already negative intrapleural pressure (normally -5 cm H_2O) more negative. In accordance with *Boyle law* ($P_1V_1 = P_2V_2$), the alveoli increase their volume, thereby lowering intra-alveolar pressure, which is equilibrated with atmospheric pressure to zero at FRC. Therefore, as intrapleural pressure becomes more negative, the transmural pressure gradient is increased and the alveoli expand. Alveolar pressure becomes subatmospheric, causing inward airflow until such time as alveolar pressure once again equilibrates with atmospheric pressure. Because only the more peripheral alveoli are subjected to the negative intrapleural pressure, the innermost alveoli are allowed to expand in concert with the outer alveoli by mechanical transmission of the transmural (transpulmonary) pressure gradient through alveolar walls by means of alveolar septae

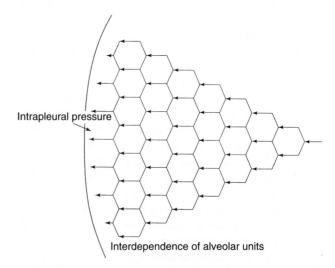

FIGURE 16.3 Schematic diagram of the structural interdependence of alveoli, by means of alveolar septae, in the mechanical transmission of changes in intrapleural pressure. (From Levitzky MG. *Pulmonary physiology*, 5th ed. New York: McGraw-Hill, 1999.)

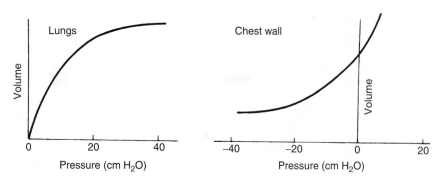

FIGURE 16.4 Individual and composite compliance curves of the lungs (**A**), chest wall (**B**), and overall thoracic compliance [balance of opposing elastic recoils of the lungs and chest wall] (**C**). TLC, total lung capacity; FRC, functional residual capacity; RV, residual volume. (From Weinberger SE. *Principles of pulmonary medicine*, 2nd ed. Philadelphia: WB Saunders, 1992; with permission.)

(Fig. 16.3). Normal expiration is entirely passive and represents a return to the normal end-tidal state of opposing elastic recoils of the chest wall and lungs upon relaxation of the muscles of inspiration (Fig. 16.4). Lung volume remaining at this point is termed the functional residual capacity (*FRC*) and is greater in the erect, as opposed to the supine, position. This is primarily because gravity pulls intra-abdominal viscera away from the diaphragm thereby increasing the outward recoil of the chest wall.

Work of Breathing
Work of breathing, generically speaking, refers to the effort required by respiratory muscles—primarily the diaphragm—to achieve adequate ventilation under varying physiologic and pathologic conditions. It is proportional to the product of the transpulmonary pressure change times the corresponding volume change in a complete V_T cycle—both inspiration and expiration. During breathing, the transpulmonary pressure change must effectively overcome the elastic recoil of the pulmonary parenchyma and chest wall as well as the resistive forces of the airway and other resistive forces of the lung and pleural tissues. Normal quiet breathing with passive expiration produces between 0.38 and 0.72 J/L of work and requires 0.25 to 0.5 mL O_2/L of ventilation, or approximately 1% to 2% of total body oxygen consumption. Increased work of breathing and muscle fatigue must be viewed with two concepts in mind: first, inspiratory muscle perfusion (and therefore aerobic metabolism) occurs during its relaxation phase; and, second, adequacy of perfusion is

inversely proportional to the intensity of contraction and to the proportion of the overall respiratory cycle during which contraction occurs (termed the *duty cycle*). *Dyspnea* is a clinical indicator of inadequate inspiratory muscle perfusion and impending muscle fatigue. *Hyperpnea* is seen with greater degrees of chemoreceptor stimulation and is manifested as a less rapid, deeper forced inspiration and expiration in an effort to eliminate the excess CO_2 produced by anaerobic metabolism.

Inspiratory muscle *strength* is best assessed by maximum static inspiratory pressure (P_{Imax}), better known as *negative inspiratory force* (NIF), which is -100 cm/H_2O in a normal adult. Inspiratory muscle *efficiency* is expressed by the inspiratory pressure index (P_{breath}/P_{Imax}; normally <0.1), where the inspiratory pressure of normal quiet breathing is -5 to -10 cm/H_2O. Inspiratory muscle *fatigue* is assessed by the *inspiratory pressure-time index or tension-time index* (TTI), which is the product of the inspiratory pressure index (efficiency of inspiratory muscle contraction) and the ratio of the duration of inspiration (i.e., duration of inspiratory muscle—mainly diaphragm—contraction) to that of the total breath, that is, the duty cycle (T_I/TTOT; normally 0.4). Fatigue generally develops when the P_{breath}/P_{Imax} exceeds 0.4. This may occur if increased airway resistance or decreased compliance of the lung or chest wall substantially increases P_{breath}, and/or if respiratory muscle weakness substantially decreases P_{Imax} (15).

Inspiratory muscle endurance is related to the TTI and there exists a threshold below which respiratory fatigue

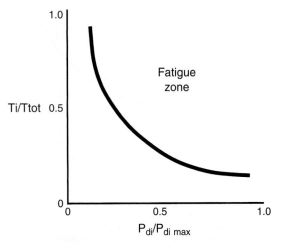

FIGURE 16.5 Graphic depiction of the tension-time index (TTI) as it relates to diaphragmatic muscle fatigue. The greater the percent of maximal transdiaphragmatic pressure developed ($P_{di}/P_{di\ max}$), the less the "duty cycle" (Ti/Ttot) must be to avoid fatigue. (From Celli B. The diaphragm and respiratory muscles. *Chest Surg Clin N Am* 1998;8:207–224; with permission.)

will not occur, and above which it will (Fig. 16.5). Hence, the greater the pressure change developed by diaphragmatic contraction, the shorter the duty cycle must be in order to avert eventual respiratory failure (16). Endurance, also being a function of inspiratory muscle perfusion, is additionally influenced by systemic perfusion pressure and RR. Hypotension decreases muscle perfusion; increased RR, by increasing oxygen consumption, increases perfusion in a linear manner. Therefore, for a given TTI, hypertension and increased RR (*tachypnea*) increase inspiratory muscle endurance. *Tachypnea*, therefore, is a compensatory mechanism for inspiratory muscle fatigue that is manifested as rapid, shallow breathing, which tends to minimize inspiratory muscle fatigue and maximize endurance by decreasing the inspiratory pressure index and increasing oxygen consumption. However, tachypnea also reduces dynamic compliance. This occurs because smaller alveoli supplied by higher resistance bronchioles have less time to fill, leading to progressive alveolar closure, and inflated alveoli have inadequate time to empty, leading to progressive alveolar hyperinflation as alveolar air is redistributed to alveoli of lower resistance or higher compliance.

Tachypnea and hyperpnea eventually lead to increased work of breathing. Hyperpnea exacerbates this by causing high lung volumes leading to decreased lung compliance, by creating increased airway resistance as a result of airway turbulence due to greater intrapleural pressures being generated, and by causing dynamic compression of smaller airways. In the final analysis, respiratory failure is imminent if the TTI exceeds 0.15 to 0.20.

Pressure–Volume Relations
During normal quiet breathing, increased breathing, or in pathologic states, the changes in thoracic volume that

determine changes in transmural (transpulmonary) pressure gradients are influenced by several factors. Among these are chest wall and pulmonary compliance, airway resistance, and the regional distribution of alveolar ventilation. *Compliance* is defined as a change in volume divided by a corresponding change in pressure and, in the case of thoracic compliance, denotes the ease with which the lung and chest wall can be adequately expanded for effective ventilation. The usual adult has a normal thoracic compliance of 100 mL/cm H_2O, normalized per kilogram of body weight. This represents a normal lung compliance of 200 mL/cm H_2O and a normal chest wall compliance of 200 mL/cm H_2O (a centimeter of pressure must be generated for each component of the thoracic compliance). Compliance is the opposite of *elasticity*, which refers to properties of the lung or chest wall that tend to oppose such facile expansion. Lung compliance is not a linear relation, but rather is volume dependent and exhibits *hysteresis*. In essence, this means that compliance is greater at low lung (alveolar) volumes and less at high lung volumes. The pressure–volume relation at any given point during inspiration is different from that same point in expiration. These phenomena are the result of several factors: (i) the inherent elastic properties of the lung parenchyma, (ii) the varying transmural pressure requirements for alveolar expansion and collapse at different radii, (iii) the effects of pulmonary surfactant on these pressure requirements, (iv) the recruitment/de-recruitment of alveoli throughout the respiratory cycle. At low lung volumes, the collagen and elastin that compose the alveolar walls and septae are minimally stretched such that small increases in transpulmonary pressure result in relatively large increases in alveolar volume. With increasing stretch to their elastic limits, progressively increasing pressure is required for correspondingly smaller increases in volume. These two phases inscribe the middle steep slope and the later plateau of the inspiratory lung compliance curve (Fig. 16.6). The relatively flat initial phase of this sigmoid curve reflects the increasing transmural pressure gradient required for recruitment of closed alveoli at FRC.

Because the lung is composed of alveoli of different sizes, higher pressures in smaller alveoli should cause them to collapse into larger alveoli with inspiration, according to the *Law of Laplace* ($T = Pr/2$) (Fig. 16.7). Were this to occur, lung compliance would decrease as fewer alveoli would reach their high-volume elastic limits earlier and the cohesive forces of the liquid–liquid interface of collapsed alveoli would require greater distending pressures to open them. This is prevented by *pulmonary surfactant*, which tends to equilibrate pressure within alveoli of varying sizes by lowering surface tension in alveoli of smaller surface area. This favorably influences the overall slope of the compliance curve. The progressively less negative intrapleural pressure opposing the relatively constant inward alveolar elastic recoil of the lung primarily determines the shape of the expiratory lung compliance curve. Therefore, progressively greater negative changes in lung volume occur with passive

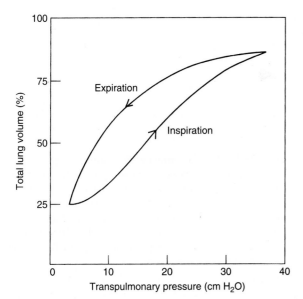

FIGURE 16.6 Pressure–volume curve for isolated lung. (From Levitzky MG. *Pulmonary physiology*, 5th ed. New York: McGraw-Hill, 1999; with permission.)

expiration, with increasing alveolar elastic recoil being the driving force of exhalation.

Several factors other than lung and chest wall compliance must be overcome to move air in and out of the lungs. These include the inertia of the respiratory system as a whole, frictional resistances of the lung and chest wall tissues, and frictional resistances of the airways to airflow. Inertia, friction between pleural surfaces, and the indigenous friction of the chest wall are generally negligible in nonpathologic situations. Pulmonary tissue resistance as the lung expands accounts for approximately 20% of the total pulmonary resistance. Airway resistance is responsible for the other 80%. *Poiseuille Law* governs airflow resistance as follows:

$$R = 8\acute{\eta}l/\pi r^4$$

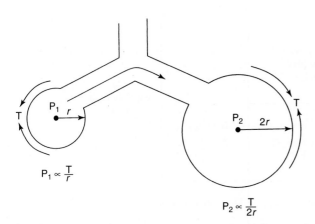

FIGURE 16.7 Schematic diagram of two alveoli of different radii connected to a common airway, illustrating the Law of Laplace regarding equal surface tensions. (From Levitzky MG. *Pulmonary physiology*, 5th ed. New York: McGraw-Hill, 1999.)

Therefore, longer airways of smaller total cross-sectional area offer the greatest resistance to flow. During normal respiration, 25% to 40% of airway resistance is contributed by the nasopharynx, larynx, and trachea, the higher figure occurring with nasal breathing. The resistances of smaller airways, the acinii of which are arranged in parallel and comprise the vast majority of the total cross-sectional area of the airways, are added as reciprocals and contribute very little to total airway resistance. Therefore, most airway resistance normally resides in the medium bronchi and bronchioles.

Airway resistance decreases with increasing lung volume. Distensible, nonsupported, small airways have their radii increased (and, therefore, have their corresponding resistances decreased in proportion to the fourth power of the radius) with increasing transmural pressure gradients. Furthermore, the mechanical interdependence of these airways, by virtue of common alveolar septae, results in increased outward traction on these smaller airways as lung volume increases. This further increases their radii. With forced expiration, especially past FRC, PIP compresses these smaller, nonsupported airways decreasing their radii and exponentially increasing airway resistance inside the small airways (*dynamic compression*). At some point between FRC and residual volume (RV), intrapleural pressure may exceed pressure within some small airways (i.e., the transmural pressure gradient becomes negative) and these nonsupported, small airways collapse, trapping air in the alveoli. This trapped volume in excess of the RV is termed the *closing volume*. It is greater in *COPD* because destruction and coalescence of alveolar septae increases the diameters of alveoli and reduces their elastic recoil as well as their radial support. Alveolar pressure is therefore less, according to the Law of Laplace, and airway closure occurs sooner at lower PIPs. Additionally, intrapleural pressure becomes positive earlier in expiration to overcome the increased resistance of small airways. Therefore, FRC and RV are both markedly increased.

The distribution of alveolar ventilation varies within the lung. The effects of gravity as well as propitious changes in chest wall mechanics sequentially favoring upper versus lower thorax on intrapleural pressure make it less negative in the lower, dependent regions of the thorax than in upper, nondependent regions. Accordingly, transpulmonary pressure gradients are greater in the upper regions of the lung and alveoli have greater volume and are less compliant at FRC than are those in the lower regions. Therefore, any change in transpulmonary pressure gradient within the normal respiratory cycle will result in a greater change in volume for alveoli in the dependent regions of the lung resulting in greater ventilation (Fig. 16.8). With forced expiration to residual lung volume, however, the pleural pressures in the more dependent regions of the lung are more positive and the elastic recoil tendency to keep alveoli open is less, resulting in closure of airways in these more dependent regions. Therefore, an inspiration taken from RV will result in air initially entering more compliant,

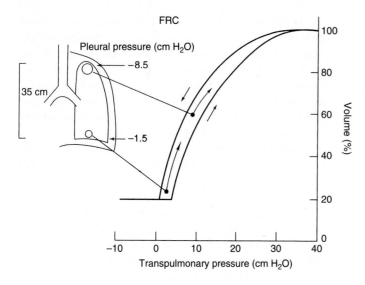

FRC

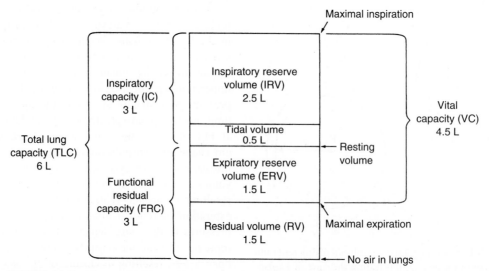

FIGURE 16.8 Diagrammatic illustration of the gravitationally influenced intrapleural pressure gradient from cephalad to caudad within the thoracic cavity, and its affect on the distribution of inspired gas at functional residual capacity. FRC, functional residual capacity. (From Milic-Emili J. Pulmonary statics. In: Widdecombe JG, ed. *MTP international review of sciences: respiratory physiology*. London: Butterworth, 1974:105–137; with permission.)

nondependent regions of the lung that are on the steeper portion of the pressure–volume curve.

Lung Volumes and Capacities

Lung volumes vary according to age, sex, and body surface area. Comparing a patient's lung volumes to standardized normal volumes (or predicted volumes) permits one to determine degrees of change that may be associated with restrictive or obstructive pathology (see Appendix C). There are four standard lung volumes and four standard lung capacities, each of the latter comprising of two or more of the aforementioned lung volumes (Fig. 16.9). V_T is the volume of air inspired and expired through the nose or mouth with each breath. It is determined by the respiratory control center and the mechanics of breathing, and is normally 500 mL (all examples are for a normal 70-kg adult). RV represents the volume of gas remaining in the lung after a maximal forced expiration. It is important in maintaining

alveolar expansion at low lung volumes and is normally 1.5 L. *The inspiratory reserve volume* (IRV) represents that volume above the usual tidal inspiration that can be achieved with additional maximal forced inspiratory effort (2.5 L). Conversely, the *expiratory reserve volume* (ERV) is that volume of gas that is expelled from the lungs forcefully at the end of tidal expiration. It represents the difference between FRC, that is, that volume of gas remaining in the lung at the end of tidal expiration, and the RV. It is 1.5 L. The combination of the normal tidal volume and the inspiratory reserve volume is the inspiratory capacity (V_T + IRV = IC). The *total lung capacity* (TLC) represents the volume of air that can be contained in the lungs at maximal inspiration with expansion of the entire alveolar and airway spaces and consists of all four lung volumes. *Vital capacity* (VC) is that volume of gas forcefully expelled from the lungs starting from maximal forced inspiration. It is the TLC minus the RV and is approximately 4.5 L.

FIGURE 16.9 The standard lung volumes and capacities for a 70-kg adult. (From Levitzky MG. *Pulmonary physiology*, 5th ed. New York: McGraw-Hill, 1999; with permission.)

Alveolar Ventilation

V_E is the total amount of air moved in and out of the nose and mouth per minute and is the product of the tidal volume and the respiratory rate ($V_E = V_T \times RR$). *Alveolar ventilation* is less than the V_E because the last part of each inspiration (approximately 150 mL with eupneic breathing) remains in the conducting airways during inspiration and expiration. This is referred to as the *anatomic dead space*. Furthermore, a certain portion of air reaching the alveoli may not undergo gas exchange because a variable percentage of alveoli may not be perfused for various physiologic or pathologic reasons. These alveoli constitute the *alveolar dead space*. The anatomic dead space and the alveolar dead space together constitute the *physiologic dead space* (V_{DCO_2}). The relative proportion of physiologic dead space ventilation varies under different physiologic and pathologic circumstances and is difficult to measure directly. The high-solubility and high-diffusion capability of CO_2 (which is 20 times that of O_2) coupled with the concept that any volume of CO_2 found in mixed expired gas must come from alveoli that are both ventilated and perfused, make its determination possible by means of the *Bohr equation*. The Bohr equation relies on the partial pressures of CO_2 in expired air and arterial blood, and the V_T for calculation of the alveolar dead space (see Appendix A).

Arterial CO_2 levels are in equilibrium with alveolar CO_2 levels and are inversely proportional to the effectiveness of alveolar ventilation. A significant arterial-alveolar CO_2 difference means there is significant alveolar dead space, generally indicating a $\dot{V}/\dot{Q}$ mismatch. Contrarily, a significant alveolar-arterial oxygen difference (A-aDO_2,) which is normally 10 to 20 mm Hg, may represent either a $\dot{V}/\dot{Q}$ mismatch or may be due to one of several other causes. Among them are diffusion blocks, pathologic shunts, low mixed-venous PO_2, hyperoxic ventilation, or shifts in the oxyhemoglobin dissociation curve (Table 16.1).

Alveolar oxygen partial pressure (P_{AO_2}) is determined by the *alveolar gas equation*:

$$P_{AO_2} = [F_{IO_2}(P_B - P_{H_2O})] - P_{ACO_2}/RER$$

TABLE 16.1

Causes of Increased Alveolar-Arterial Oxygen Partial Pressure Gradient

Increased right-to-left shunt
  Anatomic
  Intrapulmonary
Increased ventilation–perfusion mismatch
Impaired diffusion
Increased inspired partial pressure of oxygen
Decreased mixed venous partial pressure of oxygen
Shift of oxyhemoglobin dissociation curve

From Marshall BE, Wyche MQ. Hypoxemia during and after anesthesia. *Anesthesiol* 1972;37:178–209; with permission.

It is, therefore, that fraction of the total pressure of inspired dry air [i.e., barometric pressure (P_B) less water vapor partial pressure] that is oxygen (F_{IO_2}), minus the alveolar partial pressure of carbon dioxide, divided by the respiratory exchange ratio (RER). *RER* is a metabolic term referring to the ratio of carbon dioxide production relative to oxygen consumption (V_{CO_2}/V_{O_2}) as measured at the mouth or nose. It is distinguished from *respiratory quotient* (RQ), which denotes similar but not necessarily equal values at the cellular level. Under normal, resting circumstances, 250 mL of carbon dioxide is produced for every 300 mL of oxygen consumed for an RQ (or RER) of approximately 0.8. This remains in a relatively constant relation with increasing metabolic demands under *aerobic* conditions and a typical diet. It can, therefore, generally be assumed to be 0.8 under ordinary circumstances in calculating alveolar P_{AO_2}.

Room air, being approximately 21% oxygen, equates to a usual P_{AO_2} of 100 mm Hg. As may be surmised from the alveolar gas equation, the two means of increasing alveolar oxygen concentration would be to increase the inspired oxygen fraction or to decrease the carbon dioxide concentration, and thereby its partial pressure. Acute conditions of relative alveolar hypoxia are translated as hypoxemia that is sensed by the peripheral arterial chemoreceptors. Hyperventilation is initiated, which decreases the concentration of carbon dioxide in the alveoli thereby allowing an increased concentration, and thus partial pressure, of oxygen. This response under circumstances of chronic hypoxia, referred to as the *hypoxic ventilatory drive,* supersedes hypercapnia as the stimulus for ventilatory control. Although controversial, it has been postulated that the chemoreceptors become relatively desensitized to hypercapnia as a stimulus for ventilation under such conditions (17). Administration of oxygen sufficient to suppress this hypoxic drive could result in excessive, perhaps even life-threatening, hypercapnia and respiratory acidosis (18).

A balance between respiratory frequency and V_T is necessary to achieve alveolar ventilation with minimal work of breathing. For any given V_E, a higher respiratory frequency *(tachypnea)* results in less effective alveolar ventilation because much of the respiratory effort is expended in moving air through the physiologic dead space. At the same minute volume, slower and deeper inspirations result in greater alveolar ventilation, albeit at a cost of greater elastic work of breathing. The normal ratio of dead space to V_T is 0.2 to 0.3; when it becomes greater than 0.4, respiratory failure may eventually occur.

Gas Exchange

Ventilation–Perfusion Relations

Alveolar ventilation is normally 4 to 6 L/min and pulmonary blood flow (which equals cardiac output) is approximately the same. Therefore, the ratio of ventilation to perfusion for the lung ($\dot{V}/\dot{Q}$) is normally within the range of 0.8 to 1.2. The alveolar partial pressures of both oxygen and carbon dioxide are, in part, determined by this ratio. If ventilation increases relative to perfusion within the alveolar-capillary unit, the delivery of oxygen relative to its removal from the

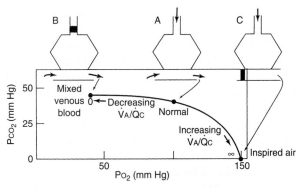

FIGURE 16.10 Effect of ventilation–perfusion mismatch on arterial P_{O_2} and arterial P_{CO_2} as expressed along a continuum (*ventilation–perfusion ratio line*) from ventilated, unperfused alveoli (*B*) to optimally ventilated and perfused alveoli (*A*) to unventilated, perfused alveoli (*C*). $\dot{V}_A/\dot{Q}$, ventilation–perfusion ratio. (From West JB. *Ventilation/blood flow and gas exchange*, 5th ed. Oxford: Blackwell Science, 1990; with permission.)

alveolus will increase, as will the removal of carbon dioxide relative to its delivery. Alveolar P_{O_2} will rise and alveolar P_{CO_2} will fall. The reciprocal is also true. Therefore, units with high $\dot{V}/\dot{Q}$ ratios will have relatively high P_{O_2} and low P_{CO_2} and units with low $\dot{V}/\dot{Q}$ ratios will have relatively low P_{O_2} and high P_{CO_2} (Fig. 16.10). Desaturated, mixed-venous pulmonary arterial blood leaving alveolar-capillary units where the alveolus is collapsed or where ventilation is otherwise severely restricted relative to its perfusion constitutes an *absolute intrapulmonary shunt*. This, together with other areas of very low $\dot{V}/\dot{Q}$ and with the anatomic shunt, constitutes the *physiologic shunt* and can be calculated by the shunt equation (see Appendix A).

There are normal regional perfusion differences in the upright lung which, when considered within the context of the regional ventilation differences previously discussed, constitute the physiologic basis for intrinsic $\dot{V}/\dot{Q}$ mismatch within the normal lung. These regional perfusion differences are primarily a consequence of gravity acting on a column of blood in the lung above or below the left atrium (pulmonary veins), and result in greater blood flow per unit volume in the more dependent regions of the lung. Because the pressure is higher in these lower lung regions, resistance is less owing to recruitment and distension of vessels there. In the upper regions of the lung, perfusion is least and actually ceases in areas where alveolar pressure exceeds capillary perfusion pressure. These regional differences in ventilation and perfusion allow one to conceive of the normal lung as having three distinct zones, the absolute demarcations of which are highly variable depending on intrinsic and extrinsic factors such as pulmonary artery pressure, patient position, positive pressure ventilation, exercise, etc. (Fig. 16.11). *Zone one* consists of larger, less compliant, and less-well ventilated alveoli supplied by nonperfused capillaries such that, in essence, it constitutes alveolar dead space. *Zone three* is composed of smaller, more compliant, and more effectively ventilated alveoli that are luxuriantly perfused with high pressure, rapid-transit pulmonary blood flow, the driving pressure of which is determined by the difference between pulmonary artery and pulmonary vein pressures. Alveoli in *zone two* have intermediate compliance. Pulmonary artery pressure is higher than the alveolar pressure, which is higher than pulmonary vein pressure; therefore, the difference between pulmonary artery pressure and alveolar pressure determines the effective driving force of perfusion.

The gradient for perfusion from the bottom of the upright lung to the top is greater than the gradient for ventilation (Fig. 16.12). Therefore, although $\dot{V}/\dot{Q}$ ratios and P_{O_2} are higher the more cephalad in the thoracic cavity one proceeds, gas exchange is most optimal in the more dependent regions

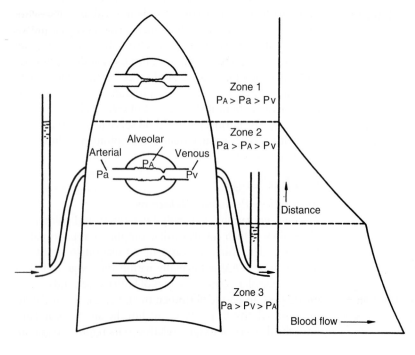

FIGURE 16.11 Schematic diagram of the effects of gravity and alveolar pressure on perfusion of the lung, and their subsequent effect on ventilation–perfusion matching: The *Zones of the Lung.* P_A, alveolar pressure; Pa, arterial pressure; Pv, venous pressure. (Redrawn from West JB, Dollery CT, Naimark A. Distribution of blood flow in isolated lung: relation to vascular and alveolar pressures. *J Appl Physiol* 1964;19:713–734; with permission.)

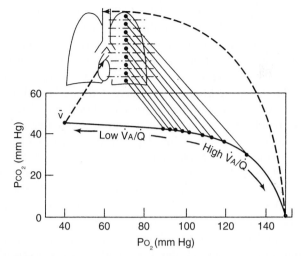

FIGURE 16.12 Schematic diagram of the effect of gravity on relative ventilation–perfusion matching within the vertical lung. $\dot{V}_A/\dot{Q}$, ventilation–perfusion ratio. (From West JB. *Ventilation/blood flow and gas exchange*, 5th ed. Oxford: Blackwell Science, 1990; with permission.)

of the lung where there is greater blood flow. Conversion of portions of zone one to zone two, and zone two to zone three occurs with increasing pulmonary artery pressure and decreasing FRC. This further optimizes $\dot{V}/\dot{Q}$ matching and gas exchange. Hypovolemia or positive-pressure ventilation causes an opposite effect.

$\dot{V}/\dot{Q}$ matching is further facilitated by an intrinsic, graded compensatory mechanism termed the *hypoxic pulmonary vasoconstrictive response* (HPV) that is independent of the central nervous system and occurs locally in areas of alveolar hypoxia. It is felt to be mediated either directly by the effects of hypoxia on pulmonary vascular smooth muscle or, less likely, by a decreased local release of nitric oxide or an increased local release of a vasoactive substance from mast cells, such as serotonin, histamine, or prostaglandins (19,20). Precapillary arterioles are affected within alveolar P_{O_2} ranges of 20 to 150 mm Hg, and dilate or constrict in an effort to minimize perfusion to atelectatic or otherwise compromised respiratory units. This response helps to minimize potentially serious intrapulmonary shunting and facilitates the maintenance of adequate arterial P_{O_2}.

Diffusion and Transport of Gases

According to the *Dalton Law* for mixed gases, the pressure exerted by each gas in a mixture is independent of the partial pressures of the other gases in the mixture (see Dalton Law, Glossary). Same gases of differing partial pressures equilibrate by random molecular motion through a gradient, a process termed *diffusion*, resulting in a net movement of gas from an area of higher partial pressure to an area of lower partial pressure. Oxygen reaches the alveoli, first by bulk flow of air through the tracheobronchial tree. The linear velocity of bulk flow progressively falls to zero as it approaches the level of the alveoli because of the tremendous cross-sectional area of the terminal bronchioles, and it then moves

through the gas phase in the alveoli according to its own partial pressure gradient. It then must make a transition through the alveolar-capillary interface from a gaseous phase to a liquid phase. In so doing, it must dissolve in and diffuse through a layer of pulmonary surfactant, the alveolar epithelium and basement membrane, the interstitium, the capillary endothelium and basement membrane, the plasma, and the erythrocyte membrane, and ultimately combine with hemoglobin. It is then distributed by bulk circulatory flow to other tissues of the body where essentially the reverse process occurs, with oxygen molecules diffusing into the mitochondria of the specific cells of the tissue to which it was delivered. A similar process in the opposite direction occurs for carbon dioxide. The *Fick Law for diffusion* determines the rate, or volume per time (V), at which gas diffuses through the alveolar-capillary barrier as follows:

$$V = A \times D \times (p_1 - p_2)/T$$

This is directly proportional to the surface area (A) available for diffusion and the partial pressure gradient for the gas and inversely proportional to the thickness of the barrier (or the diffusion distance) (T). This rate of diffusion is further influenced by a diffusion coefficient specific for the barrier (D), which itself is directly proportional to the solubility of the gas in the barrier and inversely proportional to the square root of the molecular weight of the molecule. Therefore, in nonpathologic circumstances where the physical characteristics of the alveolar-capillary barrier are constant and relatively nonrestrictive, the amount of a specific gas absorbed in blood (which otherwise does not combine chemically with any of the constituents) is proportional to its solubility and the partial pressure gradient of the gas (see *Henry Law, Glossary*).

Oxygen and carbon dioxide have relatively similar molecular weights such that the diffusion rate of oxygen in its gaseous phase is only 1.2 times that of CO_2. However, the solubility of CO_2 is 24 times that of oxygen. Therefore, the diffusion rate of CO_2 in blood (or alveolar-capillary interstitial fluid) is 20 times that of oxygen. Carbon dioxide diffuses out of blood along a continuously diminishing alveolar partial pressure gradient until it equilibrates with the partial pressure of carbon dioxide within the alveoli. Oxygen on the other hand, diffuses into blood where it rapidly chemically combines with hemoglobin, thereby maintaining the higher original pressure gradient until the hemoglobin is nearly completely saturated. This latter phenomenon, along with the fact that the original alveolar-arterial diffusion gradient for oxygen is 12 times greater than that for carbon dioxide, offsets the greater diffusion capability of CO_2 and allows adequate and metabolically proportional volumes of the gases to be exchanged per unit of time. This occurs within the first third of the approximately 0.75 seconds that blood is in transit through the alveolar-capillary unit, after which time partial pressures of the gases are usually equilibrated and no further net exchanges of volume occurs. Alveolar-capillary movement of these gases is said to be *perfusion limited* in that the rate of blood flow would have to be increased, thereby decreasing the transit time and allowing a greater volume of blood to be exposed to the alveolus per unit of time for more gas exchange to occur.

Oxygen is transported both physically dissolved in plasma and chemically combined with hemoglobin within erythrocytes. Dissolved oxygen amounts to 0.3 mL O_2/100 mL blood at a Po_2 of 100 mm Hg. This is hardly enough to meet even the resting oxygen consumption demands of approximately 300 mL O_2/ min of an adult at a normal cardiac output of 4 to 6 L/min. The remainder is bound with hemoglobin (Hb) in a rapidly reversible chemical association with hemoglobin molecules, each carrying four oxygen molecules. This *oxygen-carrying capacity* of hemoglobin amounts to 1.34 mL of O_2/g of hemoglobin. Therefore, the *oxygen content* (Cao_2) of 100 mL blood may be determined as follows:

$$Cao_2 = [Hb(g\%) \times 1.34 \times O_2 \text{ sat } (\%)] + 0.003(Pao_2)$$

The equilibrium point of this reversible reaction with Hb is dependent on the specific partial pressure of oxygen in plasma and the *oxyhemoglobin dissociation curve*. The oxyhemoglobin dissociation curve is simply a graphic plot relating the availability of oxygen in plasma (expressed as its partial pressure) to the amount of hemoglobin that has undergone this reversible reaction (expressed as percent saturation) (Fig. 16.13). This curve, as are those of most physiologic relations, is sigmoidal in configuration and is a function of hemoglobin's changing affinity for oxygen as it changes configuration with each successive release or acceptance of an oxygen molecule. The functional (and clinical) significance of this is that within a broad range of partial pressures, between 60 and 100 mm Hg, the affinity of hemoglobin for oxygen changes little, thereby allowing blood

to be highly saturated at relatively hypoxemic levels—that is, the "plateau" phase of the curve. Likewise, at levels of severe tissue hypoxia, in the range of 10 to 40 mm Hg, hemoglobin's affinity for oxygen rapidly diminishes, allowing for expeditious release of oxygen molecules to tissues—that is, the "steep" portion of the curve. Other chemical and physical influences, which represent physiologic changes that require alterations in the amount of oxygen available to tissues, also affect the slope of the oxyhemoglobin dissociation curve. High temperatures, low pH, high Pco_2, and elevated levels of 2,3-diphosphoglycerate (2,3-DPG) (a product of erythrocyte anaerobic glycolysis that decreases the affinity of hemoglobin for oxygen) shift the curve to the right. These alterations provide greater availability of oxygen for a low partial pressure of oxygen within the tissue. Low temperatures, high pH, low Pco_2, and decreased levels of 2,3-DPG shift the curve to the left. Physiologically, this is important centrally at the pulmonary capillary level where enhanced hemoglobin loading is required.

Arterial blood is 97.4% saturated at a normal Po_2 of 100 mm Hg, carrying 19.6 mL O_2/100 mL blood (assuming 15 gm Hb/100 mL blood). Arterial blood is 100% saturated at a Po_2 of 250 mm Hg, carrying 20.1 mL O_2/100 mL blood. Therefore, thanks to the phenomenon represented by the oxyhemoglobin dissociation curve, there exists little phylogenetic advantage to increasing partial pressures of oxygen to levels that could otherwise be toxic. Mixed venous blood is 75% saturated at a Po_2 of 40 mm Hg, carrying 15.1 mL O_2/100 mL blood. Cyanosis occurs when more than 5 gm/100 mL of arterial hemoglobin is in the unsaturated state. Clinically, this may be a sign of inadequate bulk circulatory transport of hemoglobin in blood, caused by increased oxygen extraction from hemoglobin. However, this may be misleading in an anemic state in which there is not enough hemoglobin to manifest cyanosis, or with polycythemic states where cyanosis may be apparent without hypoxemia.

Carbon dioxide is transported in blood largely as bicarbonate (80%–90%), but also in physical solution (5%–10%), and as a carbamino compound attached to blood proteins, predominantly deoxyhemoglobin (5%–10%). Carbonic anhydrase, present in erythrocytes, rapidly catalyzes the reversible conversion of carbon dioxide to bicarbonate at the tissue level in accordance with its partial pressure in plasma, giving off a hydrogen ion in the process. This hydrogen ion acidifies deoxyhemoglobin, shifting the oxyhemoglobin dissociation curve to the right and lowering the affinity of hemoglobin for oxygen. This *isohydric shift* occurs in reverse at the pulmonary capillary level and facilitates the efficient transport of CO_2 out of the body. Carbon dioxide transported as the carbamino radical is dissociated from oxyhemoglobin more readily than deoxyhemoglobin such that its dissociation curve is favorably influenced by higher oxygen saturations. Therefore, the carbon dioxide dissociation curve is shifted to the right at the pulmonary capillaries facilitating off-loading of CO_2, and to the left at the tissue level facilitating loading of CO_2.

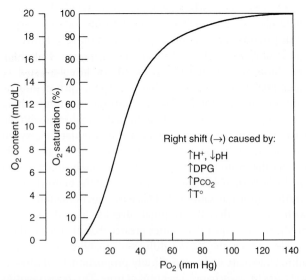

FIGURE 16.13 The oxyhemoglobin dissociation curve and factors affecting it as it relates to Po_2, oxygen saturation, and oxygen content. DPG, diphosphoglycerate. (From Miller A, Anderson OS. Blood acid-base alignment nomogram: scales for pH, Pco_2, base excess for whole blood of different hemoglobin concentrations, plasma bicarbonate, and plasma total-CO_2. *Scand J Clin Lab Invest* 1963;15:211; with permission.)

Pulmonary Acid–Base Balance

Buffering Systems

The primary regulators of acid–base homeostasis in the body are the lungs and the kidneys, the former being the acute-response mediator to abnormal changes in pH and the latter being the chronic-response mediator. Maintenance of plasma pH within the relatively strict range of 7.35 to 7.45 is important in maintaining the usual spatial configurations of most metabolically active proteins within the body. Their important functions are progressively impaired above or below this range. Maintenance of pH occurs through various *buffer* systems within the body, the major ones being the bicarbonate, protein, and phosphate buffer systems. These buffer systems accept hydrogen ions (H^+) that are created as a by-product of energy metabolism. The greatest source of H^+ is from the dissociation of carbonic acid, a volatile acid formed by the hydration of carbon dioxide following oxidation of glucose and fatty acids during aerobic metabolism. It accounts for more than 99% of the total acid production of the body. Another 0.2% of acid production comes from fixed acids, the result of anaerobic metabolism of glucose and oxidation of proteins and phospholipids that have been ingested as food.

The largest buffer system is the bicarbonate (HCO_3) buffer system, which consists of its weak acid—carbonic acid, and its conjugate base—bicarbonate. Its efficiency as a buffer for both volatile and fixed acids results from three characteristics. First, bicarbonate is in rapid equilibrium with CO_2 as follows:

$$\underset{\text{Gas}}{CO_2} \Longleftrightarrow \underset{\text{solution}}{CO_2} + H_2O \underset{\text{carbonic anhydrase}}{\Longleftrightarrow}$$

$$H_2CO_3 \Longleftrightarrow H^+ + HCO_3$$

Second, carbon dioxide is constantly and rapidly removed from the body through the lungs, thereby maintaining this reversible equilibrium in a leftward direction and creating additional bicarbonate to combine with fixed acid. Finally, the buffering capacity of bicarbonate per unit of pH for volatile acids (i.e., CO_2) is enhanced four to five times in

the presence of hemoglobin. This occurs because of the imidazole-buffering group within the histidine residues of most plasma and blood proteins that act as weak acids, hemoglobin being the protein in greatest quantity. The dissociation constant (pK) of a histidine residue depends upon the specific plasma protein of which it is a part, and has a generally broad pK range of 5.5 to 8.5. The pK for hemoglobin ranges between 7 and 8, with deoxyhemoglobin exhibiting the higher pK. Therefore, hemoglobin can accept much of the hydrogen ion created by CO_2 production and the subsequent dissociation of carbonic acid, thereby freeing the bicarbonate ion and increasing the overall buffering capacity.

There are other buffer systems of less importance. The major inorganic phosphate buffer system, dihydrogen phosphate, has a pK of approximately 6.8 and has little extracellular buffering function within the usual pH range of blood and interstitial fluid. However, many organic phosphates have pK within +/− 0.5 pH units of 7.0 and, therefore, may have an important role in intracellular acid–base homeostasis. They also act in a chronic buffering capacity as the phosphate salt of hydroxyapatite in bone.

Acidosis and Alkalosis

Acid–base disorders may be divided into four major categories: respiratory acidosis, respiratory alkalosis, metabolic acidosis, and metabolic alkalosis. These primary acid–base disorders may occur singly or in combination (mixed), or may be compensated by homeostatic mechanisms of the body (Table 16.2). Values for arterial blood pH, P_{CO_2}, and HCO_3 may be measured and the base deficit (excess) calculated. Application of these values to various available acid–base nomograms may assist one in determining the type of derangement and the degree of compensation for a particular clinical circumstance (Fig. 16.14).

Respiratory acidosis is manifested as an increase in arterial P_{CO_2} and a decrease in arterial pH and is the result of a relatively short-term impairment in alveolar ventilation. Bicarbonate ion is usually slightly increased as a result of dissociation of carbonic acid and buffering of

TABLE 16.2

Acid–Base Disturbances

	pH	P_{CO_2}	HCO^-_3
Uncompensated respiratory acidosis	↓↓	↑↑	↑
Uncompensated respiratory alkalosis	↑↑	↓↓	↓
Uncompensated metabolic acidosis	↓↓	—	↓↓
Uncompensated metabolic alkalosis	↑↑	—	↑↑
Partially compensated respiratory acidosis	↓	↑↑	↑↑
Partially compensated respiratory alkalosis	↑	↓↓	↓↓
Partially compensated metabolic acidosis	↓	↓↓	↓↓
Partially compensated metabolic alkalosis	↑	↑↑	↑↑
Respiratory and metabolic acidosis	↓↓	↑↑	↓
Respiratory and metabolic alkalosis	↑↑	↓↓	↑

From Levitzky ME. *The regulation of acid-base status. Pulmonary physiology*, 5th ed. New York: McGraw-Hill, 1999:182; with permission.

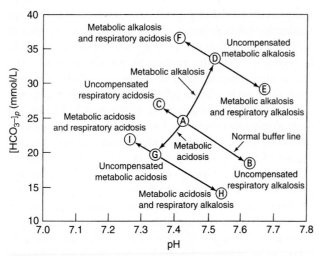

FIGURE 16.14 Acid–base relations in compensated and uncompensated pathologic states as they relate to the norm (*A*). (From Davenport HW. *The ABCs of acid-base chemistry*, 6th ed. Chicago: The University of Chicago Press, 1974:3–49; with permission.)

the hydrogen ion is therefore produced by nonbicarbonate anions. There are several causes of respiratory acidosis. They generally fall into the categories of restrictive pathology, parenchyma infiltrative disease, neuromuscular disorders, airway obstruction, or depression of the respiratory control center. One of the more common causes in the perioperative period or following trauma is "splinting" associated with pain.

Respiratory alkalosis is associated with conditions that promote hyperventilation, or overventilation, and is manifested as a decrease in P_{CO_2} and an increase in pH. Bicarbonate ion is slightly decreased. Predominant reasons for respiratory alkalosis include hypoxia from a variety of causes, hyperthermia, anxiety, and toxic or neurogenic triggers. A very common cause in the perioperative period is overventilation of the patient on a ventilator.

Metabolic acidosis, although a nonrespiratory acidosis, does have a respiratory compensatory mechanism; specifically, hyperventilation in an effort to "blow off" excessive CO_2 formed by neutralization of the hydrogen ion by bicarbonate. It has several causes: the ingestion, infusion or production of *fixed acids*; decreased renal excretion of hydrogen ions; intracellular to extracellular exchange of hydrogen ions; or loss of bicarbonate ions from the extracellular compartment. It is recognized by a decrease in pH *and* bicarbonate ion despite a relatively normal P_{CO_2}. Common problems producing metabolic acidosis include tissue hypoxia (lactic acidosis produced by shock, ischemic organs, etc.), ketogenesis (ketoacidosis produced by diabetic stress, overfeeding, etc.), fistulae and diarrhea (loss of bicarbonate), renal dysfunction, and ethanol or salicylate poisoning.

Because electrical neutrality is required among the major electrolytes (Na^+, K^+, Cl^- and $HCO3^-$) within plasma, an *anion gap* greater than 12 ± 4 (which represents the *plasma protein anion* contribution) suggests that a fixed acid

anion is likely the reason for existing acidosis. Immediate, temporary correction is accomplished by administration of bicarbonate according to the formula: mM $HCO_3 =$ (base deficit × kilogram body weight) (0.3), where 0.3 equals percent extracellular fluid volume.

Metabolic alkalosis is also a nonrespiratory acid–base derangement. It is present when pH is high and bicarbonate is elevated in the presence of a relatively normal P_{CO_2}. When not caused by direct hydrogen ion losses, as with nasogastric suction or vomiting, its occurrence is closely tied to sodium and potassium flux mediated through the kidney. Volume contraction caused by diuretic therapy activates the renin–aldosterone mechanism in an effort to retain sodium and fluid. Electrical neutrality of this large flux of sodium is accomplished by chloride and bicarbonate at the expense of potassium and hydrogen ion. Because chloride is the major anion accompanying the loss of these latter anions, bicarbonate is the predominant anion retained. Through a similar mechanism, chronic, high-dose steroid administration may also result in metabolic alkalosis (21).

Pulmonary compensation involves chemoreceptor mechanisms to decrease alveolar ventilation and increase CO_2 production, thereby shifting the equilibrium of the bicarbonate buffer system to the right, producing H^+ to neutralize $HCO3^-$. This has obvious implications (i.e., induction of hypoventilation) when attempting to wean a patient from a ventilator. Ultimate correction of metabolic alkalosis requires volume re-expansion with sodium and, more importantly, potassium chloride containing fluids. Total body potassium deficit is therefore corrected through intracellular exchange of H^+ for K^+ with neutralization of excess $HCO3^-$. Extracellular volume correction with sodium chloride suppresses the renin–aldosterone system with subsequent normalization of ion exchange at the kidney.

PULMONARY FUNCTION ASSESSMENT

Pulmonary Function Testing

Assessment of pulmonary function is basic to most interventions undertaken in surgical practice, whether it is determining the feasibility of surgical resection of the lung, the ability to achieve adequate pulmonary toilet postoperatively, or the ability to wean patients from a ventilator. Basic pulmonary function tests are derived from dynamic considerations of the basic lung volumes previously discussed and are primarily determined by means of *spirometric* testing. The best measure of overall ventilatory function is the *maximal voluntary ventilation* (MVV). This is the largest volume of air (achieved by forced hyperventilation) that can be moved in and out of the lungs in 1 minute. It is a qualitative measure of overall aerobic conditioning and indirectly assesses lung volumes, airway resistance, and respiratory muscle strength and stamina. It is determined by eliciting maximal inspiratory and expiratory effort consistently for 15 seconds during spirometric testing and subsequently extrapolating this volume to 1 minute. Normal MVV in an adult is 125 to 170 L/min. Values less than 50% of predicted for body surface area are predictive of increased risk for major abdominal or thoracic surgery. Values less than 50 L/min place a patient at an extremely high risk of postoperative complications.

Forced vital capacity (FVC) is the difference between the TLC (maximal inspiration) and the RV (maximal expiration) and, indirectly, is an assessment of inspiratory and expiratory muscle strength, thoracic compliance, and airway resistance. From a clinical perspective, it is an indication of a patient's ability to inspire deeply and cough postoperatively. It is the same as *forced expiratory volume* (FEV) when exhalation is complete. When determined by spirometry, an asymptotic curve is inscribed toward RV over time. The slope of this curve is steepest within the first second (FEV$_1$), during which time between 70% and 80% of VC is exhaled by a normal

individual (Fig. 16.15). Airway resistance is most susceptible to changes within this first second because intrapleural pressures affecting compressible small airways, as well as airflow turbulence is greatest during that time. Because vital capacities vary for different body sizes and various restrictive pathologic or physiologic conditions, a more accurate means of expressing airway resistance is to index FEV within the first second (FEV$_1$) to the patient's own FVC. A ratio less than 0.7 would be considered abnormal, and a ratio less than 0.5 would be considered predictive of increased risk for major surgery.

The inflection point of the FEV curve occurs much more quickly within the first second in patients with airway obstruction and continues over a longer period of time as increased airway resistance must be overcome. Under these circumstances, a more precise quantification of airway

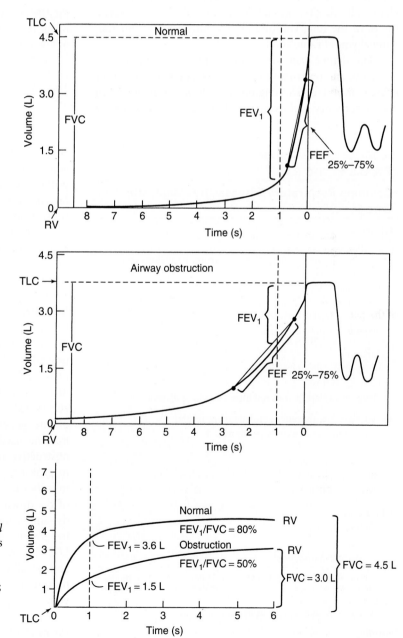

FIGURE 16.15   A and B: Tracing from a *water-filled spirometer* illustrating the segment of a forced vital capacity (FVC) acquisition analyzed for forced expiratory volume (FEV$_1$) and FEV$_{25-75}$ determinations. **C:** A more contemporary *rolling seal spirometer* tracing illustrating similar determinations in a normal individual (*upper trace*) and an individual with chronic obstructive pulmonary disease (COPD) (*lower trace*). FEF, described in text; RV, residual volume. (From Levitzky MG. *Pulmonary physiology*, 5th ed. New York: McGraw-Hill, 1999; with permission.)

resistance would be the FEV during the middle 50% of expiration (FEV_{25-75}). This is also called *maximal mid-expiratory flow rate* (MMFR). Reductions in FEV_1: FVC and MMFR reflect significant airway obstruction that may be related to bronchospasm, secretions, compression, or an intraluminal mass. Most often, however, a reduced FEV_1 reflects the reactive airway disease of COPD, which may have an active component (bronchospasm) as well as a fixed, irreversible component. Therefore, measurements of FEV_1 are usually obtained with and without bronchodilators to help clarify therapeutic possibilities.

Whereas obstructive disease interferes with airflow, restrictive disease interferes with lung expansion. Restrictive lung diseases, therefore, will frequently have a normal FEV_1/FVC, but a reduction in VC, TLC, RV, and FRC. Restrictive diseases include those for which work of breathing must be increased to overcome either the elastic recoil of the chest wall (obesity, skeletal deformities, etc.), or the elastic forces of the lung (fibrotic or infiltrative diseases of lung parenchyma) (Table 16.3).

Flow-volume loops are useful in differentiating between restrictive and obstructive lung disease, and between certain subsets of obstructive lung disease. Flow-volume loops are both inspiratory *and* expiratory FVC curves where airflow

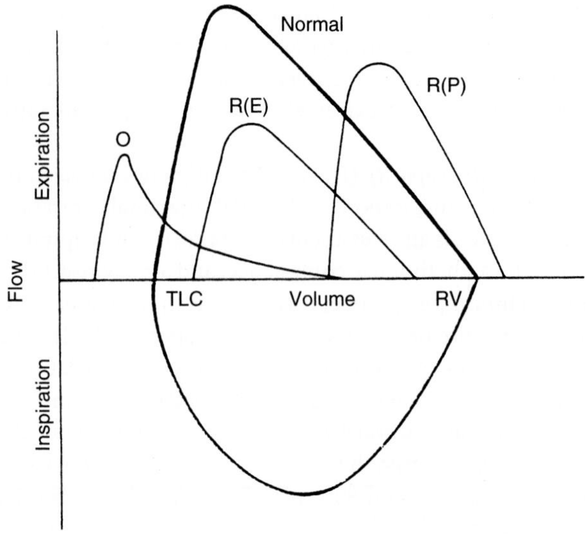

FIGURE 16.16 Schematic flow-volume loops qualitatively comparing the norm with those of restrictive and obstructive categories of lesions. O, obstructive parenchymal disease; R(E), extraparenchymal restrictive disease; R(P), parenchymal restrictive disease; TLC, total lung capacity; RV, residual volume. (From Weinberger SE. *Principles of pulmonary medicine*, 2nd ed. Philadelphia: WB Saunders, 1992; with permission.)

TABLE 16.3

Common Respiratory Diseases by Diagnostic Categories[a]

Obstructive
Asthma
Chronic obstructive lung disease (chronic bronchitis and emphysema)
Bronchiectasis
Cystic fibrosis
Bronchiolitis

Restrictive: parenchymal
Sarcoidosis
Idiopathic pulmonary fibrosis
Pneumoconiosis
Drug- or radiation-induced interstitial lung disease

Restrictive: extraparenchymal, neuromuscular
Diaphragmatic weakness/paralysis
Myasthenia gravis[b]
Guillain-Barre syndrome[b]
Muscular dystrophies[b]
Cervical spine injury[b]

Chest wall
Kyphoscoliosis
Obesity
Ankylosing spondylitis[b]

[a]From Weinberger SE, Drazen JM. Disturbances of respiratory function. *Harvey textbook of medicine*. Philadelphia: WB Saunders, 1990:389, with permission.

[b]Can have inspiratory and expiratory limitation.

is plotted against a patient's lung volume (Fig. 16.16). The inscribed expiratory curve consists of an *effort-dependent* portion (upslope) where transpulmonary pressure gradient *exceeds* airway resistance and an *effort-independent* portion (downslope) where intrapleural pressure *equals* the pressure inside compressible airways and the transpulmonary pressure gradient becomes zero. At this inflection point, intrapleural pressure equals the resistive forces of the smaller, collapsible airways and the intrinsic elastic recoil of the lung becomes a passive, and the only, driving force of exhalation—that is, effort-independent. Because flow-volume loops cycle between RV and TLC, neither of which is measurable by spirometry, quantitative flow-volume loops are not possible without deriving these volumes by means of one of several sophisticated methods (body plethysmography, nitrogen-washout technique, etc.). Fortunately, individual curves exhibit specific characteristics that are indicative of the general category of pathology in question, and may be used *qualitatively*. Although both restrictive and obstructive diseases usually exhibit a substantial *decrease* in peak expiratory flow, obstructive lung disease uniquely inscribes a signature *concave* (effort-independent) portion of the down slope of the expiratory curve. This represents dynamic compression of unsupported terminal bronchioles by alveolar septae that seriously retards passive airflow. Likewise, as will be discussed later, various intrathoracic and extrathoracic upper airway lesions may be characterized by uniquely truncated inspiratory and/or expiratory flow-volume loops.

Diffusing capacity for carbon monoxide (D_{LCO}) is a means for assessing the integrity of the alveolar-capillary barrier.

As previously discussed, certain factors limit the diffusion of a gas through the alveolar-capillary barrier. These factors are: (i) diffusion coefficient of the gas, (ii) the thickness and surface area of the barrier; and (iii) the difference in partial pressures between the alveolus and capillary plasma. Carbon monoxide (CO), like oxygen, binds with hemoglobin. Because of the low alveolar concentrations necessary for safety, the content of CO in hemoglobin never reaches full saturation. Furthermore, because CO—unlike oxygen—chemically binds irreversibly with hemoglobin, its partial pressure in plasma is virtually zero. Therefore, equilibration of CO does not occur essentially eliminating its partial pressure influence in plasma. Therefore, the gradient for its diffusion remains constant and its hemoglobin concentration steadily continues to rise for the entire time that erythrocytes traverse the alveolar-capillary unit. The content of CO in blood is thereby limited only by the properties of the alveolar-capillary barrier and is said to be *diffusion limited*. Clinically, comparison of the D_{LCO} of an individual with pulmonary disease, as a percentage of his normal predicted diffusion capacity, is indicative of a proportionate restriction by the alveolar-capillary barrier to other gases—in particular, oxygen. Diseases that increase the thickness or density of the interstitium, infiltrate the alveoli, limit surface area for diffusion, or promote $\dot{V}/\dot{Q}$ mismatch may decrease D_{LCO}. Because the transfer of CO from plasma to hemoglobin is required to maintain its constant partial pressure, anemia, low cardiac output, or significant hypovolemia may also decrease D_{LCO}. A D_{LCO} value less than 50% of predicted is considered to be predictive of an increased risk for major surgery.

Significant diffusion block may also be assessed by a simpler method that consists of comparisons of preexercise and postexercise partial pressures of oxygen in standard arterial blood gases. Ordinarily, partial pressures of O_2 rapidly equilibrate between plasma and hemoglobin within the first one third (0.25 second) of pulmonary capillary blood transit time through the alveolar-capillary unit. Arterial *desaturation* following exercise suggests, therefore, that diffusion is so impaired that any decrease in transit time across the alveolar-capillary membrane abolishes all reserve for O_2 equilibration, and results in an increased right-to-left intrapulmonary shunt. The amount of arterial desaturation is proportional to the severity of the diffusion block. A fall in arterial saturation below 90% is considered indicative of a severe degree of alveolar-capillary block. A resting arterial P_{O_2} of 60 mmHg or saturation of 90% or less places an individual at the limit of reserve on his oxyhemoglobin dissociation curve and is predictive of substantially increased morbidity and mortality after an operation. Similarly, another indicator of alveolar-capillary block is *elevation* of the partial pressure of CO_2 in arterial blood. The diffusion of CO_2 is 20 times that of oxygen. Homeostatic chemoreceptor and medullary control centers are so sensitive to changes in CO_2 that it is normally kept within a tight range approximately 40 ± 5 mm Hg. Therefore, a resting arterial blood gas P_{CO_2} in excess of 45 mm Hg in an otherwise nonsedated individual should alert one to the possibility that substantial impairment of the alveolar-capillary barrier may exist. Further compromise of available alveolar-capillary units for gas exchange, either by resection of pulmonary parenchyma or by exclusion as a result of atelectasis or consolidation, would seriously impair oxygen delivery to tissues.

Pulmonary stress testing is a sophisticated method of *quantitatively* assessing the overall aerobic conditioning of a patient. It is based on the premise that carbon dioxide production and elimination is proportionate to oxygen consumption with increasing exercise up to a certain level, after which the capacity for *aerobic metabolism* is exceeded. To meet subsequent increasing energy demands, *anaerobic metabolism* must then be initiated through the Emden-Meyerhoff glycolytic pathway. The end product of this pathway is lactic acid, which increases CO_2 production *without* an increase in oxygen consumption ($V_{O_{2max}}$). When measured with a capnometer during progressive treadmill exercise, this inflection in the CO_2 curve—the *anaerobic threshold*—represents the point of maximal oxygen consumption, and is an estimate of overall oxygen delivery to the patient (22). Although many factors influence the anaerobic threshold, including one's cardiovascular status and oxygen carrying capability (hemoglobin level), a substantial decrease in oxygen consumption at anaerobic threshold may be attributed to predominantly pulmonary factors if these other conditions are minimal or absent. Clinical correlation has shown that V_{O_2}max greater than 20 mL O_2/ kg body weight/min at anaerobic threshold, or at symptom limitation, is associated with the least postoperative morbidity and mortality. On the other hand, $V_{O_{2max}}$ less than 10 mL O_2/kg/min is associated with very high postoperative morbidity and substantial mortality (23).

Quantitative lung perfusion radionuclide scanning is useful in predicting postresection lung volumes and diffusing capacity, and has been shown to correlate with postoperative morbidity and mortality. Its usefulness relies on the distribution of I^{131} radiolabeled albumin to various perfused areas of the lung where relative count densities can be quantified by radionuclide scintigraphy. Its predictive accuracy is predicated upon the phenomenon that ventilation essentially matches perfusion, largely due to local hypoxic vasoconstriction. Therefore, that percentage of lung that manifests radionuclide uptake remaining after resection should approximate a similar percentage of the preresection functioning lung. This method is most useful in predicting morbidity and mortality following pneumonectomy where a predicted postresection FEV_1 of less than 0.8 L or a predicted postoperative DLCO of 40% or less has been shown to be associated with excessive risk (24). It is also useful in lesser resections where poor pulmonary function occurs with heterogeneous parenchymal disease as determined by computed tomography (CT) scanning. In the absence of heterogeneous pulmonary parenchymal disease, postresection predicted pulmonary function may be similarly screened without quantitative perfusion scanning by assuming that each of 19 *functional* bronchopulmonary segments (the left apical-posterior segment counts as two segments) equally contributes approximately 5.26% of functioning lung volume. The predicted postresection FEV_1 (PPFEV$_1$) is then calculated as follows: PPFEV$_1$ = FEV_1 × [1 − (segments resected × 0.0526)].

In summary, correlation of various pulmonary function tests can guide one to the basic physiologic deficits involved in patients being evaluated for major surgical intervention (see Appendix C). Acceptable risks for the development of pulmonary complications following major elective surgery may be expected when the following preresection pulmonary function values are exceeded: mandatory minute ventilation (MMV) greater than 50%, FEV_1 greater than 1.8 L for pneumonectomy and greater than 1.0 for lobectomy, PPFEV$_1$ ± 0.8 L, D$_{LCO}$ greater than 60% or PPD$_{LCO}$ greater than 40%, V$_{O2max}$ greater than 15 mL/kg/min and exercise O_2 saturation greater than 90%. *Relative* contraindications to major elective surgery or pulmonary resection include a resting arterial P$_{O2}$ less than 65 mm Hg, a resting arterial P$_{CO2}$ greater than 45 mm Hg, and an MMV less than 35% (25).

Clinical Assessment

Pulmonary performance may be estimated by clinical assessment as well as through formal testing, and both should be taken into account in the surgical decision making process. As previously alluded to, morbidly obese patients, elderly patients, and patients with skeletal muscle deformities such as kyphoscoliosis generally have a substantial restrictive thoracic component to their pulmonary function as a result of decreased chest wall compliance. A history of sarcoidosis, pneumoconiosis-related employment (miner, shipbuilder, chemical worker, etc.), or chemoradiation therapy usually implies further restrictive pulmonary parenchymal disease.

Resting tachypnea is a sensitive indicator of substantial, usually acute or subacute, deficit in respiratory reserve and generally is a harbinger of eventual respiratory failure. It may be secondary to several factors, such as compliance or diffusion problems related to congestive heart failure or pneumonia, obstructive problems associated with bronchospasm and hyperinflation, or excessive CO_2 production resulting from lactic or ketoacidosis, or caloric overfeeding (Table 16.4). *Conversational dyspnea*, similarly, is sometimes seen in patients with more chronic and very marginal pulmonary function, and is manifested by an inability to complete a sentence without requiring a second or third breath. Supraclavicular and intercostal space retraction, recruitment of accessory muscles of respiration, elevated shoulder girdles, and *paradoxical breathing* in which the thoracic and abdominal compartments move opposite one another, are all indicative of pathologically increased intrapleural pressure swings suggesting significant obstructive airway disease. Asthenic body habitus or frank muscle wasting may suggest chronically increased energy requirements dedicated to work of breathing. A prolonged expiratory phase of respiration and associated end-expiratory wheezing indicate increased small airway resistance. These can be found accompanying active bronchospasm or the peribronchiolar

---

TABLE 16.4

Major Factors Determining Balance between Ventilatory Supply and Demand[a]

Factors limiting ventilatory supply[b]

Respiratory muscle weakness (e.g., fatigue)

Unfavorable length–tension relation (e.g., due to lung hyperinflation)

Airway obstruction (e.g., asthma)

Restricted obstruction (e.g., pneumonia)

Factors raising ventilatory demand[c]

High physiologic dead space:tidal volume ratio (V$_D$:V$_T$, e.g., emphysema)

Elevated minute oxygen consumption and hence CO_2 production (e.g., sepsis)

Respiratory quotient (RQ) >1.0 (e.g., excessive carbohydrate feeding)

Maintaining arterial P$_{CO2}$ <36 mm Hg (e.g., due to metabolic acidosis)

[a]From Lanken PN. Mechanical ventilatory support. In: Wilson JD, Baunwald E, Isselbacher KJ, et al. eds. *Harrison's principles of internal medicine*, 12th ed. New York: McGraw-Hill, 1991:1125. Reprinted by permission.

[b]The maximal sustainable ventilation (MSV), which is usually equal to—*frac*12 maximal voluntary ventilation (MVV).

[c]The spontaneous minute ventilation (V$_E$) needed to maintain a certain arterial P$_{CO2}$ set by the patient's central neuronal drive. If this V$_G$ is greater than the patient's MSV, the patient will develop respiratory muscle fatigue at that V$_G$.

"cuffing" of interstitial pulmonary edema. *Stridor* indicates large airway obstruction, usually involving the larynx, trachea, or a mainstem bronchus.

Increased anterior-posterior diameter of the chest wall, outwardly flared costal margins, distant breath sounds on auscultation and hyper resonance to percussion, along with chest radiographic findings of a flattened diaphragm, increased intercostal spacing, hyperlucent lung fields, and an increased anterior retrosternal space on lateral view should alert one to the presence of advanced stages of obstructive pulmonary disease with associated severe hyperinflation. Because these patients begin tidal respirations from very high functional residual capacities, many would be incapable of recruiting adequate inspiratory or expiratory reserves or of generating adequate intrapleural pressures to overcome increased airway resistance that would be required to create necessary airflow within the perioperative period. Total thoracic compliance is also decreased at very high lung volumes and inspiratory muscles are weaker by virtue of their inefficient tension–length relations. Therefore, work of breathing rapidly increases with exercise, producing early dyspnea. This is the basis of the simple two-flight stair climbing test sometimes used to screen patients for major surgery.

Finally, a patient's overall physiologic fitness level may be assessed by one of several semiquantitative performance status scales that relate a patient's particular level of physical ability or fitness to a predicted risk of morbidity or mortality.

The *Karnofsky Performance Scale* is one of the more enduring of these, and ranks a patient between 1 and 100 in increments of 10 as to his or her need for assistance or ability to perform normal activities or do active work (see Appendix B) (26). A score below 60 generally suggests increased risk and/or marginal benefit from a major intervention.

Physiologic Variations in Respiration

Exercise

Exercise increases the metabolic demand of working muscles, thereby increasing the demand for oxygen and increasing the production of carbon dioxide. Excessive exercise, surpassing the anaerobic threshold, induces anaerobic glycolysis and the production of lactic acid. In order to meet these increasing oxygen demands, the cardiorespiratory system must modify accordingly. Much larger V_{TS} are induced as a result of the effects of increased P_{CO_2} and hydrogen ions on chemoreceptors, and V_E may increase up to 25-fold. Greater intrapleural pressures and airflow turbulence and decreased lung compliance contribute to increased airway resistance and work of breathing. Mouth breathing occurs to lessen that portion of airway resistance contributed by the nasopharynx, and lip-pursing sometimes occurs to sustain auto-positive end-expiratory pressure (PEEP) and increase FRC.

Cardiac output may increase four to six times that of resting cardiac output with exercise. The resultant increased pulmonary blood flow and pressure results in recruitment of capillaries, primarily in zones one and two, thereby minimizing $\dot{V}/\dot{Q}$ mismatching and alveolar dead-space. Furthermore, alveolar-capillary unit transit time is decreased and, in conjunction with better $\dot{V}/\dot{Q}$ matching, substantially increases partial pressure gradients for diffusion. A further factor enhancing alveolar diffusion gradients is an increased *extraction ratio for oxygen* (ER_{O_2}). This is, in essence, the ratio of oxygen consumption (V_{O_2}) relative to oxygen delivery (D_{O_2}), both being determined, in part, by cardiac output (Q) as follows:

$$ER_{O_2} = V_{O_2}/D_{O_2} = Q \times (Ca_{O_2} - Cv_{O_2})/Q \times Ca_{O_2}$$

This relation is constant until oxygen demand exceeds oxygen supply, at which time anaerobic metabolism increases the production of carbon dioxide. Because cardiac output, rather than ventilation, is normally the limiting factor in meeting the metabolic demands of exercise, mixed-venous blood returning to the lungs will have an exaggeratedly low P_{O_2} and high P_{CO_2}. This is because, at the tissue level, the factors of increased heat production as a result of exercise, lactic acidosis, hypercapnia, and increased erythrocyte levels of 2,3 DPG (a result of anaerobic glycolysis) shift the oxyhemoglobin dissociation curve to the right, facilitating oxygen off-loading to the tissues.

As exercise levels further increase, particularly to extremes, the *alveolar-arterial* P_{O_2} *difference* (A-a D_{O_2}) increases from approximately 5 to 15 mm Hg at normal rest in a normal, untrained, healthy individual to 20 to 30 mm Hg. This is due to a number of factors: intrapulmonary shunting as a result of pulmonary hypertension, increased oxygen extraction resulting in more desaturation of shunted blood at the central level, and *relative* diffusion limitation of oxygen transfer at the alveolar level. This relative desaturation serves to restrict progressively more intense activity and therefore mitigate the development of adverse effects such as pulmonary edema and certain other physically detrimental effects that might result from continuation to extreme exhaustion.

Altitude

The effects of altitude on respiration are primarily the result of effects of lowered barometric pressure in determining partial pressures of oxygen and carbon dioxide in the alveoli vis-à-vis the alveolar gas equation. Ambient air at any elevation contains oxygen at a concentration of 21%. Therefore, as one ascends, the barometric pressure decreases and the partial pressure of inspired oxygen (P_{IO_2}) also decreases. The amount of oxygen absorbed in blood is therefore decreased because mixed-venous partial pressure remains relatively unchanged (i.e., there exists a decreased partial-pressure gradient).

HPV is an adaptive mechanism to localized areas of under ventilated lung that is thought to result from a local oxygen-sensitive, K^+/CA^+ voltage-gated mechanism of arteriolar smooth muscle (27). This tends to redistribute pulmonary arteriolar blood flow to better-ventilated alveolar-capillary units and therefore minimize pulmonary venous desaturation. If these areas are extensive such as might be encountered at high altitudes involving the entire lung, ubiquitous vasoconstriction substantially elevates pulmonary artery pressure. This may overwhelm localized HPV as well as increase pulmonary hydrostatic pressure resulting in increased physiologic shunting and pulmonary edema.

Certain early compensatory mechanisms occur to reverse high-altitude hypoxemia. The hypoxic ventilatory drive increases V_E resulting in hypocapnia and a reciprocal increase in Pa_{O_2}. Hypoxia also causes reflex bronchoconstriction, which may reduce $\dot{V}/\dot{Q}$ mismatch by increasing mean airway pressure in distal bronchioles (*auto-PEEP*) and FRC. Work of breathing also increases with the need to increase V_E. Cardiac output is increased through chemoreceptor-mediated sympathetic reflexes and hypoxic pulmonary vasoconstriction leads to increased pulmonary arteriolar pressure, both of which minimize zone one $\dot{V}/\dot{Q}$ mismatch by augmenting capillary recruitment. An increased extraction ratio augments diffusion at the alveolar level, and hyperventilation respiratory alkalosis favors a higher saturation of central hemoglobin by virtue of a leftward shift in the oxyhemoglobin dissociation curve.

Hypoxia stimulates erythropoietin during acclimatization, and a later increase in hemoglobin occurs resulting in increased oxygen carrying capacity. Unfortunately, increased blood viscosity secondary to an elevated hematocrit and chronic pulmonary vasoconstriction also increase right ventricular work. Early respiratory alkalosis is ultimately alleviated by increased renal excretion of bicarbonate.

Immersion and Diving

The effects of immersion and diving are largely secondary to the physical laws pertaining to gravity and density acting on a column of water. Specifically, for every 33 ft of salt water (or 34 ft of fresh water), the ambient pressure is increased by one atmosphere (760 mm Hg). Accordingly, the volume of compressible gases in the alveolar spaces is proportionately decreased as the partial pressures and densities are reciprocally increased (*Boyle and Dalton Laws*). Similarly, the amount of gas dissolved in tissues is increased (*Henry Law*, see Glossary).

Immersion to the neck subjects the chest wall to greater than atmospheric pressure, which opposes the outward elastic recoil of the thorax and substantially reduces the FRC by approximately 50%. It also creates less negative intrapleural pressure. In addition, venous pooling in gravity-dependent regions is minimized and hypothermia-induced peripheral vasoconstriction occurs, increasing both the central venous and atrial pressures. The net result is a 60% increase in work of breathing and a 30% increase in cardiac output. $\dot{V}/\dot{Q}$ matching is enhanced by virtue of increased pulmonary arteriolar pressures and capillary recruitment, and "immersion-diuresis" is induced as the result of hormonal modulation through pressure-sensitive atrial receptors.

Below-surface breath-holding initiates additional physiologic changes. Bradycardia and increased systemic vascular resistance, the "diving reflex," limits oxygen consumption by restricting blood flow to most vascular beds with redistribution to auto-regulated vital organs. Alveolar partial pressures of oxygen and carbon dioxide are increased thereby facilitating oxygen saturation of hemoglobin, albeit tending to restrict off-loading of carbon dioxide to the alveolus. Hyperventilating before a dive increases dive efficiency by blowing off CO_2. By reducing P_{CO_2} in such a manner, the P_{AO_2} is increased and the oxyhemoglobin dissociation curve is shifted leftward, both augmenting hemoglobin saturation. Furthermore, the gradient for CO_2 diffusion is enhanced.

Diving at relatively great depths, as with SCUBA gear below 100 ft, elicits certain additional unique phenomena. *Nitrogen narcosis* develops as the result of increasing partial pressures of nitrogen with increasing depth, in accordance with Dalton Law, leading to increased solution of this gas within the blood. The effects of this are diminished neuronal function manifested as confusion and loss of judgment—so-called "rapture of the deep"—as well as loss of dexterity. Other phenomena particular to the ascent also may occur. Densely compressed gases isolated within the lung and tissues of the body may rapidly expand and come out of solution with rapid ascent in accordance with Boyle and Henry laws. Without means for equilibration, rupture of alveoli into capillaries, or "effervescence," of usually insoluble nitrogen can result in macro- or microemboli, respectively, with subsequent microvascular occlusion—so-called "bends."

With *breath-hold* deep dives, ascent causes lung volume expansion and a further decrease in partial pressure of already reduced oxygen within the alveolus. Sufficient hypoxemia may occur at a shallow depth causing loss of consciousness, termed *shallow-water blackout*. Alveolar oxygen partial pressure equilibration may be partially achieved with exhalation during the ascent, and is involuntarily facilitated by the Hering-Breuer inflation reflex.

PATHOPHYSIOLOGIC RESPIRATION

As must be apparent by now, precise interaction of components of the respiratory system at many levels must occur for adequate gas exchange to be accomplished. Efficient lung function depends on a balance between the inward elastic recoil of the lung parenchyma and the outward elastic recoil of the chest wall. Conditions that alter the balance between inward and outward forces, either by violation of the integrity of the thorax or the lung, or by alteration in the elastic characteristics of either, will adversely affect one's ability to ventilate. Neurologic diseases that affect the chest wall musculature or the diaphragm can affect the patient's ability to expand the intrathoracic space and create sufficient negative pressures to adequately ventilate. Diseases that result in deformity of the chest wall or cause fibrosis of the lung decrease the compliance, thereby requiring increased work of breathing to expand the lung. Voluntary or involuntary "splinting" secondary to pain may also limit the degree of chest expansion and, secondarily, contribute to $\dot{V}/\dot{Q}$ abnormalities. Major obstruction of the upper airways impedes the flow of air into the lungs, although the lungs and thorax themselves may be functioning normally. Causes of this may be trauma, tumor, inflammation, foreign body, or secretions. Inflammatory diseases of the lung, extrinsic compression of the lung, or occlusive pulmonary arterial pathology, among other causes, can contribute to abnormal $\dot{V}/\dot{Q}$ relations. Sepsis, extracorporeal perfusion, and destructive processes of the alveolar-capillary unit illustrate a few of the pathologic conditions that can interfere with diffusion of gases across the alveolar-capillary barrier. The CO created with smoking and certain other toxins interfere with oxygen transport in the blood.

In this section, categories of respiratory pathology will be broadly examined with respect to specific defects in ventilation or respiration. Where applicable, the appropriate interventions to correct or prevent the problem, and relevant information useful in decision making in this regard, will be discussed. It should be realized that, while specifically categorized, many of these pathologic conditions may also manifest several other categories of impairment to a greater or lesser degree.

Airway Obstruction

Large Airway Obstruction

The primary pathophysiologic impairment in airway obstruction is an increase in airway resistance, necessitating greater intrapleural pressure swings to provide adequate pressure gradients for airflow and passive alveolar expansion.

Forced expiration is also required to prevent hyperinflation and maintain acceptable thoracic compliance. Large airway obstructions are either fixed (foreign body, tumor, extrinsic compression, stricture) or variable (tracheomalacia, obstructive sleep apnea, etc.), the distinction being made by whether or not the diameter of the large airway is significantly affected by changes in transpleural pressure. Cartilaginous rings support the trachea such that its diameter is virtually uninfluenced by changes in intrapleural pressure. Therefore, when intraluminal obstruction or extrinsic compression substantially narrows the lumen (fixed obstruction), effort-dependent airflow is limited at some point during both inspiration and expiration. This results in a flow-volume loop that is truncated with a constant plateau—in accordance with Poiseuille Law (see Glossary)—before the inspiratory and expiratory peaks, normalizing only after effort-independent airflow reaches the equal pressure point (Fig. 16.17).

In pathologic circumstances where cartilaginous tracheal support is lacking (i.e., tracheomalacia) or pharyngeal muscles are either flaccid (neurologic) or restricted from full contraction because of fatty deposition (obstructive sleep apnea), the diameter of the airway is influenced by changes in intrapleural pressure. These "variable obstructions" are further diagnostically separable as to whether they are intrathoracic or extrathoracic by examining their flow-volume loops. With *extrathoracic* variable obstruction, such as with obstructive sleep apnea, forced expiration increases the diameter of the airway and inscribes a normal expiratory curve. With inspiration, however, the intrapleural, alveolar, and upper airway pressures fall below atmospheric pressure and partial closure of the pharynx may occur unless reflex contraction of pharyngeal muscles adequately supports this part of the upper airway. Equal pressure point airflow dynamics would then cause truncation of the inspiratory flow curve. Conversely, with *intrathoracic* variable obstruction, as might be seen with tracheomalacia, opposite dynamics occur. Negative intrapleural pressure and an increasing transmural pressure gradient keep the tracheal lumen open. Unimpeded inspiratory airflow inscribes a normal inspiratory flow curve during spirometric testing. With forced expiration, the nonsupported trachea collapses with increasingly positive intrapleural pressure inscribing a truncated expiratory flow curve. Continued effort-independent exhalation maintains the curve's plateau until decreasing transpleural pressure eventually reaches equal pressure point with atmospheric pressure and the flow loop tends to normalize.

Postpneumonectomy syndrome is another rare and unusual form of upper airway obstruction usually associated with right pneumonectomy, and generally occurring in young patients or patients with high lung volumes such as emphysema. This syndrome is characterized clinically by dyspnea and stridor and is associated with a marked posterior rotational displacement of the mediastinum to the side of the pneumonectomy. It generally appears approximately a year following resection. Its etiology is felt to be the result of hyperinflation of the contralateral lung with anterior herniation before the operated hemithorax can fill with fluid to adequately counterbalance the shifting mediastinum. The distal trachea and left mainstem bronchus may be angulated and compressed across the descending aorta or spine. Symptoms may not appear until the cartilaginous support of the trachea disappears leading to the development of tracheomalacia and subsequent narrowing of the airway. Although treatment is directed toward repositioning the mediastinum toward the midline by placement of inflatable prostheses within the affected hemithorax, chronic fixation of the mediastinum and the extent of residual tracheomalacia may adversely affect the ultimate result (28). Self-expandable stent insertion utilizing fiberoptic bronchoscopy/fluoroscopy or rigid bronchoscopy may be a therapeutic alternative under these circumstances (29).

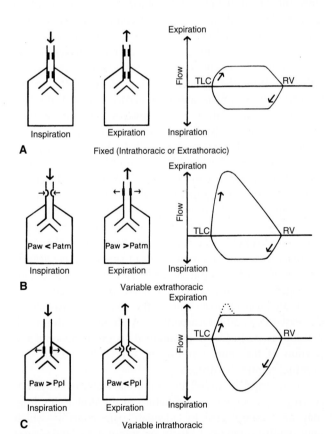

FIGURE 16.17 Flow-volume loops representing patterns of intrathoracic and extrathoracic upper airway obstruction: **A:** fixed extrathoracic obstruction; **B:** variable extrathoracic obstruction; **C:** variable intrathoracic obstruction. TLC, total lung capacity; RV, residual volume; PAW, airway pressure; PATM, atmospheric pressure; PPL, intrapleural pressure. (From Burrows B, Knudson RJ, Qwan SF, et al. *Respiratory disorders: a pathophysiological approach*, 2nd ed. Chicago: Year Book Medical Publishers, 1983; with permission.)

Small Airway Obstruction

Major causes of small airway obstruction include asthma, COPD (of which emphysema and chronic bronchitis are the most predominant), and pulmonary edema. Asthmatic airway disease is associated with hypertrophy and hypersensitivity of smooth-muscle cells of the distal bronchioles and hyperplasia of their cellular and glandular elements, especially mast cells and mucus producing goblet cells. There occurs thickening of the airway and narrowing of its lumen, hyper-responsiveness of smooth muscle to accentuated production of locally produced inflammatory mediators, and obstruction of the terminal airways with secretions and mucus. Treatment has traditionally consisted primarily of β_2 agonists and theophyllines that enhance cyclic adenosine monophosphate (cAMP) concentrations and promote smooth-muscle relaxation, corticosteroids—primarily inhaled—that decrease inflammation, and hydration, which lessens viscosity and helps to increase mobilization of secretions. More recent attention has been given to the additional therapeutic role of inflammatory mediator (particularly leukotrienes, prostanoids, etc.) suppression for intractable asthma, and the use of immunoglobulin (IgE) monoclonal antibody immunotherapy for the treatment of allergic asthma (30,31).

Pulmonary edema may be the result of either hydrostatic changes within capillaries (congestive failure, iatrogenic fluid overload, etc.) or permeability changes within the alveolar-capillary barrier [acute respiratory distress syndrome (ARDS), extracorporeal circulation, etc.]. An early consequence of interstitial pulmonary edema, which occurs before the capacitance of the interstitium is exceeded and alveolar transudation occurs, is extrinsic compression of terminal bronchioles—peribronchiolar "cuffing"—with increase in airway resistance. This is clinically manifested early by end-expiratory wheezing in a patient with other signs of volume overload, congestive heart failure, or protein depletion. Initial therapy consists of diuresis and fluid restriction as well as appropriate treatment of the precipitating cause. Although still controversial, there is some evidence to support enhancement of intravascular colloid oncotic pressure with supplemental albumin in malnourished individuals in which acute lung injury resulting from capillary membrane permeability is a component of their critical illness (32). Significant increases in diuresis, weight loss, and oxygen saturations seem to be achieved, although without improved lengths of stay or survival.

Small airway obstruction with emphysema results from the destruction of terminal bronchioles, which increases airway resistance in a reciprocal manner by decreasing total cross-sectional area; the destruction of alveolar septae, which diminishes the effect of the outward transpleural pressure gradient transmitted through alveoli that support remaining bronchioles; and increased intrapleural pressure at end expiration, which tends to further collapse these bronchioles. Fixed resistance to expired airflow, therefore, occurs that limits expiration time. Therefore, V_E must increase by increasing RR and inspiratory flow rate (PI_{breath}/PI_{max}), the latter by using accessory muscles of inspiration. Furthermore, the high FRC and early closing volumes in these patients create positive end-expiratory alveolar pressures (*auto-PEEP*) that must be overcome with the earliest portion of the inspiratory effort so that an effective transpulmonary pressure gradient for passive inspiratory airflow can develop.

These factors, as well as a decrease in thoracic compliance and the unfavorable length–tension relation of the diaphragm at very high lung volumes, substantially increase the work of breathing.

The aim of *lung-volume reduction surgery* for diffuse emphysema is to decrease the overall lung volume (FRC and RV), in particular by eliminating the pathologically increased alveolar dead-space in zone one, thereby optimizing overall thoracic compliance and the diaphragmatic length–tension relation, and minimizing intrapleural pressure swings (33). The smaller closing volumes and more efficient respiratory mechanics that result facilitate the recruitment of more normal and underutilized alveoli (primarily in zone III), and thereby decrease the work of breathing.

Pathophysiologic Compliance States

A segment of the chest wall consisting of two or more ribs broken in two or more places that become unstable, generally the result of trauma, is termed a *flail chest*. In response to the inward elastic recoil of the lung beneath the flail segment, the affected portion of the chest wall moves paradoxically inward with inspiration, becoming effectively uncoupled from the remainder of the thorax. This results in decreased regional lung volume and compliance. This can be further exacerbated by splinting secondary to pain associated with rib fractures with a further decrease in respiratory effort and subsequent loss of lung volume. Alveolar air will flow from the smaller, less compliant alveoli to the larger, more compliant alveoli in accordance with the Law of Laplace, especially if rapid, shallow breathing ensues. When large segments of underlying lung are involved, bulk airflow may be directed preferentially to the more compliant lung in the opposite hemithorax, resulting in progressive atelectasis of the involved lung segments. Furthermore, changes in transpulmonary pressure associated with the flail segment will be opposite those of the nonflail areas, leading to a pressure differential at the confluence of the mainstem bronchi. As a result, a "to-and-fro" exchange of hypoxic, hypercapnic anatomic dead-space air (*pendelluft*) may occur with inspiration and expiration (34,35). This homogenization of inspired and dead-space air produces a less than ideal environment in the alveolus consisting of decreased P_{O_2} and increased P_{CO_2}. A physiologic shunt will develop as perfusion is maintained to the hypoventilated portion of the lung, resulting in arterial hypoxemia and eventual respiratory distress.

Assuming the underlying pulmonary contusion is not severe, improvement in ventilation of the underlying lung may be accomplished by adequate pain control—which may require intercostal blocks or epidural analgesia—and aggressive pulmonary toilet such as coughing and incentive spirometry. If these fail, pneumatic stabilization of the chest wall by continuous positive airway pressure (CPAP) by mask [CPAP, biphasic positive airway pressure (BiPAP)] or positive-pressure ventilation may be necessary to stent open alveoli until such time as recoupling of the flail segment and underlying lung is able to occur with chest wall healing (36).

Early operative stabilization of the flail segment may also be an option. And although this may avert subjecting some patients to the complications of intubation and pneumatic stabilization of the chest wall or reduce the ventilation time required for others, it does not address the almost ubiquitous problem of underlying pulmonary contusion, which may still mandate sustained ventilatory support in many of the more severely injured patients.

Pneumothorax represents another instance of variable uncoupling of the lung and chest wall wherein a decrease in lung volume and compliance occurs as a result of its inward elastic recoil being incompletely opposed by the outward expansion of the chest wall. The consequences are similar to those listed earlier. This is particularly true if the chest wall defect is large, as with a "*sucking chest wound,*" or if the source is persistent, as with a ruptured and unsealed bullous or a traumatic puncture of the lung parenchyma. Air will continue to enter the pleural space until the lung is completely collapsed. As some of this parenchyma is still perfused but not ventilated, a substantial $\dot{V}/\dot{Q}$ mismatch results in significant physiologic shunting and hypoxemia. With persistent parenchymal air leak from the lung or a "ball-valve mechanism at the site of chest wall injury, air may continue to progressively accumulate in the pleural space with each negative inspiratory effort, thereby creating excessively positive pressure during expiration—a *tension pneumothorax*. The diaphragm and the mediastinal structures become displaced inferiorly and toward the contralateral pleural space, respectively, following complete collapse of the lung. Subsequently, the contralateral lung becomes compressed and venous return to the heart and myocardial diastolic compliance becomes severely compromised as intrapleural pressures exceed cardiac end-diastolic filling pressures.

Evacuation of intrapleural air to decompress the pleural space and reestablish coupling of the lung and chest wall is therapeutic. This will not only restore the mechanics of breathing, but it will usually facilitate elimination of the source of the pneumothorax by allowing the visceral and parietal pleurae to fuse. This is generally accomplished by placement of a pleural tube to dependent *water-seal drainage*. Classically, this consisted of connecting the chest tube to a vented bottle, the connection port of which was a tube extending a short length (generally 2 cm) beneath water. The distance beneath the water determined the PIP that had to be generated to evacuate any retained air. If significant drainage of fluid from within the pleural space was anticipated, a separate, nonvented bottle was interposed and connected directly to the chest tube instead, and subsequently connected in series with the water-seal receptacle (Fig. 16.18). Otherwise, fluid would drain directly into the water-seal bottle and elevate its level, thereby increasing the hydrostatic pressure. Progressively increasing positive pleural pressure would then be required with expiration to evacuate the pleural space. In the event of a substantial parenchymal air leak (*bronchopleurocutaneous fistula*) or rapid intrapleural fluid accumulation (bleeding),

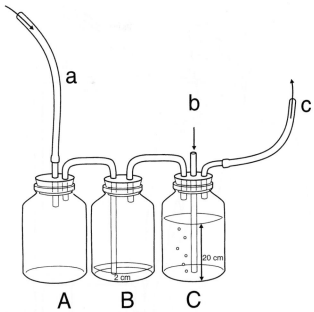

FIGURE 16.18 Schematic representation of the classic three-bottle pleural drainage system (see text for explanation): (*A*) fluid collection bottle; (*B*) water-seal bottle; (*C*) suction regulation bottle; (*a*) chest tube from patient; (*b*) atmospheric pressure; (*c*) unregulated wall suction.

a consistently more negative end-tidal intrathoracic pressure may be required to facilitate emptying. A third bottle was then connected in series to a now nonvented water-seal bottle and utilized to adjust the intrapleural pressure to the negative pressure desired. This was accomplished by venting the third bottle by way of a perpendicular tube the end of which was immersed a variable depth below the water with high suction placed to this bottle. The distance that the tube was immersed below the water determined the negative pressure transmitted to the pleural space as the column of water in the tube would be evacuated by the suction until the negative pressure in this bottle was stabilized with in-rushing atmospheric air. Contemporary pleural drainage systems are now compact, self-contained, compartmentalized, plastic devices that utilize similar principles as the old three-bottle system. One must realize that this is a *closed* system such that a tension pneumothorax may develop when a substantial air leak exists unless adequate suction is applied or steps are taken to vent the system to the atmosphere. This can generally be accomplished by disconnecting the suction tubing. Furthermore, clamping the chest tube of such a patient during prolonged transport is ill advised for similar reasons.

In rare instances when an air leak is quite large but deemed otherwise surgically unapproachable at the time, suction may be removed and the leak vented to the atmosphere through a deeper water-seal that renders the intrapleural space slightly more positive. Otherwise inspired air, by taking the path of least resistance through the fistula, could prevent adequate expansion of alveoli and result in progressively decreasing lung compliance as smaller alveoli empty to the fistula. This

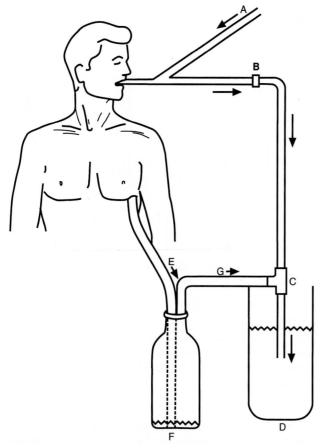

FIGURE 16.19 Pleural drainage configuration for control of a large bronchopleural fistula with the concomitant use of positive-pressure ventilation. Connection of the chest tube (*E*) and water-seal bottle (*F*) in series with a positive end-expiratory pressure (PEEP) regulation bottle (*D*) allows adjustment of positive intrapleural pressure by adjusting the length of the tube (*C*) below the water level. The PEEP-regulation bottle is connected in series through tube *C* with the exhalation valve (*B*) of the ventilation circuit thereby allowing equilibration of intrapleural pressure with end-expiratory pressure. (From Downs JB, Chapman RL Jr. Treatment of bronchopleural fistula during continuous positive pressure ventilation. *Chest* 1976;69:363–366; with permission.)

would eventually lead to atelectasis of the involved lung with increasing V̇/Q̇ mismatch and physiologic shunting. Unfortunately, continued end-expiratory leakage at FRC, because of unopposed inward elastic lung recoil toward RV, usually results in a progressive pneumothorax despite being adequately vented and generally requires frequent voluntary generation of PIP (as with coughing or valsalva maneuver) by a cooperative patient to evacuate this accumulated air in order for this application to be practical.

Very large air leaks become especially problematic in the case of positive-pressure ventilated patients such that pleural drainage should be coupled with the ventilator circuit so as to equilibrate end-expiratory ventilator and intrapleural pressures (*balanced pleural drainage*) to minimize end-expiratory leakage and maintain lung expansion (Fig. 16.19) (37). As an alternative, *high-frequency jet ventilation* (HFJV) may be

helpful in maintaining alveolar expansion and minimizing V̇/Q̇ mismatch. This is accomplished by limiting expiration time thereby increasing mean airway pressure and FRC; however, the air leak may in fact increase under these circumstances (38). Furthermore, with HFJV, as compared with conventional ventilation, laminar airflow in distal small airways may be more efficient and less influenced by compliance (elastic recoil) properties of the lung parenchyma, thereby allowing smaller V̇ts and peak airway pressures to achieve comparable results. This could have a beneficial effect in diminishing fistula leakage.

Smaller stable pneumothoraces estimated at less than 20% of the volume of the hemithorax or less than 3 cm from the chest wall by chest radiograph, for which chest tube drainage or aspiration is not deemed necessary, may be treated by allowing the patient to breath hyperoxic (usually approaching 100% O_2) concentrations of gas, thereby increasing the alveolar concentration of oxygen (39). Maximizing the partial pressure of oxygen in turn minimizes the partial pressures of other gases in the alveoli and pulmonary capillary blood, particularly nitrogen. Although the partial pressure of oxygen in pulmonary capillary blood is then quite high at the alveolar-capillary unit, it rapidly diminishes well below that which is found within the intrapleural air of a pneumothorax as a result of tissue utilization. Therefore, the overall reduction of the total partial pressure of gases in a pleural capillary increases the pressure gradient favoring more rapid absorption of intrapleural air, particularly nitrogen, from the pleural space. Although theoretically this may seem appropriate, it should be realized that only +/− 2% of the volume of the pneumothorax will resolve within 24 hours, although this represents a fourfold increase of resolution of an otherwise observed, untreated, stable pneumothorax (40). Therefore, it may be more practical to allow such a pneumothorax in an otherwise asymptomatic patient to gradually resolve without specific treatment, but with close outpatient follow-up (41).

Restrictive parenchymal (intrinsic) lung diseases are many and varied, but basically have in common some inflammatory process that causes collagen buildup and scarring within the interstitium, thereby increasing the elasticity (or decreasing the compliance) of the lung. This limits the optimal expansion and utilization of alveoli—particularly in zones two and three—ultimately leading to V̇/Q̇ mismatch, physiologic shunting, and hypoxemia (42). Among others, the more common causes are those of infectious (tuberculosis, etc.), autoimmune (sarcoidosis, collagen vascular, etc.), occupational (pneumoconiosis, silicosis, etc.), drug-induced (cytotoxic chemotherapy), and idiopathic (idiopathic pulmonary fibrosis) etiologies. It should be noted that, in most cases, variable degrees of diffusion block also account for much of the hypoxemia associated with these intrinsic, restrictive lung diseases. *Extrinsic* causes, which do not involve the lung parenchyma but rather the chest wall and pleura, yet lead to similar lung pathophysiology, are generally those due to the following: skeletal abnormalities (kyphoscoliosis, surgical thoracoplasty, etc.); neuromuscular disorders (muscular dystrophy, amyotrophic lateral sclerosis, etc.); pleural diseases (pleural effusions, loculated hemothorax, fibrothorax, etc.); and, more commonly, morbid obesity.

Pathophysiologic Diffusion/Transport States

Diffusion abnormalities, as previously described, are largely divided into disease processes that either limit the surface area available for gas exchange or physically impede the diffusion of a gas across the alveolar-capillary barrier. The former category is represented predominantly by *emphysema* wherein alveolar septae are destroyed thereby resulting in coalescence of alveoli, which form intraparenchymal air sacs—and, ultimately, bullae—leading to a drastic reduction of diffusion surface. This may be caused by smoking or by, among other less common causes, the congenital absence of α_1 antitrypsin—a protein that inhibits the breakdown of elastin and other structural proteins within the interstitium of the alveolar septae (43). When surface area is therefore reduced to such an extent that even the diffusion of carbon dioxide is impaired, the prognosis of such a patient is quite poor.

Extensive inflammatory exudative processes such as pneumonia that obliterate alveoli, likewise, result in elimination of surface area for diffusion. This mechanism, however, may be only a minor cause of hypoxemia in these circumstances as $\dot{V}/\dot{Q}$ mismatch and physiologic shunting likely play a more important role.

Pathologic processes that affect the alveolar-capillary barrier are many and varied. *Pulmonary contusion* occurs as the result of blunt trauma to the chest wall. Acutely, the concussive wave traveling through differing media (blood versus air) with different inertial forces causes disruption of the alveolar-capillary barrier and interstitial hemorrhage. Additionally, implosive forces within the air-filled alveoli may cause over distension or disruption of the alveolar-capillary membrane adding intra-alveolar hemorrhage to interstitial edema or hemorrhage, thereby also reducing surface area for diffusion. Initial efforts aimed at minimizing hydrostatic forces that might exacerbate this alveolar-capillary leak, such as fluid restriction, are helpful. Under these circumstances, fluids such as albumin or hetastarch solutions are not indicated for resuscitation or maintenance in an effort to increase vascular oncotic pressure and limit pulmonary capillary leakage as these will translocate to the interstitium and increase oncotic forces in that direction (44). With ultimate resolution and healing, fibrosis may result in significant scarring of the interstitium resulting in some degree of permanent alveolar-capillary block as well as diminished parenchymal compliance (45).

As mentioned in the previous section, occupational diseases of the pulmonary parenchyma such as silicosis, beryllium-induced pulmonary fibrosis, and other pneumoconioses result in destruction of alveoli and cause irreversible interstitial fibrosis. Certain chemotherapeutic agents such as bleomycin and cyclophosphamide may result in extensive interstitial fibrosis and subsequent hypoxemia due to alveolar-capillary block. Treatment with steroids and immunosuppressive drugs (i.e., azothioprine, etc.) may limit to a variable extent the diffusion restriction caused by these drugs (46). Extensive granulomatous diseases and autoimmune or idiopathic pulmonary fibrotic etiologies are among other causes of alveolar-capillary diffusion block.

Pulmonary interstitial edema from any cause, that is, congestive heart failure, overhydration, acute capillary leak syndromes and so on reversibly increases the thickness of the alveolar-capillary barrier and, eventually, may also diminish alveolar surface area as interstitial Starling forces are exceeded and alveoli are flooded. An unusual form of unilateral pulmonary edema, so-called re-expansion pulmonary edema, may occur following reinflation of a lung after it has been collapsed or compressed for an extended period of time. Although several theories have been proposed as to its cause, it is generally recognized that this represents a form of ischemic-reperfusion injury to the lung mediated by various inflammatory cytokines as well as oxygen-free radical peroxidation of cell membranes, which lead to increased capillary endothelial permeability (47). A similar mechanism is also likely to be responsible for the *reperfusion pulmonary edema* seen following cardiopulmonary bypass or shunt surgery for cyanotic congenital heart disease (48). *Postpneumonectomy pulmonary edema* occurs as a result of multiple factors. Iatrogenic fluid overload that increases pulmonary capillary hydrostatic pressure, critical reduction in lymphatic sump capacity that occurs more often with right pneumonectomy, and a generalized systemic inflammatory response syndrome (SIRS) response—especially to multiple blood transfusions—may play significant roles. However, ischemic-reperfusion injury due to hypoxic pulmonary vasoconstriction as a consequence of upside and, to a lesser extent, downside lung re-expansion is, once again, felt to be the primary etiology (49,50).

ARDS is a particularly devastating cause of diffusion impairment hypoxemia and is associated with unusually high mortality, approaching 40%. It seems to represent an exaggerated form of the SIRS to sepsis, trauma, shock, or extracorporeal perfusion, among other causes (51). It may also be induced by less systemic insults such as aspiration, toxic inhalation, or toxicity to certain drugs (e.g., amiodarone) (52). A specific risk factor for the development of ARDS is tobacco use (53). ARDS represents an inflammatory endothelial and epithelial permeability abnormality, unrelated to increased hydrostatic forces within the pulmonary capillary bed, which results in interstitial pulmonary edema and a loss of pulmonary surfactant. Impairment of alveolar expansion and oxygen diffusion occurs leading to $\dot{V}/\dot{Q}$ mismatching and physiologic shunting, which culminates in severe hypoxemia. Later occurrence of microvascular disseminated intravascular coagulopathy (DIC) is felt to be the mechanism of subsequent *multisystem organ failure* (MSOF), especially when associated with sepsis (54). These pathologic changes are mediated by complex humoral and cellular interactions. Granulocyte aggregation and adherence to endothelial surfaces release toxic cytokines, leukotrienes, and prostenoids that promote oxygen-free radical generation and toxic nitrite production, leading to the increased endothelial and epithelial permeability. Macrophage release of tumor necrosis factor (TNF) further propagates this inflammatory response. Cytokine release of platelet-activating factor and plasminogen activator inhibitor 1 (PAI-1) promotes microvascular coagulation, the suspected underlying cause of MSOF.

ARDS is manifested by three generally distinct phases that are heterogeneous in their timing and distribution throughout the lung. The initial *exudative phase* occurs within 48 to 72 hours of insult and consists of the extravasation of proteinaceous fluid and migration of inflammatory cellular elements into the interstitium and alveoli. The *proliferative phase* follows with destruction of alveoli and type I pneumocytes and is associated with hyaline membrane replacement, increasing fibroblast proliferation, collagen deposition, and capillary obliteration. The final *fibrotic phase* evolves after 10 days to 2 weeks with extensive fibrotic organization of the respiratory unit. This final stage is generally felt to be irreversible.

Specific therapeutic options aimed at eliminating the inciting cause of ARDS include minimizing oxygen toxicity, minimizing mechanical barotrauma to remaining functioning alveoli, and preventing the fibroproliferative organization of respiratory units. Oxygen toxicity results in superoxide-free radical generation through the cytochrome-oxidase chain of the Kreb cycle. Subsequent lipid peroxidation of cell membranes leads to cellular dysfunction and increased cellular permeability. Although the exact concentrations of oxygen and the associated time courses to lung damage are unclear, high concentrations of oxygen for longer than 48 hours are felt to be progressively detrimental (55).

Repetitive opening and closing (tidal recruitment), overexpansion of alveoli, and elevated mean airway pressures exacerbate barotrauma, so-called ventilator-induced lung injury (VILI). Low V_T (5–8 mL/kg; <40 mm Hg PIP; I:E = 1 : 1), permissive hypercapnia (P_{CO_2} = 60–100 mm Hg; pH >7.25), "best PEEP" (<0.6 F_{IO_2}; O_2 saturation >88%) ventilation delivered within the inflection points of a patient's particular compliance curve (usually at a PEEP 15 mm Hg or greater) has proved most optimal in preserving respiratory units (56,57). Because gravity affects $\dot{V}/\dot{Q}$ matching, alternating supine and prone positioning, where feasible, enhances oxygenation. RRs approximately 25 to 30/ min reverse and progressively increase theI:E ratio to greater than 1.5:1 and contribute to auto-PEEP, thereby increasing mean airway pressure and barotrauma.

Although still very controversial, earlier evidence seemed to support the use of low dose, long-term tapered steroids (2 mg/kg – 0.125 mg/kg, divided every 6–8 hours over 30 ± days) begun during the general onset of the proliferative phase (± day 7) in an effort to minimize irreversible fibrotic lung pathology and, hopefully, increase survival (58). However, more recent preliminary evidence of an ongoing prospective, randomized trial by the National Heart, Lung, and Blood Institute (NHLBI) ARDSNet consortium suggests

that, although there is early improvement in oxygenation with steroid use, overall survival does not seen to be affected (59). Past investigation suggests that early reversal of DIC by plasminogen activators (e.g., r-tpa, urokinase, etc.) may enhance oxygenation and, otherwise, favorably affect the prognosis of ARDS (60). More recent evidence suggests that recombinant protein C, important in mitigating microvascular coagulopathy, favorably affects the mortality of patients with multiorgan system failure (MOSF) due to sepsis (61). Whether this translates to similar efficacy in treating patients with ARDS of nonseptic etiology is the goal of ongoing phase III clinical trials.

Chemical reactions with hemoglobin in blood that are detrimental to oxygen transport are those related to smoking and the use of the antihypertensive drugs, nitroglycerin, and nitroprusside. CO is a gaseous by-product of tobacco combustion, as well as being an industrial and urban pollutant. Its affinity for the iron in hemoglobin is much greater than that of oxygen such that it is essentially irreversibly bound, thereby excluding oxygen uptake by those sites of hemoglobin molecules so affected. Another deleterious effect of chemically bound CO is to shift the oxyhemoglobin dissociation curve to the left, effectively impeding the off-loading of oxygen from sites of the hemoglobin molecule that are saturated with oxygen. Concentration of this *carboxyhemoglobin* may attain levels as high as 5% to 8% in urban smokers, substantially limiting oxygen delivery to tissues. This effect is accentuated by the presence of anemia, blood loss, or impaired diffusion capacity. The life span of red blood cells is approximately 120 days. Cessation of smoking at least 4 weeks before elective surgery has been shown to minimize postoperative complications by, among other mechanisms, allowing turnover of much of that fraction of ineffective carboxyhemoglobin with efficiently functioning hemoglobin (62). Nitroglycerin is an intravenous antihypertensive drug frequently used for the control of hypertension, cardiac preload and afterload reduction, and the medical management of acute cardiac ischemic syndromes. When used in high concentrations for long durations, significant amounts of *methemoglobin* (MetHb) may be formed when the nitrite oxidizes the ferrous iron (Fe^{2+}) in hemoglobin to ferric iron (Fe^{3+}). Ferric iron is incapable of binding with oxygen. Fortunately, most individuals usually endogenously counteract this by converting MetHb back to oxyhemoglobin as the result of an enzyme, MetHb reductase (63). On the other hand, nitroprusside reacts with hemoglobin to form MetHb *and* five cyanide ions, the latter which can inhibit the cytochrome oxidase electron transport chain phase of the Kreb cycle. MetHb neutralizes only one of the five cyanide ions, forming cyan-MetHb. Therefore, if prolonged use of high-dose nitroprusside is contemplated, concomitant use of nitroglycerin may mitigate the risk of cyanide poisoning. Unfortunately, cyan-MetHg still remains dysfunctional as regards its ability to transport oxygen (64).

Pathophysiologic Ventilation–Perfusion Mismatch

Most lung pathology involves some degree of $\dot{V}/\dot{Q}$ mismatch as part of its overall pathophysiology. This is particularly true of infiltrative processes of the lung such as pneumonia, restrictive conditions of the chest wall, or space-occupying conditions of the pleural space that diminish the volume of the thoracic cavity relative to the volume of contained lung. Included in the latter two categories, among others, are pleural effusions, pulmonary atelectasis as the result of hypoventilation due to pain and splinting, phrenic nerve paralysis with *eventration* (cephalad paralytic displacement) of the diaphragm, major bullous disease of the lung, and pneumothorax. These cause reduction of chest wall compliance or an uncoupling and/or displacement of a portion of the lung vis-à-vis the chest wall resulting in inward elastic lung recoil and closure of alveoli.

Pleural effusions, aside from the consequences of their potentially septic complications, are also a cause of $\dot{V}/\dot{Q}$ mismatch. Pleural effusions are basically the result of an imbalance in hydrostatic and oncotic pressures and/or increased capillary permeability. There are six mechanisms potentially responsible for excessive pleural fluid: (i) an increase in microvascular hydrostatic pressure (e.g., congestive heart failure), (ii) a decrease in serum oncotic pressure (malnutrition or cachectic patients with low serum albumin), (iii) decreased (more negative) pressure in the pleural space, (lung collapse or pneumonectomy, which shifts the pressure gradient favoring fluid formation), (iv) an increase in the permeability of the microvascular circulation (various inflammatory mediators), or toxins (such as a parapneumonic effusion, *empyema*, or malignant pleural effusion), (v) impaired drainage of the pleural lymphatics (fibrosis or tumor infiltration), and (vi) transcompartment movement of ascitic fluid (through lymphatics or diaphragmatic defects). Pleural effusions are categorized as *transudative* (e.g., congestive heart failure) or *exudative* (e.g., parapneumonic, malignant, etc.) based on three criteria: (i) a pleural fluid to serum protein ratio greater than 0.5; (ii) a pleural fluid to serum lactate dehydrogenase (LDH) ratio greater than 0.6; and (iii) an absolute pleural fluid LDH greater than two thirds the upper limit of normal for serum. Other criteria for exudates of an inflammatory nature include a pleural fluid leukocytosis greater than $10,000/\mu L$, a pH less than 7.30, and a glucose less than 60 $\mu g/dL$, indicating a metabolically active inflammatory process.

Treatment of effusions, if transudative and small, may be noninvasive, using diuresis to decrease capillary hydrostatic pressure and concentrated albumin (or chronically, nutritional repletion) to increase serum oncotic pressure. However, if they are large, exudative, or recurrent, then invasive methods are generally necessary. If the fluid is homogeneous and nonloculated on imaging studies, thoracentesis may be the initial approach. If recurrent or grossly exudative, as with empyema, tube thoracostomy with negative pressure drainage for several days to allow symphysis of the visceral and parietal pleurae is more appropriate. Should the effusion be chronic and/or loculated, especially if associated with nonhomogeneity on imaging studies suggesting an organized pleural peel, direct surgical empyemectomy or decortication of the lung may be necessary. This may be accomplished by *video-assisted thoracoscopic techniques* (VATS) if the process is less than 10 to 14 days old, the most consistent results being accomplished if the procedure is performed within 7 days (65). Otherwise, thoracotomy may be necessary. In the case of recurrent or persistently draining malignant pleural effusions or recalcitrant, nonloculated transudative effusions, chemical *pleuradesis* may be necessary. Temporary intrapleural instillation of a solution containing a sterile, inflammatory-inciting agent such as doxycycline, or talc followed by several days of negative pressure drainage can result in a 70% incidence of control of the effusion through the mechanism of sterile inflammatory symphysis of the visceral and parietal pleurae. When this is unsuccessful, VATS talc or abrasive surgical pleuradesis is generally effective in controlling the effusion.

Major bullous disease of the lung, other than causing respiratory impairment and dyspnea through mechanisms of compliance and diffusion abnormalities, may significantly contribute to major $\dot{V}/\dot{Q}$ abnormalities. This is especially likely if the bullous involvement occupies more than one third of the hemithorax and is associated with otherwise homogeneous lung parenchyma as determined by CT scanning. Re-expansion of compressed lung and recruitment of closed alveoli can be expected with resection of such an area of lung involvement, which generally requires upper lobectomy. Severe hypoxemia or hypercapnia, very low DLCO or FEV_1, or extreme heterogeneity of emphysematous air spaces involving the entire lung suggest destruction rather than compression of lung parenchyma as the cause of symptoms, and implies a worse prognosis with surgery (66). Furthermore, one-lung anesthesia and/or decubitus positioning may not be well tolerated under these circumstances necessitating other approaches to this problem (67,68)

Pulmonary embolus, although strictly classified as a $\dot{V}/\dot{Q}$ defect, also has clinical aspects of a diffusion abnormality. This is because ventilated but nonperfused lung acts as alveolar dead space. When substantial pulmonary vessel obstruction occurs, this effectively eliminates a variable amount of surface area available for diffusion. Furthermore, pulmonary arteriolar J-receptors are stimulated, ultimately leading to hypoventilation and tachypnea, which further increases dead-space ventilation and decreases alveolar ventilation (69). Increased right ventricular work and pulmonary arterial pressure tends to maintain cardiac output by distending unobstructed pulmonary arterioles and decreasing blood transit time through functioning alveolar-capillary units. This combination of hypoventilation and decreased transit time may result in an increased physiologic shunt, further increasing hypoxemia. When pulmonary arterial pressure is high enough to raise pulmonary hydrostatic pressure, interstitial pulmonary edema may further contribute to the diffusion defect. Massive embolus, involving greater than one half of the pulmonary arterial tree generally overwhelms the circulation's capacity for compensation by recruitment and distension such that right heart failure and inadequate left ventricular filling and cardiac output occur.

The principles of treatment include increasing alveolar concentrations of oxygen to maximize partial pressure diffusion gradients for those remaining functioning alveolar-capillary units, and anticoagulation to minimize propagation of thrombus and allow the intrinsic fibrinolytic system to dissolve acute thrombus and thereby reclaim nonfunctioning alveolar-capillary units. If hemodynamic compromise occurs and cannot be maintained with pharmacologic support to allow natural degradation of thrombus over time, selective pulmonary arterial administration of extrinsic fibrinolytics (recombinant tissue plasminogen activator, urokinase, etc.), catheter suction-extraction of the thrombus, or, infrequently, direct surgical removal of thrombus may be indicated (70,71). Chronic, recurrent pulmonary embolism may occur in certain conditions of deranged coagulation such as proteins C and S deficiencies, antiphospholipid syndrome, and antithrombin III deficiency resulting in fibrotic occlusion and/or narrow recanalization of pulmonary arteries proximal to more distal arterial and arteriolar perfusion beds. The absolute reduction of cross-sectional area of the proximal pulmonary vascular bed as well as loss of the ability for recruitment and distensibility within this bed often leads to secondary pulmonary hypertension and, eventually, *cor pulmonale* with dire prognostic implications. Pulmonary thromboendarterectomy utilizing cardiopulmonary bypass may be indicated in appropriate cases where occlusion is located more proximal in the pulmonary vascular bed (72).

Assisted Ventilation

It is inevitable in the care of surgical patients that utilization of various forms of assisted ventilation will be required in many cases, whether in their postoperative management or during critical care management of complications. Although it is beyond the scope of this chapter to exhaust the topic of assisted ventilation, it is hoped that the following section will provide the basic concepts adequate to provide one with a working knowledge of the subject.

Assisted ventilation may be classified as *invasive*, requiring placement of an endotracheal tube for airway access and control, or *noninvasive* as exemplified by closed-mask, nasal CPAP support. In either case, the mode of assist is almost always *positive pressure ventilation* working against the inward elastic recoil of the pulmonary parenchyma or the restrictive compliance of the chest wall, as compared with the normal circumstance of *negative pressure ventilation* that occurs with natural breathing.

Noninvasive Assisted Ventilation

Noninvasive assisted ventilation offers certain distinct advantages over invasive methods when applicable (73).

Predominant among these is the maintenance of natural airway defenses against infection such as cough, mobility, and competence of the glottis against aspiration. Other advantages include maintenance of speech, oral alimentation, and patient comfort. The major disadvantages are imprecise and less secure control of the airway, of the amount of positive pressure, and of the gas mixture delivered, as well as an inherent requirement for patient cooperation. The primary method of applying noninvasive positive pressure ventilation (NPPV) is through a tightly secured closed face mask covering the mouth and nose, in order to preclude any possibility of leakage around the mask or through the mouth that would negate the positive pressure or dilute the gas mixture delivered. There are two distinct modes of positive pressure ventilation: (i) CPAP, and (ii) BiPAP.

CPAP is a passive assist mode and applies to spontaneously breathing individuals. It is characterized by the maintenance of a positive end-expiratory airway pressure of varying degrees above atmospheric pressure in patients with *adequate*, although impaired, respiratory mechanics. This mode of assisted ventilation tends to increase FRC and decrease closing volume. The beneficial results are enhanced lung compliance by virtue of greater lung volume, increased $\dot{V}/\dot{Q}$ matching secondary to atelectatic alveolar recruitment, decreased airway resistance because of larger and better supported terminal bronchioles, decreased pulmonary edema as a result of positive pressure opposition to adverse hydrostatic or interstitial pressure gradients, and, ultimately, an overall decrease in the work of breathing. This mode of assisted ventilation is most efficacious in restrictive and neuromuscular lung diseases characterized by hypoventilation and hypercapnia, obstructive sleep apnea where collapse of pharyngeal musculature requires extrinsic support, respiratory failure secondary to severe $\dot{V}/\dot{Q}$ mismatch (e.g., atelectasis, pulmonary contusion, etc.), and pulmonary edema. It is less effective and less well tolerated in hyperinflation lung diseases such as emphysema.

BiPAP is an active, noninvasive form of assist-control ventilation utilized in patients with *inadequate* respiratory mechanics who are still spontaneously breathing. A volume-cycled ventilator delivers assisted positive-pressure ventilation with inspiration and maintains a separate PEEP at expiration. This form of assisted ventilation is more effective and better tolerated by patients with hyperinflation-type lung disease and greater initial increased work of breathing. However, this method is rather labor intensive from a therapist's viewpoint, and precautions must be taken to ensure that the positive pressure delivered through the nose is not vented through the mouth if only a nose mask is used—usually a difficult task.

Invasive (Mechanical) Assisted Ventilation

Mechanical ventilation, in its most practical application, requires three basic components: (i) a blended mixture of compressed air and oxygen delivered by an insufflation

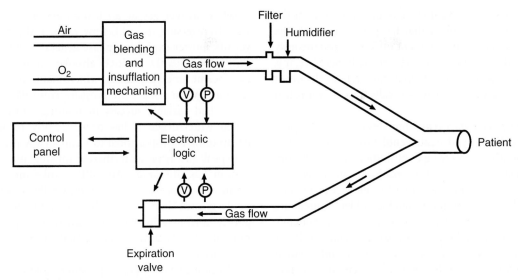

FIGURE 16.20 Schematic illustration of the basic elements of a ventilation circuit. V, volume; P, pressure. (Reproduced from Smith RA. Principles of mechanical ventilation. In: Ayers SM, ed. *Textbook of critical care medicine*, 3rd ed. Philadelphia: WB Saunders, 1995:858–867; with permission.)

mechanism (the ventilator), (ii) a breathing circuit, and (iii) airway access through an endotracheal tube or tracheostomy (Fig. 16.20). The ventilator consists primarily of a bellows mechanism to deliver gas at a constant pressure, two electromechanical valves to precisely blend compressed air and oxygen in any desired concentration from 0.21 to 1.0, and an electronic logic which modulates inspiratory and expiratory valves within the breathing circuit to achieve various gas flows, breathing circuit pressures, and time parameters as selected from a control panel. The breathing circuit consists of an inspiratory limb connected at one end to the insufflation mechanism by means of an inspiratory valve, and an expiratory limb connected in continuity with the inspiratory limb at the patient's airway access. The inspiratory limb is equipped with filtration and humidification capability while the expiratory limb contains its own expiration valve to regulate airway pressure. The electronic logic controls the inspiratory and expiratory valves through a servomechanism in accordance with variables selected by the operator through the control panel. These may include V_T, rate, inspiration: expiration ratio, insufflation time, inspiratory and expiratory pressures, gas flow characteristics, and mechanism of initiation and termination of gas flow.

Volume-controlled ventilation refers to a method wherein a gas mixture is delivered at a specifically determined volume regardless of circuit (and therefore, airway) pressure, within upper-limit safeguards. Inasmuch as the breathing circuit adds substantial dead-space, the volume selected to be delivered as V_T (normally approximately 7 mL/kg) is increased to between 10 to 12 mL/kg depending on the thoracic compliance of the patient and compliance of the circuit. In contrast, *pressure-controlled* ventilation delivers gas flow in accordance with a constant, preselected *peak inspiratory airway pressure* (PAP) such that the volume delivered is variable, depending on the thoracic compliance characteristics of the patient and the resistance of the circuit. This gas flow may be time-cycled over a set inspiratory interval or flow-cycled wherein insufflation ceases when gas flow drops below a certain percentage of initial flow. When using pressure-controlled ventilation, the optimal peak airway pressure must be regulated so as to deliver adequate V_T yet minimize barotrauma resulting from alveolar distension. Barotrauma is more directly related to mean airway pressure than to peak airway pressure, and experience in patients with ARDS suggests that a mean airway pressure under 30 cm H_2O is safe. Peak airway pressures generally exceed mean airway pressures by 5 to 10 cm H_2O, depending on thoracic compliance. Therefore, a peak airway pressure as high as 35 to 40 cm H_2O is generally acceptable when adjusting ventilator settings while treating pathologic conditions, although detrimental hemodynamic sequelae may occasionally result.

Mechanical ventilation is frequently applied along a continuum of support ranging from controlled ventilation in patients without intrinsic inspiratory effort, to CPAP in patients being weaned from the ventilator (74). Inasmuch as completely controlled ventilation is detrimental to respiratory muscle strength and coordination over time, several techniques of partial ventilatory support have been developed that allow varying degrees of patient participation. *Assisted mechanical ventilation* is a modality that allows the least participation by the patient in that a patient's inspiratory effort acts merely as the trigger for deliverance of a predetermined positive pressure breath. It was developed to allow better synchronization of ventilation between the patient and the ventilator in that the patient controls the ventilatory rate. However, a patient must be spontaneously breathing for this for this mode to be utilized; therefore, it is generally paired with a backup controlled rate in the event that a patient becomes apneic—so-called assist-controlled ventilation.

Intermittent mandatory ventilation (IMV) allows the most flexibility in delivering adequate ventilation in concurrence with the patient's own varying contributions to respiration. Predetermined positive pressure breaths are delivered at a predetermined rate while the patient is allowed to breathe spontaneously in the interim. When the predetermined rate is synchronized so that it may be initiated by a patient's own inspiratory effort, thereby optimizing patient-ventilator coordination, it is known as *synchronized intermittent mandatory ventilation* or SIMV. Adjustment of the rate allows a 0% to 100% range of ventilation control and is most effective as a means of weaning a patient from ventilatory support.

MMV is a ventilation mode that acts much as does a cardiac pacemaker in that a predetermined minute volume is set as gas flow to two, independent reservoirs; one the ventilator, and the other for spontaneous breathing. As long as a patient's spontaneous ventilation diverts the minute volume through the spontaneous ventilation circuit, no positive pressure assisted breaths are delivered. If, however, a patient becomes apneic or hypoventilates, the remaining preset minute volume is diverted to the ventilator circuit and is delivered as a positive pressure cycle once a threshold is met, which compensates for the loss of spontaneous ventilation. In an apneic patient, this would be indistinguishable from controlled ventilation.

Pressure support ventilation (PSV) is a patient-triggered, pressure-limited, flow-cycled mode, which can be used in spontaneously breathing patients only. It differs from other modes, particularly assisted mandatory ventilation, in that the positive pressure volume delivered with each breath is different depending on several patient variables. With each patient-triggered breath, gas flow is delivered at a variable rate to maintain a predetermined airway pressure until airflow is 25% of peak inspiratory flow, at which point airflow ceases. V_T depends on the preset pressure level, the inspiratory effort of the patient, the airway resistance, and the thoracic compliance. At high-pressure limits, usually greater than 20 cm H_2O, it acts in a manner similar to assisted mandatory ventilation. At low-pressure limits (<10 cm H_2O) it acts similar to CPAP, except that the work of breathing imposed by the endotracheal tube and the ventilator circuitry is eliminated.

Inverse ratio ventilation is a specialized mode of ventilation developed for particular use in patients with ARDS in an effort to recruit more alveoli without generating high airway pressures. In the usual setting, the respirator is set to deliver gas at an inspiration/expiration ratio of 1:3. By reversing the—I:E flow ratio, PAPs are kept low, yet the shorter expiratory phase generates significant *auto-PEEP* (persistently positive alveolar pressure caused by insufficient emptying time), which maintains alveolar distension. When used with pressure-controlled ventilation, it has had variable success in limiting barotrauma associated with ARDS. It has been recently recognized that barotrauma is proportional to *mean* airway pressure rather than peak airway pressure, thereby making this mode of ventilation less utilitarian. Auto-PEEP substantially increases mean airway pressure. This is especially so when the ratio is greater than 3:1. Furthermore, I:E flow reversal is poorly tolerated by patients, generally requiring neuromuscular blockade in order to facilitate patient-ventilator coordination.

Deciding when to place a patient on assisted ventilation is largely determined by subjective assessment of the patient's work of breathing, especially when associated with arterial blood gases in which the Po_2 and Pco_2 begin to merge at 50 to 55 mm Hg or so. However, weaning a patient from the ventilator requires assessment of certain parameters in a more objective way, especially when a patient has been ventilated for an extended period of time. Multiple factors come into play in chronically ventilated patients such that not only gas exchange, but also the status of the respiratory pump (inspiratory muscles) and the respiratory load (thoracic compliance, and parenchymal and airway resistance) must be taken into consideration. Chronically ill patients who are ventilated frequently exhibit respiratory muscle atrophy and neuromuscular weakness from numerous causes. Chronic illness results in a hypermetabolic, catabolic state with net protein loss despite adequate nutrition. As much as a third of diaphragm muscle mass may be lost in patients who are chronically malnourished at or below 25% of their ideal body weight.

Chronic or high-dose steroid administration, especially when given concomitantly with neuromuscular blocking agents, may induce a reversible "steroid myopathy." The mechanism is poorly understood but may be related to its mineralocorticoid effect, which promotes intracellular potassium loss leading to skeletal muscle dysfunction, atrophy, and destruction. Use of nonfluorinated corticosteroids seems to mitigate this (75).

Chronic illness may also produce a "euthyroid sick state" where T_3 levels are low as a consequence of metabolic diversion of the T_4 precursor toward production of the inactive rT_3 metabolite. These changes result in unsaturated nuclear receptors and subsequent diminished synthesis of neuromuscular protein mediators (76,77). Excessive diuresis or malnutrition may result in substantial intracellular potassium depletion and chronic renal insufficiency may result in chronic hypophosphatemia, both of which can contribute to severe respiratory muscle weakness.

Other associated conditions or circumstances may also affect one's ability to wean a patient from the ventilator. Among others, these include abdominal distension due to ileus or ascites or hyperinflation of the lungs due to bullous disease or bronchospasm which lead to a mechanical disadvantage of the length–tension relation of the diaphragm; increased airway resistance as a result of increased deadspace of the ventilator circuitry or inordinate length of or inspissated secretions within an endotracheal tube; overfeeding, especially with carbohydrate-rich elemental diets, which promotes gluconeogenesis and the overproduction of CO_2 that may increase the RQ substantially above 1.0 thereby increasing the respiratory load; (78) and any ongoing acute process, that is, congestive failure, sepsis, and pain, that might limit respiratory muscle perfusion and/or optimal ventilation mechanics and gas exchange. Having eliminated or corrected the above-mentioned impediments to weaning, the following criteria, in general, should be met to ensure successful extubation: (i) Pao_2 greater than 65, $Paco_2$ less than 50 on an Fio_2 of 0.4; (ii) tidal volume (V_T) greater than 5 mL/kg, or FVC greater than 10 mL/kg; (iii) NIF greater than −25 cm H_2O; (iv) RR less than 20 to 25/ min, V_D/V_T less than 0.4.

Anesthesia and Lateral Decubitus One-Lung Ventilation

Anesthesia and positioning during surgery substantially influences $\dot{V}/\dot{Q}$ matching and intrapulmonary shunting. The lungs are subjected to the same hydrostatic and gravitational forces in the supine and decubitus positions as they are in the upright position. Therefore, in the lateral decubitus position, the dependent lung receives most perfusion (approximately 60%) and the nondependent lung receives most ventilation (with some variation, depending on whether right or left side is down). With muscle paralysis, FRC is reduced as the diaphragm is displaced cephalad by intra-abdominal pressure and the mediastinum is displaced downward, decreasing overall compliance of the lung. Decreased compliance, especially in the dependent lung, along with high oxygen concentrations used for ventilation tends to promote atelectasis with further $\dot{V}/\dot{Q}$ mismatch. With thoracotomy, the now unrestricted, nondependent lung becomes more compliant and receives a greater proportion of the V_T, most of it dead-space ventilation. This results in hypoventilation of the dependent lung and further exacerbates $\dot{V}/\dot{Q}$ mismatch and intrapulmonary shunting. Unless averted by increasing V_T and PEEP, important hypoxemia could develop.

During one-lung ventilation, the nondependent lung is excluded from ventilation and all ventilation is directed to the dependent lung. Although intuitively, this may seem to have a salutary effect in optimizing $\dot{V}/\dot{Q}$ matching of the dependent lung, it is more than offset by the substantial increase in intrapulmonary shunting produced by the perfused, but unventilated, nondependent lung. This potentially serious problem is ameliorated to a great degree by the *HPV* response (79). This compensatory response is influenced by several factors and performs most optimally at normal pulmonary artery pressures and cardiac outputs (Svo_2). Significant deviations from this may blunt the HPV response and increase the intrapulmonary shunt (80). Inhalation anesthetics progressively inhibit HPV at increasing alveolar concentrations; most intravenous anesthetics have no effect (81). Vigorous manipulation of the operative lung may also variably inhibit HPV. Nitric oxide delivered to the dependent, ventilated lung under hypoxemic conditions, or conditions of pulmonary hypertension, may augment HPV of the nondependent lung.

Another detriment of "decubitus positioning" to ventilation of the downside lung is the artificial restrictive change in chest wall compliance caused by the operating table and the gravitational forces on the mediastinum that result in loss of FRC. Although this is not of much concern in patients with adequate pulmonary function, it may result in significant hypoxemia in patients with marginal pulmonary reserve when the upside lung is collapsed. Increasing PEEP may mitigate this to some extent, although in patients with more severe pulmonary dysfunction, supine positioning and/or two-lung ventilation may be required if surgery is deemed necessary.

GLOSSARY

Laws Governing the Behavior of Gases and Liquids

Boyle Law At constant temperature, the volume of a gas is inversely proportional to the absolute pressure;

$$P_1V_1 = P_2V_2$$

Charles Law At constant pressure, the volume of a gas is directly proportional to its temperature (Kelvin degrees);

$$V_1/V = T_1/T_2$$

Dalton Law In a gas mixture, the pressure exerted by each individual gas is independent of the pressures exerted by the other gases in the mixture;

$$P_A = P_{H_2O} + P_{O_2} + P_{CO_2} + P_{N_2}$$

Graham Law The rate of diffusion (v) of a gas (in the gaseous phase) is inversely proportional to the square root of its molecular weight or mass (m);

$$(\sqrt{m_1}/\sqrt{m_2}) = v_2/v_1$$

Henry Law The concentration of a solute gas (c) absorbed within a liquid is directly proportional to the pressure

(p) of that gas to which that liquid is exposed;

$$p = k'_c(c)$$

k'_c = Henry's Law constant on the molar concentration scale

Ideal Gas Law   The volume (V) of an *ideal gas* (one whose molecules are uninfluenced by intermolecular attractive forces) is *directly* proportional to its molar concentration (n) and temperature (T), and *inversely* proportional to its pressure (P);

$$V = nRT/P;$$

R = universal gas constant

Fick Law of Diffusion   The volume of gas per unit time (V) diffusing through a barrier is *directly* proportional to the surface area available for diffusion (A), the diffusivity (diffusion coefficient) of the particular gas within the barrier (D), and the partial pressure difference of the gas across the barrier, and is *inversely* proportional to the thickness of the barrier or *the diffusion distance* (T);

$$V = \frac{A \times D \times (P_1 - P_2)}{T}$$

$D \propto$ solubility/$\sqrt{\text{molecular wt}}$

Poiseuille Law   The resistance (R) of a fluid (gaseous or liquid) is *directly* proportional to its viscosity ($\acute{\eta}$) and the length (l) of the conduit in which it flows, and is *inversely* proportional the *fourth* power of the radius (r) of the conduit;

$$R = 8\acute{\eta}l/\pi r^4$$

APPENDIX A

Formulas of Ventilation and Respiration

Minute Ventilation (V_E):

$$V_E = V_T \times RR \quad V_T = \text{tidal volume;}$$

$$RR = \text{respiratory rate}$$

Physiologic dead-space (V_{DCO_2}):

$$V_{DCO_2}/V_T = (Pa_{CO_2} - Pe_{CO_2})/Pa_{CO_2}$$

$$E = \text{mixed expired}$$

Arterial blood O_2 content (Ca_{O_2}):

$$Ca_{O_2} = \text{Hb concentration} \times 1.34 \times \% \text{ saturation}$$
$$+ (0.003 \times \%P_{O_2})$$

Shunt equation:

$$Q_S/Q_T = (Cc'_{O_2} - Ca_{O_2})/(Cc'_{O_2} - Cv_{O_2})$$

$$c' = \text{pulmonary capillary;}$$

$$v = \text{mixed venous;}$$

$$Cc'_{O_2} \sim Ca_{O_2}, \text{ where \% saturation derived from } Pa_{O_2}$$

Alveolar gas equation:

$$Pa_{O_2} = Fi_{O_2}(P_B - P_{H_2O}) - Pa_{CO_2}/R$$

$$A = \text{alveolar;}$$

$$B = \text{barometric;}$$

$$R = \text{respiratory exchange ratio} = 0.08$$

Oxygen consumption (Fick principle):

$$V_{O_2} = Qt \times (Ca_{O_2} - Cv_{O_2})$$

$$V_{O_2} = \text{oxygen consumption;}$$

$$Qt = \text{cardiac output;}$$

$$v = \text{mixed venous}$$

Diffusion capacity (D_{LCO}):

$$D_{LCO} = V_{CO}/Pa_{CO}$$

$$V_{CO} = \text{Carbon monoxide consumption;}$$

$$A = \text{alveolar}$$

Henderson-Hasselbalch relationship for HCO_3 buffer system:

$$pH = 6.1 + \log([HCO_3]p/0.03 \times P_{CO_2});$$

$$[HCO_3]p = \text{plasma concentration of bicarbonate}$$

APPENDIX B

Karnofsky Performance Scale

Percent Capable (%)	Activity Level	Degree Impaired
100	Normal activity and work	No limitations
90	Same	Active; minor symptoms
80	Same	Some effort involved; moderate symptoms
70	Unable to work; cares for self at home	Inactive lifestyle; self-sufficient
60	Same	Sedentary; occasional assistance required
50	Same	Considerable assistance and medical care
40	Requires institutional care or home equivalent	Disabled; special care requirements
30	Same	Severely disabled; frequent hospitalization
20	Same	Hospitalized; supportive intervention
10	Same	Moribund; terminal
0	Same	Dead

Modified from Karnofsky DA, Burchenal JH. Chemotherapy of Cancer. Macleod, CM, ed. Columbia University Press, 1949:191–205; with permission.

APPENDIX C

Pulmonary Function Test Decision Tree

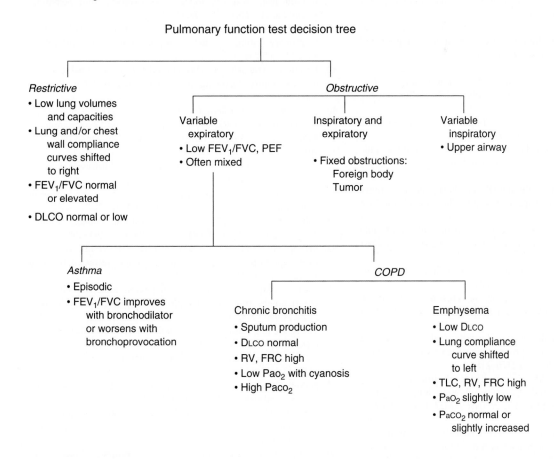

REFERENCES

1. Will JA, DiAugustine RP. Lung neuroendocrine cells and regulatory peptides: distribution, functional studies, and implications. A symposium. *Exp Lung Res* 1982;3:185.
2. King K, Torday J, Sunday M. Bombesin and {Leu8}phyllolitorin promote fetal mouse lung branching morphogenesis via-receptor mediated mechanism. *Dev Biol* 1995;92:4357–4361.
3. Blobel GA, Gould GE, Moll R, et al. Co-expression of neuroendocrine markers and epithelial cytoskeletal proteins in bronchopulmonary neuroendocrine neoplasms. *Lab Invest* 1985;52: 39.
4. Abraham SN, Thankavel K, Malaviya R. Mast cells as modulators of host defense in the lung. *Front Biosci* 1997;2:d78–d87.
5. Widdicombe JG, Pack RJ. The Clara cell. *Eur J Respir Dis* 1982;63:202.
6. Hawgood S, Clements JA. Pulmonary surfactant and its apoproteins. *J Clin Invest* 1990;86:1–6.
7. Goldstein E, Bartlema HC. Role of alveolar macrophage in pulmonary bacterial defense. *Bull Eur Physiopathol Respir* 1977;13:57–67.
8. Lee KF, Olak J. Anatomy and physiology of the pleural space. In: Rusch VW, ed. *Chest surgery clinics of North America*, Vol. 4. Philadelphia: WB Saunders, 1994:391–403.
9. Miserocchi G. Physiology and pathophysiology of pleural fluid turnover. *Eur Respir J* 1997;10:219–225.
10. Epstein SK. An overview of respiratory muscle function. *Clin Chest Med* 1994;15:619–139.

11. Polkey MI, Moxham J. Clinical aspects of respiratory muscle dysfunction in the critically ill. *Chest* 2001;119:926–939.
12. Hopkins PM. Skeletal muscle physiology. *Contin Educ Anaesth Crit Care Pain* 2006;6:1–6.
13. Downs JB, Douglas ME, Sanfelippo PM, et al. Ventilatory pattern, intrapleural pressure, and cardiac output. *Anesth Analg* 1977;56:88–96.
14. Cherniak NS, Longobardo GS. Cheyne-stokes breathing: instability in physiologic control. *N Engl J Med* 1973;288:952–957.
15. Roussos C, Fixley M, Gross D, et al. Fatigue of inspiratory muscles and their synergistic behavior. *J Appl Physiol* 1979;46:897–904.
16. Bellemare FD, Grassino A. Effect of pressure and timing of contraction on human diaphragmatic fatigue. *J Appl Physiol* 1982;53:1190–1195.
17. Weil JV, Byrne-Quinn V, Sodal IE, et al. Hypoxic ventilatory drive in normal man. *J Clin Invest* 1970;49:1061–1072.
18. Robinson TD, Freiberg DB, Regnis JA, et al. The role of hypoventilation and ventilation-perfusion redistribution in oxygen-induced hypercapnia during acute exacerbations of chronic obstructive pulmonary disease. *Am J Respir Crit Care Med* 2000;161:1524–1529.
19. Platoshyn O, Brevnova EE, Burg ED, et al. Acute hypoxia selectively inhibits KCNA5 channels in pulmonary artery smooth muscle. *Am J Physiol Cell Physiol* 2006;290:C907–C916.
20. Chabot F, Schrijen F, Saunier C. Role of NO pathway, calcium and potassium channels in the peripheral pulmonary vascular tone in dogs. *Eur Respir J* 2001;17:20–26.
21. Giebish G, Macleod MB, Pitts RF. Affect of adrenal steroids on renal tubular absorption of bicarbonate. *Am J Physiol* 1955;183:377–386.

22. Wasserman K, Koike A. Is the anaerobic threshold truly anaerobic? *Chest* 1992;101:211S–218S.

23. Wyser C, Tultz P, Soler M, et al. Prospective evaluation of an algorithm for the assessment of lung resection candidates. *Am J Respir Crit Care Med* 1999;159:1450–1456.

24. Kearney DJ, Lee TH, Reilly JJ, et al. Assessment of operative risk in patients undergoing lung resection: importance of predicted pulmonary function. *Chest* 1994;105:753–759 pgsendash.

25. Bechard DE. Pulmonary function testing. In: LoCicero J, ed. *Chest surgery clinics of North America*, Vol. 2. Philadelphia: WB Saunders, 1992:565–586.

26. Anderson F, Downing GM, Hill J. Palliative performance scale (PPS): a new tool. *J Palliat Care* 1996;12:5–11.

27. Aaronson PI, Robertson TP, Knock GA, et al. Hypoxic pulmonary vasoconstriction: mechanisms and controversies. *J Physiol* 2006;570(Pt 1):53–58.

28. Grillo HC, Shepard JA, Mathieson DJ, et al. Post pneumonectomy syndrome: diagnosis, management, and results. *Ann Thorac Surg* 1992;54:638–650.

29. Murgu SD, Colt HG. A 68 year old man with intractable wheezing and dyspnea 45 years after pneumonectomy. *Chest* 2006;129:1107–1111.

30. Barnes N, Dahlen SE, Sampson A, et al. Asthma: the role of leukotrienes. *Pharm J* 1999;263:600–601.

31. Milgrom H, Fick RB, Su JQ, et al. Treatment of allergic asthma with monoclonal antigen IgE antibody. *N Engl J Med* 1999;342:1966–1973.

32. Martin GS, Mangailardi RJ, Wheeler AP, et al. Albumin and furosemide therapy in hypoproteinemic patients with acute lung injury. *Crit Care Med* 2002;30:2175–2182.

33. Sciurba FC, Rogers RM, Keenan RJ, et al. Improvement in pulmonary function and elastic recoil after lung reduction surgery for diffuse emphysema. *N Engl J Med* 1995;334:1095–1099.

34. Safanoff I, Emmanuel GE. The effect of pendelluft and dead space on nitrogen clearance: mathematical and experimental models and their application to the study of the distribution of ventilation. *J Clin Invest* 1967;46:1683–1693.

35. Harada K, Saoyama N, Izumi K, et al. Experimental pendulum air in the flail chest. *Jpn J Surg* 1983;133:219–226.

36. Davignon K, Kwo J, Bigatello LM. Pathophysiology and management of flail chest. *Minerva Anestesiol* 2004;70:193–199.

37. Downs JB, Chapman RL. Treatment of bronchopleural fistula during continuous positive pressure ventilation. *Chest* 1976;69:363–366.

38. Turnbull AD, Carlton G, Howland WS, et al. High frequency jet ventilation in major airway or pulmonary disruption. *Ann Thorac Surg* 1981;32:468.

39. Northfield TC. Oxygen therapy for spontaneous pneumothorax. *Br Med J* 1971;4:86–88.

40. Flint K, Al-Hillawi AH, Johnson NM. Conservative management of spontaneous pneumothorax. *Lancet* 1984;2:687–688.

41. Henry M, Arnold T, Harvey J, et al. BTS guidelines for the management of spontaneous pneumothorax. *Thorax* 2003;58:ii39.

42. Sharma S. Restrictive Lung Disease. E-Medicine Specialties/Pulmonology at WebMD, June 5, 2006: www.emedicine.com/med/topic2012.htm.

43. Lee P, Gildea TR, Stoller JK. Alpha-1 emphysema in non-smokers: Alpha-1 antitrypsin deficiency and other causes. *Cleve Clin J Med* 2002;69:928–946.

44. Doweiko JP, Nompleggi DJ. Use of albumin as a volume expander. *JPEN J Parenter Enteral Nutr* 1991;15:484–487.

45. Kishikawa M, Yoshioki T, Shimazu T, et al. Pulmonary contusion causes-long term respiratory dysfunction with decreased functional residual capacity. *J Trauma* 1991;31:1203–1208.

46. Grande NR, Peao MND, de Sa CM, et al. Lung fibrosis induced by bleomycin: structural changes and overview of recent advances. *Scanning Microsc* 1998;12:487–494.

47. Jackson RM, Veal CF. Review: re-expansion, re-oxygenation, rethinking. *Am J Sci* 1989;298:44–50.

48. Chai PJ, Williamson AJ, Lodge AJ, et al. Effects of ischemia on pulmonary dysfunction after cardiopulmonary bypass. *Ann Thorac Surg* 1999;67:731–735.

49. Jordan S, Mitchell JA, Quinlan GJ, et al. The pathogenesis of lung injury following pulmonary resection. *Eur Respir J* 2000;15:790–799.

50. Deschamps C, Pairolero PC. Post-pneumonectomy pulmonary edema. In: Wilson RS, Trastek VF, eds. *Chest Surgery clinics of North America*, Vol. 2. Philadelphia: WB Saunders, 1992:785–791.

51. Ware LB, Matthay MA. The acute respiratory distress syndrome. *N Engl J Med* 2000;342:1334–1349.

52. Ashrafian H, Davey P. Is amiodarone an unrecognized cause of acute respiratory failure in the ICU? *Chest* 2001;120:275–282.

53. Iribarren C, Jacobs DR, Sydney S. Cigarette smoking, alcohol consumption, and risk of ARDS. *Chest* 2000;117:163–168.

54. Bernard GR, Hudson LD, Thompson BT. NIH NHLBI ARDSNetwork: report on ongoing clinical trials. *Annual Meeting of American Thoracic Society*. Orlando, May 24, 2004.

55. Sevitt S. Diffuse and focal oxygen pneumonitis. A preliminary report on the threshold of pulmonary oxygen toxicity in man. *J Clin Pathol* 1974;27:21.

56. The Acute Respiratory Distress Syndrome Network. Ventilation at lower tidal volumes as compared with traditional tidal volumes for acute lung injury and the acute respiratory distress syndrome. *N Engl J Med* 2000;342:1301–1308.

57. Hirvela ER. Advances in the management of acute respiratory distress syndrome. *Arch Surg* 2000;135:126–135.

58. Meduri GU, Headley AS, Golden E, et al. Effect of prolonged methylprednisolone therapy in unresolving acute respiratory distress syndrome. *JAMA* 1998;280:159–165.

59. NHLBI Acute Respiratory Distress Syndrome Clinical Trials Network. Efficacy and safety of corticosteroids for persistent acute respiratory distress syndrome. *N Engl J Med* 2006;354:1671–1684.

60. Hardaway RM, Harke H, Tyroch AH, et al. Treatment of severe respiratory distress syndrome: a final report on a phase one study. *Am Surg* 2001;6:377–382.

61. Bernard GR, Vincent JL, Laterre PF, et al. Efficacy and safety of recombinant activated protein C for severe sepsis. *N Engl J Med* 2001;344:699–709.

62. Nakagawe M, Tanaka H, Tsukuma H, et al. Relationship between the duration of the post-operative smoke-free period and the incidence of post-operative pulmonary complications after pulmonary surgery. *Chest* 2001;120:705–710.

63. Williams RS, Mickell JJ, Young ES, et al. Methemoglobin levels during combined nitroglycerine and nitroprusside infusions in infants after cardiac surgery. *J Cardiothorac Vasc Anesth* 1994;8:658–662.

64. Michenfelder JD. Cyanide release from sodium nitroprusside in the dog. *Anesthesiology* 1977;46:196–201.

65. Light RW. Parapneumonic effusions and empyema. *Proc Am Thorac Soc* 2006;3:75–80.

66. Mehran RJ, Deslauriers J. Indications for surgery and patient work-up for bullectomy. In: Faber LP, ed. *Chest surgery clinics of North America*, Vol. 7. Philadelphia: WB Saunders, 1997:801–814.

67. Goldstraw P, Petrou M. The surgical treatment of emphysema: the brompton approach. *Chest Surg Clin N Am* 1995;5:777.

68. Asaph JW, Handy JR, Grunkemeier GL, et al. Median sternotomy vs. Thoracotomy to resect primary lung cancer: analysis of 815 cases. *Ann Thorac Surg* 2000;70:373–379.

69. Stratmann G, Gregory GA. Neurogenic and humoral vasoconstriction in acute pulmonary thromboembolism. *Anesth Analg* 2003;97:341–354.

70. Turpie AGG, Chin BSP, Lip GYH. Venous thromboembolism: treatment strategies. *Br Med J* 2002;325:948–950.

71. Leacche M, Unic D, Goldhaber SZ, et al. Modern surgical treatment of massive pulmonary embolism: results in 47 consecutive patients after rapid diagnosis and aggressive surgical approach. *J Thorac Cardiovasc Surg* 2005;129:1018–1023.

72. Thistlewaite PA, Kemp A, Du L, et al. Outcomes of endarterectomy for treatment of extreme thromboembolic pulmonary hypertension. *J Thorac Cardiovasc Surg* 2006;131:307–313.

73. Hill N. Non-invasive ventilation. *Pulm Perspect* 1997;14:1–4.

74. Badar T, Bidani A. Mechanical ventilatory support. *Chest Surg Clin N Am* 2002;12:265–299.

75. van Balkan RH, van der Heijden HAF, van Herwaarden CL, et al. Corticosteroid-induced myopathy of the respiratory muscles. *Neth J Med* 1994;45:114–122.

76. Safakas NM, Salesiotou V, Filaditaki V, et al. Respiratory muscle strength in hypothyroidism. *Chest* 1992;102:189–194.

77. Wartofsky L, Burman KD. Alterations in thyroid function in patients with systemic illness: the "euthyroid sick syndrome". *Endocr Rev* 1982; 164–217.

78. Liposky JM, Nelson LD. Ventilatory response to high caloric loads in critically ill patients. *Crit Care Med* 1994;22:796–802.

79. Benumof JL. Mechanism of decreased blood flow to atelectatic lung. *J Appl Physiol* 1979;46:1047–1048.

80. Benumof JL, Pirlo AF, Trousdale FR. Inhibition of hypoxic pulmonary vasoconstriction by decreased PVO2: a new indirect mechanism. *J Appl Physiol* 1981;51:871–874.

81. Benumof JL. One-lung ventilation and hypoxic pulmonary vasoconstriction: implications for anesthetic management. *Anesth Analg* 1985;64:821.

SELECTED READINGS

Bouhuys A. *The physiology of breathing*. New York: Grune & Stratton, 1977:26–42.

Boyd AD, Glassman LR. Trauma to the lung. In: Mansour KA, ed. *Chest surgery clinics of North America*, Vol. 7. Philadelphia: WB Saunders, 1997:263–284.

Celli B. The diaphragm and respiratory muscles. In: Moores D, ed. *Chest surgery clinics of North America*, Vol. 8. Philadelphia: WB Saunders, 1998:207–224.

Cohen E. Physiology of the lateral decubitus position and one-lung ventilation. In: Wilson RS, ed. *Chest surgery clinics of North America*. Philadelphia: WB Saunders, 1997:753–771.

Cooper JD, Patterson GA. Lung-volume reduction surgery for severe emphysema. In: Deslauriers J, LeBlanc P, eds. *Chest surgery clinics of North America*, Vol. 5. Philadelphia: WB Saunders, 1995:815–831.

Davenport HW. *The ABC of acid-base chemistry*, 6th ed. Chicago: University of Chicago Press, 1974:3–49.

Hlastala MP, Berger AJ. *Physiology of respiration*. New York: Oxford Unversity Press, 1996:162–208.

Jackson RM. Oxygen therapy and toxicity. In: Ayers SM, ed. *Textbook of critical care*. Philadelphia: WB Saunders, 1995:784–789.

Karnofsky DA, Burchenal JH. The clinical evaluation of chemotherapeutic agents in cancer. In: Macleod CM, ed. *Chemotherapy of cancer*. New York: Columbia University Press, 1949:191–205.

Kreit JW, Rogers RM. The work of breathing. In: Ayers SM, ed. *Textbook of critical care*. Philadelphia: WB Saunders, 1995:643–649.

Levitzky MG. *Pulmonary physiology*, 5th ed. New York: McGraw-Hill, 1999.

Levitzky MG. *Pulmonary physiology*, 6th ed. New York: McGraw-Hill, 2003.

Levitzky MG, Cairo JM, Hall SM. *Introduction to respiratory care*. Philadelphia: WB Saunders, 1990.

Loiacono J, Cunneen C. Mechanical ventilation of the postoperative patient. In: Wilson RS, ed. *Chest surgery clinics of North America*, Vol. 7. Philadelphia: WB Saunders, 1997:801–814.

Mayberry JC, Trunkey DD. The fractured rib in chest wall trauma. In: Mansour KA, ed. *Chest surgery clinics of North America*, Vol. 7. Philadelphia: WB Saunders, 1997:239–261.

Milic-Emili J. Pulmonary statics. In: Widdicombe JG, ed. *MTP international review of sciences: respiratory physiology*. London: Butterworth-Heineman, 1974:105–137.

Mili-Emili J. Ventilation. In: West JB, ed. *Regional differences in the lung*. New York: Academic Press, 1977:167–199.

Miller A, Anderson OS. Blood acid-base alignment nomogram: scales for pH, pCO2, base excess for whole blood of different hemoglobin concentrations, plasma bicarbonate, and plasma total-CO2. *Scand J Clin Lab Invest* 1963;15:211.

Moulton A, Greenburg G. The pulmonary system. In: O'Leary JP, ed. *The physiologic basis of surgery*, 2nd ed. Philadelphia: Lippincott-Raven, 1996:376–405.

Murray JF. *The normal lung*, 2nd ed. Philadelphia: WB Saunders, 1986:83–138.

Nunn JF. *Nunn's applied respiratory physiology*, 4th ed. Oxford: Butterworth-Heinemann, 1993.

Rasanen J, Downs JB. Airway pressure therapy. In: Ayers SM, ed. *Textbook of critical care*. Philadelphia: WB Saunders, 1995:867–879.

Rochester DF, Truwit JD. Respiratory muscle failure in critical illness. In: Ayers SM, ed. *Textbook of critical care*. Philadelphia: WB Saunders, 1995:637–642.

Russell JA. Pathophysiology of acute respiratory failure. In: Todd TRJ, ed. *Chest surgery clinics of North America*, Vol. 1. Philadelphia: WB Saunders, 1991:209–237.

Sanders MH, Stiller RA, Strollo PJ. Positive-pressure ventilation without tracheal intubation. In: Ayers SM, ed. *Textbook of critical care*. Philadelphia: WB Saunders, 1995:932–943.

Sandler AN. Anesthesia. In: Pearson FG, Deslauriers J, Ginsberg RJ, et al. eds. *Thoracic surgery*. New York: Churchill Livingstone, 1995:85–112.

Sessler CN, Fowler AA. The structural basis of pulmonary function. In: Ayers SM, ed. *Textbook of critical care*. Philadelphia: WB Saunders, 1995:628–636.

Smith RA. Principles of mechanical ventilation. In: Ayers SM, ed. *Textbook of critical care*. Philadelphia: WB Saunders, 1995:858–867.

Taylor AE, Adkins WK, Wilson P. Regulation of capillary exchange of fluid and protein. In: Ayers SM, Grenvik A, Holbrook P, et al. ed. *Textbook of critical care*. Philadelphia: WB Saunders, 1995:659–667.

TenHoor T, Mannino DM, Moss M. Risk factors for ARDS in the united states: analysis of the 1993 national mortality follow-up study. *Chest* 2001;119:1179–1184.

Trottier SM, Taylor RW. Adult respiratory distress syndrome. In: Ayers SM, ed. *Textbook of critical care*. Philadelphia: WB Saunders, 1995:811–820.

Viner AM, Stein KL. High-frequency ventilation and oscillation. In: Ayers SM, ed. *Textbook of critical care*. Philadelphia: WB Saunders, 1995:880–886.

Weibel ER. *Morphometry of the human lung*. Berlin: Springer-Verlag, 1963.

Weibel ER, Taylor CR. Functional design of the human lung for gas exchange. In: Fishman AP, ed. *Pulmonary diseases and disorders*, 3rd ed. New York: McGraw-Hill, 1998:21–61.

Weinberger SE. *Principles of pulmonary medicine*, 2nd ed. Philadelphia: WB Saunders, 1992.

West JB. *Respiratory physiology—the essentials*, 6th ed. Baltimore: Lippincott Williams & Wilkins, 2000.

West JB. *Ventilation/blood flow and gas exchange*, 5th ed. Oxford: Blackwell Science, 1990.

West JB, Dollery CT, Naimark A. Distribution of blood flow in isolated lung: relation to vascular and alveolar pressures. *J Appl Physiol* 1964;19:713–724.

Yusen RD, Lefrak SS. Evaluation of patients with emphysema for lung volume reduction surgery. In: Cox JL, ed. *Seminars in thoracic and cardiovascular surgery*, Vol. 8. Philadelphia: WB Saunders, 1996:83–93.

Yusen RD, Trulock EP, Pohl MS, et al. Results of lung volume reduction surgery in patients with emphysema. In: Cox JL, ed. *Seminars in thoracic and cardiovascular surgery*, Vol. 8Philadelphia: WB Saunders, 1996:99–109.

Zebrowski BK, Yano S, Liu W, et al. Vascular endothelial growth factor levels and induction of permeability in malignant pleural effusions. *Clin Cancer Res* 1999;5:3364–3368.

CHAPTER 17

The Digestive System

Dai H. Chung and B. Mark Evers

The gastrointestinal (GI) tract represents a magnificent paradigm of efficiency and economy. The critically important task of the GI tract is the digestion and eventual absorption of liquids and nutrients that are ingested on a daily basis. This remarkable process begins in the mouth with the initial breakdown of the dietary components. The act of swallowing propels the bolus of food through the esophagus and into the stomach, where the food is further broken down in a highly acid environment. The chyme is then released into the small intestine, where almost complete digestion and absorption of the ingested nutrients occurs secondary to the well-orchestrated release of GI hormones and neural innervation, which regulate secretion, motility, and eventual absorption. Approximately 1.5 L of fluid passes through the ileocecal valve into the colon, where all but 100 mL is absorbed and the wastes are eliminated. This chapter presents an overview of GI function, including a discussion of the GI hormones, the physiology of swallowing, GI secretions, digestion, absorption, and eventual elimination.

GASTROINTESTINAL HORMONES, RECEPTORS, AND SIGNALING PATHWAYS

Gastrointestinal Hormones

GI hormones are chemical messengers that regulate intestinal and pancreatic function. These hormones are secreted by endocrine cells, which are widely distributed and localized to specific regions of the intestinal mucosa and pancreas (1–4). In fact, the gut represents the largest endocrine organ in the body (5). Although initially described as "endocrine" products, subsequent studies showed that these chemical messengers can act in a true endocrine manner (i.e., discharged into the bloodstream and act on a distant site), a paracrine manner to stimulate cells in close proximity, or an autocrine manner to stimulate the function of the cell of origin. In addition, hormones may serve as transmitting agents for nervous impulses or discharged into blood vessels

following nervous stimulation in a true neurocrine manner (Fig. 17.1). These hormones control many of the functions in the GI tract, including regulation of secretion, motility, absorption, digestion, and, in some instances, growth of the gut mucosa and pancreas (4,6–8).

The history of GI hormones dates back to January 1902 with the discovery of secretin by Bayliss and Starling (9), which was postulated based on the brisk secretion of pancreatic juice following the irrigation of a denervated loop of small bowel with dilute hydrochloric acid. The discovery of secretin was followed in short order by the discovery of gastrin by Edkins (10). However, the true physiologic and pathologic implications of these hormones were not realized for another 50 years, until radioimmunoassay became available to identify and characterize these peptides (11). The first GI hormone isolated was gastrin, which was described by Gregory and Tracy (12) in 1964. Before this, two surgeons, Zollinger and Ellison (13), described the pathologic implications of hypergastrinemia in their landmark article of 1955. After gastrin, secretin and cholecystokinin (CCK) were isolated and chemically characterized (14). To date, a variety of hormones and related peptides have been identified and physiologic functions elucidated (1–8). The further characterization of these hormones has been greatly facilitated by the molecular cloning of the genes encoding the GI hormones and their respective receptors (1,8,15–17).

The GI hormones are synthesized as inactive precursors that are converted to final secreted forms by posttranslational modifications. The most potent stimulus for hormone release and secretion is food, with the composition of the chyme dictating the timing and specific hormone released. Activation of either extrinsic or intrinsic nerves is also important in release (18). Inhibition of hormone release is mediated by removal of the stimulus, negative feedback inhibitory loops, or other peptides, such as the inhibitory hormone somatostatin, which can block the release of all known GI peptides. An overview of some of the more important GI hormones will be presented in this section. The location and major stimulants of release

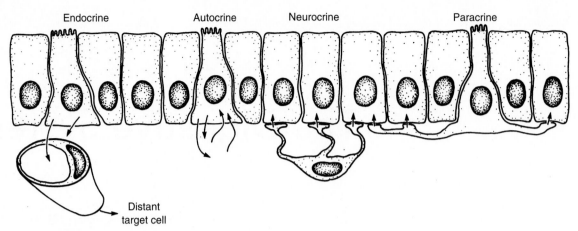

FIGURE 17.1   Actions of intestinal hormones may occur through endocrine, autocrine, neurocrine, or paracrine effects. (Adapted from Miller LJ. Gastrointestinal hormones and receptors. In: Yamada T, Alpers DH, Laine L, et al. eds. *Textbook of gastroenterology*, 3rd ed, Vol. 1. Philadelphia: Lippincott Williams & Wilkins, 1999.)

and primary action are summarized in Table 17.1. [For a more in-depth discussion of the structure, molecular biology, and physiologic functions of these hormones, the reader is referred to *references* (1–3,15,16,19)].

Gastrin

Gastrin is synthesized and stored in G cells located in the antral mucosa and in the mucosa of the proximal part of the small intestine. Gastrin is released by chemical, mechanical, or neural stimuli that act on the G cell. Proteins, peptones, and amino acids have all been demonstrated to release significant amounts of gastrin. Other stimulants of release include antral distention, vagus stimulation, and gastrin-releasing peptide (GRP). The release of gastrin is suppressed by acidification of the antral mucosa, certain prostaglandins, somatostatin, and members of the secretin family of hormones, such as secretin and glucagon. The major physiologic action of gastrin is to stimulate acid secretion from the stomach through three separate mechanisms: (i) a direct activation of the parietal cell, (ii) a potentiating interaction with histamine, and (iii) possibly the release of histamine. Gastrin also causes electrolyte and water secretion by the stomach, pancreas, liver, and Brunner glands. Gastrin stimulates motility in the stomach, small intestine, colon, and gallbladder, and it inhibits contraction of the pylorus and the sphincter of Oddi. Gastrin stimulates synthesis of protein by the fundic mucosa and amino acid uptake in the duodenal mucosa. In addition, gastrin has been shown to have a trophic effect on the fundic mucosa, pancreas, and possibly the colon, as well as certain GI and pancreatic cancers that possess gastrin receptors.

Cholecystokinin

CCK is present throughout the small intestine, with the highest concentrations in endocrine cells (I cells) of the duodenum and jejunum. CCK was purified as a 33-amino acid peptide; however, both smaller and larger forms have been described and characterized. Products of fat and protein digestion within the intestinal lumen initiate release of CCK. The concentration of intraluminal trypsin and bile acids inversely regulates CCK release. CCK and gastrin share identical carboxyl terminal tetrapeptides, which explains many of the similarities in their actions. The principal physiologic actions of CCK are stimulation of gallbladder contraction and pancreatic enzyme secretion. In addition, CCK stimulates pancreatic bicarbonate secretion and insulin release from the pancreas. Conversely, CCK inhibits contraction of the lower esophageal sphincter (LES) and the sphincter of Oddi. CCK has a trophic effect on the pancreas as well as CCK receptor—positive GI cancers.

Secretin

Secretin is a 27-amino acid peptide that is localized to specialized cells of the duodenal and proximal jejunal mucosa (S cells). Secretin is released by duodenal acidification or by contact with bile and perhaps fat. The primary role of secretin is to stimulate the release of water and bicarbonate from pancreatic ductal cells. This action facilitates the entry of pancreatic enzymes and provides a pH favorable for fat digestion. Secretin also acts to stimulate the flow of bile and to inhibit gastrin release, gastric acid secretion, and GI motility.

Somatostatin

Somatostatin is a tetradecapeptide that has been localized to various areas in the central nervous system, the antrum and fundus of the stomach, small bowel, colon, and pancreas. Simply put, somatostatin can be thought of as the universal "off switch" that inhibits the release of many hormones, as well as pancreatic and GI secretions and intestinal motility. Important clinical applications of somatostatin include its use as an inhibitory agent to decrease secretion from various fistulas (most notably pancreatic fistulas) and in the treatment of esophageal variceal bleeding. In addition, somatostatin can ameliorate many of the symptoms

TABLE 17.1

Location, Stimulants of Release, and Primary Effects of Gastrointestinal Hormones

Hormone	Location	Stimulants of Release	Primary Effects
Gastrin	Antrum, duodenum (G cells)	Peptides, amino acids, antral distension, vagal and adrenergic stimulation, gastrin releasing peptide (bombesin)	Stimulates gastric acid and pepsinogen secretion Stimulates gastric mucosal growth
Cholecystokinin (CCK)	Duodenum, jejunum (I cells)	Fats, peptides, amino acids	Stimulates pancreatic enzyme secretion Stimulates gallbladder contraction Relaxes sphincter of Oddi Inhibits gastric emptying
Secretin	Duodenum, jejunum (S cells)	Fatty acids, luminal acidity, bile salts	Stimulates release of water and bicarbonate from pancreatic ductal cells Stimulates flow and alkalinity of bile Inhibits gastric acid secretion and motility and inhibits gastrin release
Somatostatin	Pancreatic islets (D cells), antrum, small bowel, colon Pancreas: glucose, amino acids, CCK	Gut: fat, protein, acid, other hormones (e.g., gastrin, CCK)	Universal "off" switch Inhibits release of gastrointestinal (GI) hormones Inhibits gastric acid secretion Inhibits small bowel water and electrolyte secretion Inhibits secretion of pancreatic hormones
Gastrin-releasing peptide (GRP) (mammalian equivalent of bombesin)	Antrum, small bowel	Vagal stimulation	Universal "on" switch Stimulates release of all GI hormones (except secretin) Stimulates GI secretion and motility Stimulates gastric acid secretion and release of antral gastrin Stimulates growth of intestinal mucosa and pancreas
Gastric inhibitory polypeptide (GIP)	Duodenum, jejunum (K cells)	Glucose, fat, protein adrenergic stimulation	Inhibits gastric acid and pepsin secretion Stimulates pancreatic insulin release in response to hyperglycemia
Motilin	Duodenum, jejunum	Gastric distension, fat	Stimulates upper GI tract motility May initiate the migrating motor complex

(continued)

TABLE 17.1

(Continued)

Hormone	Location	Stimulants of Release	Primary Effects
Vasoactive intestinal peptide (VIP)	Neurons throughout GI tract	Vagal stimulation	Primarily functions as a neuropeptide Potent vasodilator
Pancreatic polypeptide (PP)	Pancreas	Vagal stimulation (protein, fat, carbohydrate) Hormones (gastrin, CCK, secretin, GRP)	Inhibits pancreatic exocrine secretion
Neurotensin	Small bowel (N cells)	Fat	Stimulates pancreatic water and bicarbonate secretion Inhibits gastric secretion Stimulates growth of small and large bowel mucosa
Glucagon	Pancreas (A cells), stomach, small bowel	Hypoglycemia, amino acids (alanine, arginine)	Glycogenolysis
Enteroglucagon	Small bowel (L cells)	Glucose, fat	Glucagon-like peptide 1 (GLP-1) Stimulates insulin release Inhibits pancreatic glucagon release Glucagon-like peptide 2 (GLP-2) Potent enterotrophic factor
Peptide YY	Distal small bowel, colon	Fatty acids, CCK	Inhibits gastric and pancreatic secretion Inhibits gallbladder contraction
Ghrelin	Stomach, small bowel	Fasting	Stimulates growth hormone release Stimulates appetite Controls gastric motility and secretion Cardiovascular effects

associated with hormone overproduction by endocrine tumors. A role for somatostatin as an inhibitory agent on the growth of various solid cancers has been postulated and shown experimentally; however, results in clinical trials have been disappointing.

Gastrin-Releasing Peptide

GRP, the mammalian equivalent of bombesin, is present in the gastric antrum and small bowel mucosa, where it serves as a universal "on switch" to stimulate the release of all GI hormones (except possibly secretin) and stimulate GI secretion and motility. The most important functions of GRP appear to be the stimulation of gastric acid secretion and the release of antral gastrin. This peptide also stimulates the growth of small and large bowel mucosa and pancreas, as well as various GI and pancreatic cancers.

Gastric Inhibitory Polypeptide

Gastric inhibitory polypeptide (GIP) is a 43-amino acid peptide member of the secretin/glucagon family that is released by fat and glucose. GIP cells (i.e., K cells) are identified in the duodenum and, to a lesser extent, in the jejunum. Actions of GIP include inhibition of gastric acid

secretion and stimulation of insulin release. In fact, the major action of GIP may be its insulinotropic action. In addition, GIP strongly influences hepatic glucose metabolism.

Motilin

Motilin is a 22-amino acid peptide found predominantly in the duodenum and jejunum. Release of motilin is probably mediated by vagal tone and passage of nutrients through the duodenum. In the GI tract, motilin appears to be a physiologic modulator (probably the chief modulator) of interdigestive motility, clearing the intestine between meals and preparing it for another nutritional bolus. In addition, motilin probably serves to coordinate motor activity of the LES and stomach with that of the small intestine during fasting.

Vasoactive Intestinal Peptide

Vasoactive intestinal peptide (VIP) is present throughout the central nervous system and the entire length of the gut in all of the layers, as well as around blood vessels. The major actions of VIP include dilation of most vascular beds, including the peripheral systemic vessels as well as the splenic, coronary, cerebral, extracranial, and pulmonary vessels. VIP is a potent stimulator of intestinal secretion in humans and stimulates pancreatic and biliary bicarbonate secretion in many mammals. VIP inhibits the resting tone of the LES, antagonizes the contractual effect of gastrin in several species, and inhibits gastric acid secretion. In addition, VIP is involved in the regulation of pituitary secretion, where it appears to act specifically on prolactin secretion and stimulates growth hormone (GH) release. VIP is the chief agent in the watery diarrhea syndrome, which is caused by pancreatic endocrine tumors (i.e., VIPomas).

Pancreatic Polypeptide

Pancreatic polypeptide (PP) is localized predominantly to the pancreas. Plasma PP levels rise after ingestion of protein, fat, and carbohydrate. Vagal cholinergic stimulation is probably the major regulator in the primary rapid phase of PP secretion after a meal. Also, a number of hormones, including gastrin, CCK, secretin, and GRP, have been shown to stimulate PP release in humans. The physiologic role of PP has not been entirely established. The intravenous administration of PP produces a broad spectrum of biologic actions on the GI tract, the most important of which is assumed to be an inhibitory effect on pancreatic exocrine secretion.

Neurotensin

Neurotensin (NT) is a tridecapeptide that is distributed throughout the entire small intestine, with the greatest concentration of NT-producing cells (N cells) in the distal ileum. The primary stimulant of NT release is intraluminal fat. NT is an important intestinal hormone that stimulates water and bicarbonate secretion from the pancreas, inhibits gastric secretion, facilitates fatty acid absorption in the proximal intestine, and exerts a trophic effect for small bowel and colonic mucosa, as well as certain GI tumors.

Glucagon

Glucagon, a 29-amino acid polypeptide, is synthesized in the A cells of the pancreatic islets of Langerhans and is found by radioimmunoassay in mucosal extracts of stomach and intestine. Glucagon release is stimulated by hypoglycemia, as well as by amino acids, particularly alanine and arginine. Free fatty acids, in excess, depress glucagon secretion. The classic action of glucagon is that of glycogenolysis; insulin inhibits these actions of glucagon on the liver. Glucagon also relaxes and dilates the stomach and duodenum, induces rapid transit through the small intestine, and suppresses exocrine pancreatic secretion.

Enteroglucagon

Enteroglucagon is a term designating the *family of peptides* that react with glucagon antibodies and were thought to have a trophic effect on small bowel mucosa based on a report of an enteroglucagon-secreting tumor in the kidney associated with massive small bowel hyperplasia. It has been shown that glucagon-like peptide (GLP-2), a 33-amino acid peptide, is a potent trophic factor for small bowel mucosal growth and is a member of the enteroglucagon family of peptides. Another

GLP-1, which is secreted in response to meals, stimulates insulin secretion and inhibits pancreatic glucagon release.

Peptide YY

Peptide YY (PYY) is a 36-amino acid peptide that is localized predominantly to the distal small bowel and proximal colon. PYY is released by perfusion of the colon with fat. PYY inhibits gastric and pancreatic secretions, inhibits gallbladder contraction, and exhibits trophic effects on small bowel mucosa.

Ghrelin

Ghrelin is a 28-amino acid peptide which is predominantly produced in the stomach. Ghrelin has strong GH-releasing activity. In addition, this hormone plays a role in appetite stimulation, control of energy balance, gastric motility and acid secretion, and regulation of pancreatic exocrine and endocrine function and glucose metabolism. Cardiovascular effects and modulation of neoplastic cell proliferation are other functions of ghrelin.

Therapeutic and Clinical Uses of Gastrointestinal Hormones

Various GI hormones are useful as both diagnostic and therapeutic agents (Table 17.2). For example, the gastrin analog, pentagastrin, is used to measure gastric acid secretion. CCK has been useful to stimulate gallbladder

TABLE 17.2

Diagnostic and Therapeutic Uses of Gastrointestinal Hormones

Hormone	Diagnostic/Therapeutic Uses
Gastrin	Pentagastrin (gastrin analogue) used to measure maximal gastric acid secretion
Cholecystokinin	Biliary imaging of gallbladder contraction
Secretin	Provocative test for gastrinoma
	Measurement of maximal pancreatic secretion
Glucagon	Suppresses bowel motility for endocrine spasm
	Relieves sphincter of Oddi spasm
	Provocative test for insulin, catecholamine, and growth hormone release
Somatostatin analogs	Treatment of carcinoid diarrhea and flusing
	Decrease secretion from pancreatic and intestinal fistulas
	Ameliorate symptoms associated with hormone-overproducing endocrine tumors
	Treatment of esophageal variceal bleeding

contractions to evaluate for gallbladder dysfunction. Secretin is used in patients with suspected hypergastrinemia to elicit a paradoxical increase in serum gastrin levels after administration. Glucagon acts to suppress bowel motility and has been used by endoscopists to paralyze the bowel for hypotonic studies of the duodenum and colon. In addition, glucagon has been used to relieve spasm of the sphincter of Oddi and as a provocative stimulation test for insulin release in the investigation of fasting hypoglycemia, catecholamine release in pheochromocytoma, and GH release in the assessment of pituitary function.

Perhaps the hormone with the most widespread therapeutic use is somatostatin. As previously mentioned, somatostatin can best be described as the universal "off switch." The general inhibitory function of somatostatin is wide ranging and affects a number of organ systems (20). Clinical trials have shown impressive efficacy of somatostatin and its analogs in a variety of hypersecretory disorders resistant to standard therapy, including acromegaly, pancreatic ascites, and pancreatic cholera. Somatostatin analogs have proved useful in the symptomatic treatment of GI neoplasms of endocrine origin, including Zollinger-Ellison (ZE) syndrome, insulinoma, VIPomas, glucagonoma, and carcinoid tumors. Somatostatin also acts to inhibit GI and pancreatic secretions, and, in this role, the longer-acting somatostatin analogs (e.g., octreotide) have been useful in the adjuvant treatment of pancreatic and enterocutaneous fistulas. Finally, somatostatin analogs have been used as a treatment to decrease bleeding from esophageal varices.

Pathologic Conditions Associated with Gastrointestinal Hormones

Endocrine Tumors

Probably the most clear-cut and well-recognized pathologic conditions of GI hormones are the syndromes associated with hormone overproduction. These include (i) insulin overproduction in the insulinoma syndrome, (ii) gastrin overproduction in patients with ZE syndrome, (iii) VIP overproduction in the watery diarrhea (Verner-Morrison) syndrome, (iv) glucagon overproduction in the glucagonoma syndrome, and (v) somatostatin overproduction in the somatostatinoma syndrome (21,22). Although these tumors originate predominantly in the pancreas, they will be discussed briefly as examples of pathologic conditions of hormone overproduction.

Insulinoma Syndrome

Insulinoma is the most common functioning tumor of the pancreas. Affected patients present with a constellation of symptoms referable to hypoglycemia, mental confusion, and obtundation. The diagnostic hallmark of the syndrome is the so-called Whipple triad, namely, symptoms of hypoglycemia, low blood glucose level (40–50 mg/dL), and relief of symptoms after intravenous administration of glucose. The pathognomic finding is an inappropriately high level of serum insulin during symptomatic hypoglycemia. The best way to induce hypoglycemia is with fasting. Two thirds of patients with insulinoma will experience hypoglycemic symptoms in 24 hours, and nearly all of the patients experience symptoms by 72 hours of fasting.

Zollinger-Ellison Syndrome

Gastrinoma is the second most common islet cell tumor and is the most common symptomatic, malignant, endocrine tumor of the pancreas. Approximately half of gastrinomas arise in the duodenum. The hallmark of ZE syndrome is a virulent ulcer diathesis, massive gastric hypersecretion, and an islet tumor of the pancreas. In 75% of patients with ZE syndrome, the gastrinoma is sporadic; the other 25% of patients have an associated multiple endocrine neoplasia type 1 syndrome. The main symptoms are those of peptic acid hypersecretion, with abdominal pain as a chief complaint in approximately 75% of patients. Nearly two thirds of the patients have diarrhea, and 10% to 20% of the patients present with diarrhea alone. Most patients have peptic ulcers, with duodenal ulcers being the most common, but jejunal ulceration may also be found. Current clinical clues to the diagnosis of patients with ZE syndrome include the presence of a virulent peptic ulcer or gastroesophageal reflux disease diathesis; absence of *Helicobacter pylori* or failure of the peptic ulcer to heal after either anti-*H. pylori* therapy or H_2 receptor blockade; secretory diarrhea that persists; or signs and symptoms of the multiple endocrine neoplasia type 1 syndrome.

Watery Diarrhea (Verner-Morrison) Syndrome

VIPomas are endocrine tumors that usually arise from pancreatic islets that secrete VIP and cause a syndrome of profound watery diarrhea, hypokalemia, and achlorhydria. The diarrhea, which sometimes reaches 3 to 5 L/d, persists despite fasting and nasogastric aspiration. The diagnostic triad in Verner-Morrison syndrome is a secretory diarrhea, high levels of circulating VIP, and a pancreatic tumor.

Glucagonoma Syndrome

Glucagonoma, a tumor of islet α cells, causes a syndrome with a characteristic skin rash (i.e., necrolytic migrating erythema), diabetes mellitus, anemia, weight loss, and elevated circulating levels of glucagon. Most patients are initially recognized by their skin lesions and referred to surgeons by dermatologists.

Somatostatin Syndrome

Somatostatinomas are exceedingly rare, with fewer than 60 cases reported in the literature. The full syndrome includes steatorrhea, diabetes mellitus, hypochlorhydria, and gallstones. However, the clinical presentation is unpredictable, with variable features of the syndrome present in the reported cases.

Celiac Disease and Nontropical Sprue

GI hormones may be involved in diseases of malabsorption associated with celiac disease and nontropical sprue. These diseases are associated with sensitivity to gluten. Diagnosis is established by evidence of malabsorption, small bowel mucosal atrophy, and improvement of symptoms when the patient is on a gluten-free diet (23). There is associated decreased pancreatic enzyme secretion as well as decreased gallbladder motility. Meal-stimulated and duodenal mucosal CCK concentrations are diminished in this disease. Although a number of hormones have been measured and found to be altered, the only hormone that has been consistently noted to be decreased is GIP.

Chronic Pancreatitis

Chronic pancreatitis can result in decreased pancreatic enzyme secretion and malabsorption due to loss of functional pancreatic tissue. The possible roles of GI hormones in the etiology or pathogenesis of chronic pancreatitis has been speculated, but the results have been conflicting. An increase in CCK has been postulated to contribute to the pain of chronic pancreatitis.

Carcinoid Syndrome

Carcinoid tumors have been reported in a number of organs, including most commonly the GI tract (i.e., appendix, small bowel, and colon), lungs, and bronchi (24). Carcinoid tumors have a variable malignant potential. They are composed of multipotential cells that have the ability to secrete numerous humoral agents, the most prominent of which are serotonin and substance P. The malignant carcinoid syndrome is a relatively rare disease, occurring in fewer than 10% of patients with carcinoid tumors. The classic description of the carcinoid syndrome includes vasomotor, cardiac, and GI manifestations. A number of humoral factors are produced by carcinoid tumors, but the factors considered to contribute to the carcinoid syndrome include serotonin, 5-hydroxytryptophan (a precursor of serotonin synthesis), histamine, dopamine, kallikrein, substance P, prostaglandin, and neuropeptide K. Common symptoms and signs include cutaneous flushing, diarrhea, hepatomegaly, cardiac lesions, and asthma. The diarrhea associated with carcinoid syndrome is episodic (usually occurring after meals), watery, and often explosive. Increased circulating serotonin levels are thought to be the cause of diarrhea.

Receptors and Signaling Pathways

Peptide hormones exert their effects by interacting with their specific membrane-bound receptors. Once bound to its receptor, a cascade of signaling events results in the hormone effect. There are three known classes of surface receptors: (i) the G protein—coupled receptors with seven transmembrane domains; (ii) the enzyme-linked receptors with a single transmembrane domain; and (iii) the ion channels, which are anchored to the plasma membrane with multiple domains (17).

G Protein—Coupled Receptors

The G protein—coupled receptors represent the largest known group of receptors for signaling molecules. This family includes receptors for hormonal and neuropeptides; receptors for small, nonpeptide signaling molecules, such as acetylcholine, dopamine, and serotonin; and receptors for inflammatory mediators, such as the prostaglandins (25–31). These receptors are characterized by seven hydrophobic domains that span the membrane and are functionally coupled to heterotrimeric G proteins composed of α, β, and γ subunits (Fig. 17.2) (28). Agonist binding to the receptor with seven transmembrane domains is thought to cause a conformational change in the receptor that allows it to interact with the G proteins (25–27,31).

In general, binding to the receptor sets in motion a cascade of intercellular events initiated by the action of the G protein, which ultimately results in altered levels of various intracellular messengers, such as cyclic adenosine monophosphate (cAMP), cyclic guanosine monophosphate (cGMP), and calcium. cAMP is synthesized by the enzyme adenylyl cyclase and can be rapidly degraded by cAMP phosphodiesterase. Intracellular calcium is stored in the endoplasmic reticulum and released into the cytoplasm upon stimulation. Some G proteins activate adenylyl cyclase, whereas others inhibit this enzyme. G proteins also can activate phospholipase C (PLC), leading to the release of inositol-1,4,5-triphosphate (IP$_3$) and 1,2-diacylglycerol (DAG), which increases intracellular calcium concentrations and activation of protein kinase C (PKC), respectively.

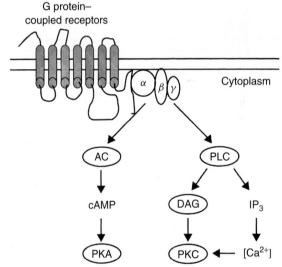

FIGURE 17.2 G protein-coupled receptor signaling pathway. G protein-coupled receptors are seven transmembrane domain proteins that are activated by the binding of ligands. Activated receptors initiate a cascade of events leading to amplification of the original signal. First, the receptor activates a trimer G protein, which consists of α, β, and γ subunits. G proteins can activate adenylyl cyclase (AC) to generate cyclic adenosine monophosphate (cAMP) or phospholipase C (PLC), which leads to the release of 1,2-diacylglycerol (DAG) or inositol-1,4,5-triphosphate (IP$_3$), respectively. Increased IP$_3$ stimulates intracellular calcium [Ca^{2+}], and both DAG and [Ca^{2+}] can activate protein kinase C (PKC). cAMP can activate protein kinase A (PKA). (Adapted from Ko TC and Evers BM. Molecular and cell biology. In: Townsend CM Jr, Beauchamp RD, Evers BM, et al. eds. *Sabiston textbook of surgery.* Philadelphia: WB Saunders, 2001.)

Changes in cAMP, calcium, and PKC, in turn, activate cascades of downstream mediators specific for different cell functions. The end result is altered biologic activity of these target proteins, leading to a specific biologic response to the initial signaling molecule.

A single peptide can interact with multiple receptors with varying affinities. One example is the CCK-A and CCK-B receptors, which exist in high-affinity, low-affinity, and very low—affinity states, with regard to binding their natural ligands (32,33). This is important because the ability of a receptor to interact with its ligand is determined by the affinity state of the receptor. Alterations in the proportion of these receptors in a particular affinity state govern how a cell responds to CCK and are therefore physiologically important.

Enzyme-Linked Receptors

Similar to the G protein—coupled receptors, the enzyme-linked receptors bind to agonists in the extracellular fluid; however, instead of interacting with G proteins, the cytoplasmic regions of the receptors are either directly associated with an enzyme or possess intrinsic enzyme activity (Fig. 17.3). The term *tyrosine kinase receptor*

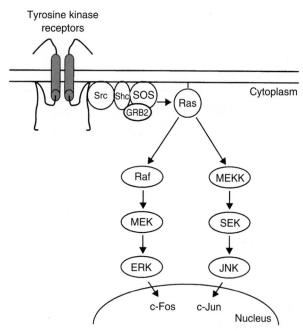

FIGURE 17.3 Tyrosine kinase receptor signaling pathway. Tyrosine kinase receptors are single transmembrane proteins that form a dimer upon ligand binding. The activated receptors bind to several proteins (Src, Shc, SOS, GRB2) to form a multiprotein signal complex. This protein complex can activate Ras, which can initiate several kinase cascades. One kinase cascade includes the Raf, MEK, and ERK members, whereas another includes the MEKK, SEK, and JNK proteins. ERK and JNK enter the nucleus to activate downstream transcription factors (e.g., c-Fos and c-Jun). (Adapted from Ko TC and Evers, BM. Molecular and cell biology. In: Townsend CM Jr, Beauchamp RD, Evers BM, et al. eds. *Sabiston textbook of surgery.* Philadelphia: WB Saunders, 2001:20, with permission.)

is traditionally applied to receptors that have a single membrane-spanning domain and are activated by growth factors, cytokines, or other hormones (31,34). Tyrosine kinase receptors include those for insulin, epidermal growth factor, transforming growth factor-α, fibroblast growth factor, and most cytokines. Stimulation of tyrosine kinase pathways is not an exclusive property of these receptors, as G protein—coupled receptors can also stimulate tyrosine phosphorylation.

Once bound, a conformational change in the receptor occurs that causes the enzymatic portion of the intracellular domain to become active. The activated enzyme phosphorylates tyrosine residues on specific target proteins, including other enzymes, factors important in regulation of gene transcription and the tyrosine kinase itself. The prototype receptor tyrosine kinase target protein is Ras, a guanosine triphosphatase (GTPase) associated with the plasma membrane. The Ras proteins serve as crucial links in the signaling cascade. On activation, Ras proteins initiate a cascade of serine and threonine phosphorylation that converges on mitogen-activated protein kinases [e.g., extracellular signal-related kinase ERK and JNK], which relay signals to downstream transcription factors (e.g., c-Fos and c-Jun) and eventually culminate in the regulation of gene expression (35–40). The Ras/mitogen-activated protein kinase pathway has been best described in its role in the control of cell proliferation (35–38). This pathway is not exclusive to the enzyme-coupled receptors, as it is well known that G protein—coupled receptors can also activate these proteins.

Ion Channel—Linked Receptors

The ion channel—linked receptors are found most commonly in cells of neuronal lineage and usually bind specific neurotransmitters (31). Examples include receptors for excitatory (acetylcholine and serotonin) and inhibitory (γ-aminobutyric acid, glycine) neurotransmitters. These receptors undergo a conformational change upon binding of the mediator, which allows passage of ions across the cell membrane and results in changes in voltage potential.

SWALLOWING AND ESOPHAGEAL PHYSIOLOGY

Swallowing

Swallowing requires a coordinated activity of the tongue, oropharynx, and upper esophagus and is divided into three phases: (i) an oral phase, which initiates the swallowing process; (ii) a pharyngeal phase, which propagates the passage of food through the pharynx into the esophagus; and (iii) the esophageal phase.

Oral Phase

The oral phase of swallowing is the transport phase of propelling a liquid or solid food bolus posteriorly into the oral cavity. It consists of both voluntary and involuntary

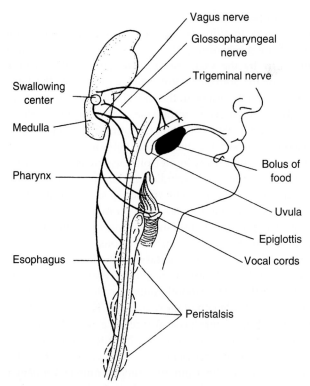

FIGURE 17.4 The swallowing mechanism. As the food bolus reaches the oropharynx, sensory impulses from cranial nerves mediate the pharyngeal phase of swallowing by a reflex mechanism through the swallowing center in the brainstem. (From Guyton AC. Transport and mixing of food in the alimentary tract. In: Guyton AC, Hall JE, eds. *Textbook of medical physiology*, 10th ed. Philadelphia: WB Saunders, 2000:729, with permission.)

components. The voluntary component of the oral phase of swallowing involves mastication, mixing with saliva, and positioning the food bolus on the dorsum of the tongue (Fig. 17.4). The involuntary phase involves glossopalatal expulsion and clearing of the food bolus into the oropharyngeal cavity (41). A food bolus coming in contact with a large number of sensory receptors from the areas of tongue and pharynx initiates the pharyngeal phase of swallowing.

Pharyngeal Phase

The pharyngeal phase of swallowing begins as a food bolus is propelled into the posterior oral cavity by the tongue. This action is mediated principally by a reflex mechanism receiving sensory impulses from vagal and glossopharyngeal afferents to the swallowing center in the brainstem (Fig. 17.4). The swallowing center in the medulla coordinates activities of several individual muscular actions as follows (42–44):

1. The soft palate is pulled upward by levator veli palatini and tensor veli palatini muscles to close the openings of the pharynx to nasal cavities.
2. The palatopharyngeal folds on either side of the pharynx are pulled medially to create a sagittal slit through which the food bolus must pass into the posterior pharynx.

3. The vocal cords are closed and the larynx is displaced upward and anteriorly by contractions of neck muscles for the posterior positioning of the epiglottis over the opening of the larynx.
4. The pharyngeal chamber shortens and widens to allow easier passage of the food bolus into the upper esophagus.
5. The contraction of the superior constrictor and the palatopharyngeus muscles of the larynx generate a propulsive peristaltic wave that propels food into the esophagus. This craniocaudal sequential contraction through the middle and inferior pharyngeal constrictor muscles is followed by an opening of the upper esophageal sphincter (UES) to allow passage of the food bolus into the esophagus. The entire passage of the food bolus through the pharynx into the esophagus takes less than 1 to 2 seconds.

Swallowing Center

The swallowing center is made up of a network of neurons in the brainstem lying mainly in the dorsal region in and adjacent to the nucleus tractus solitarius and the ventral region around the nucleus ambiguus, with extensive involvement of the reticular formation (45–47). The pharyngeal opening area contains highly sensitive receptors that transmit impulses through the sensory portions of the trigeminal and glossopharyngeal nerves to the medulla (Fig. 17.4) (48,49). This center is responsible for integrating the swallowing reflex activity of the oral cavity, pharynx, and esophagus when the food bolus is propelled to the back of the mouth (50). The swallowing center also interacts with other areas of the brainstem controlling emesis and respiration to coordinate the activity of inhibiting respiration and converting the pharynx from a respiratory to a swallowing pathway (51).

Esophageal Physiology

The esophagus serves as a conduit to propel the food bolus to the stomach. The propulsive function is accomplished by contractions of the two muscle layers (inner circular and outer longitudinal) of the esophageal wall. Both muscle layers are made up of striated muscle fibers in the upper one third to one half of the esophagus; the lower one half of the esophagus is comprised of smooth muscle. The UES consists of thickened circular striated muscles and the LES represents a 1- to 2-cm zone of increased pressure at the gastroesophageal junction.

Upper Esophageal Sphincter

The UES refers to an *anatomic zone* of high intraluminal pressure that exists between the hypopharynx and the upper esophagus. It is comprised of the muscular cartilaginous hypopharynx along with the cricoid cartilage ventrally and the cricopharyngeus muscle attached in a "C" configuration making up the lateral and dorsal walls. The inferior pharyngeal constrictor joins with the cricopharyngeus to form the UES, creating a 1- to 2-cm high-pressure zone (52). The musculature of the UES is tonically contracted at rest. The pressure profile of the UES shows axial asymmetry with a sharp ascent in its upper part as well as marked radial asymmetry (53,54). The UES pressures are higher in the anteroposterior than in the lateral orientation, and this is thought to be due to rigid cartilages of the larynx forming the anterior wall of the UES (54). Resting sphincter tone reflects the passive elastic properties of the sphincter and surrounding pharyngeal structures (55). The level of tonic contraction is based on activity of the somatic nerves innervating both the cricopharyngeus and caudal aspect of the inferior pharyngeal constrictor muscles (55). This tonic contraction of the UES is depressed during deep sleep or anesthesia (56) and shows fluctuation with respiration (55).

Esophageal Phase of Swallowing

During swallowing, the UES relaxes by a reflex mechanism coordinated through the swallowing center by contractions on the anterior sphincter wall of the suprahyoid and infrahyoid muscles. This is followed by contraction of the lower pharyngeal muscles with the arrival of the peristaltic pharyngeal contraction. As the food bolus enters the esophagus, the UES contracts to prevent reflux and entry of air. The esophagus exhibits two types of peristaltic movements: primary and secondary. Primary peristalsis is a continuation of the peristaltic wave that begins in the pharynx, spreading into the esophagus and down to the stomach (Fig. 17.5) (57). This wave of contractions, originating in the pharynx, moves to the stomach at a rate of 2 to 6 cm/s; a bolus takes approximately 8 to 10 seconds to reach the stomach. When interruption of primary peristalsis occurs, the esophagus can generate its own involuntary contractions called *secondary peristalsis*. These waves are initiated by esophageal distention largely through vagal reflexes, but myenteric nerve plexuses can also generate secondary peristaltic waves without the involvement of vagal fibers (58).

Esophageal Body

Esophageal motility is regulated by both central and peripheral mechanisms. The esophageal body is innervated primarily by the vagus nerve. These nerve fibers consist partly of the somatic motor type, arising from the lower motor neurons located in the rostral nucleus ambiguus, and partly of the visceral motor type, arising from the dorsal motor nucleus (59). The somatic motor fibers innervate the region of the striated muscles of the esophagus to control peristalsis. The sensory input from the striated muscle arises in part from the muscle spindles and sensory receptors in the ganglia of the myenteric plexus acting as tension receptors (60). Visceral motor fibers arise from the dorsal motor nucleus of the vagus as preganglionic parasympathetic motor neurons to the smooth muscle regions of the esophagus (61). These preganglionic parasympathetic fibers innervate ganglion cells of the myenteric plexus. Postganglionic fibers then innervate the smooth muscle cells of both muscle layers along the length of the esophagus. The smooth muscle portion of the esophagus also receives a sympathetic nerve supply from the cell bodies in the intermediolateral cell columns of spinal segments T-1 through T-10 (62). The afferent innervation from the smooth muscle segment is both sympathetic and parasympathetic (63).

Peristaltic contractions that accompany swallowing in the striated muscle segment of the esophagus reflect the sequential firing of somatic lower motor neurons activated in a craniocaudal sequence along the esophageal body. Sensory afferent signals triggered by distension of the esophagus regulate peristaltic contractions of the striated muscle component of the esophagus through vagal output (64). Primary peristalsis in the esophagus, initiated by the swallowing center, is a stripping wave that empties the esophagus from its proximal to distal end (Fig. 17.5) (57). The swallowing center fires vagal signals by a reflex mechanism

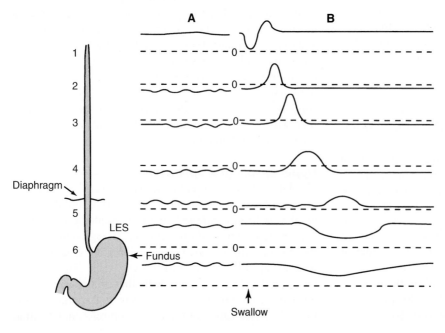

FIGURE 17.5 Manometric recordings from the esophagus and proximal stomach. *A* Between swallows, both the upper esophageal sphincter (UES) and lower esophageal sphincter (LES) are closed, as indicated by the greater than atmospheric pressures. *B* During swallowing, the UES relaxes before passage of the bolus. This is followed by peristaltic contractions in the body of the esophagus. The LES and proximal stomach relax before arrival of the primary peristaltic contraction. (From Weisbrodt NW. Swallowing. In: Johnson LR, Gerwin TA, eds. *Gastrointestinal physiology*, 6th ed. St. Louis: Mosby, 2001:31, with permission.)

and is responsible for initiating secondary peristalsis as well as altering the intensity of contractions in the smooth muscle region of the esophagus. However, the network of intrinsic myenteric plexuses coordinates the organization of these waves.

Lower Esophageal Sphincter

The LES is a 3- to 4-cm long segment of tonically contracted smooth muscle at the distal end of the esophagus. These circular muscles have irregular surfaces and evaginations due to the tonically contracted state of the sphincter muscle (65). The LES is innervated by vagal preganglionic and sympathetic postganglionic efferents, which largely innervate neurons in the myenteric plexus (66). Similar to the UES, the high-pressure LES shows axial as well as radial asymmetry. Pressures tend to be higher in the more distal segment of the LES, and both diaphragmatic and gastric sling fibers on the left side of the LES further contribute to higher pressure in this region.

The LES relaxes in response to swallowing ahead of the arrival of peristaltic waves at the distal esophagus. The LES relaxation generally lasts 5 to 10 seconds and is followed by transient contraction, which appears to be a continuation of the primary peristaltic wave sweeping the esophageal body (67). In addition to the reflexive relaxation of the LES induced by esophageal distention, LES tone is also under the control of vagal innervation. The resting tone of the LES, which ranges from 10 to 30 mm Hg, reflects a balance between two distinct regulatory influences of excitatory and inhibitory vagal fibers. LES tone is also regulated by a number of chemical and hormonal influences. For example, LES tone is increased by cholinergic agonists and decreased by prostaglandin E and isoproterenol (Table 17.3).

The primary function of the LES is to prevent reflux of gastric contents into the esophagus. Acidic gastric contents are highly caustic to the esophageal mucosa and produce symptoms of pain. Chronic exposure can also lead to other significant clinical problems, such as esophageal stricture and metaplastic transformation of the mucosal lining (i.e., Barrett esophagus).

Pathologic Conditions of Altered Swallowing and Esophageal Physiology

Oropharyngeal Dysphagia

Coordinated contraction of the pharyngeal muscles is required for proper movement of food from the oral cavity into the cervical esophagus. The etiology for oropharyngeal dysphagia varies considerably, but is largely due to inability of the pharyngeal muscles to coordinate swallowing (68). Patients with neurologic deficits (e.g., cerebrovascular accidents) or myogenic conditions (such as myasthenia gravis) may exhibit dysfunctional contractions of the oropharynx. Additionally, oropharyngeal dysfunction can result from idiopathic or secondary causes, such as the presence of a diverticulum (pharyngoesophageal) or injury to nerves. Motility studies are helpful in identifying UES abnormalities as well as distal esophageal pathology that

TABLE 17.3

Factors that Affect Lower Esophageal Sphincter Pressures

Factors	Increase LES Pressure	Decrease LES Pressure
Hormonal	Gastrin	Secretin
	Motilin	Cholecystokinin
	Substance P	Glucagon
	Bombesin	Somatostatin
		Vasoactive intestinal polypeptide
		Progesterone, estrogen
Drug related	α-Adrenergic agonists	α-Adrenergic antagonists
	Norepinephrine	Phentolamine
	Phenylephrine	β-Adrenergic agonists
		Isoproterenol
	Cholinergics	Anticholinergics
	Acetylcholine	Atropine
	Bethanechol	Theophylline
	Anticholinesterase	
	Edrophonium	
	Histamine	Barbiturates
	Metoclopramide	Prostaglandins E_1, E_2, A_2, I_2
		Serotonin
	Prostaglandin $F_{2\alpha}$	Meperidine
		Morphine
		Nitroglycerin
		Calcium channel blockers
Food related	Protein	Fat
		Chocolate
		Ethanol
		Tobacco
		Caffeine

LES, lower esophageal sphincter.

potentially contribute to oropharyngeal dysphagia. Contrast studies can also demonstrate oropharyngeal dysfunction and may be valuable diagnostic tests to consider when evaluating this condition.

Achalasia

Failure of the LES to relax in response to swallowing, along with the absence of peristalsis of the esophageal body, produce symptoms of dysphagia and regurgitation of ingested food or liquid (69). This condition is thought to be due to degeneration or absence of ganglion cells of the Auerbach plexus in the esophagus. An esophagogram can demonstrate a dilated esophageal body with its distal segment projecting a beak-like narrowing. Esophageal manometry studies can further confirm the diagnosis. In response to swallowing, abnormal simultaneous contractions occur in the esophageal body instead of normal coordinated peristaltic waves. The LES pressure, at rest, is increased and fails to relax after ingestion of food. Nonsurgical treatment options consist of pharmacotherapy and enodoscopic balloon dilatation.

Botulinum neurotoxin injections cause a sustained inhibition of neurotransmitter release at cholinergic terminals, and therefore, block excitatory acetylcholine release. A single injection of botulinum neurotoxin has been shown to be effective (70). Endoscopic pneumatic dilatation of LES, forcefully rupturing muscular fibers, is considered to be the most effective nonsurgical treatment for achalasia. Recently, minimally invasive laparoscopic Heller myotomy, in which the muscles of LES and cardia are cut, has become the standard surgical approach. The beneficial role of concomitant antireflux procedures (i.e., partial versus complete fundoplication) at the time of surgical myotomy remains controversial.

Diffuse Esophageal Spasm

This condition results from simultaneous contractions of the esophagus of unknown etiology. Contractions of high amplitude are long in duration and produce symptoms of substernal pain and dysphagia (69). These intermittent symptoms may be elicited by eating or occur spontaneously, and they frequently mimic symptoms of cardiac origin. Motility studies demonstrate simultaneous, repetitive, prolonged contractions, which are nonpropulsive, particularly in the distal two thirds of the esophagus. An esophagogram may further show simultaneous segmental contractions of the esophagus. Treatment options focus on relieving symptoms. Calcium channel blockers can decrease the amplitude of contractions. Extended myotomy of the abnormal esophagus can provide relief if medical management fails.

Gastroesophageal Reflux Disease

Idiopathic gastroesophageal reflux disorder is the most frequent condition encountered in the esophagus. As a result of an incompetent LES, gastric and/or biliary secretions can reflux into the distal esophagus and cause symptoms of heartburn. Pain is the most common symptom of this condition; however, chronic esophagitis can lead to the development of an esophageal stricture or even Barrett esophagus. A comprehensive evaluation is crucial to ensure appropriate treatment. Medical treatment consists of an H_2 blocker (e.g., cimetidine) and metoclopramide, a prokinetic agent that sensitizes the GI tract smooth muscles to the actions of acetylcholine. Various antireflux operations are considered for patients with refractory reflux disease despite appropriate medical treatment. Complete fundoplication, which can be performed using a minimally invasive laparoscopic approach, is the most commonly used technique for the effective control of symptoms. Recently, endoscopic therapy for gastroesophageal reflux disease has received considerable interest (71).

GASTROINTESTINAL SECRETION

Secretory glands are located throughout the entirety of the GI tract and serve two primary functions: (i) mucous glands provide lubrication allowing for passage of food and protection of the underlying mucosa; and (ii) digestive enzymes, which are located from the mouth to the distal small intestine, are critical for the breakdown and eventual absorption of dietary components (72). The presence of food in the GI tract is the primary stimulus for secretion. In addition, epithelial stimulation activates the enteric nervous system of the intestinal wall. Parasympathetic stimulation, predominantly in the upper part of the GI tract from vagal innervation and in the distal portion of the large intestine from pelvic parasympathetic fibers, results in increased glandular secretion. The secretion in the remainder of the small intestine and proximal portion of the colon occurs mainly in response to segmental neural and hormonal stimuli. Sympathetic stimulation can produce a slight increase in secretion; however, the predominant effect appears to be inhibition of secretion by vasoconstriction. This chapter will primarily discuss GI secretions from the mouth to the large intestine. Pancreatic and biliary secretion will be discussed further in Chapter 18.

Salivary Secretion

The salivary glands include the parotid, submandibular, and sublingual glands, which provide both mucous and serous secretions, and numerous small buccal glands located in the oral cavity that secrete only mucin. Saliva performs two important functions: (i) the mucous secretion provides lubrication; and (ii) the serous secretion contains ptyalin (an α amylase), which is important for the initial digestion of starches (72–75). Ptyalin cleaves internal α-1,4-glycosidic bonds producing maltose, maltotriose, and α-limit dextrins. A second digestive enzyme secreted in saliva is lingual lipase, which plays a role in the hydrolysis of lipids. The daily secretion of saliva ranges from 800 to 1,500 mL. The optimal pH range for saliva is between 6 and 7.4, which is favorable for the digestive action of ptyalin (72,73,76). Saliva contains a high concentration of K^+ and bicarbonate (HCO_3^-) ions and a relatively low concentration of Na^+ and Cl^- compared with plasma. Regulation of salivary secretion is controlled mainly by parasympathetic nervous signals, although sympathetic branches also result in some stimulation of secretion. In addition to these functions, salivary secretion contains antibacterial properties that are important for oral hygiene. Saliva contains a lysozyme that attacks bacterial cell walls; lactoferrin, which chelates iron, thereby preventing its use by bacteria that require iron for multiplication; and the binding glycoprotein for immunoglobulin A (IgA), which, in combination with IgA, provides an important defense against viruses and bacteria.

Esophageal Secretion

Secretions from the esophagus are entirely mucoid and provide lubrication for the process of swallowing. Simple glands are located in the body of the esophagus. Compound mucous glands are located in the upper esophagus and the gastroesophageal junction, which serve to protect the esophageal mucosa from newly digested food and the highly acidic gastric fluid, respectively.

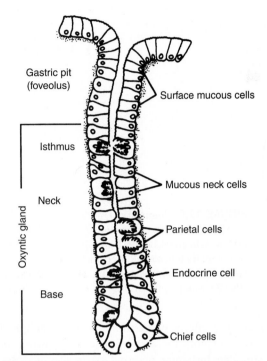

FIGURE 17.6 Schematic illustration of a typical gastric gland. (From Pandol SJ, et al. Salivary, gastric, duodenal, and pancreatic secretions. In: West JB, ed. *Physiological basis of medical practice*, 12th ed. Baltimore: Williams & Wilkins, 1990:652, with permission.)

Gastric Secretion

The critical function of the stomach is the initial breakdown of food. The stomach contains two important glands, the oxyntic (or gastric) and pyloric glands (72,77–80). Typically, the oxyntic glands, localized in the proximal 75% of the stomach, contain three main cell types: (i) mucous neck cells that secrete mucus, which, together with HCO_3^-, protect the stomach wall from acid and pepsin digestion; (ii) the peptic (or chief) cells that secrete large quantities of pepsinogen; and (iii) the parietal cells that secrete hydrochloric acid and intrinsic factor (Fig. 17.6). The pyloric glands, localized predominantly in the distal (i.e., antral) portion of the

stomach, secrete gastrin (from G cells) and a small amount of pepsinogen.

Production of Hydrochloric Acid

Hydrochloric acid, which is produced by parietal cells, facilitates the initial digestion and breakdown of food. The pH of this acid solution is approximately 0.8, which requires very high concentrations of H^+ in the lumen of the stomach. The cellular mechanisms responsible for hydrochloric acid production (Fig. 17.7) include the following: (i) The active transport of Cl^- from the cytoplasm into the lumen with active transport of Na^+ out of the lumen, thereby creating a negative potential that leads to the passive diffusion of K^+ from the cell cytoplasm into the canaliculus. (ii) Water is dissociated into H^+ ions, which are actively secreted into the canaliculus in exchange for K^+. The enzyme H^+/K^+-adenosine triphosphatase (ATPase) catalyzes this active transport of H^+ in exchange for K^+. This provides for a highly concentrated solution of hydrochloric acid. Inhibition of the H^+/K^+-ATPase completely blocks gastric acid secretion; therefore, the protein pump inhibitor agents (e.g., omeprazole) represent the most potent types of acid secretory inhibitors (81,82). (iii) CO_2 combines with the hydroxyl ions (OH^-) to form HCO_3^-, which diffuse into the extracellular fluid in exchange for Cl^-. This process is catalyzed by carbonic anhydrase. Inhibition of this enzyme decreases the rate but does not block gastric acid secretion. (iv) Water passes through the parietal cell by a process of osmosis and enters the canaliculus, providing for a final concentration of approximately 155 mEq/L of hydrochloric acid (72,79,80).

Secretion and Function of Pepsinogen and Intrinsic Factor

In addition to hydrochloric acid, pepsinogen and intrinsic factor are secreted predominantly from the oxyntic glands. Pepsinogen, which has no digestive activity, is broken down to its active form, pepsin, at pH concentrations between 1.8 and 3.5 and is inactivated with pH concentrations greater

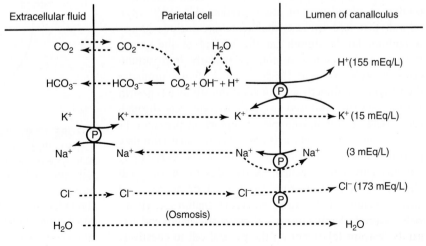

FIGURE 17.7 Postulated mechanism for the secretion of hydrochloric acid. Points labeled *P* indicate active pumps. *Dashed lines* represent free diffusion and osmosis. (From Guyton AC, Hall JE. Secretory functions of the alimentary tract. In: Guyton AC, Hall JE, eds. *Textbook of medical physiology*, 10th ed. Philadelphia: WB Saunders, 2000:743, with permission.)

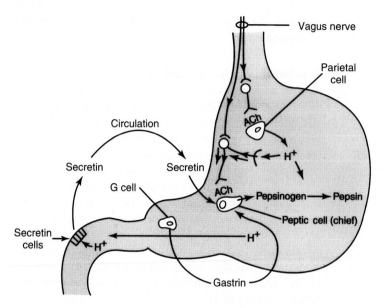

FIGURE 17.8 Summary of mechanisms for stimulating pepsinogen secretion and activation to pepsin. Ach, acetylcholine. (From Johnson LR. Gastric secretion. In: Johnson LR, Gerwin TA, eds. *Gastrointestinal physiology*, 6th ed. St. Louis: Mosby, 2001:89, with permission.)

than 5 (83). The rate of pepsinogen secretion is highly dependent on the amount of acid in the stomach. Secretion of pepsinogen occurs as a result of the stimulation of the chief cells by acetylcholine from the vagus or enteric nerves and stimulation of peptic secretion in response to acid in the stomach. The hormones gastrin and secretin can also stimulate pepsinogen release, albeit much less so than acetylcholine. A summary of factors that stimulate pepsinogen secretion and the activation of pepsin is shown in Figure 17.8.

Intrinsic factor is a mucoprotein that is secreted by the parietal cells. The combination of vitamin B_{12} with intrinsic factor is essential for absorption of this vitamin in the ileum. Patients with chronic gastritis or after massive gastric resections can develop pernicious anemia due to the absence of vitamin B_{12} and subsequent failure of maturation of the red blood cells.

Regulation of Gastric Secretion

Gastric secretion is regulated primarily by acetylcholine from nervous (i.e., vagal and local enteric reflexes) stimulation, gastrin, and histamine, which bind to their specific receptors on the parietal cells to activate various second messengers leading to stimulation of acid secretion (Fig. 17.9) (84). Stimuli that lead to acetylcholine release include gastric distention, tactile stimuli on the surface of the gastric mucosa, and chemical stimuli, particularly from amino acids, peptides, or acid (85,86). Acetylcholine stimulates the parietal cell directly and, in addition, stimulates gastrin release. Gastrin produced in antral G cells acts through cell surface G protein—coupled receptors on parietal cells to stimulate acid secretion (87,88). Factors that stimulate gastrin release include peptides, amino acids (particularly the aromatic amino acids), gastric distension (through cholinergic stimulation from vagal or enteric nerves), and GRP. Histamine is found in enterochromaffin-like (ECL) cells within the lamina propria of the gastric glands and acts on its receptor (H_2 type) on the parietal cell to effectively

potentiate the effects of gastrin and acetylcholine. ECL cells have receptors for acetylcholine and gastrin, which both stimulate histamine release. Gastrin also increases the synthesis and growth of ECL cells.

A number of surgical and pharmacologic methods to inhibit acid secretion have been developed based on the

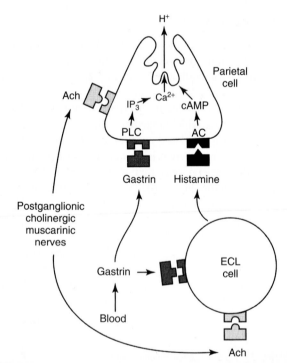

FIGURE 17.9 The parietal cell contains receptors for gastrin, acetylcholine (Ach), and histamine. In addition, gastrin and Ach release histamine from the enterochromaffin-like (ECL) cell. IP_3, inositol-1,4,5-triphosphate; cAMP, cyclic adenosine monophosphate; PLC, phospholipase C; AC, adenylyl cyclase. (From Johnson LR. Gastric secretions. In: Johnson LR, Gerwin TA, eds. *Gastrointestinal physiology*, 6th ed. St. Louis: Mosby, 2001:82, with permission.)

fact that these three agents are the predominant mediators of acid secretion. For example, H$_2$ receptor blockers [such as cimetidine and famotidine (Pepcid)] are quite effective in decreasing acid secretion (87,89,90). Surgical treatments include vagotomy (either highly selective or truncal), which limits acetylcholine secretion, and antrectomy, which removes the antrum of the stomach that contains the gastrin-secreting G cells.

The inhibition of gastric secretion occurs when the pH falls below 3, which inhibits gastrin release through a negative feedback mechanism. In addition, somatostatin, released by the drop in gastric pH, directly inhibits the parietal cells and inhibits gastrin release. Other hormones that contribute to the inhibition of acid secretion, as well as gastric emptying, include GIP, secretin, and CCK.

Three Phases of Gastric Secretion

Stimulation of gastric secretion has been arbitrarily broken down into three phases: a cephalic phase, a gastric phase, and an intestinal phase. The mechanisms for the coordinated stimulation of gastric secretion during these three "stages" are shown in Figure 17.10. The cephalic phase occurs as a result of the sight, smell, thought, or taste of food and originates from the cerebral cortex in the appetite centers of the amygdala or hypothalamus. The afferent nerve impulses are relayed through the vagal nucleus and vagal efferent fibers to the stomach. The vagus acts directly on the parietal cells to stimulate acid secretion and acts indirectly, through the release of GRP, to stimulate gastrin release. The cephalic phase accounts for less than one fifth of the gastric secretion associated with eating a meal. The gastric phase accounts for most of the gastric secretions, totaling

approximately 1,500 mL/d. Secretion is initiated by food entering the stomach that triggers release of acetylcholine from vagal and local enteric reflexes, gastrin from G cells, and histamine from ECL cells, which act in concert to potently stimulate gastric secretion. The intestinal phase accounts for a small portion (<5%) of the gastric secretion and is due to the presence of food in the upper portion of the small intestine and possibly absorbed amino acids. However, the predominant effect of chyme (particularly acid, fat, and protein) entering the small intestine is a feedback inhibition to inhibit further gastric secretion by initiating an enterogastric reflex transmitted through the enteric nervous system, which causes the release of several intestinal hormones (e.g., secretin, CCK, somatostatin, and GIP) and serves to inhibit gastric secretion.

Secretions of the Small Intestine

The small intestine secretes approximately 1,800 mL of fluid on a daily basis. Secretions from the small intestine provide mucus for lubrication as well as digestive enzymes, which aid in the complete digestion of dietary components. Brunner glands, located in the proximal duodenum, secrete mucus and protect the duodenal wall from the high acid content of the gastric juices. The Lieberkühn crypts, located through the remainder of the small intestine, provide most of the secretions for the small intestine. These secretions have a slightly alkaline pH and are pure extracellular fluid, which is rapidly absorbed when it comes in contact with the villi. The digestive enzymes of the small intestine are produced in the brush border of the villi and include peptidases for splitting small peptides into amino acids; enzymes to split disaccharides into monosaccharides (i.e., sucrase, maltase,

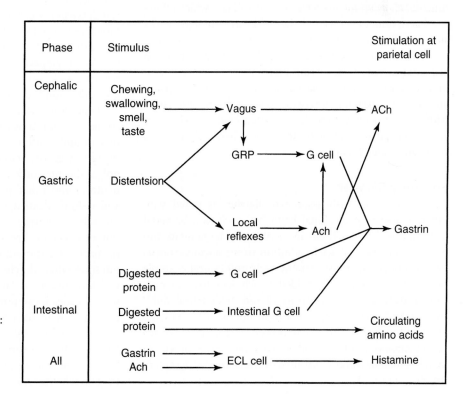

FIGURE 17.10 Mechanisms for stimulating acid secretion. Ach, acetylcholine; GRP, gastrin-releasing peptide; ECL, enterochromaffin-like cell. (From Johnson LR. Gastric secretions. In: Johnson LR, Gerwin TA, eds. *Gastrointestinal physiology*, 6th ed. St. Louis: Mosby, 2001:87, with permission.)

isomaltase, and lactase); and small amounts of intestinal lipase, which splits neutral fats into glycerol and fatty acids. Regulation of intestinal secretion is predominantly controlled by local neural reflexes initiated by tactile or irritative stimuli. In addition, GI hormones, such as secretin and CCK, contribute to the stimulation of small bowel secretion.

Secretions of the Large Intestine

Glands in the large intestine predominantly secrete mucus, which protects the colonic wall from excoriation and provides an adherent matrix for holding fecal matter together. The rate of secretion is regulated principally by direct tactile stimulation and local nervous reflexes.

Pathologic Conditions of Altered Secretion

Peptic Ulcer Disease

The causes of peptic ulcer disease are multifactorial, but it is clear that the presence of acid and pepsin is an important cofactor in the development of duodenal ulcer disease (91,92). An ulcer forms when damage from acid and pepsin overcomes the ability of the mucosa to protect itself. It has been shown that patients with duodenal ulcer disease have a somewhat higher maximal acid output than normal, and certainly the dictum "no acid, no ulcer" still applies to patients with duodenal ulcer disease. Perhaps the most drastic change in our view of peptic ulcer disease has been the association of *H. pylori* and its role in the pathogenesis of peptic ulcer (93,94). There is now a substantial body of evidence to support a causal role for *H. pylori* in this disease process. *H. pylori* is a slow-growing, highly mobile, gram-negative, spiral organism that can colonize the gastric mucosa. *H. pylori* metabolizes urea into NH_4^+, which allows the bacterium to withstand the acid environment of the stomach. The production of NH_4^+ is believed to be a major cause of cytotoxicity, as this ion directly damages epithelial cells and increases the permeability of the mucosa due to breakdown of the mucosal barrier. In addition, *H. pylori* appears to cause the increased acid secretion associated with duodenal ulcers. Medications that eradicate *H. pylori* are associated with ulcer healing and a markedly reduced recurrence rate (95,96).

Secretory Diarrhea

Altered secretion with associated diarrhea is noted with different forms of intestinal irritation, such as a bacterial infection, which can result in secretion of large quantities of water and electrolytes in addition to the alkaline mucus (91). Probably the most extreme and prototypical example of altered secretion is provided by cholera toxin, which can produce as much as 10 to 12 L/d of diarrheal fluid, specifically by increasing active transport of Cl^- into the Lieberkühn crypts of the small bowel, which, in turn, leads to this massive fluid loss. Other less severe forms of watery diarrhea include infections caused by the colon and dysentery bacilli.

DIGESTION AND ABSORPTION

The digestion of dietary components is initiated in the mouth and completed in the small intestine (97–100). The small bowel and colon perform a remarkable task in absorbing the bulk of the fluid either ingested or secreted by the digestive tract on a daily basis. This total fluid content is approximately 8 to 9 L, of which all but approximately 1.5 L is absorbed in the small intestine. Most of this 1.5 L is absorbed in the proximal colon, leaving less than 100 mL of fluid to be excreted.

The intricate morphology of the small intestinal mucosa is specifically designed for efficient absorption (Fig. 17.11) (101,102). There are millions of small finger-like projections called *villi*, which line the small bowel mucosa and greatly enhance its absorptive capacity. Moreover, each intestinal epithelial cell possesses a brush border consisting of approximately 600 microvilli, which further enhance the absorptive capacity. The combination of the villi and the brush border increases the absorptive capacity of the small bowel approximately 600-fold, allowing for a total area of approximately 250 m^2 (103). The small bowel is primarily responsible for absorption of the dietary components (carbohydrates, proteins, and fats), as well as ions, vitamins, and water. Some electrolyte absorption occurs in the proximal colon.

Carbohydrates

An adult consuming a normal Western diet will ingest approximately 300 to 350 g/d of carbohydrates, with approximately 50% consumed as starch, 30% as sucrose, 6% as lactose, and the remainder as maltose, trehalose, glucose, fructose, sorbitol, cellulose, and pectins. Dietary starch is a polysaccharide consisting of long chains of glucose molecules. Amylose makes up approximately 20% of starch in the diet and consists of glucose linked by α-1,4-glycosidic bonds. Amylopectin, making up approximately 80% of the dietary starch, consists of the α-1,4-linkages as well as α-1,6-glycosidic bonds occurring every 20 to 30 glucose units.

Digestion of starches begins in the mouth when food comes in contact with saliva that contains the α-amylase ptyalin and continues in the stomach until inactivation of ptyalin by gastric acidity (72–75). Ptyalin hydrolyzes starch only at the interior α-1,4-bonds, resulting in the disaccharide, maltose, and other polymers of glucose (e.g., maltotriose and α-limit dextrins) (Fig. 17.12). Before inactivation of the salivary amylase, approximately 30% to 40% of the starches will be broken down mainly to maltose in the stomach. Digestion of carbohydrates continues in the small intestine, where the chyme is mixed with pancreatic secretion, which contains a large quantity of α amylase that is several times more powerful than salivary amylase. As with ptyalin, pancreatic amylase attacks only the interior α-1,4-bonds, yielding maltose, maltotriose, and α-limit dextrins (oligosaccharides form because the α-1,6-bonds and α-1,4-bonds near the α-1,6-linkages are resistant to amylase). In general, the starches are almost totally converted into

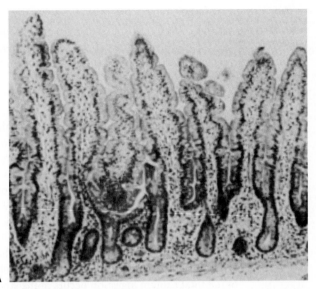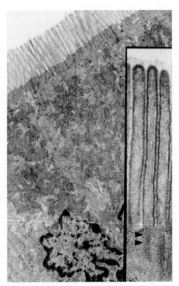

FIGURE 17.11 **A:** Light micrograph of a section of human jejunal mucosa obtained by biopsy (original magnification, ∼ × 93). (From Keljo DJ, Squires RHJ. Anatomy and anomalies of the small and large intestine. In: Feldman M, Sleisenger MH, Scharschmidt BF, eds. *Sleisenger & Fordtran's gastrointestinal and liver disease, Pathophysiology/diagnosis/management, Vol. 2*, 6th ed. Philadelphia: WB Saunders, 1998:1424, with permission.) **B:** Transmission electron micrographs of villous absorptive cells (original magnification ×6,000). (From Madara JL. The functional morphology of the epithelium of the small intestine. In: Shultz S, ed. *The handbook of physiology. Alimentary tract volumes.* Washington, DC: American Physiological Society, 1991, with permission.) **Inset:** Microvilli containing parallel arrays of acting microfilaments that plunge as a "rootlet" *(arrowheads)* into the terminal web of structural proteins (original magnification ×69,000.)

maltose and other very small glucose polymers before they have passed beyond the duodenum or upper jejunum. The remainder of carbohydrate digestion occurs as a result of brush border enzymes of the small intestine.

The brush border lining the villous epithelial cells of the small intestine contains the enzymes lactase, maltase, sucrase-isomaltase, and trehalose, which split the disaccharides, as well as other small glucose polymers, into their constituent monosaccharides (Table 17.4). Lactase hydrolyzes lactose into glucose and galactose. Maltase acts on maltose to produce glucose monomers. Sucrase-isomaltase possesses two subunits of the same molecule, each with distinct enzyme activity. Sucrase hydrolyzes sucrase to yield glucose and fructose; whereas isomaltase hydrolyzes the α-1,6-bonds in α-limit dextrins to yield glucose. Trehalose hydrolyzes trehalose, which makes up an insignificant portion of the diet, into glucose. Glucose represents

more than 80% of the final products of carbohydrate digestion with galactose and fructose, usually representing no more than 10% of the products of carbohydrate digestion.

The carbohydrates are absorbed in the form of monosaccharides, with only a small fraction of a percent being absorbed as disaccharides. Transport of the released hexoses (glucose, galactose, and fructose) is carried by specific mechanisms involving active transport. In humans, the major routes of absorption are by three membrane carrier systems, sodium glucose transporter 1 (SGLT-1), glucose transporter 5 (GLUT-5), and glucose transporter 2 (GLUT-2) (Fig. 17.13) (104–107). Glucose and galactose are absorbed by a carrier-mediated active transport mechanism, which involves the cotransport of Na^+ (SGLT-1 transporter); that is, absorption of both glucose and galactose depends on Na^+ movement into the cell by the Na^+/K^+-ATPase located on the basolateral

FIGURE 17.12 Action of pancreatic α amylase on linear (amylose) and branched (amylopectin) forms of starch to produce the breakdown products maltotriose, maltose, and dextrins. (Adapted from Alpers DH. Digestion and absorption of carbohydrates and proteins. In: Johnson LR, Alpers DH, Christensen J, et al. eds. *Physiology of the gastrointestinal tract, Vol. 2*, 3rd ed. New York: Raven Press, 1994:1727.)

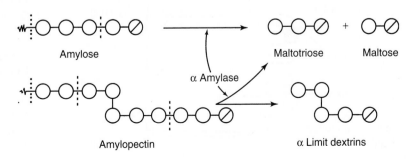

TABLE 17.4

Characteristics of Brush Border Membrane Carbohydrases

Enzyme	Substrate	Products
Lactase	Lactose	Glucose
		Galactose
Maltase (glucoamylase)	α 1–4 Linked oligosaccharides up to nine residues	Glucose
Sucrase-isomaltase (sucrose-α-dextrinase)		
Sucrase	Sucrose	Glucose
Isomaltase	α-Limit dextrin	Glucose
Both enzymes	α-Limit dextrin	Glucose
	α 1–4 Link at nonreducing end	
Trehalase	Trehalose	Glucose

From Marsh MN, Riley SA. Digestion and absorption of nutrients and vitamins. In: Feldman M, Sleisenger MH, Scharschmidt BF, eds. *Sleisenger & Fordtran's gastrointestinal and liver disease. Pathophysiology/diagnosis/management, vol. 2.* Philadelphia: WB Saunders, 1998:1480, with permission.

cell membrane. As Na$^+$ diffuses into the inside of the cell, it pulls the glucose or galactose along with it, thereby providing the energy for transport of the monosaccharide. This is often referred to as the *sodium cotransport theory* for glucose transport (also, secondary active transport of glucose). The exit of glucose from the cytosol into the intracellular space is predominantly due to a Na$^+$-independent carrier (GLUT-2 transporter) located at the basolateral membrane. Fructose, the other significant monosaccharide, is absorbed from the intestinal lumen through a process of facilitated diffusion. The carrier involved for fructose absorption is GLUT-5, which is located in the apical membrane of the enterocyte. This transport process does not depend on Na$^+$ or energy. Fructose exits the basolateral membrane by another facilitated diffusion process involving the GLUT-2 transporter.

Proteins

The dietary proteins are formed of long-chain amino acids bound by peptide linkages. Proteins are digested by a process of hydrolysis, resulting in splitting of amino acids at the peptide linkages (99,100,108–110). The digestion of dietary proteins begins in the stomach, where pepsinogen is released from chief cells of the gastric mucosa and cleaved to the active enzyme pepsin, an endopeptidase with specificity for peptide bonds involving aromatic L-amino acids. Pepsin digests collagen, which is a major constituent of the intracellular connective tissue of meats. Only approximately 10% to 20% of the total protein digestion occurs in the stomach.

Similar to carbohydrates, most of the protein is digested in the upper small intestine. When the proteins leave the stomach, they are mainly in the form of proteoses, peptones, and large polypeptides, which immediately come in contact with the proteolytic enzymes from pancreatic secretion. These proteolytic pancreatic enzymes include the endopeptidases (trypsin, chymotrypsin, and elastase) and the exopeptidases (carboxypeptidases A and B) (Table 17.5). The pancreatic proteases are all secreted into the lumen as inactive precursors. Active trypsin is formed from the proteolytically inactive trypsinogen by the action of enterokinase, a brush border enzyme in the duodenum. Trypsin then acts to activate the other pancreatic proenzymes. Trypsin, chymotrypsin, and elastase split protein molecules at interior peptide bonds into small polypeptides, and the carboxypeptidases cleave individual amino acids from the carboxyl end polypeptides. This results in splitting the complex proteins into dipeptides, triglycerides, and some larger proteins,

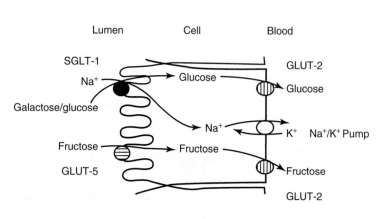

FIGURE 17.13 Model for glucose, galactose, and fructose transport across the intestinal epithelium. Glucose and galactose are transported into the enterocyte across the brush border membrane by the Na$^+$/glucose cotransporter (SGLT-1) and then transported out across the basolateral membrane down their concentration gradients by glucose transporter 2 (GLUT-2). The low intracellular Na$^+$ driving uphill sugar transport across the brush border is maintained by the Na$^+$/K$^+$ pump on the basolateral membrane. Glucose and galactose therefore stimulate Na$^+$ absorption across the epithelium. Fructose is transported across the cell down the concentration gradient across the brush border and basolateral membranes. Glucose transporter 5 (GLUT-5) is the brush border fructose transporter, whereas GLUT-2 handles fructose transport across the basolateral membrane. (From Wright EM, Hirayama BA, Loo DDF, et al. Intestinal sugar transport. In: Johnson LR, Alpers DH, Christensen J, et al. eds. *Physiology of the gastrointestinal tract*, 3rd ed. New York: Raven Press, 1994:1752, with permission.)

TABLE 17.5

Principal Pancreatic Proteases

Enzyme	Primary Action
Endopeptidases	Hydrolyze interior peptide bonds of polypeptides and proteins
Trypsin	Attacks peptide bonds involving basic amino acids; yields products with basic amino acids at C-terminal end
Chymotrypsin	Attacks peptide bonds involving aromatic amino acids, leucine, glutamine, and methionine; yields peptide products with these amino acids at C-terminal end
Elastase	Attacks peptide bonds involving neutral aliphatic amino acids; yields products with neutral amino acids at C-terminal and
Exopeptidases	Hydrolyze external peptide bonds of polypeptides and protein
Carboxypeptidase A	Attacks peptides with aromatic and neutral aliphatic amino acids at C-terminal end
Carboxypeptidase B	Attacks peptides with basic amino acids at C-terminal end

From Castro GA. Digestion and absorption. In: Johnson LR, ed. *Gastrointestinal physiology*. St. Louis: CV Mosby, 1991:108–130, with permission.

which are digested further by enzymes in the brush border and in the cytoplasm of the enterocytes (Table 17.6). These peptidase enzymes include amino peptidases and several dipeptidases, which split the remaining larger polypeptides into tripeptides and dipeptides and some amino acids. The amino acids, dipeptides, and tripeptides are easily transported through the microvilli into the epithelial cells where, in the cytosol, additional peptidases hydrolyze the dipeptides and tripeptides into single amino acids, which then pass through the epithelial cell membrane into the blood.

Most proteins are absorbed in the proximal small bowel in the form of dipeptides, tripeptides, and a few free amino acids involving an Na^+-mediated active transport mechanism (111–113). That is, most peptide or amino acid molecules bind with a specific transport protein that also requires Na^+ binding before transport can occur. The sodium ion then moves down its electrochemical gradient into the interior of the cell and pulls the amino acid or peptide along with it, in a similar manner as glucose and galactose. A few amino acids do not require this sodium cotransport mechanism and are absorbed by a process of facilitated diffusion.

Fats

Emulsification of Fats

Most adults in North America consume approximately 60 to 100 g/d of fat. Triglycerides, the most abundant fats, are composed of a glycerol, nucleus, and three fatty acids; small

quantities of phospholipids, cholesterol, and cholesterol esters also are found in the normal diet. Essentially all fat digestion occurs in the small intestine, where the first step is the breakdown of fat globules into smaller sizes so as to facilitate further breakdown by water-soluble digestive enzymes, a process called *emulsification* (99,100,114–120). This process is facilitated by bile from the liver that contains bile salts and the phospholipid lecithin. The polar parts of the bile salts and lecithin molecules are soluble in water, whereas the remaining portions are soluble in fat. Therefore, the fat-soluble portions dissolve in the surface layer of the fat globules and the polar portions, projecting outward, are soluble in the surrounding aqueous fluids. This arrangement renders the fat globules more accessible to fragmentation by agitation in the small intestine. Therefore, a major function of bile salts, and especially lecithin in the bile, is to allow the fat globules to be readily fragmented by agitation in the intestinal lumen (114,117).

Actions of Pancreatic Lipase

With the increase in surface area of the fat globules resulting from the action of the bile salts and lecithin, the fats can now be readily attacked by pancreatic lipase, which is the most crucial enzyme in the digestion of triglycerides. The triglycerides are split into free fatty acids and 2-monoglycerides. The presence of colipase, secreted by the pancreas with lipase, is critical in approximating lipase to triglyceride. In the absence of colipase, bile salts on the surface of the emulsion droplet inhibit lipase activity.

Micelle Formation

Fat digestion is further accelerated by bile salts, which, secondary to their amphipathic nature, can form micelles (99,100,114,115). Micelles are small spherical globules composed of 20 to 40 molecules of bile salts with a sterol nucleus, which is highly fat soluble, and a hydrophilic polar group that projects outward. The mixed micelles thus formed are arrayed so that the insoluble lipid is surrounded by the bile salts oriented with their hydrophilic ends facing outward. Therefore, as quickly as the monoglycerides and free fatty acids are formed from lipolysis, they become dissolved in the central hydrophobic portion of the micelles, which then act to carry these products of fat hydrolysis to the brush borders of the epithelial cells, where absorption occurs.

The cholesterol esters and phospholipids in the diet are hydrolyzed by other pancreatic lipases (i.e., cholesterol esterase and phospholipase A_2). Bile salts also play a key role in transporting the cholesterol and phospholipids to the brush borders of the epithelial cells, where they are absorbed. Therefore, the products of phospholipid and cholesterol hydrolysis utilize the same route to the brush border membrane as the fatty acids and monoglycerides.

Intracellular Processing

The monoglycerides and free fatty acids, which are dissolved in the central lipid portion of the bile acid micelles, are absorbed through the brush border due to their highly

TABLE 17.6

Peptidases found on the Brush Border Membrane and in the Cytoplasm of Villous Epithelial Cells

Peptidase	Action	Products
Brush border membrane peptidases		
Amino-oligopeptidases (at least two types)	Cleave amino acids from carboxy terminus of 3–8 amino acid peptides	Amino acids and dipeptides
Amino peptidase A	Cleaves dipeptides with acidic amino acids at amino terminus	Amino acids
Dipeptidase I	Cleaves dipeptides containing methionine	Amino acids
Dipeptidase III	Cleaves glycine-containing dipeptides	Amino acids
Dipeptidyl amino peptidase IV	Cleaver proline-containing peptides with free α-amino groups	Peptides and amino acids
Carboxypeptidase P	Cleaves proline-containing peptides with free carboxyl terminus	Peptides and amino acids
γ-Glutamyl transpeptidase	Cleaves γ-glutamyl bonds and transfers glutamine to amino acid or peptide acceptors	γ-Glutamyl amino acid or peptide
Folate conjugase	Cleaves pteroyl polyglutamates	Monoglutamate
Cytoplasmic peptidase Dipeptidases	Cleave most dipeptides	Amino acids
Aminotripeptidase	Cleaves tripeptides	Amino acids
Proline dipeptidase	Cleaves proline-containing dipeptides	Proline and amino acids

From Marsh MN, Riley SA. Digestion and absorption of nutrients and vitamins. In: Feldman M, Sleisenger MH, Scharschmidt BF, eds. *Sleisenger & Fordtran's gastrointestinal and liver disease. Pathophysiology/diagnosis/management, vol. 2.* Philadelphia: WB Saunders, 1998:1484, with permission.

lipid soluble nature and simply diffuse into the interior of the cell (115–117,120). After disaggregation of the micelle, bile salts remain within the intestinal lumen to enter into the formation of new micelles and act to carry more monoglycerides and fatty acids to the epithelial cells. The released fatty acids and monoglycerides in the cell reform into new triglycerides. This reformation of a triglyceride occurs in the cell through the interactions of intracellular enzymes that are associated with the endoplasmic reticulum. The major pathway for resynthesis involves synthesis of triglycerides from 2-monoglycerides and coenzyme A (CoA)-activated fatty acids. Microsomal acyl-CoA lipase is necessary to synthesize acyl-CoA from the fatty acid before esterification. These reconstituted triglycerides then combine with cholesterol, phospholipids, and apoproteins to form chylomicrons that consist of an inner core containing triglycerides and a membranous outer core of phospholipids and apoproteins. The chylomicrons pass from the epithelial cells into the lacteals, where they pass through the lymphatics into the venous system. Approximately 80% to 90% of all fat absorbed from the gut is absorbed in this manner and transported to the blood by way of the thoracic lymph in the form of chylomicrons. Small quantities of short- to medium-chain fatty acids

may be absorbed directly into the portal blood rather than being converted into triglycerides and absorbed into the lymphatics. These shorter-chain fatty acids are more water soluble, which allows for the direct diffusion into the bloodstream. Figure 17.14 summarizes the process of fat digestion and absorption.

Enterohepatic Circulation

The proximal intestine absorbs most of the dietary fat (117). Although the unconjugated bile acids are absorbed into the jejunum by passive diffusion, the conjugated bile acids that form micelles are absorbed in the ileum by active transport and are reabsorbed from the distal ileum. The bile acids then pass through the portal venous system to the liver for resecretion as bile. The total bile salt pool in humans is approximately 2 to 3 g, and it recirculates approximately six times every 24 hours (the enterohepatic circulation of bile salts). Almost all of the bile salts are absorbed, with only approximately 0.5 g lost in the stool every day; this is replaced by resynthesis from cholesterol.

Water, Electrolytes, and Vitamins

Water

Water is absorbed through the intestinal membrane by the process of simple diffusion. Most of the water and electrolytes

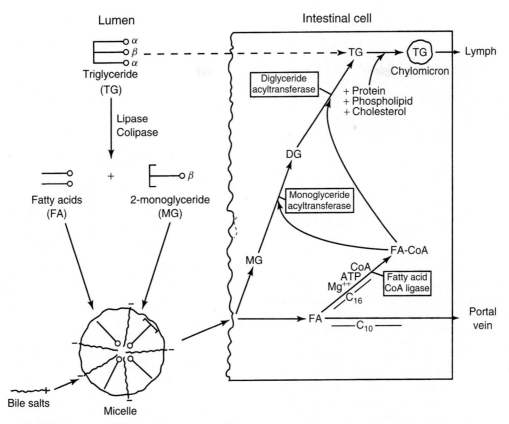

FIGURE 17.14 Schematic representation of fat digestion and absorption. DG, diglyceride; CoA, coenzyme A; ATP, adenosine triphosphate. (From Evers BM. Small bowel. In: Townsend CM Jr, Beauchamp RD, Evers BM, et al. eds. *Sabiston textbook of surgery*, 16th ed. Philadelphia: WB Saunders, 2001:878, with permission.)

from the chyme is absorbed in the small bowel; however, the proximal colon also absorbs water and ions but almost no nutrients (99,121,122). Water is absorbed through the intestinal mucosa into the blood by a process of osmosis following the osmolar gradients. Therefore, when the chyme is dilute, water is absorbed from the intestine into the bloodstream. In contrast, water can also be transported in the opposite direction (i.e., from the plasma into the intestine) when hyperosmolar solutions are discharged from the stomach.

Electrolytes

Electrolytes can be absorbed in the small bowel by active transport or by coupling to organic solutes (108,121–123). There is approximately 25 to 35 g of Na^+ each day that the small intestine must absorb. Normally less than 0.5% of the intestinal sodium is lost in the feces each day. Na^+ is absorbed by active transport through the basolateral membranes. Cl^- is absorbed in the upper part of the small intestine by a process of passive diffusion. Large quantities of HCO_3^- must be reabsorbed, and this is accomplished in an indirect manner. As the Na^+ is absorbed, H^+ is secreted into the lumen of the intestine. It then combines with HCO_3^- to form carbonic acid, which then dissociates to form water and carbon dioxide. The water remains in the chyme, but the carbon dioxide is readily

absorbed in the blood and subsequently expired. Figure 17.15 summarizes the mechanisms of NaCl absorption in the small bowel.

Calcium ions are actively absorbed, especially from the duodenum, by a process of active transport. Absorption appears to be facilitated by an acid environment and is enhanced by vitamin D and parathyroid hormone (124,125). That is, parathyroid hormone activates vitamin D in the kidneys, and this activated vitamin D stimulates the synthesis of a cytoplasmic Ca^{2+}-binding protein, which enhances calcium absorption from the proximal small intestine (Fig. 17.16) (126). Iron is absorbed as either a heme or nonheme component in the duodenum by an active process. Potassium, magnesium, phosphate, and other ions can also be actively absorbed throughout the mucosa.

Vitamins

Vitamins are classified as either fat soluble (e.g., vitamins A, D, E, and K) or water soluble [e.g., ascorbic acid (vitamin C), biotin, nicotinic acid, folic acid, riboflavin, thiamine, pyridoxine (vitamin B_6), and cobalamin (vitamin B_{12})] (99,127–129). The fat-soluble vitamins are carried in mixed micelles and transported in chylomicrons of lymph to the thoracic duct and into the venous system (Table 17.7). The absorption of water-soluble vitamins appears to be more

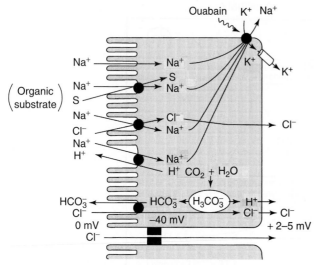

FIGURE 17.15 Mechanism of NaCl absorption in the small intestine. Sodium enters passively, following the electrochemic gradient, by cotransport with nutrients such as glucose or amino acids, or by neutral cotransport with Cl^- or in exchange for protons through a countertransport process. Chloride also is absorbed by neutral exchange with HCO_3^-. Sodium exit from the cell is through the energy-dependent Na^+ pump, and Cl^- follows passively. The electrical potential difference (PD) across the apical membrane is -40 mV, and across the entire cell is $+3$ to $+5$ mV with reference to the luminal side. Ouabain is an inhibitor of Na^+/K^+-adenosine triphosphatase (ATPase). (From Johnson LR. Fluid and electrolyte absorption. In: Johnson LR, Gerwin TA, eds. *Gastrointestinal physiology*, 6th ed. St. Louis: Mosby, 2001:146, with permission.)

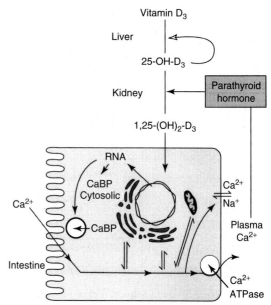

FIGURE 17.16 Calcium absorption by an enterocyte within a larger scheme of Ca^{2+} homeostasis. Vitamin D_3, $1,25-(OH)_2-D_3$, stimulates Ca^{2+} transport by interacting with nuclear receptors to effect the synthesis of calcium bending protein (CaBP). Ca^{2+} enters the cell facilitated by brush border CaBP and exits through two mechanisms. It is speculated that CaBP in the cytosol stimulates Ca^{2+}-adenosine triphosphatase (ATPase). Binding proteins in the Golgi, endoplasmic reticulum, and (possibly) mitochondria prevent an increase in intracellular Ca^{2+} during the absorptive process. RNA, ribonucleic acid. (From Johnson LR. Fluid and electrolyte absorption. In: Johnson LR, Gerwin TA, eds. *Gastrointestinal physiology*, 6th ed. St. Louis: Mosby, 2001:150, with permission.)

complex than originally thought (Table 17.8). Vitamin C is absorbed by passive processes and by an active transport process that incorporates a Na^+-coupled mechanism as well as a specific carrier system. Vitamin B_6 appears to be rapidly absorbed by simple diffusion into the proximal intestine. Thiamine (vitamin B_1) is rapidly absorbed into the jejunum by a Na^+-dependent active process, whereas, at high concentrations, passive diffusion predominates. Riboflavin (vitamin B_2) is absorbed into the proximal intestine by facilitated transport. The absorption of vitamin B_{12} (cobalamin) occurs primarily in the terminal ileum (129). Vitamin B_{12} is freed from the binding proteins (R protein) in the duodenum by pancreatic proteases and then binds to intrinsic factor, a glycoprotein secreted by parietal cells in the stomach. Receptors in the terminal ileum take up the vitamin B_{12}–intrinsic factor complex, probably by translocation. In the cell, free vitamin B_{12} is bound to an ileal pool of transcobalamin II, which transports it into the portal circulation (Fig. 17.17).

Pathologic Conditions Associated with Altered Absorption

Pathologic conditions associated with altered absorption include disease processes that destroy or damage the small intestinal mucosa. In addition, massive resections of the small bowel can lead to the "short bowel" syndrome, with the end result being lack of nutrient absorption.

Nontropical Sprue

Nontropical sprue, also known as *gluten enteropathy* or *celiac disease* (in children), results from the toxic effects of gluten present in certain types of grains (91). Gluten has a direct destructive effect on the intestinal villi, thereby effectively decreasing the absorptive surface area of the small bowel. Absorption of fat is more impaired than absorption of other digestive products. In severe cases, absorption of all nutrients is impaired, and, as a result, the patient suffers severe nutritional deficiencies, inadequate blood coagulation caused by lack of vitamin K, and macrocytic anemia secondary to diminished vitamin B_{12} and folic acid absorption.

Short Bowel Syndrome

Short bowel syndrome results from a total small bowel length that is inadequate to support nutrition (130). Approximately three fourths of the cases of short bowel syndrome occur from massive intestinal resections. In the adult, mesenteric occlusion, midgut volvulus, and traumatic disruption of the superior mesenteric vessels are the most frequent causes. Multiple sequential resections, most commonly associated with recurrent Crohn disease, account for 25% of patients. In

TABLE 17.7

Fat-Soluble Vitamin Absorptive Mechanisms

Vitamin	Reference nutrient Intake[a]	Mechanism of Absorption
Vitamin A (retinol)	700 μg/d	Passive diffusion
Vitamin D (cholecalciferol)	10 μg/d[b]	Passive diffusion
Vitamin E (α-tocopherol)	>4 mg/d[b]	Passive diffusion
Vitamin K (phytomenadione [K$_1$] and menaquinones [K$_2$])	1 μ/kg/d[c]	K$_1$ carrier-mediated uptake K$_2$ passive diffusion

[a]Reference nutrient intakes quoted are calculated at 2 SD above the average intake of normal adult males.

[b]Normal adults with normal exposure to sunlight do not require any dietary intake of vitamin D.

[c]Figures for vitamins E and K are "safe intake" values that provide safe and adequate amounts for normal nutrition. Excessive intake of vitamins A and D produce toxic effects, and the figures quoted are safe in normal men, but not necessarily in infants.

From Marsh MN, Riley SA. Digestion and absorption of nutrients and vitamins. In: Feldman M, Sleisenger MH, Scharschmidt BF, eds. *Sleisenger & Fordtran's gastrointestinal and liver disease. Pathophysiology/diagnosis/management,* vol. 2. Philadelphia: WB Saunders, 1998:1488, with permission.

neonates, the most common cause of short bowel syndrome is bowel resection secondary to necrotizing enterocolitis. The clinical hallmarks of the short bowel syndrome include diarrhea, fluid and electrolyte deficiency, and malnutrition. Other complications include an increased incidence of

gallstones due to the disruption of enterohepatic circulation and of nephrolithiasis from hyperoxaluria. Although there is considerable variation, resection of up to 70% of the small bowel can be tolerated if the terminal ileum and ileocecal valve are preserved. Length alone, however, is not the only determining factor of complications related to small bowel resection. For example, if the distal two thirds of the ileum, including the ileocecal valve, are resected, significant abnormalities of absorption of bile salts and vitamin B$_{12}$ may occur, resulting in diarrhea and anemia. Proximal bowel resection is tolerated much better than is distal bowel resection, because the ileum can adapt and increase its absorptive capacity more efficiently than can the jejunum.

GASTROINTESTINAL MOTILITY

Gastric Motility

The motor activity of gastric smooth muscles function to (i) store large quantities of food, (ii) mix food with gastric secretions to form chyme, and (iii) propel food into the duodenum at a rate for proper digestion and absorption. These functions require coordinated activities of smooth muscles of the stomach. The stomach has three layers of smooth muscles: an outer longitudinal, a middle circular, and an inner oblique layer. The circular layer is the most prominent layer, and it gradually increases in thickness toward the pylorus.

Innervation of the Stomach

Similar to other parts of the GI tract, myenteric and submucosal plexuses are the two major intrinsic innervations

TABLE 17.8

Water-Soluble Vitamins

Vitamin	Reference Nutrient Intake[a]	Transport Mechanism
Ascorbic acid	40 mg/d	Active: Na-dependent process at BBM
Folic acid	200 mg/d	Hydrolysis of dietary polyglutamates by folate conjugase at BBM; Na-dependent active transport or facilitated diffusion of monoglutamate at BBM
Cobalamin (B$_{12}$)	Intrinsic factor binding; uptake of intrinsic factor/B$_{12}$ complex at BBM by way of specific receptor	Instrinsic factor binding; uptake of intrinsic factor/B$_{12}$ complex at BBM by way of specific receptor
Thiamine	1 mg/d	Na-dependent active transport
Riboflavin	1.3 mg/d	Thiamine and riboflavin absorption includes hydrolytic and phosphorylation steps
Pantothenic acid	3–7 mg/d	
Biotin	10–200 μg/d[b]	
Pyridoxine	1.5 mg/d	Simple diffusion
Niacin	18 mg/d	?

[a]Reference nutrient intakes quoted are calculated at 2 SD above the estimated average intake for normal adult males. These figures provide an adequate intake for nonpregnant adults.

[b]Nutrient intakes for pantothenic acid and biotine are given as "safe intake" because insufficient data are available on human needs. These values provide a range over which there is no risk of deficiency or toxicity.

BBM, brush border membrane; ?, not known.

From Marsh MN, Riley SA. Digestion and absorption of nutrients and vitamins. In: Feldman M, Sleisenger MH, Scharschmidt BF, eds. *Sleisenger & Fordtran's gastrointestinal and liver disease. Pathophysiology/diagnosis/management,* vol. 2. Philadelphia: WB Saunders, 1998:1486, with permission.

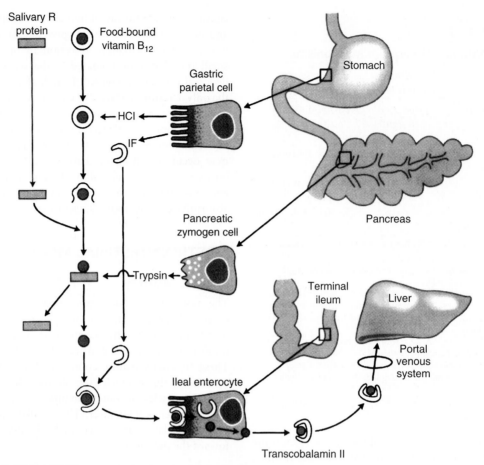

FIGURE 17.17 Steps in the chain leading to the binding of vitamin B_{12} to intrinsic factor (IF). Food-bound B_{12} is released by gastric acid and picked up preferentially by salivary R protein in the stomach. Proteolysis of R protein by duodenal trypsin releases B_{12} for binding to IF. The subsequent binding and uptake of the IF–B_{12} complex occurs through a specific receptor-mediated process on the brush border membrane of ileal enterocytes. Vitamin B_{12} is released at an intracellular site, transported across the basolateral membrane, and taken up there by transcobalamin II for transport into the portal circulation. HCl, hydrogen chloride (From Marsh MN, Riley SA. Digestion and absorption of nutrients and vitamins. In: Feldman M, Sleisenger MH, Scharschmidt BF, eds. *Sleisenger & Fordtran's gastrointestinal and liver disease, Pathophysiology/diagnosis/management, Vol. 2*, 6th ed. Philadelphia: WB Saunders, 1998:1487, with permission.)

in the stomach that contribute to sensory and motor functions. The major control for gastric motor function is dependent on extrinsic innervation of the stomach, which largely includes the vagus nerve and fibers originating from the celiac plexus of the sympathetic nervous system (131). Vagal afferents involve chemosensitive receptors, which detect physical and chemical properties of the luminal contents, and mechanosensitive receptors, which respond to distention and contractions of the stomach (131). Vagal afferents project centrally to the medulla and terminate primarily in the nucleus tractus solitarius (132). They also connect to other brainstem nuclei (dorsal motor nucleus of the vagus, nucleus ambiguus) and higher centers, such as the hypothalamus, thalamus, and insular cortex (132). Gastric splanchnic afferents also respond to chemoreceptor and mechanoreceptors and travel to the prevertebral ganglia before reaching the spinal cord (131). They have significant

peptidergic components and converge with vagal fibers at the brainstem and midbrain (131).

Vagal efferents are parasympathetic cholinergic fibers that increase fundic tone and antral contraction and constrict the pylorus. The vagal efferents also have an inhibitory component, which consists of nonadrenergic, noncholinergic fibers producing relaxation of the fundus, antrum, and pylorus (133). Sympathetic efferents travel through the celiac ganglia to inhibit gastric contractility (134).

Functions of the Stomach
Proximal Stomach
The orad or proximal region of the stomach is responsible for storage of ingested food. The resting pressure of this region is equal to intra-abdominal pressure and decreases during a swallow, before arrival of the food bolus. The proximal portion of the stomach can accommodate

volumes of as much as 1,500 mL by a process known as *receptive relaxation* (135). This mechanism is mediated by vagovagal reflexes and can be induced by swallowing as well as distension of the stomach. Vagotomy can lead to inhibition of fundic relaxation, leading to an increase in postprandial tone. The proximal gastric contractile activity is weak and serves to only partially mix ingested food contents.

Distal Stomach

In contrast to the proximal stomach, the distal or caudad region of the stomach exhibits marked contractile activity. Peristaltic contractions begin in the midstomach and propagate the food bolus toward the gastroduodenal junction (136). The duration of each contraction ranges between 2 and 20 seconds, with the maximum frequency of approximately 3 contractions per minute. However, the intensity and frequency increase near the gastroduodenal junction, resulting in propelling gastric contents back into the body of the stomach. Particles greater than 1 to 2 mm in diameter encounter a relatively closed pylorus and are propelled back into the proximal stomach. This activity has been termed *retropulsion* and results in mixing of the gastric contents as well as reducing the size of particles. Contractions of the distal region of the stomach are regulated by intrinsic activities of the smooth muscle cells.

Gastric Motor Patterns
Basic Electrical Rhythm

Smooth muscle cells from all regions of the stomach have the capability of generating periodic cell membrane depolarization from the resting potential. Basic electrical rhythms are cyclic fluctuations; they are also called *slow waves* or *pacesetter potentials* (137). These slow waves are always present even if they are not of significant magnitude to produce contractions. Slow waves originate from an area near the border of the proximal and distal areas (referred to as the *gastric pacemaker*) and spread toward the gastroduodenal junction, increasing in amplitude and frequency (Fig. 17.18). These proximal-to-distal phase lag contractions allow the stomach to propulse food from the fundus to antropyloric region. They are markedly influenced by nervous and humoral mechanisms.

Migrating Motor Complex

During the fasting state, the stomach demonstrates a cyclic pattern of intrinsic motor activity called the *migrating motor complex* (MMC). The stomach exhibits alternating periods of quiescence (phase I) and intense activity (phases II and III) of MMC during fasting (138). The quiescence period is characterized by the stable tonic contraction of the proximal stomach; the intense motor activity is demonstrated by phasic contractions. The mechanism for the initiation of the gastric MMC is not entirely known, but motilin, a gut hormone released from endocrine cells in the proximal gut, has been implicated as the triggering signal. Following food ingestion, a rapid and profound

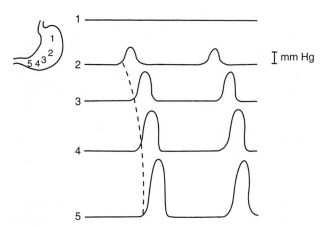

FIGURE 17.18 Gastric intraluminal pressure recordings. The orad region of the stomach has little phasic activity. Contractions begin in the midstomach and progress toward the gastroduodenal junction. The contractions increase in force and velocity near the gastroduodenal junction. (From Wiesbrodt NW. Gastric emptying. In: Johnson LR, Gerwin TA, eds. *Gastrointestinal physiology*, 6th ed. St. Louis: Mosby, 2001:38, with permission.)

change in the motor pattern of the stomach occurs. The tonic contraction of the proximal stomach is reduced, resulting in expansion of the fundus, and the antrum generates continuous and regular peristaltic activity at the maximal intrinsic rate. The regulation of switching of gastric motor patterns from the fasting to the postprandial state involves a mechanoreceptor in the proximal stomach to detect distention and postprandial release of gut hormones, such as CCK and gastrin (139).

Chemical Control of Gastric Motility

Nutrient contents in the duodenum stimulate the secretion of several gut hormones that act in both an endocrine and paracrine manner to regulate gastric motor function. CCK, which is released in response to lipids in the duodenum, is thought to be a primary inhibitory hormone for gastric emptying (140). CCK released from duodenal mucosa inhibits the motility of the proximal stomach through a vagovagal reflex pathway but stimulates pyloric contractile activity by an endocrine mechanism of action.

Regulation of Gastric Emptying

The propulsive function of gastric emptying is largely under the vagal and myenteric reflex mechanisms triggered by gastric volume and particle size. In general, the greater the volume, the more rapidly the contents empty. Liquids empty faster than solids. Solids must also be reduced in size to particles of 1 to 2 mm in diameter. The steady-state emptying of food contents, which normally takes approximately 3 hours, is also regulated by negative feedback mechanisms involving chemoreceptors and mechanoreceptors in the duodenum (141). Both hypotonic and hypertonic saline empties slowly. The addition of calories, especially in the form of lipids, or acid further slows gastric emptying.

Small Intestinal Motility

The primary function of the small intestine is the digestion and absorption of nutrients and the absorption of electrolytes. The motility functions of the small intestine are largely to support these vital activities and to propel luminal contents into the large intestine. The smooth muscle layer of the small intestine is made up of inner circular and outer longitudinal muscles, and its thickness gradually decreases toward the ileocecal junction.

Innervation of the Small Intestine

Similar to other parts of the GI tract, neural control involves both extrinsic and intrinsic nerves to innervate intestinal smooth muscle cells. The intrinsic nervous system, which consists of the myenteric and submucosal plexuses, are arranged in complex networks to transmit signals. The myenteric plexus plays a more prominent role in propulsion of intraluminal contents and involves many neurotransmitters, such as acetylcholine, VIP, and nitric oxide. The vagus nerve provides parasympathetic extrinsic innervation, and the sympathetic innervation is provided from the thoracic spinal cord through celiac and superior mesenteric ganglia. The vagal nerve responds to distension and contraction of the small intestine, and its efferent fibers synapse on both cholinergic excitatory nerves and nonadrenergic, noncholinergic inhibitory nerves (142).

Types of Contractions
Segmental Contractions

Similar to gastric smooth muscle cells, small intestinal smooth muscle cells always demonstrate slow-wave activity (basic electrical rhythm); however, unlike the stomach, they do not themselves trigger contractions (143). Contractions of the smooth muscles occur, resulting from a second electrical event (i.e., spike potential) that occurs during the depolarization phase of the slow wave. If a contraction is not coordinated with activities of adjacent smooth muscle cells, segmental contractions occur. Segmental contractions lead to thorough mixing of luminal contents and do not play a significant role in propagation of the intestinal contents.

Propulsive Contractions

The small intestine is capable of eliciting a highly coordinated contraction to produce propulsive movement. Spike potentials can recruit and coordinate depolarization of adjacent muscle cells to produce proximal-to-distal phase lag of the slow wave, thereby allowing proper aboral movement of luminal contents. This motor response is known as the *peristaltic reflex* and is thought to sequentially propel nutrients the entire length of the small intestine. However, peristalsis involving a long distance is seldom seen in normal individuals.

Patterns of Contractions
Migrating Motor Complex

During the fasting state, the motility of the small intestine is characterized by the presence of MMC (143). The MMC cycles spontaneously to conduct aboral peristaltic contractions and occurs at intervals of approximately 90 minutes (Fig. 17.19) (138). MMC activity typically originates in the smooth muscle cells of the distal stomach and propagates down to the distal ileum at a rate of 2 to 4 cm/min; however, the exact site of origin as well as the

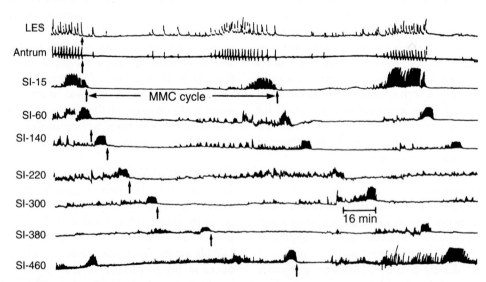

FIGURE 17.19   Migrating motor complex (MMC). Cyclic motor activity in the small intestine has four well-defined phases. Phase I has little or no contractile activity (quiescent phase). Phase II has intermittent and irregular contractions. The contractions during phase III activity occur at their maximal rate (shown by the *arrows*). Phase IV represents a brief period of intermittent contractions. Distances indicated on small intestinal strain gauges are measured from the pylorus. LES, lower esophageal sphincter; SI, small intestine. (From Sarna SK. Cyclic motor activity; migrating motor complex: 1985. *Gastroenterology* 1985;89:896, with permission.)

distance and the velocity of migration are highly variable. It takes approximately 90 minutes for contractions to move from the distal stomach to the ileocecal junction, sweeping undigested contents from the bowel. The MMC has four distinct phases of activity in the small intestine. Phase I is a period of quiescence. Phase II is characterized by irregular bursts of myoelectrical activity. During phase III, intense bursts of myoelectrical activities occur resulting in regular, high-amplitude contractions. Phase IV demonstrates short periods of irregular myoelectrical activity and contractions similar to those seen in phase II. Motilin, which is found at its peak plasma level during phase III of MMCs, plays an important role in regulating small intestinal MMC activity.

After a meal, the MMCs disappear and contractions are spread more uniformly over time. Slow waves of the small intestine do not initiate contractions, and forceful contractions are induced by spike potentials during the depolarization phase of the slow wave (144). However, the slow-wave frequency dictates the rate of contractions. Its frequency gradually decreases toward the terminal ileum, but it is constant at any one point, ranging from 11 to 12 cycles/min in the duodenum to 8 to 9 cycles/min in the ileum. These phasic contractions allow aboral movement of luminal contents during the fed state. In addition to the intrinsic mechanism of peristalsis, phasic contractions are triggered by other reflex mechanisms that are mediated by the enteric nervous system and circulating chemicals.

Giant Migrating Contractions
Giant migrating contractions (GMCs) are highly propulsive contractions that occur in greater amplitude and duration than MMCs and empty the contents of the distal intestine into the colon (143). GMCs are also called *prolonged propagated contractions* and are frequently initiated by luminal short-chain fatty acids. They may be essential to complete the propagation of luminal contents into the colon because the MMCs do not always reach the end of the terminal ileum. After administration of opioids or erythromycin, GMCs are more frequent and originate more proximally in the small intestine (145). In patients with irritable bowel syndrome, GMCs are associated with cramping (146).

Regulation of Small Intestinal Motility
Small intestinal motility is greatly influenced by neural and hormonal controls to smooth muscle cells. In general, parasympathetic innervation is stimulatory for intestinal contractions and sympathetic innervation is inhibitory. Various gut hormones affect intestinal motility. Gastrin, CCK, and motilin stimulate contractions, whereas secretin and glucagon tend to inhibit them. Motilin is also involved in regulation of the MMC cycle. In addition, calcitonin-releasing gene-related peptide and nitric oxide cause intestinal muscle cell relaxation.

Ileocecal Valve
The principal function of the ileocecal valve is to prevent backflow of fecal contents from the colon into the terminal ileum. The ileocecal sphincter mechanism is normally contracted and contributes to slowing of emptying ileal contents into the cecum (147). Following gastric emptying, peristalsis in the terminal ileum intensifies. This results in the movement of ileal contents into the cecum and is called the *gastroileal reflex*. The degree of ileocecal sphincter contraction is also under the influence of myenteric plexuses and sympathetic innervation of the cecum (147). Contraction of the ileocecal sphincter increases, and ileal peristalsis is inhibited with cecal distention.

Colonic Motility
Colonic contractions serve to maintain aboral propagation of luminal contents at rates that allow important functions of the colon, such as absorption of water and electrolytes. Colonic motility also contributes significantly to the defecatory functions.

Structure of the Colon
The large intestine is made up of inner circular and outer longitudinal muscles. The longitudinal muscle of the large intestine is concentrated into three thick bands, called *teniae coli*, throughout the entire length of the colon (142). The colonic wall bulges between the teniae during the segmental contractions, resulting in haustral formation. The circular muscle layer gradually increases in thickness down to rectum, where it forms the internal anal sphincter.

Innervation of the Colon
Intrinsic innervation of the colon involves myenteric and submucosal plexuses, where they receive inputs from the extrinsic nervous system as well as from mechanoreceptors and chemoreceptors located in the colonic wall. The intrinsic nerve plexuses form complex networks to coordinate colonic motor activity. Extrinsic innervation comes from both parasympathetic and sympathetic branches of the autonomic nervous system. Parasympathetic innervation of the colon is supplied by the vagus nerve in the proximal half of the colon and pelvic nerves from the sacral region of the spinal cord in the distal half. The efferent fibers of the vagus synapse only on postganglionic cholinergic neurons and generally are excitatory for contractile activity. In contrast, pelvic fibers synapse on both cholinergic and noncholinergic postganglionic excitatory neurons. The sympathetic fibers innervate through superior and inferior mesenteric plexuses as well as the hypogastric plexus and result in inhibition of colonic motility (142).

Types of Contractions
Individual Phasic Contractions
Similar to the small intestine, slow electrical wave activities of the smooth muscle coordinate colonic contractions, and the spike potential in the smooth muscle cells initiates colonic contractions (148). However, these spike potentials in the colon are more irregular, and correlation with contractile activity is not as well defined as in the small intestine. Phasic contractions of the colon are also not coordinated with

adjacent smooth muscle cells; therefore, the contractions are segmental and the luminal contents move back and forth. These segmental contractions, particularly notable in the right colon, allow for the mixture and prolonged exposure of the mucosa for absorption of water and electrolytes. Occasionally, these clusters of phasic contractions become coordinated to achieve slow aboral propagation of luminal contents over short distances.

Giant Migrating Contractions

Most propulsion in the colon occurs during GMCs. These contractions produce a mass movement, resulting in significant propagation of luminal contents toward the rectum (148). They are greater in amplitude and longer in duration than phasic contractions. They can occur anywhere in the colon, but are most notable in the transverse colon or descending colon. They only occur approximately three times a day, and each contraction moves the luminal contents approximately one third of the length of the colon (149).

Regulation of Colonic Motility

Many chemicals influence colonic motility. Atropine and other anticholinergic agents generally produce inhibition of colonic longitudinal muscle contractions; however, they have no significant effect on the spontaneous contractions of the circular muscle layer (148). Substance P is also known to be a major excitatory mediator of colon motility, particularly in the circular muscle layer. Nitric oxide and VIP serve as major inhibitory mediators in the colon. Adenosine triphosphate also acts as an inhibitory agent by reducing the reflex contractions induced by distension. Morphine can cause an increase in contractions in the left colon. A wide variety of laxatives are thought to act by altering colonic motility, but there are little data to support this mechanism of action.

Conditions Associated with Altered Gastrointestinal Motility

Gastroparesis

Delayed gastric emptying can occur as a result of systemic medical conditions, such as diabetes mellitus and hypothyroidism. Gastric ulcer of chronic duration can decrease normal gastric motility function. Motility is also diminished after surgical vagotomy for peptic ulcer conditions. Denervation of vagal fibers impairs gastric emptying of solids; therefore, this surgical procedure is usually coupled with a pylorus-emptying procedure (i.e., pyloroplasty) or creation of a new gastric outlet (i.e., gastroenterostomy).

Paralytic Ileus

The most common GI motility disorder occurs as a result of postoperative paralytic ileus. This usually is self-limited, but affects the colon more significantly than the stomach or small bowel. Various systemic conditions can significantly influence the motility of the GI tract. The presence of an inflammatory process in the abdominopelvic cavity can cause a prolonged ileus. Electrolyte disturbance (e.g., hypokalemia) can also negatively affect GI motility.

Irritable Bowel Syndrome

Exaggerated segmental contractions of the colon are demonstrated by motility studies in patients with irritable bowel syndrome. Frequently induced by stress or medications, such as morphine, patients experience abdominal pain and altered bowel habits. Although the exact cause is unknown, conditioning of autonomic responses to repeated exposure of stress and altered myoelectrical activities of the colon are thought to be the underlying pathophysiology of this condition.

Diverticulosis of the Colon

Most frequently noted in the sigmoid colon, this clinical entity of outpouchings of colonic mucosa through the muscular wall of the colon is considered to be a consequence of disordered colonic motility. Thickened circular muscles adjacent to the diverticula along with increased intraluminal pressures suggest abnormal colonic motility, but direct correlation cannot always be demonstrated.

Hirschsprung Disease

This congenital disorder of colonic motility is represented by the absence of ganglion cells in both myenteric and submucosal plexuses, resulting in a contracted state of the involved colon. The sigmoid colon and rectum are the most commonly involved segments of the colon. This condition is most frequently recognized when newborns demonstrate abdominal distension with delayed meconium passage. The diagnosis is confirmed by the absence of ganglion cells along with hypertrophy of the nerve trunks, as assessed by acetylcholinesterase staining. Treatment is surgical resection of the aganglionic segment of colon with anastomosis of the histologically confirmed normal colon to anus.

DEFECATORY MECHANISM

Defecatory function is controlled by a complex array of extrinsic and intrinsic nerves. Striated muscles of the external anal sphincter are under voluntary control, and circular smooth muscles of the internal anal sphincter function involuntarily by reflex mechanisms.

Structure of the Anorectum

Levator ani striated muscle forms the floor of the pelvis and expands diaphragm-like muscle fibers medially surrounding the rectum down to the external anal sphincter muscle. At rest, the puborectalis muscle forms an acute angle between the anal canal and the rectum, called the *anorectal angle*. The external anal sphincter muscle is made up of striated parasagittal fibers that meet anteriorly and posteriorly at the distal anal canal. The internal anal sphincter muscle is composed of thickening terminal circular smooth muscles of the rectum at the level of the dentate line, surrounding the proximal anal canal (150).

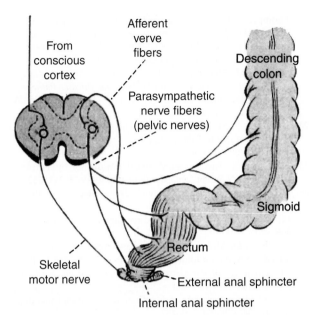

FIGURE 17.20 Afferent and efferent pathways of parasympathetic innervations for defecatory mechanism. Impulses from rectal distention are transmitted into the spinal cord, and parasympathetic nerve fibers (pelvic fibers) regulate peristaltic contractions of the rectum as well as relaxation of the internal anal sphincter. (From Guyton AC. Propulsion and mixing of food in the alimentary tract. In: Guyton AC, Hall JE, eds. *Textbook of medical physiology,* 10th ed. Philadelphia: WB Saunders, 2000:736, with permission.)

Innervation of the Anorectum

Parasympathetic innervation from the sacral region acts as inhibitory motor nerves to the rectum and receives sensation of rectal distention through mechanoreceptors located in the smooth muscle (Fig. 17.20) (142). Lumbar ganglia and the preaortic plexuses provide sympathetic innervation. They form the hypogastric plexuses that join the pelvic ganglion and function as inhibitors of anal sphincter muscle. The myenteric plexuses from the internal anal sphincter control relaxation of the internal anal sphincter induced by rectal distention. Somatic innervation to the voluntary muscle group receives innervation from the anterior roots of the third and fourth sacral nerves. The pudendal nerve, from the second through fourth sacral nerves, also innervates the levator ani and puborectalis muscles.

The distal anal canal, including a zone of approximately 1 cm proximal to the dentate line, is sensitive to various stimuli of pain, temperature, touch, and pressure. The proximal anal canal is sensitive only to rectal distention through proprioceptive receptors in the smooth muscles. The receptors in the anorectal region function in the complex task of discriminating among intraluminal gas, fluid, and solid fecal materials.

Mechanism of Anal Continence

Anal continence is achieved by a variety of factors, such as the anorectal high-pressure zone, the anorectal angle, rectal compliance, and colonic motility (151). The anorectal high-pressure zone, acting as a flap valve, is regulated by extrinsic and intrinsic pressure factors. Increased intra-abdominal pressure, compressing the distal rectum, contributes to the extrinsic pressure factor. Intrinsic pressure is created by the normal tonic contraction of the internal anal sphincter at rest. This smooth muscle tone produces a marked anteroposterior angulation (i.e., anorectal angle) at the anorectal junction and further contributes to anal continence. Decreasing colonic motility also prevents rapid rectal distention and contributes to control of anal continence. Complete anatomic disruption of the internal anal sphincter muscle can result in incontinence; however, preservation of a minimum of one fourth to one third may be enough to maintain continence.

During Valsalva, the anorectal angle becomes less acute along with the perineal descent (152). This process, which results in increasing the distance between the pubococcygeal line and the internal anal canal by 2 to 4 cm, facilitates defecation. Normal rectal capacity is low, and urgency occurs with approximately 200 mL of rectal distention. Anal incontinence occurs frequently with rectal volumes greater than 400 mL despite normal pelvic musculature and innervation.

Defecation Reflexes

The rectum is normally kept empty by segmental contractions, and the internal anal sphincter muscle sustains tonic contraction of the anal canal. As fecal material is forced into the rectum, rectal distention is mediated by mechanoreceptors in the rectum (153). The rectosphincteric reflex then leads to contraction of the rectum and relaxation of the internal anal sphincter (Fig. 17.20). Under convenient circumstances, the external anal sphincter relaxes voluntarily and defecation occurs as the rectum and distal colon contract. If defecation is not convenient, the external anal sphincter remains contracted, the internal anal sphincter regains its tone, and the urge to defecate subsides.

Conditions Associated with Abnormal Defecatory Mechanisms

Anal Incontinence

Anal incontinence usually results from abnormal innervation of the musculature of the pelvic floor as a consequence of systemic neurologic conditions or local injury to the nerves. Direct injury to the musculature of the internal as well as the external anal sphincter (e.g., after fistulotomy or sphincterotomy) can also result in incontinence. Surgery involving extended dissection of the deep pelvis (e.g., low anterior resection or ileoanal pull-through procedures) are at risk for disrupting complex neural networks controlling anal continence.

Diarrhea and Constipation

Abnormal transit of luminal contents through the colon results in diarrhea or constipation. Although the exact mechanisms of how altered motility of the colon contributes to diarrhea or constipation are not known, left colonic contraction recordings demonstrate decreased activity during diarrhea and increased activity with constipation. This is in distinct contrast to the common assumption that diarrhea is a result of increased motility of the colon.

REFERENCES

1. Greeley GH Jr. *Gastrointestinal endocrinology*. Totowa: Human Press, 1999.
2. Walsh JH. Gastrointestinal hormones. In: Johnson LR, Alpers DH, Christensen J, et al. eds. *Physiology of the gastrointestinal tract*, 3rd ed. New York: Raven Press, 1994: 1–128.
3. Thompson JC, Marx M. Gastrointestinal hormones. *Curr Probl Surg* 1984;21: 1–80.
4. Johnson LR. Regulation: peptides of the gastrointestinal tract. In: Johnson LR, Gerwin TA, eds. *Gastrointestinal physiology*, 6th ed. St. Louis: Mosby, 2001: 1–16.
5. Schmidt WE. The intestine, an endocrine organ. *Digestion* 1997;58(Suppl 1): 56–58.
6. Dockray GJ. Physiology of enteric neuropeptides. In: Johnson LR, ed. *Physiology of the gastrointestinal tract*, 3rd ed, Vol. 1. New York: Raven Press, 1994: 169–210.
7. Podolsky DK. Peptide growth factors in the gastrointestinal tract. In: Johnson LR, ed. *Physiology of the gastrointestinal tract*, 3rd ed, Vol. 1. New York: Raven Press, 1994: 129–168.
8. Walsh JH, Dockray GJ, eds. *Gut peptides: biochemistry and physiology*. New York: Raven Press, 1994.
9. Bayliss WM, Starling EH. The mechanisms of pancreatic secretion. *J Physiol (London)* 1902;28: 325.
10. Edkins JS. The chemical mechanism of gastric secretion. *J Physiol* 1906;34: 133–144.
11. Yalow RS, Berson SA. General principles of radioimmunoassay. In: Hayes RL, Goswitz FA, Pearson Murphy B, eds. *Radioisotopes in medicine: in vitro studies*. Oak Ridge: U.S. Atomic Energy Commission, 1968: 7–41.
12. Gregory RA, Tracy HJ. The constitution and properties of two gastrins extracted from hog antral mucosa. Part I. The isolation of two gastrins from hog antral mucosa. Part II. The properties of two gastrins isolated from hog antral mucosa. *Gut* 1964;5: 103.
13. Zollinger RM, Ellison EH. Primary peptic ulcerations of the jejunum associated with islet cell tumors of the pancreas. *Ann Surg* 1955;142: 709.
14. Jorpes JE. The isolation and chemistry of secretin and cholecystokinin. *Gastroenterology* 1968;55: 157–164.
15. Dockray GJ, Varro A, Dimaline R. Gastric endocrine cells: gene expression, processing, and targeting of active products. *Physiol Rev* 1996;76: 767–798.
16. Merchant JL, Dickinson CJ, Yamada T. Molecular biology of the gut: model of gastrointestinal hormones. In: Johnson LR, Alpers DH, Christensen J, et al. eds. *Physiology of the gastrointestinal tract*, 3rd ed. New York: Raven Press, 1994: 295–350.
17. Thompson JC, Cooper CW, Greeley GH Jr, et al. *Gastrointestinal endocrinology: receptors and post-receptor mechanisms*. San Diego: Academic Press, 1990.
18. Surprenant A. Control of the gastrointestinal tract by enteric neurons. *Annu Rev Physiol* 1994;56: 117–140.
19. van der Lely AJ, Tschop M, Heiman ML, et al. Biological, physiological, pathophysiological, and pharmacological aspects of ghrelin. *Endocr Rev* 2004;25: 426–457.
20. Evers BM, Parekh D, Townsend CM Jr, et al. Somatostatin and analogs in the treatment of cancer. A review. *Ann Surg* 1991;213: 190–198.
21. Perry RR, Vinik AI. Endocrine tumors of the gastrointestinal tract. *Annu Rev Med* 1996;47: 57–68.
22. Thompson JC, Townsend CM Jr. Endocrine pancreas. In: Townsend CM Jr, Beauchamp RD, Evers BM, et al. eds. *Sabiston textbook of surgery*. Philadelphia: WB Saunders, 2001: 646–661.
23. Riley SA, Marsh MN. Maldigestion and malabsorption. In: Feldman M, Sleisenger MH, Scharschmidt BF, eds. *Sleisenger & Fordtran's gastrointestinal liver and disease, Pathophysiology/diagnosis/management, Vol. 2*, 6th ed. Philadelphia: WB Saunders, 1993: 1501–1522.
24. Evers BM. Small bowel. In: Townsend CM Jr, Beauchamp RD, Evers BM, et al. eds. *Sabiston textbook of surgery*. Philadelphia: WB Saunders, 2001: 873–916.
25. Birnbaumer L, Birnbaumer M. Signal transduction by G proteins: 1994 edition. *J Recept Signal Transduct Res* 1995;15: 213–252.
26. Hepler JR, Gilman AG. G proteins. *Trends Biochem Sci* 1992;17: 383–387.
27. Lefkowitz RJ. G protein-coupled receptor kinases. *Cell* 1993;74: 409–412.
28. Logsdon CD. Molecular structure and function of G-protein-linked receptors. In: Johnson LR, Alpers DH, Christensen J, et al. eds. *Physiology of the gastrointestinal tract*, 3rd ed. New York: Raven Press, 1994: 351–380.
29. Neer EJ. Heterotrimeric G proteins: organizers of transmembrane signals. *Cell* 1995;80: 249–257.
30. Strader CD, Fong TM, Tota MR, et al. Structure and function of G protein-coupled receptors. *Annu Rev Biochem* 1994;63: 101–132.
31. Bunnett NW, Walsh JH. Gastrointestinal hormones and neurotransmitters. In: Feldman M, Sleisenger MH, Scharschmidt BF, eds. *Sleisenger & Fordtran's gastrointestinal and liver disease, Pathophysiology/diagnosis/management, Vol. 1*, 6th ed. Philadelphia: WB Saunders, 1998: 3–18.
32. Talkad VD, Fortune KP, Pollo DA, et al. Direct demonstration of three different states of the pancreatic cholecystokinin receptor. *Proc Natl Acad Sci USA* 1994;91: 1868–1872.
33. Huang SC, Fortune KP, Wank SA, et al. Multiple affinity states of different cholecystokinin receptors. *J Biol Chem* 1994;269: 26121–26126.
34. Heldin CH. Protein tyrosine kinase receptors. *Cancer Surv* 1996;27: 7–24.
35. Campbell SL, Khosravi-Far R, Rossman KL, et al. Increasing complexity of Ras signaling. *Oncogene* 1998;17: 1395–1413.
36. Seger R, Krebs EG. The MAPK signaling cascade. *FASEB J* 1995;9: 726–735.
37. Wilkinson MG, Millar JB. Control of the eukaryotic cell cycle by MAP kinase signaling pathways. *FASEB J* 2000;14: 2147–2157.
38. Schaeffer HJ, Weber MJ. Mitogen-activated protein kinases: specific messages from ubiquitous messengers. *Mol Cell Biol* 1999;19: 2435–2444.
39. Davis RJ. Signal transduction by the JNK group of MAP kinases. *Cell* 2000;103: 239–252.
40. Whitmarsh AJ, Davis RJ. Transcription factor AP-1 regulation by mitogen-activated protein kinase signal transduction pathways. *J Mol Med* 1996;74: 589–607.
41. Miller AJ. Deglutition. *Physiol Rev* 1982;62: 129–184.
42. Logemann JA, Kahrilas PJ, Cheng J, et al. Closure mechanisms of laryngeal vestibule during swallow. *Am J Physiol* 1992;262: G338–G344.
43. Kahrilas PJ, Logemann JA, Lin S, et al. Pharyngeal clearance during swallowing: a combined manometric and videofluoroscopic study. *Gastroenterology* 1992;103: 128–136.
44. Kahrilas PJ, Dodds WJ, Dent J, et al. Upper esophageal sphincter function during deglutition. *Gastroenterology* 1988;95: 52–62.
45. Kessler JP, Jean A. Inhibitory influence of monoamines and brainstem monoaminergic regions on the medullary swallowing reflex. *Neurosci Lett* 1986;65: 41–46.
46. Kessler JP, Cherkaoui N, Catalin D, et al. Swallowing responses induced by microinjection of glutamate and glutamate agonists into the nucleus tractus solitarius of ketamine-anesthetized rats. *Exp Brain Res* 1990;83: 151–158.

47. Sessle BJ, Henry JL. Neural mechanisms of swallowing: neurophysiological and neurochemical studies on brain stem neurons in the solitary tract region. *Dysphagia* 1989;4: 61–75.

48. Miller AJ. Significance of sensory inflow to the swallowing reflex. *Brain Res* 1972;43: 147–159.

49. Jean A. Control of the central swallowing program by inputs from the peripheral receptors. A review. *J Auton Nerv Syst* 1984;10: 225–233.

50. Miller AJ. The search for the central swallowing pathway: the quest for clarity. *Dysphagia* 1993;8: 185–194.

51. McFarland DH, Lund JP. An investigation of the coupling between respiration, mastication, and swallowing in the awake rabbit. *J Neurophysiol* 1993;69: 95–108.

52. Goyal RK, Martin SB, Shapiro J, et al. The role of cricopharyngeus muscle in pharyngoesophageal disorders. *Dysphagia* 1993;8: 252–258.

53. Castell JA, Castell DO. Modern solid state computerized manometry of the pharyngoesophageal segment. *Dysphagia* 1993;8: 270–275.

54. Welch RW, Luckmann K, Ricks PM, et al. Manometry of the normal upper esophageal sphincter and its alterations in laryngectomy. *J Clin Invest* 1979;63: 1036–1041.

55. Asoh R, Goyal RK. Manometry and electromyography of the upper esophageal sphincter in the opossum. *Gastroenterology* 1978;74: 514–520.

56. Kahrilas PJ, Dodds WJ, Dent J, et al. Effect of sleep, spontaneous gastroesophageal reflux, and a meal on upper esophageal sphincter pressure in normal human volunteers. *Gastroenterology* 1987;92: 466–471.

57. Kahrilas PJ, Dodds WJ, Hogan WJ. Effect of peristaltic dysfunction on esophageal volume clearance. *Gastroenterology* 1988;94: 73–80.

58. Janssens J, Vantrappen G, Hellemans J. Neural control of primary esophageal peristalsis. *Gastroenterology* 1978;74: 801–803.

59. Bieger D, Hopkins DA. Viscerotopic representation of the upper alimentary tract in the medulla oblongata in the rat: the nucleus ambiguus. *J Comp Neurol* 1987;262: 546–562.

60. Asaad K, Abd-El Rahman S, Nawar NN, et al. Intrinsic innervation of the oesophagus in dogs with special reference to the presence of muscle spindles. *Acta Anaesthesiol* 1983;115: 91–96.

61. Collman PI, Tremblay L, Diamant NE. The central vagal efferent supply to the esophagus and lower esophageal sphincter of the cat. *Gastroenterology* 1993;104: 1430–1438.

62. Weisbrodt NW. Neuromuscular organization of esophageal and pharyngeal motility. *Arch Intern Med* 1976;136: 524–531.

63. Christensen J, Percy WH. A pharmacological study of oesophageal muscularis mucosae from the cat, dog and American opossum (*Didelphis virginiana*). *Br J Pharmacol* 1984;83: 329–336.

64. Janssens J, Valembois P, Hellemans J, et al. Studies on the necessity of a bolus for the progression of secondary peristalsis in the canine esophagus. *Gastroenterology* 1974;67: 245–251.

65. Seelig LL Jr, Goyal RK. Morphological evaluation of opossum lower esophageal sphincter. *Gastroenterology* 1978;75: 51–58.

66. Biancani P, Zabinski M, Kerstein M, et al. Lower esophageal sphincter mechanics: anatomic and physiologic relationships of the esophagogastric junction of cat. *Gastroenterology* 1982;82: 468–475.

67. Reynolds JC, Ouyang A, Cohen S. A lower esophageal sphincter reflex involving substance P. *Am J Physiol* 1984;246: G346–G354.

68. Galmiche JP, Clouse RE, Balint A, et al. Functional esophageal disorders. *Gastroenterology* 2006;130:1459–1465.

69. Adler DG, Romero Y. Primary esophageal motility disorders. *Mayo Clin Proc* 2001;76: 195–200.

70. Davletov B, Bajohrs M, Binz T. Beyond BOTOX: advantages and limitations of individual botulinum neurotoxins. *Trends Neurosci* 2005;28: 446–452.

71. Falk GW, Fennerty MB, Rothstein RI. AGA Institute technical review on the use of endoscopic therapy for gastroesophageal reflux disease. *Gastroenterology* 2006;131: 1315–1336.

72. Guyton AC, Hall JE. Secretory functions of the alimentary tract. In: Guyton AC, Hall JE, eds. *Textbook of medical physiology*, 10th ed. Philadelphia: WB Saunders, 2000: 738–753.

73. Johnson LR. Salivary secretion. In: Johnson LR, Gerwin TA, eds. *Gastrointestinal physiology*, 6th ed. St. Louis: Mosby, 2001: 65–74.

74. Cook DI, Van Lennep EW, Roberts ML, et al. Secretion by the major salivary glands. In: Johnson LR, Alpers DH, Christensen J, et al. eds. *Physiology of the gastrointestinal tract*, 3rd ed. New York: Raven Press, 1994: 1061–1118.

75. Kukuruzinska MA, Tabak LA. *Salivary gland biogenesis and function.* New York: Academy of Science, 1997.

76. Petersen OH. Electrophysiology of salivary and pancreatic acinar cells. In: Johnson LR, Alpers DH, Christensen J, et al. eds. *Physiology of the gastrointestinal tract*, 3rd ed. New York: Raven Press, 1994: 1025–1060.

77. Davenport HW. *Physiology of the digestive tract*, 5th ed. Chicago: Year Book Medical, 1982.

78. Feldman M. Gastric secretion: normal and abnormal. In: Feldman M, Sleisenger MH, Scharschmidt BF, eds. *Gastrointestinal and liver disease*, 6th ed, Vol. 1. Philadelphia: WB Saunders, 1998: 587–603.

79. Hersey SJ, Sachs G. Gastric acid secretion. *Physiol Rev* 1995;75: 155–189.

80. Johnson LR. Gastric secretion. In: Johnson LR, Gerwin TA, eds. *Gastrointestinal physiology*, 6th ed. St. Louis: Mosby, 2001: 75–94.

81. Sachs G. The gastric H, K ATPase: regulation and structure/function of the acid pump of the stomach. In: Johnson LR, Alpers DH, Christensen J, et al. eds. *Physiology of the gastrointestinal tract*, 3rd ed. New York: Raven Press, 1994: 1119–1138.

82. Maton PN. Omeprazole. *N Engl J Med* 1991;324: 965–975.

83. Hersey SJ. Gastric secretion of pepsins. In: Johnson LR, Alpers DH, Christensen J, et al. eds. *Physiology of the gastrointestinal tract*, 3rd ed. New York: Raven Press, 1994: 1227–1238.

84. Soll A, Berglindh T. Receptors that regulate gastric acid-secretory function. In: Johnson LR, Alpers DH, Christensen J, et al. eds. *Physiology of the gastrointestinal tract*, 3rd ed. New York: Raven Press, 1994: 1139–1170.

85. Kent Lloyd KC. Peripheral regulation of gastric acid secretion. In: Johnson LR, Alpers DH, Christensen J, et al. eds. *Physiology of the gastrointestinal tract*, 3rd ed. New York: Raven Press, 1994: 1185–1226.

86. Tache Y. Central nervous system regulation of gastric acid secretion. In: Johnson LR, Christensen J, Jackson MJ, et al. eds. *Physiology of the gastrointestinal tract*, 2nd ed, Vol. 2. New York: Raven Press, 1987: 911–930.

87. Debas HT, Mulholland MW. Drug therapy in peptic ulcer disease. *Curr Probl Surg* 1989;26: 1–54.

88. Sawada M, Dickinson CJ. The G cell. *Annu Rev Physiol* 1997;59: 273–298.

89. Meurer LN. Treatment of peptic ulcer disease and nonulcer dyspepsia. *J Fam Pract* 2001;50: 614–619.

90. Wolfe MM, Sachs G. Acid suppression: optimizing therapy for gastroduodenal ulcer healing, gastroesophageal reflux disease, and stress-related erosive syndrome. *Gastroenterology* 2000;118: S9–S31.

91. Guyton AC, Hall JE. Physiology of gastrointestinal disorders. In: Guyton AC, Hall JE, eds. *Textbook of medical physiology*, 10th ed. Philadelphia: WB Saunders, 2000: 764–771.

92. Hojgaard L, Mertz Nielsen A, Rune SJ. Peptic ulcer pathophysiology: acid, bicarbonate, and mucosal function. *Scand J Gastroenterol Suppl* 1006;216: 10–15.

93. Wilkinson M. *Helicobacter pylori*: an overview. *Br J Biomed Sci* 2001;58: 59–60.

94. Chaun H. Update on the role of *H. pylori* infection in gastrointestinal disorders. *Can J Gastroenterol* 2001;15: 251–255.

95. Williamson JS. *Helicobacter pylori*: current chemotherapy and new targets for drug design. *Curr Pharm des* 2001;7: 355–392.

96. Axon AT. Treatment of *Helicobacter pylori*: an overview. *Aliment Pharmacol Ther* 2000;14(Suppl 3): 1–6.

97. Ballard ST, Hunter JH, Taylor AE. Regulation of tight-junction permeability during nutrient absorption across the intestinal epithelium. *Annu Rev Nutr* 1005;15: 35–55.

98. Ferraris RP. Regulation of intestinal nutrient transport. In: Johnson LR, Alpers DH, Christensen J, et al. eds. *Physiology of the gastrointestinal tract*, 3rd ed. New York: Raven Press, 1994: 1821–1844.

99. Guyton AC, Hall JE. Digestion and absorption in the gastrointestinal tract. In: Guyton AC, Hall JE, eds. *Textbook of medical physiology*, 10th ed. Philadelphia: WB Saunders, 2000: 754–763.

100. Johnson LR. Digestion and absorption. In: Johnson LR, Gerwin TA, eds. *Gastrointestinal physiology*, 6th ed. St. Louis: Mosby, 2001: 119–142.

101. Madara JL, Trier JS. The functional morphology of the mucosa of the small bowel. In: Johnson LR, Alpers DH, Christensen J, et al. eds. *Physiology of the gastrointestinal tract*, 3rd ed. New York: Raven Press, 1994: 1577–1622.

102. Keljo DJ, Squires RHJ. Anatomy and anomalies of the small and large intestine. In: Feldman M, Sleisenger MH, Scharschmidt BF, eds. *Sleisenger & Fordtran's gastrointestinal and liver disease, Pathophysiology/diagnosis/management, Vol. 2*. Philadelphia: WB Saunders, 1998: 1419–1436.

103. Snipes RL. *Absorptive surface in mammals of different sizes*. Berlin: Springer, 1997.

104. Ferraris RP, Diamond J. Regulation of intestinal sugar transport. *Physiol Rev* 1997;77: 257–302.

105. Hediger MA, Rhoads DB. Molecular physiology of sodium-glucose cotransporters. *Physiol Rev* 1994;74: 993–1026.

106. Wright EM. The intestinal Na^+/glucose cotransporter. *Annu Rev Physiol* 1993;55: 575–589.

107. Wright EM, Hirayama BA, Loo DDF, et al. Intestinal sugar transport. In: Johnson LR, Alpers DH, Christensen J, et al. eds. *Physiology of the gastrointestinal tract*, 3rd ed. New York: Raven Press, 1994: 1751–1772.

108. Alpers DH. Digestion and absorption of carbohydrates and proteins. In: Johnson LR, Alpers DH, Christensen J, et al. eds. *Physiology of the gastrointestinal tract*, 3rd ed. New York: Raven Press, 1994: 1723–1750.

109. Freeman HJ, Kim YS. Digestion and absorption of protein. *Annu Rev Med* 1978;29: 99–116.

110. Sleisenger MH, Kim YS. Protein digestion and absorption. *N Engl J Med* 1979;300: 659–663.

111. Ganapathy V, Brandsch M, Leibach FH. Intestinal transport of amino acids and peptides. In: Johnson LR, Alpers DH, Christensen J, et al. eds. *Physiology of the gastrointestinal tract*, 3rd ed. New York: Raven Press, 1994: 1773–1794.

112. Gardner MLG. Absorption of intact proteins and peptides. In: Johnson LR, Alpers DH, Christensen J, et al. eds. *Physiology of the gastrointestinal tract*, 3rd ed. New York: Raven Press, 1994: 1795–1820.

113. Leibach FH, Ganapathy V. Peptide transporters in the intestine and the kidney. *Annu Rev Nutr* 1996;16: 99–119.

114. Borgstrom B. Fat assimilation. In: Bockus HL, ed. *Gastroenterology*, 4th ed. Philadelphia: WB Saunders, 1985: 1510–1519.

115. Davidson NO. Cellular and molecular mechanisms of small intestinal lipid transport. In: Johnson LR, Alpers DH, Christensen J, et al. eds. *Physiology of the gastrointestinal tract*, 3rd ed. New York: Raven Press, 1994: 1909–1934.

116. Hofmann AF. Fat absorption and malabsorption: physiology, diagnosis, and treatment. *Viewpoints Dig Dis* 1977;9: 4.

117. Hofmann AF. Intestinal absorption of bile aids and biliary constituents: the intestinal component of the enterohepatic circulation and the integrated system. In: Johnson LR, Alpers DH, Christensen J, et al. eds. *Physiology of the gastrointestinal tract*, 3rd ed. New York: Raven Press, 1994: 1845–1866.

118. Hofmann AF, Small DM. Detergent properties of bile salts: correlation with physiological function. *Annu Rev Med* 1967;18: 333–376.

119. Ockner RK, Isselbacher KJ. Recent concepts of intestinal fat absorption. *Rev Physiol Biochem Pharmacol* 1974;71: 107–146.

120. Tso P. Intestinal lipid absorption. In: Johnson LR, Alpers DH, Christensen J, et al. eds. *Physiology of the gastrointestinal tract*, 3rd ed. New York: Raven Press, 1994: 1867–1908.

121. Chang EB, Rao MC. Intestinal water and electrolyte transport: mechanisms of physiological and adaptive responses. In: Johnson LR, Alpers DH, Christensen J, et al. eds. *Physiology of the gastrointestinal tract*, 3rd ed. New York: Raven Press, 1994: 2027–2082.

122. Johnson LR. Fluid and electrolyte absorption. In: Johnson LR, Gerwin TA, eds. *Gastrointestinal physiology*, 6th ed. St. Louis: Mosby, 2001: 143–154.

123. Sellin JH. Intestinal electrolyte absorption and secretion. In: Feldman M, Sleisenger MH, Scharschmidt BF, eds. *Sleisenger & Fordtran's gastrointestinal and liver disease, Pathophysiology/diagnosis/management, Vol. 1*. Philadelphia: WB Saunders, 1998: 1451–1470.

124. Civitelli R, Avioli LV. Calcium, phosphate, and magnesium absorption. In: Johnson LR, Alpers DH, Christensen J, et al. eds. *Physiology of the gastrointestinal tract*, 3rd ed. New York: Raven Press, 1994: 2173–2182.

125. Rucker RB, Lonnerdal B, Keen CL. Intestinal absorption of nutritionally important trace elements. In: Johnson LR, Alpers DH, Christensen J, et al. eds. *Physiology of the gastrointestinal tract*, 3rd ed. New York: Raven Press, 1994: 2183–2202.

126. Brasitus TA, Sitrin MD. Absorption and cellular actions of vitamin D. In: Johnson LR, Alpers DH, Christensen J, et al. eds. *Physiology of the gastrointestinal tract*, 3rd ed. New York: Raven Press, 1994: 1935–1956.

127. Alpers DH. Absorption of water-soluble vitamins, folate, minerals and vitamin D. In: Sleisenger MH, Fordtran JS, eds. *Gastrointestinal disease: pathophysiology, diagnosis, management*, 3rd ed. Philadelphia: WB Saunders, 1983: 830–843.

128. Marsh MN, Riley SA. Digestion and absorption of nutrients and vitamins. In: Feldman M, Sleisenger MH, Scharschmidt BF, eds. *Sleisenger & Fordtran's gastrointestinal and liver disease, Pathophysiology/diagnosis/management, Vol. 2*, 6th ed. Philadelphia: WB Saunders, 1998: 1471–1500.

129. Seetharam B. Gastrointestinal absorption and transport of cobalamin (vitamin B_{12}). In: Johnson LR, Alpers DH, Christensen J, et al. eds. *Physiology of the gastrointestinal tract*, 3rd ed. New York: Raven Press, 1994: 1997–2026.

130. Scolapio JS, Fleming CR. Short bowel syndrome. *Gastroenterol Clin North Am* 1998;27: 467–479, viii.

131. Blair RW. Convergence of sympathetic, vagal, and other sensory inputs onto neurons in feline ventrolateral medulla. *Am J Physiol* 1991;260: H1918–H1928.

132. Sawchenko PE. Central connections of the sensory and motor nuclei of the vagus nerve. *J Auton Nerv Syst* 1983;9: 13–26.

133. Holzer HH, Raybould HE. Vagal and splanchnic sensory pathways mediate inhibition of gastric motility induced by duodenal distension. *Am J Physiol* 1992;262: G603–G608.

134. Furness JBCM. *Sympathetic influences on gastrointestinal function*. London: Churchill Livingstone, 1987.

135. Barker MC, Cobden I, Axon AT. Proximal stomach and antrum in stomach emptying. *Gut* 1979;20: 309–311.

136. Burks TF, Galligan JJ, Porreca F, et al. Regulation of gastric emptying. *Fed Proc* 1985;44: 2897–2901.

137. Sanders KM, Vogalis F. Organization of electrical activity in the canine pyloric canal. *J Physiol* 1989;416: 49–66.

138. Sarna SK. Cyclic motor activity; migrating motor complex: 1985. *Gastroenterology* 1985;89: 894–913.

139. Weisbrodt NW, Copeland EM, Kearley RW, et al. Effects of pentagastrin on electrical activity of small intestine of the dog. *Am J Physiol* 1974;227: 425–429.

140. Debas HT, Farooq O, Grossman MI. Inhibition of gastric emptying is a physiological action of cholecystokinin. *Gastroenterology* 1975;68: 1211–1217.

141. Gulsrud PO, Taylor IL, Watts HD, et al. How gastric emptying of carbohydrate affects glucose tolerance and symptoms after truncal vagotomy with pyloroplasty. *Gastroenterology* 1980;78: 1463–1471.

142. Johnson LR. Motility. In: Johnson LR, ed. *Essential medical physiology*, Philadelphia: Lippincott Williams & Wilkins, 1998: 429–443.

143. Otterson MF, Sarna SK. Neural control of small intestinal giant migrating contractions. *Am J Physiol* 1994;266: G576–G584.

144. Otterson MF, Sarr MG. Normal physiology of small intestinal motility. *Surg Clin North Am* 1993;73: 1173–1192.

145. Otterson MF, Sarna SK, Moulder JE. Effects of fractionated doses of ionizing radiation on small intestinal motor activity. *Gastroenterology* 1988;95: 1249–1257.

146. Kellow JE, Phillips SF. Altered small bowel motility in irritable bowel syndrome is correlated with symptoms. *Gastroenterology* 1987;92: 1885–1893.

147. Bogers JJ, Van Marck E. The ileocaecal junction. *Histol Histopathol* 1993;8: 561–566.

148. Sarna SK. Colonic motor activity. *Surg Clin North Am* 1993;73: 1201–1223.

149. Bassotti G, Gaburri M. Manometric investigation of high-amplitude propagated contractile activity of the human colon. *Am J Physiol* 1988;255: G660–G664.

150. Stonesifer GJ, Murphy GP, Lombardo CR. The anatomy of the anorectum. *Am J Surg* 1960;10: 666–671.

151. Bielefeldt K, Enck P, Erckenbrecht JF. Sensory and motor function in the maintenance of anal continence. *Dis Colon Rectum* 1990;33: 674–678.

152. Infantino A, Masin A, Pianon P, et al. Role of proctography in severe constipation. *Dis Colon Rectum* 1990;33: 707–712.

153. Schuster MM, Hendrix TR, Mendeloff AI. The internal anal sphincter response: manometric studies on its normal physiology, neural pathways, and alteration in bowel disorders. *J Clin Invest* 1963;42: 196–207.

CHAPTER 18

Liver, Biliary Tract, and Pancreas

Robert E. Glasgow and Sean J. Mulvihill

EMBRYOLOGY

To fully understand the anatomy of the liver, biliary tract, and pancreas, one must understand the embryology of these organs. As is the case with the entire gastrointestinal tract, the liver, biliary tree, and pancreas are derived from a combination of the primitive endoderm which gives rise to the epithelium and glands of the digestive tract and the splanchnic mesenchyme with gives rise to the muscular, connective tissue, and other layers and tissue of the developing gut. The liver, biliary tree, and pancreas are derived from the primitive foregut.

Early in the fourth week in the development of the human embryo, a projection appears in the ventral wall of the primitive foregut. This ventral projection off the developing duodenum is the hepatic diverticulum. From this diverticulum, three buds can be recognized. The large, cranial bud of proliferating and branching endoderm expands into the septum transversum, a mass of splanchnic mesoderm between the pericardial cavity and the yolk stalk in an area called the *ventral mesentery*. This aggregate of the endoderm and mesoderm develops into two lobes of the liver. The developing biliary tract, including the intrahepatic and extrahepatic bile ducts, is derived from the endoderm from the foregut while the hemopoietic cells, fibrous tissue, suspensory ligaments of the liver, and Kupffer cells are derived from the mesoderm of the septum transversum. The small caudal bud, arising in close proximity to the larger cranial bud, becomes the gallbladder and its stalk, the cystic duct (Fig. 18.1) (1).

At the base of the ventral projection near the bile duct insertion into the duodenum, the ventral pancreatic bud develops which gives rise to part of the head and uncinate process of the pancreas. Just proximal to the ventral projection, a dorsal projection arises from the developing duodenum. This larger dorsal pancreatic bud grows rapidly into the dorsal mesentery of the developing gut and gives rise to the remainder of the head, body, and tail of the pancreas. As the duodenum rotates to the right at the 12-mm stage, the ventral pancreatic bud is carried dorsally with the origin of the bile duct to lie posterior to the dorsal pancreatic

bud. In most humans, these structures then merge giving rise to a pancreas with a single dominant ductal system by the sixth to seventh week of gestation. The main pancreatic duct derives from the duct of the ventral pancreatic bud and the distal two thirds of the dorsal pancreatic duct. In some people, a persistent extension of the dorsal duct to the duodenum persists called the *minor* or *accessory duct*. Pancreatic parenchyma, including acinar and islet cells, is derived from the endoderm while the fibrous structure and septations of the gland are mesenchymal in origin (1).

Within another week, the lumen of the developing gallbladder, bile ducts, and pancreatic ducts becomes canalized as a result of vacuolization and degeneration of the endodermal cells centrally located in the ducts. The right and left ducts, which also begin as solid outgrowths from the original diverticulum, likewise canalize and drain bile from the liver. By the 12th week of fetal life, the liver begins to secrete bile, and the pancreas secretes fluid that flows through the extrahepatic biliary tree and pancreatic ducts, respectively, into the duodenum.

Anomalies in the development of this complex array of ducts, organ rotation and fusion, and proliferation of tissue gives rise to many variations in normal anatomy and congenital anomalies. Although congenital anomalies of the liver are rare, variations in bile duct anatomy are common. Biliary atresia results from failure of canalization of the developing bile ducts. Malrotation of the pancreas gives rise to annular pancreas, where a thin band of pancreatic tissue surrounds the descending duodenum. Failure of fusion of the pancreatic ducts results in pancreatic divisum, seen in approximately 9% of people.

ANATOMY AND HISTOLOGY

Liver

Anatomy

The liver is a large, wedge-shaped organ that occupies the right upper quadrant of the abdomen under the

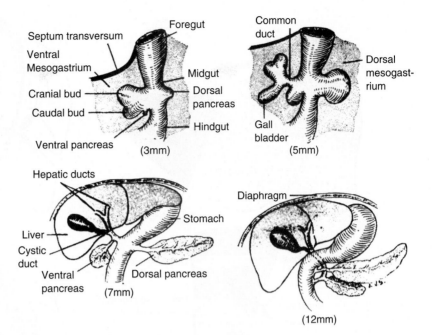

FIGURE 18.1   Development of the liver, biliary tract, and pancreas from the 3-mm to 12-mm stage. (From Lindner HR. Embryology and anatomy of the biliary tract. In: Way LW, Pellegrini CA, eds. *Surgery of the gallbladder and bile ducts.* Philadelphia: WB Saunders, 1987:4, with permission.)

right hemidiaphragm. The left lobe extends beyond the midline into the left upper quadrant. In the adult, the liver ranges in weight from 1,200 to 1,600 g and is the single largest organ in the body. The average adult liver measures 23 cm transversely, 15 cm anteroposteriorly, and 6 cm vertically. The liver's anterior and superior diaphragmatic surfaces are covered with visceral peritoneum. Posteriorly, the peritoneum becomes fused with the visceral peritoneum of the underside of the diaphragm at the coronary and triangular ligaments leaving exposed or "bare areas" on the right and left void of a true peritoneal cover.

The appearance of the anterior and superior surfaces of the liver as seen *in situ* is interrupted only by the falciform ligament emanating from the umbilical fissure. Early descriptions of anatomy used the falciform ligament to divide the liver on its superior surface into a large right and small left lobe (Fig. 18.2A). In this perspective, the quadrate lobe was defined as the area between the umbilical fissure and the gallbladder fossa. The caudate lobe was defined as the portion of liver wedged between the groove of the inferior vena cava, transverse hilar fissure, and umbilical fissure. However, these lobar divisions, based on surface topography of the liver, do not coincide with the course of the intrahepatic vasculature and bile ducts and, therefore, are not relevant to our current understanding of surgical anatomy of the liver.

A more anatomically correct description of the surgical anatomy of the liver was defined by Couinaud (2,3). This schema is based on the sequential branching of the portal vein, hepatic artery, and biliary tree as they enter the parenchyma at the hilum and the corresponding drainage patterns of the hepatic veins. All three of the inflow structures follow roughly parallel courses and bifurcate just before entering the liver. This major bifurcation divides the liver into left and right lobes. According to the Couinaud classification,

the caudate lobe is segment I, segments II to IV are on the left, and segments V to VIII are on the right (Fig. 18.2B). The left portal vein, hepatic artery, and hepatic duct run along the surface of the liver for several centimeters before entering the liver parenchyma. After entering the liver on the left, these structures bifurcate with one branch, continuing directly into the segment II and III and another to Couinaud segment IV. On the left, segments II and III reside to the left of the falciform ligament or umbilical fissure. Segment IV is defined as the area between the umbilical fissure and the main scissura that is loosely identified on the surface of the liver as a vertical line drawn between the long access of the gallbladder and the middle of the inferior vena cava. The main scissura or Cantlie line separates the true left and right lobe of the liver.

The right portal vein, hepatic artery, and hepatic duct bifurcate into anteromedial and posterolateral branches shortly after entering the parenchyma. In the Couinaud classification, segments V and VIII originate from the anteromedial branch, and segments VI and VII arise from the posterolateral branch. Anomalies of the main portal veins are unusual. In comparison, the so-called normal "standard" anatomy of the hepatic arteries is present in only 55% to 65% of the population. Generally, the common hepatic artery arises from the celiac axis and gives rise to the right and left hepatic arteries. The two most common arterial anomalies are a right hepatic artery originating from the superior mesenteric artery and a left hepatic artery arising from the left gastric artery. These vessels may account for all arterial input to their respective lobes, in which case they are called *replaced hepatic arteries* or be an accessory to the standard anatomy.

Three hepatic veins drain the liver. Unlike the portal veins and hepatic arteries, the hepatic veins do not correlate with or arise from the center of hepatic segments, but instead run in intersegmental planes within the liver (Fig. 18.2B). The

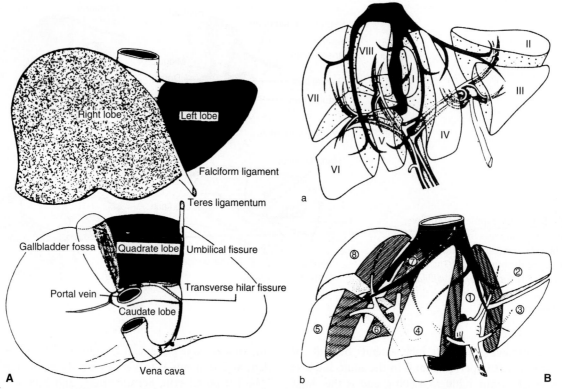

FIGURE 18.2 **A:** Historical lobar anatomy of the liver. **B:** Functional segments of the liver according to Couinaud's classification in the (*a*) *ex vivo* and (*b*) *in situ* positions. (From Bismuth H. Surgical anatomy of the liver. In: Bengmark S, Blumgart LH, eds. *Liver surgery.* New York: Churchill Livingstone, 1986:3, with permission.)

left hepatic vein runs in the left vertical scissura separating segments II and III or lateral segment from segment IV or medial segment of the liver and drains most of the left lobe. The right hepatic vein runs in the right vertical scissura separating the right lobe into the anteromedial (segments V and VIII) and posterolateral (segments VI and VII) sectors and drains most of the right lobe. The middle hepatic vein runs in the main scissura corresponding to the Cantlie line and drains both lobes. The three hepatic veins enter the inferior vena cava at the superior aspect of the liver just below the diaphragm. In two thirds of people, the middle vein will join the left vein as a common trunk before entering the vena cava. Multiple lesser retrohepatic veins also enter the vena cava directly from the hepatic parenchyma and the caudate lobe.

Histology

The surface of the liver is covered by a single layer of mesothelial cells. Immediately beneath this layer is the Glisson capsule, which is a layer of collagen, fibroblasts, and blood vessels. At the hepatic hilum, the Glisson capsule is joined by connective tissue surrounding the intrahepatic projection of the portal veins, hepatic arteries, and bile ducts. Within the liver, this dense tissue is replaced by a more delicate reticular tissue that serves to aid in liver regeneration.

Hepatocytes constitute approximately 80% of the liver mass with the remainder consisting of hemopoietic cells, fibrous tissue, suspensory ligaments of the liver, and Kupffer cells. The functional unit of the liver is the hepatic acinus, which is loosely characterized as an oval collection of hepatocytes oriented around a portal triad (portal vein, bile duct, and hepatic artery) at the apices of the acinus and the terminal branches of the hepatic vein at the axis of the acinus. Hepatocytes nearest the portal structures are in Zone 1 of the acinus and those nearest the hepatic venules Zone 3 with the midacinar cells termed *Zone 2* (Fig. 18.3) (4). The term *hepatocyte heterogeneity* refers to the differential processing of substrate depending on the location of the hepatocyte within the acinus. Zone 1 cells more readily engage in absorption by simple diffusion whereas Zone 2 cells require receptor-mediated uptake or endocytosis. Zone 1 cells are the first to receive nutrients, regenerate in response to injury, and the last to die because of the higher oxygen content in their local milieu. In contrast, Zone 3 cells are relatively susceptible to damage and ischemia.

Biliary Tract

Anatomy

The biliary tract extends from the intrahepatic ducts, the right and left hepatic ducts, the common hepatic duct (CHD), and the common bile duct (CBD) to the sphincter of Oddi with the cystic duct and gallbladder arising as adjoining structures. As a rule, the intrahepatic ducts drain the liver segments from which they are derived and are separated into right and left lobar branches (Fig. 18.2B).

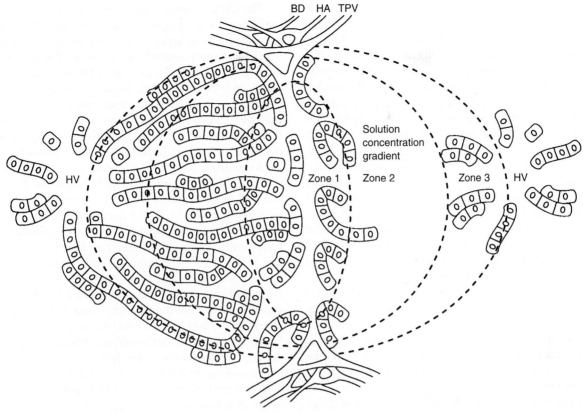

FIGURE 18.3 The hepatic acinus. Unidirectional perfusion of the hepatocytes within the acinus causes a gradient of solute concentration as blood moves from the terminal portal venule (TPV) to the hepatic venule (HV). Hepatocytes nearest the portal tract are labeled Zone 1, mid-acinar cells are labeled Zone 2, and centriolobular cells are Zone 3. The TPV to HV oxygen gradient is 50 mmol/L. This implies that Zone 1 cells have a higher oxygen tension that Zone 3 cells and are less susceptible to ischemia and toxic injury. BD, bile ductule; HA, hepatic arteriole. (From Raper SE, Hepatic physiology. In: Greenfield LJ, Mulholland M, Oldham KT, et al. eds. *Surgery: scientific principles and practice*, 2nd ed. Philadelphia: Lippincott-Raven Publishers, 1997.)

Normal variations in the anatomy of the extrahepatic bile ducts are common. Most patients have a bifurcation where the right and left hepatic ducts join to form the CHD. This junction may occur as a wide or an acute angle, or the two hepatic ducts may run parallel to each other before joining. In some patients, three hepatic ducts will join to form the CHD, including a left duct and separate right anterior and posterior sectoral branches. Usually, the hepatic ducts meet just outside of the liver parenchyma, with the cystic duct entering 2 to 3 cm distally. Occasionally, the two hepatic ducts do not unite until after the cystic duct has joined the right hepatic duct.

The cystic duct is generally approximately 0.5 to 4 cm in length depending on its mode of junction with the hepatic duct. The cystic duct usually runs downward, backward, and to the left in the hepatoduodenal ligament, usually joining the CHD at an acute angle on its right side. Variations in cystic duct anatomy are very common. The cystic duct may (i) enter the right hepatic duct or posterior sectoral duct, (ii) join the CHD at a right angle, (iii) parallel the CHD, (iv) enter the CHD dorsally, (v) enter the CHD on its left side, (vi) enter the CHD behind the duodenum, or (vii) join

the CHD as it enters the duodenal wall (1). The entrance of the cystic duct into the CHD may be spiral as well as angular or parallel. The cystic duct usually has four to ten crescentic folds known as the *spiral valves of Heister*. The cystic duct, CHD, and hilum of the liver form the hepatocystic triangle, an important landmark during cholecystectomy.

The gallbladder is a pear-shaped organ that lies on the inferior surface of the liver at the junction of the left and right hepatic lobes between Couinaud segments IV and V (Fig. 18.2B). The gallbladder varies from 7 to 10 cm in length and from 2.5 to 3.5 cm in width. Gallbladder volume varies considerably, being large during fasting states and small after eating. A moderately distended gallbladder has a capacity of 50 to 60 mL of bile but may become much larger with certain pathologic states. The gallbladder has been divided into four areas: the fundus, body, infundibulum, and neck. The Hartmann pouch is an asymmetric bulge of the infundibulum that lies close to the neck of the gallbladder. The neck points in a cephalad and dorsal direction to join the cystic duct.

The CBD begins at the junction of the cystic duct with the CHD. The average CBD length is approximately 7.5 cm, but this figure varies considerably, depending on the site of union of the cystic duct with the CHD. The normal CBD diameter is usually less than 1.0 cm, but this figure increases with age and increases dramatically when the CBD is obstructed. The diameter of the CBD varies according to the observer—to the ultrasonographer, it averages 5 to 6 mm in internal diameter, but to the surgeon looking at the external dimensions, it is usually 2 to 3 mm larger. The CBD dilates somewhat after cholecystectomy, but is still usually less than 10 mm in diameter (by ultrasonography). The CBD can be separated into the (i) supraduodenal, (ii) retroduodenal, (iii) pancreatic, and (iv) intraduodenal-intramural portions (Fig. 18.4A). The CBD opens into the ampulla of Vater and usually, but not always, unites with the pancreatic duct just within the bowel wall (Fig. 18.4B). The CBD enters the duodenum near the junction of the second and third portions in approximately 90% of the population (1).

The entire sphincteric system of the distal bile duct and the pancreatic duct is commonly referred to as the *sphincter of Oddi.* This term is imprecise because the sphincter is subdivided into several sections and contains both circular and longitudinal fibers. The sphincter mechanism functions independently from the surrounding duodenal musculature and has separate sphincters for the distal bile duct, pancreatic duct, and ampulla. In more than 90% of the population, the common channel, where the biliary and pancreatic ducts join, is less than 1 cm in length and lies within the ampulla. In the rare situation in which the common channel is longer than 1 cm or the biliary and pancreatic ducts open separately into the duodenum, pathologic biliary or pancreatic problems may develop.

The CBD, common hepatic artery, and portal vein lie in the hepatoduodenal ligament. Normally, the CBD is on the right, the common hepatic artery is on the left, and the portal vein is in a dorsal position between the two. The right hepatic artery usually passes dorsal to the CHD and ventral to the portal vein. When the right hepatic artery is replaced and originates from the superior mesenteric artery, it lies to the right and dorsal to the CBD and to the right and just ventral to the portal vein. The blood supply to the extrahepatic biliary tree arises from the right and left hepatic, common hepatic, gastroduodenal, and pancreatoduodenal arteries. Within the CHD and CBD, longitudinal vessels run in the 3-o' clock and 9-o' clock positions. The cystic artery arises from the right hepatic artery in 95% of the population but may arise from any of the other adjacent arteries. The gallbladder and biliary ducts receive nerve fibers from both the sympathetic and parasympathetic nervous systems. These nerves begin at the celiac plexus and travel through the hepatic plexus along the hepatic artery and portal vein. The hepatic plexus contains fibers from the posterior vagus and is joined just inferior to the liver by branches from the anterior vagus. The lymphatic drainage from the gallbladder may go directly into the liver or toward the cystic duct. Lymph drainage from here and along the CBD courses toward the liver and into a deep pancreatic group of nodes, which eventually drain back to the celiac nodes.

Histology

The extrahepatic biliary tree, including the gallbladder and cystic duct, consists of a columnar mucosa surrounded by

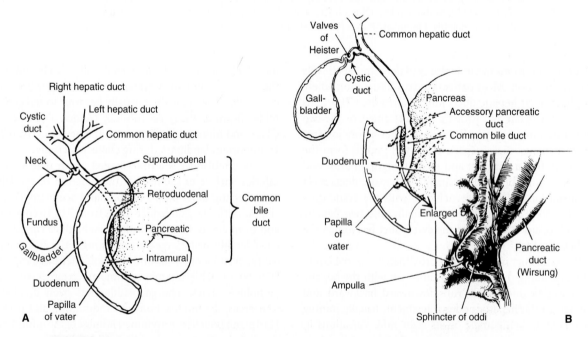

FIGURE 18.4 **A:** Anatomic division of the extrahepatic biliary tract. **B:** Relation of the gallbladder and bile ducts to the duodenum. (From Gadacz TR. Anatomy, embryology, congenital anomalies, and physiology of the gallbladder and extrahepatic biliary ducts. In: Zuidema GD, Turcotte JG, eds. *Shackelford's surgery of the alimentary tract,* 3rd ed. Philadelphia: WB Saunders, 1991:139, with permission.)

a connective tissue layer. The most distal bile duct mucosa has mucin-secreting glands not apparent in more proximal ducts. The bile ducts have a fibromuscular wall consisting of discontinuous and sparse smooth muscle cells. As a result of this lack of an organized muscular wall, the bile duct lacks motility seen in other viscera. At the level of the terminal bile duct, the smooth muscle cells become more prominent with a well-defined circular and longitudinal layer at the level of the sphincter of Oddi. The gallbladder wall consists of five layers: mucosa, lamina propria, smooth muscle, perimuscular subserosal connective tissue, and serosa. Unlike the main extrahepatic bile duct, the cystic duct contains the spiral valve of Heister, which is a transversely oriented bundle of smooth muscle thought to play a role in filling and emptying of the gallbladder.

Pancreas

Anatomy

The pancreas is a retroperitoneal organ extending in an oblique, transverse position from the duodenal C-loop to the hilum of the spleen. The pancreas is covered with a fine connective tissue but lacks a true serosal surface or capsule. The pancreas lies anterior to the right renal vessels, vena cava, portal vein, aorta, superior mesenteric artery, splenic vein, and left renal vessels. The celiac axis, hepatic artery, and splenic artery run along its cephalad edge, and the transverse mesocolon borders the pancreas inferiorly. The stomach and greater omentum cover most of the pancreas anteriorly. The

normal pancreas weighs 70 to 110 g and is approximately 12 to 20 cm in length. The body of the pancreas measures approximately 4 to 5 cm in width and 1.5 to 2 cm in thickness.

The pancreas is divided into five parts: the head, uncinate, neck, body, and tail. The pancreatic head lies adjacent to the second lumbar vertebra and is intimately attached to the C-loop of the duodenum. The distal CBD passes through the pancreatic head (Fig. 18.4B), although in approximately 15% of people, the CBD lies in a groove on the posterior aspect of the pancreas. The uncinate process lies adjacent to the third and fourth portions of the duodenum and next to the superior mesenteric vein (SMV). The uncinate process also extends behind the SMV and portal vein to the right edge of the superior mesenteric artery.

The neck of the pancreas joins the head and the body. The pancreatic neck overlies and is grooved by the junction of the SMV and splenic veins as they become the portal vein. Usually, no anterior venous tributaries of the SMV or portal vein extend from the pancreatic neck. The communication of the gastroduodenal artery with the right gastroepiploic artery lies on the anterior surface of the pancreatic neck (Fig. 18.5). These vessels run between the pancreatic neck and the pylorus, which also covers the pancreatic neck anteriorly.

The body of the pancreas extends to the left of the neck beyond the superior mesenteric vessels. The body usually crosses the vertebral column at the level of the first lumbar vertebra. Superiorly, the pancreatic body lies adjacent to the

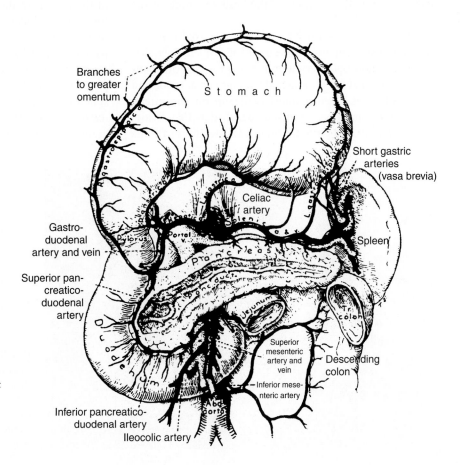

FIGURE 18.5 Blood supply of the pancreas and duodenum. The stomach is shown reflected upward, and the pancreatic duct is exposed. (From Jones T, Shepard WC. *A manual of surgical anatomy.* Philadelphia: WB Saunders, 1950, with permission.)

celiac axis and splenic arteries, whereas the ligament of Treitz and the proximal jejunum are related inferiorly. The splenic vein lies in a groove posteriorly, and multiple small veins enter it from the pancreas. The inferior mesenteric vein also joins the splenic vein to the left of the ligament of Treitz and along the inferior border of the body of the pancreas. No specific landmark defines the merger of the body and tail of the pancreas. Normally, the pancreatic tail extends into the splenic hilum. However, this relation is variable with some patients having the tail terminate inferior and, less likely, superior to the splenic hilum.

The pancreas has two ducts draining into the duodenum: the main duct of Wirsung and the accessory duct of Santorini (Fig. 18.4B). The main pancreatic duct extends from the tail of the pancreas toward the head. In the body of the pancreas, the main duct usually runs midway between the superior and inferior borders and closer to the posterior than to the anterior surface. The main pancreatic duct normally measures 3 to 4.5 mm in diameter. After passing into the neck of the pancreas, the main pancreatic duct extends in a caudal and posterior direction before joining the distal bile duct at the ampulla. The accessory pancreatic duct usually drains the anterior and superior portions of the pancreatic head through a minor papilla, which enters the duodenum approximately 2 cm proximal and slightly anterior to the ampulla of Vater. The accessory duct is patent in approximately 70% of autopsy specimens and usually communicates with the main duct. In 90% of the population, the main and accessory pancreatic ducts join near the junction of the head and neck of the pancreas.

The pancreas has a rich blood supply derived from the gastroduodenal, superior mesenteric, and splenic arteries. The gastroduodenal artery terminates as the superior pancreaticoduodenal artery, which divides into an anterior and posterior branch. The first branch of the superior mesenteric artery is the inferior pancreaticoduodenal artery that divides into an anterior and posterior branch collateralizes with the

superior arcade to supply the pancreatic head and duodenum (Fig. 18.5). The neck, body, and tail of the pancreas receive blood from the splenic artery as the dorsal pancreatic artery arising near the celiac trunk, the great pancreatic or pancreatic magna to the body, and the caudal pancreatic artery supplying the tail. These usually arise from the splenic artery and run within the substance of the gland. When the right hepatic artery arises from the superior mesenteric, it usually runs along with the portal vein posterior to the neck of the pancreas. The venous blood from the pancreas drains into the portal system through the superior mesenteric or splenic veins or directly into the portal vein. Lymphatic drainage extends in all directions but concentrates in pancreatoduodenal and preaortic nodes near the origins of the superior mesenteric artery and the celiac axis.

The pancreas is innervated by both sympathetic fibers from the splanchnic nerves and parasympathetic fibers from the vagus. The preganglionic efferent fibers of splanchnic nerves pass through the celiac ganglion before reaching the pancreas. Afferent pain fibers have cell bodies in the dorsal root ganglia of T-5 to T-12. The efferent and afferent parasympathetic fibers also have cell bodies in the brain and pass through the posterior vagus through the celiac ganglion without synapsing before entering the pancreas.

Histology

The pancreas has both an exocrine and endocrine component. The exocrine pancreas comprises approximately 85% of the volume of the gland; 10% of the gland is accounted for by extracellular matrix and 4% by blood vessels and the major ducts, leaving only 2% of the volume for the endocrine pancreas. The functional unit of the exocrine pancreas is the acinus and its associated duct system. Each acinus is composed of a single layer of acinar cells assuming a roughly spheroid or tubular configuration surrounding a draining ductule. Acinar cells (Fig. 18.6) contain abundant zymogen granules in their narrow, centrally located apical portion

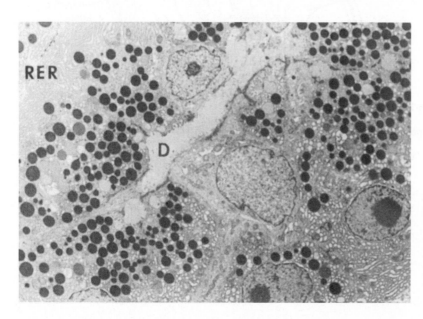

FIGURE 18.6 Electron micrograph of multiple acinar cells and a section of terminal duct (*D*). The acinar cells contain extensive rough endoplasmic reticulum (*RER*) and numerous electron-dense spherical zymogen granules (uranyl acetate and lead citrate, original magnification × 2,000.)

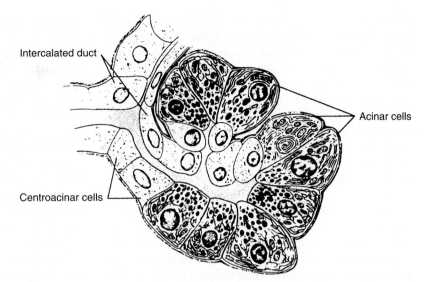

FIGURE 18.7 Schematic representation of the relations between acinar cells and the cells of the pancreatic ductal system, including centroacinar cells and intercalated duct cells. (From Bloom W, Fawcett DW. *A textbook of histology,* 10th ed. Philadelphia: WB Saunders, 1975:738, with permission.)

responsible for storing digestive enzymes; they also have a large nucleus, abundant endoplasmic reticulum, and an active Golgi complex to support extensive protein synthesis. The basolateral surface is rich in receptors for hormones and neurotransmitters that control pancreatic secretion. The pancreatic ductal system originates within each acinus as a draining ductule closely associated with the centroacinar cells. As these ducts leave the acinar units, they incorporate with other small intercollated ducts. The intercollated ducts join to form interlobular ducts which form secondary ducts that drain into the main excretory duct of the pancreas (Fig. 18.7). Centroacinar cells contain sparse cytoplasm and a small Golgi complex and are devoid of zymogen granules, yet they contain high concentrations of the enzyme carbonic anhydrase. Centroacinar cells contain carbonic anhydrase and other enzymes necessary for the formation of bicarbonate and electron transport and secretion.

The endocrine pancreas consists of the nearly spheroid collections of endocrine cells scattered throughout the pancreatic parenchyma, termed the *islets of Langerhans*. Each islet contains approximately 3,000 cells and range from 40 to 900 μm. Up to 1 million islets are located within each gland. Each islet is composed of several distinctive cell types. The centrally located insulin-producing cells or B cells (β) cells make up 50% to 70% of the islet population. The glucagon-producing cells or A (α) cells make up approximately 10% of each islet are generally located at the periphery of each islet. Also located in the periphery of each islet are the somatostatin-producing cells (5%) or D (δ) cells and pancreatic polypeptide (PP)-secreting F cells (15%). B and D cells are distributed evenly across the pancreas whereas islets in the uncinate are rich in F cells and poor in A cells. Islets in the body and tail are rich in A cells and poor in F cells.

HEPATIC PHYSIOLOGY

The liver is a remarkable organ with a spectrum of functions including energy metabolism, protein synthesis, bile production, clearance of toxins, and host defense. The liver takes up nutrients absorbed in the gut, modifies them for storage as energy sources, and modulates their systemic availability (5). In the fasted state, the liver is able to release stored energy sources and synthesize new protein. Regulation of these processes is subject to close interplay between neurohumoral reflexes from the endocrine pancreas, thyroid gland, and adrenal gland. The liver is unique in its dual circulation input through the hepatic artery and the portal vein and is especially positioned to both metabolize nutrients from the gut and also serve as the first line of defense against invading organisms. According to Ambrose Pierce, the famous American writer: "It was at one time considered the seat of life; hence its name—liver." The liver is known in folklore for its unusual ability to regenerate, illustrated in the parable of Prometheus, who was punished by Zeus for his defiance of the gods and defense of man by being chained to a mount, where an eagle would each day eat his liver, which regenerated each night. Now we have a much better understanding of the functions of the liver, as summarized in subsequent text.

Carbohydrate Metabolism

Glucose is the primary energy source for the central nervous system as well as erythrocytes, muscle, and the renal cortex. The liver stores approximately a 2-day supply of glucose in the form of glycogen. In addition, the liver provides glucose through gluconeogenesis, the generation of glucose from nonoxidative metabolites such as lactate and pyruvate as well as amino acid precursors. Insulin upregulates glycolytic gene expression in the liver and downregulates genes for enzymes responsible for gluconeogenesis. In contrast, glucagon, epinephrine, cortisol, and growth hormone contribute to enhanced gluconeogenesis.

In the fed state, glucose enters the hepatocyte through the low-affinity, high-capacity glucose transporter-2 independent of metabolic conditions and insulin levels. During fasting, when serum glucose levels are relatively low, hepatocytes absorb glucose through a high-affinity, low-capacity glucose transporter-1. Within the hepatocyte in the fed state, glucose is rapidly converted to glucose-6-phosphate by glucokinase. Glucokinase is activated by insulin and inhibited by glucagon. Glucose-6-phosphate is the substrate for three independent metabolic pathways within the hepatocyte: (i) glycogen synthesis, (ii) anaerobic glycolysis through the Embden-Meyerhof pathway to produce pyruvate and/or lactate (substrates for the Kreb cycle in mitochondria), and (iii) the pentose-phosphate shunt. Conversely, in the starved state, glucose-6-phosphate is converted to glucose by glucose-6-phosphatase within the endoplasmic reticulum.

The liver also metabolizes other carbohydrates, such as galactose and fructose. Lactose in milk is split into galactose and glucose by intestinal brush border disaccharidases such as lactase. Galactose is metabolized within the hepatocyte by galactokinase to galactose-1-phosphate and subsequently to glucose-1-phosphate and then glucose-6-phosphate. Fructose is converted to fructose-1-phosphate by fructokinase with subsequent steps allowing its use in gluconeogenesis and glycogen synthesis or glycolysis to lactate.

Lipid Metabolism

Lipids produce more than twice the energy per gram than carbohydrates and are an important energy source for both the liver and the rest of the body. The liver regulates fatty acid levels through storage, oxidation, conversion to lipoproteins, and synthesis from glucose. Fatty acids are synthesized in the hepatocyte from acetyl-coenzyme A (CoA) derived from glucose. Acetyl-CoA carboxylase converts acetyl-CoA to malonyl CoA, which is subsequently elongated in two carbon fractions by fatty acid synthase to a variety of fatty acid chains. These fatty acids are esterified with glycerol to form triglycerides. Triglycerides are ordinarily transported by lipoproteins to storage sites within the body for later use. In the setting of excess triglyceride synthesis, reduced transport, or decreased oxidation, triglycerides can accumulate within hepatocytes, resulting in steatosis. This is particularly seen in settings when much of the daily caloric intake is from ethanol.

The liver synthesizes apolipoproteins, particularly apoB-100, which transports triglycerides in the blood. The apoC is also synthesized in the liver and functions to inhibit uptake of chylomicron remnants by the liver. The apoE similarly is synthesized by the liver and functions to remove lipoprotein remnants from the serum, bind to low density lipoprotein (LDL) receptors, and target lipoproteins on specific cell surface receptors. Absence of apoE is associated with reduced chylomicron clearance, increased very low density lipoproteins (VLDLs), and increased risk of atherosclerosis. These apolipoproteins, after synthesis in the liver, combine with triglycerides and cholesterol, and phospholipids to form circulating lipoproteins. Lipoproteins are classified according to their density from chylomicrons, the lowest density products, to VLDL through high density lipoproteins (HDLs). Peripheral tissues use cholesterol in lipoproteins as a structural component of cell membranes and as a steroid

precursor. Triglycerides in lipoproteins are used largely as an energy source and as structural components of membranes. The liver is the key site for receipt of dietary fatty acids and cholesterol from the intestine and packaging of them into lipoproteins for transport into the circulation. The liver also synthesizes cholesterol from precursors through the action of HMG-CoA-reductase.

Protein Synthesis

The liver produces approximately 90% of plasma proteins and 15% of the total protein mass of the body. This is one of the most important specialized functions of the hepatocyte (Table 18.1). The hepatocyte exhibits a remarkable array of gene expression events in response to stimuli. Gene expression is initiated by transcription of DNA into messenger ribonucleic acid (mRNA) by RNA polymerase II in the nucleus. The mRNA fragments are transported out of the nucleus to the cytoplasm, where it binds to the 40s ribosomal subunit. Protein synthesis takes place through translation on the ribosome, a subcellular structure located in the cell cytoplasm. In general, secretory protein synthesis occurs on ribosomes anchored to the rough endoplasmic reticulum, and intracellular proteins are translated on free ribosomes. This distinction is thought to be related to the presence of a hydrophobic N-terminus sequence of extra amino acids, a feature common among secretory proteins, which as a group are first synthesized as precursor molecules. The initial N-terminus sequence, which is actually translated on free ribosomes, subsequently facilitates attachment to the rough endoplasmic reticulum. The extra amino acids of the precursor are then cleaved from the parent peptide before being secreted from the hepatocyte.

Albumin is the protein produced in largest quantity by the human liver. Albumin is a single-polypeptide chain composed of 581 amino acid residues organized into three relatively equal-sized domains. A healthy adult synthesizes approximately 10 g of albumin daily, and the half-life of this protein is roughly 22 days. Albumin binds to a variety of other molecules, including bilirubin, thyroid hormone, cortisol, testosterone, metals, and pharmaceutical agents, and it plays an important role in the transport of these substances. Other transport or carrier proteins synthesized and secreted by the liver are transferrin, haptoglobin, ferritin, hemopexin, and

TABLE 18.1

Plasma Proteins Synthesized by the Liver

α-Fetoprotein	Fatty acid–binding protein
α_1-Antitrypsin	Ferritin
α_2-Macroglobulin	Haptoglobin
Apoproteins	Hemopexin
Albumin	Serum amyloid A protein
Ceruloplasmin	Transferrin
C-reactive protein	
Complement components	

TABLE 18.2

Coagulation Factors and Inhibitors of Hepatic Origin

Fibrinogen (I)	Factor XI
Prothrombin (II)	Hageman factor (XII)
Proaccelerin (V)	Fibrin-stabilizing factor (XIII)
Proconvertin (VII)	α_2-Antiplasmin
Factor IX	Antithrombin (III)
Stuart-Prower factor (X)	C_1 inhibitor

ceruloplasmin. Albumin belongs to a family of proteins that share structural homology, including α-fetoprotein and the vitamin D— binding protein (6).

The liver is responsible for the production of more than 20 major plasma proteins, including those responsible for coagulation (7). Fibrinogen is a large dimeric protein synthesized exclusively by the hepatocyte, which, in the presence of thrombin, gives rise to fibrin monomers, the building blocks of fibrin. Thrombin itself is derived from prothrombin, a glycoprotein that is also of hepatic origin. These and other coagulation factors synthesized by the liver are listed in Table 18.2. Protein turnover occurs daily at a rate of 3%, or 200 to 300 g for an average 70-kg adult. Under stable conditions, the amount of protein synthesis equals protein breakdown. Most of the amino acids delivered to the liver in the portal circulation come from dietary protein; other sources include exfoliated gut cellular protein and degraded plasma proteins.

Metabolism of Drugs and Toxins

The body is exposed to toxic endogenous and exogenous substances, which, if not processed and eliminated from the circulation, may cause considerable damage. Xenobiotics refer to agents, such as drugs and toxins, which are not used in normal metabolic pathways to maintain the integrity of a cell or tissue. In some instances, detoxification is a misnomer because the products of xenobiotic metabolism may be more potent or harmful than the parent compound. Detoxification occurs primarily in the liver but can also occur in the kidney, lung, and intestines. The metabolic reactions involved consist primarily of oxidation, reduction, hydrolysis (phase I reactions), and conjugation (phase II reactions), depending on the specific substrate. In addition to the generation of a biologically less active compound, many of these reactions tend to promote conversion of a chemical to a more polar and hence more water-soluble molecule, which then can be excreted by the kidneys.

The phase I enzyme system in humans, which is most important in xenobiotic metabolism, is the cytochrome P-450 system located on hepatocyte microsomes. Following exposure to an inducing agent, P-450 catalytic activity increases within hours to days and returns to baseline levels within a similar time frame after removal of the inducing agent. The phase II reactions comprise a heterogeneous group of transferase enzymes that catalyze the combination of the target molecule with an endogenous agent to yield compounds of decreased activity. The same biochemical reactions that reduce the toxic load from certain xenobiotic agents may actually increase the potency of others with a positive (cyclophosphamide to aldophosphamide) or negative (parathion to paraoxon) therapeutic impact.

The detoxification of endogenous substances is also an important function of a healthy liver. Ammonia is the nitrogen-containing waste product of amino acid and nucleic acid catabolism. Substantial amounts of ammonia are also derived from the action of intestinal bacteria upon dietary protein. Within the liver, ammonia is detoxified to urea through enzymes of the urea cycle. Methionine, its metabolite mercaptan, and aminobutyric acid are also products of protein degradation, which, if not processed by the liver, are thought to exert neurotoxic effects.

Hepatocyte Bile Formation

Bile is produced by the hepatocyte to serve as the route of excretion for organic solids, such as bilirubin and cholesterol, and to facilitate intestinal absorption of lipids and fat-soluble vitamins. Bile secretion results from the active transport of solutes into the bile canaliculus from the lateral canalicular surface of the hepatocyte followed by the passive flow of water. Water constitutes approximately 85% of the volume of bile. The major organic solutes in bile are bilirubin, bile salts, phospholipids, and cholesterol. Bilirubin, the breakdown product of spent red blood cells, is conjugated with glucuronic acid by the hepatic enzyme glucuronyl transferase and is excreted actively into the adjacent canaliculus. Normally, a large reserve exists to handle excess bilirubin production, which might exist in hemolytic states.

Bile salts are steroid molecules synthesized by the hepatocyte. The primary bile salts in humans, cholic and chenodeoxycholic acid, account for more than 80% of those produced. The primary bile salts, which are conjugated with either taurine or glycine, can undergo bacterial alteration in the intestine to form the secondary bile salts, deoxycholate and lithocholate. Bile salts serve to solubilize lipids and facilitate their absorption from the intestinal mucosa.

Phospholipids are synthesized in the liver in conjunction with bile salt synthesis. Lecithin is the primary phospholipid in human bile, constituting more than 95% of the total. The final major solute of bile is cholesterol, which is also produced primarily by the liver with little contribution from dietary sources. It is important to recognize that biliary cholesterol concentrations are unassociated with serum cholesterol levels.

The normal volume of bile secreted daily by the liver is 500 to 1,000 mL. Bile flow depends on neurogenic, humoral, and chemical control. Vagal stimulation increases bile secretion. Splanchnic stimulation causes vasoconstriction with decreased hepatic blood flow and, thereby, diminished bile secretion. Gastrointestinal hormones, including secretin, cholecystokinin (CCK), gastrin, and glucagon, all increase bile flow, primarily by increasing water and electrolyte secretion. This action probably occurs at a site distal to the hepatocyte. Finally, the most important factor in regulating the volume of bile flow is the rate of bile salt synthesis by the hepatocyte. This rate is regulated by the return of bile salts to the liver by the enterohepatic circulation.

Micelle Formation

Cholesterol is nonpolar and insoluble in water or bile. Cholesterol is maintained in solution through the formation of micelles, a bile salt-phospholipid-cholesterol complex. Bile salts are amphipathic compounds containing both a hydrophilic and hydrophobic portion. In aqueous solutions, bile salts are oriented with the hydrophilic portion outward. Phospholipids are incorporated into the micellar structure, allowing cholesterol to be added to the hydrophobic central portion of the micelle. In this way, cholesterol can be maintained in solution in an aqueous medium. Recently, the concept of mixed micelles as the only cholesterol carrier has been challenged by the demonstration that much of the biliary cholesterol exists in a vesicular form. Structurally, these vesicles are made up of lipid bilayers of cholesterol and the phospholipid lecithin. In their simplest and smallest form, the vesicles are unilamellar, but aggregation may take place, leading to multilamellar vesicles. Present theory suggests that in states of excess cholesterol production, these large vesicles may exceed their capability to transport cholesterol, and crystal precipitation may occur.

Cholesterol solubility depends on the relative concentration of cholesterol, bile salts, and phospholipids (8). By plotting the percentages of each component on triangular coordinates, the micellar zone in which cholesterol is completely soluble can be demonstrated (Fig. 18.8). In a solution composed of 10% solutes similar to bile, the area under the curve represents the concentration at which cholesterol is maintained in solution. In the area above the curve, bile is supersaturated with cholesterol, and precipitation of cholesterol crystals can occur.

A mathematic model of cholesterol solubility has been developed (9). It is influenced by the relative concentrations of lipid components and the total lipid composition. A numerical value, known as the *cholesterol saturation* (or *lithogenic*) *index*, is derived that expresses the relative degrees of cholesterol saturation. When the cholesterol saturation index is greater than 1.0, the solution is supersaturated with cholesterol. Changes in the relative concentrations of bile salts, cholesterol, or phospholipids alter the capacity of micelles, thereby changing the cholesterol saturation index of the solution.

Bilirubin Metabolism

The breakdown of senescent erythrocytes is the source of approximately 80% to 85% of the bilirubin produced daily. The remaining 15% to 20% is derived largely from the breakdown of hepatic hemoproteins. Both enzymatic and nonenzymatic pathways for the formation of bilirubin have been proposed. Although both may be important physiologically, the microsomal enzyme heme-oxygenase, which is found in high concentration throughout the liver, spleen, and bone marrow, plays a major role in the initial conversion of heme to biliverdin. Biliverdin is then reduced to bilirubin by the cytosolic enzyme biliverdin reductase in a reduced nicotinamide adenine dinucleotide (NADH)-dependent reaction before being released into the circulation. In this "unconjugated" form, bilirubin has a very low solubility. Bilirubin is bound avidly to plasma proteins, primarily albumin, before uptake and further processing by the liver. The liver is the sole organ capable of removing the albumin–bilirubin complex from the circulation and esterifying the potentially toxic bilirubin to water-soluble, nontoxic monoconjugated and deconjugated derivatives. Conjugated bilirubin is the form excreted into the bile.

Bile Acids and the Enterohepatic Circulation

Bile acids are synthesized and conjugated in the liver, secreted into bile, stored temporarily in the gallbladder, emptied

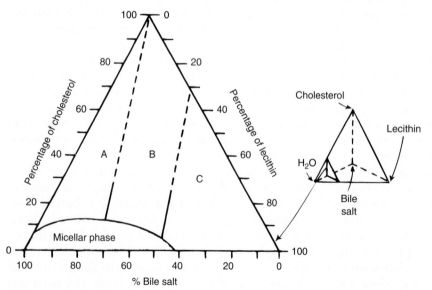

FIGURE 18.8 Solubility of cholesterol in bile. The graph demonstrates the relations of the three major constituents of bile: bile salts, lecithin, and cholesterol. The area enclosed by the triangular coordinates can be divided into four zones that represent the physical state of the solutes in bile: crystals of cholesterol plus liquid (*A*); cholesterol crystals plus cholesterol liquid crystals plus liquid (*B*); liquid crystals plus liquid (*C*); and the micellar zone, in which cholesterol is in water solution through the formation of cholesterol-lecithin-bile salt micelles. The *solid line* is the 10% solute line. (From Admirand WH, Small DM. The physiochemical basis of cholesterol gallstone formation in man. *J Clin Invest* 1968; 47:1043, with permission.)

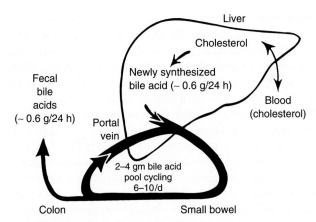

FIGURE 18.9 Enterohepatic circulation of bile salts. Cholesterol is taken up from plasma by the liver. Bile acids are synthesized at a rate of 0.6 g per 24 hours and are excreted through the biliary system into the small bowel. Most of the bile salts are reabsorbed in the terminal ileum and are returned to the liver to be extracted and re-excreted. (Modified from Dietschy JM. The biology of bile acids. *Arch Intern Med* 1972;130:473–474.)

from the gallbladder into the duodenum in response to meal stimulation, absorbed throughout the small intestine but especially in the ileum, and returned to the liver through the portal vein. This cycling of bile acids between the liver and the intestine is referred to as the *enterohepatic circulation* (Fig. 18.9). The total amount of bile acids in the enterohepatic circulation is defined as the circulating bile pool. In this highly efficient system, approximately 95% of bile salts are reabsorbed. Therefore, of the total bile salt pool of 2 to 4 g, which recycles through the enterohepatic cycle six to ten times daily, only approximately 600 mg of bile salt is actually excreted into the colon. Bacterial action in the colon on the two primary bile salts, cholate and chenodeoxycholate, results in the formation of the secondary bile salts, deoxycholate and lithocholate. Although the colon reabsorbs some deoxycholate passively, the remainder is lost in fecal waste.

The enterohepatic circulation provides an important negative feedback system on bile acid synthesis. Should the recirculation be interrupted by resection of the terminal ileum or by primary ileal disease, abnormally large losses of bile salts can occur. This situation increases bile acid production to maintain a normal bile salt pool. Similarly, if bile salts are lost by an external biliary fistula, increased bile acid synthesis is necessary. However, except for those unusual circumstances in which excessive losses occur, bile acid synthesis matches losses, maintaining a constant pool size. During fasting, approximately 90% of the bile acid pool is stored in the gallbladder.

Reticuloendothelial Function

Approximately 80% to 90% of the fixed macrophages in the body reside in the liver as Kupffer cells, where they function as part of the reticuloendothelial system (RES). These cells serve to remove particulate matter and toxins

from the portal circulation, but their abnormal function has been implicated in the pathogenesis of a variety of liver diseases (10). Kupffer cells are likely derived from bone marrow stem cells or monocytes. They reside in the sinusoidal lumen adjacent to sinusoidal endothelial cells. In addition to its ability to phagocytize and destroy infectious agents, the Kupffer cell functions to clear the circulation of old or damaged blood cells, cellular debris, fibrin degradation products, and endotoxin. Recently, the significant role played by Kupffer cells in the elaboration and regulation of prostaglandins, interleukins (ILs), oxygen-free radicals, tumor necrosis factor (TNF), and other signalling molecules has been appreciated. They can increase under conditions of sepsis or decrease when exposure to toxins is low. It is now recognized that there is close interaction between hepatocytes and Kupffer cells during normal physiologic periods and periods of sepsis. The spleen and lung also display clinically significant levels of RES activity.

Stellate Cell Function

It has recently been recognized that a unique population of mesenchymal cells within the liver, lung, pancreas, kidney, and intestine function to regulate the microvascular environment of these organs. In the liver, stellate cells are found at the interface between the basolateral membranes of hepatocytes and sinusoidal endothelial cells and are characterized by the presence of lipid-rich, vitamin A containing droplets. It is estimated that they represent 5% to 8% of all liver cells. Stellate cells appear to be important paracrine regulators of hepatocyte and endothelial cell function. Importantly, hepatic stellate cells are activated in states of liver injury and this activation is a central event in hepatic fibrosis (11). The overall number of hepatic stellate cells increases in fibrosis, probably due to inhibition of apoptosis. Exciting recent studies suggest that this fibrosis may be reversible, opening up new avenues of possible treatment for cirrhosis (12).

Hepatic Regeneration

The liver is an unusual organ in its ability to respond to injury with regeneration. Normal hepatocytes divide infrequently. In response to reduced liver volume after resection, however, proliferation occurs in a finely regulated way, resulting in a "restorative hyperplasia" that produces a liver mass nearly identical to baseline within weeks in animal models. The initial response in this process is activation of gene expression for protooncogenes such as c-fos, c-jun, and c-myc and transcription factors such as nuclear factor kB (NFkB) (13,14). These early gene expression events are followed by induction of cytokines such as IL-6 and TNF and stimulation of the liver by growth factors such as hepatocyte growth factor (HGF), transforming growth factor α (TGF-α). Apoptotic mechanisms finely tune the regenerative response, resulting in restoration of normal liver volume. Abnormalities of this regenerative response contribute to the development of cirrhosis.

Measurement of Liver Function

Synthetic Function

No one test is available that adequately assesses all aspects of hepatic function. Synthetic function of the liver is best estimated by serum albumin levels and prothrombin time. All clotting factors (except factor VIII, which is synthesized in vascular endothelium and reticuloendothelial cells) are synthesized by hepatocytes. The prothrombin time estimates liver function because it measures the function of the extrinsic coagulation pathway including factors II, V, VII, and X, all synthesized by the liver. Of these, factor VII has the shortest half-life in serum of approximately 6 hours and can also be specifically measured and monitored in liver failure. In hepatic insufficiency, albumin production also declines rapidly, resulting in hypoalbuminemia. Serum albumin has a relatively long serum half-life of approximately 20 days. Therefore, albumin levels are a better estimate of function in chronic liver disease than acute liver failure. Prealbumin is also synthesized by the liver and has a shorter half-life in serum than albumin. It should be recognized that albumin and protime can be influenced by nonhepatic factors and may be abnormal even in the setting of a normal liver. Albumin, for example, is lowered in the setting of malnutrition, renal failure, and enteropathy. Protime can be influenced by vitamin K deficiency, use of coumadin for anticoagulation, or in disseminated intravascular coagulopathy (DIC). Therefore, use of albumin and protime in the assessment of liver function must be taken in the context of these other potentially confounding factors.

Hepatocyte Injury

Hepatocyte injury can be assessed by measurement of serum aminotransferases, including aspartate aminotransferase [(AST), also known as *serum glutamic oxaloacetic transaminase* or (SGOT)] and alanine aminotransferase [(ALT), also known as *serum glutamic pyruvic transaminase* or (SGPT)]. These enzymes function within hepatocytes to form oxaloacetic acid and pyruvic acid during gluconeogenesis. Hepatocellular injury, such as is seen in hepatitis, ischemia, and toxin ingestion, result in leakage of AST and ALT into the serum. ALT is found almost exclusively within the liver, but AST is present in many extrahepatic sites, including myocardium and skeletal muscle. Therefore, vigorous exercise with muscle injury or myocardial infarction may be associated with elevation of serum AST, but generally not ALT. Transaminase elevations correlate poorly with the severity of liver injury and do not predict prognosis. The degree of elevation can provide a clue to the underlying mechanism of injury, however, with mild degrees of elevation of transaminases typically seen in hepatic steatosis, moderate degrees of elevation in alcoholic hepatitis and biliary obstruction, and severe degrees of elevation in viral hepatitis and acetaminophen toxicity. An AST/ALT ratio greater than 1 is suggestive of alcoholic liver disease.

Secretory Function

The secretion of bile by the liver is altered in many forms of liver disease, resulting in cholestasis, or impaired bile flow. Alkaline phosphatase (APase) is an enzyme highly expressed in hepatocytes and biliary epithelium. Its serum levels correlate with all forms of biliary obstruction (e.g., bile duct stones and tumors, sclerosing cholangitis, biliary cirrhosis) and infiltrative processes within the liver (e.g., liver tumors and granulomatous disease). The degree of elevation, however, does not correlate well with the extent of disease. Unlike transaminase elevations, which appear to be due to leakage of enzymes from hepatocytes into the serum, elevations in APase in biliary obstruction appear to be due to increased synthesis (15). APase is expressed in many tissues other than liver and the biliary tract, including bone, placenta, kidney, and intestine. Therefore, elevations in serum APase are not specific to hepatobiliary disease. Levels of other enzymes, including γ glutamyl transpeptidase (GGT) and 5′-nucleotidase, rise in serum in response to hepatobiliary disease much like APase but are more specific. GGT expression, for example, is not present in bone; therefore, GGT can be used to differentiate the source of an abnormally elevated APase. Serum bilirubin is a sensitive indicator of hepatic secretory function. Bilirubin can be fractionated as direct, a water-soluble, conjugated form, or indirect, a lipid-soluble, unconjugated form. In the normal setting, more than 90% of serum bilirubin is in the unconjugated, indirect form. In biliary obstruction, serum levels of direct, or conjugated bilirubin rise and, because this form is water soluble and not attached to serum albumin as a carrier, it may be excreted in the urine. Rises in unconjugated bilirubin in the serum are seen in states of increased production (e.g., hemolytic anemia, muscle injury, and resolving hematoma) or decreased hepatic uptake and conjugation (e.g., hepatic injury). Elevated serum conjugated bilirubin occurs because of biliary obstruction at any level from the bile canaliculus to the ampulla of Vater. The degree of serum bilirubin elevation correlates with prognosis in patients with cirrhosis and acute liver failure (16,17). Typically, patients with acute biliary obstruction, such as choledocholithiasis, will present earlier in the course of their illness and have total bilirubin levels less than 10 mg/dL whereas disorders with more insidious onset of obstruction, such as in malignant stricture, may lead to delayed presentation with levels greater than 10 mg/dL.

Prognostic Tests in Liver Failure

In the setting of chronic liver disease, decisions regarding surgical treatment depend on knowledge of prognosis of the underlying disease and estimation of the impact of that disease on surgical risk (18,19). Operative risk is increased in patients with chronic liver insufficiency and is dramatically elevated in those with acute liver failure, even for relatively minor procedures such as hernia repair and cholecystectomy. In chronic liver disease, the Child-Turcotte-Pugh score (Table 18.3) has proven utility in predicting operative risk. Originally described to predict operative mortality in

TABLE 18.3

Child-Turcotte-Pugh Classification of Prognosis in Portal Hypertension

	Numerical Score		
	1	*2*	*3*
Ascites	None	Slight	Moderate/severe
Encephalopathy	None	Slight/moderate	Moderate/severe
Bilirubin (mg/dL)	<2.0	2–3	>3.0
Albumin (g/dL)	>3.5	2.8–3.5	<2.8
Protime (seconds increased)	13	4–6	>6
Total numerical score	*Child-Turcotte-Pugh class*		
5–6	A		
7–9	B		
10–15	C		

procedures for portal hypertension, the Child-Turcotte-Pugh score has subsequently undergone several modifications and has been shown to correlate with operative mortality and morbidity for a variety of procedures (13,20). More recently, the Model for End-Stage Liver Disease (MELD) has been developed to estimate prognosis in chronic liver disease and has been applied by the United Network for Organ Sharing (UNOS) as an objective criteria for organ allocation in liver transplantation (16,17). The MELD score is dependent on bilirubin, protime, and creatinine values. Convenient on-line calculators are available from a number of sources.

(http://www.unos.org/resources/MeldPeldCalculator .asp, http://www.mayoclinic.org/meld/mayomodel17.html)

Recent individual studies and systematic reviews suggest that the Child-Turcotte-Pugh and MELD scores are approximately equivalent in assessing prognosis in liver failure outside the setting of transplantation (21,22).

Quantitative Tests of Liver Function

Many attempts have been made to develop a dynamic, quantitative test of liver function that would predict prognosis in liver failure, assess operative risk in patients with chronic liver insufficiency, and predict survival after liver resection. Indocyanine green clearance, galactose elimination capacity, lidocaine metabolism to monoethylglycinexylidide (MEGX), and the aminopyrine breath test all in some way correlate with the degree of functional capacity of the liver. Their expense, technical complexity, and lack of availability have hindered their clinical application. Furthermore, comparative studies have not shown clear-cut superiority of any of these tests over conventional biochemical assessment such as the Child-Turcotte-Pugh score (23,24). Liver biopsy with histologic evaluation can be useful to assess the degree of liver injury in hepatitis, steatohepatitis, and cirrhosis.

BILIARY PHYSIOLOGY

Gallbladder Absorption and Secretion

Bile is essential for normal intestinal digestion and absorption of fats and fat-soluble vitamins and drugs. As noted earlier, bile is secreted by the hepatocyte in a form initially isosmotic with plasma (Table 18.4). The composition and rate of secretion of bile from the hepatocyte is dependent on dietary factors and general homeostatic mechanisms such as blood flow to the liver. During fasting, bile is stored and concentrated approximately 10-fold in the gallbladder (25). The gallbladder absorbs water from hepatic bile with passive absorption of sodium and chloride ions across an electrochemical gradient between the gallbladder lumen and surface epithelial cells. In addition, these epithelial cells have an active sodium transporter system carrying ions from the cell lumen across the basolateral cell membrane into the intercellular space. Chloride transport is coupled to this active sodium transport to maintain electrical neutrality. Water follows this active ion exchange, further reducing gallbladder volume.

TABLE 18.4

Composition of Bile

	Hepatic	Gallbladder
Na^+ (mEq/L)	140–159	220–340
K^+ (mEq/L)	4–5	6–14
Ca^{2+} (mEq/L)	2–5	5–32
Cl^- (mEq/L)	62–112	1–10
Bile acids (mEq/L)	3–55	290–340
Cholesterol (mg/dL)	60–70	350–930

(Adapted from Davenport HW. *Physiology of the digestive tract*, 4th ed. Chicago: Year Book Publishers, 1977.)

The gallbladder epithelium secretes mucin and glycoproteins that may serve as a nidus for cholesterol gallstone formation. In chronic obstruction of the cystic duct, absorbed bile may be replaced with mucinous fluid, so-called "white bile." A minor degree of water and solute secretion from gallbladder mucosa has been identified experimentally (26).

Gallbladder Motility

Gallbladder motility is dependent on both hormonal and neural regulation. The gallbladder passively fills with bile during fasting, likely due to increased biliary pressures from sphincter of Oddi contraction. In the fasting state, approximately 90% of secreted hepatic bile enters the gallbladder. In response to fat and protein in a meal, CCK is released from the duodenal mucosa, perhaps through the action of an intermediary releasing factor (Fig. 18.10). CCK acts hormonally on specific smooth muscle CCK receptors in the gallbladder to cause contraction (27,28). This effect is calcium dependent. Gallbladder contraction is stimulated to a lesser degree by vagal cholinergic agonists. Gallbladder contraction is inhibited by somatostatin that reduces both vagal and CCK-stimulated gallbladder contraction. This is the likely mechanism for gallstone formation in patients with somatostatinoma and those treated for long periods with somatostatin analogs (29).

Sphincter of Oddi Function

The intact sphincter of Oddi functions to separate duodenal contents from the biliary tree. Flow of bile between the gallbladder and the duodenum is dependent on the relaxation of this sphincter and the differential pressure between the two lumens generated by gallbladder contraction. Simultaneous to meal-induced gallbladder contraction, CCK induces an indirect relaxation effect on the sphincter of Oddi. This is a neurohumoral reflex mediated by vasoactive intestinal peptide (VIP). VIP is a neuropeptide present throughout the gut that acts as a neurotransmitter to cause smooth muscle relaxation. This coordinated gallbladder contraction

with sphincter relaxation allows gallbladder emptying. Classification and treatment of disorders of sphincter of Oddi function has been reviewed (30).

Effect of Surgical Procedures on Biliary Physiology

Cholecystectomy

Although the gallbladder serves as a storage organ for bile, its removal has minimal impact on the total rate of bile acid production (31). After cholecystectomy, a larger fraction of the total bile acid pool resides in the intestine and minor changes in the composition of the bile acid pool have been reported. These changes do not appear to be sufficient to cause significant alteration in digestion. An occasional patient with postcholecystectomy diarrhea may have bile acid malabsorption due to a relative increase in the ileal bile acid pool. This effect is usually transient and can be aided by a bile acid sequestrant such as cholestyramine.

Small Bowel Resection

Bile acids are reabsorbed in the ileum. With increasing extent of small bowel resection, especially with inclusion of the ileocecal valve, depletion of the bile acid pool from malabsorption may occur. This effect is mitigated in part by increased hepatic bile acid synthesis; however in some patients, diarrhea, fat malabsorption, and deficiencies in fat-soluble vitamins may ensue. This may also occur in diseases affecting the ileum, such as Crohn disease or radiation enteritis.

PANCREATIC PHYSIOLOGY

Exocrine Function

The main functional unit of the exocrine pancreas is the acinus and associated draining ducts. These structures give rise to pancreatic juice that is rich in organic and inorganic constituents. The acinar cells give rise to the organic components of pancreatic juice, digestive enzymes. The inorganic component of pancreatic secretions include water, sodium, potassium, chloride, and bicarbonate. These constituents are derived from the intercollated duct and centroacinar cells. The final product is a clear isotonic solution with a pH of 7.6 to 9.0 and a specific gravity that varies between 1.007 and 1.035. Basal secretory rates of the exocrine pancreas average 0.2 to 0.3 mL/min; maximal rates approach 5 mL/min with appropriate stimulation. The total daily volume of pancreatic secretion is 2.5 L. The anion composition of exocrine pancreatic juice varies with the rate of pancreatic secretion (Fig. 18.11) (32). At low secretory rates, the concentrations of chloride and bicarbonate ions are nearly equivalent to plasma. With neurohumoral stimulation, the bicarbonate component increases in concentration whereas the chloride concentration falls. In contrast, the composition of sodium and potassium in the pancreatic exocrine effluent remains constant; the concentrations of these cations are roughly equivalent to plasma.

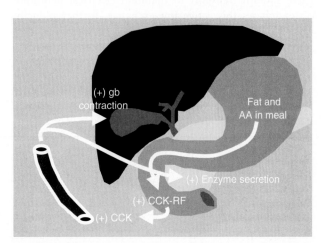

FIGURE 18.10   Cholecystokinin (CCK) acts to stimulate pancreatic exocrine secretion, gallbladder contraction, and sphincter of Oddi relaxation. AA, amino acids; RF, releasing factor.

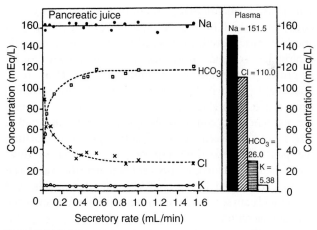

FIGURE 18.11 Relation between the rate of secretion and the concentration of electrolytes in pancreatic juice compared with the electrolyte concentration of plasma. (From Bro-Rasmussen F, Killmann SA, Thaysen JH. The composition of pancreatic juice as compared to sweat, parotid saliva and tears. *Acta Physiol Scand* 1956;37:97–113, with permission.)

TABLE 18.5

Pancreatic Acinar Cell Products

Enzymes	Amylase
	Lipase
	Carboxylesterase
	Sterol esterase
	Dnase
	Rnase
Proenzymes[a]	Cationic trypsinogen
	Anionic trypsinogen
	Mesotrypsinogen
	Chymotrypsinogen (A, B)
	Kallireinogen
	Procarboxypeptidase A (1,2)
	Procarboxypeptidase B (1,2)
	Prelastase

[a]Proenzymes are stored in the pancreas and released into the duodenum in an inactive form where they are activated. If these enzymes were secreted in an active form in the pancreas, autodigestion may occur. Other enzymes are stored and secreted in their active form, including amylase and lipase.

(Adapted from Gorelick F, Pandol SJ, Topazian M. *Pancreatic physiology, pathophysiology, acute and chronic pancreatitis.* Gastrointestinal Teaching Project. American Gastroenterological Association. 2003.)

The principal stimulant for pancreatic water and electrolyte secretion is the hormone secretin. Secretin is derived from mucosal S cells of the crypts of Lieberkühn of the proximal small bowel. It is released into the blood in the presence of a duodenal luminal pH of less than 3.0 and bile. Secretin is the principal stimulant of pancreatic water and electrolyte secretion. Secretin stimulates pancreatic water and electrolyte secretion by binding to pancreatic ductal cell receptors and effecting signal transduction through the adenyl cyclase second messenger system. The result is an increase in intracellular cyclic adenosine monophosphate (cAMP). CCK, gastrin, and acetylcholine are also weak stimulants of bicarbonate secretion. CCK and cholinergic innervation appear to play a permissible role potentiating secretin-mediated secretion. Several endogenous inhibitors of pancreatic water and electrolyte secretion have been identified; however, their physiologic roles remain to be defined. In particular, somatostatin, PP, and glucagon may play a humoral or paracrine role in the reduction of pancreatic water and electrolyte secretion.

The pancreas has a tremendous capacity for the synthesis and excretion of digestive enzymes from pancreatic acinar cells. Acinar cells are programmed to direct more than 90% of their biosynthetic effort toward the production and storage of a mixture of approximately 20 different digestive enzymes and enzyme precursors (Table 18.5). These enzymes can be characterized as having proteolytic, amlyolytic, lipolytic, or nuclease activity. Within the acinar nucleus, DNA is transcribed to yield mRNA, which travels to the cytoplasm where it is translated on the microsomes of the rough endoplasmic reticulum into proenzymes. These proenzymes subsequently pass to the Golgi apparatus, where they are packaged within a glycoprotein vesicular membrane. Zymogen granules formed at the level of the Golgi apparatus contain a full complement of the digestive enzymes. Zymogen granules then migrate to the cell apex, where the granule's membranes fuse with the acinar cell membrane, leading to extrusion of the zymogen granule contents into the centroacinar luminal space by exocytosis. All peptidases synthesized by acinar cells are released into the pancreatic ductal system in an inactive form. Duodenal mucosal enterokinase serves to activate trypsinogen to the active enzyme trypsin, which further activates the other peptidases. Some enzymes are secreted by acinar cells in their active form, including amylase and lipase. In addition to the proteolytic enzymes, acinar cells also secrete a trypsin inhibitor, pancreatic secretory trypsin inhibitor, that protects the pancreas from trypsin that is prematurely activated within the pancreas.

Pancreatic enzyme secretion by the acinar cells is regulated by neural and hormonal factors. This neurohumoral regulation is mediated by secretogogue binding the G protein–coupled receptors on the basolateral surface of the acinar cell. Two categories of receptors have been characterized. The first category of agonists includes receptors for gastrin-releasing peptide (GRP), acetylcholine, and CCK. The main secretogogue for acinar cell secretion is CCK. These agonists stimulate acinar cell secretion by a stimulating intracellular calcium mobilization by receptor-mediated hydrolysis of phosphatidylinositol-4,5-bisphosphate, generating two intracellular messengers: inositol-1,4,5-triphosphate and diacylglycerol. The formation of inositol-1,4,5-triphosphate leads to the release of Ca^{2+} from intracellular stores. The generation of diacylglycerol activates protein kinase C, an ubiquitous calcium- and phospholipid-dependent phosphorylating enzyme, which has been implicated in the mediation of a number of intracellular processes, including exocytotic secretion, changes in ion channel conductance, receptor affinity, and cell proliferation. The second category of receptors are those that stimulate enzyme release by activation of adenylyl cyclase, giving rise to intracellular cAMP. These include the receptors for VIP and secretin.

Unlike nonhuman species, dispersed human acinar cells lack the CCK receptor (33,34). This indicates that CCK mediates acinar cell secretion through its interaction with sensorineural pathways, thereby illustrating the importance of both humoral and neural regulatory mechanisms. CCK is released in response to a meal activates vagal afferent pathways which project to the dorsal vagal complex (35). Vagal efferents are then activated that synapse with the pancreatic ganglia releasing the neurotransmitters acetylcholine, GRP, and VIP which trigger enzyme secretion. Vagotomy and atropine infusion attenuate meal-mediated pancreatic enzyme release and release of enzymes in response to exogenous CCK infusion, thereby confirming the importance of a brain–gut interaction in the regulation of pancreatic enzyme release (36,37).

The most important aspect of pancreatic exocrine secretion involves the response of the gland to an ingested meal. The functional reserve of the pancreas is enormous. A total of 80% to 90% of the functional acinar mass must be absent for clinical evidence of malabsorption to appear. Therefore, normal digestion is associated with an excess of pancreatic enzymes. In addition to the enzyme products, the exocrine pancreas also secretes water, bicarbonate, and electrolytes, which help to neutralize acidic gastric chyme and maintain the pH in the optimal range for the activity of most pancreatic enzymes.

The physiologic control of pancreatic secretion lacks a fine-tuning mechanism, is overwhelmingly stimulatory, and is controlled by interacting neurohormonal mechanisms. Like gastric acid secretion, pancreatic exocrine secretion is divided into three phases: a cephalic, gastric, and intestinal phase. During the cephalic phase of digestion, stimuli activate vagal efferent signals, which follow parasympathetic pathways to stimulate pancreatic exocrine secretion and account for one fourth to one third of the maximal pancreatic response (38,39). In addition, cephalic phase stimulation of gastric acid secretion, both by direct cholinergic influence on parietal cells and through the release of antral gastrin, leads to duodenal acidification. This acidification releases secretin, which stimulates pancreatic bicarbonate secretion. During the gastric phase of digestion, antral distention and the presence of protein in the antrum stimulate the release of gastrin. Gastrin itself serves as a weak stimulator of pancreatic enzyme secretion because of the sequence homology between gastrin and the C-terminus pentapeptide-amide sequence of CCK. In addition, gastric distension triggers pancreatic enzyme release through a vasovagal response. These two processes act primarily on the acinar cells themselves giving rise to an enzyme-rich secretion during the gastric phase (40).

The intestinal phase of pancreatic exocrine secretion commences when chyme reaches the upper small intestine.

This phase is quantitatively the most important, involving both neural and hormonal mechanisms. Duodenal acid and bile cause secretin release, which stimulates pancreatic bicarbonate secretion from duct cells. The presence of fat or protein in the duodenum stimulates CCK release from duodenal I cells, which causes pancreatic enzyme secretion from acinar cells (Fig. 18.10). Current evidence supports the existence of considerable overlap and potentiating interactions between secretin and CCK in stimulating the pancreatic exocrine response. In addition to these hormonally mediated events, enteropancreatic vagovagal reflexes stimulated by luminal bile salts, fatty acids, and amino acids can serve as an important stimulus for pancreatic exocrine secretion.

As in other organ systems, a feedback mechanism exists to turn off the pancreatic enzyme secretion. It is hypothesized that trypsin itself regulates CCK release from the I cells in the duodenum. Two substances, the monitor peptide and luminal CCK-releasing factor [luminal cholecystokinin-releasing factor (LCRF)], are released by the pancreas and duodenal mucosa (41,42). During a meal, trypsin is occupied with digestion, thereby allowing the monitor peptide and LCRF to stimulate the I cells to release CCK which, through its neurohumoral mechanism, stimulates the acinar cells to release more enzymes. Between meals, these substances are degraded by luminal trypsin and are not available to stimulate I cell CCK release. This decreases pancreatic exocrine secretion.

Recent evidence has clarified the role of different dietary constituents in postprandial pancreatic enzyme secretion. Diets high in carbohydrate (50%–80%) are associated with the lowest postprandial amylase, lipase, and trypsin outputs, whereas diets high in fat (40%) are associated with the highest postprandial output of these enzymes. Furthermore, diets rich in medium-chain triglycerides and/or elemental diets stimulate pancreatic secretion to a lesser extent than long-chain triglyceride or complex formula diets (43,44). The variations in pancreatic enzyme secretion associated with different dietary constituents may have important implications in the pathogenesis and treatment of human diseases of the pancreas. For example, the risk of developing chronic alcoholic pancreatitis has been related to the amount of protein in the diet, and a diet that minimally stimulates pancreatic secretion may be most beneficial in patients convalescing from acute pancreatitis.

Endocrine Pancreas

The principal endocrine function of the pancreas involves maintenance of glucose homeostasis. The pancreatic islets of Langerhans are the main functional unit responsible for this process. As in the case with pancreatic exocrine secretion, glucose homeostasis involves a complex interplay between neuronal and humoral factors within the islet. The main humoral factors include the hormones released from individual islet cell subtypes, including insulin, glucagon, PP, and somatostatin. There is likely cross communication among the different cell types of an islet through an intraislet circulation. Blood flows from the centrally located B cells within an islet in a centripetal manner towards the more peripherally located A, D, and F cells in the mantle of the islet whereas other vessels originate in the periphery and travel to the core. Therefore, insulin release regulates glucagon and somatostatin release and vice versa. Paracrine interactions are also important, as is the case with somatostatin inhibition of insulin release. To a lesser extent, the islets are also under neuronal control with cholinergic and β-sympathetic fibers stimulating insulin release and α-sympathetic fibers inhibiting release. In addition to the earlier mentioned hormones, islet cells secrete VIP, serotonin, pancreastatin and the neuropeptides, calcitonin gene–related peptide (CGRP), neuropeptide Y, and GRP which likely have local regulatory effects on endocrine and exocrine function.

Insulin

Insulin is the principal product of the islets and is derived from the islet B cells. The human insulin gene is located near the end of the short arm of chromosome 11, in band p15.5. The insulin molecule consists of two polypeptide chains joined by two disulfide bridges. Within the B cell, insulin is translated as a proenzyme precursor, proinsulin, which consists of the insulin molecule and a C-peptide extension. The induction of proinsulin synthesis is achieved by enhancement of the translation efficiency of proinsulin mRNA on the membrane-bound polysomes (translational control). When the B cell is stimulated, the proinsulin molecule is transported from the endoplasmic reticulum to the Golgi where it is packaged into granules. At this point, the C-peptide is cleaved giving rise to the active insulin molecule which is then released by the islet into the intravascular space. Insulin promotes glucose uptake in all cells, except hepatocytes, central nervous system cells, and B cells. Insulin inhibits glycogenolysis and fatty acid breakdown and stimulates protein synthesis.

The actual release of insulin from the cell into the portal blood is under a variety of controls, including not only the level of glycemia but also vagal interactions and local concentrations of inhibitory peptides. Insulin release occurs in two phases. The first lasts approximately 5 minutes and represents release of stored insulin. The second phase is sustained and is a product of ongoing synthesis. Although glucose is the main stimulant, certain amino acids, including arginine, lysine, and leucine, and free fatty acids regulate insulin release. Oral glucose stimulates insulin release to a greater extent than intravenous glucose. This is the result of an enteroinsular axis that is likely mediated by gastric inhibitory peptide (GIP) (45). Insulin release is also influenced by other hormones, including glucagon and CCK which stimulate release and somatostatin, pancreastatin, and amylin that inhibit release.

Glucagon

Glucagon is a single-chain peptide with 29-amino acid residues, synthesized and released from islet cells. Glucagon is a member of a family of homologous peptides that includes secretin, vasoactive intestinal polypeptide, gastric inhibitory polypeptide, and growth hormone-releasing factor. Glucose is a potent inhibitor of glucagon release. Therefore, insulin and glucagon have a reciprocal effect on glucose homeostasis. Like insulin, glucagon release is also influenced by neuronal factors as well. The biologic properties of glucagon can be divided into four categories: (i) *effects on metabolism,* including stimulation of glycogenolysis, gluconeogenesis, and ketogenesis in the liver, stimulation of lipolysis in adipose tissue, and stimulation of insulin secretion; (ii) *effects on gastrointestinal secretion,* including inhibition of gastric acid and pancreatic exocrine secretion; (iii) *effects on intestinal motility,* including inhibition of intestinal peristaltic activity; and (iv) *effects on the cardiovascular system,* including increase in heart rate and the force of cardiac contraction.

Somatostatin

Initially isolated in 1973 from the hypothalamus, somatostatin is now known to have widespread distribution throughout the body. Somatostatin is a cyclic tetradecapeptide synthesized and released from islet cells and many other brain-gut sources. In the pancreas, somatostatin is present mainly in the 14-amino acid form, whereas a 28-amino acid precursor of somatostatin, called *prosomatostatin,* predominates in other tissues. Somatostatin receptors have been found on pancreatic acinar cell membranes and on the secretory vesicles of pancreatic islet cells. Somatostatin has a broad spectrum of gastrointestinal activity, including inhibition of gastric acid, pepsin, and pancreatic exocrine secretion; inhibition of gastrointestinal motor activity and ion secretion; reduction of gastrointestinal blood flow; and inhibition of pancreatic islet insulin, glucagon, and PP release. The intracellular mechanisms of somatostatin action involve primarily the activation of the inhibitory G protein in the adenylyl cyclase system, whereby somatostatin binding inhibits the activation of adenylyl cyclase and reduces intracellular cAMP levels. However, all inhibitory actions of somatostatin cannot be explained solely by cAMP-dependent cell activation mechanisms, and some may involve regulation of intracellular Ca^{2+} turnover.

Pancreatic Polypeptide

PP is a 36-amino acid peptide localized exclusively in the islet cells of the pancreas. The PP family of homologous peptides includes PP, neuropeptide Y, and peptide YY. PP cell densities increase from the tail of the gland to the head of the gland; concentrations of PP are five to eight times higher in the pancreatic head than in the tail. In humans, total pancreatectomy results in undetectable levels of PP in both basal and postprandial sera, supporting the notion that the pancreas is the only significant site of PP secretion. The mechanisms of release of PP after a meal are complex and include a characteristic biphasic pattern with an early peak followed by a long plateau. PP release following a meal is stimulated during the cephalic, gastric, and intestinal phases of digestion and appears to depend on both cholinergic and adrenergic modulation. The most likely physiologic role for PP involves inhibition of pancreatic exocrine secretion. Multiple pharmacologic effects of PP have been reported, including modulation of gastric acid secretion, alterations in intestinal motility, and suppression of islet insulin release. In humans, PP has also been used as a marker for pancreatic endocrine tumors. However, the clinical importance of the identification of elevated PP levels remains to be established convincingly.

Islet–Acinar Interactions

The islets of Langerhans are dispersed throughout the acinar and ductal tissues of the exocrine pancreas. Structural and functional evidence suggests a close integration of the exocrine and endocrine portions of the pancreas. For example, the presence of specific islet hormone receptors on the plasma membranes of pancreatic acinar cells gives support to the notion of direct regulation of the function of the acinar cells by islet hormones. Furthermore, insulin-binding sites in the acinar parenchyma are not distributed evenly. Rather, the acinar cells located around the islets (peri-insular region) show higher densities of receptor labeling than those at a distance from the islets (teleinsular regions). Morphometric studies have demonstrated that the peri-insular acinar cells are twice as large as those found in the teleinsular regions. Determination of volume densities of the different cellular organelles has shown that peri-insular cells contain many more zymogen granules than teleinsular cells. Despite these differences in zymogen granule numbers, the actual content and type of enzymes in the granules of cells from the two regions are similar. However, the pattern of response to secretagogues differs between peri-insular and teleinsular cells. For example, during vagal stimulation, the release of zymogen granules by peri-insular acinar cells is slow, whereas teleinsular cells are rapidly depleted of zymogen granules.

Further evidence in support of the theory of islet–acinar interaction comes from the existence of an insuloacinar portal blood system. Arterial branches that penetrate the pancreas travel along the interlobular and intralobular septa and eventually contribute to the arterioles that penetrate the islets, giving rise to an extensive capillary network (46). After supplying the endocrine tissue, the collecting vessels radiate from the islets to supply the surrounding acinar tissue. Therefore, the acinar cells located around the islets of Langerhans may be exposed to very high levels of islet hormones.

HEPATIC PATHOPHYSIOLOGY

Cirrhosis

Laennec first described the characteristic clinical and patho-logic features of cirrhosis in 1826. Cirrhosis is a chronic liver disease characterized by destruction of hepatic parenchyma, with replacement by fibrosis and regenerative nodules. A wide variety of insults may result in this hepatic response, including alcohol ingestion, viral infections, toxin exposure,

metabolic disorders such as hemochromatosis, chronic biliary obstruction, and nutrient deficiency. Fibrogenesis and collagen deposition, inhibition of collagen degradation, infiltration of inflammatory cells, and an abnormal hepatic regenerative response to injury all participate in the process. Hepatic stellate cells play an important role in the pathophysiology of these processes, as described earlier in this chapter (11,12). A current hypothesis suggests that the fibrosis seen in cirrhosis may not be fixed, but is possibly reversible. A better understanding of the dynamics of collagen synthesis and degradation in the liver and the mechanisms of control by stellate cells and other factors give the promise of new strategies in treatment.

Portal Hypertension

The venous drainage of the gut depends on intact flow in the portal vein towards the liver and normal sinusoidal drainage at the level of the hepatocytes into the hepatic veins. Obstruction of flow at any of these levels (presinusoidal, sinusoidal, or postsinusoidal) leads to increased portal vein pressures with decompression and flow back to the heart through collaterals (Table 18.6). These varices and collaterals are likely formed by dilatation of small, preexisting venules. They are typically thin-walled, fragile, and rupture easily with ensuing bleeding. Reduction in the pressure gradient between the portal and hepatic veins to less than 12 mm Hg reduces the risk of bleeding (47).

Mesenteric blood flow in the gut is under close neurohumoral control. A hallmark of portal hypertension is a relative decrease in intrahepatic nitric oxide (NO) production, leading to intrahepatic vasoconstriction and an increase in splanchnic NO production leading to mesenteric vasodilatation (48). The functional unit controlling sinusoidal pressure in cirrhosis is the action of hepatic stellate cells acting as myofibroblasts and causing contraction around sinusoidal endothelial cells. Early in the course of cirrhosis, this increased sinusoidal vascular resistance may be reversible, but as fibrosis and regenerative nodules develop later in the illness, a fixed increased resistance to sinusoidal blood flow develops.

TABLE 18.6

Venous Collaterals in Portal Hypertension

Collateral	Decompression
Esophageal varices	Left gastric vein to azygos vein
Hemorrhoids	Inferior rectal vein to external iliac veins
Caput medusae	Umbilical vein to epigastric veins
Veins of Retzius	Retroperitoneal veins to vena cava
Veins of Sappey	Liver capsule to diaphragm
Splenophrenic veins	Splenic and short gastric veins to phrenic veins

Portal hypertension has a number of secondary effects systemically. Portal hypertension may result in vasodilatation, decreased peripheral vascular resistance, renal sodium retention, ascites formation, renal vasoconstriction, and renal failure. Hepatic encephalopathy may result from portosystemic shunting through collaterals and failure of hepatic clearance of neurotoxins such as ammonia (49).

Acute Liver Failure

Acute liver failure is the sudden loss of liver metabolic functions resulting in coagulopathy and encephalopathy. This severe liver injury may result from a variety of infectious, immunologic, metabolic, vascular, and infiltrative disorders, but common causes currently include acute viral hepatitis and acetaminophen toxicity. Acute necrosis of a large volume of hepatocytes leads to cerebral edema and hepatic encephalopathy, leading to high mortality rates of up to 80% in reported series (50). Coagulopathy and acidosis are common and are associated with a poor prognosis. Hypoglycemia may occur from impaired hepatic gluconeogenesis; renal failure is common. Systemic hypotension may occur, even in the setting of high cardiac output, because of low systemic vascular resistance. Severely affected patients should be considered for liver transplantation (51).

BILIARY PATHOPHYSIOLOGY

Gallstone Formation

Gallstone disease is one of the most common disorders of the gastrointestinal tract, present in an estimated 10% of the U.S. population. The prevalence in women is about twice that of men, and certain ethnic groups, such as the Pima Indians of Arizona are at higher risk. Gallstones can be divided into three types: (i) the most common cholesterol stones, comprised of cholesterol, mucin glycoproteins, and a small amount of bile pigments; (ii) black pigment stones, comprised of calcium bilirubinate with some mucin glycoproteins; and (iii) brown pigment stones, comprised of calcium salts with some cholesterol, protein, and often, bacteria. Pigment stones are seen in the setting of increased hemolysis, such as hemolytic anemia. Brown pigment stones are associated with biliary infection and are typically seen in patients with recurrent pyogenic cholangitis, also known as *Oriental cholangiohepatitis*.

Cholesterol gallstone formation depends on three main factors: (i) cholesterol supersaturation in bile, (ii) a nucleating event, and (iii) incomplete gallbladder emptying. As shown in Figure 18.12, cholesterol is normally maintained in solution in bile in equilibrium with bile salts and phospholipids (8). Changes in the relative concentrations of cholesterol, bile salts, and phospholipids in bile allow crystals of cholesterol to precipitate around a nucleating agent such as mucin or epithelial debris. In the face of incomplete gallbladder emptying in response to a meal, cholesterol

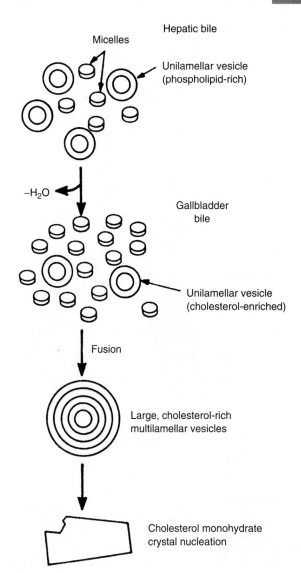

FIGURE 18.12 Concentration of bile leads to net transfer of phospholipid and cholesterol from vesicles to micelles. Phospholipids are transferred more efficiently than cholesterol, leading to cholesterol enrichment of the remaining (remodeled) vesicles. Aggregation of these cholesterol-rich vesicles to form multilamellar liquid crystals may be followed by precipitation of excess cholesterol as solid crystals of cholesterol monohydrate. (From Vessey DA. Metabolism of drugs and toxins by the human liver. In: Zakin D, Boyer TD, eds. *Hepatology: a textbook of liver disease*, 2nd ed. Philadelphia: WB Saunders, 1990:1492, with permission.)

gallstones may form and enlarge over time. Excellent reviews of this subject are available (52,53).

Acute Cholangitis

Cholangitis is an acute bacterial infection of the biliary tree and liver, first recognized by Charcot in 1877. He postulated that the condition was caused by "stagnant bile," usually associated with an obstructed bile duct. His original report described the triad of fever, jaundice, and right upper quadrant pain. The Reynold pentad includes the addition of mental status changes and sepsis. It is now recognized that

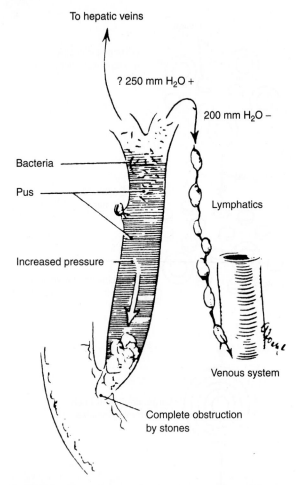

FIGURE 18.13 Cholangitisis caused by the combination of biliary obstruction, often attributable to distally impacted stones and bactibilia. Bacteria then reflux into the hepatic veins and perihepatic lymphatics, resulting in systemic bacteremia. (From Pitt HA, Longmire WP Jr. Suppurative cholangitis. In: Hardy JM, ed. *Critical surgical illness*, 2nd ed. Philadelphia: WB Saunders, 1980:380, with permission.)

the pathophysiology of cholangitis requires a combination of three factors: bile duct obstruction, increased intraluminal biliary pressure, and bacterial contamination of the bile (Fig. 18.13). The resulting increased intraductal pressure causes the reflux of bacteria up the biliary tree, across biliary canaliculi, and into the hepatic veins and perihepatic lymphatics, resulting in bacteremia. In addition, increased biliary pressure affects host defense mechanisms including the integrity of hepatic tight junctions, Kupffer cell function, bile flow washout of the biliary tree, and immunoglobulin A (IgA) production making the liver more susceptible to infection (54).

CBD stones are the most common cause of biliary obstruction resulting in cholangitis. Malignant biliary obstruction rarely presents with cholangitis unless the patient has had biliary manipulation. The advances in invasive biliary tract procedures, however, have changed the spectrum of this disease. Manipulations of the biliary tract, either

percutaneously or transampullary, can be associated with both the introduction of bacteria and sudden increases in biliary tract pressure, which may result in cholangitis.

Although the bile normally is sterile, positive cultures are found in up to 90% of patients with choledocholithiasis and in virtually all patients with acute cholangitis. Blood cultures are also positive in 40% to 50% of patients with cholangitis. The most common organisms associated with acute cholangitis are gram-negative coliforms, including *Escherichia coli* and *Klebsiella* species. *Enterococcus* is the next most common organism in most series. Anaerobic bacteria, particularly *Bacteroides fragilis*, are also important pathogens, especially in elderly patients with choledocholithiasis and patients with indwelling biliary stents. Infections may be polymicrobial. In recent years, a change in the spectrum of bacterial infection has occurred as an increasing number of cases of cholangitis are seen following biliary tract manipulations. In such cases, previously uncommon gram-negative rods, such as *Pseudomonas* sp and *Enterobacter* sp, and yeast are now being isolated. The increasing frequency with which patients are treated with indwelling biliary stents for unresectable biliary or pancreatic malignancies has been accompanied by an increased incidence of cholangitis with resistant organisms.

The spectrum of disease of acute cholangitis can range from a mild self-limited illness to a life-threatening condition with septic shock. The therapy for cholangitis must be individualized on the basis of the severity of the disease. Virtually all patients require rehydration and prompt institution of broad-spectrum antibiotics. The vast majority of patients with cholangitis will respond to antibiotics and intravenous fluids without the need for urgent biliary decompression. However, emergency biliary decompression may be necessary in the small subset of patients with septic shock. Currently, the preferred route of biliary decompression depends on the likely cause of obstruction and available expertise in percutaneous biliary drainage and endoscopic sphincterotomy.

PANCREATIC PATHOPHYSIOLOGY

Acute Pancreatitis

Acute pancreatitis is an acute inflammatory process of the pancreas with varying involvement of other regional tissues and remote organ system (55). The spectrum of acute pancreatitis ranges from mild or interstitial pancreatitis to severe or necrotizing pancreatitis. Most patients with interstitial pancreatitis experience mild-to-moderate symptoms and show pathologic changes of mild interstitial edema and inflammatory cells within the parenchyma, but no gross necrosis. Unless the pancreatitis recurs, normal pancreatic function and morphology can be expected following recovery. Less than 10% of patients develop a severe life-threatening illness associated with severe necrotizing destruction of the pancreas. These patients will have gross necrosis of pancreatic and peripancreatic tissue

TABLE 18.7

Causes of Acute Pancreatitis

Obstructive causes
    Gallstones (stones, biliary sludge, microlithiasis)
    Tumors (duodenum, pancreas, bile duct)
    Duodenal diverticulum
    Congenital obstruction (choledochocele, annular pancreas,
        pancreas divisum)
Toxin
    Alcohol
    Scorpion venom
    Organophosphate insecticides
Drugs and medications
Metabolic causes
    Hypertriglyceridemia
    Hyperparathyroidism/hypercalcemia
Infections
    Direct infection (viral, bacteria, fungal, parasitic)
    Ductal obstruction (parasitic)
Vascular causes
    Systemic vasculitis
    Hypotension
    Emboli to pancreatic vessels
Trauma
    Blunt and penetrating trauma
    Postprocedure (ERCP, Surgery)
Pregnancy
Idiopathic
Hereditary/genetic/familial causes
    PRSS1, CFTR, SPINK1 mutations
Controversial
    Pancreas divisum
    Sphincter of Oddi dysfunction

ERCP, endoscopic retrograde cholangiopancreatography; CFTR, cystic fibrosis transmembrane conductance regulator, SPINK1, serine protease inhibitor Kazal type 1.

with signs of remote organ system compromise. Mortality in these patients occurs either as a consequence of mutiple system organ failure, usually in the first week, or as a result of infection of necrotic pancreatic and peripancreatic debris, usually in the second to third week. Multiple causes of acute pancreatitis exist (Table 18.7) (56). In the United States, alcohol-related pancreatitis and gallstone pancreatitis account for more than 80% of all cases.

Although a variety of insults can give rise to acute pancreatitis, the pathogenesis is the same. The initial pathogenesis results from intracellular activation of trypsinogen to active trypsin with the acinar cell. Normally, cellular proteases and phospholipases are synthesized in an inactive form. They are sequestered into zymogen granules and directed towards the apical membrane for exocytosis into the pancreatic ductal system along with endogenous protease inhibitors to protect the pancreas from premature activation. In acute pancreatitis, this orderly process is disrupted. Trypsinogen and other proteolytic enzymes are prematurely activated within the cells, likely as a consequence of fusion of the zymogen granules

with lysosomes containing hydrolases such as cathepsin B which can activate trypsinogen to trypsin. The autophagic cytoplasmic vacuoles that are formed move preferentially to the basolateral surfaces of the acinar cell rather than to the apical surface. As a result of this loss in acinar cell polarity, the contents are released into the interstitium of the pancreas resulting in tissue digestion and injury. Disruption of acinar paracellular barrier and intralobular pancreatic duct cells soon follows, which facilitates a local inflammatory response with recruitment of inflammatory cells that along with inflammatory mediators derived from the pancreatic acinar cells and tissue macrophages enhances the process.

The pathophysiologic mechanisms responsible for the development of pancreatitis stem from this process. These include direct injury to pancreatic and peripancreatic tissue from activated pancreatic enzymes, microcirculatory impairment, leukocyte chemoattraction, release of proinflammatory cytokines, oxidative stress, and late in the process, bacterial translocation, infection, and sepsis. Microcirculatory impairment includes vasoconstriction, capillary stasis, shunting, and ischemia. Activation of complement early in the course of pancreatic tissue injury causes release of C5a with resultant recruitment of macrophages and leukocytes. This enhances the inflammatory process by release of TNF, interleukins (IL-1, IL-6, and IL-8), platelet activating factor, and proteolytic enzymes. Other mediators released in the pancreatic tissue include arachidonic acid metabolites, NO, and oxygen metabolites that induce an oxidative stress. The mechanisms that limit this inflammatory process to interstitial edema in some patients but progress to pancreatic necrosis in others are not understood.

Patients with severe pancreatitis manifest remote organ system involvement, including fever, adult respiratory distress syndrome, renal insufficiency, myocardial depression, metabolic disturbances including loss of glucose and electrolyte homeostasis, and shock. Remote organ system impairment results from direct organ injury from circulating activated pancreatic enzymes and inflammatory cytokines. This process is accentuated by the activation of hepatic Kupffer cells, which release more cytokines into the circulation. The lung and renal capillary beds are particularly sensitive to circulating pancreatic enzymes and damage from inflammatory cytokines. Bacterial infection occurs as a consequence of direct hematogenous spread or translocation resulting from a loss of the normal gut mucosal barrier.

The two most common causes of acute pancreatitis are ethanol and gallstones. Alcohol consumption is thought to trigger acute pancreatitis by several mechanisms. These include direct toxic effects on acinar cells by acetaldehyde, the hepatic by-product of ethanol metabolism, and triglycerides, increased proteolytic enzyme production and release with a decrease in the trypsin inhibiting capacity, microtubule disruption, increased acinar cell permeability, and decreased blood flow. Alcohol may also affect sphincter of Oddi function, which along with increased flows in response to elevations in secretin resulting from increased gastric acid production, cause pancreatic ductal hypertension.

TABLE 18.8

Causes of Chronic Pancreatitis

Alcoholic
Obstructive
   Benign stricture (traumatic, postpancreatitis stricture,
     pancreas divisum, sphincter of Oddi stricture or
     dysfunction)
   Malignant stricture (pancreatic, duodenal, biliary neoplasm)
Metabolic
   Hypercalcemia
   Hyperlipidemia (hypertriglyceridemia, lipoprotein lipase
     deficiency, apolipoprotein C-II deficiency)
Genetic
   Autosomal dominant
     Hereditary pancreatitis (PRSS1 mutations)
   Autosomal recessive or modifier genes
     CFTR, SPINK1 mutations, others
Autoimmune pancreatitis
Postnecrotic chronic pancreatitis
Idiopathic
   Early onset
   Late onset
Tropical
   Tropical calcific pancreatitis, fibrocalculous pancreatic
     diabetes
Other
   Old age
   Chronic renal failure
   Diabetes
   Radiotherapy

CFTR, cystic fibrosis transmembrane conductance regulator, SPINK1, serine protease inhibitor Kazal type 1.

Gallstones are thought to trigger acute pancreatitis by transient obstruction at the ampulla of Vater by a stone passing into the duodenum. This may allow for reflux of bile into the pancreas or transient pancreatic duct hypertension. Experimental evidence supports a possible role for each mechanism in the pathogenesis of gallstone pancreatitis.

Chronic Pancreatitis

Chronic pancreatitis is characterized by irreversible parenchymal destruction with histologic evidence of chronic inflammation, fibrosis, and loss of exocrine and endocrine cells. Common causes of chronic pancreatitis are shown in Table 18.8 (57). The two most common categories of chronic pancreatitis are chronic calcific pancreatitis that is usually attributed to alcohol abuse and chronic obstructive pancreatitis from pancreatic ductal obstruction from tumors.

As is the case with acute pancreatitis, the various etiologies that cause chronic pancreatitis produce a similar pathologic finding. Histologically, chronic pancreatitis is characterized by fibrosis of the interlobular areas of the pancreas with gradual involvement of the acinar cells and ducts. The inciting event is usually repeated acinar cell injury. Initially, areas of chronic inflammation surround areas of normal glandular architecture. There is loss of ductal epithelium, acinar tissue, and precipitation of proteinaceous material within the ducts. This deposition of proteinaceous plugs within the ducts is exacerbated by the increased enzyme secretion seen in response to alcohol and a loss of pancreatic stone protein, lithostathine, which normally suppresses nucleation of calcium carbonate in pancreatic juice. Pancreatic juice is rich in calcium. A loss of lithostathine allows for precipitation of calcium and calcific stone formation within the ducts. Although islets are usually spared early in the course of the disease, they are eventually involved as the pancreatic parenchyma and ducts are replaced by fibrosis. Ductal involvement leads to stricture and dilatation, which is the hallmark of chronic calcific pancreatitis seen in alcoholic patients. Therefore, chronic calcific pancreatitis is thought to arise as a consequence of toxic-metabolic effects as seen in chronic alcohol use, ductal obstruction from stones, and necrosis-fibrosis of the gland.

These processes are not unique to alcohol use. Stone formation is also seen in hereditary chronic pancreatitis, tropical pancreatitis, and idiopathic chronic pancreatitis as well. In these diagnoses, a genetic predisposition is thought to be important. In patients with idiopathic pancreatitis, an increased rate of cystic fibrosis transmembrane conductance regulator (CFTR) mutations has been identified leading to a decrease in bicarbonate secretion, ductal debris deposition, and atrophy (58). In patients with hereditary pancreatitis, a mutation in the cationic trypsinogen gene (*PRSS1*) has been identified (59,60). This is a gain of function mutation in which activated trypsinogen is resistant to inactivation. A mutation in the serine protease inhibitor Kazal type 1 (*SPINK1*) gene has been observed in idiopathic, hereditary, and tropical pancreatitis (58,60–64). This results in a loss of trypsin inhibitor activity. Therefore, the development of chronic pancreatitis may be both environmental and genetic in origin.

In obstructive chronic pancreatitis, the pancreatic duct is blocked by tumor, congenital anomalies, previous trauma, or at the level of the ampulla. In this case, the gland upstream from the blockage becomes fibrotic and the duct dilated. The duct epithelium remains normal, however. Calcifications and protein plugs are uncommon. Relief of the obstruction can cause reversal of the fibrosis and atrophy, unlike other forms of chronic pancreatitis.

REFERENCES

1. Linder HR. Embryology and anatomy of the biliary tree. In: Way LW, Pellegrini CA, eds. *Surgery of the gallbladder and bile ducts.* Philadelphia: WB Saunders, 1987:322.
2. Sutherland F, Harris J. Claude Couinaud: a passion for the liver. *Arch Surg* 2002;137:1305–1310.
3. Couinaud C. Surgical anatomy of the liver. Several new aspects. *Chirurgie* 1986;112:337–342.
4. Rappaport AM, Wanless JR. Physioanatomic considerations. In: Schiff L, Schiff ER, eds. *Diseases of the liver.* Philadelphia: JB Lippincott Co, 1993:1.

5. Felber JP, Golay A. Regulation of nutrient metabolism and energy expenditure. *Metabolism* 1995;44:4–9.
6. Nishio H, Dugaiczyk A. Complete structure of the human alpha-albumin gene, a new member of the serum albumin multigene family. *Proc Natl Acad Sci USA* 1996;93:7557–7561.
7. Miller LL, Bale WF. Synthesis of all plasma protein fractions except gamma globulins by the liver; the use of zone electrophoresis and lysine-epsilon-C14 to define the plasma proteins synthesized by the isolated perfused liver. *J Exp Med* 1954;99:125–132.
8. Admirand WH, Small DM. The physicochemical basis of cholesterol gallstone formation in man. *J Clin Invest* 1968;47:1043–1052.
9. Carey MC. Critical tables for calculating the cholesterol saturation of native bile. *J Lipid Res* 1978;19:945–955.
10. Bilzer M, Roggel F, Gerbes AL. Role of Kupffer cells in host defense and liver disease. *Liver Int* 2006;26:1175–1186.
11. Rockey DC. Hepatic fibrosis, stellate cells, and portal hypertension. *Clin Liver Dis* 2006;10:459–479, vii–viii.
12. Henderson NC, Iredale JP. Liver fibrosis: cellular mechanisms of progression and resolution. *Clin Sci (Lond)* 2007;112:265–280.
13. Pahlavan PS, Feldmann RE Jr, Zavos C, et al. Prometheus' challenge: molecular, cellular and systemic aspects of liver regeneration. *J Surg Res* 2006;134:238–251.
14. Fausto N, Campbell JS, Riehle KJ. Liver regeneration. *Hepatology* 2006;43:S45–S53.
15. Seetharam S, Sussman NL, Komoda T, et al. The mechanism of elevated alkaline phosphatase activity after bile duct ligation in the rat. *Hepatology* 1986;6:374–380.
16. Kamath PS, Wiesner RH, Malinchoc M, et al. A model to predict survival in patients with end-stage liver disease. *Hepatology* 2001;33:464–470.
17. Wiesner R, Edwards E, Freeman R, et al. Model for end-stage liver disease (MELD) and allocation of donor livers. *Gastroenterology* 2003;124:91–96.
18. Keegan MT, Plevak DJ. Preoperative assessment of the patient with liver disease. *Am J Gastroenterol* 2005;100:2116–2127.
19. Friedman LS. The risk of surgery in patients with liver disease. *Hepatology* 1999;29:1617–1623.
20. Mansour A, Watson W, Shayani V, et al. Abdominal operations in patients with cirrhosis: still a major surgical challenge. *Surgery* 1997;122:730–735; discussion 735–736.
21. Papatheodoridis GV, Cholongitas E, Dimitriadou E, et al. MELD vs Child-Pugh and creatinine-modified Child-Pugh score for predicting survival in patients with decompensated cirrhosis. *World J Gastroenterol* 2005;11:3099–3104.
22. Cholongitas E, Papatheodoridis GV, Vangeli M, et al. Systematic review: the model for end-stage liver disease–should it replace Child-Pugh's classification for assessing prognosis in cirrhosis? *Aliment Pharmacol Ther* 2005;22:1079–1089.
23. Zoedler T, Ebener C, Becker H, et al. Evaluation of liver function tests to predict operative risk in liver surgery. *HPB Surg* 1995;9:13–18.
24. Albers I, Hartmann H, Bircher J, et al. Superiority of the Child-Pugh classification to quantitative liver function tests for assessing prognosis of liver cirrhosis. *Scand J Gastroenterol* 1989;24:269–276.
25. Nervi F, Marinovic I, Rigotti A, et al. Regulation of biliary cholesterol secretion. Functional relationship between the canalicular and sinusoidal cholesterol secretory pathways in the rat. *J Clin Invest* 1988;82:1818–1825.
26. Wood JR, Saverymuttu SH, Heintze K. Gallbladder secretion. *Gastroenterology* 1977;73:629.
27. Lilja P, Fagan CJ, Wiener I, et al. Infusion of pure cholecystokinin in humans. Correlation between plasma concentrations of cholecystokinin and gallbladder size. *Gastroenterology* 1982;83:256–261.
28. Rehfeld JF. Clinical endocrinology and metabolism. Cholecystokinin. *Best Pract Res Clin Endocrinol Metab* 2004;18:569–586.
29. McKeage K, Cheer S, Wagstaff AJ. Octreotide long-acting release (LAR): a review of its use in the management of acromegaly. *Drugs* 2003;63:2473–2499.
30. Behar J, Corazziari E, Guelrud M, et al. Functional gallbladder and sphincter of oddi disorders. *Gastroenterology* 2006;130:1498–1509.
31. Berr F, Stellaard F, Pratschke E, et al. Effects of cholecystectomy on the kinetics of primary and secondary bile acids. *J Clin Invest* 1989;83:1541–1550.
32. Bro-Rasmussen F, Killmann SA, Thaysen JH. The composition of pancreatic juice as compared to sweat, parotid saliva and tears. *Acta Physiol Scand* 1956;37:97–113.
33. Miyasaka K, Shinozaki H, Jimi A, et al. Amylase secretion from dispersed human pancreatic acini: neither cholecystokinin a nor cholecystokinin B receptors mediate amylase secretion *in vitro*. *Pancreas* 2002;25:161–165.
34. Ji B, Bi Y, Simeone D, et al. Human pancreatic acinar cells do not respond to cholecystokinin. *Pharmacol Toxicol* 2002;91:327–332.
35. Li Y, Hao Y, Owyang C. High-affinity CCK-A receptors on the vagus nerve mediate CCK-stimulated pancreatic secretion in rats. *Am J Physiol* 1997;273:G679–G685.
36. Owyang C. Physiological mechanisms of cholecystokinin action on pancreatic secretion. *Am J Physiol* 1996;271:G1–G7.
37. Singer MV, Solomon TE, Grossman MI. Effect of atropine on secretion from intact and transplanted pancreas in dog. *Am J Physiol* 1980;238:G18–G22.
38. Katschinski M, Dahmen G, Reinshagen M, et al. Cephalic stimulation of gastrointestinal secretory and motor responses in humans. *Gastroenterology* 1992;103:383–391.
39. Anagnostides A, Chadwick VS, Selden AC, et al. Sham feeding and pancreatic secretion. Evidence for direct vagal stimulation of enzyme output. *Gastroenterology* 1984;87:109–114.
40. Kreiss C, Schwizer W, Erlacher U, et al. Role of antrum in regulation of pancreaticobiliary secretion in humans. *Am J Physiol* 1996;270:G844–G851.
41. Liddle RA. Regulation of cholecystokinin secretion by intraluminal releasing factors. *Am J Physiol* 1995;269:G319–G327.
42. Spannagel AW, Green GM, Guan D, et al. Purification and characterization of a luminal cholecystokinin-releasing factor from rat intestinal secretion. *Proc Natl Acad Sci USA* 1996;93:4415–4420.
43. Symersky T, Vu MK, Frolich M, et al. The effect of equicaloric medium-chain and long-chain triglycerides on pancreas enzyme secretion. *Clin Physiol Funct Imaging* 2002;22:307–311.
44. O'Keefe SJ, Lee RB, Anderson FP, et al. Physiological effects of enteral and parenteral feeding on pancreaticobiliary secretion in humans. *Am J Physiol Gastrointest Liver Physiol* 2003;284:G27–G36.
45. Ebert R, Creutzfeldt W. Gastrointestinal peptides and insulin secretion. *Diabetes Metab Rev* 1987;3:1–26.
46. Bonner-Weir S, Orci L. New perspectives on the microvasculature of the islets of Langerhans in the rat. *Diabetes* 1982;31:883–889.
47. D'Amico G, Garcia-Pagan JC, Luca A, et al. Hepatic vein pressure gradient reduction and prevention of variceal bleeding in cirrhosis: a systematic review. *Gastroenterology* 2006;131:1611–1624.
48. Langer DA, Shah VH. Nitric oxide and portal hypertension: interface of vasoreactivity and angiogenesis. *J Hepatol* 2006;44:209–216.
49. Garcia-Tsao G. Portal hypertension. *Curr Opin Gastroenterol* 2006;22:254–262.
50. Khan SA, Shah N, Williams R, et al. Acute liver failure: a review. *Clin Liver Dis* 2006;10:239–258, vii–viii.
51. O'Grady JG, Alexander GJ, Hayllar KM, et al. Early indicators of prognosis in fulminant hepatic failure. *Gastroenterology* 1989;97:439–445.
52. Portincasa P, Moschetta A, Palasciano G. Cholesterol gallstone disease. *Lancet* 2006;368:230–239.
53. Strasberg SM. The pathogenesis of cholesterol gallstones a review. *J Gastrointest Surg* 1998;2:109–125.
54. Sung JY, Costerton JW, Shaffer EA. Defense system in the biliary tract against bacterial infection. *Dig Dis Sci* 1992;37:689–696.
55. Bradley EL III. A clinically based classification system for acute pancreatitis. Summary of the International Symposium on Acute Pancreatitis, Atlanta, Ga, September 11 through 13, 1992. *Arch Surg* 1993;128:586–590.

56. Steinberg WM. Acute pancreatitis. In: Feldman M, Friedman LS, Brandt LJ, eds. *Sleisenger and Fordtran's gastrointestinal and liver disease*. Philadelphia: WB Saunders, 2006:1245.

57. Forsmark CE. Chronic pancreatitis. In: Feldman M, Friedman LS, Brandt LJ, eds. *Sleisenger and Fordtran's gastrointestinal and liver disease*. Philadelphia: WB Saunders, 2006:1274.

58. Whitcomb DC. Genetic predisposition to alcoholic chronic pancreatitis. *Pancreas* 2003;27:321–326.

59. Etemad B, Whitcomb DC. Chronic pancreatitis: diagnosis, classification, and new genetic developments. *Gastroenterology* 2001;120:682–707.

60. Schmid RM, Whitcomb DC. Genetically defined models of chronic pancreatitis. *Gastroenterology* 2006;131:2012–2015.

61. Witt H, Luck W, Hennies HC, et al. Mutations in the gene encoding the serine protease inhibitor, Kazal type 1 are associated with chronic pancreatitis. *Nat Genet* 2000;25:213–216.

62. Threadgold J, Greenhalf W, Ellis I, et al. The N34S mutation of SPINK1 (PSTI) is associated with a familial pattern of idiopathic chronic pancreatitis but does not cause the disease. *Gut* 2002;50:675–681.

63. Schneider A, Suman A, Rossi L, et al. SPINK1/PSTI mutations are associated with tropical pancreatitis and type II diabetes mellitus in Bangladesh. *Gastroenterology* 2002;123:1026–1030.

64. Drenth JP, te Morsche R, Jansen JB. Mutations in serine protease inhibitor Kazal type 1 are strongly associated with chronic pancreatitis. *Gut* 2002;50:687–692.

CHAPTER 19

Hemostasis, Thrombosis, Anticoagulation, Hematopoiesis, and Blood Transfusion

Kent Choi, Richard K. Spence, Aryeh Shander, and Carol E. H. Scott-Conner

This chapter begins with an overview of hematopoiesis and the coagulation system. Common disorders, pharmacologic agents, and other interventions are then discussed. The chapter concludes with an introduction to transfusion medicine and a brief discussion of current work on blood substitutes.

OVERVIEW OF THE HEMOSTATIC SYSTEM

Surgeons could not operate if blood did not clot and if the body did not have the ability to replenish lost blood, platelets, and white cells. When the vascular endothelium is breached, a complex, interdependent set of events forms a stable clot.

Clotting begins when platelets adhere to exposed subendothelial collagen, assisted by von Willebrand factor (vWF) (Fig. 19.1). These adherent platelets release substances that recruit more platelets into the growing clot. They also cause vasoconstriction by releasing vasoactive amines (serotonin and thromboxane A_2). In a counter-regulatory manner, endothelial cells synthesize prostacyclin, a vasodilator and inhibitor of platelet aggregation, as well as endothelial-derived relaxing factor. Platelets also release platelet-derived growth factor (PDGF).

Primary hemostasis denotes the events leading to the formation of this fragile initial hemostatic plug. It requires the presence of adequate numbers of normally functioning platelets, collagen and vWF synthesized by endothelial cells, and products of the coagulation cascade (thrombin and fibrinogen). Deficits of primary hemostasis are recognized in the operating room when normal avascular planes continue to ooze as numerous small capillaries continue to bleed, despite the application of pressure and the passage of time (1).

The platelet plug is stabilized and a mechanically strong clot composed of fibrin, platelets, and erythrocytes forms through the mechanism of *secondary hemostasis (the*

coagulation cascade). Receptors on platelet membranes activate this cascade. Cross-linking of fibrin further strengthens the clot, which then contracts as a result of the activity of the contained platelets.

Propagation of thrombus beyond the site of injury is limited by several major regulatory mechanisms (Table 19.1) that downregulate an amplifying system, which would otherwise culminate in massive intravascular coagulation.

Chemotactic factors stimulate phagocytic leukocytes to migrate to the region of injury to clean up the debris. Substances such as PDGF, released by degranulating platelets, stimulate vascular repair. Finally, when healing and restoration of endothelial continuity has occurred, the *fibrinolytic system* is activated and the occluding thrombus lysed. This system also helps localize the thrombus to the area of need. When the fibrinolytic system is activated prematurely, clots form normally but lyse prematurely. The result is delayed rebleeding after initial satisfactory hemostasis.

TABLE 19.1

Regulatory Mechanisms that Control Procoagulant Pathways and Limit Clot Formation

Phase of Coagulation	Control Mechanism
Initiation	Tissue factor pathway inhibitor (TFPI) inhibits tissue thromboplastin-induced coagulation by inhibiting the interaction of factors VIIa, Xa, and tissue factor complex on a cell membrane
Amplification	Protein C pathway, activated by complex of thrombomodulin and thrombin on an endothelial cell surface
Propagation	Antithrombin III

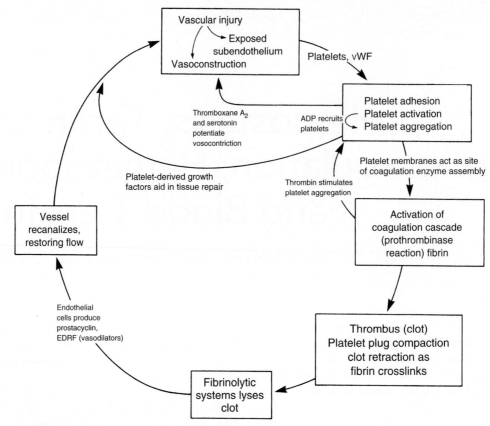

FIGURE 19.1   Overview of the hemostatic system. Vascular injury triggers platelet aggregation with subsequent activation of the coagulation cascade and formation of a clot composed of platelets, erythrocytes, and fibrin. Plasminogen is bound to fibrin within the clot; the active form, plasmin, initiates clot lysis when healing has occurred. vWF, von Willebrand factor.

Hemostasis therefore may be thought of as a tightly regulated system of interdependent factors. In the sections that follow, each of the major elements will be briefly explored. Congenital and acquired defects of each element leading to pathologic hemorrhage or a thrombotic diathesis will be considered, and the effects of pharmacologic interventions will be detailed.

The Platelet and Formation of the Primary Hemostatic Plug

Platelets are disc-shaped fragments of megakaryocyte cytoplasm. As shown in Figure 19.2, platelets adhere to a site of injury, become activated, and stimulate further aggregation (2,3). During platelet activation, platelets change shape, extrude the contents of their granules, and expose receptor sites that provide a surface for activation and assembly of coagulation enzyme complexes, culminating in the generation of fibrin.

Platelet Production and Destruction

Platelets are released into the bone marrow sinusoids as large cytoplasmic fragments termed *proplatelets*, which then break into individual platelets. Thrombopoietin regulates platelet production (2). Production can be increased up to sixfold in response to increased platelet destruction. In states of rapid

platelet release, platelets vary in size, and a preponderance of relatively large platelets may be noted. Because these large platelets would, under normal circumstances, have been further subdivided, they possess significantly greater hemostatic capability.

The average life span of a platelet is 8 to 12 days. Senescent platelets are destroyed in the bone marrow, spleen, and liver. A fixed loss of 7 to 10×10^9 platelets per day may reflect the role that platelets play in maintaining vascular integrity.

Approximately 33% of the platelet pool is sequestered in the spleen. In the normal situation, these sequestered platelets are freely exchangeable with those in the blood and are released in large numbers in response to epinephrine (EPI) and exercise. In hypersplenism, increased splenic sequestration of platelets may result in thrombocytopenia.

After splenectomy, the entire platelet pool resides in the circulation. Therefore, thrombocytosis occurs immediately after splenectomy and persists to a varying extent thereafter, and the platelet count no longer rises in response to EPI or exercise (3).

Disorders of Platelet Number

The normal platelet count ranges from 150,000 to 400,000, corresponding to 6 to 10 platelets per high-power field. Because platelets vary in size or may clump in the presence

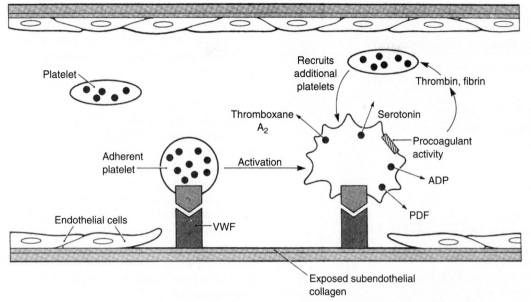

FIGURE 19.2   The three phases of platelet function are adherence, activation, and aggregation. Platelets adhere to the exposed subendothelium with the aid of von Willebrand factor (vWF), which is synthesized and released by endothelial cells. Adherent platelets become activated, changing shape and releasing the contents of their granules. This recruits more platelets into the growing thrombus (platelet aggregation). Thrombin activation of platelets exposes binding sites for Xase and the prothrombinase complex (procoagulant effect). Therefore, the growing platelet thrombus acts as a site for assembly of enzymes of the coagulation reaction as well as a scaffold upon which the fibrin clot forms. ADP, adenosine diphosphate; PDF, platelet derived factor.

of ethylene diaminetetraacetic acid (EDTA) anticoagulant, a falsely low automated count is sometimes encountered, requiring verification by visual inspection of a blood smear. Examination of the smear also provides information on platelet size and may reveal additional evidence, such as the characteristic red cell fragmentation of microangiopathic hemolytic anemia [seen in disseminated intravascular coagulation (DIC) or thrombotic thrombocytopenic purpura (TTP)].

Decreased production, or increased destruction, or both may cause *thrombocytopenia*, a decrease in the number of circulating platelets. Many conditions may decrease the platelet count, particularly in critically ill patients (Table 19.2). Decreased platelet production occurs when functioning marrow is replaced by tumor, leukemic cells, or fibrosis and in response to myelosuppressive drugs and radiation. Several drugs and toxins exhibit a selective and generally temporary effect on platelet production. Chronic alcohol ingestion causes thrombocytopenia in some patients, and rebound thrombocytosis may accompany alcohol withdrawal.

Bone marrow examination will reveal a normal or increased number of megakaryocytes when thrombocytopenia is the result of increased platelet destruction. Immunologically mediated platelet destruction occurs in idiopathic or autoimmune thrombocytopenic purpura, posttransfusion purpura, and heparin-induced thrombocytopenia (HIT) (4–10). Consumption of platelets and other clotting factors results in thrombocytopenia in DIC (discussed later in this chapter). Paroxysmal nocturnal hemoglobinuria

is a stem cell disease for which platelet production is reduced and platelets are consumed by inappropriate thrombus formation, resulting in profound thrombocytopenia.

Platelet transfusion (generally with single-donor apheresis packs) is used when profound thrombocytopenia complicates surgical hemostasis. As a rule of thumb, transfusion of 6 to 10 single apheresis U will raise the platelet count by 17,000 to 31,000 (9).

TABLE 19.2
Causes of Thrombocytopenia
Spurious
Underproduction
Drugs and toxins
Infiltrative disease of the bone marrow
Aplastic marrow
Paroxysmal nocturnal hemoglobinuria
Overdestruction
Immunologically mediated
Idiopathic thrombocytopenic purpura
Posttransfusion purpura
Heparin-induced throbocytopenia
Thrombotic thrombocytopenic purpura
Disseminated intravascular coagulation
Hypersplenism

TABLE 19.3

Causes of Reactive Thrombocytosis

Chronic inflammatory disorders
    Most of the so-called rheumatoid disorders
    Crohn disease
    Chronic ulcerative colitis

Recovery from acute infection
Acute hemorrhage
Hemolytic anemia
Iron deficiency anemia
Malignancy
Postsplenectomy
Response to drugs
    Vincristine
    Epinephrine

Rebound phenomenon
    After discontinuation of myelosuppressive agents
    Alcohol withdrawal

Thrombocytosis is an excess of circulating platelets (Table 19.3). *Primary thrombocytosis* sometimes occurs in association with polycythemia vera or other myeloproliferative disorders (11). These patients are aptly described as being in double jeopardy; they are prone to abnormal bleeding, but may also manifest a thrombotic diathesis. It is extremely important to recognize this increased surgical risk, particularly when the platelet count is greater than $1,500,000/\text{mm}^3$.

Hemostatic abnormalities rarely occur in *secondary or reactive thrombocytosis* (in contrast to primary thrombocytosis). Reactive thrombocytosis in surgical patients is most commonly seen after splenectomy. Because of fear of thrombosis, many clinicians treat platelet counts greater than $1,000,000/\text{mm}^3$ with antiplatelet drugs. These complications are rare, except in patients with hemolytic anemia; and even there, the incidence of thrombosis correlates poorly with the platelet count.

Platelet Granules, Receptors, and Intrinsic Contractile System

Cytoplasmic granules (dense bodies and α-granules) comprise approximately 20% of platelet volume. These contain PDGF, adenosine triphosphate (ATP), adenosine diphosphate (ADP), guanosine pyrophosphate (GTP), guanosine diphosphate (GDP), pyrophosphate, orthophosphate, calcium, serotonin, and other substances (3).

Platelet-specific proteins are released only by platelets during degranulation; hence detection of one of these substances in the serum is presumptive evidence for platelet activation. Thrombin is physiologically the most important platelet agonist. It stimulates degranulation and activates phospholipase A_2, which stimulates synthesis and release of thromboxane A_2 and its precursors. ADP stimulates platelet shape change and aggregation. It requires the ability of the platelet to synthesize prostaglandins and is

hence inhibited by aspirin. Platelets also release serotonin, a vasoconstrictor that may aid in primary hemostasis by causing small vessels to go into spasm. It may also contribute to the pulmonary vasoconstriction accompanying pulmonary embolism.

Growth factors released by platelets include PDGF, transforming growth factor-β (TGF-β), and connective tissue-activating peptide (CTAP-III).

Study of rare individuals deficient in platelet granules has provided important insights platelet function in normal hemostasis (12).

In addition to release of preformed substances, activated platelets synthesize and release prostaglandins, the most important of which is thromboxane A_2. This pathway is altered by aspirin and other similar inhibitors. Thromboxane A_2, PGG_2 and PGH_2 function as vasoconstrictors and strong stimulants of platelet aggregation. Other arachidonic acid metabolites are strong chemotaxis substances for neutrophils (13).

Proteins of the cytoskeleton—actin and myosin, as well as microtubules, microfilaments, and intermediary filaments—are responsible for the maintenance of platelet structural stability and the conformational changes accompanying platelet activation (14).

Receptors on platelet membranes form a critical part of the hemostatic mechanism. A platelet agonist, such as thrombin, binds to a specific receptor on the surface of a platelet. A second messenger is generated on the cytoplasmic side of the membrane, transmitting the message to the inside of the platelet, increasing intracellular calcium or cyclic adenosine monophosphate (cAMP) (14,15). Receptors which bind fibrinogen, vWF, calcium, thrombospondin, and fibronectin contribute to platelet adhesion to surfaces and stabilization of the platelet thrombus by fibrinogen. VWF acts as a bridge between glycoprotein Ib and IIb/IIIa sites on platelets and binding sites on collagen in the subendothelium, thereby producing adhesion of platelets to the site of injury (15,16). Membrane receptors for fibrinogen, only active when platelets form a clot, are critically important for the formation of a stable clot. The identification of a "platelet-type" bleeding diathesis in patients with abnormal fibrinogen or congenital hypofibrinogenemia or afibrinogenemia underscores the importance of this mechanism.

Platelets are responsible for the phenomenon of clot retraction observed *in vitro*. Platelet membranes provide a surface on which elements of the coagulation cascade form enzyme complexes that culminate in the formation of thrombin. In addition, platelets release significant amounts of some clotting factors, including factor V, an enzyme crucial in the coagulation cascade. Approximately 20% of factor V is located within platelet α-granules, and patients lacking in serum factor V, but having adequate platelet factor V, have minimal bleeding problems. Defects in platelet membrane receptors (Glanzmann thrombasthenia, Bernard-Soulier syndrome) produce predictable alterations in hemostasis (12).

Assessment of Platelet Function

The bleeding time was for many years the standard method for assessing primary hemostasis, but it is subject to many problems in technique and interpretation (17). However, the bleeding time procedure has fallen from favor in recent years. Many hospitals are no longer offering it, and several national organizations have issued position statements against its routine use as a presurgical screen. The bleeding time is not sensitive or specific. It is poorly reproducible, can be affected by aspirin ingestion and by the skill of the person performing the test, and frequently leaves small thin scars on the forearm.

The PFA-100 (Platelet Function Analyzer-100) is a testing device that many hospitals are using as a platelet function screen, in place of the bleeding time, to mimic the clotting process. A blood sample is put into a test cartridge. Vacuum is then used to draw blood through a very thin glass tube that has been coated with collagen and with either EPI or ADP. This coating activates the platelets in the moving sample and promotes platelet adherence and aggregation. The time it takes for a clot to form inside the glass tube and prevent further blood flow is measured as a closure time (CT). An initial screen is done with collagen/EPI. If the CT is normal, it is unlikely that a platelet dysfunction exists. The collagen/ADP test is run to confirm an abnormal collagen/EPI test. If both tests are abnormal, it is likely that the patient has a platelet dysfunction and further testing for inherited or acquired bleeding disorders is indicated. If the collagen/ADP test is normal, then the abnormal collagen/EPI test may be due to aspirin ingestion. This is the most frequently encountered abnormal collagen/EPI result as a single dose of aspirin can affect platelet function for approximately 10 days.

Although the PFA-100 test has gained acceptance as a useful screen for platelet dysfunction, there is no consensus that it is the replacement test for the bleeding time. The PFA-100 has not been shown to be able to predict the likelihood that a patient will bleed excessively during surgery and its full clinical utility has yet to be established.

Platelet aggregometry (PAA) is considered the gold standard for platelet function analysis. It is widely used in academic centers and large hospitals. One or two tubes of blood are drawn from a vein, and the response of either whole blood or platelet-rich plasma to specific agents known to induce aggregation of platelets is studied. In such a test, a beam of light passes through a suspension of stirred platelets and the percent transmission is measured. When an agonist such as thrombin is added, a small initial drop in light transmission typically occurs as platelets change shape from discs to spheres. As platelet aggregation occurs, light transmission increases (Fig. 19.3). Platelet aggregation tests use a battery of agonists such as ADP, collagen, ristocetin, and arachidonic acid. This test is used to diagnose inherited and acquired platelet function disorders. It is affected by aspirin and a variety of other drugs that alter platelet function.

There are many other platelet function tests that measure particular aspects of platelet aggregation or clot formation. Some are still only being used for research, whereas others are being used by some doctors for specific purposes. The VerifyNow Aspirin Assay [formerly Ultegra rapid platelet function assay-aspirin (RPFA-ASA)], for instance, is a test that may be ordered to help detect platelet dysfunction due to aspirin ingestion; VerifyNow IIb/IIIa Assay is a test that may be used to monitor abciximab (an antiplatelet therapy); and Plateletworks is a testing method used to monitor changes in platelet function by measuring aggregation ability.

An older test that is staging a comeback is thromboelastography or (TEG), which measures clot strength and has been used to monitor platelet function and coagulation during cardiovascular surgery and to predict bleeding and monitor blood transfusion effectiveness during cardiopulmonary surgery. It should be noted that because most samples for platelet function testing are only stable for a very short period of time, testing choices are often limited to what is locally available.

The Coagulation Cascade and Formation of the Fibrin Clot

During secondary hemostasis, the fragile platelet plug becomes a mechanically strong clot. The coagulation system is now thought of as one central reaction (18) in which a serine protease and a nonenzymatically active protein cofactor assemble on cell membranes in the presence of calcium ions, speeding up critical reactions by a factor of 10^4 to 10^5.

The enzymes and cofactors of the coagulation system are numbered with Roman numerals in order of discovery; therefore, the numbers do not relate to the order in which they appear in the reaction. Eponyms and descriptive terms are encountered occasionally and are listed in Table 19.4.

Most of these enzymes and factors are synthesized in the liver. Factors which require vitamin K for synthesis are termed *vitamin K–dependent factors* (Table 19.5) (19). Although some vitamin K is synthesized by gastrointestinal flora, an additional dietary intake of 1 to 3 $\mu g/kg/d$ is required. A normal person will develop vitamin K deficiency 1 to 2 weeks after cessation of oral vitamin K intake. Two of the vitamin K–dependent factors, protein C and protein S, form part of a critical anticoagulant system that limits the formation of thrombosis, discussed later in this chapter.

Fibrinogen is produced in large quantities by the liver and has a serum half-life of 3 days. Hepatic output is increased in response to inflammatory stimuli, including a number of monokines, and therefore fibrinogen is one of the so-called acute phase reactants. Fibrinogen is the stable precursor of fibrin, the monomer from which fibrin clots are built.

Thrombin cleaves fibrinogen into fibrin, which then polymerizes into long strands to glue platelets and erythrocytes together in the growing clot. Circulating enzymes and cofactors of the coagulation cascade provide a mechanism for controlled generation of thrombin through the prothrombinase reaction (Fig. 19.4) (20–29). "The prothrombinase complex catalyzes in 2 minutes what free factor Xa would catalyze in 1 year (30)." Platelets probably form

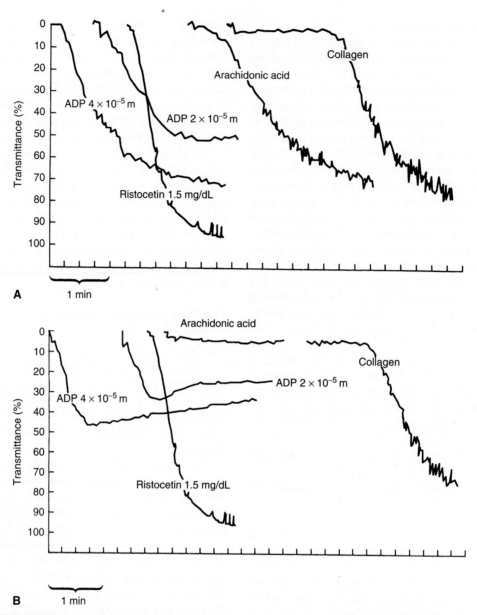

FIGURE 19.3 Platelet aggregometer tracings. The response of normal platelets is shown in the *top tracing*. Aspirin significantly impairs the response to all aggregating agents with the exception of ristocetin (*bottom tracing*). The aspirin effect is irreversible and lasts for the lifetime of the platelet. ADP, adenosine diphosphate.

the most important site of prothrombinase assembly during *in vivo* clotting.

Prothrombin accumulates on membrane surfaces in the vicinity of the prothrombinase complex. Factor Va increases this reaction speed by 10,000 times. Thrombin accelerates the conversion of factor V, the circulating and relatively inactive form, to factor Va. Factor V is inactivated by protein C; a genetic polymorphism (factor V Leiden) may render factor V resistant to protein C inactivation, resulting in a hypercoagulable state (20,31).

The activity of the prothrombinase complex is carefully modulated by thrombin, the inactivation of factor Va by activated protein C, and inhibition by the antithrombin III system (30).

The primary activator of blood coagulation is a complex of tissue factor (TF) and activated factor VII complex (TF-VIIa). This is inhibited by tissue factor pathway inhibitor (TFPI), sufficient factor Xa is left to generate thrombin. The small amount of thrombin left over is sufficient to activate cofactors V and VIII. The activation of VIII with factor IX proceeds to convert factor X to factor Xa and to continue the generation of thrombin and eventually the fibrin for the fibrin clot. Therefore, factor XII, prekallikrein, and high molecular weight kininogen (HMWK) deficiencies prolong the aPTT but do not cause bleeding (30).

Thrombin not only produces fibrin but also downregulates the coagulation cascade by binding to thrombomodulin on the endothelial cell surface. It is a potent platelet agonist,

TABLE 19.4

Names Associated with Coagulation Enzymes and Cofactors

Factor	Name
I	Fibrinogen
II	Prothrombin
III	Tissue factor
IV	Ionized calcium
V	Proaccelerin
VII	Proconvertin
VIII	Antihemophilic factor
IX	Christmas factor
X	Stuart-Prower factor
XI	Plasma thromboplastin antecedent
XII	Hageman factor
XIII	Fibrin stabilizing factor

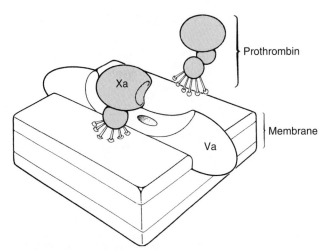

FIGURE 19.4 The prothrombinase complex consists of factors Xa and Va on a suitable phospholipid membrane surface in the presence of calcium ions. Platelet activation by thrombin results in exposure or steric change in membrane receptors, which act as binding sites for Xase and the prothrombinase complex.

stimulating platelet aggregation, and it acts as a chemoattractant for monocytes. By binding to monocytes, thrombin induces the release of interleukin 1(IL-1), causing a number of substances [including plasminogen-activator inhibitor 1 (PAI-1), which depresses activity of the fibrinolytic system] to be synthesized (30).

As fibrin polymerization progresses, a small amount of thrombin is incorporated within the growing clot. This may serve to limit the spread of thrombin outside the region of thrombus formation but may also yield a burst of procoagulant material when clot lysis occurs.

Factor XIIIa stimulates cross-linkage of fibrin to produce a mechanically stable clot. In its absence, the clot is weak and wound healing is impaired. Fibrin enhances the rate of activation of factor XIII.

Assessment of Coagulation In vitro

Two measures of *in vitro* coagulation, the prothrombin time [reported as International Normalized Ratio(INR)] and partial thromboplastin time (PTT), are used as screening tests for disorders of the coagulation cascade and to monitor anticoagulant therapy (Fig. 19.5). These tests are relatively crude and are generally not prolonged until factor levels fall below 30% of normal.

In the one-step *prothrombin time* test, a mixture of calcium and thromboplastin is added to citrated blood and the time to clot formation is measured. The PT value reflects the coagulation ability of the extrinsic coagulation

pathway. It is commonly used in monitoring the therapeutic effect of warfarin. The PT is prolonged by deficiencies in factors VII (activated by TF on a phospholipid surface in the presence of calcium), X (converted to Xa by VIIa), factor V, prothrombin, and fibrinogen. It is used clinically to monitor oral anticoagulation with coumarin-type drugs.

Tissue thromboplastin is a mixture of TF, a necessary cofactor in the extrinsic Xase system, and phospholipid membrane fragments on which the system assembles. Depending on the laboratory, normal PT averages 12 ± 2 seconds, but because tissue thromboplastins vary, PT results vary between laboratories. The INR, defined as the ratio of the patient's PT to the individual laboratory standard, provides a standardized way to report the prothrombin time relative to control.

The *PTT* measures the slower intrinsic pathway. *In vitro*, this requires all of the clotting factors with the exception of factor VII. Normal levels of Hageman factor (factor XII), prekallikrein, and HMWK are required for a normal PTT, but do not appear to be important *in vivo* because individuals lacking these factors do not bleed abnormally. The PTT is used commonly to monitor anticoagulation with heparin (31).

The lupus anticoagulant is an acquired anticardiolipin antibody that prolongs the PTT by inhibiting the activity of the phospholipid used in the test. Clinical bleeding is rare. This rare antibody has been identified in a wide variety of autoimmune disorders, in association with drugs, in acute infections, and in patients with neoplasia. Despite the elevated PTT, an increased risk of venous thrombosis or spontaneous abortions may be seen in some patients (26,28,32).

The *thrombin time* (TT) measures the thrombin-induced conversion of fibrinogen to fibrin and is prolonged in states of decreased fibrinogen or by the presence of an abnormal form

TABLE 19.5

Vitamin K-Dependent Coagulation Factors

II (prothrombin)	X
VII	Protein C
IX	Protein S

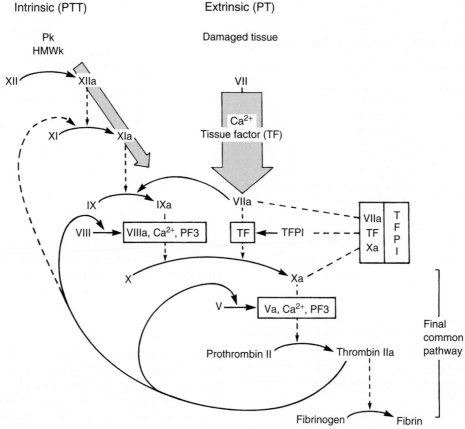

FIGURE 19.5 Overview of the coagulation cascade showing components assessed by prothrombin time (PT) and partial thromboplastin time (PTT). The path of primary *in vivo* significance is the so-called "extrinsic" pathway, initiated by tissue damage. Components along this pathway are assessed using PT. Components along the "intrinsic" pathway are assessed using PTT. Thrombin exerts feedback effects at various points in the cascade, as shown by the loops. Tissue factor pathway inhibitor (TFPI) has an inhibitory effect that modulates the response. TF, tissue factor.

of fibrinogen, or circulating anticoagulants, includingfibrin degradation products (FDPs). This test is a useful screen for hypofibrinogenemia when a quantitative fibrinogen is not available. Its marked sensitivity to heparin rules out this test for most hospitalized patients with keep-open arterial lines.

The *activated clotting time* (ACT) is a measurement of the ability of whole blood to clot. This test is commonly applied to monitor heparin levels intraoperatively to adjusted the dose of anecdote (Protamine). The ACT measurement corresponded in a linear manner with increase or decrease heparin doses, as well as Protamine dosing. It is commonly accepted that ACT of 360 to 600 seconds are adequate for extracorporeal bypass whereas it is kept at 250 seconds or greater for the majority of vascular procedures. At the end of the operative procedures, or coming off extracorporeal bypass, most surgeons want to correct the ACT value to less than 150 seconds to minimized postoperative bleeding.

Disorders of the Coagulation Cascade

In the congenital disorders of coagulation, individual clotting factors are produced in decreased numbers or in abnormal forms. These are conventionally grouped according to the

factor that is diminished or abnormal (e.g., factor VIII in hemophilia A). Factor levels must be significantly below normal before screening tests such as the PT and PTT are prolonged. Affected individuals vary in the severity of bleeding problems, depending on how much of the factor is present or how abnormal it is. For example, in hemophilia A, the PTT remains normal until factor VIII falls below 30% of normal levels. A personal or family history of spontaneous bleeding, especially bleeding into joints, soft tissues, or body cavities, or a history of abnormal bleeding after surgery or trauma are important clues (33–36).

When surgery is necessary in individuals with coagulation disorders, replacement therapy is guided by serum factor levels. The amount of required factor and its half-life *in vivo* vary considerably. These patients are best managed in cooperation with an experienced hematologist. Factor levels must be typically maintained (although at a lower level) until all sutures and drains are out, or the risk of complications is passed. Additional factor replacement at the time of suture removal may be required. In some disorders, wound healing is delayed. This should be anticipated and sutures should be left in for a longer period than usual. Topical hemostatic agents and fibrin glue may be useful but cannot replace meticulous hemostasis (36).

Hemophilia A, or classic hemophilia (factor VIII deficiency) is a sex-linked recessive genetic condition that is by far the most commonly inherited coagulation disorder, occurring in approximately 1 of 10,000 male births and accounting for 80% of all congenital factor deficiencies. Clinical manifestations correlate with factor VIII levels, which vary from less than 1% in severely affected individuals to as high as 40% in those with mild hemophilia. Patients with factor VIII levels greater than 5% rarely bleed spontaneously but will have bleeding problems after surgery or trauma. Most carriers of hemophilia A have factor VIII levels that are greater than 50% and have no difficulty with spontaneous bleeding or with abnormal bleeding after surgery (37,38). 1-Deamino-8-D-arginine vasopressin (DDAVP) causes release of endogenous factor VIII from liver sinusoids and endothelial cells, and also releases vWF resulting in a transient increase in factor VIII levels—because the response is variable it should be monitored [bleeding time and activated partial thromboplastin time (aPTT)] (38,39). Sterilized factor VIII concentrates were not available until 1984, and at present, approximately 90% of severely affected multiple transfused hemophiliacs have chronic active or chronic persistent hepatitis. The same percentage is human immunodeficiency virus (HIV) positive (40). Anti–factor VIII antibodies (factor VIII inhibitors) develop in 10% to 15% of severely affected hemophiliacs, usually in response to prior factor VIII infusion. Management of these patients is complicated, and patients with hemophilia A should be screened for factor VIII inhibitors before surgery so that appropriate treatment can be used (41). Factor VIII inhibitors occasionally occur in nonhemophiliac patients and can cause a clinical bleeding diathesis with prolonged PTT and decreased factor VIII levels clinically similar to classic hemophilia (37,38). Factor VIII levels are also decreased in patients with von Willebrand disease because vWF acts as a carrier molecule for factor VIII.

Hemophilia B (Christmas disease or factor IX deficiency) was identified when it was observed that blood from one hemophiliac corrected the prolonged clotting time of another patient with hemophilia. The pattern of inheritance and clinical manifestations are similar. Generally, the PT is normal and the PTT is prolonged; however, factor IX activity must be less than 30% of normal for prolongation to occur. Heat-treated, concentrated preparations of factor IX are available; dosage is important because excessive administration has been associated with venous and arterial thromboses (37,40,41).

Hereditary deficiencies of factor V (parahemophilia), factor VII, factor X (Stuart-Prower factor), and factor XI occur. All are extremely rare. Most are inherited as autosomal recessives, and a great deal of heterogeneity exists within each disorder.

Hageman factor (factor XII) deficiency highlights the difference between coagulation *in vivo* and *in vitro*. Decreased factor XII levels prolong the PTT, but even complete absence of factor XII does not cause abnormal bleeding. Patients deficient in Hageman factor are asymptomatic and are generally identified on screening PTT. The diagnosis is confirmed by specific factor XII assays. No treatment is indicated, as abnormal bleeding does not occur after surgery. Hageman factor is also a component of the intrinsic system for the conversion of plasminogen to plasmin, which causes clot lysis. Whether deficiency of factor XII predisposes to thrombosis is uncertain.

Prekallikrein (Fletcher factor) deficiency and deficiency in HMWK produce clinical syndromes similar to Hageman factor deficiency. The PTT is prolonged, but abnormal bleeding does not occur. Prekallikrein and HMWK are also components of the intrinsic plasminogen activation system.

Several forms of congenital and acquired combined factor deficiency syndromes have been identified. Some of these are caused by deficient enzymes in the vitamin K–dependent carboxylation system. The mechanisms of the other syndromes are unknown. Patients with amyloidosis, the nephrotic syndrome, and Gaucher disease may develop an acquired coagulation disorder owing to increased clearance and/or binding of coagulation factors.

Endothelial Cells and the Regulation of Coagulation

Endothelial cells form a continuous barrier that contains and maintains the fluidity of blood. In a 70-kg adult, the total endothelial cell surface area exceeds 1,000 m^2. More than a simple passive barrier, endothelial cells modulate the hemostatic response by several mechanisms (42–47).

Blood flow in normal vessels is laminar, with the fastest flow in the center of the channel. Erythrocytes and larger formed elements tend to channel in the center. Platelets are found in the slower-moving layers immediately adjacent to the endothelium, and their function is inhibited by substances secreted by endothelial cells.

Stasis, the first element of the Virchow triad, occurs more commonly in larger vessels such as the deep veins of the calf. Here, platelet aggregates may form and transient activation of coagulation enzymes may occur. Reestablishment of blood flow rapidly disperses these aggregates. Regions of abnormal blood flow, such as bifurcations and stenoses, produce turbulence that may contribute to endothelial cell damage and thrombosis (46,47).

Endothelial cells secrete the subendothelial matrix on which they lie. Healthy endothelium forms a functionally seamless coating over this thrombogenic subendothelium. Endothelial cells are joined by intercellular adhesion molecules (ICAMs) which form tight junctions and limit the permeability of the endothelium to plasma and cells. Cells that normally pass through the capillary wall, such as neutrophils, monocytes, basophils, and eosinophils, first adhere to endothelial cell adhesion molecules (ELAMs) by specialized receptors and then pass between endothelial cells. Platelets probably play an important role in the maintenance of capillary integrity. Thrombocytopenia is associated with increased capillary fragility and a measurable increase in permeability to erythrocytes and carbon particles.

Endothelial cells and their basement membrane (subendothelium) constitute the intima of large vessels. This provides an additional mechanical barrier against blood loss after injury and acts as a potent stimulus for platelet aggregation. In vitamin C deficiency, abnormal collagen is formed in the subendothelium and petechial bleeding results despite normal platelet function (47).

Prostacyclin is probably the most important platelet-inactivating substance secreted by endothelial cells. PGI_2 synthesis requires the enzyme cyclo-oxygenase (COX) (which is blocked by aspirin). Despite initial concerns, this aspirin effect does not appear to be clinically significant and is overshadowed by the therapeutic effect on thromboxane A_2 synthesis. Endothelial cells also inactivate ADP, a potent platelet agonist (47).

Endothelial cells have an extremely important role in modulating the coagulation system. Two primary mechanisms have been identified: (i) the presence of cell-surface molecules similar to heparin that bind antithrombin III, inactivating coagulation enzymes; and (ii) thrombomodulin on endothelial cell surfaces binds thrombin, inactivating it and forming a powerful activator of protein C. Endothelial cells also secrete tissue-type plasminogen activator (tPA) that converts fibrin-bound plasminogen to plasmin, initiating clot lysis (46).

Antithrombin (formerly antithrombin III), produced by the liver, forms a complex with thrombin and neutralizes it. Activation of antithrombin by endothelial cells increases the rate of complex formation 1,000-fold. Activated antithrombin is a major inhibitor of thrombin and factor Xa, with some inhibition of factors IX, XI, and XII. Antithrombin is a necessary cofactor for the pharmacologic agent *heparin*, which binds to antithrombin and increases its activity 1,000 to 10,000 times (48–53). Both congenital and acquired states of antithrombin deficiency occur and are associated with pathologic thrombosis. Approximately 2% of patients with idiopathic venous thrombosis have been found to have decreased antithrombin. Specific replacement therapy is available (50–53).

Thrombomodulin is located in high concentration on endothelial cells of all organs except the brain. Thrombin loses its procoagulant properties, including fibrinogen cleavage, factor V activation, and platelet activation, when it is bound by thrombomodulin (54,55). Thrombomodulin provides a means for localizing thrombin effect to the site of injury by limiting its effect in proximity to intact endothelial cells.

Protein C and *protein S* are synthesized in the liver and require vitamin K for carboxylation. Thrombin slowly activates protein C (56). The rate of activation is increased 1,000 times by the binding of thrombin to thrombomodulin on endothelial cell surfaces (Fig. 19.6). Protein S is a necessary cofactor. Activated protein C is a potent inactivator of factors Va and VIIIa (critical enzymes of the coagulation cascade)

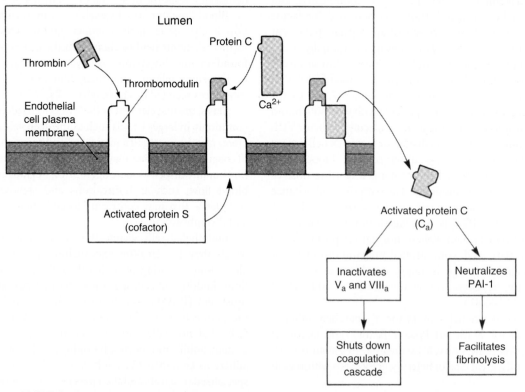

FIGURE 19.6 Thrombomodulin–protein C system. The system is activated when thrombomodulin and thrombin form a complex on the endothelial cell plasma membrane. In addition to shutting down the coagulation cascade, the system contributes to the initiation of fibrinolysis by neutralizing plasminogen activator inhibitor 1 (PAI-1).

and also neutralizes PAI-1 (facilitating fibrinolysis). The protein C pathway provides a link to inflammatory mediators and is important in host defense.

A total of 10% to 15% of patients with unexplained venous thrombosis have been identified as having either protein C or protein S deficiency. Screening of large numbers of blood donors has demonstrated that asymptomatic protein C deficiency is relatively common in the general population, suggesting that an additional factor may be necessary to produce thrombosis. Thrombotic complications (e.g., warfarin-induced skin necrosis) sometimes occur early in the course of oral anticoagulation with vitamin K antagonists and may be more likely in patients deficient in protein C or protein S (57,58). (See further discussion in Pharmacology section.)

Disorders of the Endothelial Cell

Endothelium exposed to endotoxin, IL-1, or tumor necrosis factor (TNF) loses thrombomodulin function. The resulting loss of downregulatory function may contribute to the development of widespread intravascular thrombosis characteristic of DIC. DIC is part of a spectrum of consumptive thrombohemorrhagic disorders, in which inappropriate uncontrolled activation of the hemostatic mechanism occurs, with deposition of thrombus in areas where no local injury exists, resulting in widespread areas of local ischemia, tissue dysfunction, and possibly cellular death. DIC is discussed in more detail with other complex disorders of coagulation.

von Willebrand disease should be suspected in any individual with an increased bleeding time despite a normal platelet count and normal clot retraction. In the more common form of this heterogeneous group of relatively common disorders, endothelial cells do not produce enough vWF, causing a platelet type bleeding diathesis (59,60).

vWF is synthesized by endothelial cells. It is released as multimers of varying molecular weight. Larger multimers have more binding sites and hence function better (60).

The common forms of von Willebrand disease are mostly inherited as autosomal dominants. Because many individuals are only mildly affected, the true incidence in the population is unknown. Ristocetin, an antibiotic that was withdrawn from clinical use because it produced thrombocytopenia, causes platelet agglutination through enhanced binding of plasma vWF to platelet receptors. This ability may be used as a test for von Willebrand disease. This indirect test has been largely superseded by direct measurement of vWF antigen and multimers.

Desmopressin (DDAVP) is a vasopressin analog that causes release of vWF and factor VIII from endothelial cells, resulting in a transient increase in these (61). It is useful in mild forms of von Willebrand disease and is also used in a wide variety of other clotting defects (39,62). Clinical response varies (63).

Many drugs inhibit platelet function, either by design or as a side effect. Mechanisms by which such drugs might act include blocking COX or thromboxane synthetase, blocking the thromboxane A2 receptor, increasing intraplatelet cAMP

or guanosine monophosphate (GMP), or directly blocking platelet receptors. They are discussed in a subsequent section of this chapter.

TTP is a rare disorder in which there is widespread occlusion of the microvasculature with hyaline thrombi. The characteristic triad consists of fluctuating neurologic signs, thrombocytopenia, and microangiopathic hemolytic anemia. Renal dysfunction and fever are often present as well. The primary laboratory hemostatic abnormality is thrombocytopenia. Endothelial cell abnormalities have been identified (64). Plasmapheresis is the most effective treatment and probably acts by removing toxic substances and replacing an inhibitor by infused fresh frozen plasma (FFP). Despite thrombocytopenia, platelet transfusion is not indicated, as this may worsen formation of microthrombi. *Hemolytic-uremic syndrome* is a closely related disorder of infancy and childhood and is occasionally seen in adults. Renal symptoms predominate and neurologic dysfunction is rare. A genetic predisposition seems to exist, but as with TTP, the inciting factor appears to be endothelial cell damage (64).

Thrombosis and Hypercoagulable States

Hypercoagulable states reflect a problem with the third element of the Virchow triad—an imbalance between procoagulant and anticoagulant tendencies (32,65). Specific conditions associated with a thrombotic tendency are listed in Table 19.6. *Factor V Leiden, protein C* and *protein S* deficiencies have previously been discussed. *Antiphospholipid antibody syndrome*, mentioned earlier with the so-called "lupus anticoagulant" is a marker for a thrombotic diathesis whose mechanism is poorly understood (3,26,28).

HIT, an acquired thrombotic diathesis, will be discussed in a subsequent section.

The Fibrinolytic System and Healing

The fibrinolytic system limits thrombus formation to the site of injury (66) and dissolves clot during wound healing, allowing vessels to recanalize. It is tightly regulated by a complex series of activators and inhibitors (Fig. 19.7). When activity of the fibrinolytic system is depressed, a thrombotic diathesis ensues; conversely, overactivity of this system results in bleeding (67,68).

TABLE 19.6

Conditions Associated with Thrombotic Diatheses

Factor V Leiden
Antithrombin deficiency
Protein C deficiency
Protein S deficiency
Hypofibrinolysis
Antiphospholipid antibodies
    "Lupus anticoagulant"
    Anticardiolipin antibodies
Heparin-induced thrombocyptopenia

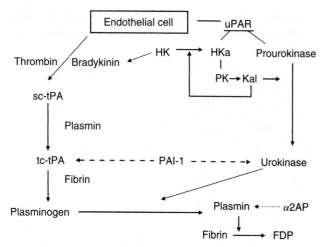

FIGURE 19.7 Fibrinolysis. *Lines* indicate bindings; *thin arrows* indicate transformation or stimulation; *filled arrows* indicate transformation of zymogens to active enzymes; *dashed arrows* indicate inhibition of active enzymes. PAR, HK, high molecular weight kininogen; Hka, kini-free kininogen; PK, prekallikrein; Kal, kallikrein; sc-tPA, single-chain tissue plasminogen activator; tc-tPA, two-chain tissue plasminogen activator; PAI-1, plasminogen activator inhibitor 1; α2AP, α_2-antiplasmin; FDP, fibrinogen deposition products. (From Colman RW, Hirsh J, Marder VJ, et al. Overview of coagulation, fibrinolysis, and their regulation. In: Colman RW, Hirsh J, Marder VJ, et al. eds. *Hemostasis and thrombosis: basic principles and clinical practice*, 4th ed. Philadelphia: Lippincott Williams & Wilkins, 2001:19.)

Plasminogen and Plasmin

Plasminogen (synthesized by the liver) is the circulating precursor of plasmin, the active form of the enzyme. Plasmin can degrade both fibrin and fibrinogen. Normally there is essentially no ongoing fibrinolytic activity (69).

Rare congenital disorders in which an abnormal plasminogen (dysplasminogenemia) or depressed level of normal plasminogen (hypoplasminogenemia) are associated with a thrombotic diathesis, as would be predicted (67,68).

Plasminogen Activators

tPA and urokinase-type plasminogen activator (uPA) both cleave plasminogen, generating plasmin.

The intrinsic tPA is produced by endothelial cells and released into the circulation. High local concentrations of thrombin and conditions of venous stasis stimulate tPA release, which is rapidly cleared by the liver (half-life ~5 minutes). tPA binds avidly to fibrin, bringing it into close proximity to fibrin-bound plasminogen and increasing the enzymatic activity of tPA. This highly clot-specific property of tPA appears to enhance its dose-predictable activity when administered as a therapeutic agent, but it does not enhance its efficacy or safety compared with other agents. (See later discussion in Pharmacology section.)

uPAs are found in limited amounts in the blood. Urokinase is one such uPA that is responsible for the fibrinolytic activity of urine. uPAs lack the fibrin affinity of tPA and do not exhibit a greater enzymatic activity for plasminogen in the presence of fibrin. Urokinase is extremely effective and dose predictable as a thrombolytic agent. (See later discussion in Pharmacology section.)

Inhibitors of Fibrinolysis

The two major physiologic *inhibitors of fibrinolysis* are α_2-antiplasmin and PAI-1. α_2-*Antiplasmin* binds avidly to circulating plasmin and irreversibly inactivates it, preventing a generalized fibrinolytic state in the circulating blood. Within a thrombus, the situation is more complex. During clot formation, small amounts of α_2-antiplasmin are incorporated within the fibrin mesh and are bound covalently to fibrin as factor XIIIa stimulates fibrin cross-linkage. Mature clots in which fibrin cross-linkage has occurred are much more resistant to plasmin than fresh thrombi for this reason. When plasmin is subsequently generated within the thrombus, it must saturate the binding sites of this inhibitor before clot lysis occurs. This prevents premature clot lysis. Plasmin bound to fibrin is relatively resistant to inactivation by α_2-antiplasmin, however, and once the small amount of inhibitor bound within the fibrin is saturated, additional plasmin generated within the thrombus is protected from the effects of circulating inhibitor.

PAI-I is synthesized by endothelial cells and released into the blood and extracellular matrix. It is one of the IL-1 mediated acute phase reactants; therefore, the synthesis and release of PAI-I can occur in response to a variety of stimuli, including bacterial endotoxin. PAI-I binds to and inhibits tPA, preventing cleavage of plasminogen to plasmin and inhibiting fibrinolysis. PAI-I is elevated in patients with acute myocardial infarction, and elevation of PAI-I may represent the most common abnormality of the hemostatic system that predisposes to thrombosis (70).

PAI-II can be isolated from the trophoblastic epithelium of the placenta during pregnancy and occurs in increasing amounts in maternal plasma. A corresponding decrease in fibrinolytic activity occurs, which peaks at the time of separation of the placenta and then rapidly returns to normal. This protective mechanism helps prevent exsanguinating hemorrhage from the raw surface of the uterus, but it accounts in part for the increased incidence of venous thromboembolism and may contribute to the pathophysiology of eclampsia (70,71).

Hyperfibrinolysis

Hyperfibrinolysis, or pathologic activation of the fibrinolytic mechanism, occurs in response to severe stress, heat stroke, and in association with certain neoplasms. Currently, it occurs most often as a side effect of fibrinolytic therapy (70–73).

Complex Disorders of Hemostasis and Thrombosis

In complex disorders, an abnormality of more than one component of the hemostatic mechanism exists. DIC and the bleeding diathesis associated with uremia and liver disease are all commonly encountered in surgical practice. The

TABLE 19.7

Causes of Disseminated Intravascular Coagulation

Sepsis
  Gram-negative bacteria
  Gram-positive bacteria
Viruses
Hemolysis (massive)
  Transfusion of incompatible blood
Ischemia
Hypotension
Hypoperfusion
Trauma
  Brain injury
Systemic inflammatory response syndrome (SIRS)
Obstetrical emergencies
  Abruptio placentae
  Amniotic fluid embolism
  Pre-eclampsia
Snake bite
Localized disseminated intravascular coagulation
  Aneurysms
  Hemangiomas
Allograft rejection
Glomerulonephritis
Malignancy
  Prostate cancer
  Acute promyelocytic leukemia

Adapted from Bick RL. Disseminated intravascular coagulation: objective clinical and laboratory diagnosis, treatment, and assessment of therapeutic response. *Semin Thromb Hemost* 1996; 22:69–88.

TABLE 19.8

Laboratory Abnormalities in Disseminated Intravascular Coagulation

Decresed platelets
Decreased fibrinogen
Decreased prothrombin
Decreased levels of factors V, VIII, XII
Increased fibrin degradation products
  Fibrin D-dimers

mucinous adenocarcinoma) may develop a characteristic migratory thrombophlebitis.

The laboratory abnormalities and clinical manifestations in DIC reflect consumption of clotting elements and enhanced fibrinolysis (Table 19.8). The combination of D-dimer and FDPs provides a rapid and specific test (1).

Therapy is primarily directed at correcting the underlying condition while supporting the patient with transfusion of specific hemostatic elements. In surgical patients, a vigorous search for sepsis should be considered. Supportive care with replacement of platelets and clotting factors is appropriate in the bleeding patients, and concern that this will "fuel the fire" of DIC-associated thrombosis seems to be unwarranted. Treatment with heparin may be appropriate for the patients with DIC and primarily thrombotic manifestations. Even when fibrinolysis is a prominent component, treatment with inhibitors of the fibrinolytic system is fraught with hazard as it may cause widespread deposition of thrombus throughout the microcirculation. For this reason, antifibrinolytic agents such as ε-aminocaproic acid (EACA) should not be given alone but always accompanied by the administration of heparin (77,78).

consequences of massive transfusion, including coagulopathy, are discussed in a subsequent section of this chapter.

Disseminated Intravascular Coagulation

DIC is the manifestation of an underlying disease process (Table 19.7) and may be classified as acute or chronic. The clinical picture may be dominated primarily by bleeding or by thrombosis. Classic causes of acute DIC, usually with hemorrhagic manifestations, include obstetrical emergencies (abruptio placentae and amniotic fluid embolism), infection, and massive brain trauma (74,75). Acute DIC in surgical patients is heralded frequently by bleeding, with oozing from all tubes, wounds, and vascular access sites. Shock, ischemia, and infection are the most common precipitating factors. Severe acidosis and multiple blood transfusions often complicate the picture (76).

Less commonly in surgical practice, DIC causes microcirculatory thrombosis. Manifestations include dermal ischemia, renal failure, focal neurologic signs, delirium and coma, and gastrointestinal ulcerations. These are more commonly seen in patients with the chronic forms of DIC. Localized deposition of fibrin with laboratory evidence of DIC may occur in allograft rejection and proliferative glomerulonephritis. Patients with malignancy (particularly

Uremia

Uremia may cause a complex bleeding diathesis characterized by abnormal platelet function and improved by dialysis. In some patients, thrombocytopenia is present and contributes to the problem. However, transfused platelets are ineffective and rapidly become abnormal. Platelet adherence to subendothelial collagen is impaired. Although the total amount of circulating vWF may be normal, the largest vWF multimers (which may be most important for platelet adhesion) are decreased. Platelet synthesis of thromboxane A$_2$ is decreased, and uremic platelets have lower than normal concentrations of serotonin, ADP, and vWF. Endothelial prostacyclin production increases and, paradoxically, levels of endothelially derived vWF increase (79). Fibrinogen and several of the clotting factors may be decreased. Antithrombin and protein C are decreased, and the fibrinolytic system is impaired, probably the result of circulating inhibitors.

The main treatment for uremic bleeding is adequate dialysis and elevation of the hematocrit (Hct). The effects of dialysis last 2 to 3 days. Cryoprecipitate infusion and DDAVP may also correct the bleeding problem. Conjugated estrogens shorten the bleeding time in uremia by an unknown mechanism, providing an effect that lasts 10 to 15 days (80,81). They have been most useful in patients with gastrointestinal bleeding and telangiectasias (82).

Liver Disease

Severe liver disease produces a coagulopathy by several mechanisms. Synthesis of all coagulation factors, with the exception of factor VIII, is decreased. Vitamin K deficiency may result from decreased oral intake, malabsorption, or biliary obstruction, resulting in deficiency of the vitamin K–dependent procoagulant and anticoagulant factors. Fibrinogen synthesis is decreased in severe liver failure, and an abnormal fibrinogen may be produced. This hypofibrinogenemia may also adversely affect platelet function. Thrombocytopenia is common in patients with portal hypertension and secondary hypersplenism (82).

Endotoxin absorbed from the gut is poorly cleared from the portal circulation and may spill over into the systemic circulation, resulting in chronic low-grade DIC. Poor hepatic clearance of plasminogen activators results in a state of systemic fibrinolysis.

Peritoneovenous shunting for ascites (LeVeen or Denver shunt) causes direct infusion of procoagulant material into the venous circulation, again triggering DIC (82). Treatment of these multifactorial abnormalities involves replacement of clotting factors with FFP, cryoprecipitate, and vitamin K as needed (83).

Multiple Myeloma and Other Hematologic Malignancies

Surgeons have known for decades that patients with plasma cell dyscrasias and other hematologic malignancies are prone to bleed. In multiple myeloma, acquired vWF and factor X deficiencies have been reported. Inhibition of fibrin polymerization, the presence of a circulating heparin-like anticoagulant, as well as thrombin inhibitors have all been described (84–90). The details of these various mechanisms and their implications for surgical hemostasis are still being elucidated.

Pharmacologic Manipulation of Coagulation

Antiplatelet Agents

The protocol agent is acetyl salicylic acid (Aspirin, ASA). It is commonly classified as a nonsteroidal anti-inflammatory drug, rather than an antiplatelet agent. Aspirin differs from other antiplatelet agents by also exerting a strong antithrombotic effect and preventing clot propagation in vessels.

Aspirin noncompetitively and irreversibly inhibits COX, thereby suppressing the production of prostaglandins and thromboxanes. Inhibition of this enzyme blocks the formation of thromboxane A2 from arachidonic acid, thereby reducing platelet aggregation, shape changes, and release reactions. The platelet inhibitory effect appears within 1 to 7.5 minutes after oral administration. The duration of action is 4 to 6 hours. Aspirin is hydrolyzed by hepatic esterases and to a lesser extent in plasma and erythrocytes.

Aspirin has significant antithrombotic effects when compared to other antiplatelet agents. When used alone, it significantly reduces the incidence of transient ischemic attacks and postoperative venous thromboembolism. In combination with other antiplatelet agents, aspirin can reduce reocclusion rates of coronary artery bypass grafts and has been used successfully in TTP. Selective thromboxane synthetase inhibitors may be necessary to reduce thromboxane levels without also decreasing prostacyclin generation.

Aspirin passes the placental barrier, but fetal levels are generally lower than maternal because of placental esterase. Aspirin is generally not recommended during the last trimester of pregnancy; however, randomized clinical trials have demonstrated that low-dose aspirin can help prevent toxemia of pregnancy.

Other nonsteroidal anti-inflammatory drugs, such as indomethacin and ibuprofen, apparently bind to the same COX inhibitory site as aspirin. This binding blocks the acetylation of COX by aspirin; therefore concomitant indomethacin or ibuprofen administration with aspirin can reduce the long-lasting effect of aspirin on platelet aggregation.

Other antiplatelet agents include clopidogrel (Plavix), ticlopidine (Ticlid), and dipyridamole (Persantine). Their mechanism of action is slightly different from Aspirin. Reversal of the effects of these agents requires transfusion of new platelets or by de novo platelet production as the serum drug level declined.

Clopidogrel's mechanism of action is selective, irreversible inhibition of ADP-induced platelet aggregation; with no significant effect on thromboxane A2 or prostacyclin synthesis, or phospholipase A activity (91). With use of clopidogrel, complete recovery of platelet function did not occur till 7 days after ingestion of the last dose of drug. Clopidogrel is an analog of ticlopidine. ADP-induced platelet aggregation was inhibited to a similar degree by clopidogrel 75 mg once daily, and ticlopidine 250 mg twice daily (92).

Ticlopidine is an inhibitor of platelet function with a mechanism which is different from other antiplatelet drugs. The antiplatelet effect of ticlopidine is not apparent in vitro. When the drug is studied in vivo, it appears that inhibition results from a direct effect on platelets, rather than a plasma component, but that ticlopidine itself does not act directly on circulating platelets. Another possibility is that ticlopidine exerts an effect on platelets as they are formed in the bone marrow (93–96). This mechanism, however, is perhaps unlikely based on the demonstration of antiplatelet activity so soon (4 hours) after an oral dose.

Dipyridamole inhibits phosphodiesterase to increase levels of cAMP in the platelet. This effect potentiates the platelet deaggregating effects of prostacyclin, which also increases cAMP (97). The effect of dipyridamole may not be due only to its effect on phosphodiesterase, but also on its ability to increase prostacyclin production (98) and by its ability to inhibit adenosine metabolism (99–103) or to inhibit erythrocyte uptake of adenosine (104–107). Dipyridamole also potentiates the inhibitory effects of aspirin on platelet aggregation, but the effect of aspirin in blocking cyclo-oxygenase activity may prevent the dipyridamole-induced increase in prostacyclin release (108).

Antithrombin Agents

Unfractionated heparin (UFH) and low molecular weight heparin (LMWH) are the most commonly used antithrombin agents in clinical practice. Heparin is a mucopolysaccharide organic acid composed of the sulfated units, α-D-glucuronic acid and 2-amino-2-deoxy-α-D-glucose. Its molecular weight ranges from 6,000 to 20,000. Heparin can be found in the mast cells of many animal tissues, including the lung, liver, and intestine. The commonly used products are extracted either from bovine lung or porcine gut mucosa. There does not appear to be a clinically significant difference between these two sources.

The anticoagulant properties are a direct result of heparin's strong electronegative charge, which enables it to combine with many different proteins. Heparin is generally thought to work primarily through the intrinsic clotting system (109). The effect is mediated directly by inhibiting thrombin-activated conversion of fibrinogen to fibrin (110–113). It blocks the activation of factor IX and neutralizes activated factor X by activating factor X inhibitor (114). Heparin may also enhance the effects of an α-2 globulin molecule which inhibits thrombin and blocks conversion of fibrinogen to fibrin (114). The α-2 globulin molecule is thought to be the same as antithrombin III, a potent inhibitor of factor X (115). Therefore, inhibition of factor X, which is central to both clotting systems, will block the formation of relatively large amounts of later reaction products. This helps explain why only small amounts of heparin are needed to prevent thrombosis, while large amounts are needed to actively treat it.

Standard heparin must be administered parenterally. Commercially available heparin contains molecular weights ranging from 4,000 to 40,000 Da. The low molecular weight fractions are rapidly absorbed orally (although this is not clinically used at present). Intramuscular absorption is unpredictable and associated with pain and hematoma formation. Subcutaneous administration is also variable, but clinically useful.

Intravenous administration produces an immediate on-set of action. ACT values peaked within 2 minutes and lost 25.7% within 2 to 20 minutes of bolus administration in one study (116). An effect can be detected within 20 to 30 minutes of subcutaneous injection. Heparin binds to low-density lipoprotein, globulins (including the α-globulin antithrombin III), and fibrinogen. It does not cross the placenta. Heparin is metabolized by N-desulfation and may be cleared by resident phagocytes. Half-life after UFH administration is unchanged in patients with abnormal renal function, suggesting that renal clearance is not a significant mechanism. In contrast, LMWH clearance from the plasma is renal dependent and the dose must be adjusted in renal dysfunction.

There is no evidence that heparin is active on formed thrombi. It does serve, however, to present distal propagation of further thrombus and the thrombin-mediated platelet aggregation which follows. Heparin also promotes clearance of lipids from plasma by stimulating the release of lipoprotein lipase. It also suppresses secretion of aldosterone; however, this effect is probably only important in patients on extended heparin therapy and potassium supplementation. Long-term heparin administration (10,000 U daily for 6–12 months) can produce osteoporosis.

Heparin is the parental anticoagulant of choice for treatment and prophylaxis of deep venous thrombosis (DVT) and pulmonary embolism. It is also used for treatment of DIC (see previous sections). It is used to prevent blood from clotting in extracorporeal circuits and to maintain patency of indwelling intravenous catheters. Heparin is preferred over warfarin in pregnant patients because warfarin (see subsequent section) crosses the placental barrier and can cause fetal malformation and hemorrhage. Low-dose subcutaneous heparin is used for prophylaxis for thrombosis in high-risk patients such as the elderly following orthopaedic surgery.

Full-dose heparin therapy is usually the initial treatment of deep vein thrombosis or pulmonary embolus, because of its immediate onset of anticoagulation. Warfarin requires 3 to 5 days to achieve full therapeutic effects, and should therefore be started as soon as possible while the patient is still receiving heparin. Subcutaneous heparin has been tested as an alternative to warfarin therapy with mixed results. It may be associated with less bleeding than warfarin, but has not been proved to be as effective. In addition, frequent injections, increased cost, and risk of thrombocytopenia make chronic heparin therapy somewhat less desirable than warfarin.

LMWHs (e.g., enoxaparin 1 mg/kg subcutaneously) are largely comparable to UFH in producing anticoagulation for prophylaxis and treatment of DVT and during hemodialysis. Preliminary data suggests that LMWH may be useful in patients with a history of HIT (see subsequent text), but more clinical trials are needed.

Although being a weak anticoagulant, protamine sulfate is an effective antidote for heparin overdose. It binds heparin in a 1:1 ratio, thereby preventing heparin from enhancing the anticoagulant effect of antithrombin III. Heparin reversal is frequently required in cardiovascular surgery, especially when coming off extracorporeal bypass. Protamine is dosed based on ACT measurement. Protamine affects only circulating heparin; therefore, initial reversal might not be adequate as extravascular heparin reenters the circulation,—a so-called heparin rebound (117). The heparin neutralization occurs 5 minutes after Protamine administration and its elimination half-life is 7.4 minutes (118–120) The major side effects of Protamine administration include pulmonary vasoconstriction and systematic hypotension (121–123).

Heparin-Associated Thrombocytopenia

The etiology of heparin-associated thrombocytopenia (HAT) is not clearly understood. It may involve other risk factors such as comorbid disease states, pulmonary catheter use, transfusions, and length of stay in intensive care.

Two distinct types of thrombocytopenia have been described. The first type occurs in 1% to 30% of patients receiving heparin, and is a result of temporary platelet aggregation, margination, and peripheral sequestration (124). The degree of platelet count reduction is usually mild and transient, occurring after 2 to 4 days of heparin therapy. Thrombocytopenia resolves despite the continued administration of heparin.

The second type of thrombocytopenia is thought to be mediated by a heparin-dependent IgG antibody that induces thromboxane-B2 synthesis, ^{14}C-serotonin release, and platelet aggregation (121,123–125). An incidence of 0.6% to 10% has been reported in patients receiving heparin (126). A rapid reduction in the platelet count generally occurs on the fourth to eighth day of heparin therapy. This type of thrombocytopenia will not resolve with continued therapy. Patients with this form of thrombocytopenia are predisposed to thromboembolic events that may result in limb amputation or death. This paradoxical phenomenon of heparin-induced thrombosis is also known as the *white clot syndrome*. The clot consists almost entirely of fibrin and platelet aggregates that give it the characteristic white color.

The clinical picture is rather characteristic. A patient receiving heparin for several days develops petechiae, purpura, melena, or some other manifestations of a diffuse hemorrhagic disorder and is found to have profound thrombocytopenia (127). Other major features of this disorder include increase in heparin tolerance, and recurrent myocardial, cerebral, pulmonary, and/or peripheral arterial thromboembolism (127). There is no relation between the amount of heparin administered and the severity of thrombocytopenia (126). If the heparin is discontinued, the platelet count will increase rapidly within 48 to 72 hours (128). Thrombocytopenia may recur if the individual is rechallenged with heparin as reported in one study (129). Heparin therapy should be withdrawn if thrombocytopenia is severe or if thrombocytopenia and an acute thrombotic event occur during therapy (130). The development of new thrombosis and thrombocytopenia during heparin administration warrants immediate withdrawal and substitution with alternative therapy. The etiology of HAT is not clearly understood and may involve other risk factors such as comorbid disease states, pulmonary catheter use, transfusions, and length of stay in the intensive care unit (ICU). HAT often appears within 48 to 72 hours of heparin initiation with smaller declines in platelet count than HIT (131).

HAT is usually diagnosed by assays employing either PAA and/or carbon-14-serotonin release assay (SRA). A new assay, heparin-induced platelet activation (HIPA), is faster, and is just as accurate as SRA (132). HIPA can also test for cross reactivity with other types of heparin. This may allow patients with HAT who need to remain on anticoagulant therapy to be switched to a better-tolerated heparin product thereby providing uninterrupted therapy and improving clinical outcome.

HIT, similar but different from HAT type II, is also an immune, IgG-mediated condition that occurs rarely in patients treated with UFH or, less commonly, LMWH (129). HIT is considered an immune reaction involving newly developed antibodies to heparin-platelet factor IV complexes. This typically manifests 5 to 10 days after heparin initiation or earlier if recently exposed to heparin. An SRA and enzyme-linked immunosorbent assay are currently available for diagnosis of HIT. One of the serious sequelae of HIT is paradoxical thrombosis.

Heparin-induced thrombocytopenia associated with thrombosis (HITT), the white clot syndrome, is a serious complication of heparin therapy which may lead to death or major morbidity (133). The incidence of HITT is below 1%; much less common than HIT. Aggressive screening of patients with heparin-associated antiplatelet antibodies, and early diagnosis of HIT decreased morbidity and mortality (7.4% and 1.1% respectively) in a group of 100 patients with positive platelet aggregation tests.

Low Molecular Weight Heparin

There are many different brands of LMWH available on the market, corresponding to different methods of heparin depolymerization. These agents have numerous differences from UFH (**Table 19.9**). The equivalence of different preparations with similar molecular weights but different preparation methods has not been established. Because LMWH can be given subcutaneously and does not require aPTT monitoring, it permits outpatient management of conditions that previously required hospitalization. The use of LMWH must be monitored closely in patients at extremes of weight or with renal dysfunction. LMWH may not be feasible in patients with end-stage renal disease. Anti–factor Xa activity may be useful for monitoring anticoagulation during LMWH therapy. The therapeutic target should be a 4-hour postinjection anti-Xa level of 1.0 IU/mL.

Hirudin

Hirudin, isolated from salivary glands of the medicinal leech, is the most potent noncovalent inhibitor of thrombin. It

---

TABLE 19.9

Differences between Low Molecular Weight Heparin (LMWH) and Unfractionated Heparin (UFH)

- LMWH averages 3,000 Da compared to an average of 20,000 Da for UFH
- LMWH is dosed once daily rather than by continuous infusion
- It is not necessary to monitor aPTT for LMWH
- The risk of bleeding may be lower with LMWH
- The risk of osteoporosis associated with long-term use may be reduced for LMWH
- The risk of HIT is smaller with LMWH

aPTT, activated partial thromboplastin time; HIT, heparin-induced thrombocytopenia.

is a natural anticoagulant with a single peptide chain of 65 amino acids; its molecular weight is 7,000. It selectively binds thrombin in a 1:1 manner at each of two sites on the enzyme: (i) the domain that recognizes fibrinogen, and (ii) the catalytic domain. Because of the specificity of binding, hirudin does not inhibit other enzymes in the coagulation or fibrinolytic pathways, such as factor Xa, factor IXa, kallikrein, activated protein C, plasmin or tPA.

Hirudin produces a dose-dependent increase in the aPTT, prothrombin time and TT. Unlike heparin, which commonly produces wide fluctuations in the aPTT measurement, hirudin maintains a stable aPTT during its infusion period. The ability to achieve a more stable aPTT may be an important benefit because it avoids periods of inadequate anticoagulation. In addition to a dose-dependent increase in the aPTT, hirudin achieves a very consistent level of anticoagulation. In contrast to heparin, hirudin (i) does not require antithrombin as a cofactor, (ii) is not inactivated by anti-heparin protein, (iii) has no direct effect on platelets, and (iv) may also inactivate thrombin bound to clots or to subendothelium.

Hirudin has a very narrow therapeutic window. The hirudin–thrombin complex circulates in the blood for 4 to 6 hours, after which it is cleared by the reticuloendothelial system. Circulating free hirudin is excreted by the kidneys and, therefore, dose adjustment must be made in the setting of renal dysfunction. The dose-dependent elimination half-life is 1 to 2 hours. Because it is a foreign polypeptide, hirudin may elicit an immunologic response.

Hirudin and synthetic analogs of hirudin are being developed using recombinant deoxyribonucleic acid (DNA) technology. *Bivalirudin*, a synthetic congener of hirudin, is currently available in Europe and pending U.S. Food and Drug Administration (FDA) approval in the united States. These drugs are alternatives to heparin for the treatment of (i) unstable angina, (ii) abrupt closure and restenosis following coronary angioplasty, and (iii) prevention of deep vein thrombosis after major orthopaedic surgery. They are also used as adjunct to fibrinolytic therapy. They are also choices for the anticoagulant treatment of patients with HIT with thromboembolic complications.

The primary adverse effect of hirudin is bleeding. Most bleeding events occur at invasive sites. An antidote is not yet available.

Argatroban

Argatroban is a small molecule direct thrombin inhibitor. It is approved for prophylaxis or treatment of thrombosis in patients with HIT, and for use during percutaneous coronary interventions in patients who have or at risk for developing HIT. Argatroban is given intravenously. Time to peak concentration with intravenous infusion is 1 to 3 hours. Argatroban is metabolized in the liver and has a half-life of 30 to 50 minutes. Its therapeutic effect is monitored by the aPTT. It may be used in patients with renal dysfunction, and can be removed through dialysis.

Vitamin K Antagonists

Warfarin is the only FDA-approved vitamin K antagonist available in the United States. In some countries, other coumarins are used instead of warfarin, such as aceno-coumarol and phenprocoumon. These have a shorter (aceno-coumarol) or longer (phenprocoumon) half-life, and are not completely interchangeable with warfarin. Coumarins decrease blood coagulation by interfering with vitamin K metabolism, and hence preventing complete synthesis of active II, VII, IX and X in the liver. Body stores of previously produced active factors degrade and inactive factors take their place; hence the anticoagulation effect takes several days to become apparent. Warfarin is absorbed rapidly and predictably from the gastrointestinal tract. Vitamin K is the antidote of choice in case of warfarin overdose.

Treatment is usually initiated with heparin, as previously mentioned. The therapeutic effect of warfarin is monitored using the INR. The target INR will vary from case to case and according to clinical indication, but tends to be 2 to 3 in most situations. In patients with mechanical heart valves, a target INR of 2.5 to 3.5 may be appropriate. Higher INRs are associated with increased risk of bleeding, and lower INRs may not produce the desired therapeutic effect.

Skin necrosis, sometimes resulting in amputation or death, has been reported as a serious side effect of warfarin therapy. The estimated incidence is 0.01% to 0.1%. This typically manifests between 1 to 10 days after initiation of therapy. It frequently begins with paresthesia, associated with poorly demarcated erythema. The lesions are painful and initially hemorrhagic or edematous. Petechiae and hemorrhagic bullae form over the next 24 hours. Eschar forms, and when the eschar sloughs a defect deep into the subcutaneous tissue is revealed. Protein C deficiency is a major predisposing factor, and extreme care must be taken when initiating warfarin therapy in these patients. To minimize risk, concomitant administration of heparin and warfarin for 3 to 6 days is recommended.

Warfarin is not used in pregnant women, or women who may become pregnant. It crosses the placenta and has been associated with fetal abnormalities.

Interactions with food, herbal supplements, and drugs have been reported. A recent publication by Holbrook et al. provided a systematic overview of warfarin and its drug and food interaction (134). Many foods contain vitamin K and may alter the anticoagulant effect of warfarin. Excessive use of alcohol may affect warfarin metabolism, and patients with liver damage or alcoholism are usually treated with heparin instead. Moderate drinking usually has little or no effect on the INR. Herb supplements in common use (ginkgo, St John's wort, ginseng, garlic, and ginger) may also interact with warfarin. Potential drug interactions require careful review of any medications the patient may be taking.

Plasminogen Activators

Plasminogen activators cleave plasminogen, the circulating inactive form, into plasmin, an enzyme capable of degrading both fibrin and fibrinogen. Alteplase is a recombinant human tissue-type plasminogen activator (rtPA), which specifically cleaves the Arg-Val bond of plasminogen resulting in the formation of plasmin. Alteplase differs from streptokinase in that it is fibrin specific. tPA binds avidly to fibrin, thereby bringing it into close proximity to fibrin-bound plasminogen and increasing the enzymatic activity of tPA. Therefore, tPA produces plasmin within the thrombus, with little activation of circulating plasminogen (135–137). The highly clot-specific property of tPA appears to enhance its dose-predictable activity when administered as a therapeutic agent, but it does not enhance its efficacy or safety compared with other thrombolytic agents, nor does it prevent the potential bleeding complications associated with all thrombolytic agents.

Single-chain form rtPA has a plasma half-life of approximately 5 minutes. More than 50% of alteplase is cleared within 5 minutes of the infusion has been terminated, and approximately 80% is cleared within 10 minutes. The rtPA is also inactivated by circulating PAI-1, whose concentration may vary among patients.

Fibrin-bound tPA will initiate thrombolysis with equal efficacy in undesirable locations where hemostasis is essential (e.g., arterial puncture sites and spontaneous internal hemorrhages) and in desirable, or therapeutic, locations (e.g., coronary arteries and vascular grafts) and is the most expensive currently available thrombolytic agent (70–73,137,138).

In some situations, lysis of thrombus in native arteries or grafts may be the only acute therapy needed to revascularize severely ischemic organs; however, in most cases, it is a temporary remedy that is of greatest benefit in allowing accurate radiographic diagnosis of underlying pathology for appropriate treatment (135–138).

The euglobulin lysis time is used to evaluate systemic fibrinolysis and is believed to reflect primarily the level of plasminogen activators. Acidified, diluted plasma (the euglobulin fraction) is relatively free of inhibitors of fibrinolysis. The euglobulin fraction is allowed to form a fibrin clot, and the time to subsequent clot lysis (90 minutes to 6 hours) is measured. A more rapid lysis (<1 hour) implies that circulating activators are present.

Measurement of the TT is more useful in monitoring the systemic fibrinolytic state achieved during fibrinolytic therapy because it is quicker and more widely available. A satisfactory fibrinolytic state is achieved when the TT is two times normal (70–73,135–139). Plasminogen, fibrinogen, fibrin, FDPs and D-dimer can be measured directly. Most bleeding complications related to fibrinolytic therapy occur when fibrinogen levels have diminished to less than 50 to 100 mg/dL. The thrombolytic infusion rate should be reduced by 50% if the fibrinogen level is less than 150 mg/dL, discontinued if the fibrinogen level is less than100 mg/dL, and FFP should be administered prophylactically to replenish fibrinogen if the level is less than 80 mg/dL (70,138).

Fibrinolytic agents are absolutely contraindicated when significant risk of producing fatal hemorrhagic complications exists, such as after recent intracranial hemorrhage or trauma, pregnancy, or recent liver or spleen injury (135–138).

There are currently six FDA-approved plasminogen-activators, with more under development. Half-life, antigenicity, potency, cost, and incidence of side effects vary. Concomitant administration of heparin is often used to minimize the risk of catheter-associated thrombosis or rethrombosis.

Urokinase is an enzyme found in human urine and isolated from tissue culture of human kidney cells. Urokinase is also found in limited amounts in the blood. Urokinase is one of the uPA that is responsible for the fibrinolytic activity of urine. uPAs lack the fibrin affinity of tPA and do not exhibit a greater enzymatic activity for plasminogen in the presence of fibrin. Urokinase is extremely effective and dose predictable as a thrombolytic agent, has no immunologic side effects, and is intermediate in cost. Urokinase was the most widely used thrombolytic agent for intra-arterial infusion into the peripheral arterial system and grafts (135–138). However, its clinical usage has largely been replaced by alteplase (tPA).

Streptokinase, a glycoprotein produced by β-hemolytic streptococci, is not a proteolytic enzyme and does not convert plasminogen to plasmin. Instead, it complexes with plasminogen, and this complex is then capable of activating other plasminogen molecules. The affinity of streptokinase for fibrin is low, hence, like uPA, streptokinase is not selective for fibrin-bound plasminogen. Because streptokinase is a nonhuman protein, it may elicit profound allergic (febrile) responses, which limits its clinical utility. Preformed antibodies to streptokinase may also bind and inactivate it, but in clinically administered doses this effect is usually overwhelmed and a thrombolytic state is achieved easily. Some dose–response unpredictability may occur because the streptokinase–plasminogen complex resists inactivation by α-antiplasmin and because degradation products are multiple and maintain variable activity (79,140).

Reteplase (Retavase) and tenecteplase (TNKase) are still commercially available. Reteplase is a recombinant nonglycosylated form of human tPA, which has been modified to contain 357 of the 527 amino acids of the original protein. It is produced in the bacterium *Escherichia coli*. Reteplase is similar to rtPA (alteplase), but the modifications give reteplase a longer half-life of 13 to 16 minutes. Reteplase also binds fibrin with lower affinity than alteplase, improving its ability to penetrate into clots. Tenecteplase is produced by recombinant DNA technology using an established mammalian cell line (Chinese Hamster Ovary cells). In the presence of fibrin, *in vitro* studies demonstrate that tenecteplase conversion of plasminogen to plasmin is increased relative to its conversion in the absence of fibrin. This fibrin specificity decreases systemic activation of plasminogen and the resulting degradation of circulating fibrinogen as compared to a molecule lacking this property.

Inhibitors of Thrombolytic Agents

The pharmacologic agents, EACA and tranexamic acid (AMCA), inhibit fibrinolysis by competitive binding to plasminogen. The resulting complex is unable to bind to and cleave fibrin. AMCA is more potent than EACA and has less renal excretion (79). Both agents accumulate in tissues (141). Aprotinin, a serine protease inhibitor, has been used to decrease bleeding associated with cardiopulmonary bypass (142–146).

Activated Factor VIIa

Local hemostasis may be induced with the use of recombinant human coagulation factor VIIa (rF VIIa) through the extrinsic pathway of the coagulation cascade in which rF VIIa, complexed with TF, can activate coagulation factors IX and X to factors IXa and Xa, respectively (147). Activated factor X (factor Xa), complexed with other factors, converts prothrombin to thrombin and fibrinogen to fibrin to form a hemostatic plug.

Factor VIIa initiates coagulation at the site of tissue injury by complexing with TF; the factor VIIa-TF complex activates factor X (and factor IX) in the presence of calcium, resulting in activation of the final common pathway of the coagulation cascade independent of factor VIII: protein C (148,149). Activation of factor X may also occur with high concentrations of factor VIIa in the absence of TF (150,151). There is evidence that factor VII binding to TF enables autoactivation of factor VII to factor VIIa (152). An *in vitro* study also found that high-dose coagulation factor VIIa binds to activated platelets and initiates thrombin generation independent of TF (153).

Recombinant human factor VIIa [NovoSeven, eptacog alfa (activated)] was initially introduced for use in uncontrollable bleeding in hemophilia patients with acquired inhibitors of replacement coagulation factors. It is being increasingly used in uncontrollable hemorrhage (154). The rationale for its use in hemorrhage is that it will only induce coagulation in those sites where TF is present. However, an increased risk of DVT, pulmonary embolism, and myocardial infarction has been reported (155,156).

BASIC HEMATOPOIESIS

The formed elements of the blood (erythrocytes, granulocytes, lymphocytes, and platelets) derive from pluripotent stem cells (157). A relatively small number of these long-lived stem cells form the basic pool from which all other cells are derived. In a process that has been termed *death by differentiation,* offspring of these stem cells undergo progressive differentiation. They lose proliferative ability with each cell division until the mature form, incapable of replication, is produced and released into the circulation.

Stem cells first undergo an initial differentiation into lymphopoietic or hematopoietic progenitor cells. Lymphopoietic progenitor cells are the origin of both T and B lymphocytes. Lymphopoiesis is a complex process, involving the initial formation of T and B lymphocyte progenitor cells within the thymus and bone marrow, with subsequent processing of lymphocytes within aggregates of lymphoid tissue, such as lymph nodes. It will not be discussed further here.

The term *hematopoiesis* is conventionally used to cover the genesis of all nonlymphocyte blood cell lines. Hematopoietic progenitor cells undergo further differentiation into progenitor cells of granulocyte (neutrophil, basophil, and eosinophil), erythrocyte, or megakaryocyte lineage (Fig. 19.8). Initial production of blood cells occurs in the yolk sac of the growing embryo. By the second month of fetal life, the liver has become an important hematopoietic organ, joined during later fetal development by the spleen. Hematopoietic cells first appear in the bone marrow at about the fifth month of gestation. The center of hematopoietic activity gradually shifts until, at birth, the marrow is active and hematopoiesis has virtually ceased in extramedullary (outside of the bone marrow) locations. However, for the next several years, the volume required by the hematopoietic cell mass nearly approximates the volume available within the marrow cavities. Hence, under conditions of stress, extramedullary hematopoiesis may again occur in the liver and spleen in normal children. The hematopoietic cells gradually recede and become localized within the central marrow locations of the vertebrae, skull, ribs, and pelvis. Fat cells occupy the remaining space in the long bones of the extremities (158–160).

In the adult, hematopoietic activity normally occurs only within the marrow. Nests of hematopoietic cells corresponding to different cell lines occupy the extravascular spaces, tending to cluster in characteristic locations of the marrow sinusoids. The marrow cavity forms a complex microenvironment in which endothelial cells, fibroblasts, macrophages, and other stromal cells interact with hematopoietic cells. Mature cells exit the marrow by pushing through endothelial cells into the marrow sinusoids (157,161).

Erythropoiesis

The average erythrocyte lives for approximately 120 days. The bone marrow must release 3×10^9 new red blood cells (RBCs), or reticulocytes, each day to maintain a normal Hct. Marrow response requires a structurally intact microenvironment, the presence of erythrocyte precursor cells that are sensitive to erythropoietin (EPO), an optimal iron supply, and adequate levels of functional EPO. Disruption or malfunction of any of these components can lead to decreased red cell production and anemia (160).

The differentiating cells of the erythroid line are collectively referred to as the *erythron*. Three functional compartments are recognized: early progenitor cells (recognizable only by their capacity to give rise to erythroid colonies *in vitro*); erythroid precursors (proerythroblasts and marrow reticulocytes); and reticulocytes/erythrocytes. As differentiation progresses, cells become recognizable as erythroid precursors and gain sensitivity to their specific growth factor, EPO. EPO stimulates transformation to proerythroblasts, which subsequently multiply and mature (161–163). Reticulocytes lose their nucleus within the bone marrow and exit the marrow by passing through the endothelial cells. This appears to require a pressure gradient from within the marrow

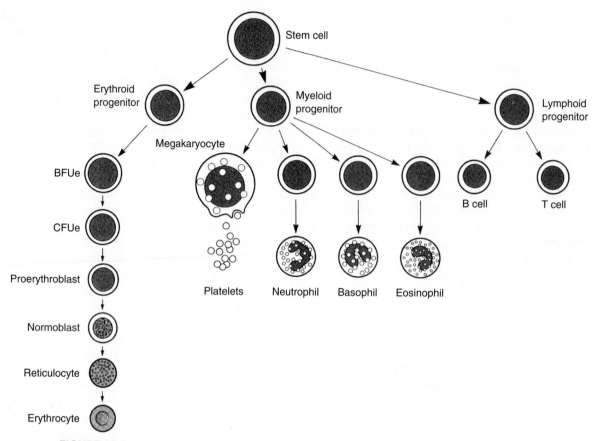

FIGURE 19.8   Overview of hematopoietic cell lines.

and considerable deformation of the reticulocyte. The reticulocyte continues its maturation within the bloodstream.

Hematopoietic growth factors (originally called *colony-stimulating* and *burst-stimulating factors*) function as trophic hormones for stem and progenitor cells. Most growth factors are stimulatory for more than one cell line but have predominant activity for one. In the absence of specific growth factors, progenitor cells fail to differentiate and die (161). These growth factors form part of a tightly controlled system that maintains cell counts within relatively small tolerances and adapts to changing needs. The bone marrow of the average adult generates 2.4 million erythrocytes per second and twice as many platelets (161). Bleeding, stress, and infection are stimuli for an increase of up to 6 to 10 times in output of the appropriate cell line, which is promptly shut off when the abnormal demand ceases. Inhibitors of hematopoiesis include steroids, interferons, TNFs, lactoferrin, transferrin, ferritin, and arachidonic acid metabolites (162–164).

EPO is a glycoprotein hematopoietic growth factor that primarily stimulates erythroid precursors but has secondary effects on megakaryocytes. In the fetus, the liver is the major source of production of EPO. After birth, more than 90% of EPO is produced in the kidney, and only approximately 10% is made in the liver. Anemia of prematurity may be related to failure to switch from hepatic to renal production of EPO.

Hepatic production of EPO becomes important in anephric patients (162–164).

EPO is synthesized in cells adjacent to the proximal renal tubules. It is increased by tissue hypoxia caused by anemia, hypoxemia, ischemia, and abnormal hemoglobin (increased affinity for oxygen, hence less delivery of oxygen at the tissue level) (Fig. 19.9). Hypoxia stimulates the release of EPO with a 5- to 6-hour delay. EPO then binds to specific receptors on erythroid progenitor cells (160–165).

Normal levels of EPO (10 to 20 U/L or ~2 pmol) are sufficient for replacement of worn-out erythrocytes in the healthy patient. EPO rises as the Hct falls, reaching 100 times normal at a Hct of 20% and causing the release of large, immature "stress" reticulocytes (166).

Anemia

Blood loss is the most common cause of anemia in surgical patients. Patients with an intact bone marrow will respond rapidly to the rise in endogenous EPO described earlier, and transfusion is less often used than previously (see subsequent text).

A different problem exists in patients with anemia of chronic disease, as well as in surgical intensive care unit (SICU) patients, in whom both low EPO levels and a functional iron deficiency have been implicated (167). In functional iron deficiency, iron stores are normal or increased but not enough is available for erythropoiesis. Low *serum*

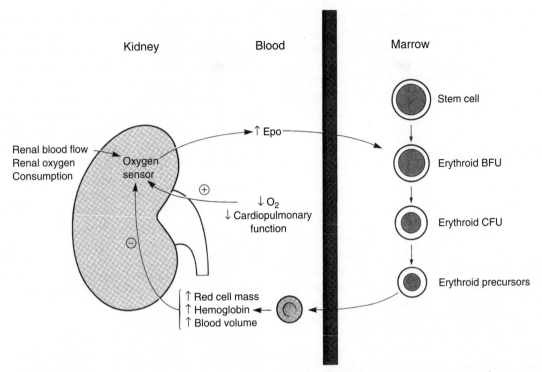

FIGURE 19.9   Control of erythropoiesis. Epo, erythropoietin; BFU, burst forming unit; CFU, colony forming unit.

iron, total iron binding capacity (TIBC) and the Fe/TIBC ratio may all be involved. Serum ferritin may be elevated but available ferritin receptors are decreased. EPO varies and may be low or mildly elevated. Bone marrow response to circulating EPO is blunted.

Functional iron deficiency may be due to release of inflammatory cytokines. These activate macrophages leading to increased production of TNF-α, IL-1 and IL-6. TNF-α and IL-1 increase expression of ferritin synthesis and iron storage in macrophages and hepatocytes. INF-γ depresses transferrin expression in an attempt to keep Fe out of macrophages. On a cellular level, nitroxide (NO) and H_2O_2 decrease ferritin synthesis through interactions with messenger ribonucleic acid (mRNA). Renal production of EPO is decreased through these same mechanisms. Decreased availability of iron to the marrow causes iron deficiency anemia and the release hypochromic microcytic erythrocytes.

Standard laboratory tests of iron levels, serum ferritin, and transferrin saturation do not reflect this diagnosis accurately. One can measure the percentage of hypochromic RBCs (Hgb <28 g/dL) with flow cytometry but this is time consuming and expensive. Measurements of the hemoglobin content of reticulocytes (CHR) have been used both to establish a diagnosis and to guide treatment (168,169). CHR values of less than 26 to 28 pg predicts Fe deficiency (170). These patients respond rapidly to intravenous iron therapy of 500 to 1,000 mg i.v. with increases in CHR and reticulocyte counts by greater than 1% within 24 hours.

The perceived risks of intravenous iron therapy have limited its use by some clinicians (171). In experimental animals, increases in Fe-binding protein increase risk of infection. The clinical importance of these findings is controversial. An increase in infections was noted in a small group of nutritionally depleted children treated with intravenous iron. However, this group (a mixture of kwashiorkor and marasmus) had ample other reasons to develop infections. Studies of intravenous iron therapy in dialysis patients have shown no increased risk of infection (172).

Short-term risks of intravenous iron do exist and are related to preformed dextran antibodies and the rate of administration. Iron dextran preparations can produce type I IgE-mediated anaphylaxis. All patients should receive a test dose of 0.5 mL to look for this response before starting infusion of iron. The incidence of these reactions has been reported to be approximately 0.7% (172–176). Anaphylactoid reactions can occur with either iron dextran or iron polysaccharide compounds if they are infused rapidly. Transient overload of transferrin with release of free Fe induces either a histamine or immune mediated response that produces respiratory symptoms, pain, nausea and vomiting, and hypotension. Infusions of iron should be given over several hours to avoid this complication.

Recombinant human EPO (rHuEPO, Procrit, Ortho Biotech, Raritan, NJ) provides a means of restoring red cells without either autologous or allogeneic transfusion. Several, large-scale, prospective, studies of this drug in both orthopaedic and cardiac surgical patients have proved its value as an alternative to allogeneic transfusion (177,178). RHuEPO has been used successfully in Jehovah's Witness patients to restore red cell mass, in both the preoperative and postoperative periods (179,180). Standard dosing regimens for rHuEPO or Procrit are 600 IU/kg given subcutaneously once a week or 300 IU/kg given daily for 1 week before surgery. It is important when using EPO to make sure that the patient's iron stores are replenished, since existing iron is rapidly depleted (181–183).

BLOOD TRANSFUSION

Basic Principles

Erythrocytes carry surface antigens for more than 30 different systems. Leukocytes carry human leukocyte antigens (HLAs), and platelets carry both HLA and platelet-associated antigens. Blood is typed and cross-matched only for red cell antigens, because the leukocytes and platelets that are incidentally infused with packed red blood cells (PRBCs) are normally well tolerated. Although any of the red cell surface antigens are capable of producing reactions, the two most important systems are the ABH (ABO) and Rh (181,182).

Two genes determine the ABH genotype; there are six possible genotypes but only four phenotypes. Blood type O (corresponding to the H antigen) is the most common (47% of the general population in the United States). These individuals have antibodies to A and B and will react to blood from A or B (or AB) donors. Because H is a weak antigen, most people can accept blood from an O donor regardless of their blood type.

Type A is almost as common (41% of the U.S. population). The genotype may be either AA or AH. These individuals possess antibodies to B. Types B (genotype BB or BH) and AB are rare, occurring in 9% and 3% of the population, respectively. A separate *secretor* gene (80% of Western Europeans) determines whether these antigens are water soluble and hence are found in secretions such as saliva (183).

The most immunogenic blood group antigens are A and B (184,185). Antibodies to A and B are found in virtually all individuals who lack the corresponding antigens, regardless of previous transfusion history (186).

ABO incompatibility reactions occur when a patient receives RBCs of a different ABO, for example, A cells transfused into a B patient. Complement activation can cause membrane lysis and liberation of free hemoglobin within the vascular system. The degree of resulting hemolysis depends on the quantity of donor red cells, antigen specificity, immunoglobulin (Ig) type (IgM versus IgG), antibody subclass, antibody thermal amplitude, antibody titer and the clinical condition of the recipient (186). It may be catastrophic.

PRBC units currently available for transfusion contain either citrate, phosphate, dextrose, and adnenine (CPDA) or these chemicals plus additional dextrose, adenine, and mannitol (Adsol). Approximately 20 to 30 mL of residual plasma containing anti-A and anti-B antibodies remain in most red cell concentrates resuspended in additive solutions.

However, erythrocytes prepared in CPDA-1 anticoagulant-preservative solutions may contain as much as 50 to 80 mL of residual plasma. Plasma in this quantity from individuals with high titer anti-A and/or anti-B has been known to cause significant hemolysis (187). Therefore, Group O CPDA-1 RBC is less desirable than Adsol units for non–Group O recipients. After determination of the patient's blood type, type-specific CPDA-1 RBCs may be used. These factors should be remembered when using non—type-specific blood in massive transfusion and resuscitation.

Transfusion Risks

The risks of allogeneic RBC transfusion include transfusion reactions, transfusion-related acute lung injury (TRALI), transfusion-transmitted infectious disease (TTD), immunomodulation [including graft versus host disease (GVHD)], and problems related to erythrocyte storage defects. Each topic will be considered briefly here.

Transfusion reactions

There are three main types of transfusion reactions: (i) acute intravascular immune hemolytic reactions from ABO incompatibility, (ii) delayed immune hemolytic reactions, and (iii) febrile reactions (188–190). Reactions are estimated to occur in approximately 5% of transfusion recipients (191). The risk of a fatal hemolytic reaction is less than 1:1,000,000; those of nonfatal hemolytic reactions and febrile reactions 1:25,000 and 1:100, respectively. Fortunately, most blood group antigens are only weakly immunogenic, and fewer than 1% of patients who receive RBC transfusions will subsequently develop antibodies (192). (Table 19.10)

The most common cause of ABO incompatibility reactions is human error. Symptoms depend upon the volume of incompatible cells transfused. Patients may experience hemoglobinuria, fever, chills, coagulopathy, chest pain, and circulatory collapse. In the unconscious, anesthetized, euvolemic patient, acute reactions may present either as sudden, hypotension and/or unexpected bleeding secondary to DIC (184). Treatment consists of immediate cessation of the transfusion, circulatory support, and saline diuresis to minimize renal tubule obstruction.

Delayed hemolytic reactions are caused by non-ABO antigen–antibody incompatibilities, primarily RhD. Although called *naturally occurring*, these antibodies are virtually all produced following RBC transfusion 44 (186,192–194).

Blood group alloantibodies are detected by testing donor serum against two or three different Group O reagent cells of known phenotype. Clinically significant antibodies of this type may cause acute and/or delayed hemolytic transfusion reactions. *In vitro* agglutination and/or hemolysis are determined at room temperature, at 37°C and in the antihuman globulin (AHG) phase. Reactions at room temperature usually indicate the presence of cold agglutinins (IgM antibodies) with little or no clinical significance. Reactions at 37°C or in the AHG phase indicate the presence of clinically significant (IgG) antibodies.

TABLE 19.10

Transfusion Reactions: Symptoms, Causes, and Incidence

Reaction	Symptoms	Cause	Incidence
Febrile nonhemolytic acute transfusion reaction	Temperature rise >1°C, chills, rigors, shivering	Leukotrienes and cytokines from infused blood	1/100–1/200 transfusions
Mild allergic urticarial	Urticaria, erythema, cutaneous flushing, hoarseness, stridor	Antigen or allergen in transfused blood, donor drug, cytokines, leukotrienes, passive transfer of IgG antibodies, cold	Common; 1%–2% (179)
Severe allergic anaphylactic	Hypotension, tachycardia, loss of consciousness, arrhythmia, shock, cardiac arrest, death	IgA in transfused blood given to patient with IgA deficiency	Rare
Acute hemolytic	Hemolysis, fever, chills, nausea, vomiting, pain, dyspnea, tachycardia, hypotension, unexplained intraoperative bleeding, hemoglobinuria, death	ABO-incompatible blood, or IL-1, IL-6, IL-8, TNF-α infusions	Rare; estimaed 1/33,000 transfusions. Fatalities estimated 1/600,000 units (143). SAnGUIS study estimates 0.8% of surgical patients transfused (180)
Delayed hemolytic	Hemolysis at least 24 h pottransfusion and up to 6 wk; symptoms may recur	Donor antibodies to recipient red blood cells	2.9% of transfused patients; only 1 patient with clinical symptoms (181); more common in multitransfused patients, e.g., sickle cell
Bacterial contamination	Fever, chills, nausea, vomiting, shock, death	Bacterial contamination of unit during collection with overgrowth during storage. *Yersinia enterocolitica and Pseudomonas* genus most common organisms	Unknown
Transfusion-related acute lung injury	Acute noncardiogenic pulmonary edema within hours of transfusion, dyspnea, fever, hypoxemia	Antibodies in transfused plasma against human leukocyte antigens or granulocyte antigens mediated by lipid inflammatory agents	Unknown; probably misdiagnosed and underreported
Posttransfusion purpura	Thrombocytopenia, bleeding, purpura from 5–10 d posttransfusion up to 3 wk	Patient's alloantibody against antigen in transfused blood that reacts with platelets	Unknown
Hypotensive reaction	Hypotension in absence of other symptoms	Release of bradykinin through coagulation pathway activation from platelet transfusion	unknown; associated with platelet and plasma transfusion; increased incidence in patients taking ACE inhibitor drugs
Nonimmune hemolysis	Acute or delayed mild hemolysis, hemoglobinuria	Improper storage or handling of blood	Rare
Circulatory overload	Acute pulmonary edema	Iatrogenic volume overload	Unknown
Hypothermia	Aggravation of hypothermia; hemolysis in patient with circulating cold agglutinins	Iatrogenic administration of cold blood	Common in massive transfusion and trauma if blood warmer not used
Hyperkalemia	Cardiac arrhythmias	Iatrogenic transfusion of old, stored blood	Rare; seen in massive transfusion and trauma in renal failure patients and children
Acidosis	Shock, cardiac arrhythmias	Iatrogenic transfusion of old, stored blood	Rare; seen in massive transfusion

Ig, immunoglobulin; IL, interleukin; SAnGUIS, Safe and Good Use of Blood in Surgery; TNF, tumor necrosis factor; ACE, angiotensin–converting enzyme.

The risk of significant unexpected antibodies in men with a negative history of transfusion or in women with no history of transfusion or pregnancy is 0.04% (194). The risk of unexpected antibodies increases to 1.0% in men and women who are the recipients of previous transfusions or in women who have been pregnant. For women who have been both pregnant and have been the recipients of transfusions, the risk of unexpected antibodies increases to approximately 3.0% (195). Clinically significant antibodies have been identified in 1% to 4% of patients requiring massive transfusion (196,197).

Patients with life-threatening blood loss may need transfusion before antibody identification or screening for antigen-negative units. In this situation, it is necessary to determine if the medical benefits of immediate transfusion justify the risk of a hemolytic transfusion reaction. Physicians and nursing personnel must be attentive to the signs and symptoms of acute hemolysis. In the massively transfused or anesthetized patient, the clinical manifestations of an acute hemolytic reaction may be difficult to recognize.

Delayed reactions occur when ABO-compatible red cells containing a specific antigen, for example, Rh D or Kell, are transfused into a patient who has preformed alloantibodies. Symptoms appear within 3 to 10 days and include fever, malaise, hyperbilirubinemia or a falling Hct. A decline in Hct during the immediate postoperative period in a recently transfused patient is often attributed to recurrent or continued bleeding, rather than to a transfusion reaction. A real danger exists in continuing to transfuse such patients with incompatible blood. An acute hemolytic reaction can be precipitated if blood has not been re-crossmatched since the original transfusion. Delayed hemolytic reaction should be ruled out by appropriate antibody testing in any patient with a falling postoperative Hct and no overt evidence of ongoing bleeding (198,199).

Febrile reactions, the most common type, have been attributed in the past to circulating recipient antibodies to donor leukocyte or platelet contaminants. Recent evidence suggests that cytokines with pyrogenic, proinflammatory, and leukocyte-activating properties are produced in both hemolytic and febrile reactions (200). In addition, cytokines released by leukocytes accumulate in blood components during storage. Transfusion of such units produces both hemolytic and febrile transfusion reactions (201–203). Although patients usually only experience minor symptoms, serious leukocyte-mediated pulmonary infiltrates and insufficiency have been reported (204,205).

Transfusion-Related Acute Lung Injury

A working group of the National Heart, Lung, and Blood Institute (NHLBI) has defined TRALI as a "new acute lung injury occurring during or within 6 hours of a transfusion, with a clear temporal relation to the transfusion" (197). TRALI is difficult to distinguish clinically from circulatory overload. It mimics and can develop into the adult respiratory distress syndrome (206). Neutrophil-derived inflammatory chemokines and cytokines are believed to be involved in the pathogenesis of both entities (207–210). HLA class I, HLA class II, and neutrophil-specific antibodies in the plasma of both blood donors and recipients have been implicated in the pathogenesis of TRALI. TRALI can be demonstrated by donor antibody- recipient antigen reaction through crossmatching the donor plasma against the recipient's leukocytes.

There are two proposed pathophysiologic mechanisms for TRALI: the antibody hypothesis and the two-event hypothesis. In the first, antibody–antigen interaction causes complement-mediated pulmonary sequestration and activation of neutrophils [pulmonary neutrophils (PMNs)]. The two-event model presupposes that the clinical condition of the patient has led to pulmonary endothelial activation and PMN sequestration. Transfusion of a biologic response modifier (including antigranulocyte antibodies, lipids, and CD40 ligand) then activates these adherent PMNs resulting in endothelial damage, capillary leak, and TRALI. The final common pathway in all of the proposed pathogenic mechanisms of TRALI is increased pulmonary capillary permeability, which results in movement of plasma into the alveolar space causing pulmonary edema.

Serologic workup for TRALI consists of tests for HLA class I and II and neutrophil-specific antibodies. Flow cytometry and HLA-coated microbeads are recommended for detection of HLA antibodies in plasma of implicated blood donors, and a combination of the granulocyte agglutination test and granulocyte immunofluorescence test for detection of neutrophil-specific antibodies. Genotyping for class I and II HLA and for a limited number of neutrophil antigens may also be helpful in establishing antibody–antigen concordance.

Transfusion-Transmitted Infectious Diseases

Blood can carry and transmit a wide variety of viral, parasitic, rickettsial, and bacterial diseases. The estimated risk of contracting a specific disease from transfusion of blood products varies and depends upon many factors including the organism, patient risk factors, screening processes, country of origin, and overall vigilance of the blood provider (211,212) (Table 19.11). State-of-the-art HIV testing (including screening of high-risk patients, p-24 HIV antigen analysis, and antibody testing) has all but eliminated the risk of transmitting this virus by transfusion, but at an enormous cost (213). Hepatitis C virus currently accounts for 98% of the risk to patients, both in terms of disease transmission and mortality (214).

Some viruses are common in blood donors but do not present a serious infectious risk. Cytomegalovirus (CMV) is present in up to one half the units of transfused allogeneic blood (215,216). It presents a small but troublesome risk, especially to specific groups of patients, including premature infants less than 1,200 g, pregnant CMV-seronegative mothers, and seronegative adults who may need multiple transfusions, for example, liver transplant recipients or blunt trauma victims. Symptoms include pulmonary, gastrointestinal, or systemic manifestations. Exposure can be reduced by eliminating unnecessary transfusions, screening

TABLE 19.11

Transfusion-Transmitted Diseases: Agent, Clinical Impact and Risk

Agent	Disease or Clinical Impact	Risk	Year
HIV	Acquired immunodeficiency syndrome (AIDS)	1/1,000,000	2000
HBV	Hepatitis B	1/600,000	2000
		Antibodies found in 32.8% of multitransfused children	1997
HCV	Hepatitis C	1/600,000	
		Antibodies found in 31.3% of multitransfused children	2000
HDV	Superinfection in hepatitis B patients, may lead to fulminant hepatic failure	Antibodies found in 1.6% of multitransfused children	1997
HEV	Hepatitis	2.8% of blood donors positive	1999
HGV	Hepatitis?, may increase risk of hepatitis C	9% of transfused cardiac surgery patients seroconverted to antibody positive postoperatively	1996
TTV	Hepatitis?	28%–53% of long-term HDV patients seropositive	1999
		81.7% of 120 blood donors positive	
		5.3% of blood donors positive	
HTLV-I, HTLV-II	Adult T-cell leukemia and lymphoma; myelopathies; tropical spastic paresis	1/64,000	1997
CMV	Ranges from no disease to lethal pneumonitis in immunocompromised patients	Seroprevalence ranges from 40%–100%	1999
Parvo B19	Spontaneous abortions	Antibodies found in 7.5% of donors	1999
Plasmodium falciparum	Malaria	Antibodies found in 4.1% of healthy donors in Nigeria	1998
		103 reported cases in United States over last 40 years	
Trypanosoma cruzi	Chagas disease	1.3%–1.9% of donors in Brazil, Mexico, and Argentina	1999
Borrelia burgdorferi	Lyme disease	Transmission found only in isolated cases	1994
Treponema pallidum	Syphilis	Fresh blood greatest risk	
Prion	New variant CJD	Unproven	2001
Toxoplasma gondii	Toxoplasmosis in immunocompromised patients	36% antibody positive in 392 plasmapheresis donors	1989
Epstein-Barr virus	Mononucleosis; lymphomas	?	
Babesia microti	Babesiosis	0.17% of 155 multitransfused patients	1994
Herpes 6 virus	Lymphoma; marker for CMV?	Unknown	1999
Borna disease virus	Psychiatric illnesses	1.09% of blood donors' antibody positive 8%–50% of psychiatric patients' antibody positive	1999

HIV, human immune deficiency virus; HBV, hepatitis B virus; HCV, hepatitis C virus; HDV, hepatitis D virus; HEV, hepatitis E virus; HGV, hepatitis G virus; TTV, transfusion transmitted virus; HTLV-I and HTLV-II, human lymphotropic virus I and II; CMV, cytomegalovirus; CJD, Creutzfeldt-Jakob disease.

for antibodies, and filtering leukocyte (213). Hepatitis G virus is common in donors but no causal relation between its transmission by transfusion and clinical hepatitis has been established (187,217).

Many other diseases can be transmitted by transfusion including malaria, Chagas disease, Q fever, and Lyme disease (218,219). Although new variant Creutzfeldt-Jacob disease (human bovine spongiform encephalopathy) has been produced in animals by the injection of contaminated blood, there is no evidence at this time that supports transfusion as a vector for this disease. Overgrowth of bacteria not typically identified as pathogens, such as *Yersinia enterocolitica*, may occur, particularly in units stored for prolonged periods of time or in platelet transfusions. Administration of such contaminated blood produces overwhelming sepsis and death (220). In summary, allogeneic blood has the potential to transmit infectious disease in spite of our best efforts and a zero-risk blood supply is not possible at this time. Agents that kill or inactivate bacteria and viruses may provide a generic solution to this difficult problem in the future (221–223).

Immunomodulation

RBC transfusion can produce systemic immunomodulation through poorly understood mechanisms (224,225). Both cellular and humoral factors appear to play a role. Immunomodulatory effects associated with allogeneic transfusions include the greater subsequent allograft survival, earlier recurrence of malignancy, increased susceptibility to bacterial infection, the prevention of recurrent abortions, the suppression of inflammatory bowel disease such as Crohn disease, the reactivation of latent viral infection, and GVH disease (226). The immunomodulatory effect can occur following a single-unit transfusion, but does demonstrate a dose–response relations (227).

Beneficial effects are related to the generation of specific immunologic tolerance to donor antigens. Deleterious effects may be related to the suppression of the normal host immune response. Donor leukocytes might mediate clonal deletion of cytotoxic T-cell precursors in some recipients. Another theory is that transfusion can induce development of recipient suppressor cells, which then inhibit the proliferation of immunocompetent cells. Soluble major HLA class I and Fas-ligand molecules have been identified in supernatants of blood components. These molecules inhibit mixed lymphocyte responses and cytotoxic T-cell activity and induce apoptosis in Fas-positive cells (228).

Macrophage function is altered following transfusion resulting in decreased migratory capability and both eicosanoid and IL-2 production. Lymphocyte responses to both antigen and mitogen are suppressed; suppressor cell activity is increased with concomitant declines in helper-suppressor cell ratios. Decreased numbers of CD4+ cells and a decreased CD4+/CD8+ ratio have been found in recipients of allogeneic blood transfusions.

Another observed effect in transfused recipients is reducednatural killer (NK) cell activity. Studies in patients undergoing surgery for colorectal malignancy have shown that NK cell activity is not reduced when they are transfused with leukocyte-depleted blood. It may be that donor leukocytes are able to downregulate NK cell activity in the recipient. Additionally, allogeneic transfusion may affect the production of cytokines in the recipient in such a manner as to induce tolerance. Finally, soluble substances produced in donor blood units might cause immunomodulatory effects in recipients.

GVHD results from the engraftment of immunocompetent donor T lymphocytes, typically in an immunosuppressed recipient. Donor lymphocytes recognize recipient HLA as foreign and produce a characteristic immune response. Eight to 10 days after transfusion, fever, skin rash, and gastrointestinal symptoms may appear. The disease is almost always fatal within 3 to 4 weeks. GVHD is most commonly associated with preexisting immunodeficiency or following bone marrow and stem cell transplantation. However, it has been reported in otherwise healthy patients following directed donations from immediate family members (first-degree relatives or those sharing an HLA haplotype). Pretransfusion irradiation eliminates the offending lymphocytes without damaging erythrocytes.

RBC transfusions can also produce a microchimeric population of lymphocytes in the recipient (222,229). This may be associated with one or more symptoms of GVH. The long-term consequences are unknown.

Of greatest concern are multiple reports of an increased susceptibility to bacterial infection, increased cancer-related mortality and shortened disease-free interval following allogeneic transfusion (222,226,230–236). The evidence regarding these findings comes primarily from observational studies with a handful of randomized, controlled trials, and cohort analyses. Most investigators have found statistical support for either a causal relation or an association between allogeneic blood transfusion and increased postoperative morbidity/mortality (203,237–241).

Although the precise mechanism is not yet known, the surgeon should be aware of the potential risks to patients. Reduction of leukocytes by filtration is an effective way to decrease the clinical impact (242).

Leukoreduction at the time of collection of the blood appears to be more beneficial than bedside leukofiltration, by preventing the release and accumulation of biologically active cytokines and soluble cellular mediators that accumulate during prolonged storage.

Storage Defects

During the preparation of PRBCs, erythrocytes are centrifuged and resuspended in an additive solution that extends cell viability and improves flow. Units currently available for transfusion contain either CPDA or these chemicals plus additional dextrose, adenine and mannitol (Adsol). Usually, 450 mL of whole blood is mixed with 60 mL of additive, providing a total volume of 510 mL. This extends storage time up to 42 days depending on the product used (Table 19.12). Typical units of packed RBCs contain approximately 250 mL of volume with a Hct in the 55% to 65% range.

When transfusion is initiated, 0.9% sodium chloride should be used concomitantly or as a diluent for PRBC. Ringers lactate will cause clotting (due to 2.7 mEq/L per liter of calcium) and should not be used. Red cells in the nutrient/preservative solution Adsol may not need additional dilution.

Massive transfusion can also cause citrate toxicity. Excess citrate is used to bind calcium in stored blood to prevent clotting. CPDA-1 and Adsol red cell concentrates contain 5 mg/mL and 2 mg/mL of citrate, respectively. However, the plasma from Adsol units contains approximately 30 mg/mL of citrate from the citrate phosphate dextrose (CPD) anticoagulant used in the initial collection (243). During massive transfusion, plasma-containing blood products (FFP, platelets) are the major source of citrate. Citrate is

TABLE 19.12

Storage Defects: Effect of Additives and Storage on Erythrocytes

	CPDA	CPDA	Adsol
Variable	Fresh	35 d	35 d
In vivo survival (at 24 h/%)	100	71.0	88.0
pH	7.5	6.7	6.7
ATP (% initial)	100	45	76
2,3-diphosphoglycerate (% initial)	100	<10.0	<10.0
Plasma K^+ (mEq/L)	5.1	78.5	49.5

CPDA, citrate, phosphate, dextrose, and adenine; Adsol, additional dextrose, adenine, and mannitol.

From Ness PM, Rothko K. Principles of red blood cell transfusion. In: Hoffman R, et al., eds. *Hematology: basic principles and practice*, 2nd ed. New York: Churchill and Livingstone, 1995:1981–1986, with permission.

excreted in the urine and metabolized rapidly by the liver in normal patients, yielding bicarbonate. Citrate infusion causes a transient decrease in ionized calcium, which is restored by mobilization of skeletal calcium. In patients who have limited ability to metabolize citrate (severe hypotension, hypothermia, hepatic injury or preexisting hepatic disease) citrate toxicity can cause muscle tremors, increased myocardial irritability and decreased cardiac output (244). Irreversible ventricular fibrillation may occur at citrate levels of 60 mg/mL.

Potassium leaks from RBCs during storage. Hyperkalemia may occur during rapid blood transfusion in patients with severe shock or renal dysfunction, and in patients with extensive muscle necrosis. In recent years, the ability to infuse large volumes of stored blood rapidly using high-capacity blood warmers has increased the risk. This metabolic load is transient, as potassium reenters erythrocytes within a few hours of transfusion. In actual practice, patients may experience a paradoxical hypokalemia resulting from the metabolism of citrate to bicarbonate and increased urinary excretion of potassium (245). Because hyperkalemia and hypokalemia are associated with cardiac dysfunction, close monitoring of potassium levels is recommended in the massively transfused patient.

Storage of red cells also leads to changes in cellular membrane, shape changes, phospholipid content, phospholipid asymmetry, and antigenic markers (246). Levels of integrin-associated protein CD47, Annexin V, a cytosolic component of blood cells and a global marker of cellular injury and fragmentation and phosphatidylserine all decline with storage. Absence of CD47, a "self-recognition" marker on circulating RBCs, leads to increased phagocytosis by macrophages and accelerated clearance of transfused RBCs by the spleen (247,248).

Prolonged storage of RBCs decreases levels of 2,3 d iphosphoglycerate (2,3-DPG) (249). The ability of RBCs to bind and release oxygen is dependent on the ability of

2,3-DPG to bind and stabilize deoxyhemoglobin. During red cell storage normal levels of 2,3-DPG are maintained for approximately 10 days. The subsequent precipitous loss of 2,3-DPG causes the oxygen-dissociation curve to shift to the left. Stored red cells therefore have a greater affinity for oxygen and are less likely to release oxygen. Following transfusion, transfused red cells require 3 to 8 hours to regenerate half of their 2,3-DPG levels. Recovery of sufficient 2,3-DPG levels to correct this problem may take 24 to 48 hours, depending on the length of pretransfusion storage (250). The clinical effect of low 2,3-DPG levels in transfused blood has never been determined but is likely offset by other *in vivo* variables including increases in cardiac output, vasodilation, and local acidosis (251).

The ability of RBCs to deform during passage through capillaries, which is important in determining resistance of blood to flow, is dependent on cellular ATP levels. During storage the red cell changes shape from a biconcave disc to a sphere as ATP levels decrease. The loss of ATP is anticoagulant dependent. Whole blood in CPDA-1 at 35 days of storage retains only 45% of initial ATP levels. Adsol has effectively reduced ATP loss (60%–65% of initial levels are retained) and increased red cell storage to 42 days (252,253). Photographs from capillary microscopy in an anemic patient before and after transfusion of stored red cells show the decrease in blood flow and stasis of deformed RBCs that result from the storage lesion (Fig. 19.10).

High oxygen affinity and lack of deformability caused by storage lesions combine to decrease tissue oxygen consumption. This may explain the lack of effect from stored allogeneic RBCs seen in critical care populations. Transfusing a critically ill patient creates a false sense of security. Oxygen delivery calculated from increased hemoglobin makes it appear that more oxygen is being delivered to the tissues then may actually be the case. The desired benefit from transfusion of increased oxygen consumption during acute tissue ischemia may not be immediately attainable with transfusion of stored allogeneic or autologous blood. (Fig. 19.11)

Platelets also develop a progressive storage lesion during their 5-day residence in the blood bank, but this does not usually result in impaired effectiveness (254,255). In stored whole blood, platelet function is virtually lost after 48 hours of storage at 4°C. Similarly, there is progressive loss of the labile coagulation factors; namely, factors V and VIII. Factor VIII is most unstable and decreases to 50%, 30% and 6% of baseline values after 1, 5, and 21 days of storage, respectively. Factor V is also labile and decreases to 50% of baseline values after storage for 14 days (256).

Indications for Transfusion

In 1988, the National Institutes of Health consensus conference on perioperative red cell transfusion produced recommendations for a new transfusion trigger of 8 gm/dL (257). These guidelines included use of clinical need and symptoms rather than numbers alone (258,259). Subsequent investigators have focused on defining an acceptable hemoglobin level

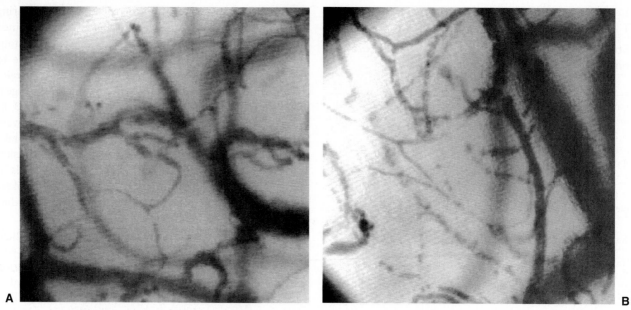

FIGURE 19.10 **A:** Capillary circulation in an anemic patient before transfusion of stored allogeneic blood. **B:** Capillary circulation in an anemic patient after transfusion of sotred allogeneic blood.

for transfusion, deriving a trigger from oxygen transport or metabolic variables, and describing the effect of transfusion in specific clinical settings.

The primary function of RBCs is the transport of oxygen to tissues. Therefore, any red cell transfusion should be physiologic, that is, to provide the additional oxygen delivery needed to correct or protect against the development of tissue hypoxia.

Current policies that focus on the use of physiologic transfusion decisions state that blood should be transfused only when there is a documented need to increase oxygen delivery in those patients who are unable to meet demands through normal cardiopulmonary mechanisms (260).

Physiologic Response to Anemia and Transfusion

Acute blood loss accompanied by hypovolemia stimulates an adrenergic response and release of vasoactive and metabolic substances (261). Vasopressin and angiotensin have effects on both the peripheral circulation and the heart. Venules and arterioles constrict, forcing blood into the central circulation. Resultant vasoconstriction, as well as increases in extracellular glucose concentrations mediated

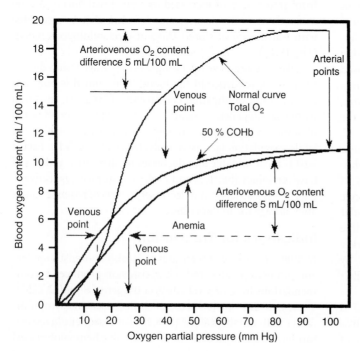

FIGURE 19.11 Oxygen-hemoglobin dissociation curve.

TABLE 19.13

O_2 Values: Hemoglobin and Oxygen Transport Relationships

Parameter	Formula	Normal range
Cardiac output (CO)	Stroke volumes (SV) × heart rate (HR)	4–6 L/min
Cardiac index (CI)	CO/body surface area in m^2	3.2 L/min/m^2
Arterial oxygen content (CaO_2)	$(1.34 \times Hgb \times SaO_2) + (0.003 \times PaO_2)$	15–22 mL/dL
Mixed venous oxygen content (CvO_2)	$(1.34 \times Hgb \times SvO_2) + (0.003 \times PvO_2)$	12–17 mL/dL
Oxygen delivery (DO_2)	$CO \times CaO_2 \times 10$	500–750 mL/min/m^2
Oxygen consumption (VO_2)	$CO \times (CaO_2 - CvO_2) \times 10$	100–300 mL/min/m^2
Oxygen extraction ratio (O_2ER)	VO_2/DO_2	0.23–0.30

Hgb, hemoglobin.

by EPI, cortisol, and glucagons, promotes flow of interstitial fluid into the intravascular space. Concomitant release of endorphins aids in directing blood flow away from splanchnic beds to critical organs. Fluid shifts in peripheral vessels lead to increase in central and stroke volumes.

Cardiac output increases, through either an increase in heart rate or an increase in stroke volume, providing the primary response (262,263). Release of adrenergic substances produces acute increases in heart rate. Changes in peripheral fluid distribution increase stroke volume. Because the heart extracts approximately 80% of the oxygen delivered under normal conditions, its ability to increase output is determined by its ability to increase its own oxygen consumption. Cardiac oxygen extraction is enhanced by coronary artery dilatation, which increases coronary flow. In the presence of coronary artery disease, the heart may be unable to provide the work needed to increase total body oxygen delivery without risk to the myocardium. Continued demands on the stressed heart to provide oxygen in the face of anemia may produce an anaerobic myocardium and infarction (244,264,265).

Peripheral tissues may also compensate for anemia by increasing oxygen delivery, either by recruiting more capillaries or by increasing blood flow through existing beds. Some tissues, particularly those that are supply dependent, may compensate by increasing oxygen extraction (266). Laser-Doppler flow studies of the skin, muscle and splanchnic bed microcirculation suggest that these compensatory mechanisms are limited and dependent upon not only red cell mass but also circulating volume (267).

In the chronically anemic patient, increases in stroke volume and, therefore, in cardiac output, are supplemented by increased levels of 2,3-DPG. These intracellular changes shift the oxyhemoglobin curve to the right, facilitating oxygen off-load and increasing oxygen delivery.

Oxygen transport and delivery also depend on blood oxygen content. Although a small amount of oxygen can be dissolved in plasma, the primary molecule responsible for oxygen transport is hemoglobin, contained in the RBC. Arterial oxygen content equals the product of hemoglobin concentration, oxygen saturation, the amount of oxygen dissolvable in one gram of hemoglobin (1.39 times hemoglobin), plus the amount of oxygen physically dissolved

in plasma (calculated as the partial pressure of oxygen times the constant 0.0031). Oxygen delivery and consumption are derived in turn from this equation (Table 19.13). Because of compensatory changes in cardiac output and oxygen extraction, oxygen consumption (VO_2) is relatively independent of hemoglobin level across a wide range of oxygen delivery (DO_2) (Table 19.13). As DO_2 decreases through a loss of hemoglobin, oxygen extraction should increase from a baseline of 15% to 25% to maintain a constant consumption. Hence any increase in circulating volume that improves cardiac output will also improve oxygen delivery regardless of hemoglobin level.

However, an improvement in DO_2 from transfusion does not necessarily lead to an increase in oxygen consumption. Wilkerson et al. have shown in the exchange-transfused baboon that VO_2 is maintained down to an Hct of 4% if left atrial pressure is held constant (268). These animals survived by increasing their oxygen extraction ratio (O_2ER) significantly. Under these conditions, coronary blood flow is shifted from the endocardium to the epicardium, thereby placing subendocardial tissue at an increased risk of ischemia. The investigators detected a conversion to anaerobic metabolism at a 10% Hct level, which correlated with an O_2ER of 50%, suggesting these two numbers might be useful as transfusion guidelines. The addition of an experimental coronary stenosis to this model results in depressed cardiac function at hemoglobin levels of 7 to 10 g/dL. Spahn et al. found somewhat different results in a similar model of acute normovolemic hemodilution (ANH) in dogs with a critical coronary artery stenosis (269). Their 19 dogs exhibited evidence of regional myocardial dysfunction at hemoglobin levels below 7.5 g/dL. The dysfunction was corrected by raising hemoglobin by 2 g/dL, the equivalent of a two-unit transfusion of packed RBCs. A recent experimental analysis of critical oxygen delivery using stepwise hemodilution in rats shows the difficulty in identifying which parameters to follow (270). The authors found that multiple variables estimated critical delivery, including lactate, bicarbonate, base excess, O_2ER, expired CO_2, pulse pressure, cardiac index, and systolic pressure. Their data suggest that a multivariable analysis of critical delivery may be needed. These studies serve to guide us but should not be taken as proof for one side or the other in the transfusion argument because of substantial differences between laboratory dogs and the human. As important is the use of fresh, whole blood for transfusion as opposed to stored red cells with their defects. The justification for blood transfusion instead of nonsanguinous volume resuscitation is based on the theoretic ability of hemoglobin to restore oxygen delivery directly. Unfortunately, this may be more theoretic than real, with a basis in mathematics rather than scientific or experimental evidence. For example, assuming a cardiac output of 5 L/min, an oxygen saturation of 98% and a PaO_2 of 80 mm Hg, raising hemoglobin from 10 to 15 g/dL by transfusion mathematically increases oxygen content from 14.7 mL/min to 20.7 mL/min. Evidence documenting that calculated increases actually translate into clinical increases in oxygen consumption and patient benefit are for the most part lacking. Rapid restoration of oxygen delivery and elimination of the oxygen debt, in part through transfusion to Hct levels of 30% to 33%, have been proposed as part of a regimen designed to prevent the development of posttraumatic organ tissue failure (271). Brazzi and Gatinoni's recent review of the studies of supranormal values in critically ill patients points out conflicting results in the treatment or prevention of multisystem organ failure (272). Spence et al. summarized several studies that have been conducted to evaluate the effect of transfusion on oxygen transport in a variety of clinical settings (273). Pretransfusion O_2ERs ranged between 24% to 48%, with the highest values seen in patients with cardiogenic shock. The effect of transfusion to a hemoglobin level of 10 g/dL on O_2ER was minimal in most patients.

More unsettling is recent evidence that demonstrates no clinical benefit from increasing hemoglobin from 8 to 10 g/dL by transfusion. Carson et al.'s large-scale study of transfusion-related outcomes in 8,787 hip fracture patients showed that a liberal transfusion policy to a peak hemoglobin of 10 g/dL did not improve either 30- or 90-day survival when compared to a policy of restricting transfusion to a maximum hemoglobin of 8 g/dL (274). Hebert et al.'s cohort analysis of 4,470 patients admitted to ICUs with a variety of diagnoses showed that anemia increased the risk of death in critically ill patients and that blood transfusion appeared to decrease this risk (275). However, a concomitant multicenter, randomized, controlled pilot study of two transfusion triggers—one restrictive, 7 to 9 g/dL; one liberal, 10 to 12 g/dL—in the treatment of similar patients showed no difference in ICU 30-day and 120-day mortality (276). Corwin et al. had the same results in a similar study (277).

A subgroup of Hebert's patients with severe ischemic heart disease had a higher mortality if transfused to 10 g/dL, although this group of 257 patients did not reach statistical significance (278). These results suggest that there may be dangers in overtransfusing patients, perhaps in this case from increases in blood viscosity that may increase cardiac work. Hebert's findings echo those of the Multicenter Study of Perioperative Ischemia Research group on the effect of transfusion in 2,202 patients undergoing coronary artery bypass surgery (279). Q-wave infarction and overall mortality

rates were significantly greater in those patients with Hcts greater than or equal to 34% when compared to the medium-Hct (25%–33%) group and the low-Hct (24% and below) group. Mortality rate increased directly with Hct. Initial Hct remained the most significant independent predictor of poor outcome [relative risk = 2.22 for low versus high; confidence interval (CI) 1.04 to 4.76] when all groups were combined in a multivariate analysis. This may be a marker for subsequent transfusion and the possible deleterious effect of stored blood.

Because humans tolerate anemia surprisingly well, symptoms and signs caused by decreased red cell mass have limited usefulness as transfusion triggers (280–284). Healthy individuals do not develop exertional dyspnea until hemoglobin concentration reaches 7 g/dL. Even at this and lower levels, symptoms and signs vary. In several studies, Hgb levels as low as 5 or 6 g/dL produced only variable symptoms of tachycardia, hypotension, dyspnea, or impaired levels of consciousness. Adults were more likely to show symptoms than children.

The minimally acceptable Hgb may be that beyond which coronary artery blood flow cannot increase enough to meet myocardial oxygen demands, but this level has yet to be defined in useful clinical terms. Several retrospective analyses of Jehovah's Witness patients have shown that these patients can tolerate perioperative hemoglobin values below 8 g/dL safely (235). Unfortunately, most of these had small numbers preventing stratification by hemoglobin value and failed to control for confounding variables. Carson et al. have reported the largest retrospective study conducted to date of the effect of transfusion on mortality in the hope of defining both the benefits of and the appropriate hemoglobin level for transfusion in the surgical patient (285). They concluded that most patients without underlying cardiopulmonary disease tolerated surgery well without transfusion across a wide range of hemoglobin values. Mortality curves began to rise at 8 g/dL in those who had any clinical evidence of cardiopulmonary disease, for example, a history of angina or an abnormal electrocardiogram. Robertie and Gravlee recommend accepting a transfusion trigger of 6 gm/dL in well-compensated patients with no heart disease and no postoperative complications (286). A higher trigger of 8 g/dL should be used in patients with stable cardiac disease and when blood loss of approximately 300 mL is expected. Older patients and those with postoperative complications who cannot increase cardiac output to compensate for hemodilution should be transfused when Hgb reaches 10 g/dL.

There have been few clinical studies of the effect of coexisting medical conditions on the ability of the heart to compensate for moderate or severe anemia in surgical patients. In Carson's study of mortality and hemoglobin level in Jehovah's Witnesses, preoperative cardiac disease as defined by the Multifactorial Cardiac Risk Index appeared to worsen outcome (287) (Fig. 19.12). In a smaller study of 47 patients with more severe anemia (mean Hgb = 4.6 + .2 g/dL), a history of cardiac, pulmonary, or renal disease had

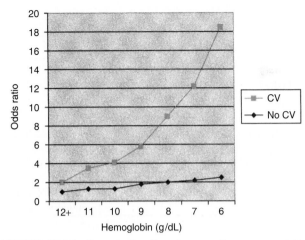

FIGURE 19.12 Impact of cardiopulmonary disease on mortality in the nontransfused Jehovah's Witness. CV, cardiovascular disease.

no association with adverse outcome (288,289). Two reports of an increased incidence of electrocardiographic evidence of myocardial ischemia in postoperative vascular patients with Hcts below 29% suggest that patients with cardiac disease may need hemoglobin levels higher than 8 g/dL, although neither accounted for the presence or severity of underlying heart disease (290). This is corroborated by a retrospective, cohort study of 1958 adult Jehovah's Witnesses by Carson et al. (290). This work, in demonstrating that the nontransfused Jehovah's Witness patient with cardiopulmonary disease is at increased risk of dying as hemoglobin drops below 10 g/dL, is the first to provide solid data regarding the relation between information derived from the history and physical examination, that is, symptoms and hemoglobin level.

The earlier studies show that hemoglobin values significantly lower than an optimal level of 10 g/dL is tolerated by many patients. This does not necessarily mean that a *tolerable* Hgb level should automatically be considered an *acceptable* level for use as a transfusion trigger in all patients (291). Conversely, it is unnecessary and potentially risky to transfuse all patients to an optimal Hgb of 10 g/dL. The main problem with a hemoglobin-based trigger is its lack of generalizability. Some patients can tolerate very low perioperative Hgb levels; whereas others will require supranormal values to survive, depending upon diagnosis and clinical condition.

The decision to transfuse should be related to the specific patient's condition, assessing need on a case-by-case basis. This assessment should include a history and physical examination, a review of pertinent laboratory data, consideration of the operation planned and expectant blood loss, and analysis of risk factors that may contribute to increased morbidity and mortality. The history and physical examination should focus on preexisting diseases or conditions that may increase the risk of blood loss or the need for increased oxygen delivery. The presence of cardiac, pulmonary, and other atherosclerotic disease processes should be assessed and quantified when possible. Surgical

patients with coronary artery disease and pulmonary hypoxia will most likely require higher perioperative hemoglobin levels than those with normal hearts and lungs to avoid ischemia and undue cardiac stress.

In the ICU patient, the first postoperative 24 to 48 hours are the most critical. The controlled setting of the operating room, where the patient is ventilated and anesthetized, is replaced by a period of increased stress and pain. Oxygen consumption, which was reduced intraoperatively by both anesthesia and ventilation, increases and may become directly dependent on delivery. Hemoglobin fluctuates as intravascular and interstitial fluid volumes shift. Neither hemoglobin concentration nor oxygen-derived parameters are completely reliable as transfusion triggers. Increased cardiac work puts demands on myocardial oxygen delivery, such that patients with quiescent coronary artery disease may develop arrhythmias or subendocardial ischemia. In this setting, the surgeon may chose to maintain the most critically ill patients in an anesthetized, ventilated state to lessen oxygen consumption. Measures should be taken to prevent shivering, because the latter can increase oxygen consumption 35% to 40%.

Transfusion in Acute Blood Loss

A classification of hemorrhagic shock based on clinical symptoms is currently in use. (Table 19.14)

Class I hemorrhage is considered to be a loss of less than 15% total blood volume and has the clinical manifestations of a normal pulse rate, blood pressure, and pulse pressure and no changes in signs of tissue perfusion (292). In class II hemorrhage (15%–30% blood volume loss) the pulse rate is increased and systolic blood pressure is normal, but pulse pressure decreases in response to vasoconstriction and tachycardia, which compensate for decreased perfusion. Capillary refill, which reflects tissue perfusion, is tested easily by pinching and releasing the fingertip while observing how quickly and completely the tissues revert from a blanched to a perfused appearance. Capillary refill may be delayed in class II hemorrhage and the respiratory rate may be slightly elevated (293). At this point, patients demonstrate some signs of anxiety as a result of decreased cerebral perfusion. Patients with class III (30%–40% blood loss) present with tachycardia in excess of 120 beats per minute, a decrease in systolic blood pressure and pulse pressure, delayed capillary refill and a progressively increasing respiratory rate. Urine output may become decreased and the patient may become confused at this level. In class IV hemorrhage (>40% blood loss), clinical signs are those of shock: tachycardia, hypotension, oliguria, and lethargy or coma. Clinical assessment of the patient in severe hemorrhagic shock is usually obvious. It is the patient with class I or class II hemorrhagic shock that is difficult to identify.

The primary indication for the transfusion of blood and blood products in the trauma or emergency surgical patient is shock from ongoing blood loss. The decision to transfuse emergently requires a detailed clinical analysis that must include a combination of factors such as the patient's clinical

TABLE 19.14

Classes of Hemorrhage

Class of Hemorrhage	Blood Loss (% TBV)	Heart Rate	Blood Pressure	Tissue Perfusion	Other Clinical Signs	Fluid Therapy
I	<15	Normal or increased	Normal	Normal	None	None
II	15–30	Increased	Normal or decreased	Decreased	Decreased	Crystalloid/colloid Blood ±
III	30–40	Increased	Decreased	Decreased	Oliguria, confusion	Crystalloid/colloid Blood +
IV	>40	Increased	Decreased	Decreased	Lethargy, coma	Crystalloid/colloid Blood +

TBV, total blood volume.

condition, initial hemoglobin concentration, response to fluid resuscitation, coexisting respiratory, cardiac and vascular conditions, and measurements of tissue oxygenation obtained by cardiac and peripheral monitors.

The primary purpose of emergency transfusion is to restore perfusion and reverse the effects of shock by assuring adequate oxygen delivery. Rush et al. (294,295) have shown that a loss of up to 25% of a patient's blood volume can be replaced by a balanced salt solution, with volume replacement calculated as approximately three times the amount of the blood loss. A low hemoglobin in the acutely bleeding patient with signs of shock is evidence of ongoing hemorrhage and should not be misinterpreted as chronic, compensated anemia (296). Conversely, a normal hemoglobin level in an acutely bleeding patient does not mean that red cell mass is normal but may reflect hemoconcentration from volume loss and a lack of replenishment of plasma volume.

Massive Transfusion

Massive transfusion is commonly defined as transfusion approximating or exceeding the patient's blood volume within a 24-hour period (297). However, in many trauma victims, this volume is administered within a shorter time interval. In this setting, blood losses of between 30% to 50% of total blood volume may be defined as massive hemorrhage. Essential to the definition of massive transfusion is an understanding of the principles of exchange transfusion and the concept of a dilutional coagulopathy. The kinetics of exchange transfusion predict that approximately 37% of the original blood volume remains following the loss of a single blood volume (10 units in a 70-kg adult) (298,299). With two or three volume exchanges, the remaining coagulation factors and platelets will drop to levels of approximately 15% and 5%, respectively. Not surprisingly, trauma patients receiving massive transfusion may develop coagulation problems.

Coagulation factor and platelet depletion is not as common a cause of intraoperative hemorrhage as many surgeons think. Hypothermia may be a contributing factor (300). It may be difficult to directly correlate the clinical observation

of bleeding with prolongation of the PT and aPTT, which are reagent and temperature dependent (301). Because coagulation testing is routinely performed at 37°C, rather than at the patient's actual *in vivo* temperature, normal coagulation tests can be obtained even in the presence of clinical evidence of a coagulopathy (302). Normal test results in this setting suggest that sufficient clotting factors are available for coagulation if normothermia is restored (303–313).

Dilutional coagulopathy may be mistaken for or aggravated by the development of DIC (314,315). DIC in the setting of massive transfusion is reported to occur in 5% to 30% of trauma patients and is associated with mortality rates approaching 70% (300). Tissue injury and hemolysis with release of cytokines and tissue thromboplastin into the circulation may cause immediate activation of both the coagulation and the fibrinolytic systems, resulting in severe DIC (316). At the present time no single laboratory test can be used to confirm or exclude the diagnosis of DIC. However, the combination of a low platelet count, a low fibrinogen, an elevated D-dimer and the presence of soluble fibrin monomers in the context of the patient's underlying condition are the most helpful indicators of DIC.

Coagulation factors and platelets can be replaced as needed by infusing FFP or platelets. Stored, allogeneic blood maintains sufficient levels of all coagulation factors needed to prevent bleeding except V and VIII, which decrease over time (317). If available, whole blood obtained through ANH can be used to restore coagulation factors and platelets.

Alternatives to Allogeneic Blood

Directed Donor Blood

Patient preference is strong for the use of directed donor blood, but its use does not reduce the risks associated with allogeneic transfusion (318–325). Directed donor blood carries significant risks including disease transmission and graft versus host disease. The use of directed donor blood may be an acceptable option in specific settings, for example, neonatal or pediatric surgery, but for the most part, surgeons should discourage its use and should instruct patients about potential dangers.

Autologous Predonation

Autologous predonation (PAD) is an alternative that has been proved to reduce dependence on allogeneic blood in multiple studies of a variety of surgical procedures (326). Successful PAD depends on (i) adequate time for donation (ii) a hemoglobin level greater than 11.0 g/dL, (iii) absence of significant disease, that is, severe aortic stenosis or active angina, (iv) selection of appropriate patients based on anticipated blood loss and transfusion need, and (v) both patient and physician cooperation. The ideal patient for predonation is one who has an anticipated need for blood transfusion with a window of two or more weeks before surgery to donate. Relative contraindications to predonation include a history of congestive heart failure, valvular heart disease, recent myocardial infarction, angina, dysrhythmias, and hypertension requiring multiple drug therapy, seizures, or cerebrovascular disease. An increased incidence of reactions is associated with donor age younger than 17 years, weight more than 110 lbs., female gender and a history of previous reactions. Approximately 10% to 15% of patients are unable to reach the acceptable hemoglobin level of 11 g/dL for predonation. Male gender and higher initial Hct are independent factors associated with successful completion of a four-unit order. Treatment with RHuEPO can facilitate predonation in mildly anemic patients scheduled for orthopaedic surgery.

Autotransfusion

The value of autotransfusion, or collection and reinfusion of shed blood, in reducing the need for allogeneic blood transfusion has been documented in multiple retrospective analyses. Reports from more than 20,000 patients during a variety of elective surgical procedures show reduction in allogeneic blood use by up to 75% (327). Intraoperative autotransfusion can be performed with systems that either collect blood directly, anticoagulate it and reinfuse it through filters or systems that collect the blood, wash it and reinfuse a packed red cell product (328). Systems without washing capability collect shed blood through a suction wand that simultaneously adds either heparin or citrate-phosphate-dextrose anticoagulant into a collection chamber (329). Collected blood is returned to the patient through a filter, which is the only means of preparing the blood. Filters are capable of removing large debris such as bone chips and smaller particulate matter such cellular fragments. Following filtration, the salvaged blood represents "red cells suspended in plasma," containing platelets, fibrinogen, and clotting factors.

Unwashed blood may contain vasoactive contaminants, activated clotting factors, FDPs, and free hemoglobin, all of which can be dangerous. Bartels, et al. analyzed differences in hemostatic, hemolytic, and hematologic parameters after autotransfusion of washed cell saver blood versus unprocessed, shed whole blood during major aortic surgery in 32 patients (330). Levels of bilirubin, free hemoglobin, lactic dehydrogenase, D-dimers, and FDPs were significantly higher before transfusion in whole blood compared to cell saver blood. Moreover, patients who received unprocessed

whole blood had significantly higher circulating levels of these products and of D-dimers after autotransfusion. High postoperative serum levels of creatine kinase (CK) and lactate dehydrogenase (LDH) enzymes have been measured after infusion of blood shed from the mediastinum, leading to the possible misinterpretation of these enzymes as evidence of new myocardial infarction (331). Febrile transfusion reactions in patients who receive filtered, unwashed blood may be caused by leukocyte-derived vasoactive contaminants (332). Washing shed blood reduces but does not completely eliminate leukocytes from the infused product (333).

Dzik has thoroughly reviewed the current literature on the controversy over whether or not to wash shed blood before autotransfusion, concluding that washing of shed blood is preferable to not washing (328,334–336). However, he points out that clinical studies of unwashed blood show that its use is safe under specific circumstances (321). Safety depends on limiting infusion to small quantities, restricting collection and reinfusion times to 6 hours or less, and reduction of toxicities by avoiding skimming, using a second suction wand for blood unsuitable for reinfusion and avoidance of chemical agents, that is, topical hemostatics, and biological substances, that is, urine (337).

Systems that wash blood and concentrate the red cells have the advantage of providing a cleaner product, free of the contaminants found in unwashed blood. With these devices, blood is collected from the operative field, filtered, anticoagulated and temporarily stored in a reservoir. The blood is transferred to a centrifuge bowl that spins at approximately 5,000 revolutions per minute, separating the red cells from plasma. The cells are washed and resuspended in saline to attain a Hct of 40% to 60% before reinfusion (333). Disadvantages of these systems include the loss of the plasma component; as well as the need for expert help, setup time and expense.

Relative contraindications to the use of autotransfused blood, whether washed or not, include the presence of infection or bowel contamination, malignancy and obstetric procedures contaminated with amniotic fluid (338,339). In these situations the surgeon must weigh the potential benefit obtainable from autotransfusion against the risks. Autotransfusion has been used successfully and without increased infectious risk with potentially contaminated blood (340). Washing the blood appears to reduce the bacterial load; prophylactic antibiotics provide additional protection (341,342). Autotransfusion has been used safely in cancer surgery in the Jehovah's Witness when the real risk of death from blood loss outweighed the theoretic one of tumor cell dissemination (343). An answer to the problem of reinfusing cancer cells with shed blood may be found in the use of leukocyte reduction filters which appear to eliminate viable cancer cells from shed blood (344).

Acute Normovolemic Hemodilution

ANH is an anesthetic procedure that first reduces the patient's RBC mass by removing whole blood and replacing it with colloid, crystalloid, or a combination of both (295). The intention is to reduce the amount of RBC loss during the intra- or immediate postoperative period by having a large portion of RBC present in the "ANH" container, and thereby losing dilute blood from the surgical field. The concentrated blood is returned to the patient at any point that the patient meets the clinician's criteria for transfusion. This method of RBC conservation will result in the patient ending up having the highest hemoglobin level postoperatively, and therefore reducing or eliminating the patient's exposure to allogeneic blood. The return of the patient's blood without a storage lesion provides all functional components in the plasma as well as the oxygen-carrying RBC's.

ANH is well described in the anesthesia and surgical intraoperative blood management literature (345,346). It was endorsed as an effective blood conservation technique by the National Institutes of health (NIH) consensus panel, as well as by the American Society of Anesthesiologists (347–352). Despite these endorsements, use of ANH has been limited mostly to cardiac surgery. Only in the last two decades has ANH been applied with success to patients undergoing other surgical procedures (353,354).

Physiology

Depending on the amount of blood removed, ANH can produce a rapid and sometimes severe acute anemia. This in itself may be the initial reason for the poor acceptance of the procedure by many clinicians. The concept of intentionally producing acute anemia raises the concern of reduced oxygen delivery and the possibility of significant morbidity and possible mortality.

In fact, the compensatory mechanisms in response to ANH are protective to the individual down to hemoglobin levels thought to be inconsistent with either survival or consistent with organ and tissue injury (355). As the acutely anemic patient's circulation is replenished with colloid or crystalloid, oxygen delivery to the tissues is well maintained and oxygen demand on the myocardium may be held steady or may be reduced (284). As with patients who develop chronic anemic states, the tolerance of low hemoglobin to levels less than 4.0 g is primarily due to volume compensation. This situation persists in the chronically anemic patient and results in a high output state, with deterioration of the myocytes and congestive heart failure. Patients undergoing ANH will benefit from these compensatory mechanisms, and their exposure to anemia is too short-lived to lead to a high output state and cardiac decompensation. In Table 19.15, the compensatory mechanisms are listed in order. Failure to maintain adequate circulatory volume will negate most, if not all of the positive compensatory mechanisms (287,356,357).

Patient Selection and Limits of Acute Normovolemic Hemodilution

In our experience all patients are candidates for ANH. Mitigating factors that will be a reasonable concern are included in Table 19.16. Although no specific contraindications exist, experience in performing ANH is essential in the listed

TABLE 19.15

Compensatory Mechanisms Following Hemodilution and Creation of Acute Anemia

Increased cardiac output (CO)
Increased stroke volume
Slight increase in heart rate (not clinically significant)
Reduced blood viscosity and decreased afterload
Increased blood flow to oxygen dependent tissues beyond the CO increase
Increased oxygen extraction in end organs
Increased coronary blood flow

possible contraindications in Table 19.16. It is also important to note that some Jehovah's Witness patients may accept ANH, but others will not. Several of these complicating conditions are considered individually here.

Preexisting anemia requires the clinician to have a clear endpoint of the ending hemoglobin with ANH. Patients who have tolerated hemoglobin of 3 g and above whom present to surgery with higher hemoglobin will tolerate ANH down to the lower initial hemoglobin. Of all the many concerns the clinician may have regarding ANH, cardiac, cerebral, and renal effect of decreased oxygen delivery are the most dominant. Data on the tolerance of volume compensated anemia in humans and animals suggest that levels of normovolemic anemia to hemoglobin of 5.0 g/dL are well tolerated and individual patients may do well with hemoglobin levels below 5.0 g/dL. In the face of severe anemia tissue extraction with added capillary recruitment deliver adequate oxygen to the essential organs and tissues. One cannot underscore enough the importance of normal intravascular circulating volume.

Patients with known hemoglobinopathies may tolerate ANH, but data on RBC survivability at room temperature is not known. Therefore, other blood conservation methods should be used first, unless the patient's life is at risk and they refuse or are unable to accept transfusion of allogeneic blood.

Cardiac disease, especially ischemic cardiac disease, has been considered as a relative or absolute contraindication to ANH. Reports of patients not tolerating hemoglobins of less than 9.0 g without the onset of ischemic signs have

TABLE 19.16

Possible Contraindications to Performing Acute Normovolemic Hemodilution

Anemia with hemoglobin <7.0 g/dL
Hemoglobinopathy associated with hemolysis (sickle cell disease, etc.)
Active ischemic cardiac disease
Renal failure
Known coagulopathy associated with active bleeding

led many clinicians to avoid this procedure (358). In our experience, patients with active ischemic cardiac disease tolerate moderate amounts of ANH without difficulty. Cardiac medications such as nitrates and β blockers are first line treatment for ischemic episodes, whereas replenishing volume and red cells should be reserved as second-line treatment. Currently, ST-segment analysis is the standard monitoring tool of the patient during surgery, and will alert the clinician to the need for assessment and treatment. Patients with valvular heart disease present a more complex problem, and should have invasive monitoring and/or ongoing transesophageal echocardiography if ANH is contemplated. It is generally difficult to assess volume status and changes in patients with valvular heart disease. Introduction of ANH under these circumstances makes it more difficult and complex.

Renal failure has been thought as a contraindication for ANH, because volume to restore circulation cannot be removed effectively during the intraoperative period. For those patients whose life may depend on ANH blood because they cannot or will not receive allogeneic transfusions, ANH with continuous veno–veno hemofiltration can be performed (359–361). Maintaining blood flow as well as anticoagulation presents a problem for the anesthesiologist and the surgeon, but most cardiac and vascular surgery is performed successfully in the presence of partial or full anticoagulation. In patients with coagulation abnormalities, *in vitro* coagulation measurements are mildly abnormal and no clinical signs of bleeding are associated with ANH (362–366). Data is still sparse and one must maintain constant vigilance in patient's coagulation status. In the face of documented coagulopathy associated with bleeding, it is difficult to predict the effects of ANH on the outcome of surgery; therefore, ANH under this circumstance must be weighed against other blood conservation techniques. ANH has been performed in the parturient, the neonate, and the pediatric patient. ANH has also been used successfully in trauma and other emergency surgery.

Calculation of End Point for Acute Normovolemic Hemodilution

Controversy exists as to the end point of ANH. In one center with the largest experience in radical prostatectomy, ANH is used to reduce patients' exposure to allogeneic blood. Removal of whole blood to target hemoglobin of 9.0 g is used to limit ANH. We prefer to use the patient's vital signs is an indicator for the end point of blood withdrawal. Because no consensus exists currently, the author strongly recommends attaining a level of experience and comfort in order to develop clear and concise guidelines for those who are to perform ANH. Although formulas to guide the clinician exist, these may or may not prove to be helpful in the operating room setting. One formula commonly used is the following: $ANH_v = EBV\ Hct_i - Hct_f\ (3 - average\ Hct)$, where EBV is the estimated blood volume, ANH_v is the amount of blood to be collected through ANH and Hct_i, Hct_f are the initial and final Hct respectively.

Blood Substitutes

Two types of blood substitutes are currently under investigation: perfluorocarbon-based and hemoglobin-derived. The perfluorocarbon-based substances are under continuous developmental design and not in clinical trial. These will not be further discussed in this chapter.

Hemoglobin-based products are well into various phases of clinical trials. None of these products are FDA-approved for clinical use in the United States. The challenges that these substances must meet include availability, immunologic properties, half-life within the circulation, excessive affinity for oxygen, and vasoactive properties. Currently available products derive either from human or bovine blood, the latter source providing a potentially unlimited supply. Recombinant human hemoglobin is also under investigation.

Immunologically, early products activated the complement cascade and caused anaphylactoid reactions. This was attributed to phospholipids from residual red cell stroma, and improved ultrafiltration and purification has substantially reduced this problem. Hemoglobin itself is a very poor immunogen.

When removed from the protective erythrocyte membrane, hemoglobin has a half-life of less than 1 hour in the circulation. It breaks down readily from tetramers to monomers, and then is freely filtered by the glomerulus, causing renal toxicity and even renal failure. Cross-linking and polymerization or encapsulation of the hemoglobin molecules can extend the half-life up to 30 hours.

Circulating hemoglobin also has excessive affinity for oxygen, thought to be related to insufficient plasma 2,3-DPG and relatively alkaline pH. This is being addressed by changes in manufacturing process, and may be less of a problem with bovine hemoglobin.

Vasoactive properties remain a significant challenge. Free hemoglobin scavenges NO in interstitial tissues, potentiating vasoconstriction already induced by excess oxygen delivery. The oxidative properties of hemoglobin may potentially add to its vasoconstriction effect. Multiple phase III trials are currently ongoing and initial reports of the utility of these agents as temporary oxygen carriers that provide a "bridge to transfusion" are encouraging.

ACKNOWLEDGMENTS

The expert assistance of Tara Maurer in the preparation of this manuscript is gratefully acknowledged. Henry L Bennett, Ched Singleton, and William A Rock Jr. contributed to the prior edition of this chapter.

REFERENCES

1. Addonizio VP, Stahl R. Bleeding. In: Wimore DL, Brennan MF, Harken AH, et al. eds. *American college of surgeons care of the surgical patient.* New York: Scientific American, 1992:1–13.

2. von dem Borne AE, Folman C, Linthorst GE, et al. Thrombopoietin: its role in platelet disorders and as a new drug in clinical medicine. *Baillieres Clin Haematol* 1998;11:427–445.

3. George JN, Colman RW. Overview of platelet structure and function. In: Robert WC, Victor JM, Alexander WC, et al. eds. *Hemostasis and thrombosis basic principles and clinical practice*, 4th ed. Philadelphia: Lippincott Williams & Wilkins, 2001: 381–386.

4. Kelton JG, Warkentin TE. Heparin-induced thrombocytopenia. Diagnosis, natural history, and treatment options. *Postgrad Med* 1998;103:169–178.

5. Cancio LC, Cohen DJ. Heparin-induced thrombocytopenia and thrombosis. *J Am Coll Surg* 1998;186:76–91.

6. Pineo GF, Hull RD. Unfractionated and low-molecular-weight heparin. Comparisons and current recommendations. *Med Clin North Am* 1998;82:587–599.

7. Hirsh J, Warkentin TE, Raschke R, et al. Heparin and low-molecular-weight heparin: mechanisms of action, pharmacokinetics, dosing considerations, monitoring, efficacy, and safety. *Chest* 1998;114(Suppl 5):489S–510S.

8. Brieger DB, Mak KH, Kottke-Marchant K, et al. Heparin-induced thrombocytopenia. *J Am Coll Cardiol* 1998;31:1449–1459.

9. Drews RE, Weinberger SE. Thrombocytopenic disorders in critically ill patients. *Am J Respir Crit Care Med* 2000;162(2 Pt 1): 347–351.

10. Ananthasubramaniam K, Shurafa M, Prasad A. Heparin-induced thrombocytopenia and thrombosis. *Prog Cardiovasc Dis* 2000;42:247–260.

11. Schafer AI. Essential thrombocythemia. *Prog Hemost Thromb* 1991;10:69–96.

12. Rao AK. Congenital disorders of platelet function. *Hematol Oncol Clin North Am* 1990;4:65–86.

13. Prescott SM, McIntyre TM, Zimmerman GA. The role of platelet activating factor in endothelial cells. *Thromb Haemost* 1990; 64:899–903.

14. Ashby B, Daniel JL, Smith JB. Mechanism of platelet activation and inhibition. *Hematol Oncol Clin North Am* 1990;4:1–26.

15. Colman RW, Hisch K, Maider VJ, et al. Platelet receptors. *Hematol Oncol Clin North Am* 1990;4:27–42.

16. McEver RP. The clinical significance of platelet membrane glycoproteins. *Hematol Oncol Clin North Am* 1990;4:87–105.

17. Peterson P, Hayes TE, Arkin CF, et al. The preoperative bleeding time test lacks clinical benefit. *Arch Surg* 1998;133:134–139.

18. Roberts HR, Tabarea AH. Overview of the coagulation reaction. In: High KA, Roberts HR, eds. *Molecular basis of thrombosis and hemostasis*. New York: Marcel Decker Inc, 1995:35–50.

19. Bovill EG, Malhotra OP, Mann KG. Mechanisms of vitamin K antagonism. *Baillieres Clin Haematol* 1990;3(3):555–581.

20. Heresbach D, Pagenault M, Gueret P, et al. Leiden factor V mutation in four patients with small bowel infarctions. *Gastroenterology* 1997;113(1):322–325.

21. Leroyer C, Mercier B, Escoffre M, et al. Factor V Leiden prevalence in venous thromboembolism patients. *Chest* 1997; 111(6):1603–1606.

22. Mahmoud AE, Elias E, Beauchamp N, et al. Prevalence of the factor V Leiden mutation in hepatic and portal vein thrombosis. *Gut* 1997;40(6):798–800.

23. Eskandari MK, Bontempo FA, Hassett AC, et al. Arterial thromboembolic events in patients with the factor V Leiden mutation. *Am J Surg* 1998;176(2):122–125.

24. Bergenfeldt M, Svensson PJ, Borgstrom A. Mesenteric vein thrombosis due to factor V Leiden gene mutation. *Br J Surg* 1999; 86(8):1059–1062.

25. Dahlback B. Procoagulant and anticoagulant properties of coagulation factor V: factor V Leiden (APC resistance) causes hypercoagulability by dual mechanisms. *J Lab Clin Med* 1999;133(5): 415–422.

26. Bennett JC. Both sides of the hypercoagulable state. *Hosp Pract (Off ed)* 1997;32(11):105–108, 111–112, 119–121.

27. Martinelli I, Mannucci PM, De Stefano V, et al. Different risks of thrombosis in four coagulation defects associated with inherited thrombophilia: a study of 150 families. *Blood* 1998;92(7): 2353–2358.

28. Bick RL, Kaplan H. Syndromes of thrombosis and hypercoagulability. Congenital and acquired causes of thrombosis. *Med Clin North Am* 1998;82(3):409–458.

29. Major DA, Sane DC, Herrington DM. Cardiovascular implications of the factor V Leiden mutation. *Am Heart J* 2000;140(2):189–195.

30. Tracy PB. Regulation of thrombin generation at cell surfaces. *Semin Thromb Hemost* 1988;14(3):227–233.

31. Kearon C, Hirsh J. Management of anticoagulation before and after elective surgery. *N Engl J Med* 1997;336(21):1506–1511.

32. Brigden ML. The hypercoagulable state. Who, how, and when to test and treat. *Postgrad Med* 1997;101(5):249–252, 254–256, 259–262.

33. White GC, Marder VJ, Colman RW, et al. Approach to the bleeding patient. In: Colman RWHJ, Marder VJ, et al. eds. *Hemostasis and thrombosis: basic principles and clinical practice*. Philadelphia: JB Lippincott Co, 1994:1134–1147.

34. Hilgartner M. Factor replacement therapy. In: Hilgartner M, Pochedly C, eds. *Hemophilia in the child and adult*. New York: Raven Press, 1989:1–26.

35. Morgan CH, Penner JA. Bleeding complications during surgery: part I. Defects of primary hemostasis and congenital coagulation. *Lab Med* 1986;17:207–212.

36. Kram HB, Nathan RC, Stafford FJ, et al. Fibrin glue achieves hemostasis in patients with coagulation disorders. *Arch Surg* 1989;124(3):385–387.

37. Roberts HR, Jones MR. Hemophilia and related conditions—congenital deficiencies of prothrombin (factor II), factor V, and factors VII to XII. In: Williams WJ, William BE, Erslev AJ, et al. eds. *Hematology*, 4th ed. New York: McGraw Hill, 1990:1453–1473.

38. Berry EW. Use of DDAVP and cryoprecipitate in mild to moderate haemophilia A and von Willebrand's disease. *Prog Clin Biol Res* 1990;324:269–278.

39. Cattaneo M, Moia M, Delle Valle P, et al. DDAVP shortens the prolonged bleeding times of patients with severe von Willebrand disease treated with cryoprecipitate. Evidence for a mechanism of action independent of released von Willebrand factor. *Blood* 1989;74(6):1972–1975.

40. Radosevich M. Safety of recombinant and plasma-derived medicinals for the treatment of coagulopathies. *Hematol Oncol Clin North Am* 2000;14(2):459–470.

41. Arun B, Kessler CM. Clinical manifestations and therapy of the hemophilias. In: Colman RW, Hirsh J, Marder VJ, eds. *Hemostasis and thrombosis: basic principles and clinical practice*. Philadelphia: JB Lippincott Co, 1994:815–824.

42. Preissner KT. Anticoagulant potential of endothelial cell membrane components. *Haemostasis* 1988;18(4–6):271–300.

43. Jaffe EA. Vascular function in hemostasis. In: Williams WJ, Beutler E, Erslev AJ, et al. eds. *Hematology*, 4th ed. New York: McGraw Hill, 1990:1322–1337.

44. Wu KR. Endothelial cells in hemostasis, thrombosis and inflammation. *Hosp Pract* 1992;145–166.

45. Vanhoutte PM, Luscher TF, Graser T. Endothelium-dependent contractions. *Blood Vessels* 1991;28(1–3):74–83.

46. van Hinsbergh WWM. Regulation of the synthesis and secretion of plasminogen activators by endothelial cells. *Haemostasis* 1988;18: 307–327.

47. Brenner BM, Troy JL, Ballermann BJ. Endothelium-dependent vascular responses. Mediators and mechanisms. *J Clin Invest* 1989; 84(5):1373–1378.

48. Bauer KA, Rosenberg RD. Role of antithrombin III as a regulator of *in vivo* coagulation. *Semin Hematol* 1991;28(1):10–18.

49. Riess H. Antithrombin: mechanism of action and clinical usage. Conclusion. *Blood Coagul Fibrinolysis* 1998;9(Suppl 3):S23–S24.

50. Menache D. Antithrombin III: introduction. *Semin Hematol* 1991; 28(1):1–2.

51. Vinazzer H. Hereditary and acquired antithrombin deficiency. *Semin Thromb Hemost* 1999;25(3):257–263.

52. Jackson CM. Mechanism of heparin action. *Baillieres Clin Haematol* 1990;3(3):483–504.

53. Rosenberg RD. Redesigning heparin. *N Engl J Med* 2001;344(9): 673–675.

54. Dittman WA, Majerus PW. Structure and function of thrombomodulin: a natural anticoagulant. *Blood* 1990;75(2):329–336.

55. Esmon NL. Thrombomodulin. *Prog Hemost Thromb* 1989;9:29–55.

56. Esmon CT. The protein C pathway. *Chest* 2003;124(Suppl 3): 26S–32S.

57. Simmonds RE, Ireland H, Lane DA, et al. Clarification of the risk for venous thrombosis associated with hereditary protein S deficiency by investigation of a large kindred with a characterized gene defect. *Ann Intern Med* 1998;128(1):8–14.

58. Chan YC, Valenti D, Mansfield AO, et al. Warfarin induced skin necrosis. *Br J Surg* 2000;87(3):266–272.

59. Miller JL. von Willebrand disease. *Hematol Oncol Clin North Am* 1990;4:107–128.

60. Sixma JJ, de Groot PG. Von Willebrand factor and the blood vessel wall. *Mayo Clin Proc* 1991;66:628–633.

61. Sutor AH. Desmopressin (DDAVP) in bleeding disorders of childhood. *Semin Thromb Hemost* 1998;24:555–566.

62. Mannucci PM. Desmopressin: a nontransfusional hemostatic agent. *Annu Rev Med* 1990;41:55–64.

63. Nolan B, White B, Smith J, et al. Desmopressin: therapeutic limitations in children and adults with inherited coagulation disorders. *Br J Haematol* 2000;109:865–869.

64. George JN, Vesely S, Rizvi M. Thrombotic thrombocytopenic purpura—hemolytic-uremic syndrome. In: Colman RW, Hirsh J, Marder VJ, et al. eds. *Hemostasis and thrombosis: basic principles and clinical practice*. Philadelphia: JB Lippincott Co, 1994:1235–1242.

65. Rosenberg RD, Aird WC. Vascular-bed–specific hemostasis and hypercoagulable states. *N Engl J Med* 1999;340(20):1555–1564.

66. Loskutoff DJ, Curriden SA. The fibrinolytic system of the vessel wall and its role in the control of thrombosis. *Ann N Y Acad Sci* 1990;598:238–247.

67. Robbins KC. Classification of abnormal plasminogens: dysplasminogenemias. *Semin Thromb Hemost* 1990;16(3):217–220.

68. Leebeek FW, Knot EA, Ten Cate JW, et al. Severe thrombotic tendency associated with a type I plasminogen deficiency. *Am J Hematol* 1989;30(1):32–35.

69. Bachmann F. Plasminogen-plasmin enzyme system. In: Colman RW, Hirsh J, Maider VJ, et al. eds. *Hemostasis and thrombosis basic principles and clinical practice*, 4th ed. Philadelphia: Lippincott Williams & Wilkins, 2001:275–320.

70. Conrad J, Samama M. Theoretic and practical considerations on laboratory monitoring of thrombolytic therapy. *Semin Thromb Hemost* 1987;13:212–222.

71. Stump DC, Taylor FB, Nesheim ME, et al. Pathologic fibrinolysis as a cause of clinical bleeding. *Semin Thromb Hemost* 1990; 16(3):260–273.

72. Wiman B, Hamsten A. The fibrinolytic enzyme system and its role in the etiology of thromboembolic disease. *Semin Thromb Hemost* 1990;16(3):207–216.

73. Bonnar J, Daly L, Sheppard BL. Changes in the fibrinolytic system during pregnancy. *Semin Thromb Hemost* 1990;16(3):221–229.

74. Levi M, Ten Cate H. Disseminated intravascular coagulation. *N Engl J Med* 1999;341(8):586–592.

75. Yu M, Nardella A, Pechet L. Screening tests of disseminated intravascular coagulation: guidelines for rapid and specific laboratory diagnosis. *Crit Care Med* 2000;28(6):1777–1780.

76. Jagneaux T, Taylor DE, Kantrow SP. Coagulation in sepsis. *Am J Med Sci* 2004;328(4):196–204.

77. Carvalho AC. Acquired platelet dysfunction in patients with uremia. *Hematol Oncol Clin North Am* 1990;4(1):129–143.

78. Castillo R, Lozano T, Escolar G, et al. Defective platelet adhesion on vessel subendothelium in uremic patients. *Blood* 1986;68(2):337–342.

79. Mannucci PM. Hemostatic drugs. *N Engl J Med* 1998;339(4): 245–253.

80. Bronner MH, Pate MB, Cunningham JT, et al. Estrogen-progesterone therapy for bleeding gastrointestinal telangiectasias in chronic renal failure. An uncontrolled trial. *Ann Intern Med* 1986;105(3):371–374.

81. Lethagen S, Rugarn P, Aberg M, et al. Effects of desmopressin acetate (DDAVP) and dextran on hemostatic and thromboprophylactic mechanisms. *Acta Chir Scand* 1990;156(9):597–602.

82. Joist JHGJ. Hemostatic abnormalities in liver and renal disease. In: Colman RW, Hirsh J, Marder VJ, et al. eds. *Hemostasis and thrombosis: basic principles and clinical practice*. Philadelphia: JB Lippincott Co, 1994:955–976.

83. Colwell NS, Tollefsen DM, Blinder MA. Identification of a monoclonal thrombin inhibitor associated with multiple myeloma and a severe bleeding disorder. *Br J Haematol* 1997;97(1):219–226.

84. Bendixen BH, Adams HP. Ticlopidine or clopidogrel as alternatives to aspirin in prevention of ischemic stroke. *Eur Neurol* 1996;36(5):256–257.

85. Schafer AI. Antiplatelet therapy. *Am J Med* 1996;101(2):199–209.

86. Verstraete M. New developments in antiplatelet and antithrombotic therapy. *Eur Heart J* 1995;16(Suppl L):16–23.

87. Verstraete M, Zoldhelyi P. Novel antithrombotic drugs in development. *Drugs* 1995;49(6):856–884.

88. Gachet C, Cattaneo M, Ohlmann P, et al. Purinoceptors on blood platelets: further pharmacological and clinical evidence to suggest the presence of two ADP receptors. *Br J Haematol* 1995;91(2): 434–444.

89. Roald HE, Barstad RM, Kierulf P, et al. Clopidogrel—a platelet inhibitor which inhibits thrombogenesis in non-anticoagulated human blood independently of the blood flow conditions. *Thromb Haemost* 1994;71(5):655–662.

90. Mills DC, Puri R, Hu CJ, et al. Clopidogrel inhibits the binding of ADP analogues to the receptor mediating inhibition of platelet adenylate cyclase. *Arterioscler Thromb* 1992;12(4):430–436.

91. CAPRIE Steering Committee. A randomised, blinded, trial of clopidogrel versus aspirin in patients at risk of ischaemic events (CAPRIE). *Lancet* 1996;348(9038):1329–1339.

92. Gordon JL. Overview: pharmacology of ticlopidine. *Agents Actions Suppl* 1984;15:108–115.

93. Moncada S, Korbut R. Dipyridamole and other phosphodiesterase inhibitors act as antithrombotic agents by potentiating endogenous prostacyclin. *Lancet* 1978;1(8077):1286–1289.

94. Mehta J, Mehta P, Pepine CJ, et al. Platelet function studies in coronary artery disease. X. Effect of dipyridamole. *Am J Cardiol* 1981; 47(5):1111–1114.

95. Jackson CA, Greaves M, Preston FE. A study of the stimulation of human venous prostacyclin synthesis by dipyridamole. *Thromb Res* 1982;27(5):563–573.

96. Harker LA, Kadatz RA. Mechanism of action of dipyridamole. *Thromb Res Suppl* 1983;4:39–46.

97. Neri Serneri GG, Masotti G, Poggesi L, et al. Enhanced prostacyclin production by dipyridamole in man. *Eur J Clin Pharmacol* 1981; 21(1):9–15.

98. Klabunde RE. Dipyridamole inhibition of adenosine metabolism in human blood. *Eur J Pharmacol* 1983;93(1–2):21–26.

99. Dawicki DD, Agarwal KC, Parks RE Jr. Role of adenosine uptake and metabolism by blood cells in the antiplatelet actions of dipyridamole, dilazep and nitrobenzylthioinosine. *Biochem Pharmacol* 1985;34(22):3965–3972.

100. Dawicki DD, Agarwal KC, Parks RE Jr. Potentiation of the antiplatelet action of adenosine in whole blood by dipyridamole or dilazep and the cAMP phosphodiesterase inhibitor, RA 233. *Thromb Res* 1986;43(2):161–175.

101. Heptinstall S, Fox S, Crawford J, et al. Inhibition of platelet aggregation in whole blood by dipyridamole and aspirin. *Thromb Res* 1986;42(2):215–223.

102. Gresele P, Arnout J, Deckmyn H, et al. Mechanism of the antiplatelet action of dipyridamole in whole blood: modulation of adenosine concentration and activity. *Thromb Haemost* 1986;55(1):12–18.

103. Solvay H, Kahn M, Garreyn S, et al. Glucose and erythrocyte ATP: distinctive effects of dipyridamole and of ticlopidine. *Angiology* 1987;38(11):815–824.

104. Mehta J, Mehta P. Dipyridamole and aspirin in relation to platelet aggregation and vessel wall prostaglandin generation. *J Cardiovasc Pharmacol* 1982;4(4):688–693.

105. Uotila P, Dahl ML, Matintalo M, et al. The effects of aspirin and dipyridamole on the metabolism of arachidonic acid in human platelets. *Prostaglandins Leukot Med* 1983;11(1):73–82.

106. Costantini V, Talpacci A, Cipolloni S, et al. Effect of aspirin and dipyridamole treatment on prostacyclin production by human veins. *Thromb Res* 1990;58(2):109–117.

107. Muller TH, Su CA, Weisenberger H, et al. Dipyridamole alone or combined with low-dose acetylsalicylic acid inhibits platelet aggregation in human whole blood ex vivo. *Br J Clin Pharmacol* 1990;30(2):179–186.

108. Levine MN. Nonhemorrhagic complications of anticoagulant therapy. *Semin Thromb Hemost* 1986;12(1):63–66.

109. Deykin D. Current concepts: the use of heparin. *N Engl J Med* 1969;280(17):937–938.

110. Biggs R, Denson KW, Akman N, et al. Antithrombin 3, antifactor Xa and heparin. *Br J Haematol* 1970;19(3):283–305.

111. O'Brien JR. The effect of heparin on the early stages of blood coagulation. *J Clin Pathol* 1960;13:93–98.

112. Kakkar VV, Corrigan T, Spindler J, et al. Efficacy of low doses of heparin in prevention of deep-vein thrombosis after major surgery. A double-blind, randomised trial. *Lancet* 1972;2(7768):101–106.

113. Kakkar VV, Field ES, Nicolaides AN, et al. Low doses of heparin in prevention of deep-vein thrombosis. *Lancet* 1971;2(7726):669–671.

114. Moser KM, Hajjar GC. Effect of heparin on the one-stage prothrombin time. Source of artifactual "resistance" to pro-thrombinopenic therapy. *Ann Intern Med* 1967;66(6):1207–1213.

115. Gravlee GP, Angert KC, Tucker WY, et al. Early anticoagulation peak and rapid distribution after intravenous heparin. *Anesthesiology* 1988;68(1):126–129.

116. Pifarre R, Babka R, Sullivan HJ, et al. Management of postoperative heparin rebound following cardiopulmonary bypass. *J Thorac Cardiovasc Surg* 1981;81(3):378–381.

117. Butterworth J, Lin YA, Prielipp R, et al. The pharmacokinetics and cardiovascular effects of a single intravenous dose of protamine in normal volunteers. *Anesth Analg* 2002;94(3):514–522; table of contents.

118. Fiser WP, Fewell JE, Hill DE, et al. Cardiovascular effects of protamine sulfate are dependent on the presence and type of circulating heparin. *J Thorac Cardiovasc Surg* 1985;89(1):63–70.

119. Latson TW, Kickler TS, Baumgartner WA. Pulmonary hypertension and noncardiogenic pulmonary edema following cardiopulmonary bypass associated with an antigranulocyte antibody. *Anesthesiology* 1986;64(1):106–111.

120. Culliford AT, Thomas S, Spencer FC. Fulminating noncardiogenic pulmonary edema. A newly recognized hazard during cardiac operations. *J Thorac Cardiovasc Surg* 1980;80(6):868–875.

121. Ansell JE, Price JM, Shah S, et al. Heparin-induced thrombocytopenia. What is its real frequency? *Chest* 1985;88(6):878–882.

122. Powers PJ, Cuthbert D, Hirsh J. Thrombocytopenia found uncommonly during heparin therapy. *JAMA* 1979;241(22):2396–2397.

123. Bell WR, Royall RM. Heparin-associated thrombocytopenia: a comparison of three heparin preparations. *N Engl J Med* 1980;303(16):902–907.

124. Chong BH, Pitney WR, Castaldi PA. Heparin-induced thrombocytopenia: association of thrombotic complications with heparin-dependent IgG antibody that induces thromboxane synthesis in platelet aggregation. *Lancet* 1982;2(8310):1246–1249.

125. Silver D, Kapsch DN, Tsoi EK. Heparin-induced thrombocytopenia, thrombosis, and hemorrhage. *Ann Surg* 1983;198(3):301–306.

126. Green D, Harris K, Reynolds N, et al. Heparin immune thrombocytopenia: evidence for a heparin-platelet complex as the antigenic determinant. *J Lab Clin Med* 1978;91(1):167–175.

127. Rhodes GR, Dixon RH, Silver D. Heparin induced thrombocytopenia: eight cases with thrombotic-hemorrhagic complications. *Ann Surg* 1977;186(6):752–758.

128. Kapsch DN, Adelstein EH, Rhodes GR, et al. Heparin-induced thrombocytopenia, thrombosis, and hemorrhage. *Surgery* 1979;86(1):148–155.

129. Kelton JG, Levine MN. Heparin-induced thrombocytopenia. *Semin Thromb Hemost* 1986;12(1):59–62.

130. Shalansky SJ, Verma AK, Levine M. Factors to consider before discontinuing heparin in patients who develop thrombocytopenia. *Pharmacotherapy* 1999;19(8):1011–1012.

131. Greinacher A, Michels I, Kiefel V, et al. A rapid and sensitive test for diagnosing heparin-associated thrombocytopenia. *Thromb Haemost* 1991;66(6):734–736.

132. Warkentin TE, Levine MN, Hirsh J, et al. Heparin-induced thrombocytopenia in patients treated with low-molecular-weight heparin or unfractionated heparin. *N Engl J Med* 1995;332(20):1330–1335.

133. Almeida JI, Coats R, Liem TK, et al. Reduced morbidity and mortality rates of the heparin-induced thrombocytopenia syndrome. *J Vasc Surg* 1998;27(2):309–314; discussion 315–316.

134. Holbrook AM, Pereira JA, Labiris R, et al. Systematic overview of warfarin and its drug and food interactions. *Arch Intern Med* 2005;165(10):1095–1106.

135. Collen D, Lijnen HR. Thrombolytic therapy. *Ann N Y Acad Sci* 1991;614:259–269.

136. Weitz JI. Mechanism of action of the thrombolytic agents. *Baillieres Clin Haematol* 1990;3(3):583–599.

137. Marder VJ. Thrombolytic therapy: foundations nad clinical results. In: Colman RW, Hisch K, Maider VJ, et al. eds. *Hemostasis and thrombosis basic principles and clinical practice*, 4th ed. Philadelphia: Lippincott Williams & Wilkins, 2001:1475–1495.

138. Meyerovitz MF, Goldhaber SZ, Reagan K, et al. Recombinant tissue-type plasminogen activator versus urokinase in peripheral arterial and graft occlusions: a randomized trial. *Radiology* 1990;175(1):75–78.

139. Kwaan HC, Keer HN. Fibrinolysis and cancer. *Semin Thromb Hemost* 1990;16(3):230–235.

140. Nilsson IM. Clinical pharmacology of aminocaproic and tranexamic acids. *J Clin Pathol Suppl (R Coll Pathol)* 1980;14:41–47.

141. Rich JB. The efficacy and safety of aprotinin use in cardiac surgery. *Ann Thorac Surg* 1998;66(Suppl 5):S6–S11; discussion S25–S28.

142. Tengborn L, Kjellman B, Elfstrand PO, et al. Recombinant factor VIIa in an infant with haemophilia A and inhibitors. *Acta Paediatr* 1992;81(6–7):566–567.

143. Krishnaswamy S. The interaction of human factor VIIa with tissue factor. *J Biol Chem* 1992;267(33):23696–23706.

144. Ingerslev J, Feldstedt M, Sindet-Pedersen S. Control of haemostasis with recombinant factor VIIa in patient with inhibitor to factor VIII. *Lancet* 1991;338(8770):831–832.

145. Aledort L. Inhibitors in hemophilia patients: current status and management. *Am J Hematol* 1994;47(3):208–217.

146. Komiyama Y, Pedersen AH, Kisiel W. Proteolytic activation of human factors IX and X by recombinant human factor VIIa:

effects of calcium, phospholipids, and tissue factor. *Biochemistry* 1990;29(40):9418–9425.

147. Levi M, Peters M, Buller HR. Efficacy and safety of recombinant factor VIIa for treatment of severe bleeding: a systematic review. *Crit Care Med* 2005;33(4):883–890.

148. Telgt DS, Macik BG, McCord DM, et al. Mechanism by which recombinant factor VIIa shortens the aPTT: activation of factor X in the absence of tissue factor. *Thromb Res* 1989;56(5):603–609.

149. Hoffman M, Monroe DM, Roberts HR. Human monocytes support factor X activation by factor VIIa, independent of tissue factor: implications for the therapeutic mechanism of high-dose factor VIIa in hemophilia. *Blood* 1994;83(1):38–42.

150. Nakagaki T, Foster DC, Berkner KL, et al. Initiation of the extrinsic pathway of blood coagulation: evidence for the tissue factor dependent autoactivation of human coagulation factor VII. *Biochemistry* 1991;30(45):10819–10824.

151. Pedersen AH, Lund-Hansen T, Bisgaard-Frantzen H, et al. Autoactivation of human recombinant coagulation factor VII. *Biochemistry* 1989;28(24):9331–9336.

152. Monroe DM, Hoffman M, Oliver JA, et al. Platelet activity of high-dose factor VIIa is independent of tissue factor. *Br J Haematol* 1997;99(3):542–547.

153. Roberts HR. Recombinant factor VIIa: a general hemostatic agent? Yes. *J Thromb Haemost* 2004;2(10):1691–1694.

154. O'Connell KA, Wood JJ, Wise RP, et al. Thromboembolic adverse events after use of recombinant human coagulation factor VIIa. *JAMA* 2006;295(3):293–298.

155. Till JE, McCulloch EA. A direct measurement of the radiation sensitivity of normal mouse bone marrow cells. *Radiat Res* 1961; 14:213–222.

156. Becker AG, McCulloch EA, Till JA. Cytological demonstration of the clonal nature of spleen colonies derived from transplanted mouse marrow cells. *Nature* 1963;197:452–454.

157. Erslev AJ, Lichtman MA. Structure and function of the marrow. In: Williams WJ, Beulter E, Erslev AJ, et al. eds. *Hematology*, 4th ed. New York: McGraw Hill, 1990:37–47.

158. Torok-Storb B. Cellular interactions. *Blood* 1988;72(2):373–385.

159. Quesenberry PJ, McNiece IK, Robinson BE, et al. Stromal cell regulation of lymphoid and myeloid differentiation. *Blood Cells* 1987;13(1–2):137–146.

160. Erslev AJ. Production of erythrocytes. In: Williams WJ, Beutler E, Erslev AJ, et al. eds. *Hematology*, 4th ed. New York: McGraw Hill, 1990:389–398.

161. Robinson BE, Quesenberry PJ. Hematopoietic growth factors: overview and clinical applications, Part I. *Am J Med Sci* 1990; 300(3):163–170.

162. Robinson BE, Quesenberry PJ. Hematopoietic growth factors: overview and clinical applications, Part III. *Am J Med Sci* 1990; 300(5):311–321.

163. Robinson BE, Quesenberry PJ. Hematopoietic growth factors: overview and clinical applications, Part II. *Am J Med Sci* 1990; 300(4):237–244.

164. Bunn HF. Erythropoietin: current status. *Yale J Biol Med* 1990; 63(5):381–386.

165. Erslev AJ. Erythropoietin. *N Engl J Med* 1991;324(19):1339–1344.

166. Major A, Mathez-Loic F, Rohling R, et al. The effect of intravenous iron on the reticulocyte response to recombinant human erythropoietin. *Br J Haematol* 1997;98(2):292–294.

167. Schaefer RM, Schaefer L. Hypochromic red blood cells and reticulocytes. *Kidney Int Suppl* 1999;69:S44–S48.

168. Fishbane S, Galgano C, Langley RC Jr, et al. Reticulocyte hemoglobin content in the evaluation of iron status of hemodialysis patients. *Kidney Int* 1997;52(1):217–222.

169. Mittman N, Sreedhara R, Mushnick R, et al. Reticulocyte hemoglobin content predicts functional iron deficiency in hemodialysis patients receiving rHuEPO. *Am J Kidney Dis* 1997; 30(6):912–922.

170. Weiss G. Iron and anemia of chronic disease. *Kidney Int Suppl* 1999;69:S12–S17.

171. Burns DL, Pomposelli JJ. Toxicity of parenteral iron dextran therapy. *Kidney Int Suppl* 1999;69:S119–S124.

172. Van Wyck DB. Iron management during recombinant human erythropoietin therapy. *Am J Kidney Dis* 1989;14(2 Suppl 1):9–13.

173. Faris P. Use of recombinant human erythropoietin in the perioperative period of orthopedic surgery. *Am J Med* 1996;101(2A): 28S–32S.

174. Goodnough LT. Clinical application of recombinant erythropoietin in the perioperative period. *Hematol Oncol Clin North Am* 1994;8(5):1011–1020.

175. Sowade O, Warnke H, Scigalla P, et al. Avoidance of allogeneic blood transfusions by treatment with epoetin beta (recombinant human erythropoietin) in patients undergoing open-heart surgery. *Blood* 1997;89(2):411–418.

176. D'Ambra M. Perioperative epoetin alfa reduces transfusion requirements in coronary artery bypass graft surgery. *Semin Hematol* 1997;33(2 Suppl 2):74.

177. Baron JF. Autologous blood donation with recombinant human erythropoietin in cardiac surgery: the Japanese experience. *Semin Hematol* 1996;33(2 Suppl 2):64–67; discussion 68.

178. Wolff M, Fandrey J, Hirner A, et al. Perioperative use of recombinant human erythropoietin in patients refusing blood transfusions. Pathophysiological considerations based on 5 cases. *Eur J Haematol* 1997;58(3):154–159.

179. Atabek U, Alvarez R, Pello MJ, et al. Erythropoetin accelerates hematocrit recovery in post-surgical anemia. *Am Surg* 1995;61(1):74–77.

180. Goldberg MA. Erythropoiesis, erythropoietin, and iron metabolism in elective surgery: preoperative strategies for avoiding allogeneic blood exposure. *Am J Surg* 1995;170(Suppl 6A):37S–43S.

181. Issitt PD, Anstee DJ. *Applied blood group serology*, 4th ed. Miami: Montgomery Scientific, 1998.

182. Harmening D, Pittiglio D, Flynn JC. The ABO blood group system. In: Harmening D, ed. *Modern blood banking and transfusion practices*, 2nd ed. Philadelphia: FA Davis Co, 1989:78–104.

183. Silberstein L, Spitalnik SL. Blood group antigens and antibodies. In: Rossi EC, Simon TL, Moss GS, eds. *Principles of transfusion medicine*. Baltimore: Williams & Wilkins, 1990:63–78.

184. O'Connor KL. The Rh blood group system. In: Harmening D, ed. *Modern blood banking and transfusion practices*, 2nd ed. Philadelphia: FA Davis Co, 1989:105–119.

185. Springer GF, Horton RE. Blood group isoantibody stimulation in man by feeding blood group-active bacteria. *J Clin Invest* 1969; 48(7):1280–1291.

186. Mollison PL, Engelfriet CP, Contreras M. Hemolytic transfusion reactions. *Blood transfusion in clinical medicine*, 9th ed. Oxford: Blackwell Science, 1993.

187. Ahsan N. Intravenous infusion of total dose iron is superior to oral iron in treatment of anemia in peritoneal dialysis patients: a single center comparative study. *J Am Soc Nephrol* 1998;9(4):664–668.

188. Klein HG. Allogeneic transfusion risks in the surgical patient. *Am J Surg* 1995;170(6A Suppl):21S–26S.

189. Linden JV, Kaplan HS. Transfusion errors: causes and effects. *Transfus Med Rev* 1994;8(3):169–183.

190. Jeter EK, Spivey MA. Noninfectious complications of blood transfusion. *Hematol Oncol Clin North Am* 1995;9(1):187–204.

191. Devine P, Postoway N, Hoffstadter L, et al. Blood donation and transfusion practices: the 1990 American Association of Blood Banks Institutional Membership Questionnaire. *Transfusion* 1992; 32(7):683–687.

192. Sazama K. Reports of 355 transfusion-associated deaths: 1976 through 1985. *Transfusion* 1990;30(7):583–590.

193. Agre P, Cartron JP. Molecular biology of the Rh antigens. *Blood* 1991;78(3):551–563.

194. Hsia CC. Respiratory function of hemoglobin. *N Engl J Med* 1998;338(4):239–247.

195. Schmidt PJ, Leparc GF, Samia CT. Use of Rh positive blood in emergency situations. *Surg Gynecol Obstet* 1988;167(3):229–233.

196. Schwab CW, Shayne JP, Turner J. Immediate trauma resuscitation with type O uncrossmatched blood: a two-year prospective experience. *J Trauma* 1986;26(10):897–902.

197. Seyfried H, Walewska I. Immune hemolytic transfusion reactions. *World J Surg* 1987;11(1):25–29.

198. Ramsey G. The pathophysiology and organ-specific consequences of severe transfusion reactions. *New Horiz* 1994;2(4):575–581.

199. Muylle L. The role of cytokines in blood transfusion reactions. *Blood Rev* 1995;9(2):77–83.

200. Shanwell A, Kristiansson M, Remberger M, et al. Generation of cytokines in red cell concentrates during storage is prevented by prestorage white cell reduction. *Transfusion* 1997;37(7):678–684.

201. Gu YJ, de Vries AJ, Boonstra PW, et al. Leukocyte depletion results in improved lung function and reduced inflammatory response after cardiac surgery. *J Thorac Cardiovasc Surg* 1996;112(2):494–500.

202. Lane TA. Leukocyte reduction of cellular blood components. Effectiveness, benefits, quality control, and costs. *Arch Pathol Lab Med* 1994;118(4):392–404.

203. Rapaille A, Moore G, Siquet J, et al. Prestorage leukocyte reduction with in-line filtration of whole blood: evaluation of red cells and plasma storage. *Vox Sang* 1997;73(1):28–35.

204. Toy P, Popovsky M, Abraham E, et al. Transfusion-related acute lung injury: definition and review. *Crit Care Med* 2005;33(4):721–726.

205. Shandar A, Poposvsky M. Understanding the consequences of transfusion-related acute lung injury. *Chest* 2005;128(5 Suppl 2):598S–604S.

206. Swanson K, Dwyre DM, Krochmal J, et al. Transfusion-related acute lung injury (TRALI): current clinical and pathophysiologic considerations. *Lung* 2006;184(3):177–185.

207. Zeuzem S, Teuber G, Lee JH, et al. Risk factors for the transmission of hepatitis C. *J Hepatol* 1996;24(Suppl 2):3–10.

208. Schmunis GA, Zicker F, Pinheiro F, et al. Risk for transfusion-transmitted infectious diseases in Central and South America. *Emerg Infect Dis* 1998;4(1):5–11.

209. Courouce AM, Pillonel J. Transfusion-transmitted viral infections. Retrovirus and Viral Hepatitis Working Groups of the French Society of Blood Transfusion. *N Engl J Med* 1996;335(21):1609–1610.

210. Choudhury N, Ramesh V, Saraswat S, et al. Effectiveness of mandatory transmissible diseases screening in Indian blood donors. *Indian J Med Res* 1995;101:229–232.

211. Lackritz EM, Satten GA, Aberle-Grasse J, et al. Estimated risk of transmission of the human immunodeficiency virus by screened blood in the United States. *N Engl J Med* 1995;333(26):1721–1725.

212. AuBuchon JP, Birkmeyer JD, Busch MP. Cost-effectiveness of expanded human immunodeficiency virus-testing protocols for donated blood. *Transfusion* 1997;37(1):45–51.

213. Alter HJ. Transfusion transmitted hepatitis C and non-A, non-B, non-C. *Vox Sang* 1994;67(Suppl 3):19–24.

214. Weber B, Doerr HW. Diagnosis and epidemiology of transfusion-associated human cytomegalovirus infection: recent developments. *Infusionsther Transfusionsmed* 1994;21(Suppl 1):32–39.

215. Gunter KC. Transfusion-transmitted cytomegalovirus: the part-time pathogen. *Pediatr Pathol Lab Med* 1995;15(3):515–534.

216. Friedman LI, Stromberg RR, Wagner SJ. Reducing the infectivity of blood components–what we have learned. *Immunol Invest* 1995;24(1–2):49–71.

217. Leiby DA, Read EJ, Lenes BA, et al. Seroepidemiology of Trypanosoma cruzi, etiologic agent of Chagas' disease, in US blood donors. *J Infect Dis* 1997;176(4):1047–1052.

218. Sanz C, Pereira A, Vila J, et al. Growth of bacteria in platelet concentrates obtained from whole blood stored for 16 hours at 22 degrees C before component preparation. *Transfusion* 1997;37(3):251–254.

219. Sarkodee-Adoo CB, Kendall JM, Sridhara R, et al. The relationship between the duration of platelet storage and the development of transfusion reactions. *Transfusion* 1998;38(3):229–235.

220. Ben-Hur E, Barshtein G, Chen S, et al. Photodynamic treatment of red blood cell concentrates for virus inactivation enhances red blood cell aggregation: protection with antioxidants. *Photochem Photobiol* 1997;66(4):509–512.

221. Bradley JA. The blood transfusion effect: experimental aspects. *Immunol Lett* 1991;29(1–2):127–132.

222. Tartter PI. Transfusion-induced immunosuppression and perioperative infections. *Beitr Infusionsther* 1993;31:52–63.

223. Houbiers JG, van de Velde CJ, van de Watering LM, et al. Transfusion of red cells is associated with increased incidence of bacterial infection after colorectal surgery: a prospective study. *Transfusion* 1997;37(2):126–134.

224. Blumberg N, Heal JM. Transfusion-induced immunomodulation and its possible role in cancer recurrence and perioperative bacterial infection. *Yale J Biol Med* 1990;63(5):429–433.

225. Mynster T, Christensen IJ, Moesgaard F, et al. Danish RANX05 Colorectal Cancer Study Group. Effects of the combination of blood transfusion and postoperative infectious complications on prognosis after surgery for colorectal cancer. *Br J Surg* 2000;87(11):1553–1562.

226. Klein HG. Immunologic aspects of blood transfusion. *Semin Oncol* 1994;21(2 Suppl 3):16–20.

227. Ghio M, Contini P, Puppo F, et al. The immunomodulatory effect of blood transfusions and intravenous immunoglobulins: the role of the soluble molecules of the Class-I major histocompatibility complex and of the Fas ligand. *Ann Ital Med Int* 2000;15(1):70–74.

228. Otter GH, Nathens AB, Lee TH, et al. Leukoreduction of blood transfusions does not diminish transfusion-associated microchimerism in trauma patients. *Transfusion* 2006;46:1863–1869.

229. Blajchman MA, Bordin JO. The tumor growth-promoting effect of allogeneic blood transfusions. *Immunol Invest* 1995;24(1–2):311–317.

230. Triulzi DJ, Blumberg N, Heal JM. Association of transfusion with postoperative bacterial infection. *Crit Rev Clin Lab Sci* 1990;28(2):95–107.

231. Quintiliani L, Pescini A, Di Girolamo M, et al. Relationship of blood transfusion, post-operative infections and immunoreactivity in patients undergoing surgery for gastrointestinal cancer. *Haematologica* 1997;82(3):318–323.

232. Heiss MM, Fasol-Merten K, Allgayer H, et al. Influence of autologous blood transfusion on natural killer and lymphokine-activated killer cell activities in cancer surgery. *Vox Sang* 1997;73(4):237–245.

233. Donohue JH, Williams S, Cha S, et al. Perioperative blood transfusions do not affect disease recurrence of patients undergoing curative resection of colorectal carcinoma: a Mayo/North Central Cancer Treatment Group study. *J Clin Oncol* 1995;13(7):1671–1678.

234. Gorog D, Toth A, Weltner J, et al. The effect of blood transfusion on the late results of the surgical treatment of rectal cancer. *Orv Hetil* 1996;137(31):1693–1698.

235. Carson JL, Altman DG, Duff A, et al. Risk of bacterial infection associated with allogeneic blood transfusion among patients undergoing hip fracture repair. *Transfusion* 1999;39(7):694–700.

236. McAlister FA, Clark HD, Wells PS, et al. Perioperative allogeneic blood transfusion does not cause adverse sequelae in patients with cancer: a meta-analysis of unconfounded studies. *Br J Surg* 1998;85(2):171–178.

237. Jensen LS, Hokland M, Nielsen HJ. A randomized controlled study of the effect of bedside leukocyte depletion on the immunosuppresive effect of whole blood transfusion in patients undergoing elective colorectal surgery. *Br J Surg* 1996;83:973–977.

238. Riggert J, Schwartz DW, Wieding JU, et al. Prestorage inline filtration of whole blood for obtaining white cell-reduced blood components. *Transfusion* 1997;37(10):1039–1044.

239. Manno CS. What's new in transfusion medicine? *Pediatr Clin North Am* 1996;43(3):793–808.

240. Buttnerova I, Baumler H, Kern F, et al. Release of WBC-derived IL-1 receptor antagonist into supernatants of RBCs: influence of storage time and filtration. *Transfusion* 2001;41(1):67–73.

241. Wadhwa M, Seghatchian MJ, Dilger P, et al. Cytokine accumulation in stored red cell concentrates: effect of buffy-coat removal and leucoreduction. *Transfus Sci* 2000;23(1):7–16.

242. Racek J, Herynkova R, Holecek V, et al. Influence of antioxidants on the quality of stored blood. *Vox Sang* 1997;72(1):16–19.

243. Shoemaker WC, Appel PL, Kram HB. Tissue oxygen debt as a determinant of postoperative organ failure. *Prog Clin Biol Res* 1989;308:133–136.

244. Tuman K. Tissue oxygen delivery: the physiology of anemia. *Anesthesiol Clin North America* 1990;9:451–469.

245. Bessos H, Seghatchian J. Red cell storage lesion: the potential impact of storage-induced CD47 decline on immunomodulation and the survival of leucofiltered red cells. *Transfus Apheresis Sci* 2005;32(2):227–232.

246. Oldenbrog PA, Zheleznyak A, Fang YF, et al. Role of CD47 as a marker of self on red blood cells. *Science* 2000;288 (5473):2051–2054.

247. Karger R, Kretschmer V. The importance of quality of whole blood and erythrocyte concentrates for autologous transfusion. A literature survey and meta-analysis of *in vivo* erythrocyte recovery. *Anaesthesist* 1996;45(8):694–707.

248. Fitzgerald RD, Martin CM, Dietz GE, et al. Transfusing red blood cells stored in citrate phosphate dextrose adenine-1 for 28 days fails to improve tissue oxygenation in rats. *Crit Care Med* 1997;25(5):726–732.

249. Rasia RJ, Valverde J, Garcia Rosasco M. Blood preservation. Bacteriological, immunohematological, hematological and hemorrheological studies. *Sangre (Barc)* 1998;43(1):71–76.

250. Kruskall MS, Mintz PD, Bergin JJ, et al. Transfusion therapy in emergency medicine. *Ann Emerg Med* 1988;17(4):327–335.

251. Wolfe LC. The membrane and the lesions of storage in preserved red cells. *Transfusion* 1985;25(3):185–203.

252. Leach MF, AuBuchon JP. Effect of storage time on clinical efficacy of single-donor platelet units. *Transfusion* 1993;33(8):661–664.

253. Muller-Steinhardt M, Janetzko K, Kandler R, et al. Impact of various red cell concentrate preparation methods on the efficiency of prestorage white cell filtration and on red cells during storage for 42 days. *Transfusion* 1997;37(11–12):1137–1142.

254. Caggiano V. Red blood cell transfusions. In: Silver H, ed. *Blood, blood components and derivatives in transfusion therapy*. Arlington: American Association of Blood Banks, 1980.

255. Counts RB, Haisch C, Simon TL, et al. Hemostasis in massively transfused trauma patients. *Ann Chir Main Memb Super* 1979; 190(1):91–99.

256. Perioperative red cell transfusion. *NIH Consens Dev Conf Consens Statement*. Bethesda: 1988;7(4):1–19.

257. Adams RLJ. Anesthesia in cases of poor surgical risk. Some suggestions for decreasing the risk. *Surg Gynecol Obstet* 1942; 74:1011–1019.

258. Greenburg AG. Pathophysiology of anemia. *Am J Med* 1996; 101(2A):7S–11S.

259. Report of the Expert Working Group. Guidelines for red blood cell and plasma transfusion for adults and children. *Can Med Assoc J* 1997;156(Suppl 11):S5–S6.

260. Holcroft JW, Robinson MK. Shock. In: Wilmore DW, Cheung L, Harken AH, et al. eds. *Scientific American surgery*, Vol. 1. New York: Scientific American, 1997:3–37.

261. Ostgaard G. Perioperative and postoperative normovolemic anemia. Physiological compensation, monitoring and risk evaluation. *Tidsskr Nor Laegeforen* 1996;116(1):57–60.

262. Buckberg G, Brazier J. Coronary blood flow and cardiac function during hemodilution. *Bibl Haematol* 1975;41:173–189.

263. Doak GJ, Hall RI. Does hemoglobin concentration affect perioperative myocardial lactate flux in patients undergoing coronary artery bypass surgery? *Anesth Analg* 1995;80(5):910–916.

264. Kleen M, Habler O, Hutter J, et al. Effects of hemodilution on splanchnic perfusion and hepatorenal function. I. Splanchnic perfusion. *Eur J Med Res* 1997;2(10):413–418.

265. Chapler CK, Cain SM, Stainsby WN. Blood flow and oxygen uptake in isolated canine skeletal muscle during acute anemia. *J Appl Physiol* 1979;46(6):1035–1038.

266. Erni D, Banic A, Wheatley AM, et al. Haemorrhage during anaesthesia and surgery: continuous measurement of microcirculatory blood flow in the kidney, liver, skin and skeletal muscle. *Eur J Anaesthesiol* 1995;12(4):423–429.

267. Wilkerson DK, Rosen AL, Sehgal LR, et al. Limits of cardiac compensation in anemic baboons. *Surgery* 1988;103(6):665–670.

268. Spahn DR, Smith LR, Veronee CD, et al. Acute isovolemic hemodilution and blood transfusion. Effects on regional function and metabolism in myocardium with compromised coronary blood flow. *J Thorac Cardiovasc Surg* 1993;105(4):694–704.

269. Torres-Filho IP, Spiess B, Pittman RN, et al. Experimental analysis if critical oxygen delivery. *Am J Physiol Heart Circ Physiol* 2005;288(3):H1071–H1079.

270. Shoemaker WC. Pathophysiology, monitoring, outcome prediction, and therapy of shock states. *Crit Care Clin* 1987;3(2):307–357.

271. Brazzi LGL. Optimization of oxygen transport in the ICU patient. *TATM* 2000;2(5):20–27.

272. Spence RK, Cernaianu AC, Carson J, et al. Transfusion and surgery. *Curr Probl Surg* 1993;30(12):1101–1180.

273. Carson JL, Duff A, Berlin JA, et al. Perioperative blood transfusion and postoperative mortality. *JAMA* 1998;279(3):199–205.

274. Hebert PC, Wells G, Marshall J, et al. Canadian Critical Care Trials Group. Transfusion requirements in critical care. A pilot study. *JAMA* 1995;273(18):1439–1444.

275. Hebert PC, Yetisir E, Martin C, et al. Is a low transfusion threshold safe in critically ill patients with cardiovascular diseases? *Crit Care Med* 2001;29(2):227–234.

276. Corwin HL, Parsonnet KC, Gettinger A. RBC transfusion in the ICU. Is there a reason? *Chest* 1995;108(3):767–771.

277. Hebert PC, Wells G, Martin C, et al. Variation in red cell transfusion practice in the intensive care unit: a multicenter cohort study. *Crit Care* 1999;3(2):57–63.

278. Spiess BD, Ley C, Body SC, et al. The Institutions of the Multicenter Study of Perioperative Ischemia (McSPI) Research Group. Hematocrit value on intensive care unit entry influences the frequency of Q-wave myocardial infarction after coronary artery bypass grafting. *J Thorac Cardiovasc Surg* 1998;116(3):460–467.

279. Linman JW. Physiologic and pathophysiologic effects of anemia. *N Engl J Med* 1968;279(15):812–818.

280. Lunn JN, Elwood PC. Anaemia and surgery. *Br Med J* 1970; 3(5714):71–73.

281. Rawstron E. Anemia and surgery. A retrospecitve clinical study. *Aust NZ J Surg* 1970;39:425–432.

282. Alexiu O, Mircea N, Balaban M, et al. Gastro-intestinal haemorrhage from peptic ulcer. An evaluation of bloodless transfusion and early surgery. *Anaesthesia* 1975;30(5):609–615.

283. Spence RK, Carson JA, Poses R, et al. Elective surgery without transfusion: influence of preoperative hemoglobin level and blood loss on mortality. *Am J Surg* 1990;159(3):320–324.

284. Carson JL, Poses RM, Spence RK, et al. Severity of anaemia and operative mortality and morbidity. *Lancet* 1988;1(8588):727–729.

285. Robertie P, Gravlee G. Safe limits of hemodilution and recommendations for erythrocyte transfusion. *Int Anesthesiol Clin* 1990;28(4):197–204.

286. Spence RK, Costabile JP, Young GS, et al. Is hemoglobin level alone a reliable predictor of outcome in the severely anemic surgical patient? *Am Surg* 1992;58(2):92–95.

287. Nelson AH, Fleisher LA, Rosenbaum SH. Relationship between postoperative anemia and cardiac morbidity in high-risk vascular

patients in the intensive care unit. *Crit Care Med* 1993; 21(6):860–866.

288. Christopherson R, Frank S, Norris E, et al. Low postoperative hematocrit is associated with cardiac ischemia in high-risk patients. *Anesthesiology* 1991;75(3A):A100.

289. Carson JL, Duff A, Poses RM, et al. Effect of anaemia and cardiovascular disease on surgical mortality and morbidity. *Lancet* 1996;348(9034):1005–1060.

290. Lum G. Should the transfusion trigger and hemoglobin low critical limit be identical? *Ann Clin Lab Sci* 1997;27(2):130–134.

291. Ownings FT, Utter GH, Gosselin RC. Chapter 4-Bleeding and transfusion. In: Souba WW, Wilmore DW, eds. *ACS Surgery: principles and practice.* American College of Surgeons. 1993.

292. Schriger DL, Baraff LJ. Capillary refill–is it a useful predictor of hypovolemic states? *Ann Emerg Med* 1991;20(6):601–605.

293. Schumer W Nyhus LM, eds. G R. volume replacement: why, what and how much. *Treatment of shock.* Philadelphia: Lea & Febiger, 1974.

294. Knottenbelt JD. Low initial hemoglobin levels in trauma patients: an important indicator of ongoing hemorrhage. *J Trauma* 1991; 31(10):1396–1399.

295. NIH. Consensus conference: perioperative red cell transfusion. National Institutes of Health. *Conn Med* 1988;52(10):593–596.

296. Adverse Effects of Blood Transfusion. *Technical manual, American Association of Blood Banks,* 11th ed. Bethesda: American Association of Blood Banks, 1993.

297. Marsaglia G, Thomas ED. Mathematical consideration of cross circulation and exchange transfusion. *Transfusion* 1971;11(4): 216–219.

298. Ferrara A, MacArthur JD, Wright HK, et al. Hypothermia and acidosis worsen coagulopathy in the patient requiring massive transfusion. *Am J Surg* 1990;160(5):515–518.

299. Bush HL Jr, Hydo LJ, Fischer E, et al. Hypothermia during elective abdominal aortic aneurysm repair: the high price of avoidable morbidity. *J Vasc Surg* 1995;21(3):392–400; discussion 400–402.

300. Bick RL. Disseminated intravascular coagulation and related syndromes: a clinical review. *Semin Thromb Hemost* 1988; 14(4):299–338.

301. Rohrer MJ, Natale AM. Effect of hypothermia on the coagulation cascade. *Crit Care Med* 1992;20(10):1402–1405.

302. Nicholls MD, Whyte G. Red cell, plasma and albumin transfusion decision triggers. *Anaesth Intensive Care* 1993;21(2):156–162.

303. Valeri CR, Feingold H, Cassidy G, et al. Hypothermia-induced reversible platelet dysfunction. *Ann Surg* 1987;205(2):175–181.

304. Collins JA. Problems associated with the massive transfusion of stored blood. *Surgery* 1974;75(2):274–295.

305. Lucas CE, Ledgerwood AM. Clinical significance of altered coagulation tests after massive transfusion for trauma. *Am Surg* 1981;47(3):125–130.

306. Hewson JR, Neame PB, Kumar N, et al. Coagulopathy related to dilution and hypotension during massive transfusion. *Crit Care Med* 1985;13(5):387–391.

307. Humphries JE. Transfusion therapy in acquired coagulopathies. *Hematol Oncol Clin North Am* 1994;8(6):1181–1201.

308. Jurkovich GJ, Greiser WB, Luterman A, et al. Hypothermia in trauma victims: an ominous predictor of survival. *J Trauma* 1987; 27(9):1019–1024.

309. Gubler KD, Gentilello LM, Hassantash SA, et al. The impact of hypothermia on dilutional coagulopathy. *J Trauma* 1994; 36(6):847–851.

310. van der Sande JJ, Emeis JJ, Lindeman J. Intravascular coagulation: a common phenomenon in minor experimental head injury. *J Neurosurg* 1981;54(1):21–25.

311. Bick RL. *Disseminated intravascular coagulation. CRC Press,* 1983.

312. Mahajan SL, Myers TJ, Baldini MG. Disseminated intravascular coagulation during rewarming following hypothermia. *JAMA* 1981;245(24):2517–2518.

313. Carden DL, Novak RM. Disseminated intravascular coagulation in hypothermia. *JAMA* 1982;247(15):2099.

314. Ciavarella D, Reed RL, Counts RB, et al. Clotting factor levels and the risk of diffuse microvascular bleeding in the massively transfused patient. *Br J Haematol* 1987;67(3):365–368.

315. Gando S, Tedo I, Kubota M. Posttrauma coagulation and fibrinolysis. *Crit Care Med* 1992;20(5):594–600.

316. Lahrmann C, Hojlund K, Kristensen T, et al. Use of fresh frozen plasma in patient treatment. Indications illustrated by a literature review and a study of practice at a university hospital. *Ugeskr Laeger* 1996;158(24):3467–3470.

317. Sibrowski W, Schneider C. Possibilities of family blood donation for children and adults. *Infusionsther Transfusionsmed* 1994;21(Suppl 1):69–72.

318. Britton LW, Eastlund DT, Dziuban SW, et al. Predonated autologous blood use in elective cardiac surgery. *Ann Thorac Surg* 1989;47(4):529–532.

319. Spiess BD. Pro: autologous blood should be available for elective cardiac surgery. *J Cardiothorac Vasc Anesth* 1994;8(2):231–237.

320. D'Ambra MN, Kaplan DK. Alternatives to allogeneic blood use in surgery: acute normovolemic hemodilution and preoperative autologous donation. *Am J Surg* 1995;170(Suppl 6A):49S–52S.

321. Nelson CL, Fontenot HJ. Ten strategies to reduce blood loss in orthopedic surgery. *Am J Surg* 1995;170(Suppl 6A):64S–68S.

322. Forgie MA, Wells PS, Laupacis A, et al. International Study of Perioperative Transfusion (ISPOT) Investigators. Preoperative autologous donation decreases allogeneic transfusion but increases exposure to all red blood cell transfusion: results of a meta-analysis. *Arch Intern Med* 1998;158(6):610–616.

323. Tedesco M, Sapienza P, Burchi C, et al. Preoperative blood storage and intraoperative blood recovery in elective treatment of abdominal aorta aneurysm. *Ann Ital Chir* 1996;67(3):399–403.

324. Godet G, Canessa R, Arock M, et al. Effects of platelet-rich plasma on hemostasis and transfusion requirement in vascular surgery. *Ann Fr Anesth Reanim* 1995;14(3):265–270.

325. Mercuriali F. Epoetin alfa increases the volume of autologous blood donated by patients scheduled to undergo orthopedic surgery. *Semin Hematol* 1996;33(2 Suppl 2):10–12; discussion 13–14.

326. Spiess BD, Sassetti R, McCarthy RJ, et al. Autologous blood donation: hemodynamics in a high-risk patient population. *Transfusion* 1992;32(1):17–22.

327. Giordano GF, Giordano DM, Wallace BA, et al. An analysis of 9,918 consecutive perioperative autotransfusions. *Surg Gynecol Obstet* 1993;176(2):103–110.

328. Lagana S, Cattaneo F, Hackenbruch W. Autologous blood transfusion: results with routine use of autologous blood transfusion, normovolemic, hemodilution and postoperation retransfusion of drainage blood salvaged with the Solcontrans system. *Swiss Surg* 1996;2(6):244–251.

329. Bartels C, Bechtel M, Winkler C, et al. Quality of retransfused blood: whole blood versus cell separateion [Letter]. *Ann Thorac Surg* 1996;61:279–280.

330. Nguyen DM, Gilfix BM, Dennis F, et al. Impact of transfusion of mediastinal shed blood on serum levels of cardiac enzymes. *Ann Thorac Surg* 1996;62(1):109–114.

331. Connall TP, Zhang J, Vaziri ND, et al. Leukocyte CD11b and CD18 expression are increased in blood salvaged for autotransfusion. *Am Surg* 1994;60(10):797–800.

332. Perttila J, Leino L, Poyhonen M, et al. Leukocyte content in blood processed by autotransfusion devices during open-heart surgery: postoperative inflammatory response after autologous and allogeneic blood transfusion. *Acta Anaesthesiol Scand* 1995;39(4):511–516.

333. Dzik WH, Sherburne B. Intraoperative blood salvage: medical controversies. *Acta Anaesthesiol Scand* 1990;4(3):208–235.

334. Trubel W, Gunen E, Wuppinger G, et al. Recovery of intraoperatively shed blood in aortoiliac surgery: comparison of cell washing with simple filtration. *Thorac Cardiovasc Surg* 1995;43(3):165–170.

335. Valbonesi M, Carlier P, Florio G, et al. Intraoperative blood salvage (IOBS) in cardiac and vascular surgery. *Int J Artif Organs* 1995;18(3):130–135.

336. Patra P, Sellier E, Chaillou P. Blood salvage: decisive progress in vascular surgery. *J Mal Vasc* 1996;21(Suppl A):13–21.

337. Tawes R, Duvall T. Autotransfusion in cardiac and vascular surgery: overview of a 25-year experience with intraoperative autotransfusion. In: Tawes R, ed. *Autotransfusion: therapeutic principles and trends*, Vol. 1. Detroit: Gregory Appleton, 1997:147–148.

338. Boudreaux JP, Bornside GH, Cohn I Jr. Emergency autotransfusion: partial cleansing of bacteria-laden blood by cell washing. *J Trauma* 1983;23(1):31–35.

339. Ozmen V, McSwain NE Jr, Nichols RL, et al. Autotransfusion of potentially culture-positive blood (CPB) in abdominal trauma: preliminary data from a prospective study. *J Trauma* 1992;32(1):36–39.

340. Wollinsky KH, Oethinger M, Buchele M, et al. Autotransfusion—bacterial contamination during hip arthroplasty and efficacy of cefuroxime prophylaxis. A randomized controlled study of 40 patients. *Acta Orthop Scand* 1997;68(3):225–230.

341. Atabek U, Spence RK, Pello M, et al. Pancreaticoduodenectomy without homologous blood transfusion in an anemic Jehovah's Witness. *Arch Surg* 1992;127(3):349–351.

342. Bengtsson A, Johansson S, Hahlin M, et al. Autotransfusion of blood cells made surgery of a Jehovah's Witness possible. *Lakartidningen* 1992;89(37):2955–2957.

343. Kongsgaard UE, Wang MY, Kvalheim G. Leukocyte depletion filter removes cancer cells in human blood. *Acta Anaesthesiol Scand* 1996;40(1):118–120.

344. Goodnough LT, Monk TG, Brecher ME. Acute normovolemic hemodilution in surgery. *Hematology* 1998;2:413–420.

345. A report by the American Society of Anesthesiologists Task Force on Blood Component Therapy. Practice guidelines for blood component therapy. *Anesthesiology* 1996;84(3):732–747.

346. Goodnough LT, Brecher ME, Kanter MH, et al. Transfusion medicine. Second of two parts–blood conservation. *N Engl J Med* 1999;340(7):525–533.

347. Monk TG, Goodnough LT, Brecher ME, et al. Acute normovolemic hemodilution can replace preoperative autologous blood donation as a standard of care for autologous blood procurement in radical prostatectomy. *Anesth Analg* 1997;85(5):953–958.

348. Monk TG, Goodnough LT, Birkmeyer JD, et al. Acute normovolemic hemodilution is a cost-effective alternative to preoperative autologous blood donation by patients undergoing radical retropubic prostatectomy. *Transfusion* 1995;35(7):559–565.

349. Goodnough LT, Grishaber JE, Monk TG, et al. Acute preoperative hemodilution in patients undergoing radical prostatectomy: a case study analysis of efficacy. *Anesth Analg* 1994;78(5):932–937.

350. Ness PM, Bourke DL, Walsh PC. A randomized trial of perioperative hemodilution versus transfusion of preoperatively deposited autologous blood in elective surgery. *Transfusion* 1992;32(3):226–230.

351. Weiskopf RB, Viele MK, Feiner J, et al. Human cardiovascular and metabolic response to acute, severe isovolemic anemia. *JAMA* 1998;279(3):217–221.

352. Aly Hassan A, Lochbuehler H, Frey L, et al. Global tissue oxygenation during normovolemic haemodilution in young children. *Paediatr Anaesth* 1997;7(3):197–204.

353. Van der Linden P, Wathieu M, Gilbart E, et al. Cardiovascular effects of moderate normovolemic haemodilution during enflurane-nitrous oxide anaesthesia in man. *Acta Anaesthesiol Scand* 1994;38(5):490–498.

354. Hogue CW Jr, Goodnough LT, Monk TG. Perioperative myocardial ischemic episodes are related to hematocrit level in patients undergoing radical prostatectomy. *Transfusion* 1998;38(10):924–931.

355. Carson JL, Spence RK, Poses RM. A pilot randomized trial comparing symptomatic vs. hemoglobin-level-driven red blood cell transfusions following hip fracture. *Transfusion* 1998;38:522–529.

356. Meyer MM. Renal replacement therapies. *Crit Care Clin* 2000;16(1):29–58.

357. Sherman LA, Lippmann MB, Ahmed P, et al. Effect on cardiovascular function and iron metabolism of the acute removal of 2 units of red cells. *Transfusion* 1994;34(7):573–577.

358. Hensel M, Wrobel R, Volk T, et al. Changes in coagulation physiology and rheology after preoperative normovolemic hemodilution. *Anasthesiol Intensivmed Notfallmed Schmerzther* 1996;31(8):481–487.

359. McLoughlin TM, Fontana JL, Alving B, et al. Profound normovolemic hemodilution: hemostatic effects in patients and in a porcine model. *Anesth Analg* 1996;83(3):459–465.

360. Cliville X, Bofill C, Joven J, et al. Hemorheological, coagulative and fibrinolytic changes during autologous blood donation. *Clin Hemorheol Microcirc* 1998;18(4):265–272.

361. Hobisch-Hagen P, Wirleitner B, Mair J, et al. Consequences of acute normovolemic haemodilution on haemostasis during major orthopaedic surgery. *Br J Anaesth* 1999;82(4):503–509.

362. Scott MG, Kucik DF, Goodnough LT, et al. Blood substitutes: evolution and future applications. *Clin Chem* 1997;43(9):1724–1731.

363. Riess JG, Krafft MP. Advanced fluorocarbon-based systems for oxygen and drug delivery, and diagnosis. *Artif Cells Blood Substit Immobil Biotechnol* 1997;25(1–2):43–52.

364. Greenburg AG, Kim HW. Current status of stroma-free hemoglobin. *Adv Surg* 1997;31:149–165.

365. Gould SA, Moss GS. Clinical development of human polymerized hemoglobin as a blood substitute. *World J Surg* 1996;20(9):1200–1207.

366. Messmer K. Hemodilution. *Surg Clin North Am* 1975;55(3):659–678.

SUGGESTED READINGS

1. Borghi B, Oriani G, Bassi A. Blood saving program: a multicenter Italian experience. *Int J Artif Organs* 1995;18(3):150–158.

2. Keeling MM, Gray LA Jr, Brink MA, et al. Intraoperative autotransfusion. Experience in 725 consecutive cases. *Ann Surg* 1983;197(5):536–541.

3. Williamson K, Taswell H. Intraoperative autologous transfusion (IAT): experience in over 8000 surgical procedures. *Transfusion* 1988;28:11S.

CHAPTER 20

The Musculoskeletal System

Martha Meaney Murray, Henry J. Mankin, and Julie Glowacki

BONE

Physiologic Function

Bone tissue serves two major roles in vertebrates, *mechanical* and *metabolic*. The extracellular matrix of bone is a composite material comprised of mineral and organic phases with combined characteristics to fulfill these roles.

As a tissue, bone furnishes important *mechanical* properties to the skeleton. The mechanical roles of the skeleton are to provide for support of the organism, locomotion, and protection of vital organs, such as the brain and heart. These mechanical demands require stiffness to resist large forces. The strength of bone tissue is approximately one tenth that of steel. The mineral structure of bone makes up 70% of its weight and provides its compressive strength. Bone mineral is similar to calcium and phosphate-containing hydroxyapatite crystal, but has substitutions with carbonate, sodium, magnesium, and other ions. The amount of mineral per volume of bone matrix contributes to the stiffness of bone. The organic phase of bone matrix is primarily collagen fibers (90% of organic dry weight) that are generally aligned parallel to the axis of the bone and furnish tensile strength. Therefore, as a material, bone tissue provides strength, rigidity, and flexibility because of its composition.

Bones have different material properties in axial and transverse directions because of two factors. Foremost is the parallel orientation of collagen fibers (anisotropic), making the bone stronger in compression along its axis than transverse to this axis.

Second, at a higher level of organization, the architecture of different bones varies to serve their specific mechanical requirements and displays directional differences. There are two extremes of porosity in bone: dense cortical and porous trabecular bone. Cortical bone, exemplified by the midshafts of long bones, is the stronger but more brittle form, whereas trabecular (or cancellous) bone, exemplified by the bulk of the vertebral bodies, is lighter and weaker but more compliant. Although there is actually a continuum

of porosity, the average thickness of trabecular struts is 100 to 300 μm and the spaces between them range from 300 to 1,500 μm. Regarding this internal architecture, Julius Wolff observed 100 years ago that the delicate trabeculae in cancellous bone were organized in obvious lines that can be described in mathematical terms similar to the compression and tension trajectories familiar to engineers of his day (commonly referred to as *Wolff Law*). Furthermore, pathologic specimens of rickets or of fractures that healed with deformity suggested to Wolff that the internal architecture conformed to the mathematical description of the new static loading circumstances. For such changes in architecture to happen, he reasoned, bone must be adapting to the changes in stress. Current literature continues to elucidate the mechanisms of bone tissue remodeling, how these forces are disturbed in pathologic situations, and how they can be manipulated surgically and pharmacologically.

The *metabolic* role of bone is its contribution to calcium homeostasis (Fig. 20.1). Constancy in serum calcium levels is necessary for vital physiologic processes, including blood clotting, neuromuscular irritability, growth and regeneration, maintenance of mucous coverings, intercellular contacts, and ameboid and ciliary motion. Calcium and other ions are stored in the matrix of bone and can be mobilized when needed. Calcium homeostasis is tightly regulated in humans by parathyroid hormone (PTH), 1,25-dihydroxyvitamin D, and calcitonin. These calcitropic hormones regulate serum levels of calcium by their actions on bone, intestine, and kidney. Calcium and phosphate enter the blood from the intestine, are removed by the kidney, and are stored in bone. Each is a bidirectional process, depending upon the dietary intake, and each is modulated by the calcitropic hormones. Nutritional and lifestyle factors that strain this system's campaign for mineral homeostasis can increase the drain on skeletal reserves, and increase the risk of fracture. PTH is synthesized in the parathyroid gland and its release is regulated by serum-ionized calcium. A membrane-bound calcium-sensing receptor is activated by normal levels of extracellular calcium ions and inhibits PTH secretion. A small decrease in calcium ions results

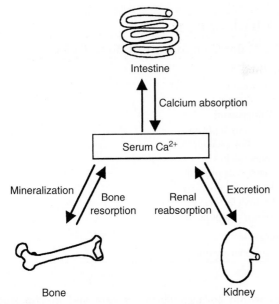

FIGURE 20.1 Schematic diagram of regulation systems for serum calcium. Intestinal absorption, bone resorption, and renal reabsorption all contribute to increased serum calcium, whereas bone mineralization and renal excretion are the main contributors to lowering serum calcium.

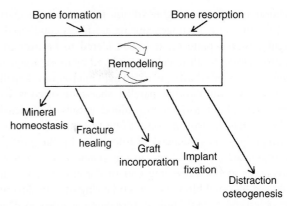

FIGURE 20.2 Bone remodeling results form cycles of resorption of old bone and formation of new bone. Remodeling activity contributes to mineral homeostasis. As a result of turnover, bone is capable of healing and incorporation of grafts and implants.

in increased secretion of PTH. The actions of PTH are to increase extracellular ionized calcium. In bone, it stimulates calcium efflux and bone resorption. In the renal distal tubule, PTH increases calcium reabsorption. It modifies intestinal absorption of calcium indirectly by stimulating the activity of vitamin D. Vitamin D is obtained through the diet and through sun-activated synthesis in skin. It is modified by hepatic 25-hydroxylation and renal 1-hydroxylation to its active circulating (hormone) form, 1,25-dihydroxyvitamin D (calcitriol). This active metabolite increases renal reabsorption of calcium and increases intestinal calcium absorption. Calcitonin can be thought of as the antihypercalcemic hormone; it inhibits resorption of bone and renal reabsorption of calcium.

Central to understanding bone growth, adaptation, pathophysiology, and orthopedic principles is the concept of skeletal *remodeling*. Adult bone undergoes a continuous process of cell-mediated internal turnover, in which packets of bone are resorbed and subsequently replaced with newly synthesized tissue. The remodeling occurs in sites known as *basic multicellular units*, activated in orchestrated cycles of resorption and formation. Because turnover occurs within small packets in bone, the overall mechanical integrity of the tissue is not compromised under normal circumstances. Cellular activity is responsible for remodeling and, in order to maintain a stable mass of tissue, the amount of formation must be equal to resorption. As a consequence, the molecular composition of the adult skeleton is not static, but it changes as new bone fills each excavation site. Two functions of remodeling are appreciated. One is to maintain mechanical strength by replacing fatigued and microfractured bone with sound tissue. The other is to renew dense mineral with more

soluble and accessible mineral for ion exchange. Therefore, remodeling is central for mineral homeostasis. Markers of the cellular activities are found in blood and urine and reflect rates of skeletal turnover (1). Useful serum markers of the magnitude of bone formation are bone-specific alkaline phosphatase, osteocalcin, and newer assays for propeptides of type I procollagen. Useful markers of bone resorption are urinary pyridinium cross-links, cross-linked peptides, and hydroxyproline and the serum levels of tartrate-resistant acid phosphatase (TRAP) and bone sialoprotein (BSP). The continuous process of internal turnover endows bone with the capacity for true scarless regeneration in response to injury (Fig. 20.2). If bone tissue did not turn over in this manner and healed by scar formation, as do other tissues, its mechanical properties would be compromised. Turnover also endows bone with the capacity for incorporation of bone grafts, for osteointegration with metallic implants, and for osteogenesis by gradual distraction. Discussion of the cells of bone and mechanisms of bone growth illuminates these phenomena.

Normal Histology and Biochemistry

The long bones of the skeleton consist of a thick, dense outer layer or cortex of compact bone. The flat bones (cranial bones, scapula, ilium, mandible) are bicortical with a variable amount of space between the two layers of dense cortical bone. These types of organization are well suited for the mechanical and protective functions of the skeleton. The internal spaces of the vertebrae, the ilium, and the ends of long bones, in particular, are filled with a network of calcified trabecula that comprise cancellous bone. Only 15% to 25% of the volume of trabecular bone is calcified tissue, the remainder being hematopoietic marrow, connective, or fatty tissue. Therefore, cancellous bone is porous and lighter than cortical bone.

At the microscopic level, two main type of osseous tissue can be distinguished, woven and lamellar. Woven bone is observed during active growth periods, in fracture callus, in heterotopic osteogenesis (such as myositis ossificans), and in osteosarcoma. It has a higher volume ratio of cells-to-matrix and the matrix is homogeneous or has fibers condensed in angular woven patterns. It is considered to be immature or provisional, to ultimately be replaced by more organized bone. When viewed with polarized light microscopy, lamellar bone shows multilayered parallel sheets or osteons with concentric plates surrounding blood vessels. Cell density is lower than in woven bone. Bone resorption in cortical lamellar bone is evidenced histologically by the presence of organized units called *cutting cones*. Bone-resorbing osteoclasts at the advancing end of the cutting cones are followed by small blood vessels and a ring of bone-forming osteoblasts filling in the hole and creating a new osteon. These are considered as the histologic unit by which remodeling occurs. Cutting cones are evident in histologic sections of adult cortical bone and are rarely seen in trabecular bone. Darkly staining cement lines bounding osteons define a unit of newly synthesized bone that has replaced older bone. Focal remodeling activity results in a mosaic of branching and interconnected osteons, partial osteons, and interstitial areas that are remnants of former osteons resorbed during the remodeling process. Not all osteons are equally mineralized. Younger osteons often contain only 70% of the mineral found in older ones. This fact helps us to understand a purpose of remodeling, namely to rejuvenate the matrix and to maintain the mineral in a more soluble and therefore more readily mobilizable form. Without this rejuvenation of mineral, thermodynamics would render the hydroxyapatite more and more crystalline, dense, and, consequently, insoluble. In cancellous bone, remodeling occurs on the surfaces of the trabeculae, leaving patterns of cement lines that demark bundles of collagen fibers in different directions.

The bones are covered by a thin, tough membrane, called the *periosteum*. Microscopically, it is composed of two layers, the outer fibrous and an inner cambium layer. It is the inner cambium that gives rise to new bone during growth and after trauma or infection. Bone tissue is characterized by a higher ratio of extracellular matrix-to-cell volume when compared with other tissue types.

Bone matrix is composed of organic and inorganic phases (Table 20.1). The organic phase accounts for one third of the dry weight of bone and is comprised of collagen type I, noncollagenous proteins, proteoglycans, and proteolipids. Some of the constituents are structural and others are more informational, providing signals for organization, mineralization, and turnover. The organic matrix is secreted by osteoblasts and is organized in an orderly manner. The organic phase, or osteoid, becomes mineralized under the control of osteoblasts. In the adult, there is normally little osteoid volume seen histologically. In calcium- or vitamin D-deficiency, however, impaired mineralization results in abundance of osteoid and reduced mechanical properties, a condition termed *rickets* in children and osteomalacia in adults.

The inorganic phase is in the form of carbonate-containing calcium phosphate similar to geologic hydroxyapatite. Mineralization of lamellar bone begins in nucleation

---

TABLE 20.1

The Major Components of Bone Tissue

Organic
  Collagen I
  Osteonectin
  Sialoproteins
      Osteopontin
      Bone sialoprotein
  Osteocalcin
  Matrix Gla protein
  Proteoglycans I and II
  Growth factors
  Serum components

Inorganic
  Carbonatoapatite

---

sites within collagen fibers. *In vitro* and *in vivo* studies showed that initial crystals are formed within the hole zones that result from the quarter-stagger of collagen molecules in fibers. Therefore, mineral nucleation occurs at multiple, independent sites in the hole zones. Once nuclei of calcium phosphate crystals are formed, however, further crystal growth is thermodynamically favored at physiologic levels of ion concentrations. This mechanism of bone mineralization is distinct from the mechanisms of cartilage mineralization, which utilizes matrix vesicles, or of dental enamel, which uses degradation of an organic anlage.

Osteoblasts are found on active bone-forming surfaces, where they first deposit the osteoid layer of organic matrix. Osteoblasts regulate mineralization of the osteoid by the action of the cell-surface enzyme alkaline phosphatase. One of the activities of the enzyme is to liberate phosphate ion from matrix organic molecules, therefore raising the local concentration of inorganic phosphate and precipitation of calcium phosphate. In the adult, trabecular surfaces are covered by inactive lining cells. When an osteoblast has completely surrounded itself within matrix, it is called an *osteocyte*. The osteocytes are organized in a network in which they are connected to each other and to surface osteoblasts by extended cytoplasmic processes through narrow canaliculi. This anatomic arrangement results in a very high surface area of interaction between the osteocytes and the mineralized matrix. This allows the osteocytes to maintain the minute-to-minute exchange of mineral between the matrix and the circulation. In addition to that metabolic function, osteocytes also serve as transducers of mechanical loading on bone. The piezoelectric property of bone matrix allows for transmission of load throughout the skeleton. The detailed mechanisms are not completely known, but the result is that the bone adapts to external forces (compression and tension) and produces changes in internal architecture of bony trabeculae to provide maximum resistance to these forces. In this way, superfluous bits of bone are removed and new bone is deposited to transform the bone's structure.

Osteoclasts are large, multinucleated cells found on the surfaces of trabeculae and in Howship lacunae. They are responsible for bone resorption. They have two specialized membrane mechanisms that, when in juxtaposition to bone, are responsible for focal bone resorption. The sealing zone is a ring of attachment to the matrix surrounding a central area of foldings called the *ruffled border*. The polarized secretion of acid into the compartment underlying the ruffled border promotes the solubilization of calcium from the bone surface. The cytoplasm of osteoclast is abundant with lysosomes that contain lytic enzymes that degrade the organic fraction of bone. Osteoclasts possess calcitonin receptors and are profoundly inhibited by this hormone. They are also directly inhibited by the class of agents known as *bisphosphonates*, which are used in Paget disease, osteoporosis, and malignancies that are associated with bony metastases or humeral hypercalcemia of malignancy (HHM).

The vascular organization of bone is divided into afferent, efferent, and intermediate systems. The afferent includes the nutrient artery, periosteal arterioles, and the metaphyseal arteries (Fig. 20.3). The nutrient artery passes through the cortex and branches within the medullary cavity into ascending and descending branches. It is an elaborate branching system in which cortical bone is fed by periosteal vessels and by endosteally derived vessels that enter the cortex through Volkmann canals. The venous efferent system is comprised of veins that accompany the afferent vessels. These veins coalesce into large exiting veins that pass through the cortex like the nutrient artery. Certain anatomic sites are vulnerable to avascular necrosis; for example, infarction of the femoral head is a common complication of a subcapital fracture of the femoral neck. One explanation of avascular necrosis with steroid therapy or with alcoholism implicates fatty microemboli, which are found in many parenchymal organs at autopy, also occuring in bones throughout the skeleton.

Growth and Development

Bone is unusual in that it can grow only by its apposition to the surface of an already existing substrate such as bone or calcified cartilage. Most of the embryonic skeleton is first formed as cartilage that undergoes mineralization through matrix vesicles associated with the hypertrophy and death of the chondrocytes. The periosteum surrounding the shaft of calcified cartilage produces a primitive bone matrix and forms a collar within which capillaries invade the calcified cartilage and osteoclasts (chondroclasts) mediate the removal of the cartilage matrix. Osteoblasts deposit bone matrix on cores of calcified cartilage. This tissue is often referred to as *primary spongiosa*. It is remodeled and reorganized into secondary spongiosa made of mature lamellar bone. The process is called *endochondral ossification*, to signify that the bone develops within the cartilaginous anlage. Bone formation also occurs in secondary centers of ossification at the ends of long bones. The physis, or growth plate, is the portion of cartilage that remains between the main part of the shaft of bone and the epiphysis or bone

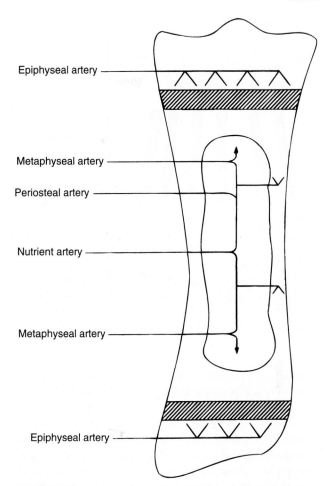

FIGURE 20.3 Schematic diagram of the blood supply to a typical long bone. The nutrient artery branches proximally and distally after entering the medullary canal. Periosteal vessels give diaphyseal and metaphyseal bone a dual blood supply by joining the medullary system. The metaphyseal arteries also anastomose with the medullary system. The epiphysis receives a direct blood supply. At maturation with physeal closure, an anastomosis forms between the medullary vascular system and the epiphyseal system.

end. The growth plate has three discrete zones (reserve, proliferative, and hypertrophic) (Fig. 20.4). In the reserve zone are resting chondrocytes. The proliferative zone has columns of chondrocytes that are actively dividing. The hypertrophic zone has chondrocytes that secrete matrix and undergo maturation, which results in the triad of cellular degeneration, provisional calcification of the matrix, and vascularization from the subchondral bone. The metaphysis is the region immediately beneath the growth plate and the diaphysis is the midshaft region between the growth plates. These terms are frequently used clinically because certain diseases have predilections for one or more of these zones. Through childhood, the growth plates become narrower and are the organizing center of bone elongation until adolescence is reached. Although growth plates are enveloped by a dense collar of cortical bone, they are vulnerable sites for displacement in athletic or overweight adolescents during periods of accelerated skeletal growth. Slipped capital

In the figure, the labels from top to bottom read: Epiphyseal artery, Metaphyseal artery, Periosteal artery, Nutrient artery, Metaphyseal artery, Epiphyseal artery.

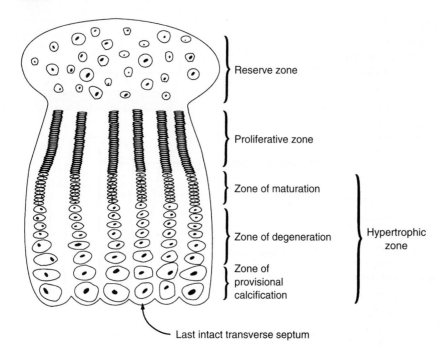

Reserve zone

Proliferative zone

Zone of maturation

Zone of degeneration

Hypertrophic zone

Zone of provisional calcification

Last intact transverse septum

FIGURE 20.4   Zonal division of the cartilaginous portion of a growth plate.

femoral epiphysis (SCFE) of the hip can occur unilaterally or bilaterally and presents with pain, limping, or limitation of mobility and often requires surgical fixation of the femoral head to prevent further motion at the growth plate. At puberty, the growth plates become obliterated, preventing further elongation. Upon radiography, a horizontal plate, the epiphyseal scar, can be identified in some bones as the site of blending of the bone from either side. A diverse group of conditions can result in premature closure of the growth plate. A bar or bridge of bone can form across the growth plate, preventing further growth or producing malalignment. Careful, narrow resection of physeal bridges in such patients leads to satisfactory results in many patients; however, early diagnosis of the formation of these bridges remains critical to successful outcomes.

The bones of the skull, some of the facial bones, and most of the clavicle form in a different manner. These bones are formed without the cartilage stage and without growth plates. Rather, they develop by intramembranous ossification. Embryologically these bones originate directly from undifferentiated mesenchymal tissue and grow by apposition of bone matrix. Changes in the shape (modeling) of these bones occur by apposition of some surfaces and resorption on others. Bone formed by the periosteal collar around long bones may be viewed as intramembranous ossification.

Innervation of bone has been documented in animal models and human fetuses. Classical studies in the 19th century showed that the femoral nerve penetrates the nutrient foramina with the nutrient artery. Afferent fibers and efferent sympathetic fibers have been demonstrated to be profusely distributed around the small vessels in bone. Innervation extends to the vessel's finest endings. A supply of nonmyelinated and myelinated fibers penetrate the cortex, enter the small foramina of the epiphyses and metaphyses,

and pass through Haversian canals. Some information suggests that perception and transmission of pain sensation is mediated by the periarterial sympathetic nerves. This is the theory of the vascular nature of bone pain. For example, it has been proposed that the intermittent pain associated with sclerotic bone is due to dilatation of the large venules and sinusoids found in those sites. The dilatation is produced by occlusion of efferent veins upon contraction of muscles around the affected bone.

Biology of Fracture Repair and Fusion

Fracture of a bone results from mechanical injury. In general, compressive loads result in oblique fractures, and torsional loads produce spiral fractures. Tensile loads cause flat fractures and are uncommon. The fracture line may be single (a simple fracture) or the bone may be broken into multiple fragments (a comminuted fracture). If the skin over the fractured bone is broken, it is considered a compound fracture, and is associated with an increased risk for infection and delayed or poor repair. Repeated stress to the bone may produce stress (or fatigue) fractures, in which accumulation of microfractures eventually results in collapse, usually without substantial antecedent trauma.

Under favorable conditions, bone can be regenerated and will function normally. There are two types of fracture healing, primary and secondary, both of which depend on the cellular processes fundamental to bone turnover. The constitutive activities of osteoclastic bone resorption and osteoblastic bone formation that are essential for mineral homeostasis also serve to repair microfractures as well as large injuries to bone (Fig. 20.2). Primary (direct or contact) repair occurs spontaneously under special circumstances in which the fracture is a partial fissure and/or stable, is aligned, and has its surfaces closely apposed. It occurs in both cortical and cancellous bone. Such repair does not often require clinical intervention. Evidence of such repair can be encountered incidentally upon x-ray. Histologic studies with experimental animals show that intracortical healing is associated with the ingrowth of vessels and osteogenic cells within cutting cones on both sides of an osteotomy. Excavating osteoclasts resorb the devitalized bone and lead capillaries across the fissure while trailing osteoblasts deposit new bone along the walls of the tunnels. Therefore, new osteons connect the two sides. Depending upon the amount of necrosis along the fissure, resorption and replacement with new woven bone may extend to irregular distances. Woven bone predominates in early stages of cancellous primary repair. Remodeling can completely obliterate the fissure or may leave a trace of dense trabeculae along the fracture surface.

The essential requirement for primary healing of a fracture is complete immobilization. Healing of bone by primary intention that is facilitated by exact reduction and compression. If the blood supply is adequate, healing is related to stability. Even wide gaps can heal by ingrowth of new bone into hematoma in the gap if stability is achieved.

There are several basic principles of fracture fixation. With weight-bearing casts and external fixators, cyclic loading can promote healing if introduced appropriately. In splinting, a stiff device is affixed to the fractured bone to minimize fracture mobility. Operative fixation can be achieved with internal rods or plates and screws. In compression fixation, two surfaces (bone-to-bone or implant-to-bone) are pressed together to apply load to the surfaces and to reduce friction. Compression devices can be static (remaining unaltered) or dynamic (providing partial loading and unloading). With optimal fixation, direct bone formation occurs with minimal resorption of fragment ends. Eccentric loading of bone may have one cortex in tension and the other in compression. Bone tissue responds to these loads in distinct ways: resorption dominates in surfaces under tension and formation dominates in surfaces under compression. The net effect of eccentric loading is modeling of the bone to achieve more balanced conditions.

More common than primary repair, secondary repair of bone involves a sequence of reactions that can result in restoration of the injured bone, even in the face of mobility. The injured part is ultimately replaced by bone and not by scar; therefore there is regeneration and not repair. The first phase is inflammation. This phase includes hematoma and fibrin clot formation. Fibroblasts, mesenchymal cells, and macrophages predominate. It is the macrophage that controls angiogenesis in the hypoxic milieu. Where the blood supply has been compromised, the bone margin undergoes necrosis followed by removal with osteoclast activity. The next phase is characterized by zones of hard and soft callus formation. Medullary precursor/progenitor cells differentiate to osteoblasts and deposit trabeculae of woven bone. Cells of the inner (cambial) layer of periosteum proliferate and differentiate into osteoblasts near the cortex. Further away, differentiation to chondrocytes and formation of hyaline cartilage results in an expansive mass around the fracture. The amount of cartilage varies, but it is avascular

and is greatest in unstable fractures. It can be said that the callus is an attempt to form a natural splint. With time, the callus undergoes endochondral ossification. Cartilage zones are invaded by capillaries and undergo mineralization of the matrix, resorption of the mineralized regions, and hypertrophy of the cells. Endochondral ossification of callus differs from that in growth plates in that the former results in the disappearance of the large mass of callus. Although foci of osteoblasts can be seen within the callus, bone is thought to emanate from the marrow and cambium.

The basic aim of fracture treatment is to achieve proper anatomic alignment. Satisfactory reduction requires the restoration of axial alignment in all three planes (frontal, sagittal, and horizontal), without causing damage to the blood supply. It has been reported that fixation occurs approximately 3 weeks after injury if there has been a robust development of soft callus.

Fractures of the femoral neck, patella, tibia, and some carpal and tarsal bones can severely compromise the local vascular supply. Avascular bone death after fractures has been referred to as *aseptic necrosis*. Small necrotic fragments can be completely resorbed by osteoclasts. Creeping repair of cortical bone occurs by osteoclastic tunneling and bone formation, but resorption can exceed formation, resulting in weak, porous bone. Dead cortical bone may remain at the site for extended periods of time and presents a risk of fracture.

Inadequate nutrition, smoking, comorbidity such as diabetes, and drugs such as glucocorticoids can compromise fracture repair. Tibial fractures constitute most healing problems, in part because of the minimal soft tissue and relatively low vascularity, both of which also increase risk for infection.

Bone Grafts, Implants, and Substitute Materials

Although bone has a remarkable capacity to regenerate itself, osseous deficiencies occur in a number of congenital, traumatic, and pathologic situations. Various surgical techniques for managing them adapt the bone tissue remodeling process to promote new bone formation or incorporation of prostheses. Small segments of bone and particles of viable bone can be transplanted from one part of the body to another and produce new bone in the new location. Larger segments can be transferred as fresh vascularized grafts. Autogenous bone grafts are the optimal choice for reconstruction of congenital and acquired bone defects. Iliac grafts are considered the gold standard because they are rich in osteoblast progenitors/precursors and the particulate quality allows for early revascularization. As an alternative to autogenous bone grafts, which are limited in availability (particularly in infants and in frail adults), allogeneic bone from surgical or cadaveric material is available in many forms from certified tissue banks. Banked segments and particles of processed allogeneic bone from screened donors or cadavers can become incorporated into the recipient site by a process that relies on the innate remodeling mechanism. Adjacent cutting cones invade the implanted segment and mediate its resorption and replacement with viable bone. Use of allogeneic demineralized bone for orthopedic applications (2–4) has increased because of wide availability through regional bone banks. Synthetic (alloplastic) bone-substitute materials have the advantages of safety and unlimited off-the-shelf supply. The rational design of bone-substitute materials requires understanding of tissue responses to implanted materials and their potential for specific applications. Ceramics such as calcium phosphates are not recognized as foreign bodies and can provide immediate rigidity and mass, at low cost. Polymers such as polylactic acid (PLA) and polyglycolic acid (PGA) are attractive as bone substitute materials because they are degradable and their chemical composition, porosity, shape, and rate of resorption can be modified. In addition, they have potential as scaffolds for tissue engineering, as carriers of cells, and for controlled delivery of drugs or factors. Metallic implants are also incorporated into bone because of their inert or compatible composition and because new bone can grow against them. Cell-based and cell-free methods of tissue engineering are being investigated for application to osseous lesions (5).

Metabolic Influences on the Skeleton

Metabolic bone diseases are fundamentally disorders of bone remodeling. Osteopenia is recognized radiographically as a decreased mineralized bone mass. Decreased density may be the result of increased bone loss, decreased bone formation, or decreased mineralization of bone (osteomalacia in adults, rickets in children). Osteomalacia may have a number of causes: nutritional deficiencies in calcium or vitamin D, gastrectomy or malabsorption, anticonvulsant medications, or inherited disorders of vitamin D metabolism. Many nations do not have widespread vitamin D supplementation in dairy products. Even in developed countries, daily intake of vitamin D can be diminished in elderly patients and others avoiding supplemented dairy and other products. Vitamin D can be synthesized by the skin but requires adequate exposure to the sun. Endogenous production can be impaired in housebound or bedridden individuals, in populations dwelling in northern latitudes, pigmented individuals, and in girls and women in veiled societies. Liver conditions like cirrhosis can impair activation of vitamin D and thereby cause osteomalacia. Dilantin therapy, chronic renal failure, renal tubular acidosis, and hypophosphatemia can result in osteomalacia. Osteomalacia also occurs in patients with hemodialysis, patients with anorexia nervosa, and patients with oncogenic phosphaturic tumors. Mineralization defects also result from aluminum toxicity and long-term treatment with first-generation bisphosphonates like etridronate. In addition to increasing the risk of nonvertebral fractures, osteomalacia can cause bone pain and is associated with muscle weakness. Radiographic findings often include lucent areas called *Looser zones* or *pseudofractures*. Histologic examination shows the characteristic increase in the amount of unmineralized bone matrix (osteoid). Chronic vitamin D deficiency can contribute to osteopenia through secondary hyperparathyroidism and ensuing activation of bone resorption. Recent studies indicate the widespread prevalence of vitamin D deficiency in children and adults in the United States (6).

Unlike osteomalacia, osteoporosis describes reduced bone tissue mass but with essentially normal extent of matrix mineralization. The pathologic mechanisms of primary osteoporosis differ from osteomalacia. Throughout adulthood, bone is continually remodeled through osteoclastic resorption of old tissue and the production and laying down of new bone matrix by osteoblasts. Into young adulthood, osteoblast activity results in overall skeletal growth. Peak bone mass is achieved during this time, after which, osteoclast activity begins to outpace that of osteoblasts. Throughout the rest of life, this imbalance results in a continuing reduction in bone density and mass with a variable degree of increased porosity. Osteoporotic bone is characterized histologically by thinned trabeculae and Haversian systems of larger diameter. Dual-energy x-ray absorptiometry (DXA) provides measures of bone mineral content (grams) and bone area (cm^2). Bone mineral density (BMD, g/cm^2) is calculated from those measures and is correlated with bone strength. A patient's BMD is expressed as a T-score, or the number of standard deviations above or below the mean value for young normal adults. The Z-score is the comparison with persons of the same age, gender, and race. Numerous studies indicate that BMD is an index of fracture risk (7). Osteoporosis is defined by the World Health Organization as a BMD T-score below -2.5. Risk for osteoporosis is increased after/with menopause, long-term steroid use, diabetes, poor nutrition, and a positive family history. Fragility fractures are those that occur with minimal or no trauma. The frequency of distal radius fractures (Colles fracture) increases rapidly after the menopause and should serve as the clinical indication of severe osteoporosis. Vertebral fractures have an earlier onset than hip fractures, but more than half of the vertebral fractures are not clinically recognized. Having had one fragility fracture increases the risk of subsequent fractures. Standard treatments include calcium and vitamin D, hormone replacement therapy, bisphosphonates, calcitonin, and selective estrogen receptor modulators (SERMs) for women with a history of breast cancer. Selection of treatment depends upon the predisposing conditions.

The Geriatric Skeleton

Bone has a remarkable capacity to renew itself. It is lamentable that this rejuvenation process is imperfect and that remodeling does not prevent skeletal aging. There is vast literature showing that the mechanical properties of bone decline with aging (8). Bone fragility with aging is in large part due to loss of bone mass (9). Another factor is the accumulation of microcracks that accompany the decreased rate of remodeling with aging (10). There are also changes in the mineral phase of bone with advancing years. On the basis of the composition of bone mineral and its x-ray diffraction characteristics, it is clear that the mineral phase of bone becomes more crystalline with age and maturation, although it never approaches the highly crystalline state of geologic hydroxyapatite. Laboratory studies show that fine powders of bone can be separated on the basis of density, revealing heterogeneity in mineral content and crystallinity. Bone mineral appears to be deposited as poorly crystalline carbonatoapatite and, with time, there is an increase in the Ca/P ratio, an increase in crystal size, and a loss of many of the impurities, generally referred to as an *increase in crystallinity* (11). Remodeling replaces the more crystalline mineral with new, more poorly crystalline mineral, but as turnover decreases with aging, there is an accumulation of the denser crystals. The metabolic consequences of this are striking. Hypermineralization of bone tissue is associated with decreased modulus of toughness though it is stiffer and more rigid (8). Second, the denser mineral is less soluble and therefore is less mobilized in calcium homeostasis (12). Finally, the remodeling processes that are essential aspects of fracture healing, bone grafting, and implant incorporation are reduced.

During aging and in states of relative calcium insufficiency, the mechanical functions of bone tissue can be compromised in the face of metabolic needs. This is evidenced, for example, by increased risk of fracture with aging. The tension between the maintenance of extracellular calcium homeostasis and the maintenance of skeletal carbonatoapatite is the basis for the effects of bone aging. Calcium nutrition and modulation of homeostatic mechanisms are pivotal in prevention and treatment of age-related bone loss. With aging, the abilities of the kidney and intestine to maintain calcium homeostasis decline, resulting in a drain of mineral from the bone without a compensatory increase in bone formation.

In the elderly, osteoporosis may coexist with osteomalacia. Vitamin D deficiency is more prevalent than expected in the United States (6). For example, in a series of community-dwelling women admitted for osteoporotic hip fractures, 50% had extreme vitamin D deficiency and 37% had secondary hyperparathyroidism (13). According to the Institutes of Medicine, current daily recommendations for vitamin D are 700 units for adults older than 70 years, although many now recommend 2,000 units as necessary and safe in adults (14). Because vitamin D deficiency is preventable, heightened awareness is necessary to ensure adequate vitamin D nutrition, especially in elderly patients with fractures.

Comorbid illness is frequent in the aged population with osteoporosis or osteoarthritis, especially hypertension and diabetes (15). Repair and reconstruction of bone can be improved in the elderly with management of systemic problems and with proper nutrition.

ARTICULAR CARTILAGE

Physiologic Function

Articular cartilage is a unique tissue that covers the bones of the joints and provides a system with a remarkable capacity

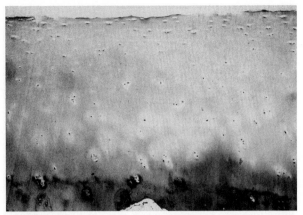

FIGURE 20.5 A low-power histologic picture of normal articular cartilage. Notice that the matrix is nonuniform and the cells very sparse in number. The cells of the radial zone are separated from the calcified layer by an irregular line, the "tidemark" (hematoxylin and eosin, original magnification × 35.)

for almost frictionless joint movement. The tissue has no blood, lymphatic or nerve supply and hence is "isolated" from the rest of the body. Nutrition fluids come from the blood stream to the synovial fluid; and then by transport across the cartilage external membrane, which limits material by both size and chemical structure. The cartilage chemical construct prevents the ingress of unwanted materials and the egress of important agents required by the cartilage for normal function. The matrix of cartilage consists of some unique collagen components and large molecules known as *aggrecan*, which consist principally of glycosaminoglycans on a protein string, which are attached to a filament of hyaluronic acid (Fig. 20.5). The aggrecan provide a major component of the cartilage structure, its relation to water content and its resiliency. Unfortunately cartilage in adults has a very limited capacity for repair and with acute or chronic injury, the cartilage can be damaged and over time develop osteoarthritis.

Normal Histology and Biochemistry

Articular cartilage has five distinct zones (Fig. 20.6) (12,13). On the surface of the cartilage is a fine acellular filamentous zone, which is called the *lamina splendens*. Beneath that is a zone occupying less than one fourth of the cartilage structure, which is rich in collagen and called the *gliding zone*. Beneath the gliding zone is the *transitional zone* in which the cells are randomly arranged and the chemical components dominate the composition. Below that component which occupies well over two thirds of the structure is the *radial zone* in which the cells are arranged in short columns at right angles to the surface. Beneath the radial zone is *the calcified zone*, which lies adjacent to the bony endplate of the subjacent osseous segment. The radial zone is separated from the calcified zone by the *tidemark*, a linear slightly wavy bluish line seen best on hematoxylin and eosin stained sections (12,14).

Articular cartilage consists of three major components: cells, matrix and water; and all have a role and relation to one

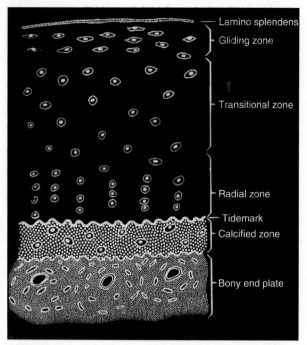

Lamina splendens
Gliding zone

Transitional zone

Radial zone

Tidemark
Calcified zone

Bony end plate

FIGURE 20.6 A diagram showing the structure of articular cartilage. Note the surface layer showing a *lamina splendens* consisting of a fine filamentous fibrillar material that stains poorly. Below that is the *gliding zone* where the cells are elongated and resemble fibroblasts. They are responsible for the synthesis and maintenance of a dense collection of collagen fibers that run parallel the surface ("the skin"). Below that is the *transitional layer*, rich in proteoglycan and collagen fibers and beneath that the *radial zone* where the cells are less active and line up in short columns perpendicular to the surface. The *tidemark* separates the radial zone from the calcified zone which is adherent to the *bony end plate*.

another (12). The number of cells is sparse by comparison with most other body tissues and the cells vary somewhat in size and shape and have no direct contact or relation to one another. The cells of the surface layer resemble fibroblasts and actually synthesize a large number of linearly placed collagen fibers in the surface layer. The cells of the intermediate zone of the cartilage are randomly arranged and moderate in size and have components suggestive of active synthetic activities. The cells of the radial zone are smaller and less active appearing; and the cells of the calcified layer seem to be dead or at least remaining dormant. Beneath this region is the subchondral bone, which in adults does not provide nutrients to the cartilage, but may affect the distribution and structure of the cartilage.

Cartilage is heavily hydrated with a 70% concentration of water, most of which is in the form of a gel (12). With pressure on the cartilage surface such as occurs with standing or especially compressive movement, the water passes off to the surface to attach to a part of the lamina splendens and forms the lubrication system. The remaining materials consist of collagen, proteoglycan and noncollagenous proteins. The collagens account for approximately 60% of the dry weight of the cartilage and include principally type II, but also

smaller concentrations of types VI, IX, X and XI, all of which play a role in cartilage structure (12). The proteoglycans consist of a core protein and negatively charged repeating disaccharides, which remain stiffly extended in space and attract cations. The glycosaminoglycans include chondroitin-4 sulfate, chondroitin-6 sulfate and keratan sulfate. These materials are fixed to protein cores with the aid of link proteins and known as *aggrecan molecules*. The aggrecan molecules in turn attach to a long filament of hyaluronic acid and these macromolecules are known as *proteoglycan aggregates*, which fill the intrafibrillar space (Fig. 20.7). There is considerable alteration in the aggrecan components with advancing age with reduction in size and alteration in structure.

Three other forms of proteoglycans are present in small concentrations: decorin, biglycan and fibromodulin all of which bind to type II collagen and seem to prevent healing of cartilage defects, by interfering with transforming growth factor β (TGF-β) activity (15). Other proteinaceous materials are present in low concentrations and these include Anchorin CII, cartilage oligomeric protein (COMP), fibronectin, thrombospondin, and tenascin, all of which bind the cells to collagen.

Despite the absence of blood supply, the low oxygen tension of articular cartilage ($\sim$8%) and the low temperature of many joints, chondrocytes are active cells in terms of production of materials and in children, cell replication. Chondrocytes synthesize proteoglycans, the link proteins and other proteinaceous materials sometimes at a fairly rapid rate. The chondrocyte produce collagen and then cleave the molecules and set up cross-links to increase the organization of the structure. Chondrocytes are also responsible for developing the degradative cascade, which includes interleukins, matrix metalloproteases, collagenase, and aggrecanase. In addition, however, the cells are responsible for producing other materials such as TGF-β, tissue inhibitors of metalloproteases (TIMPs) and insulin-like growth factors (IGFs) all of which diminish or prevent the action of the degradative materials. Weight-bearing movement and appropriate exercise activity are activators of the materials that inhibit degradation, which helps to explain the role of controlled exercise in the prevention and treatment of cartilage injuries.

Growth and Development

At 7 to 8 weeks of embryonic life, the human embryo has formed synovial joint spaces, including cellular condensations for bone, ligament, capsule, and cartilage. The immature cartilage contains abundant chondrocytes that proliferate and secrete cartilage extracellular matrix. In young animals, cellular replication occurs in both the superficial and deep zones of cartilage; however, as the animal approaches skeletal maturity, replication only occurs in the deep zone of cartilage. With aging, the cellularity of the articular cartilage decreases, and chondrocytes in mature cartilage are thought to rarely, if ever, divide.

The biochemistry of the articular cartilage changes in aging as well. Water content is highest in the immature

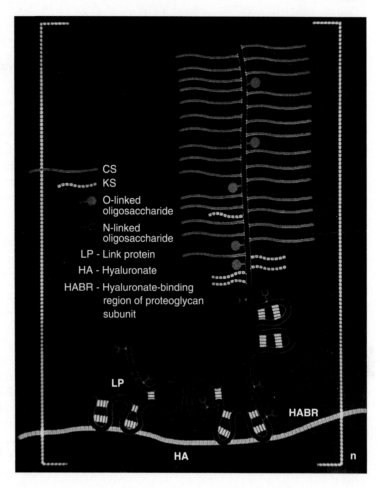

CS
KS
O-linked oligosaccharide
N-linked oligosaccharide
LP - Link protein
HA - Hyaluronate
HABR - Hyaluronate-binding region of proteoglycan subunit

LP

HABR

HA   n

FIGURE 20.7   A diagram showing the structure of aggrecan proteoglycan. Notice the chondroitin sulfate (CS) and keratan sulfate (KS) chains, the protein core, the hyaluronate-binding region (HABR) where the molecule is attached to a long filament of hyaluronic acid (HA). The link protein (LP) is responsible for holding the molecule firmly in place on the hyaluronate chain. Note the presence of two types of oligosaccharide in the molecule as well.

cartilage, and decreases during growth, then remains relatively constant throughout adulthood. Proteoglycan content mirrors the changes in water content. Collagen content begins at a low level and increases during growth until skeletal maturity is reached. With advancing age, proteoglycan size decreases, and the chondrocytes are thought to become less responsive to growth factors and other stimuli.

Cartilage Wear and Repair

Cartilage Synthesis and Response to Injury

Chondrocytes in immature individuals have the capacity to divide and enlarge the cartilaginous structure (12). There is evidence for deoxyribonucleic acid (DNA) synthesis and increased rates of synthesis of collagen, proteoglycans, and other proteins. With cessation of length growth, normal cartilage chondrocytes lose the capacity to divide. There are, however, three ways which the chondrocytes can actively synthesize new cells in support of the cartilage structure: cartilage injury, which does not enter the underlying bone; cartilage injury in which the underlying bone is damaged; and osteoarthritis.

Cartilage injuries that do not penetrate the calcified layer usually show death of cells at the sites of the injury and a modest biologic response related principally to the synovial inflammation. A modest DNA synthetic activity occurs in

the cartilage, which rarely lasts longer than 2 weeks. No remodeling occurs and the extent of the injury present initially remains the same (12).

Those cartilage injuries that penetrate into the underlying bone cause a major response in the osseous tissues, which show death of tissue followed by a marked vascular response with the development of vascular granulation tissue. Cartilage is produced but the material synthesized by the new chondrocytes seems to have too much bone-like materials and breaks down and becomes locally osteoarthritic.

Osteoarthritis is a common, progressive disorder of unknown cause, as a rule occurring late in life and principally affecting the hands and weight bearing joints. The syndrome is characterized clinically by pain, deformity, and limitation of motion and pathologically by focal erosive lesions, cartilage destruction, subchondral bony sclerosis, cyst formation, and marginal osteophytes.

There are many postulated etiologic factors for osteoarthritis including aging, genetic errors, hormonal errors, inflammatory changes, and mechanical injury.

Histologic, Biochemical, and Clinical Characteristics of Osteoarthritis

Sequential histologic alterations in osteoarthritic cartilage show initial diminished staining of the tissue, irregularity of the surface of the cartilage and clefts, which descend

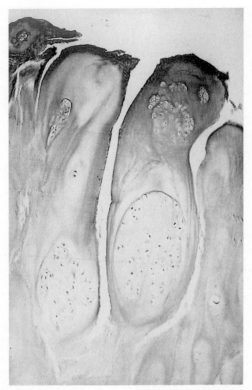

FIGURE 20.8 Histologic picture of cartilage from a severely osteoarthritic knee joint. The surface is fragmented and deep clefts are present. The matrix is irregular in structure and stains poorly. There are large numbers of cells in clones indicating the attempt at the repair process (hematoxylin and eosin, original magnification × 45.)

deeper and deeper into the cartilaginous tissue (Fig. 20.8). The tidemark is violated by blood vessels and the most striking feature is the presence of increased numbers of cells, often in clones, which appear to be attempting a restoration of the structure of the tissue. The disease worsens, the clefts get deeper and eventually the surface is left with no cartilage at all and only the underlying dense and sometimes cyst-containing and osteonecrotic bone. Cartilage and bone structures known as *osteophytes* appear at the margins of the diseased joint. Cysts may be very large and occur on both sides of the joints.

Biologically the cartilage undergoes some major changes including increased water content and cartilage swelling, diminished proteoglycans and less collagen, which however remains as type II. Materials of the degradative cascade are markedly increased in concentration and actively destructive of the cartilage. These include an array of metalloproteinases (MMPs), synovial and cartilage interleukin 1, prostromelysin, procollagenase, proaggrecanase, plasminogen activator, and prostaglandins, all of which serve to produce collagenase, aggrecanase, and other materials which destroy the matrix of the cartilage. The inhibitors of these materials include TGF-β and TIMPs, both of which attempt to reverse the action of the degradative agents.

Clinically, the joints become enlarged with fluid, become sometimes profoundly limited in motion and sometimes cause major disability. Imaging studies show the classic changes of narrow joints, dense subchondral bone sites, cysts, osteophytes and sometimes fractured segments within the joints. Computed tomography (CT), magnetic resonance imaging (MRI) and high-resolution spectroscopy are useful in defining the extent of the disease and the possibility of surgical correction without total joint replacement. A recent approach to defining the extent of the disease and the effect of treatment is the use of gadolinium [diethylenetriamine pentaacetic acid (DPTA)] 2, which is a special stain for glycosaminoglycan.

Treatment of Osteoarthritis

Numerous methods have been introduced over the years for the treatment of osteoarthritis.

1. Anti-inflammatory drug treatment: Aspirin, acetominophen, nonsteroidal anti-inflammatory drugs (Cox 1 inhibitors), Cox 2 inhibitors and corticosteroids have all been utilized with some success. The approaches depend principally on reducing the inflammatory response in the synovium.
2. Radiation treatment has been tried using approximately 60 Gy given over a prolonged period of time but seems to be of limited value.
3. Injections of corticosteroids and hyaluronic analogs have resulted in mild to moderate improvement in patient complaints.
4. Recent introduction of orally administered chondroitin sulfate and glucosamine has been tried and seems to provide some improvement for the patients.
5. Physiotherapy designed to strengthen muscles about the damaged joint has a limited success rate but is certainly an important addition to the program.
6. Arthroscopic "washout" may be temporarily successful (16).
7. Deep cartilage defects can be treated by chondroplastic procedures producing tiny defects in the underlying bone; or with autologous cartilage transplants; or with cryopreserved allogeneic periosteum; or even with cartilage incubated with TGF-β. Stem cells have also been introduced in scaffolds but thus far have shown limited success. Small segments of cartilage obtained from a condylar site in the joint may be introduced into defects, a technique known as *mosaicplasty*.
8. Allograft transplantation has had some success for condylar defects particularly in the distal femur or proximal tibia.
9. Major surgical efforts such as osteotomy have a long history with limited success unless a specific error can be corrected. In the past arthrodesis has been advocated for certain types of osteoarthritic lesions such as those affecting the feet or hand bones.
10. Total joint replacement surgery for hip, knee, or shoulder is usually successful particularly for older patients.

SKELETAL MUSCLE AND TENDON

Physiologic Function

Skeletal or striated muscle accounts for more than 40% of total body weight, making it the largest tissue mass in the body. Tendons connect the skeletal muscle to the bony skeleton, allowing for transfer of the force generated by the muscle into motion of the skeleton. The musculotendinous unit crosses a joint, thereby allowing the muscle force to translate into motion of the joint and skeleton. The musculotendinous unit can cause acceleration of limb motion when the muscle undergoes a concentric contraction, resulting in muscle shortening. Eccentric contraction of the muscle body can result in muscle lengthening and limb deceleration.

There are two major types of muscle fibers. Type I fibers are slow-twitch, oxidative fibers which function as the endurance elements. These fibers are able to maintain low strength for long periods of time, and have high aerobic capacity. The type II fibers are fast-twitch fibers, responsible for bursts of power at relatively high-energy cost. These fibers are not able to maintain sustained contraction, and are called *fatigable fibers*. They are largely dependent on anaerobic metabolism. Most skeletal muscles are composed of both types of fibers.

Normal Histology and Biochemistry

The muscle fiber is the basic cellular unit of skeletal muscle. Each fiber is a multinucleated syncytium formed by fusion of myoblasts during development. The nuclei of the muscle fibers are located in the periphery of the cell cytoplasm. The center of the muscle fiber contains a central cable of a long chain of interdigitating filaments of actin and myosin, the sarcomeres. Simultaneous contraction of the sarcomeres leads to an abrupt and forceful shortening of the muscle fiber. A muscle is composed of groups of the muscle fibers that are covered with a vascular connective tissue called *endomysium*. The connective tissue encasing the entire muscle is called the *epimysium* (Fig. 20.9). The nerves and blood vessels in both muscle and tendon are found predominantly in the connective tissue around the groups of muscle fibers.

The basic motor unit of the musculotendinous unit includes the anterior horn cell, the peripheral nerve, the myoneural junction, and the muscle fibers innervated by the nerve cell. Each motor nerve fiber branches to supply an average of 100 to 200 muscle fibers. The ends of the nerve fibers supplying skeletal muscle are embedded in the surface of the muscle fiber at the neuromuscular junction. The motor nerve fibers are surrounded by Schwann cells and a myelin sheath which ends just before the myoneural junction. The efferent nerve signal, carried by a wave of depolarization in the neuron, triggers a release of the neurotransmitter acetylcholine into the neuromuscular junction, where it triggers the opening of calcium channels in the muscle membrane. The resulting influx of calcium binds to troponin and this complex results in the release of tropomyosin from the myosin-binding sites of actin. Once the binding sites are freed, the actin and myosin fibers slide past each other, with adenosine triphosphate (ATP) driving a conformational change in the head of the myosin. The actin is anchored to the muscle cell cytoskeleton by α actinin. Therefore, when the actin filaments are brought closer together by the action of myosin, the cell cytoskeleton contracts.

Muscle contains four types of sensory nerve fibers that serve as receptors of the stretch reflex, proprioception, and pain. One type, the muscle spindle, lies parallel to the muscle fibers. With stimulation by muscle tension (as during testing of the deep tendon reflexes on physical examination), the muscle spindles trigger a reflex arc that results in contraction of the muscle fibers. Two additional types, the Golgi tendon organs and Golgi-Mazzoni corpuscles, are also stimulated by mechanical deformation, and are thought to provide proprioceptive and vibration information. The fourth type, the sensory free nerve endings in the muscle, are thought to function in pain sensation.

Tenocytes are located between the dense collagen fibers of the tendon. They are typical fibroblasts, with long cytoplasmic extensions along and among the fibers, facilitating intercellular communication. The cell density of tendons is similar to that in ligaments, and less than that of bone marrow or the viscera. The extracellular matrix of tendons is largely composed of dense, parallel bundles of collagen fibers that are oriented along the line of tension between muscle and bone insertion for maximal transmission of load. Tendons have less crimp than ligaments, allowing for greater efficiency in load transfer. The collagen component is predominantly type I (~95% of the dry weight of tendon), with the remaining organic matrix mostly composed of type III collagen and proteoglycans. Some tendons, such as the flexor tendons of the fingers, are surrounded by a synovial sheath, which facilitates gliding of the tendon. The myotendinous junction is also specialized for load transfer with a highly convoluted surface area. Tendons generally attach to bone with long, parallel fibers. The outer fibers usually blend with the periosteum, whereas the central fibers insert directly into the bone. The direct insertion site has four

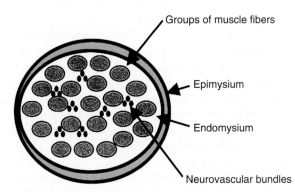

FIGURE 20.9 Schematic of the arrangement of tissue types in a skeletal muscle. Groups of muscle fibers are encased by endomysium, through which the neurovascular bundles course. The entire muscle is covered with epimysium.

zones: tendon, fibrocartilage, mineralized fibrocartilage, and bone (17). Sharpey fibers are collagen bundles that extend from the tendon or periosteum into the bone.

Growth and Development

During embryonic development, the individual muscle cells (the myoblasts) fuse to form multinucleated cells or muscle fibers. The commitment of myoblasts to fuse and become muscle fibers is thought to be dependent on signaling from neural tube and dorsal ectoderm. Satellite cells are detected after fiber maturation and are thought to contribute to muscle fiber growth and tissue regeneration during postnatal life. These myogenic cells may arise from the vasculature and become committed to myogenesis by local signaling (18). With fetal development, the number of muscle fibers and the size and length of the muscle fibers increase until birth. After birth, few new fibers form and the increase in muscle size is primarily due to hypertrophy of the existing fibers (19). New fibers can be formed after birth from undifferentiated satellite cells (20). However, most of the compensation for muscle tissue injury comes from an increase in size in the remaining muscle fibers.

Overall muscle mass decreases in most people between ages 25 to 50 years. This is largely due to an increased rate of fiber atrophy, which leads to a decrease in the total number of muscle fibers (21). The effects of muscle fiber loss can be counteracted by weight training, which increases the size of the remaining fibers. Muscle stiffness (due to increasing collagen content) also increases with age, leading to increased incidence of muscle strains in older athletes, especially associated with inadequate preactivity stretching and "warm-up." In tendons, the mean collagen fibril diameter decreases with age. Tendons increase in stiffness and failure strength until maturity, and then decrease with aging.

Both components of the muscle-tendon unit have been shown to increase in size with repetitive loading, or training. In the tendon, this is due to an increase in the number and density of smaller diameter fibrils. In skeletal muscle, "low-tension, high-repetition" training (such as distance running) leads to increased endurance by facilitating the function of type I fibers with increased capillary density and mitochondrial density in the fibers. "High-tension, low-repetition" training (such as power lifting), leads to hypertrophy of type II muscle fibers.

During immobilization, skeletal muscle atrophies. The muscle fiber number and size both decrease, and microscopic changes in the sarcomere length-tension relation occur. At the same time, the stiffness of tendons decreases. It is not known whether additional mechanical properties are also affected, and whether these changes are irreversible.

Pathophysiologic Conditions of Muscle and Tendon

Duchenne Muscular Dystrophy (DMD) is a disease that causes progressive weakness, particularly of central muscles of the trunk, hips, and shoulders. Histologically, it is characterized by muscle necrosis and fatty degeneration of the muscle

fibers. These changes result from a loss of the functional gene that codes for the protein dystrophin, found on the surface of skeletal muscle cells. In DMD, there is an "in-frame" deletion in a triplet base pair. All the downstream triplet pairs are subsequently shifted, and the resultant protein is non-functional. In Becker muscular dystrophy, the deletion occurs between base pairs, therefore a less functional, smaller dystrophin protein is produced. Becker muscular dystrophy typically has a later time of onset and slower clinical progression than DMD. As the dystrophin gene is found on the X-chromosome, this is an X-linked recessive gene that affects the male offspring of women who carry the dysfunctional gene. It is hoped that ultimately, treatment with the introduction of a normal dystrophin gene into the muscle fibers will result in normal muscle histology and function.

Myasthenia gravis is a disease that causes muscle fatigue and weakness that worsens with exercise. It initially involves the extraocular muscles and muscles of the eyelids, and progresses to larger muscle groups in the body. It is the most common defect of the neuromuscular junction and results from damage to the postsynaptic acetylcholine receptor sites. This is thought to be an autoimmune disease, where antibodies destroy the acetylcholine receptor, thereby preventing calcium influx into the muscle and muscle contraction. Current treatment methods include anticholinesterase medications, corticosteroids, immuno-suppressant drugs, thymectomy and plasmapheresis.

Muscle strains can range from microscopic fiber tears to complete ruptures of the entire muscle. Injuries most frequently happen during eccentric contraction, and often occur at the myotendinous junction. The healing response occurs in three phases: inflammatory, proliferative, and remodeling phases. The inflammatory phase is characterized by an influx of inflammatory cells into a hematoma formed at the site of injury. The hematoma is gradually invaded by myoblasts, which originate from surrounding muscle satellite cells. The myoblasts proliferate and produce a collagen scar. During the healing process the muscle is weaker than normal; strenuous activity should be avoided until the later phases of scar remodeling. However, early gentle motion of the injured muscle is thought to facilitate a return to function and to limit the size of the resultant scar.

Tendon injuries are often the result of trauma, such as a sudden tensile force or laceration. Tendons that cannot be maintained in close apposition with immobilization of the limb, such as the flexor tendons of the fingers, often require surgical reapproximation and suturing to hold the ends together while healing occurs. Tendons respond to injury and surgical reapproximation in a manner similar to that of other connective tissues. An initial phase of inflammation is followed by invasion of the repair site by fibroblastic cells, and remodeling of the scar. Controversy still exists as to whether this process is mediated by cells intrinsic or extrinsic to the tendon. The strength of the healing tendon is significantly lower than the uninjured tendon in the initial phase of healing. Strength begins to increase at 3 weeks after injury. With improved techniques of tendon suture repair, early motion is now possible after tendon lacerations, and is thought to improve the functional outcome by minimizing adhesion formation. In addition, recent work has demonstrated improved tendon to bone healing at the surface of the bone as opposed to within a tunnel of bone (22). The use of mesenchymal stem cells to improve healing has been an active field of research for tendon healing as it has for bone and cartilage (23).

LIGAMENTS

Physiologic Function

Skeletal ligaments are fibrous connective tissues that connect bone to bone and mechanically stabilize joints. Examples of ligaments are the collateral and cruciate ligaments of the knee. These connect the femur and tibia. The medial and lateral collateral ligaments are extra-articular (outside the knee), whereas the anterior cruciate ligament (ACL) is intra-articular (passing through the middle of the knee). Ligaments provide minimal resistance to normal joint motion, while providing stability against abnormal joint motion. Ligaments also provide proprioceptive feedback to the muscles surrounding the joint, which enhances the dynamic stability of the joint.

Normal Histology and Biochemistry

Ligaments are composed primarily of parallel type I collagen fibrils arranged in groups, or fibers. When the ligament is not under tension, the fibrils assume a wavy structure, or crimp (Fig. 20.10). This fiber redundancy is responsible for the relatively easy initial extensibility of the ligament. When

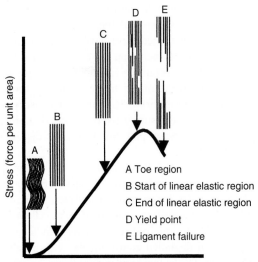

FIGURE 20.11 Schematic of the relation between the mechanical response and the histologic changes in a skeletal ligament. At rest, the ligament fibers have a wavy structure (*A*). During normal joint motion, the ligament fibers straighten (*A–B*). During additional stress, ligament fibers can break in small areas (*D*), and ligament failure will result from application of large stresses or strains across the joint (*E*).

the ligament is stretched initially, it extends easily until the crimp has been straightened, then the collagen fibrils resist further extension (Fig. 20.11). This mechanical behavior is critical to the function of the ligament in allowing normal joint motion while protecting the articular surfaces from injury. For instance, the medial collateral ligament of the knee stretches easily through a physiologic range, allowing the knee to move into slight valgus to accommodate uneven walking surfaces. However, if the stresses across the knee attempt to force the joint into too much valgus (such as during a fall), the medial collateral ligament tightens and prevents the abnormal joint motion and joint injury.

The ligament cells are typically oriented along the longitudinal axis of the tissue. The density of cells in most ligaments is slightly greater than articular cartilage and cortical bone, and far less than cell-dense organs such as liver or kidney. Although the cytoplasm of the cells of ligaments is difficult to visualize with standard light microscopic methods, recent work with low-power electron microscopy reveals extensive cytoplasmic processes that extend along the collagen fibrils. The cells within the fibers depend predominantly on diffusion of nutrients from the surrounding vascularized tissues. The bundles of collagen fibrils, or fibers, are surrounded by the endoligament. The surface of the ligament is covered by an adherent, fibrous, cellular layer called the *epiligament*, which is also well vascularized. The vascular supply for most ligaments comes from vessels that cross joints and send branches to the periarticular ligaments (24). Within the ligament, the vessels typically course with the nerves of the ligaments, as neurovascular bundles (25).

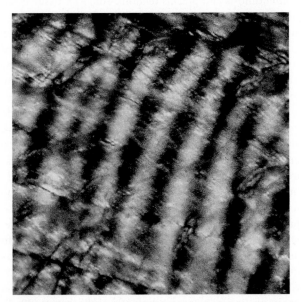

FIGURE 20.10 Photomicrograph of a human anterior cruciate ligament demonstrating the waviness, or crimp, of the collagen fibers when the ligament is not under tension (picrosirius red stain, original magnification × 200).

Ligaments contain mechanoreceptors, which are thought to signal the reflex systems of the neuromuscular system. Three types of mechanoreceptors have been identified in the ligaments of the knee, including Ruffini receptors, Pacinian receptors, and Golgi receptors (26). A fourth type of nerve supply, the free unmyelinated nerve ending, is thought to function as pain receptors (25). The neurosensory role of these receptors has been supported by studies demonstrating changes in electromyographic function after disruption of the ACL of the knee.

Collagen comprises 70% to 80% of the dry weight of ligaments. More than 90% of the collagen is fibrillar type I, with the remainder being type III collagen. This collagen is produced intracellularly, modified extracellularly, and self-assembled into microfibrils. Collagen in ligaments is synthesized and degraded continuously, with a half-life of 300 to 500 days. The factors regulating collagen turnover have yet to be determined. Proteoglycans, such as chondroitin-4-sulfate and dermatan sulfate, comprise less than 1% of the dry weight of ligaments, although the exact amounts and composition are considered ligament specific. Ligaments also contain elastin, fibronectin, and other glycoproteins. As much as 70% of the wet weight of ligaments is water, which is both structurally bound to collagen and freely associated with the interfibrillar gel.

Growth and Development

Development of ligaments begins with fibroblasts aligning between the bony attachment sites. Normal development requires joint motion, and the condensations disappear if motion is stopped (27). Collagen fibrils are deposited between the cells, in parallel with the longitudinal axis of the ligament. The cytoplasm in the fetal and young adult rat ligament cells contain abundant rough endoplasmic reticulum and a prominent Golgi apparatus, consistent with active synthetic and secretory cells. As the cells deposit more and more collagen, the bundles of matrix separate the cells, thereby forming the mature ligament with a lower cell number density and higher collagen content.

Studies of growth in the rabbit medial collateral ligament demonstrated elongation of the ligament at all locations, rather than the presence of a growth center as found in long bones (28). At the insertion of the ligament into bone, rapid cell division is noted. With growth, the collagen of the insertion site is incorporated into the adjacent bone. This active formation of the insertion site allows the insertion to remain metaphyseal rather than gradually becoming diaphyseal with bone growth. Mechanical tension has been found to accelerate the rate of ligamentous growth in immature animals (29).

Biology of Ligament Rupture and Repair

Ligament injuries account for 25% to 40% of all knee injuries (30). These injuries can be caused both by contact (i.e., a blow) or noncontact (i.e., a deceleration injury resulting in a tear of the ACL). In adults, the ligament injury is typically a midsubstance rupture, whereas in skeletally immature patients, the injury is more commonly a bony avulsion of the attachment site of the ligament.

The response to injury of the medial collateral ligament occurs in three phases: inflammatory, proliferative, and remodeling (31). During the inflammatory phase, fibrin clot forms and the surrounding tissue is invaded by mononuclear inflammatory cells. Within a few weeks, the proliferative phase ensues, in which the fibrin clot is invaded by fibroblasts that begin producing a disorganized functional scar, composed principally of type I and type III collagen. When the scar has gained sufficient strength, the remodeling phase begins, and randomly oriented scar fibers are gradually altered to an increasingly parallel structure which approaches the configuration of the original tissue. Although the scar tissue has histologic differences that distinguish it from native tissue, this process results in healing of the ligament in most cases and a return of its original function.

Therefore, extra-articular ligament injuries can be treated successfully with immobilization or primary repair. Intra-articular ligaments, however, such as the ACL, fail to heal after rupture, even with primary repair. Although the ACL is able to mount a proliferative and vascular response to rupture, the observation of the failure of formation of a provisional scaffold at the rupture site and resynovialization of the ligament remnants provide two possible reasons for the failure of ACL healing (32). Because of the failure of the ACL to heal, additional treatments, such as ligament reconstruction, have been developed for intra-articular ligament injuries. The ACL is currently treated with removal of the torn ligament and replacement with a tendon graft (either autologous or allograft) that is secured with interference screws or other fixation devices in bony tunnels (Fig. 20.12). Autograft choices include the middle third of the patellar tendon and a combined graft of the semitendinosis and gracilis tendons. Allograft tissue is used for primary ACL reconstruction, as well as in revision surgery or multiple ligament reconstruction. Once placed, autograft tissue undergoes a period of ischemic necrosis. Both autograft and allograft tissue subsequently undergo graft revascularization, which is believed to originate from synovial vessels (24). The revascularization phase is followed by a remodeling phase, during which time the tendon graft, with its straighter fibers, becomes more ligament-like, with greater fiber waviness and redundancy. However, no tendon graft has been demonstrated to have biomechanical properties similar to that of the ACL, even when studied as much as 3 years after reconstruction. The lack of restoration of the normal biomechanics of the knee may be one reason that ACL reconstruction has not been found to prevent or slow the premature onset of osteoarthritic changes after knee injuries. Multiple studies with 5-year or greater follow-up demonstrated increased radiographic changes consistent with osteoarthritis in patients with no treatment, primary repair, or surgical reconstruction of their ligaments (33–36). Whether these changes are the result of articular injury at the time of ligament rupture, or due to loss of the normal mechanics and proprioception of the ACL is unknown.

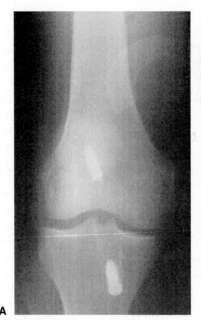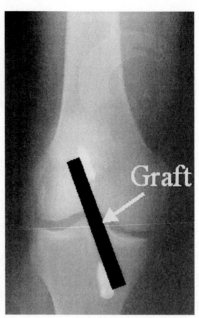

FIGURE 20.12 Postoperative anterior posterior (AP) radiograph after anterior cruciate ligament (ACL) reconstruction with interference screws. **A:** Screws and bony tunnels in femur and tibia visible. **B:** Black rectangle demonstrating course of ACL graft.

New research is focusing on the development of alternative therapies for ACL injuries, including reconstruction with allograft (37), reconstruction with silk and other proteins (38), and enhanced primary repair (39). It is hoped that one or more of these new innovations will lead to improved outcomes for the large patient population suffering each year from tears of the ACL.

MENISCUS

Physiologic Function

The knee menisci are C-shaped pieces of fibrocartilage that serve as shock absorbers in the knee. Their triangular cross section serves to increase the area of load transfer between the rounded end of the distal femur and the relatively flat tibial plateau, thereby lowering the peak stresses in the articular cartilage and subchondral bone (40). The menisci also contribute to knee joint stability, joint lubrication, and proprioception. The menisci are able to slide to the front and the back of the tibial plateau as the knee flexes and rotates, with the less constrained lateral menisci moving to a greater extent than the medial meniscus. The more limited range of motion of the medial meniscus makes it more vulnerable to tearing and injury.

Macroscopically, the meniscus has a fibrous, sponge-like structure, which is filled with a gel of proteoglycans. Initial loading of the meniscus results in deformation of the fibrous structure, and flow of the gel through the fibers. The resistance to flow of the gel provides the energy dissipation, with compressive loading of the meniscus as is seen during running or jumping. The menisci have a higher Young modulus near the anterior and posterior attachments (or horns), and a lower modulus in the midsection. The anterior and posterior horns also have the greatest degree of

parallel fibers, which suggests that the tensile properties of the meniscus are influenced by the collagen fiber arrangement.

The blood supply of the menisci originates from the medial, middle, and lateral geniculate arteries (41). These vessels give branches that supply the capillary bed of the perimeniscal tissue and penetrate the outer third of the meniscus (the "red zone"). The inner two thirds of the meniscus is avascular (the "white zone"). These zones are crucial in predicting the success of meniscal repairs. Repairs within the "red" (vascular) zone are more successful than repairs within the "white" (avascular) zone. The cells in the inner zone derive their nutritional supply from a combination of diffusion and fluid flow induced by joint loading and motion.

Normal Histology and Biochemistry

Two major types of cells have been identified in the meniscus. The first is a cell that is fusiform and fibroblast-like, and is found in the peripheral meniscus. In the inner, avascular zones of the meniscus, the cells are ovoid or polygonal. These cells are called fibrochondrocytes as they are able to synthesize fibrous extracellular proteins (including type I collagen) yet have the rounded appearance of chondrocytes. Both cell types have abundant endoplasmic reticulum and Golgi complexes, with minimal mitochondria, suggesting a dependence on anaerobic metabolism. Whether these two cell types are actually distinct or are the same cell type with modulation in phenotypic expression as a result of environmental influences is unclear.

Collagen comprises 60% to 70% of the dry weight of the menisci. More than 90% of the collagen is fibrillar type I, with types II, III, V, and VI comprising the remainder. The fibers have a complex three-dimensional arrangement, with predominantly circumferential fibers (like the staves of a barrel) and interweaving radial fibers which prevent splits between the circumferential fibers. Repairs of bucket-handle

Bucket-handle meniscal tear

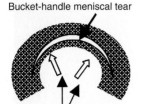
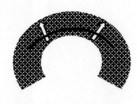

Bioresorbable arrows   Arrows transfixing tear

FIGURE 20.13 Schematic demonstrating the use of bioresorbable arrows to transfix a meniscal tear, providing a mechanically stable environment for meniscal healing.

tears (which are splits between the circumferential fibers) are performed by placement of sutures or bioresorbable arrows to replace the lost radial fibers (Fig. 20.13). Proteoglycans, such as aggrecan and chondroitin-6-sulfate, comprise approximately 1% of the dry weight of the menisci. The menisci also contain elastin, fibronectin, and other glycoproteins. As much as 70% of the wet weight of the meniscus is water, which is both structurally bound to collagen and freely associated with the interfibrillar proteoglycans.

Nerve fibers have been identified throughout the entire meniscus, with a greater concentration at the anterior and posterior horns (42). The fibers originate from the perimeniscal and synovial tissue of the knee, and radiate into the periphery of the meniscus. Many of the fibers are seen to accompany the vascular supply of the tissue. The proprioceptive function of the menisci has been inferred from the finding of three types of mechanoreceptors within the medial meniscus, including Ruffini endings, Golgi tendon organs, and Pacinian corpuscles. These nerve endings are found in the greatest concentration in the anterior and posterior horns of the menisci. They are thought to trigger a proprioceptive reflex and contribute to the functional stability of the knee.

The intervertebral discs of the spine are similar to the knee meniscus in that they are also viscoelastic and act as shock absorbers. The discs have an outer ring, the annulus fibrosus, which is constructed of layers of oriented type I collagen, and an inner section, the nucleus pulposus, which is a gelatinous material of proteoglycans and water. The cells populating the annulus fibrosus are fibroblast-like, whereas those in the nucleus pulposus are more chondrocytic in appearance and synthetic characteristics. The discs are attached to the vertebral bodies by small collagen fibers called *Sharpeys fibers*. Protrusions of the nucleus pulposus, through tears in the annulus fibrosus, are called a *herniated disc*. When this herniation compresses a spinal nerve root, sciatica (or pain which radiates down the leg) can result.

Growth and Development

The menisci form during the eighth week of embryonic development as condensations of mesenchymal cells. As the fetus develops, collagenous fibers appear and are oriented in a circumferential pattern. The increase in the organization and concentration of collagen fibers continues into early adulthood, then remains constant for the next 50 years before beginning to decrease. The proteoglycan content also shifts with age, with an increase in chondroitin-6-sulfate and a decrease in chondroitin-4-sulfate; the water content does not change. The percent of noncollagenous proteins also declines from 20% at birth to 10% in patients older than 50 years of age. Although the immature meniscus is vascular, only the outer tissue contains vessels after adolescence.

Biology of Meniscal Injury and Repair

Excision or repair of meniscal tears is one of the most commonly performed operations in orthopaedic surgery, with 45,000 cases performed each year in the United States alone (43). The decision whether to repair or partially excise a meniscal tear is based on the location of the tear (in the vascular or avascular zone). Tears within the vascularized periphery of the meniscus ("red–red" tears) have a functional blood supply. These vessels provide a fibrin clot that is revascularized and repopulated with cells capable of making fibrocartilage. Experimental studies in animal models have shown that complete radial tears (tears which begin at the inner edge of the mensicus and extend outwards to the synovial tissue) heal spontaneously with fibrovascular scar by 10 weeks after injury (44). Over time, it is thought that this scar tissue remodels to more closely resemble intact meniscal tissue, with an accompanying increase in tissue strength. In humans, tears in this region that are unstable (and cause mechanical symptoms such as locking or catching of the knee) are repaired with sutures or bioresorbable arrows to immobilize the torn area and allow healing to occur (Fig. 20.13). Many of these techniques are now performed arthroscopically with specially designed instrumentation. However, even with surgical repair, peripheral tears in ligamentously stable knees have reported clinical failure rates of 10% to 25% (45–58). These percentages are significantly higher than failure rates of healing for extra-articular tissues where nonunion rates are typically closer to 2% (59). In addition, recent work has suggested that reported clinical failure rates may underestimate the true wound healing failure rates for meniscus, and that even in asymptomatic patients (clinical successes), the meniscus may have failed to heal in as high as 45% of cases (60).

In addition, tears within the inner, avascular, zone ("white–white" tears), have been shown to be incapable of healing with simple repair, and are treated with removal of the torn tissue (partial meniscectomy). Tears at the junction of the vascular and avascular zones ("red–white" tears) can sometimes be repaired using additional techniques to provide vascularity to the torn region, such as creation of "vascular access" channels that extend to the meniscal periphery. These techniques have been developed in an attempt to extend the repairable region of the meniscus. This technique has been shown to be successful in experimental studies in dogs (44) and rabbits (61). Exogenous fibrin clot has also been used to enhance the healing of tears near the limits of meniscal vascularity ("red–white" tears) in a dog model (62).

Recent work has focused on the histology of the torn human meniscus and its possible effect on the success or failure of meniscal repair (63). The patient factors of age, time since injury, tear type and meniscus location all had significant effects on the histology of the torn meniscus. Patients older than 40 years had a decreased intrinsic and perimeniscal cellularity in the torn menisci than patients younger than 40 years. Time since injury was a significant predictor of the rate of DNA fragmentation in the midsubstance of the meniscus, decreasing histologic score of the meniscus tissue and increasing prevalence of Outerbridge II changes in the adjacent cartilage. Histologic score was related to tear type with poorer scores found in degenerative and radial tear types compared to control.

One of the main principles in meniscus surgery is preservation of as much of the meniscal tissue as possible. This is to preserve the contact area of the knee and to maintain the stresses across the articular cartilage as low as possible. Complete excision of the meniscus results in a decrease in the load transmission area of approximately 50%, and even partial meniscectomy can significantly decrease contact areas (and thereby increase peak pressures across the articular surfaces). Long-term results of total meniscectomy demonstrate an acceleration of osteoarthritis in the affected compartment. Although it has been suggested this acceleration is due to the initial trauma which caused the meniscal injury, animal studies in several species (including primates) have demonstrated the rapid progression of cartilage loss after total meniscectomy. However, there are cases where complete meniscal resection is the only option. Techniques of meniscal replacement with allograft or synthetic materials are being developed. Allograft menisci are typically cryopreserved and secured into position with peripheral sutures. With time, the allograft is thought to repopulate with cells from the surrounding synovial tissue, although recent work has shown that repopulation occurs mostly in the superficial regions of the allograft (64). Biopsies of previously implanted allograft menisci have provided histologic evidence of an immune response directed against the transplant. It is postulated that this immune reaction may affect the healing, incorporation, and revascularization of the graft.

The use of recombinant adenoviral vectors to transfer genes into meniscal fibrochondrocytes has been successfully demonstrated *in vitro* (65). Although further understanding of the genetic basis of the healing response is still in the preliminary stage, the potential exists for future transfer of genetic material that codes for cytokines, which enhance the healing response and accelerate the repair and regeneration of the meniscus after injury.

REFERENCES

1. Seibel MJ, Robins SP, Bilezikian JP. *Dynamics of bone and cartilage metabolism: principles and clinical applications.* San Diego: Academic Press, 1999.

2. Urist MR, Dawson E. Intertransverse process fusion with the aid of chemosterilized autolyzed antigen-extracted allogeneic (AAA) bone. *Clin Orthop* 1981;154:97–113.

3. Upton J, Glowacki J. Hand reconstruction with allograft demineralized bone: twenty-six implants in twelve patients. *J Hand Surg [Am]* 1992;17:704–713.

4. Rosenthal RK, Folkman J, Glowacki J. Demineralized bone implants for nonunion fractures, bone cysts, and fibrous lesions. *Clin Orthop* 1999;364:61–69.

5. Mueller S, Glowacki J. Construction and regulation of three-dimensional bone tissue *in vitro*. *Bone engineering*. Toronto: Em Squared, Inc. 2000; 473–487.

6. Glowacki J, LeBoff MS. Vitamin D insufficiency and fracture risk. *Curr Opin Endocrin Diabetes* 2004;11:353–358.

7. Miller PD, Bonnick SL, Rosen CJ, et al. Clinical utility of bone mass measurements in adults: consensus of an international panel. The Society for Clinical Densitometry. *Semin Arthritis Rheum* 1996;25:361–372.

8. Burr DB, Turner CH. Biomechanical measurements in age-related bone loss. In: Rosen CJ, Glowacki J, Bilezikian JP, eds. *The aging skeleton*, San Diego: Academic Press, 1999:301–311.

9. Smith CB, Smith DA. Relations between age, mineral density and mechanical properties of human femoral compacta. *Acta Orthop Scand* 1976;47:496–502.

10. Mori S, Harruff R, Ambrosius W, et al. Trabecular bone volume and microdamage accumulation in the femoral heads of women with and without femoral neck fractures. *Bone* 1997;21:521–526.

11. Bonar LC, Roufosse AH, Sabine WK, et al. X-ray diffraction studies of the crystallinity of bone mineral in newly synthesized and density fractionated bone. *Calcif Tissue Int* 1983;35:202–209.

12. LeGeros RZ. *Calcium phosphates in oral biology and medicine.* 'Monographs in Oral Science', Vol. 15. Basel: Karger, 1991.

13. LeBoff MS, Kohlmeier L, Hurwitz S, et al. Occult vitamin D deficiency in postmenopausal US women with acute hip fracture. *JAMA* 1999;281:1505–1511.

14. Heaney RP. The vitamin D requirement in health and disease. *J Steroid Biochem Mol Biol* 2005;97:13–19.

15. Winemaker MJ, Thornhill TS. Complications of joint replacement in the elderly. In: Rosen CJ, Glowacki J, Bilezikian JP, eds. *The aging skeleton*. San Diego: Academic Press, 1999:421–440.

16. Calvert GT, Wright RW. The use of arthroscopy in the athlete with knee osteoarthritis. *Clin Sports Med* 2005;24:133–152.

17. Cooper RR, Misol S. Tendon and ligament insertion. A light and electron microscopic study. *J Bone Joint Surg Am* 1970;52:1–20.

18. Cossu G, De Angelis L, Borello U, et al. Determination, diversification and multipotency of mammalian myogenic cells. *Int J Dev Biol* 2000;44:699–706.

19. McCall GE, Byrnes WC, Dickinson A, et al. Muscle fiber hypertrophy, hyperplasia, and capillary density in college men after resistance training. *J Appl Physiol* 1996;81:2004–2012.

20. Best TM, Hunter KD. Muscle injury and repair. *Phys Med Rehabil Clin N Am* 2000;11:251–266.

21. Lexell J. Human aging, muscle mass, and fiber type composition. *J Gerontol A Biol Sci Med Sci* 1995;50 Spec No:11–16.

22. Silva MJ, Thomopoulos S, Kusano N, et al. Early healing of flexor tendon insertion site injuries: Tunnel repair is mechanically and histologically inferior to surface repair in a canine model. *J Orthop Res* 2006;24:990–1000.

23. Krampera M, Pizzolo G, Aprili G, et al. 2006. Mesenchymal stem cells for bone, cartilage, tendon and skeletal muscle repair. *Bone* 2006;39:679–683.

24. Alm A, Stromberg B. Vascular anatomy of the patellar and cruciate ligaments. A microangiographic and histologic investigation in the dog. *Acta Chir Scand Suppl* 1974;445:25–35.

25. Halata Z, Wagner C, Baumann KI. Sensory nerve endings in the anterior cruciate ligament (Lig. cruciatum anterius) of sheep. *Anat Rec* 1999;254:13–21.

26. Johansson H, Sjolander P, Sojka P. Receptors in the knee joint ligaments and their role in the biomechanics of the joint. *Crit Rev Biomed Eng* 1991;18:341–368.

27. Ruano-Gil D, Nardi-Vilardaga J, Tejedo-Mateu A. Influence of extrinsic factors on the development of the articular system. *Acta Anat (Basel)* 1978;101:36–44.

28. Muller P, Dahners LE. A study of ligamentous growth. *Clin Orthop* 1988;229:274–277.

29. Dahners LE, Sykes KE, Muller PR. A study of the mechanisms influencing ligament growth. *Orthopedics* 1989;12:1569–1572.

30. DeHaven KE, Lintner DM. Athletic injuries: comparison by age, sport, and gender. *Am J Sports Med* 1986;14:218–224.

31. Frank C, Schachar N, Dittrich D. Natural history of healing in the repaired medial collateral ligament. *J Orthop Res* 1983;1:179–188.

32. Murray MM, Martin SD, Martin TL, et al. Histological changes in the human anterior cruciate ligament after rupture. *J Bone Joint Surg Am* 2000;82-A:1387–1397.

33. Maletius W, Messner K. Eighteen- to twenty-four-year follow-up after complete rupture of the anterior cruciate ligament. *Am J Sports Med* 1999;27:711–717.

34. Anderson AF, Snyder RB, Lipscomb AB Sr. Anterior cruciate ligament reconstruction using the semitendinosus and gracilis tendons augmented by the losee iliotibial band tenodesis. A long-term study. *Am J Sports Med* 1994;22:620–626.

35. Aglietti P, Buzzi R, D'Andria S, et al. Long-term study of anterior cruciate ligament reconstruction for chronic instability using the central one-third patellar tendon and a lateral extraarticular tenodesis. *Am J Sports Med* 1992;20:38–45.

36. Pattee GA, Fox JM, Del Pizzo W, et al. Four to ten year followup of unreconstructed anterior cruciate ligament tears. *Am J Sports Med* 1989;17:430–435.

37. Poehling GG, Curl WW, Lee CA, et al. Analysis of outcomes of anterior cruciate ligament repair with 5-year follow-up: allograft versus autograft. *Arthroscopy* 2005;21:774–785.

38. Laurencin CT, Freeman JW. Ligament tissue engineering: an evolutionary materials science approach. *Biomaterials* 2005;26:7530–7536.

39. Murray MM, Spindler KP, Devin C, et al. Use of a collagen-platelet rich plasma scaffold to stimulate healing of a central defect in the canine ACL. *J Orthop Res* 2006;24:820–830.

40. King D. The healing of semilunar cartilages. *J Bone Joint Surg* 1936;18:333–342.

41. Arnoczky SP, Warren SF. The microvasculature of the meniscus and its response to injury: An experimental study in the dog. *Am J Sports Med* 1983;11:131–141.

42. Day B, Mackenzie WG, Shim SS, et al. The vascular and nerve supply of the human meniscus. *Arthroscopy* 1985;1:58–62.

43. Praemer A, Furner S, Rice DP. *Musculoskeletal conditions in the United States.* Rosemont: American Academy of Orthopaedic Surgeons, 1999:170.

44. Arnoczky SP, Warren RF. The microvasculature of the meniscus and its response to injury. An experimental study in the dog. *Am J Sports Med* 1983;11:131–141.

45. Kotsovolos ES, Hantes ME, Mastrokalos DS, et al. Results of all-inside meniscal repair with the FasT-Fix meniscal repair system. *Arthroscopy* 2006;22:3–9.

46. Papachristou G, Efstathopoulos N, Plessas S, et al. Isolated meniscal repair in the avascular area. *Acta Orthop Belg* 2003;69:341–345.

47. Frosch KH, Fuchs M, Losch A, et al. Repair of meniscal tears with the absorbable Clearfix screw: results after 1–3 years. *Arch Orthop Trauma Surg* 2005;125:585–591.

48. Hantes ME, Kotsovolos ES, Mastrokalos DS, et al. Arthroscopic meniscal repair with an absorbable screw: results and surgical technique. *Knee Surg Sports Traumatol Arthrosc* 2005;13:273–279.

49. Tsai AM, McAllister DR, Chow S, et al. Results of meniscal repair using a bioabsorbable screw. *Arthroscopy* 2004;20:586–590.

50. Bohnsack M, Borner C, Schmolke S, et al. Clinical results of arthroscopic meniscal repair using biodegradable screws. *Knee Surg Sports Traumatol Arthrosc* 2003;11:379–383.

51. Ellermann A, Siebold R, Buelow JU, et al. Clinical evaluation of meniscus repair with a bioabsorbable arrow: a 2- to 3-year follow-up study. *Knee Surg Sports Traumatol Arthrosc* 2002;10:289–293.

52. Gill SS, Diduch DR. Outcomes after meniscal repair using the meniscus arrow in knees undergoing concurrent anterior cruciate ligament reconstruction. *Arthroscopy* 2002;18:569–577.

53. Marsolais GS, Dvorak G, Conzemius MG. Effects of postoperative rehabilitation on limb function after cranial cruciate ligament repair in dogs. *J Am Vet Med Assoc* 2002;220:1325–1330.

54. Petsche TS, Selesnick H, Rochman A. Arthroscopic meniscus repair with bioabsorbable arrows. *Arthroscopy* 2002;18:246–253.

55. Spindler KP, McCarty EC, Warren TA, et al. Prospective comparison of arthroscopic medial meniscal repair technique: inside-out suture versus entirely arthroscopic arrows. *Am J Sports Med* 2003;31:929–934.

56. Rockborn P, Messner K. Long-term results of meniscus repair and meniscectomy: a 13-year functional and radiographic follow-up study. *Knee Surg Sports Traumatol Arthrosc* 2000;8:2–10.

57. Johnson MJ, Lucas GL, Dusek JK, et al. Isolated arthroscopic meniscal repair: a long-term outcome study (more than 10 years). *Am J Sports Med* 1999;27:44–49.

58. Eggli S, Wegmuller H, Kosina J, et al. Long-term results of arthroscopic meniscal repair. An analysis of isolated tears. *Am J Sports Med* 1995;23:715–720.

59. Larsen LB, Madsen JE, Hoiness PR, et al. Should insertion of intramedullary nails for tibial fractures be with or without reaming? A prospective, randomized study with 3.8 years' follow-up. *J Orthop Trauma* 2004;18:144–149.

60. van Trommel MF, Simonian PT, Potter HG, et al. Different regional healing rates with the outside-in technique for meniscal repair. *Am J Sports Med* 1998;26:446–452.

61. Veth RP, den Heeten GJ, Jansen HW, et al. Repair of the meniscus. An experimental investigation in rabbits. *Clin Orthop Relat Res* 1983;175:258–262.

62. Arnoczky SP, Warren RF, Spivak JM. Meniscal repair using an exogenous fibrin clot. An experimental study in dogs. *J Bone Joint Surg Am* 1988;70:1209–1217.

63. Mesiha M, Zurakowski D, Nielson J, et al. Pathology of the torn human meniscus. *Am J Sports Med* 2007;35(1):103–112.

64. Rodeo SA, Seneviratne A, Suzuki K, et al. Histological analysis of human meniscal allografts. A preliminary report. *J Bone Joint Surg Am* 2000;82-A:1071–1082.

65. Goto H, Shuler FD, Niyibizi C, et al. Gene therapy for meniscal injury: enhanced synthesis of proteoglycan and collagen by meniscal cells transduced with a TGFbeta(1)gene. *Osteoarthr Cartil* 2000;8:266–271.

CHAPTER 21

Basic Neuroscience

Roger D. Smith, Robert L. Tiel, and Robert J. Johnson, Jr.

An understanding of basic principles of neuroscience will benefit all those practicing surgery, as the nervous system integrates so many bodily functions and organ systems. This chapter will outline fundamental aspects of neuroanatomy, neurophysiology, and neuropathology, and will introduce some of the newer discoveries in the neurosciences that may prove applicable to a wide variety of surgical disciplines.

CELLULAR ANATOMY AND PHYSIOLOGY

The central nervous system (CNS) contains more than 30 billion cells. These are divided morphologically and functionally into three major groups: the neurons, the neuroglial cells, and the microglia that represent the reticuloendothelial system in the brain and spinal cord. The neurons and the glia maintain a complex relation that allows for the orderly passage of information in the nervous system.

Cellular Morphology

The Neuron
The neuron is the functional unit of the nervous system. Depolarization of the neuronal membrane propagates an electrochemical impulse that is transferred to other neurons through specialized junctions called *synapses*. In this way, information is continually processed in the nervous system. The neuron is divided into the cell body or soma and the cell processes—the axon and the dendrites. The morphology of these processes allows classification of neurons into unipolar, bipolar, and multipolar neurons. Unipolar neurons have a single process arising from the soma that gives rise to both the dendrite and the axon. The dorsal root ganglion cell, which brings somatic sensation to the CNS, is the prototype of this neuronal type. Bipolar neurons with a single dendrite and an axon are found in special sensory systems such as the retina and vestibule. By far the largest group is the multipolar type. Elaboration of the dendritic tree allows for a greatly increased surface area for synaptic contact. A single Purkinje cell in the cerebellum may receive 150,000 synapses, allowing for extremely fine modulation of cell activity.

The axon is the neuronal process along which the electrochemical impulse is propagated to communicate with subsequent neurons. The axon may be long, extending 3 m from the brain or spinal cord, yet arising from a 20-μ to 40-μ soma. This is a complex structure containing microtubules and filaments that transport the axoplasm, which contains neurotransmitters and other chemicals, over great distances to and from the soma. The origin of the axon, the axon hillock, is the most electrically excitable portion of the neuron and generally gives rise to the nerve action potential (NAP).

The Glia
Glial cells include astrocytes, oligodendrocytes, ependymal cells, and microglia. Astrocytes are found throughout the CNS. They are characterized by extensive processes that completely encase the neurons, isolating them from each other, except at synapses, and separating the neuron from direct contact with the capillary by special astrocytic foot processes. Although the astrocytes are polarized to −90 mV internally, they are not electrically excitable and cannot propagate an action potential. Astrocytes may play a role in regulating the extracellular ionic environment, especially potassium that is liberated during neuronal depolarization. Astrocytes respond to ischemia and injury, initially with swelling, and subsequently with proliferation to form scarring in the brain. They give rise to most of the primary brain tumors.

Oligodendrocytes are smaller than astrocytes and are more concentrated in white matter. These cells form the myelin that electrically insulates the axons and greatly increases the rate of nerve impulse propagation. In the peripheral nervous system (PNS), this function is carried out by the Schwann cell. In both cases, the myelin is formed by concentric layers of the lipid-rich cell membrane of the glial cell (Fig. 21.1). There are varying degrees of myelination of different axons and tracts. Axonal conduction velocities are directly proportional to the degree of myelination. Unmyelinated nerve fibers indent the oligodendrocyte or Schwann cell but are not surrounded by the concentric lamellae of myelin.

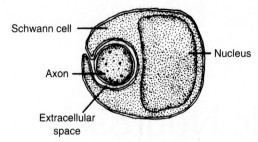

FIGURE 21.1 Concentric layers of the Schwann cell membrane encase a peripheral nerve axon as myelin. (From Morrell P. Myelin. In: Adelman G, ed. *Encyclopedia of neuroscience*, Vol. 2. Boston: Birkhauser, 1987:729, with permission.)

Ependymal cells line the cerebral ventricles; over the vascular choroid plexus they are specialized so that they can produce cerebrospinal fluid (CSF). The ependyma is a single layer of cuboidal epithelial cells that exhibits secretory and absorptive functions and provides a cellular layer between the CSF in the ventricle and the extracellular space of the brain. Ependymal cells lining the ventricle are relatively permeable to solutes, although those of the choroidal epithelium show tight junctions controlling the passage of solutes from the capillaries of the choroid plexus into the CSF.

Microglia represent the reticuloendothelial cells of the CNS and are derived from outside the brain and spinal cord. Microglial proliferation occurs in response to infectious processes, although blood-derived lymphocytes and neutrophils represent a major part of an inflammatory response in the CNS. Whether microglial cells are truly resident in the brain tissue or derived only from blood elements is still unclear.

Other Cell Types

The capillaries of the CNS are characterized by a special penta laminar interdigitation referred to as a *tight junction*. This inhibits the passage of molecules from the bloodstream into the CNS, forming a blood–brain barrier (BBB).

The meninges are mesenchymal tissues that completely envelop the brain and spinal cord. The dura mater is approximated to the skull but is more separated in the spine. It functions as a bone-forming tissue in the skull during development and provides a relatively competent barrier to encroachment of infection or tumor into the nervous system. The thin trabeculated arachnoid contains the CSF. It is approximated loosely to the spinal cord and forms cisterns at the base of the brain. Over the brain surface there is closer approximation to the pia mater, which is approximated tightly to the surface of the brain and spinal cord. The leptomeninges (the arachnoid and the pia) follow the blood vessels into the brain parenchyma for some distance as the Virchow-Robin spaces.

Synapses and Receptors

Contact between neurons occurs at a synapse, a specialized structure composed of a presynaptic axonal terminal bouton that contains neurotransmitter and a postsynaptic membrane-bound protein designated a receptor. The discovery of new neurotransmitters and the elucidation of the complex role of receptors has been one of the most exciting developments in current neuroscience.

As the action potential arrives at the axon terminal, the presynaptic membrane is depolarized, opening protein channels in the membrane that are permeable to calcium. Neurotransmitter molecules are packaged into discrete quanta by membranes. The entry of calcium into the cytoplasm causes these membranes to fuse with the presynaptic membrane and release the neurotransmitter into the synaptic cleft. There is a 200-Å distance from the presynaptic membrane to the receptor membrane. Neurotransmitter molecules migrate to the receptor proteins and bind with them, causing conformational changes that increase or decrease the permeability of the adjacent membrane channels to various ions, including potassium, sodium, and chloride. This may depolarize or hyperpolarize the postsynaptic membrane, thereby facilitating or inhibiting the propagation of further nerve impulses. Muscle cells have similar postsynaptic receptors in a specialized area of the membrane called the *motor endplate*. NAPs are translated into muscle contraction across these synapses.

The action of the neurotransmitter at the synapses must be reversed quickly to allow a new signal to arrive. Synapses may have enzymes that destroy the neurotransmitter, or reuptake of the neurotransmitter into the axon may occur for reuse. The pharmacologic effect of many agents are to (i) mimic the neurotransmitter substance, (ii) block its action at the receptor or prevent its release from the presynaptic membrane, (iii) prevent its enzymatic degradation or prevent its reuptake.

Different receptors may respond to a given neurotransmitter with different physiologic consequences. For most of the better-evaluated neurotransmitters, such as the vasoactive amines and acetylcholine (Ach), several subsets of receptors have been identified. Therefore, a neurotransmitter may be inhibitory at a given synapse but excitatory at another.

A second and extremely important concept in the function of receptors is that, rather than changing ion conductance as the primary response to the neurotransmitter–receptor interaction, biologic information may be conveyed by the release of so-called second messengers by the cell membrane. Second messengers, such as cyclic adenosine monophosphate (cAMP), phosphoinositides, and calcium, may catalyze the phosphorylation of proteins concerned with cellular metabolic processes, the increase (upregulation) or decrease (downregulation) of other membrane receptors, or even gene expression of factors such as cell growth or differentiation. Intermediate between a receptor and a second messenger are membrane-associated proteins such as the G protein that, when activated by the neurotransmitter–receptor complex, binds guanosine 5'-triphosphate (GTP) and protein kinase C, which catalyzes phosphorylation of the phosphoinositide system. As with ion permeability changes, the same neurotransmitter may be excitatory or inhibitory to the associated membrane protein catalyzing the formation of the second messenger. For example, norepinephrine stimulates adenyl cyclase to form cAMP at β-adrenergic receptors, inhibits the same enzyme at α_2-receptors, and activates phospholipase C at α_1-adrenergic receptors. A more thorough understanding of these mechanisms should open new avenues to pharmacologic therapy.

Nerve Action Potential

Selective permeability of the neuronal membrane to different ion species creates an electrical potential across the membrane that is negative on the inside of the membrane and positive on the outside. Proteins in the cell membrane act as channels to the passage of ions across the membrane, and there are specific channels for potassium, sodium, chloride, and calcium. The membrane is much more permeable to potassium than to sodium. This allows a concentration gradient to be maintained for sodium and potassium across the cell membrane. The presence of negatively charged protein molecules within the cytoplasm that cannot cross the membrane creates an opposing force to the migration of potassium ions out of the cell. Although the concentration gradients of all ionic species contribute to the resting potential of the cell membrane, the equilibrium potential of potassium contributes most to this potential. Therefore, the resting potential [electromotive force (EMF), in mV] is approximated by the Nernst equation for potassium concentration inside and outside the neuron: EMF = $-61 \times$ log concentration K$^+$ in/concentration K$^+$ out. This varies from -50 to -90 mV, depending on the type of neuron. A more complete mathematical description, the Goldman equation, accounts for the concentrations of all relevant ions (1).

The nerve impulse is generated by depolarization of the membrane that is then propagated along the axon to the synapse. Depolarization of sensory receptors or nerve endings occurs through a variety of sensory stimuli—mechanical, temperature, light, chemical, etc. Depolarization within the

nervous system is caused by the binding of neurotransmitters to receptors across synapses. The depolarization of hundreds or thousands of synapses on dendrites, soma, and even the axon is summated over time until a threshold depolarizing potential is reached in the region of the axon hillock. This is generally approximately -45 mV. When threshold is reached, a self-propagating depolarization along the axon occurs—the so-called all-or-none response—which conveys the action potential along the entire length of the axon to the synapse. Although the propagation of an impulse may occur in either direction along a cell membrane, a period of refractivity after depolarization directs propagation toward the synapse.

Depolarization occurs when molecular changes in the postsynaptic membrane allow opening of the previously gated sodium channels. Increased permeability to sodium allows an influx of sodium ions along the concentration gradient toward its equilibrium potential of $+40$ mV. The sodium channel gate quickly closes to allow the return of negativity to the inside of the membrane. An increased permeability to potassium creates a temporary period of relative refractoriness to depolarization that gradually returns toward baseline. This series of molecular exchanges is recorded as an action potential. The action potential depolarizes the adjacent membrane to propagate the impulse along the axon. Myelinated nerve fibers are insulated, except at small regular bare spots called the *nodes of Ranvier*, where sodium channels are clustered. Depolarization jumps from one node to the next, markedly accelerating the process and increasing axonal conduction velocity. This is termed *saltatory conduction* (Fig. 21.2). Sodium accumulated within the axon during depolarization is expelled by an energy-consuming protein-exchange transfer mechanism called the *sodium–potassium pump*.

A neurotransmitter may depolarize or hyperpolarize the postsynaptic membrane. These voltage changes are called *excitatory postsynaptic potentials* (EPSPs) and *inhibitory postsynaptic potentials* (IPSPs), respectively. Hyperpolarization

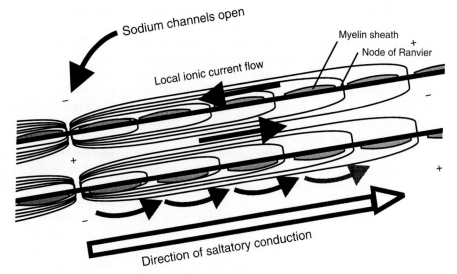

FIGURE 21.2 Saltatory conduction. Currents generated at node of Ranvier are propagated to the next node, bypassing the insulated portion of the axon and thereby accelerating nerve conduction velocity. Note that the current generated can trigger four to five nodes ahead of the active site.

may result from increased conductance of potassium ion or chloride ion that will increase the interior negativity of the cell. Depolarization is primarily a function of sodium conductance. Increasing or decreasing the number of various receptors at the synapse is a mechanism to increase or decrease its sensitivity to incoming neural connections and may form the basis for such functions as learning and accommodation.

NEUROANATOMY

The nervous system is classically divided into the CNS, the PNS, and the autonomic nervous system (ANS). The CNS is enclosed within the bone of the skull and spine and covered by the meninges: the dura mater, arachnoid, and pia. The PNS and ANS are also ensheathed in investing layers of mesenchymal tissue.

Gross Anatomy of the Central Nervous System

The Skull, Spine, and Meninges

The skull is formed of multiple plates that fuse after birth through sutures to form the calvarium and the skull base. The paired frontal, parietal, and temporal bones and the occipital bone are membranous bones that form the calvarium. Portions of the frontal bones, temporal bones, occipital bone, and the sphenoid bone are endochondral bone formed from cartilage and comprise the skull base. Small areas of the ethmoid and zygomatic bones are also in contact with the dura. Three fossae are recognized in the skull base. The anterior fossa is formed by the orbital roofs, cribriform plate, and planum sphenoidale. The middle fossa is formed by the greater wing of the sphenoid and petrous portion of the temporal bone on each side, and the posterior fossa by the clivus of the sphenoid and occipital bones and the petrous portions of the temporal bones. The tentorium cerebelli, a dural fold extending from the clinoid processes of the sella turcica and the petrous ridges of the temporal bones to the occipital bone, separates the posterior fossa or infratentorial compartment from the supratentorial compartment. The tentorial hiatus, or notch, separates the two sides of the middle fossa and allows passage of the brainstem from the supra- to the infratentorial compartment. A sickle-shaped fold of dura, the falx cerebri, extends from the crista galli of the cribriform plate to the tentorium and separates the cerebral hemispheres. The opening at the base of the clivus and occipital bone, the foramen magnum, allows the brainstem to pass through to the spinal cord. Displacements or herniations of brain tissue through these dural and bony apertures are characteristic of mass brain lesions and have important physiologic consequences.

The spine is composed of segmental vertebrae and includes 7 cervical vertebrae, 12 thoracic (rib-bearing) vertebrae, 5 lumbar vertebrae, a sacrum of 5 fused sacral vertebrae, and a coccyx of 2 to 5 vertebrae. A common variation is attachment of the fifth lumbar vertebra to the sacrum (sacralization) or nonattachment of the first sacral vertebra to the sacrum (lumbarilization). The first cervical vertebra (atlas) forms a ring to support the cranium and allow rotation. The second cervical vertebra (axis) incorporates the body of C1 as the odontoid process, or dens, through the ring of the atlas. The remainder of the cervical, thoracic, and lumbar vertebrae are composed of a body anteriorly and a dorsal arch attached to the body by pedicles and formed by the facet joints (articulating processes), laminae, and spinous processes. The sacral bones are fused into a single triangular-shaped bone but maintain foramina for the exit of sacral nerve roots. Anterior and posterior longitudinal ligaments run the length of the spine, and the intersegmental ligamenta flavum between the lamina and interspinous ligaments between the spinous processes add additional strength to the spinal column. Cartilaginous intervertebral discs from C2 to L5 allow flexibility to the spine and dissipate forces applied to the spinal column. The disc is composed of a fibrous annulus and a softer central nucleus pulposus. Degeneration of the nucleus pulposus through aging, trauma, and weakening of the annulus may lead to disc herniation into the spinal canal, a substantial cause of neurologic morbidity.

With growth of the individual prenatally through adolescence, a relative ascendancy of the spinal cord occurs in relation to the bony spine. Therefore, in adulthood, the tip of the spinal cord, the conus medullaris, ends at about the L1-2 disc space. The nerve roots continue caudally as the cauda equina and exit at their appropriate segmental bony level. The pia arachnoid continues to about S2 as the filum terminale, and the dura attaches to the coccyx. A lesion at the C7 vertebra may be associated with a T1 spinal cord lesion, and a lesion at the T11 vertebra may be associated with a L3 lesion. As the C1 nerve root exits above the atlas, there are eight cervical spinal segments but only seven cervical vertebrae. Below C8, the nerve roots exit below the pedicles of the corresponding vertebra. Thickened arachnoid bands, the dentate or denticulate ligaments, attach the spinal cord to the dura at each segmental level. These ligaments serve as a landmark for the midpoint of the spinal cord in the anterior-posterior direction.

The Brain

The brain weighs approximately 1,400 to 1,600 g in the adult (~2% of body weight). It can be divided grossly into the cerebral hemispheres, the brainstem-diencephalon, midbrain (mesencephalon), pons, medulla, and the cerebellum. The cerebral hemispheres occupy the supratentorial compartment; the brainstem passes through the tentorial notch and lies behind the clivus as it courses down to the foramen magnum, where it becomes spinal cord. The cerebellum occupies the infratentorial compartment behind and lateral to the brainstem. The cerebellum and brainstem account for approximately 15% to 20% of the brain's mass.

The cerebral hemispheres are essentially symmetrical, with their surfaces characterized by convolutions (gyri) and fissures (sulci). The neuronal cell bodies are on the

(Brain A. The broken white lines mark the boundaries between the lobes)

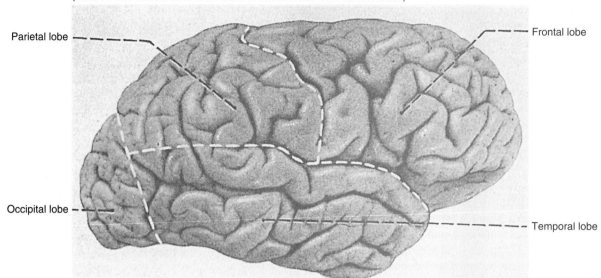

Parietal lobe

Frontal lobe

Occipital lobe

Temporal lobe

FIGURE 21.3 Lobes of the right hemisphere. (From Zuckerman S. *A new system of anatomy.* London: Oxford University Press, 1961:498, with permission.)

surface of the brain (gray matter), and the myelinated axons project internally (white matter). Deep gray nuclei are found subcortically. The cerebral hemispheres are connected by broad white matter tracts—the corpus callosum, and anterior, posterior, and hippocampal commissures. The cerebral hemispheres are divided into four lobes: frontal, temporal, parietal, and occipital, although these do not show distinct anatomic boundaries (Fig. 21.3). The frontal lobe is the portion of the cerebral hemisphere that is anterior to the central sulcus of Rolando and superior and medial to the sylvian fissure. The basal ganglia, nucleus basalis, and insula of Reil are contained within the frontal lobe. The cortex of the frontal lobe is subdivided further into the precentral gyrus (primary motor cortex) just anterior to the central sulcus and premotor cortex, including the area for conjugate eye movements just anterior to this. More frontally are the transversely oriented superior, middle, and inferior frontal gyri. The inferior gyrus, usually on the left side, contains the primary motor speech area. The orbital surface of the frontal lobe is divided by the olfactory sulcus into the gyrus rectus medially and the orbital gyri laterally. Deep to the sylvian fissure is the insular cortex covering the basal ganglia. The edges of cortex around the sylvian fissure are called *opercula*.

The temporal lobe lies inferior to the sylvian fissure. It is separated from the parietal lobe by a line running from the posterior edge of the sylvian fissure inferiorly to the preoccipital notch and on its inferomedial surface by a line from the splenium of the corpus callosum to the preoccipital notch. The mesial gyri, the uncus, contain the hippocampus. Superior, middle, and inferior temporal gyri are recognized on the surface of the temporal lobe. The transverse gyri of Heschl are contained in the temporal opercula and represent the primary auditory cortex.

The parietal lobe extends from just behind the central sulcus, which separates it from the frontal lobe, to the parieto-occipital sulcus on the mesial cerebral hemisphere, separating it from the occipital lobe. A line from the parieto-occipital sulcus to the posterior sylvian fissure to the preoccipital notch divides the parietal lobe from the temporal and occipital lobes on the surface of the hemisphere. The postcentral gyrus immediately behind the central sulcus is the primary sensory cortex. A mixture of sensory and motor functions exist in the pre- and postcentral gyri; these are sometimes termed the *sensorimotor cortex*. More posteriorly, the parietal lobe is divided into superior and inferior parietal lobules by the interparietal sulcus. The inferior parietal lobule contains the supramarginal and angular gyri, which on the left side are usually concerned with speech reception, reading, writing, and calculation. Body organization and spatial relations are important right-sided parietal lobe functions. The occipital lobe is that cortex posterior to the parietal and occipital lobes. The cortex faces primarily mesially. The deep horizontal calcarine fissure separates the cuneate gyrus superiorly from the lingual gyrus inferiorly. These form the primary visual cortex, with the central (macular) visual cortex close to the occipital pole.

On the mesial surface of the cerebral hemispheres, the hippocampus, the fornix, and the cingulate gyrus above the corpus callosum run in close proximity to the ventricular system. These, in association with the anterior subcallosal area, the amygdala of the temporal lobe, and parts of the diencephalon, subserve arousal and emotion and are sometimes termed the *limbic lobe*.

White matter tracts are divided into (i) association fibers that connect cortical neurons within the same hemisphere, (ii) commissural fibers that connect corresponding areas of cortex in opposite hemispheres, (iii) and projection fibers that run from the cerebral hemispheres to the brainstem and spinal cord. Important association fiber bundles include the arcuate fasciculus from the temporal to the frontal lobe and the optic radiations from the thalamus to the occipital cortex. The main portions of the two cerebral hemispheres are connected through the corpus callosum, the primary cerebral commissure. The anterior commissure connects the temporal lobes, and the hippocampal commissure connects the hippocampal cortex bilaterally. The posterior commissure is in the diencephalon and connects pretectal nuclei concerned with eye movements. Projection fibers include the long tracts, such as the corticospinal and extrapyramidal pathways. The white matter of the cerebral hemisphere is called the *centrum semiovale* above the basal ganglia and the internal capsule as it passes through the basal ganglia and thalamus to the brainstem.

The deep nuclei of the cerebral hemispheres include the basal ganglia—caudate, putamen, and globus pallidus—that are believed to modulate motor function but also seem to be concerned with behavior, affect, and ideation. Functionally, these are related closely to the thalamus and brainstem nuclei. The nucleus basalis of Meynert is located caudal to the basal ganglia and may play a role in cognitive function.

The diencephalon includes the paired thalami, the hypothalamus, the pineal gland, the habenular nuclei, and the subthalamus. Except for olfaction, all sensory information coming into the cerebral hemispheres is relayed through the thalamus. The thalamus maintains reciprocal connections with all areas of cerebral cortex and has been considered the key to understanding brain function. The thalami abut the ventricular system, forming the floor of the lateral ventricles and the medial walls of the third ventricle. The hypothalamus sits beneath the third ventricle and is continuous with the pituitary stalk. It has extensive hormonal and visceral functions. The pineal gland is in the roof of the third ventricle, and the subthalamus is continuous with the mesencephalon. The subthalamic area is functionally related to the basal ganglia and is sometimes included in this term.

The mesencephalon (midbrain) is characterized by the quadrigeminal plate (the superior and inferior colliculi) dorsally and the cerebral peduncles (the corticospinal and corticopontine tracts) ventrally. The cerebral aqueduct (of Sylvius) in the mesencephalic tegmentum connects the third and fourth ventricles. The tegmentum contains the nuclei of cranial nerves (CNs) III and IV; the red nuclei; the substantia nigra; the ascending long tracts, including the decussation of the superior cerebellar peduncles; and the reticular formation. CNs III and IV exit from the mesencephalon ventrally and dorsally, respectively.

A pontomedullary sulcus ventrally divides the mesencephalon from the pons. The cerebral peduncles pass through the base of the pons and are dispersed into bundles of nerve fibers. Corticospinal and corticobulbar fibers continue caudally. Corticopontine fibers synapse with pontine nuclei and project to the cerebellum as the middle cerebellar peduncles. The tegmentum of the pons contains the nuclei of CN V with its associated spinal nucleus and tract, the nuclei of

CNs VI and VII, the long ascending tracts, and the reticular formation. CN V exits the pons, and CN VI exits the pontomedullary sulcus at the caudal end of the pons. CN VII exits laterally at the pontomedullary sulcus. The fourth ventricle separates the pons from the cerebellum.

The medulla is separated from the pons by the pontomedullary sulcus. The corticospinal tracts form the pyramids on the base of the medulla, and these decussate at this level before entering the spinal cord. The medullary tegmentum contains the nuclei for CNs VIII through XII, the decussation of the posterior columns, the olivary nuclei, the long ascending tracts, and the reticular formation. The fourth ventricle ends dorsal to the medulla at the obex through a midline opening, the foramen of Magendie. The lateral openings, the foramina of Luschka, are located above the pontomedullary sulci (Fig. 21.4).

The cerebellum lies dorsal to the brainstem and is attached to it through three peduncles: the superior (brachium conjunctivum) to the mesencephalon; the middle (brachium pontis) to the pons; and the inferior (restiform body) to the medulla. The cerebellum is composed of a midline vermis and two hemispheres. Anatomically, there are multiple lobes of the cerebellum based on connections between the hemispheres and the vermis. Functionally, the cerebellum may be divided into the flocculonodular lobe (archicerebellum), concerned with vestibular function; the anterior lobe (paleocerebellum), concerned with spinal reflexes; and the posterior lobe (neocerebellum), concerned with fine-motor activity. The cerebellum functions to coordinate motor activity at an unconscious level and to set postural muscles to allow coordinated voluntary movements. The output of the cerebellum is through the superior cerebellar peduncles to the thalamus and brainstem nuclei.

The Spinal Cord

The spinal cord runs from the cervicomedullary junction to the inferior body of the L1 vertebra. It is a segmental structure composed of central gray matter surrounded by ascending and descending white matter tracts. Small rootlets are given off ventrally and dorsally, and these combine at each segmental level to give a ventral motor root and a dorsal sensory root that exit the spine. The cell bodies of the dorsal root are in the dorsal root ganglion outside the spinal cord, whereas those of the motor root are in the ventral column of gray matter cells. Autonomic fibers also contribute to the ventral root. Sensory fibers may be contained in the ventral root, a location that thereby explains the failure of dorsal rhizotomy in relieving pain.

The spinal cord diameter gradually reduces from rostral to caudal as motor tracts synapse and sensory input is added. Cervical and lumbar enlargements of the spinal cord signify neural output to the extremities. Spinal cord tracts are divided into three columns: (i) the posterior columns, conveying vibration, touch, and joint position; (ii) the lateral columns, containing the corticospinal (motor) and lateral spinothalamic (pain and temperature) tracts; and (iii) the

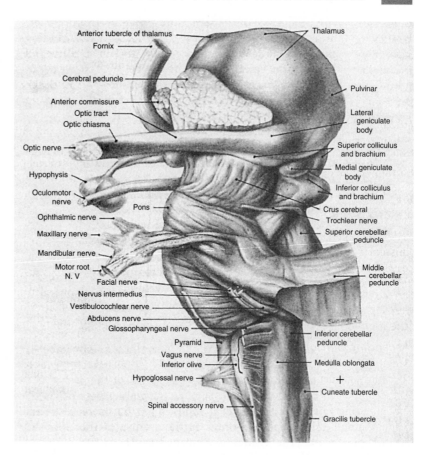

FIGURE 21.4 Drawing of the brainstem with the cerebral and cerebellar peduncles cut. (From Carpenter MB, Sutin J, eds. *Human neuroanatomy*, 8th ed. Baltimore: Williams & Wilkins, 1983:49, with permission.)

anterior columns, conveying touch sensation. Many other ascending and descending tracts share these three columns (Fig. 21.5).

Intrinsic Architecture of the Central Nervous System

Reflex Arcs

The nervous system operates through a hierarchy of reflexes from the most basic monosynaptic stretch reflex through segmental, suprasegmental, autonomic, on up to complex behavioral reflexes. The term *reflex* implies a stereotyped and unconscious or involuntary response to a sensory input. The prototype monosynaptic stretch reflex involves a specialized sensory receptor in the muscle, the muscle spindle, which, when activated by lengthening, transmits an afferent impulse over a large myelinated (Ia) fiber to an excitatory synapse on the α-motor neuron supplying that muscle. This results in contraction of the skeletal muscle

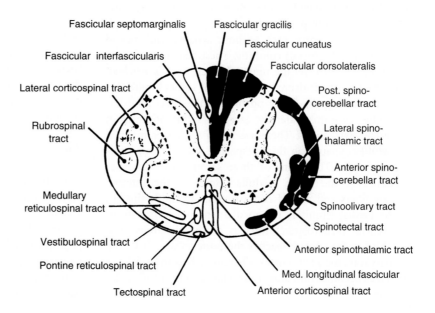

FIGURE 21.5 Diagram of the ascending and descending tracts of the spinal cord. (From Carpenter MB, Sutin J, eds. *Human neuroanatomy*, 8th ed. Baltimore: Williams & Willkins, 1983:302, with permission.)

fiber to restore the length of the muscle spindle. The resting length or tension in the muscle spindle is influenced by a τ-motor neuron that in turn receives input from segmental and suprasegmental interneurons. The same afferent fiber that excites the α-motor neuron of the stretched muscle inhibits the motor neurons of antagonistic muscles through interposed inhibitory neurons.

Increasingly complex responses, such as withdrawal of a limb in response to pain, setting of proximal muscles to allow fine movements of distal muscles, locomotion, visceral responses, and so forth, can be considered extensions of this concept, with progressively larger numbers of excitatory and inhibitory interneurons involved in the reflex. Many reflexes are genetically coded into the architecture of the nervous system, although others can be learned, modified, and forgotten over the lifetime of an individual. Understanding how responses are elicited and how they can be modified by experience is a key goal of neurosciences.

Ascending Sensory Systems

Sensation below the head is conveyed into the spinal cord through neurons located in the dorsal root ganglia. These unipolar neurons carry information received from specialized nerve endings sensitive to a variety of external stimuli into the dorsal horn of the central gray matter of the spinal cord. The central gray matter has been subdivided into ten laminae (I–X) by Rexed (2) based on cell type and functional considerations. Laminae I to VII are in the dorsal horn and intermediate area, laminae VIII to X in the ventral horn, and lamina X in the area of the central canal. A functional division of sensory information occurs at a spinal cord level, with pathways for conscious position sense, pain and temperature, touch, and unconscious position sense ascending in discrete nerve bundle tracts.

Posterior Columns

The large myelinated nerve fibers subserving pressure, vibration, and joint position (proprioception) pass through the dorsal root entry zone without synapse and ascend as the posterior (dorsal) columns. These remain ipsilateral in the spinal cord. As the upper thoracic area is reached, two ipsilateral fasciculi are recognized: the fasciculus gracilis, medially serving the lower portion of the body, and the fasciculus cuneatus, laterally carrying information from the upper extremities. These ascend to the lower medulla where they synapse on their respective nuclei, the gracilis and cuneatus. The axons of these second-order neurons decussate at the lower medullary level as the internal arcuate fibers and ascend contralaterally in the brainstem as the medial lemnisci. The medial lemnisci terminate in the ventral posterolateral nucleus of the thalamus, and the third-order neuron reaches the postcentral gyrus—the primary somatosensory cortex. Therefore, these modalities of sensation become conscious at the synapse of the third-order neuron.

Pain Pathways
Lateral Spinothalamic Tract

Smaller nerve fibers that carry the sensations of pain and temperature (nociception) enter the spinal cord through the dorsal root and ascend or descend one or two segments as Lissauer tract. These synapse primarily on neurons in laminae I, II, and V. Lamina II, the substantia gelatinosa, is composed primarily of interneurons, whereas laminae I and V are the primary projection neurons for ascending pain pathways. The nociceptive neurotransmitter, substance P, is found in high concentration in these gray matter laminae. A complex interaction between excitatory and inhibitory interneurons in the substantia gelatinosa has been suggested to modulate pain pathway transmission (gate theory), but the exact mechanisms of this remain unclear.

The projection axons from laminae I and V cross just in front of the central canal of the spinal cord as the anterior commissure and ascend contralaterally in the anterior portion of the lateral column as the lateral spinothalamic tract. Because destruction of this tract does not completely abolish pain sensation contralaterally, other ascending pathways have been postulated. The lateral spinothalamic tract ascends through the brainstem to reach the thalamus, but many of the fibers synapse with the brainstem reticular formation so that the number of fibers projecting directly to the thalamus is reduced considerably. The lateral portion of the spinothalamic tract projects to the ventral posterior thalamic nuclei and is concerned with more acute, localized pain. The medial portion projects to the medial and intralaminar thalamic nuclei, as do those fibers synapsing through the reticular formation. These may convey less localized, more chronic pain. Ventroposterior thalamic neurons project to the somatosensory cortex, although the medial and intralaminar nuclei have extensive connections with the limbic system and frontal lobes.

Although pain perception results from afferent transmission from pain-sensitive nerve endings, considerable modulation of pain pathways by other neuronal groups exist at both the spinal cord and the brainstem levels. Areas of the brainstem concerned with pain modulation include the periaqueductal gray matter, the hypothalamic periventricular gray matter, the dorsal pontine tegmentum, and the ventral medullary reticular formation. These pathways converge in the ventral medulla and travel in the spinal cord in the dorsal part of the lateral column to synapse on cells of laminae I, II, and V in the spinal gray matter dorsal horn. One system uses the amine neurotransmitters norepinephrine and serotonin from the pons and medulla, respectively, to inhibit spinal nociceptive neurons and to interconnect brainstem pain-modulating centers. Another system uses the endogenous opioid peptide neurotransmitters enkephalin, β-endorphin, and dynorphin. These peptides and their receptors are located in the periaqueductal gray matter, hypothalamus, ventral medulla, and dorsal horn of the spinal cord. The precise interconnections of these pain pathways remain to be elucidated.

Spinocerebellar Tracts

Information from muscle and joint stretch and pressure receptors, including muscle spindles and Golgi tendon organs, is conveyed through the spinal cord to the cerebellum by the spinocerebellar tracts. These transmit unconscious proprioception and are thought to function in coordinating fine-motor movements and setting postural and antagonistic muscles.

Afferent fibers from the dorsal root ganglion enter the spinal cord and may ascend or descend several segments in the posterior lamina VII (Clarke nucleus). The second-order neurons ascend on the dorsal margin of the lateral column as the posterior spinocerebellar tract. In the medulla, these join with the inferior cerebellar peduncle to terminate in the cerebellar vermis.

Neurons that give rise to the anterior spinocerebellar tract are localized less discretely in the spinal gray matter and are concentrated in the base of the dorsal and ventral horns. They receive afferents from ipsilateral and contralateral joint receptors in the lower extremities and pass with the superior cerebellar peduncle to the anterior lobe of the cerebellum. Inherited ataxias may selectively affect the spinocerebellar tracts and their connections.

Anterior Spinothalamic Tract

The sensation of light touch is conveyed through tactile receptors (Meissner corpuscles) to the dorsal root ganglion and into the dorsal horn, where synapses occur in laminae I, IV, and V. Second-order axons cross in the anterior commissure to the contralateral anterior column, where they ascend as the anterior spinothalamic tract. Itching and tickling may be sensations subserved by this tract.

Descending Motor Systems

Spinal Motor Neurons

Muscular contraction is initiated by the firing of motor neurons in the spinal cord and brainstem. These motor neurons are the only connection of the CNS to muscles and therefore represent the final common pathway of the excitatory and inhibitory motor pathways within the CNS. Two types of motor neurons are recognized: the larger α- and the smaller γ-motor neurons. The α-motor neuron innervates the skeletal muscle fibers through a specialized synaptic connection, the motor endplate, using Ach as a neurotransmitter. One motor neuron innervates a few hundred to several thousand muscle fibers. This is termed a *motor unit*. The α-motor neuron innervates the muscle spindle, a specialized receptor that sets muscle tone and monitors stretch and contraction.

Spinal motor neurons are arranged in columns in the ventral horn of spinal gray matter in laminae VIII and IX. The α-motor neurons (anterior horn cells) are arranged into medial and lateral groups, with the medial group supplying muscles attached to the axial skeleton and the lateral group supplying the muscles of the trunk and extremities. The lateral group is organized somatotopically so that the more medial neurons supply proximal muscles and the more lateral neurons, the more distal muscles. In addition, neurons supplying flexor muscles are dorsal to those supplying extensor muscles.

The α-motor neuron is termed the *lower motor neuron*. All descending neurons that modulate the activity of the lower motor neuron are called *upper motor neurons*. The lower motor neuron synapses directly to the muscle, and its loss results in atrophy of the muscle, loss of tone and stretch reflexes, and spontaneous contractions of muscle, such as fasciculations. Upper motor neuron lesions cause hypertonia, increased stretch reflexes, release of spinal reflexes, and spasticity. Spasticity refers to *tonic contraction* of antigravity muscles that will suddenly release with stretching of the muscle. The concept of upper and lower motor neuron lesions is extremely important in localizing a neurologic lesion.

Corticospinal Tracts

The corticospinal tracts include those nerve fibers that originate in the cerebral cortex and connect with motor neurons in the brainstem and spinal cord. Each corticospinal tract contains approximately 1 million axons located in the precentral and postcentral gyri and the premotor area of the frontal lobe. The large pyramidal Betz cells account for approximately 40,000 axons in each corticospinal tract. The corticospinal tract passes through the subcortical white matter (corona radiata) and the internal capsule at the level of the basal ganglia and thalamus to form the cerebral peduncle with the corticopontine fibers. The tract courses through the basis pontis to form the medullary pyramids. The corticospinal tract is also termed the *pyramidal tract* because of this formation. Fibers given to the brainstem motor nuclei are called *corticobulbar fibers*, and those that pass into the spinal cord are *corticospinal fibers*. Approximately 90% of the corticospinal fibers cross in the pyramidal decussation and travel in the dorsal half of the lateral column as the lateral corticospinal tract. The remaining 10% of fibers descend ipsilaterally in the anterior column as the anterior corticospinal tract that ends at upper thoracic cord levels. These latter fibers cross in the anterior commissure to supply contralateral anterior horn cells. The corticospinal tract is responsible for volitional movement, especially of the upper extremities, and interruption of the tract leads to paralysis.

Extrapyramidal Descending Motor Tracts

The remaining descending motor tracts originate in the brainstem and course to spinal levels. These tracts are more concerned with coordination of movements, postures, and muscle tone. Many descending motor tracts are recognized. Most important are the rubrospinal, vestibulospinal, and reticulospinal tracts.

Fibers from the red nucleus descend in the spinal cord as the rubrospinal tract to synapse upon the motor neurons supplying flexor muscles. The vestibulospinal tract originates from the lateral vestibular nucleus and synapses primarily upon extensor motor neurons. Therefore, an antagonistic role exists between the rubrospinal and vestibulospinal tracts in control of posture and tone. The reticulospinal tract descends from the lower brainstem to the spinal cord. The reticulospinal tract is involved in respiration, cardiopressor responses, bladder function, and pain modulation.

Brainstem Nuclei and Tracts

Motor Nuclei and Cranial Nerves

Muscles controlling eye movements, facial and masticatory movements, and movement of the tongue and pharyngeal muscles are subserved by motor neurons in the brainstem. These in turn are under reflex and voluntary control from cortical, brainstem, and spinal cord influences.

CNs controlling ocular movements and pupillary reflexes are the oculomotor (CN III), trochlear (CN IV), and the abducens (CN VI). These exit the brainstem, traverse the cavernous sinus, and enter the orbit through the superior orbital fissure. The abducens nerve supplies the lateral rectus muscle to abduct the eye, and the trochlear nerve innervates the superior oblique muscle to depress and intort the eye. All other ocular muscles, including lid elevators and pupillary sphincters, are supplied by the oculomotor nerve.

Eye movements are coordinated by multiple controlling influences. The medial longitudinal fasciculus (MLF) interconnects the nuclei of CN III, IV, and VI and connects these with the vestibular system and ascending and descending axons in the reticular formation. The tract extends from the cervical spinal cord to the upper mesencephalon. Damage to the MLF gives dysconjugate gaze difficulties, particularly medial rectus dysfunction on attempted lateral gaze and nystagmus. This is termed *internuclear ophthalmoplegia*. Conjugate gaze is controlled by two "gaze centers," one in the pons and one in the frontal lobe. Damage to the pontine gaze center causes the patient to look away from the side of the lesion. The gaze center in the posterior frontal lobe projects through the superior colliculus to the oculomotor complex. Damage to one cerebral hemisphere causes the patient to look toward the side of the lesion. The superior colliculi are responsible for allowing an object of interest to be brought into the center of the visual field. The pretectal area just rostral to the superior colliculi mediates the pupillary light reflex and subserves upward gaze.

The facial nerve (CN VII) is a complex nerve supplying the muscles of facial expression. It also carries parasympathetic fibers and afferent axons conveying taste and somatic sensation. The facial nerve nucleus is just beneath the floor of the fourth ventricle in the caudal pons. The fibers of the nerve course over the abducens nucleus, turn laterally, and exit the lateral pontomedullary junction just beneath the foramen of Luschka. The nerve passes with CN VIII into the internal auditory canal, runs through the temporal bone to exit the stylomastoid foramen, and branches in the parotid gland to supply facial muscles. Corticobulbar fibers cross in the pons to supply the facial nerve nucleus. The upper one third of the face has more bilateral representation, so that upper motor neuron lesions tend to affect the lower two thirds of the face primarily. These are distinguished from lower motor neuron lesions, where all ipsilateral facial muscles are weak.

The autonomic portion (nervus intermedius) passes into the internal auditory canal with the motor facial nerve but diverges in the temporal bone to send parasympathetic fibers to the pterygopalatine ganglion (lacrimal and nasal glands), through the superficial petrosal nerve, and to the submandibular ganglion (submandibular and sublingual glands), through the chorda tympani connection to the trigeminal nerve. The chorda tympani carries the afferent fibers for taste on the anterior tongue back to the geniculate ganglion in the temporal bone and with the facial nerve back to the solitary (gustatory) nucleus in the medulla.

The muscles of mastication—the masseters, pterygoids, and temporalis—are supplied by the motor division of the trigeminal nerve (CN V). This nerve exits the foramen ovale and runs with the mandibular branch of the trigeminal nerve.

The muscles of the pharynx and larynx receive innervation from the glossopharyngeal (CN IX), vagus (CN X), and spinal accessory (CN XI) nerves whose cell bodies lie in the nucleus ambiguus adjacent to the medullary reticular formation. The glossopharyngeal nerve is primarily a sensory nerve but also supplies the stylopharyngeal muscles. The cranial portion of CN XI supplies the vocal cords through the recurrent laryngeal nerve. The spinal portion of CN XI originates from cells in the upper cervical spinal cord and supplies the trapezius and sternocleidomastoid muscles. The remainder of the palatal and pharyngeal muscles are supplied by the vagus nerve. The extensive autonomic functions of these CNs will be discussed with the ANS. These three nerves exit the jugular foramen to pass to the pharynx and neck. The glossopharyngeal nerve (CN IX) courses over the internal carotid artery and beneath the styloid process and external carotid artery. It reaches the posterior tongue and pharynx beneath the hyoglossus muscle. The vagus nerve is joined by the cranial portion of the accessory nerve and first courses between and then behind the internal carotid artery and jugular vein in the carotid sheath. The spinal accessory nerve diverges from the vagus nerve in the carotid sheath, passes through the sternocleidomastoid muscle, and posteriorly enters the trapezius muscle.

The hypoglossal nerve (CN XII) innervates the muscles of the tongue. The nerve arises from cells near the midline in the lower medulla and emerges as rootlets between the pyramid and olive to coalesce into a single nerve that exits the hypoglossal foramen on the skull base. There is usually prominent bilateral corticobulbar supply, so weakness is more apparent with lower-motor neuron lesions. The strongest muscle, the genioglossus, protrudes the tongue, so with weakness deviation exists to the ipsilateral side. After exiting the hypoglossal canal, the nerve passes between the internal carotid artery and jugular vein and anterior to the external carotid and lingual arteries. It gives off the descendens hypoglossi (ansa cervicalis) nerve, passes deep to the digastric muscle, and enters the muscles of the tongue.

Sensory Nuclei and Cranial Nerves

Sensation on the face, nasal cavity, teeth, mouth, and part of the skull base is conveyed by the trigeminal nerve

(CN V). The three peripheral divisions of this nerve—the ophthalmic, maxillary, and mandibular—pass through the superior orbital fissure, foramen rotundum, and foramen ovale, respectively, to their cell bodies in the trigeminal (gasserian) ganglion, located in a trough in the temporal bone (Meckel cave). Fibers from the trigeminal ganglion carrying pain sensation enter the brainstem and descend as the spinal trigeminal tract, which continues into the cervical spinal cord. These synapse on the adjacent spinal trigeminal nucleus, which is continuous with the substantia gelatinosa of the spinal cord. Secondary axons cross the brainstem and ascend to the ventral posteromedial thalamus as the trigeminothalamic tract. Fibers conveying pain and general sensation around the ear, tonsil, and pharynx are also carried with the facial, glossopharyngeal, and vagus nerves and enter the spinal trigeminal nucleus.

Taste sensation enters the medulla from the facial nerve (anterior tongue), glossopharyngeal nerve (posterior tongue and pharynx), and a few fibers of the vagus nerve (epiglottis) to enter the lateral portion of the nucleus solitarius in the medulla. General sensation from the tongue, pharynx, larynx, and thoracic and abdominal viscera is conveyed through the glossopharyngeal and vagus nerves to the medial portion of the nucleus solitarius. Second-order neurons ascend to the ventral posteromedial nucleus of the thalamus and reticular formation. CNs I (olfactory) and II (optic) represent brain tracts and will be discussed with the thalamus.

The vestibulocochlear nerve (CN VIII) has two anatomic and functional components: the cochlear, carrying hearing, and the vestibular, carrying the sense of equilibrium and orientation in space. Both components of the nerve arise from receptors in the temporal bone: the cochlear nerve from the cochlea and the vestibular nerve from the labyrinth.

Sound waves are transmitted from the tympanic membrane through the middle ear ossicles to the oval window of the inner ear. The inner ear (organ of Corti) consists of a tectorial membrane and a basilar membrane suspended in fluid (perilymph). Sound waves oscillate the basilar membrane, distorting hair cells and propagating an impulse. These bipolar cells have cell bodies in the spiral ganglion within the cochlea. The afferent axons form the cochlear nerve and course to the medulla to synapse on the cochlear nuclei lateral to the inferior cerebellar peduncle. Axons from the cochlear nuclei form the acoustic striae that both cross and ascend uncrossed as the lateral lemnisci. The lateral lemniscus synapses primarily in the ipsilateral inferior colliculus in the midbrain, with some fibers crossing to the opposite inferior colliculus and others coursing directly to the medial geniculate body of the thalamus. All fibers eventually reach the medial geniculate body. Geniculocortical fibers project to the temporal operculum (transverse gyri of Heschl), the primary auditory cortex. Loss of the cochlear nerve or nucleus causes complete unilateral deafness. Lesions of the brainstem and cortex do not cause complete deafness but may affect localization of sound and perhaps discrimination.

Receptors in the labyrinth—the utricle, saccule, and semicircular canals—transmit impulses through the vestibular ganglion (Scarpa) along the superior and inferior vestibular nerves to the vestibular ganglia in the medulla. Vestibular connections are widespread, but particularly important connections include the flocculonodular lobe of the cerebellum, the median longitudinal fasciculus (see earlier text), and the vestibulospinal tract to motor neurons in the spinal cord. Vestibular stimulation results in vertigo (a sense of whirling and nausea) and nystagmus (rhythmic oscillations of the eyes). Vestibular tracts are concerned with oculocephalic and tonic neck reflexes and subserve decerebrate rigidity after brainstem injury.

Brainstem Reticular Formation

The central core of polysynaptic neurons in the brainstem is called the *reticular formation*. The reticular formation extends from the lower medulla to the upper mesencephalon. Descending and ascending projections arise from cells in the larger medial reticular formation. Descending reticulospinal fibers primarily facilitate deep tendon reflexes and extensor motor tone. This is effected through the τ-efferent motor neuron system. The medullary reticular formation contains the respiratory and vasomotor centers.

An ascending central reticular polysynaptic pathway, independent of the ascending lemniscal sensory systems, is responsible for generalized cortical arousal and is termed the *ascending reticular-activating system* (ARAS). This system receives collaterals from all ascending sensory systems but does not convey a specific sensory modality. It is responsible for the waking pattern onelectroencephalogram (EEG) and is believed to be the basis for consciousness.

Cerebellum

The cerebellum is responsible for coordination of muscle movements and tone. Information delivered to the cerebellum does not enter consciousness but allows the setting of postural and associated muscles, allowing smooth voluntary movement. Afferent impulses from muscle spindles, joint receptors, and tendon organs are carried to the cerebellum through the spinocerebellar tracts. These combine with the corticopontine tracts to influence cerebellar efferent neurons.

The cerebellar cortex is thrown into folds (folia) and consists of three layers: the superficial molecular layers, the Purkinje cell layer, and the granular layer (Fig. 21.6). Ascending sensory fibers entering the cerebellar cortex are modulated by neurons in the deeper granular layer before ascending to the molecular layer to synapse with Purkinje cell dendrites. Axons of the Purkinje cells course in the cerebellar white matter to the deep cerebellar nuclei and the vestibular nucleus. They use γ-aminobutyric acid (GABA) as an inhibitory neurotransmitter.

The deep cerebellar nuclei—the fastigial, globose, emboliform, and dentate—are located within the white matter close to the fourth ventricle and project as the superior cerebellar peduncle to the ventrolateral nucleus of the contralateral thalamus. The thalamocortical fibers synapse mainly on primary motor cortical areas.

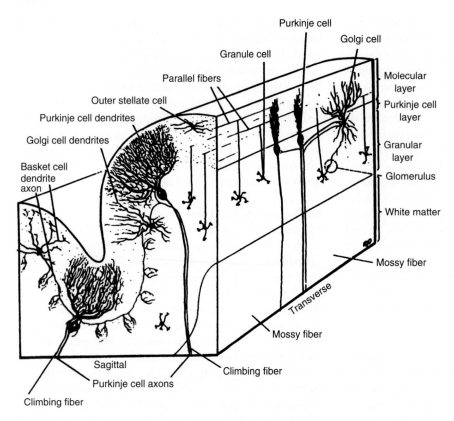

FIGURE 21.6 Diagram of the cerebellar cortex. (From Carpenter MB, Sutin J. *Human neuroanatomy*, 8th ed. Baltimore: Williams & Wilkins, 1983:458, with permission.)

Functionally, there are three cerebellar zones: a vermal (midline) cerebellar cortex, which projects the fastigial nucleus and secondarily to the vestibular nuclei, regulating extensor (postural) tone; a paravermal zone, projecting to the globose and emboliform nuclei and then to the red nucleus, facilitating flexor tone; and a lateral zone, projecting to the dentate nucleus, to the ventral lateral nucleus of the thalamus, and finally to the sensorimotor cerebral cortex to coordinate pyramidal tract function. Lesions involving the vermal and paravermal zones produce gait disturbance and imbalance (ataxia) and often cause nystagmus and speech dysfunction. Lesions involving the lateral zone (cerebellar hemisphere) include hypotonia, tremor, dysmetria, dysdiadochokinesia, and other types of muscle coordination asynergia.

Thalamus

The paired thalami, separated by the third ventricle, are large nuclear masses responsible for the integration of sensory information. All sensation except olfaction is processed in the thalamus before arriving at a cortical level. The thalamic nuclei project to all areas of the cerebral cortex and, in turn, receive input from corresponding cortical areas. Because the specific ascending sensory pathways and the ARAS converge in the thalamus, the thalamus is considered to bring sensory information into awareness.

The thalamus contains multiple nuclear groups with complex relations. The ventral nuclei convey sensation of pain, touch, vibration, position, and temperature to the primary sensory cortex (postcentral gyrus) in a topographic manner. The ventral nuclei also modulate motor activity. The lateral and medial geniculate bodies subserve vision and hearing, respectively. Anterior and dorsal nuclei are related to the limbic system concerned with the emotional and affective processing of information. The intralaminar nuclei are thought to be involved in general arousal responses and central control of pain.

Hypothalamus

The hypothalamus forms the walls of the third ventricle below the hypothalamic sulcus and is connected to the pituitary gland through the infundibulum and pituitary stalk. This small area of brain is vitally important for control of autonomic, endocrine, and behavioral functions. The hypothalamus has afferent and efferent connections to multiple areas of the nervous system, including the brainstem, spinal cord, pituitary gland, and limbic system.

The hypothalamus functions as the brain center for autonomic function. Both sympathetic and parasympathetic activity are coordinated in the hypothalamus. In general, the anteromedial area of the hypothalamus is responsible for parasympathetic functions, and the posterolateral area regulates sympathetic activity. Osmoreceptors in the anterior hypothalamus constitute a thirst center and are related to the supraoptic nucleus, where the antidiuretic hormone (ADH) vasopressin is formed. The lateral area of the hypothalamus seems concerned with hunger, and the ventromedial area with satiety. The anterior hypothalamus also controls temperature regulation by its connections with other hypothalamic areas.

Another important function of the hypothalamus is hormonal regulation. The neuropeptides vasopressin and oxytocin are secreted directly from axons in the posterior lobe of the pituitary, with their cell bodies in the supraoptic and paraventricular nuclei. The hormones of the anterior lobe of the pituitary are regulated by releasing factors from the hypothalamus that are brought to the pituitary gland through the hypophyseal portal system rather than through direct neural connections. These releasing factors regulate growth hormone, adrenocorticotropic hormone, thyroid-stimulating hormone, luteinizing hormone, follicle-stimulating hormone, prolactin, and their target organs through a complicated feedback mechanism. These factors are, in turn, acted on by afferent fibers to the hypothalamus from other brain centers.

Finally, the hypothalamus acts as a center for behavior and emotional expression. Attentiveness, somnolence, and the visceral components of rage, fear, aggressiveness, and pleasure are produced by electrical stimulation of areas of the hypothalamus in animals. The neuroanatomic connections of these complex behaviors in humans are unclear.

Basal Ganglia

The basal ganglia are located in the deep frontal lobe and diencephalon and are concerned with motor function. They consist of the corpus striatum (caudate, putamen, and globus pallidus), the claustrum, the subthalamic nuclei, and the substantia nigra. The caudate and putamen are termed *neostriatum* and seem to be a unified nucleus anatomically divided by the internal capsule. The globus pallidus is medial to the putamen and separated from the thalamus by the posterior limb of the internal capsule. The subthalamic nucleus lies just caudally in the diencephalon, and the substantia nigra lies farther caudally in the midbrain tegmentum. These nuclei form circuits that modulate and connect the motor cortex, thalamus, and descending motor pathways.

Afferents to the striatum include cerebral cortex, thalamus, and substantia nigra. All areas of the cortex project to the caudate and putamen, but the sensorimotor cortex and premotor areas are better represented. The striatum receives bilateral projections from the cortex. An important afferent input to the striatum is the substantia nigra. Melanin-containing cells in the substantia nigra convey the neurotransmitter dopamine to the putamen and caudate. Degeneration of these nigral cells is associated with parkinsonism. A reciprocal striatonigral pathway uses GABA and substance P as neurotransmitters, which are inhibitory and excitatory, respectively. Finally, there is a serotonin-transmitted pathway from the dorsal brainstem to the striatum that has been implicated in behavioral disturbances.

The primary output of the caudate and putamen (striatum) is to the globus pallidus. The globus pallidus does not receive fibers directly from the cerebral cortex, thalamus, or substantia nigra. Striatopallidal fibers use GABA as a neurotransmitter.

Lesions of the basal ganglia are associated with alterations in tone and involuntary movements. Muscular rigidity and slowness in initiating movements as well as tremor are characteristic of parkinsonism, for which the primary lesion is loss of dopamine-producing cells in the substantia nigra. Chorea (quick involuntary movements), athetosis (writhing movements), and dystonia (fixed postural movements) are found in Huntington disease and other genetic disorders and are associated with neuronal atrophy and loss of GABA in the neostriatum. Ballism (violent movements of the extremities) occurs with lesions in the contralateral subthalamic nucleus. The efferent fibers of the basal ganglia course to the thalamus and, subsequently, to the cerebral cortex but not to the lower brainstem or spinal cord. Therefore, the modulation of motor activity from the basal ganglia is thought to be mediated through the corticospinal tract.

Visual System

The visual system is concerned with the processing of visual information (light) and voluntary and reflex movements of the eyes that fix the visual image to be processed. Eye movements and tracking were discussed under brainstem nuclei. The visual world seen by each eye is termed the *visual field*. The visual fields generally are divided into superior and inferior, nasal, and temporal quadrants. The lens inverts and transposes the visual field onto the retina so that the temporal fields are on the nasal retina, the superior fields on the inferior retina, etc. The photosensitive cells, or the rods (low illumination) and cones (high illumination and color), are connected by bipolar cells to the retinal ganglion cells whose axons form the optic nerves. The optic nerves pass from the orbit through the optic foramina to the subarachnoid chiasmatic cistern, where they partially decussate as the optic chiasm. Only the fibers from the nasal retina that represent the temporal visual fields cross. Posterior to the chiasm, the fibers are called the *optic tracts*, with each tract carrying the contralateral hemivisual field. The tracts encircle the hypothalamus and synapse in the lateral geniculate body of the thalamus. Those fibers concerned with eye movements and pupillary reactions go directly to the area of the superior colliculus without entering the lateral geniculate body.

The visual fibers coursing from the thalamus to the occipital cortex are termed the *geniculocalcarine tract* or *optic radiations*. Superior fibers carrying the inferior visual field course adjacent to the ventricle to reach the occipital lobe superior to the calcarine fissure. Inferior fibers carrying the superior visual field course forward into the temporal lobe and follow the temporal horn of the ventricle posteriorly to end in the occipital lobe inferior to the calcarine fissure (Fig. 21.7). Therefore, temporal lesions give a homonymous (both eyes) superior quadrantanopsia, and parietal lesions give an inferior quadrantanopsia. Occipital lesions are associated with homonymous hemianopsia. The more posterior the lesion, the more similar (congruous) the field loss in each eye. Macular fibers end in the occipital pole, and peripheral retinal fibers end more rostrally.

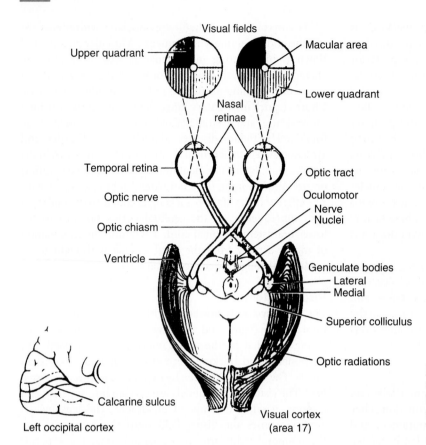

FIGURE 21.7 Diagram of the visual pathways showing the optic chiasm and optic radiations. (From Carpenter MB, Sutin J. *Human neuroanatomy*, 8th ed. Baltimore: Williams & Wilkins, 1983:541, with permission.)

Processing of visual information occurs at all levels of the visual system. In the retina, one ganglion cell receives several rods and cones. The receptive area for each ganglion cell is circular and has an excitatory center and inhibitory margin or an inhibitory center and excitatory margin. Neurons in the lateral geniculate body have a similar anatomic mechanism to enhance discrimination. Occipital (striate) cortex has a columnar arrangement of neurons; the columns are stimulated by edges of light/dark in various orientations, and the columns of cells respond more to images in one or the other eye. Interconnections between these columns of cells allow patterns to be formed and provide binocular vision. Adjacent association cortex connects these patterns to memory and recognition.

Olfactory System

Olfactory sensory cells are found in a specialized epithelium in the nasal mucosa. These are bipolar neurons that project their axons through the cribriform plate of the ethmoid bone to the olfactory bulb, where they synapse on mitral cells. Axons of mitral cells form the olfactory tract that courses posteriorly in the olfactory sulcus between the gyrus rectus and the orbital gyri and divides into medial and lateral striae. The smaller medial stria runs to the subcallosal (septal) area, although the larger lateral stria synapses in the prepiriform area of the temporal lobe. This cortex then projects to the parahippocampal gyrus (uncus and entorhinal areas) and the amygdala. Olfaction is the only sensation not processed by the thalamus.

Cerebral Cortex and Higher Cortical Functions
Cortical Architecture

The cerebral cortex is characterized by alternating layers of larger pyramidal and smaller granule cells. Typically, the adult cerebral cortex contains six layers: I, consisting mainly of dendrites; II, an external granular layer; III, an external pyramidal layer; IV, an internal granular layer; V, an internal pyramidal layer; and VI, a layer of fusiform cells. Areas of the hippocampus contain only three layers: a molecular layer, a pyramidal or granular layer, and a polymorphic layer. Six-layered cortex is called *neocortex*, and three-layered cortex is called *allocortex*. Development of these layers varies in different areas of the cortex. Efferent axons of cortical neurons are termed *association fibers* if they synapse within the same hemisphere, commissural fibers if they connect to corresponding regions of the opposite hemisphere, and projection fibers if they course to subcortical destinations. Association and commissural fibers arise mainly from cells in layers II and III, and projection fibers primarily from pyramidal cells in layer V. Cells in layer VI project to the thalamus. In addition to the horizontal layers of cells, the cortex is arranged into vertical columns that extend through all six layers and form functional physiologic units. This organization is particularly apparent in visual and sensory cortex.

Motor Areas

The precentral gyrus contains mainly pyramidal neurons, including the giant Betz cells, and is considered the primary

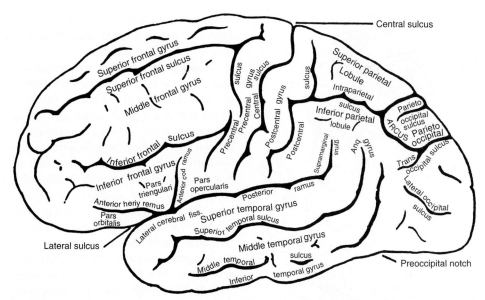

FIGURE 21.8 Lateral view of the cerebral hemisphere, showing the precentral and postcentral gyri in relation to other areas of cortex. (From Goss CM. *Gray's anatomy*, 28th ed. Philadelphia: Lea & Febiger, 1970:842, with permission.)

motor area, although it accounts for only approximately 30% of axons in the corticospinal tract (Fig. 21.8). The largest nerve fibers in the corticospinal tract originate from this area. Stimulation of this gyrus results in discrete movements of the contralateral face and limbs; the face area is closest to the sylvian fissure, the arm area is located more superiorly on the frontal lobe, and the lower extremity is on the mesial aspect of the hemisphere (Fig. 21.9). Destruction of the gyrus

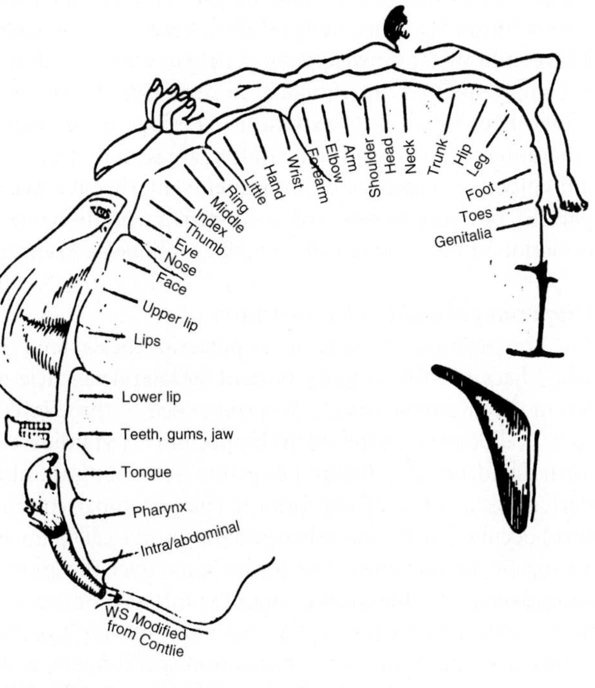

FIGURE 21.9 Motor homunculus, showing motor representation in the precentral gyrus. (From Goss CM. *Gray's anatomy*, 28th ed. Philadelphia: Lea & Febiger, 1970:849, with permission.)

causes contralateral paralysis that is initially flaccid but later shows some return of tone. Spasticity is not characteristic.

Adjacent rostrally to the primary motor area is the premotor area. Stimulation of cortex closest to the primary motor area results in similar movements but requires a greater stimulus, whereas stimulation more rostrally on the superior frontal gyrus causes aversive head and eye movements and posturing of the trunk and extremities. Bilateral movements of the face and pharyngeal muscles can be elicited. The cortex on the medial surface of the superior frontal gyrus is called the *supplementary motor area*, and stimulation results in posturing and bilateral movements. Ablation of the premotor area does not cause paralysis, but removal of the primary motor and premotor areas gives paralysis for which spasticity is a prominent feature. Approximately 40% of axons in the corticospinal tract come from neurons in the postcentral gyrus (parietal lobe), and sensations are described with stimulation of the precentral gyrus. Therefore, the precentral and postcentral gyri have overlapping functions and are together called *sensorimotor cortex*.

Sensory Areas

The postcentral gyrus represents the primary cortical sensory area. Granule cells predominate (granular cortex). The edge of the gyrus closest to the central sulcus receives the major output of the ventral posterior thalamic nuclei, and this area responds most readily to cutaneous stimuli (Fig. 21.10). The posterior edge of the gyrus receives finer fibers and responds to joint movement and deep pressure. A secondary somatic sensory area is described along the parietal operculum of the sylvian fissure.

Visual cortex is located in the occipital lobe above and below the calcarine fissure and was discussed under the visual

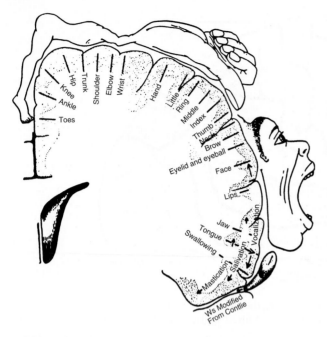

FIGURE 21.10 Sensory homunculus, showing tactile sensory representation in the postcentral gyrus. (From Goss CM. *Gray's anatomy*, 28th ed. Philadelphia: Lea & Febiger, 1970:850, with permission.)

system. Auditory cortex is composed of two transverse gyri on the superior temporal lobe buried in the sylvian fissure. The anterior gyrus is the primary auditory area and the posterior auditory association cortex. The auditory cortex receives its primary input from the medial geniculate body of the thalamus. Each ear has bilateral cortical representation, so destruction of the auditory cortex on one side does not significantly decrease hearing but does affect spatial localization of sound. Taste is represented in the parietal operculum near the somatic tongue area. Vestibular function is found on the posterior edge of the postcentral gyrus near the end of the interparietal sulcus.

Association Areas

Areas of cortex not concerned directly with primary motor and sensory functions are termed *association cortex*. This cortex integrates the primary sensory modalities with memory and experience and allows symbolic interpretation and expression of events such as language, calculation, and spatial construction. Speech function resides in the left hemisphere of most people, including left-handed individuals. Speech comprehension depends on the temporoparietal cortex at the posterior end of the sylvian fissure (Wernicke area), and, to some degree, speech production depends on cortex of the posteroinferior frontal lobe (Broca area). These areas are connected by white matter association fibers, the arcuate fasciculus. Inability to understand and form language is termed *aphasia* and is divided into receptive (fluent) aphasia, when comprehension is lost, and expressive (nonfluent) aphasia, when production is lost. Most patients with aphasia show elements of both. Characteristics of aphasia include inability

to form words, word deletions, inability to name objects, repetitive use of a word (perseveration), and inability to follow spoken commands.

Inability to recognize sensory information and assign meaning to it is called an *agnosia*. With visual agnosia, an object is seen but not recognized. Inability to read is termed *alexia* and is a type of visual agnosia. Lesions of the left hemisphere cortex between the primary visual areas and the inferior parietal lobe (angular gyrus) create visual agnosias. Similarly, auditory agnosias, for which sound is heard but not interpreted, occur with lesions of the left posterior temporal lobe and connections to the inferior parietal lobe. Receptive aphasia is basically a high-level auditory agnosia. Tactile agnosia or astereognosis is the inability to recognize objects by touch and is associated with lesions of the left supramarginal gyrus (parietal lobe). These specific agnosias involve the formulation of language, reading, and writing. They result from left hemisphere lesions, although contralateral astereognosis is present with lesions of either hemisphere. The parietal cortex of the right hemisphere seems to be concerned with spatial and constructional relations. Damage to right parietal cortex results in the inability to draw figures and recognize spatial relations. Nonrecognition and neglect of the opposite side of the body are associated with more severe damage. Nevertheless, right–left disorientation and inability to recognize fingers, in association with writing and calculation difficulties, form a specific syndrome (Gerstmann) related to damage to the left angular gyrus. Finally, some agnosias result from an inability to transfer information from the right to the left hemisphere caused by lesions in the corpus callosum; they are termed *disconnection syndromes*. Damage to the dominant supramarginal gyrus and adjacent parietal lobe can impair the execution of learned motor skills in the absence of paresis. This condition is termed *apraxia*. A patient understands what is being requested but is unable to carry out the task. The impairment involves all extremities. Lesions in the frontal lobe anterior to the primary motor areas may also cause difficulty in execution of movements in the absence of paresis, but this is more of a clumsiness or difficulty in initiation of movement. Gait apraxia would be an example.

Hippocampal and Limbic Structures

The hippocampus is found in the posterior mesial temporal lobe adjacent to the temporal horn of the lateral ventricle and lies in the choroidal fissure. It is composed of three-layered cortex (allocortex). Axons of the hippocampal pyramidal cells form the fornix, the efferent projection of the hippocampus. Partial decussation of the fornices (hippocampal commissure) occurs as they course beneath the corpus callosum and on top of the thalamus. The fornix splits over the anterior commissure near the Monro foramina into precommissural fibers, which reach the septal area and anterior hypothalamus, and more numerous postcommissural fibers, which synapse in the mammillary bodies of the posterior hypothalamus. The mammillothalamic tract projects to the anterior and intralaminar nuclei of the thalamus, which themselves project to the cingulate gyrus. This loop from cingulate gyrus to entorhinal cortex to hippocampus to mammillary bodies through the fornix to thalamus and back to cingulate gyrus is termed the *Papez circuit*. Bilateral damage to any component of this circuit causes severe impairment of short-term memory. Other components of the limbic system include the amygdala, prefrontal and orbitofrontal cortex, the septal area, and nucleus basalis (Meynert).

Limbic structures are concerned with memory, affect, emotion, and behavior. The hippocampus seems important in short-term memory and learning. Bilateral destruction results in loss of acquisition of new memories but spares long-standing memories and experiences. Damage to the mammillary bodies may cause a similar syndrome (Korsakoff). The hippocampus possibly influences the expression of emotion by connecting the cortex to the hypothalamus and brainstem through the Papez circuit. However, experimentally, stimulation of the amygdala is more consistent in producing autonomic and psychic concomitants of strong emotional states. Bilateral destruction of the amygdala seems to lessen aggressive behavior. Disconnection of the prefrontal area (prefrontal lobotomy) results in lessening of anxiety but also decreased concentration and attention span, lessening of drive and initiative, and impaired social behavior. Bilateral cingulum lesions decrease the affective components of pain without as profound an effect on attentiveness.

The Peripheral Nervous System
General Considerations
The PNS consists of 31 pairs of segmental spinal nerves and the CNs that were discussed earlier. The spinal nerves contain motor, sensory, and visceral elements. Motor (ventral) and sensory (dorsal) roots form the spinal nerve at each level. Visceral fibers travel with the ventral root and will be discussed in the next section. In the cervical and lumbar areas, the spinal nerves form plexuses, where redistribution of axons takes place to form the peripheral nerves.

The peripheral nerves are invested in a connective tissue sheath, the epineurium. Within the nerve the axons are arranged in fascicles bound by perineurium. The perineurium is the first level of a blood–nerve barrier. A regrouping of axons into different fascicles occurs along the course of a nerve such that when a segment of nerve is removed, the fascicles no longer precisely match. Connective tissue within the fascicle invests each axon as the endoneurium. Finally, the axon is surrounded by myelin, the concentric laminations of the cell membranes of Schwann cells, which increases the rate of conduction of the nerve impulse in relation to its thickness. Even unmyelinated axons are believed to be in contact with, but not invested by, Schwann cells.

Peripheral nerve fibers are classified by size in an ABC system. Size depends on the diameter of the axon and, more important, the thickness of the myelin sheath. Myelinated fibers are designated group A and may be subdivided α through δ. Diameters range from 2 to 20 μ, and nerve conduction velocities (NCVs) range from 20 to 120 m/s.

B fibers are myelinated preganglionic autonomic fibers, 2 to 5 μ in diameter, and C fibers are unmyelinated fibers, 1 to 2 μ in diameter with NCVs less than 2 m/s. Larger A sensory fibers subserve joint and tendon receptors, muscle spindles, and pressure receptors. Smaller A_δ and C fibers carry pain (nociceptive) impulses. Motor neurons to skeletal muscle are A_α and those to muscle spindles are A_τ. A similar classification system uses Roman numerals I to IV for large to small fibers.

Each motor neuron synapses with many muscle fibers. The axon and its associated muscle fibers are termed a *motor unit*. Muscle contraction represents the simultaneous firing of many motor units within the given peripheral nerve.

When a nerve is severed, the distal portion of the nerve undergoes a progressive degeneration (wallerian) that may take several days, depending on the length of the nerve. Schwann cells form tubules to allow regrowth of the nerve, but scar tissue inhibits this process. The axon also dies back a few millimeters, and the endoplasmic reticulum of the cell shows dispersion of ribonucleic acid (RNA, chromatolysis). The neuromuscular synapse dissipates, and the entire muscle fiber becomes sensitized and may spontaneously contract (fibrillation). This process is usually evident by 3 weeks after a nerve injury and forms the basis of an electromyographic examination (EMG) for nerve injury.

Anatomy of the Peripheral Nervous System
The 31 spinal nerves are divided into 8 cervical, 12 thoracic, 5 lumbar, 5 sacral, and 1 coccygeal. Shortly after exiting the intervertebral foramina, the spinal nerves divide into dorsal and ventral rami. The dorsal rami supply motor innervation to the long extensors of the back and sensation over the spine.

The cervical plexus is formed from the first four cervical segments. C2, with its dorsal ramus, supplies the occipitalis muscle and the skin of the scalp as the occipital nerves. C2–C4 supply the hyoid muscles, through the ansa cervicalis, and the diaphragm, through the phrenic nerve. The phrenic nerve is supplied primarily by C4. It runs along the lateral border of the anterior scalene muscle, passes anterior to the subclavian artery, and lies in the mediastinum in close relation to the vagus nerve. It supplies the diaphragm from its inferior surface.

The brachial plexus is formed by the spinal nerves (roots) of C5 through T1. These form upper (C5, C6), middle (C7), and lower (C8, T1) trunks (Fig. 21.11). The trunks form anterior and posterior divisions that give rise to three cords named for their relation to the axillary artery. The lateral cord is formed by the anterior divisions of the upper and middle trunks (C5–C7), the medial cord by the anterior division of the lower trunk (C8, T1), and the posterior cord from the posterior divisions of all three trunks (C5–C8). The cords then give rise to the major peripheral nerves, although nerves are given off the plexus all along their course. From the cervical spine, the plexus runs beneath the clavicle, in front of the scapula, and over the first rib. It is covered by the scalene muscles and courses behind the pectoralis minor

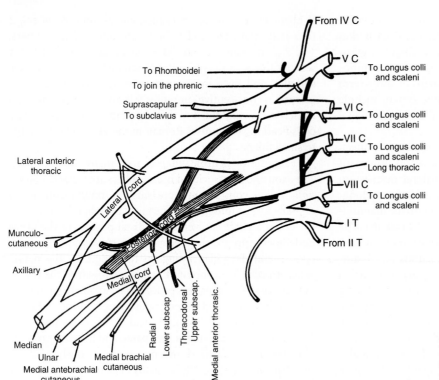

FIGURE 21.11 Diagrammatic drawing of the brachial plexus. (From Goss CM. *Gray's anatomy*, 28th ed. Philadelphia: Lea & Febiger, 1970:965, with permission.)

muscle. It is intimately related to the subclavian and axillary artery and vein.

Nerves to the scalene muscles, rhomboids (dorsal scapular nerve C5), and serratus anterior (long thoracic nerve C5–C7), are the most proximal branches of the plexus and exit at a root to trunk level. The upper trunk gives the suprascapular nerve (C5, C6) to the supraspinatus and infraspinatus muscles. At the cord level, the lateral cord gives the lateral pectoral nerve (C5–C7), the medial cord, the medial pectoral nerve (C8, T1), and the medial cutaneous nerve of the arm and forearm; the posterior cord provides the nerves to the latissimus dorsi (C6–C8) and subscapular muscles (C5–C7). The posterior cord gives rise to the axillary nerve (C5) to the deltoid muscle and becomes the radial nerve. The lateral cord divides into the musculocutaneous and lateral half of the median nerves, and the medial cord divides into the ulnar and medial half of the median nerves.

The musculocutaneous nerve (C5–C7) runs through the coracobrachialis muscle and between the biceps and brachialis muscles, which it supplies. It emerges as the lateral cutaneous nerve of the forearm on the radial side of the forearm. The median nerve (C6–T1) runs with the brachial artery on the medial side of the upper arm; passes between the heads of the pronator teres in the antecubital fossa; gives off the anterior interosseous branch, which supplies forearm muscles; and passes beneath the carpal tunnel to supply the thenar muscles and sensation to the thumb, index finger, middle finger, and median half of the ring finger. Muscles supplied by the median nerve, in order, are pronator teres; palmaris longus; flexor carpi radialis; flexor digitorum superficialis, as anterior interosseous nerve-flexor pollicis longus, flexor digitorum profundus (half), and pronator

quadratus; in the hand, abductor pollicis brevis, opponens pollicis, and flexor pollicis brevis; and the first two lumbricals.

The ulnar nerve (C8, T1) initially runs with the brachial artery but passes posteriorly between the medial epicondyle and the olecranon, courses through the flexor carpi ulnaris muscle, and runs with the ulnar artery to enter the hand, where it provides sensation to the small finger and ulnar half of the ring finger. Muscles supplied by the ulnar nerve, in order, are flexor carpi ulnaris, flexor digitorum profundus (half), palmaris brevis, hypothenar, adductor pollicis, lumbricals, and interossei. The radial nerve (C5–C8) is the continuation of the posterior cord as it passes between the heads of the triceps muscle. It winds around the humerus in the spiral groove giving off the posterior cutaneous nerve of the forearm. Coursing alongside the brachioradialis muscle, it divides near the elbow into a superficial sensory branch and a deep branch to the extensor muscles of the forearm, called the *posterior interosseous nerve*. Innervation of the extensor carpi radialis occurs before this division. The superficial sensory branch supplies the dorsum of the radial side of the hand and fingers. Muscles supplied by the radial nerve, in order, are triceps, anconeus, brachioradialis, extensor carpi radialis, extensor digitorum, extensor carpi ulnaris, extensor pollicis longus, abductor pollicis longus, extensor indicis, and extensor pollicis brevis.

The 12 thoracic segments give intercostal nerves at each level. T1 is mainly part of the brachial plexus, and T2 gives some sensory innervation to the upper inner arm. The intercostal nerves run between the pleura and the intercostal muscles on the inferior edge of the rib. On the abdominal wall, the nerves run between the internal oblique and transversus abdominis muscles and come through the posterior rectus

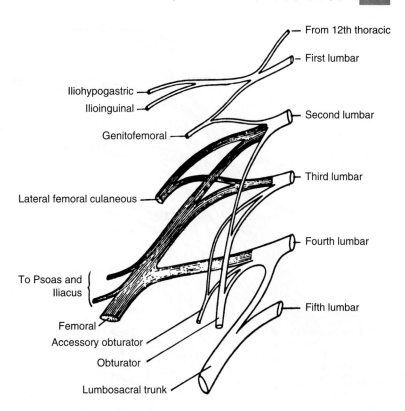

From 12th thoracic

First lumbar

Iliohypogastric

Ilioinguinal

Genitofemoral

Second lumbar

Lateral femoral culaneous

Third lumbar

Fourth lumbar

To Psoas and
Iliacus

Fifth lumbar

Femoral

Accessory obturator

Obturator

Lumbosacral trunk

FIGURE 21.12 Diagrammatic drawing of the lumbar plexus. (From Goss CM. *Gray's anatomy*, 28th ed. Philadelphia: Lea & Febiger, 1970:988, with permission.)

sheath. These nerves innervate the intercostal and abdominal wall musculature and give lateral and anterior cutaneous branches to the skin of the chest and abdomen.

The first three and the upper portion of the fourth lumbar nerves form the lumbar plexus (Fig. 21.12). Anterior divisions of the lumbar plexus give rise to the iliohypogastric (L1), ilioinguinal (L1), genitofemoral (L1, L2), and obturator (L2–L4) nerves. The first three nerves are primarily sensory nerves. The iliohypogastric and ilioinguinal nerves run from the lateral border of the psoas muscle on the quadratus lumborum muscle and behind the kidney. The nerves course in close relation to the inguinal canal and supply the pubis and scrotum or labia, respectively. The genitofemoral nerve passes through the psoas muscle beneath the ureter and runs with the spermatic cord or round ligament to supply the scrotum or labia. The nerve supplies the cremaster muscle. The obturator nerve enters the pelvis from the medial edge of the psoas muscle and supplies the obturator, gracilis, and adductor thigh muscles as well as sensation to the medial thigh.

The posterior divisions of the lumbar plexus form the iliopsoas (L2, L3), femoral (L2–L4), and lateral femoral cutaneous (L2, L3) nerves. The iliopsoas nerves arise primarily from spinal nerves L2 and L3 before dividing to supply the psoas muscle. The femoral nerve leaves the lateral edge of the psoas muscle and passes beneath the inguinal ligament with the femoral artery and vein and supplies the quadriceps femoris and sartorius muscles. It ends as the cutaneous sensory saphenous nerve, which courses all the way to the medial foot. The lateral femoral cutaneous nerve passes beneath the inguinal ligament close to the anterior

superior iliac spine to supply the lateral thigh to the knee. Entrapment results in a common painful syndrome, meralgia paresthetica.

The lumbosacral plexus (sacral plexus) arises from spinal nerves L4 to S3 (Fig. 21.13). The principal nerves formed by this plexus are the sciatic (L4–S3), the gluteals (L4–S1), and the pudendal (S2–S4). The sciatic nerve is a composite nerve of two divisions, the peroneal and the tibial, which generally diverge at mid-thigh level but may split much higher. The anterior division of the plexus forms the tibial nerve and the posterior division forms the peroneal. The sciatic nerve exits the pelvis through the greater sciatic foramen (sciatic notch) below the piriformis and gluteal muscles, and runs between the biceps femoris and semimembranosus muscles in the thigh. The peroneal nerve passes laterally under the head of the fibula and supplies the extensor muscles of the lower leg and sensation to the dorsum of the foot. The tibial nerve runs through the popliteal fossa, continues distally between the soleus and gastrocnemius muscles, and passes around the medial malleolus to supply the sole of the foot as the plantar nerves. The peroneal division of the sciatic supplies the following muscles, in order: biceps femoris (short head), peroneus longus, tibialis anterior, extensor digitorum longus, extensor hallucis longus, peroneus tertius, peroneus brevis, and extensor digitorum brevis. Muscles supplied by the tibial division, in order, are biceps femoris (long head), semimembranosus, semitendinosus, adductor magnus (part), gastrocnemius, soleus, flexor hallucis longus, flexor digitorum longus, tibialis posterior, and intrinsic foot.

The superior gluteal nerve supplies the gluteus medius and minimus muscles, and the inferior gluteal nerve supplies

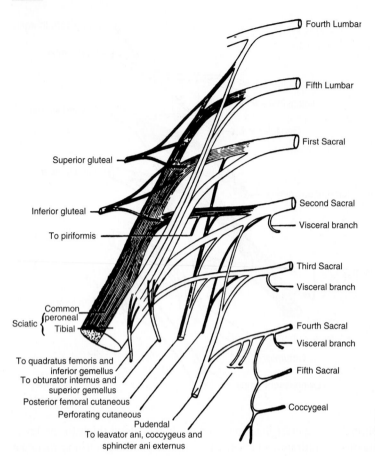

FIGURE 21.13 Diagrammatic drawing of the sacral plexus. (From Goss CM. *Gray's anatomy*, 28th ed. Philadelphia: Lea & Febiger, 1970:998, with permission.)

the gluteus maximus muscle. The nerves exit the pelvis above and below the piriformis muscle, respectively. The pudendal nerve passes into the ischiorectal fossa through the lesser sciatic foramen, where it gives rise to rectal and perineal nerves. The inferior rectal nerve supplies the external rectal sphincter, although the perineal nerve goes to the external bladder sphincter and to the genitalia.

The Autonomic Nervous System

General Considerations

The ANS refers to that part of the CNS and PNS concerned with visceral functions as opposed to somatic, by which is generally meant the innervation of blood vessels, glands, skin appendages, heart, viscera, and pupils. The central portion of the system includes the hypothalamus and reticular formation in the brain and the intermediolateral cell column in the spinal cord. The peripheral portion of the system is characterized by a two-neuron system with an interposed autonomic ganglion. The ANS is divided into two parts: a sympathetic and a parasympathetic system (Fig. 21.14). These systems generally have opposing actions on the target organ. Although central control for both systems arises in the hypothalamus and reticular formation, preganglionic nerves of the sympathetic system are found only in the thoracolumbar spinal cord, and preganglionic nerves of the parasympathetic system are found in the brainstem and sacral spinal cord. Sympathetic ganglia are generally close to the spinal cord, whereas parasympathetic ganglia tend

to be close to or within the organ supplied. Both sympathetic and parasympathetic preganglionic neurons use Ach as their neurotransmitter. Ach is also the neurotransmitter for postganglionic parasympathetic neurons and for postganglionic sympathetic neurons (sudomotor) to sweat glands, but the receptor for the neurotransmitter is different. Autonomic ganglia primarily have nicotinic receptors, which are blocked by hexamethonium, whereas smooth muscle receptors are muscarinic and are blocked by atropine. The enzyme acetylcholinesterase destroys released Ach in the synapse. The remainder of postganglionic sympathetic nerve fibers are adrenergic and use norepinephrine at synapses. Adrenal and other chromaffin tissues release epinephrine into the circulation after stimulation. Two general categories of receptors exist at adrenergic synapses, α and β, although subcategories are recognized. In general, α-receptors are excitatory and β-receptors are inhibitory, although the heart and viscera are exceptions. Norepinephrine is catalyzed by the enzymes monoamine oxidase (MAO) and catechol-O-methyltransferase (COMT), although reuptake by the nerve terminal is the most potent regulatory mechanism.

The Sympathetic System

Preganglionic cell bodies lie in the intermediolateral cell column of the spinal cord between T1 and L2. Postganglionic cell bodies are found in either the sympathetic trunks (chains) or the prevertebral ganglia. The sympathetic trunks are formed by ganglia that are interconnected but not strictly

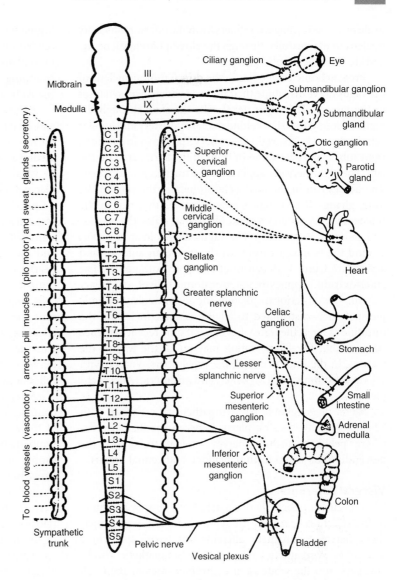

FIGURE 21.14 Diagram of the autonomic nervous system (ANS). (From Carpenter MB, Sutin J. *Human neuroanatomy*, 8th ed. Baltimore: Williams & Wilkins, 1983:211, with permission.)

segmental and run from C1 to the coccyx. The trunks lie on the anterior surface of the lateral masses in the cervical spine and transverse processes in the thoracolumbar spine and cross in front of the sacral promontory to fuse at the coccyx. There are three cervical ganglia: the superior, middle, and inferior (stellate). The nerve fibers from the spinal cord are myelinated (B fibers) as they enter the sympathetic trunks and are called *white rami communicantes*. Postganglionic nerve fibers returning to the spinal nerve are unmyelinated (C fibers) and are called *gray rami communicantes*. The preganglionic fibers run up and down in the sympathetic trunk, and some synapse with postganglionic neurons within the trunk. Others pass through to reach the prevertebral ganglia. The prevertebral ganglia are related to the abdominal aorta and its branches and are embedded in extensive plexuses, including cardiac, pulmonary, celiac, superior and inferior mesenteric, renal, and hypogastric (pelvic) plexuses. Three nerves, composed of white rami communicantes, course from the thoracic sympathetic chain as the greater, lesser, and least splanchnic nerves. The first two go to the celiac plexus and the last go to the renal plexus, where they

synapse on postganglionic neurons. Postganglionic nerve fibers reach their target organ by traveling with cranial or spinal nerves, by coursing in the adventitia of arteries, or through a combination of both.

The Parasympathetic System

Four parasympathetic ganglia are recognized in the head. The ciliary ganglion receives preganglionic fibers from the Edinger-Westphal nucleus (oculomotor) in the midbrain, through the oculomotor nerve, and sends postganglionic fibers to the pupil. It is located within the orbit. The pterygopalatine ganglion is in close relation to the maxillary division of the trigeminal nerve near the foramen rotundum. It receives preganglionic fibers from the superior salivatory nucleus in the pons, through the intermedius portion of the facial nerve, and supplies the lacrimal and intranasal glands. The submandibular ganglion at the base of the tongue receives similar input through the facial nerve and chorda tympani and supplies the submandibular and sublingual glands. Finally, the otic ganglion that is adjacent to the mandibular division of the trigeminal nerve near the foramen ovale receives preganglionic fibers from the inferior salivatory nucleus in the medulla, through the glossopharyngeal nerve, and supplies the parotid gland.

Preganglionic cell bodies in the dorsal motor nucleus of the vagus nerve distribute their fibers to widespread synapses in the viscera. The vagus nerve exits the skull through the jugular foramen and lies behind the carotid artery and jugular vein in the neck. The right vagus nerve passes in front of the right subclavian artery and in front of the aortic arch on the left. The right nerve is applied to the trachea more closely. The nerves run in the mediastinum behind the root of the lung, giving off recurrent laryngeal nerves that run in the tracheoesophageal groove and fibers that enter the cardiac and pulmonary plexuses. The vagus nerves form a plexus around the esophagus from which emerge an anterior and a posterior trunk, with contributions from both nerves. The anterior trunk supplies the anterior stomach, liver, and biliary system. The posterior trunk joins the abdominal autonomic plexus and is distributed to all the viscera, including the intestine as far as the transverse colon. Some recent evidence suggests that vagal innervation may go all the way to the rectum. In the intestinal wall, the vagal fibers synapse with cells in the submucosal (Meissner) and myenteric (Auerbach) plexuses.

Sacral preganglionic parasympathetic fibers travel with S2–S4 to the hypogastric plexus between the iliac arteries, where pelvic splanchnic nerves emerge to supply the descending colon and rectum, bladder, and genital organs.

Visceral Afferents

Visceral afferent fibers that originate from sensory receptors in the viscera course with the sympathetic and parasympathetic nerves. Sympathetic afferents travel with splanchnic and other sympathetic nerves to the sympathetic trunks and pass into the white rami communicantes to their cell bodies in the dorsal root ganglia. Although all afferent cell bodies are in the dorsal root ganglia, it is estimated that 20% of ventral root fibers represent visceral afferents and another 10% represent somatic afferents. These enter the spinal cord with the ventral root and are distributed to spinal gray matter. Parasympathetic afferents travel with the facial, glossopharyngeal, and vagus nerves with cell bodies in the geniculate, inferior glossopharyngeal (petrosal), and inferior vagal (nodose) ganglia, respectively. Sacral visceral afferents pass with the pelvic nerves to the dorsal root ganglia of S2–S4 and enter the conus medullaris.

Visceral Reflexes

The simplest autonomic reflex arc involves afferent input from a visceral or somatic afferent fiber, with its cell body in the dorsal root ganglion. This synapses on an interneuron in the spinal cord gray matter, which in turn connects to a preganglionic autonomic neuron in the intermediolateral column of the cord. The preganglionic cell synapses on a postganglionic cell in an autonomic ganglion, which is the final effector cell. Therefore, three synapses are involved, unlike the monosynaptic arc of a deep tendon reflex.

Segmental reflexes from the abdominal viscera include reddening of the skin and contraction of the abdominal musculature (guarding) from distension, inflammation, and cramping of the intestine and inhibition of intestinal motility (ileus) from peri-intestinal inflammation.

Reflexes concerning cardiac rate, cardiac contractility, and systemic arterial pressure (SAP) are mediated through the reticular formation in the medulla in what is considered a cardiovascular autonomic center. Heart rate is affected both by vagal fibers and sympathetic afferents through the cardiac nerves (T1–T5), which converge in the superficial and deep cardiac plexuses in front and behind the aortic arch, respectively, and the cardiac ganglia near the sinoatrial and atrioventricular nodes. Sympathetic input is β-adrenergic and increases heart rate. Parasympathetic input decreases heart rate through a muscarinic type receptor. β-Adrenergic sympathetic nerves also synapse directly on cardiac muscle cells, increasing contractility and, consequently, stroke volume and cardiac output. There is no direct parasympathetic effect on cardiac contractility. Cardiac visceral afferents travel with the vagus nerve to the medulla and with the sympathetic nerves to the cervicothoracic spinal cord both to monitor reflex activity and to convey cardiac pain.

Arterial blood pressure (ABP) depends on the rate and contractility of the heart but more so on vasoconstriction of the arterioles, which is mediated through α-adrenergic sympathetic receptors. There is no direct parasympathetic supply to the arterioles of the skin and muscles, but parasympathetic input to the coronary vessels and some viscera (especially the kidney) have been demonstrated. Baroreceptors in the aortic arch (vagal) and carotid sinus (glossopharyngeal) provide afferents to the nucleus solitarius in the medulla to maintain ABP. A constant secretion of epinephrine from the adrenal medulla also helps to maintain blood pressure. When blood pressure drops, there is reflex vasoconstriction of the arterioles to the skin and abdominal viscera and constriction of the venous system. This is associated with dilation of the arterioles of the brain and the coronary arteries and an increase in heart rate. With muscular activity, there is a marked dilation of blood vessels to muscle that is sympathetic but cholinergically mediated, probably through a nicotinic-type receptor. Cardiac output is increased, and there is vasoconstriction of the blood vessels to the skin and abdominal viscera. The afferent signaling of these responses is not well understood.

There is thought to be a respiratory center in the medullary reticular formation that can be divided into inspiratory and expiratory areas. These are under the control of a pontine respiratory center that, in turn, is influenced by hypothalamic, limbic, and cortical centers. Visceral and somatic afferents have their sensory endings in the epithelium of the respiratory tract from the trachea and major bronchi to the alveoli. In addition to touch, stretch, and pain receptors, some endings respond to carbon dioxide tension (chemoreceptors). Cell bodies for these fibers are in the nodose ganglion of the vagus nerve. These synapse through the medullary respirator center with motor nerves to the diaphragm and accessory muscles of respiration in the spinal cord to mediate respiratory and cough reflexes. Chemoreceptors are also found in the carotid and aortic bodies, which respond to carbon dioxide and, to a lesser extent, oxygen tension in the blood. These fibers accompany the carotid sinus nerve (glossopharyngeal) and vagus nerve, respectively.

Swallowing reflexes involve sensory (glossopharyngeal) and motor (vagal) inputs. Although the pharynx and upper esophagus are supplied by the vagus nerve, they are striated muscle and, therefore, are not considered autonomic. The esophagus gradually becomes autonomic innervated smooth muscle. The presence of food initiates the swallowing reflex and a wave of esophageal contraction. Overstimulation of the posterior pharynx causes the gag reflex. Vagal stimulation increases peristalsis in the gastrointestinal tract, relaxes sphincters, and increases secretion of hydrochloric acid and pepsin in the stomach. Sympathetic stimulation has the opposite effects and causes vasoconstriction in the intestinal vasculature. Visceral pain is conducted through the sympathetic visceral afferents. Gallbladder, biliary, and pancreatic ducts are contracted and sphincters are relaxed by parasympathetic stimulation. Sympathetic stimulation inhibits contraction of the ducts and closes the sphincters. Rectal and anal reflexes are mediated through the sacral parasympathetic system.

Parasympathetic supply to the kidney is through the vagus nerve, and sympathetic supply is through the celiac ganglion and splanchnic nerves to the renal plexus. Parasympathetic stimulation increases and sympathetic stimulation decreases renal blood flow; hence urinary output. The ureter receives parasympathetic input from both the vagus nerve and the sacral segments, and sympathetic input from the lower splanchnic nerves. Stimulation of either system has little effect on ureter function, and the kidney and ureter can be denervated as in transplantation without any functional impairment. Micturition is mediated through the parasympathetic system. Stretch receptors in the bladder wall stimulate visceral afferents that travel with the pelvic nerves to spinal cord levels S2–S4. Parasympathetic efferents over the same nerves cause contraction of the detrusor muscle and relaxation of the sphincters. These neurons are influenced by a micturition center in the pontine reticular formation, which in turn is under cortical control. Sympathetic input mildly inhibits bladder contraction but may be responsible for preventing reflux into the ureters. Erection is caused by parasympathetically (S2–S4) induced vascular engorgement of the penis. Emission of semen is a sympathetic function, and ejaculation is a combination of autonomic and somatic activities.

THE CEREBRAL CIRCULATION

Cerebrovascular Anatomy

The arterial blood supply to the brain arises from the aortic arch. The right common carotid and subclavian arteries are

the primary branches of the innominate artery. The left common carotid artery usually arises directly from the aortic arch. The vertebral arteries are proximal branches of the subclavian arteries. The common carotid arteries bifurcate at about the C3–C4 level into internal carotid arteries (ICAs), carrying blood to the brain, and external carotid arteries, carrying blood to the neck, face, mouth, jaw, scalp, and meninges. Potential anastomoses between the two systems exist, especially around the orbit and upper face, which become important with carotid artery stenosis or occlusion.

Small branches of the intracavernous ICA supply the pituitary gland and meninges and have surgical importance in cases of carotid-cavernous fistula. Intracranial branches of the ICA, in order, are the ophthalmic, which courses with the optic nerve to the orbit; the posterior communicating, which crosses the oculomotor nerve and connects to the posterior cerebral artery (PCA); the anterior choroidal, which runs between the uncus and the cerebral peduncle before entering the choroidal fissure; the small superior hypophyseal branches, which run along the pituitary stalk; and the terminal branches of the anterior and middle cerebral arteries.

The two ICA systems are interconnected through the anterior communicating artery, a channel of considerable variability. The posterior communicating artery connects each ICA to the basilar artery through the posterior cerebral arteries. This system of junctions is called the *circle of Willis*. In 10% to 15% of cases, the PCA will be supplied primarily by the ICA. Variability of size of these arterial segments is common and has relevance to the ability of diseased carotid arteries to sustain the cerebral circulation.

The anterior communicating artery courses horizontally to the skull base between the frontal lobe and optic chiasm, giving medial striate branches to the basal ganglia, cortical branches to the orbital frontal lobe, and with the anterior communicating artery, branches to the optic chiasm and hypothalamus. Distal to the anterior communicating artery, paired anterior cerebral (pericallosal) arteries ascend over the genu of the corpus callosum and remain in the callosal cistern to anastomose with smaller pericallosal branches of the posterior cerebral arteries. Cortical branches, including fronto-orbital, frontopolar, callosomarginal, and cranial, supply the mesial cerebral hemisphere. Disorders of consciousness, affect, and hypothalamic function occur with ischemia in the proximal anterior cerebral artery distribution. More distal ischemia affects the legs more than the arms because of the mesial hemisphere cortical representation. Bilateral ischemia in this distribution can cause leg weakness, gait disturbance, and bladder dysfunction, suggestive of spinal cord disease.

The middle cerebral artery (MCA) is the primary continuation of the ICA, coursing in the sylvian fissure between the frontal and temporal lobes and over the insula of Reil. Lateral striate or "lenticulostriate" branches arise before the primary bifurcation of the artery and perforate the basal frontal lobe to supply the basal ganglia and internal capsule. Because the corticospinal fibers are concentrated at the genu and posterior limb of the capsule, occlusion of a small lenticulostriate branch can cause a profound contralateral hemiplegia, often in the absence of sensory findings. At the edge of the insula, the MCA bifurcates and turns posteriorly. In general, the superior trunk supplies the frontal lobe back to the central sulcus and the inferior trunk supplies the parietal and temporal lobes, but considerable variation exists in the patterns of branching. Viewed in a sagittal plane, the MCA supplies the lateral two thirds of the cerebral hemisphere and the basal ganglia, and the anterior cerebral and PCA supply the medial one third of the hemisphere anteriorly and posteriorly, respectively. The anterior choroidal artery divides to supply the uncal area of the temporal lobe and continues between the temporal lobe and brainstem, supplying the lower diencephalon and posterior internal capsule before entering the choroidal fissure in the temporal horn of the ventricle to supply the choroid plexus.

The vertebral arteries arise from the subclavian artery on each side and ascend through the foramina transversaria of the cervical vertebrae from C6 to C2. They exit at C2, cross behind the atlas, and enter the foramen magnum anterior to the hypoglossal nerve rootlets. The vertebral arteries join at the pontomedullary junction to form the basilar artery, which continues anterior to the pons and mesencephalon and divides between the cerebral peduncles into the posterior cerebral arteries. Connection of these arteries to the ICA through the posterior communicating arteries completes the circle of Willis.

Three pairs of cerebellar arteries arise from the vertebral and basilar arteries in the posterior fossa. The posterior inferior cerebellar artery (PICA) is a branch of the vertebral artery, usually at the level of the medulla. It courses underneath CNs IX, X, and XI, supplying the lateral medulla; courses around the cerebellar tonsil; gives branches to the choroid plexus of the fourth ventricle; and divides into inferior vermian and hemispheral branches. The anterior inferior cerebellar artery (AICA) is usually the smallest of the cerebellar arteries. It arises from the basilar artery at the lower pons in close relation to the origin of CN VI. It then follows CNs VII and VIII into the cerebellopontine angle, supplying the lateral pons; loops laterally; and courses on the inferior surface of the cerebellum. The superior cerebellar artery (SCA) arises near the basilar artery bifurcation, courses around the midbrain and pons between CNs III and V, and divides into hemispheral and superior vermian branches. A reciprocal size relation generally exists among the cerebellar arteries.

The PCA is the terminal branch of the basilar artery. It courses around the midbrain anterior to CN III and supplies the thalamus and midbrain. Over the quadrigeminal plate, the artery gives branches to the hippocampal (posterior temporal) area and divides into a calcarine branch, supplying the visual cortex, and a parieto-occipital branch, going to visual and parietal association areas.

Paramedian branches of the basilar artery supply the medial brainstem. More inferiorly, the anterior spinal artery,

a common branch of the vertebral arteries, supplies the medial medulla and continues caudally to supply the spinal cord. Perforating branches to the thalamus are termed *anterior* if they arise from the posterior communicating artery and posterior if they arise from the PCA. The posterior cerebral arteries also give off medial and lateral posterior choroidal arteries, which supply the diencephalon and choroid plexus. In the spinal cord, the anterior spinal artery is reconstituted by segmental arteries, including the large lumbar radicular artery of Adamkiewicz, which serves the cord below about T10 and is important in operations on the abdominal aorta. The anterior spinal artery supplies the anterior two thirds of the cord, and the paired posterior spinal arteries supply the dorsal one third.

Cerebral veins can be divided into superficial and deep systems. The superficial system drains superiorly and inferiorly from the superficial middle cerebral veins of the sylvian fissure. Superiorly running veins drain into the superior sagittal sinus. The largest of these is called the *vein of Trolard*. Inferiorly running veins drain into the sphenoparietal, petrosal, and transverse (lateral) sinuses. The largest of these is termed the *vein of Labbé*. The veins are considered anastomotic because blood can drain through them in either direction. Veins from the mesial hemisphere drain into the falx and the inferior and superior sagittal sinuses.

The deep venous system includes the deep anterior and middle cerebral veins that form the basal vein of Rosenthal. This vein courses around the brainstem in close relation to the PCA and enters the vein of Galen in the quadrigeminal area. Subependymal veins in the ventricles drain the deep hemisphere. Septal and caudate veins join to form the internal cerebral vein. The thalamostriate vein runs on top of the thalamus in the floor of the lateral ventricle. It joins the internal cerebral vein near the foramen of Monro (venous angle), and the paired internal cerebral veins continue posteriorly in the roof of the third ventricle to drain into the vein of Galen. Posterior fossa veins drain from the cerebellum and around the brainstem toward midline to form the precentral cerebellar veins, which in turn drain into the vein of Galen. Other posterior fossa veins empty directly into the petrosal, transverse, and cavernous sinuses. Pericallosal veins from the splenium of the corpus callosum also enter the vein of Galen. The vein of Galen is therefore formed by the paired internal cerebral, basal, precentral cerebellar, and pericallosal veins. It lies dorsal to the quadrigeminal (collicular) plate and drains into the straight sinus at the junction of the falx and tentorium.

The superior sagittal and straight sinuses converge at the torcula (torcular herophili) and continue as the paired transverse (lateral) sinuses. These are joined by the superior petrosal sinuses behind the mastoid processes and descend as the sigmoid sinuses, which form the jugular bulbs at the jugular foramen, and continue into the neck as the internal jugular veins. Connections between the sigmoid, petrosal, and cavernous sinuses and the pterygoid plexus allow for collateral drainage when the internal jugular veins are blocked. The torcula may be incomplete, most often with the superior sagittal sinus and superficial system running to the right transverse sinus and the straight sinus and deep system draining to the left. This can preclude elective ligation of a major sinus.

The basal subarachnoid space is divided into a system of well-defined cisterns. These compartments allow a convenient road map for understanding vascular and CN anatomy. Especially well-developed is a sheet of arachnoid, Lilliequist membrane, extending across the tentorial notch between the unci of the temporal lobes and surrounding the pituitary stalk, effectively dividing the supratentorial and infratentorial compartments ventrally. Cisterns above this membrane include (i) the carotid cistern with the ICA and its branches, (ii) the chiasmatic cistern with the optic nerves and ophthalmic arteries, (iii) the sylvian cistern with the MCA and its branches, (iv) the crural cistern with the anterior choroidal artery and basal vein of Rosenthal, (v) the lamina terminalis cistern with the anterior cerebral and anterior communicating and recurrent arteries, and (vi) the callosal cistern with the pericallosal arteries. Cisterns around the upper brainstem include the interpeduncular cistern with the basilar bifurcation, posterior cerebral and posterior communicating arteries, and CN III; the ambient cistern with the posterior cerebral, superior cerebellar, and posterior choroidal arteries; the quadrigeminal cistern with the vein of Galen, pineal gland, and CN IV; and the velum interpositum cistern with the posterior medial choroidal artery and the internal cerebral veins. Posterior fossa cisterns include the prepontine cistern with the basilar artery, origins of the AICA, and CN VI; the cerebellopontine cistern with AICA, CNs V, VII, and VIII, and the foramen of Luschka; the premedullary cistern with the anterior spinal artery and CN XII; the cerebellomedullary cistern with the vertebral arteries, PICA, and CNs IX, X, and XI; and the cisterna magna with the distal PICA and the foramen of Magendie. These relations form the basis of a microsurgical anatomy for basal tumors and intracranial vascular surgery.

Cerebrovascular Physiology

The brain has a mass of approximately 1,500 g (2% body weight) and has a total brain blood flow of approximately 750 mL/min (15% of cardiac output). Each carotid artery carries approximately 300 mL/min, and the vertebrobasilar system carries 150 mL/min. Therefore, average cerebral blood flow (CBF) is approximately 50 mL/100 g/min. Separate gray and white matter compartments are recognized with CBF of 75 to 80 mL and 20 to 25 mL/100 g/min, respectively. Capillary density in gray matter is also approximately four times that of white matter. The metabolic rate of oxygen ($CMRo_2$) in the brain under resting conditions is approximately 3.0 to 3.5 mL/100 g/min (20% of total body oxygen consumption), and the metabolic rate of glucose (CMRGlu) is 25 to 30 mol (3.5–5.0 mg)/100 g/min. The brain depends on a continuous supply of oxygen and glucose, and with total global ischemia, unconsciousness ensues in

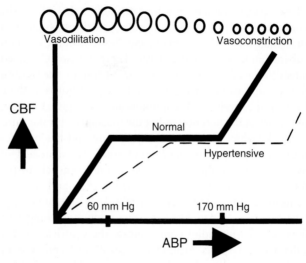

FIGURE 21.15 Graphic relation of cerebral blood flow (CBF) to arterial blood pressure (ABP) with progressive vasoconstriction being responsible for the flat portion of the curve (autoregulation). Note that the curve is shifted to the right in hypertension.

approximately 10 seconds and irreversible damage occurs in 4 to 5 minutes.

CBF remains constant over a range of systemic ABPs, generally between approximately 60 and 170 mm Hg mean ABP. This is termed *autoregulation* (Fig. 21.15). The range of autoregulation will be elevated in chronic hypertension. Autoregulation is based on the underlying vascular caliber. This caliber and therefore CBF depends greatly on the arterial tension of carbon dioxide ($Paco_2$) increasing or decreasing approximately 2.5% for each 1 mm Hg change in $Paco_2$ between 30 and 60 mm Hg.

Poiseuille Law

$$CBF = (\pi [P_1(8 - \eta LP)_2]R^4)$$

describing newtonian flow through a cylinder gives particular insight into mechanisms controlling CBF. The dependence on pressure ($P_1 - P_2$) shows a direct relation to CBF. The dependence on vessel caliber shows a fourth-power relation to vessel radius and illustrates how even minor vessel dilation may cause significant increases in CBF. The symbol for viscosity (η) shows an inverse relation. Agents such as mannitol, which decrease viscosity as well as hemodilution, will increase CBF.

Activation of brain areas causes a focal increase in CBF, $CMRo_2$, and CMRGlu. This is called *coupling of CBF to metabolism*. The precise regulatory mechanism is not clear, but adenosine is believed to be an important signal, whereas H^+, K^+, and CO_2 seem less important.

CEREBROSPINAL FLUID

CSF is contained in the ventricles and the cerebral and spinal subarachnoid spaces, and is continuous with the brain extracellular space through the ependyma and pia mater.

These spaces contain approximately 150 mL CSF in the young adult, of which 25 mL is in the ventricles, 50 mL is in the spinal subarachnoid space, and 75 mL is in the cerebral subarachnoid space and cisterns. There are two C-shaped lateral ventricles composed of an atrium in the central portion and frontal, temporal, and occipital horns in these lobes, respectively. Each communicates through a foramen of Monro at the anterior end of the thalamus with the third ventricle, which lies between the thalami and has recesses into the hypothalamus and pineal areas. The aqueduct of Sylvius in the midbrain connects the third ventricle to the fourth ventricle, which lie between the pons and medulla ventrally and the cerebellum dorsally. Two lateral openings (the foramina of Luschka) and one midline opening (the foramen of Magendie) communicate the ventricles to the subarachnoid space. Around the spinal cord and base of the brain, the subarachnoid space is large and forms cisterns, described in more detail previously. On the cortical surface, the arachnoid is more closely applied to the pia and extends into the sulci and white matter around the blood vessels as the Virchow-Robin spaces.

CSF is produced in the choroid plexus, a special vascularized epithelium that extends from the choroidal fissure in the temporal horn, where it receives the anterior and lateral posterior choroidal arteries, through the atrium to the foramen of Monro and into the roof of the third ventricle, where it receives the medial posterior choroidal artery. There is no choroid plexus in the frontal or occipital horns. Choroid plexus is also found in the roof of the fourth ventricle, where it is supplied by choroidal branches of the PICA.

Approximately 70% of CSF is generated by the choroid plexus, the other 30% from brain capillaries and metabolic water. CSF production is 0.35 mL/min, or approximately 500 mL/d. Therefore, the entire CSF volume turns over three to four times each 24 hours. Generation of CSF results from hydrostatic forces and through an active Na^+ transport system that depends on Na^+/K^+/adenosine triphosphatase (ATPase). The role of carbonic anhydrase in the Na^+ transport is unclear, but acetazolamide, a carbonic anhydrase inhibitor, decreases production of CSF. CSF production is selective with increased Mg^{2+} and Cl^-; decreased glucose, K^+, Ca^{2+}; and negligible protein secreted compared with plasma levels. CSF is absorbed at the arachnoid villi, clusters of arachnoid cells that project into the dural sinuses. These act as one-way valves, requiring a pressure of approximately 3 mm Hg to open, and preventing reflux of blood and plasma into the CSF. The villi have the capacity to absorb approximately five times normal CSF production. Resting pressure of the CSF is between 60 and 180 mm H_2O (5–13 mm Hg).

Inflammation within the meninges causes an increase in protein, appearance of white blood cells, and sometimes lowering of glucose in CSF. Subarachnoid hemorrhage is associated with ruptured cerebral aneurysms, vascular malformations, and trauma. Neoplastic cells may be seen in cases of CNS malignancy. Lumbar puncture (LP) is used to obtain CSF for diagnostic tests, measure intracranial pressure (ICP), and deliver therapeutic agents into the CSF (intrathecally).

Generally, the lumbar subarachnoid space is in communication with the cerebral subarachnoid space. When this is not the case, a pressure gradient may exist. Under these circumstances, LP will lower spinal pressure and may cause brain or spinal cord displacement (herniation), often with disastrous consequences. A focal neurologic deficit should always be viewed as a relative contraindication for LP until more precise information [computed tomography (CT)/magnetic resonance imaging (MRI)] is available. Markedly elevated protein on LP (Froin syndrome) may be an indicator of a spinal block and a precursor to an impending spinal herniation.

An imbalance in the production or absorption of CSF causes ventricular enlargement (hydrocephalus). Hydrocephalus is categorized as obstructive, meaning the ventricular system is blocked, or communicating, meaning the subarachnoid pathways or arachnoid villi are obstructed. In most cases of obstructive and acute communicating hydrocephalus, ICP is increased, resulting in headache, vomiting, visual disturbance, and decreased level of consciousness. Congenital stenoses, brain tumors, acute hemorrhage, and inflammation are common etiologic factors. In cases of chronic communicating hydrocephalus, the ICP may be normal because of a compensated ventriculomegaly. Typical symptoms in this setting are dementia, gait apraxia, and urinary incontinence. The etiology is often obscure. Sometimes, a prior history of meningitis or subarachnoid hemorrhage may be obtained, whereas in other cases it is idiopathic (normal pressure hydrocephalus).

BLOOD–BRAIN BARRIER

The brain extracellular space constitutes approximately 15% of brain volume. Although relatively free passage of solutes exists between the CSF in the ventricles, subarachnoid spaces, and the extracellular space, molecules in the blood are selectively allowed passage into the extracellular space and CSF. This is termed the *BBB* and is based on special connections between capillary endothelial cells (tight junctions). The BBB continues out into the peripheral nerve at the level of the perineurial capillaries to continue as the blood–nerve barrier. The BBB serves both to control the chemical environment of the neurons and glial cells and to protect the brain from potentially harmful substances. In general, lipid-soluble compounds pass easily through the capillary endothelium, and ionic compounds pass with difficulty. Water and diffusible gases such as oxygen and carbon dioxide are not restricted. To allow entry of important nutrients such as glucose and amino acids, specific transport systems are used. These enzymatic groups are stereospecific, saturable, and competitively inhibited. A similar process is used for returning small ionic molecules from the CSF to the bloodstream. The circumventricular organs (area postrema, median eminence, etc.) are areas where the BBB is not present and allow receptors in the brain to sense molecules in the blood.

Delivery of drugs into the CSF depends on their lipid solubility and use of carrier mechanisms. In pathologic states, the capillary endothelium can be damaged or tight junctions can be destroyed, rendering the BBB inoperable. This contributes to vasogenic edema and may allow circulating toxins to pass into the brain. However, loss of the BBB allows intravascular contrast media to enhance abnormal areas of the brain on imaging studies and allows chemotherapeutic agents and antibiotics to pass in the brain and CSF more easily. Intravenous mannitol will temporarily open the BBB and has been used to improve delivery of antineoplastic drugs.

CEREBRAL ELECTRICAL ACTIVITY

Electroencephalography

All neurons exhibit continuous generation of electrical impulses. Excitation and inhibition can be considered alterations in the rate of neuron firing. When groups of neurons, firing simultaneously, are large enough, change in potential can be recorded through the scalp as an EEG. Cortical cells, especially pyramidal cells, are oriented perpendicular to the surface and arranged in columns. Electrically, these create dipoles. Their dendritic potentials summate to create waves of depolarization and repolarization. The EEG records the differences in potential between bipolar electrodes or a unipolar electrode and a reference, amplifies the microvolt potentials, and records them on an oscilloscope or chart paper for analysis. Usually, 16 electrodes are used, and a given array of electrodes is termed a *montage*.

EEG activity is categorized by frequency. α-Waves (8–13 Hz) predominate in the occipital areas at rest. They are synchronous between the two hemispheres and are believed to be generated from thalamic and brainstem sources. β-Activity (14–30 Hz) results from arousal, eye opening, and some drugs. It predominates in the frontal and central areas. It is of lower voltage than α-activity and nonsynchronous. θ-Waves (4–7 Hz) and δ-waves (1–3 Hz) are considered pathologic in an awake adult and, when localized, suggest a structural brain lesion. Sharp voltage activity (spikes); high-frequency, high-voltage discharges; distinctive spike; and special wave patterns are associated with seizure disorders. Diffuse encephalopathies show loss of normal patterns and generalized slowing. Triphasic waves are associated with hepatic encephalopathy.

The use of EEG monitoring during carotid endarterectomy is based on the correlation of CBF with EEG. An EEG record will show slowing with ischemia and will become isoelectric with a reduction of CBF below 20 mL/100 g/min. EEG monitoring can be used to assess the need for intraoperative vascular shunting.

Evoked Potentials

Evoked potentials refer to the electrical responses obtained in cortex, brainstem, or spinal cord after stimulation elsewhere in the nervous system. Typically, responses are averaged over many repetitions to enhance the desired response and to average-out background activity. Evoked potentials demonstrate continuity in the pathways being evaluated and, when altered, suggest dysfunction specific to these pathways.

Somatosensory evoked potentials (SSEPs) use stimulation of the median or tibial nerves and record over the somatosensory cortex (postcentral gyrus). They primarily record conduction in the posterior columns, medial lemniscus, thalamus, and cortex. The principal cortical response has a latency of approximately 19 ms. Visual evoked responses (VERs) record potential changes in the occipital cortex in response to flashing lights or checkerboard patterns, and evaluate transmission through the retina, optic nerves, optic tracts, lateral geniculate body, optic radiations, and occipital cortex. Brainstem auditory evoked responses (BAERs) are obtained by stimulating with repetitive clicks in the ear and recording over the auditory cortex. Depolarizing waves are demonstrated in the cochlea, auditory nerve, and brainstem structures in addition to the cortex. These are termed *far-field potentials*. BAERs are used primarily to demonstrate brainstem abnormalities. Methods under investigation to record motor evoked potentials include electrical and magnetic stimulation of the motor cortex and spinal corticospinal tracts.

Evoked potentials have proved useful for intraoperative monitoring and diagnostic evaluations. SSEPs are used in spinal operations and operations on the abdominal aorta to monitor spinal cord function. They can be used to evaluate cerebral function in carotid surgery and in cases of subarachnoid hemorrhage. Motor evoked potentials may be more predictive of outcome in these settings. BAERs are used in operations in the posterior fossa and VERs in pituitary and other operations around the optic nerves and chiasm.

Sleep

The sleep-wake cycle is one example of circadian rhythms that seems to be genetically encoded and is found in all animals. The inherent sleep-wake cycle in humans is closer to 25 to 26 hours but is modified by environmental factors to create a 24-hour periodicity. Five stages of sleep are described based on EEG and observation. The resting individual shows α-rhythm in the occipital areas. As sleep comes, the EEG shows progressive slowing through θ- to δ-wave activity. Specific wave complexes—sleep spindles and K complexes—appear in deeper sleep. This process then reverses itself and returns to lighter sleep patterns; the cycle is repeated three or four times a night. During the earlier stages of sleep, there is a loss of muscle tone associated with rapid eye movements (REMs). REM sleep is correlated with dreaming and seems to be a necessary component of sleep. The brainstem basis for non-REM sleep is postulated to be serotonergic neurons in the raphe nuclei; for REM sleep, it is thought to be noradrenergic neurons in the locus ceruleus. Sleep is independent of coma, and destruction of the ARAS does not abolish sleep cycles.

PATHOLOGIC CONDITIONS

Decreased Levels of Consciousness

Consciousness is appreciated instinctively but not defined easily. Clinically, a person is considered fully conscious when he or she is attentive and responsive, demonstrating spontaneous purposeful activity and using coherent thought patterns. Affective abnormalities such as anxiety, fear, and depression generally are not considered disordered levels of consciousness, whereas agitation, sluggishness, or incoherence may be the earliest findings in a patient lapsing into coma. Similarly, patients with dementia and psychosis are considered to retain consciousness, although they might be immobile and unresponsive. Decreased levels of consciousness include lethargy, where a person is drowsy, needs to be stimulated to respond and often does so incompletely, but is verbal and will follow command; stupor or obtundation, where there is minimal verbalization and limited response to command but there is semipurposeful to purposeful response to pain; semicoma, where there is no verbalization and stereotyped or reflex responses to pain; and coma, where the patient is unresponsive to pain or command. These classifications form a continuum, and full description is preferred in medical communication (Table 21.1). The Glasgow coma scale is commonly used to grade levels of consciousness in patients with head injuries and gives a score from 15 (fully awake) to 3 (comatose) based on best verbal response, best motor response, and eye opening.

The physiologic basis of consciousness is considered to be the ARAS in the upper pons and midbrain and its projections through the nonspecific thalamic nuclei and hypothalamus to the limbic and prefrontal cortex and ultimately to the cerebral hemispheres, especially the left hemisphere. Isolated lesions of one hemisphere do not impair consciousness, although they may depress affect. Therefore, a patient must have either widespread damage to both hemispheres or a lesion affecting the ARAS to experience a decrease in level of consciousness.

As the brain exquisitely depends on oxygen and glucose for function, any deprivation of these—such as through anoxia, decreased CBF with hypotension, insulin overdosage, or carbon monoxide or cyanide poisoning—will lead to decreased consciousness. Similarly, a variety of metabolic and toxic alterations can lead to coma, including hyponatremia, hypocalcemia, myxedema, meningitis, uremia, hyperammonianemia, and a host of anesthetic and sedative drugs. Some of these affect the entire brain; others act more specifically on pathways concerned with consciousness.

Structural lesions in the brain cause coma if they involve the ARAS and its projections. Therefore, lesions in the upper brainstem may be associated primarily with coma. Hemispherical lesions produce coma by secondary effects on the upper brainstem (see "Herniation Syndromes").

Cerebral Ischemia

Cerebral ischemia is a common denominator of many pathologic processes, including arterial occlusion, hypotension, subarachnoid hemorrhage, head injury, local and generalized increases in brain pressure, and brain herniation syndromes. Resting CBF for the whole brain is approximately 50 mL/100 g/min. This can be lowered acutely to approximately 20 mL/100 g/min without change in function. Below this level, EEG changes are appreciated, suggesting that ischemia first affects synaptic transmission. Between 8 and 10 mL/100 g/min, there is a precipitous rise in extracellular potassium; this has been thought to signify cell death. CBF of less than 20 mL/100 g/min over a 30-minute period is often associated with cerebral infarction.

The relations between CBF, the metabolic rate of oxygen ($CMRo_2$), and the metabolic rate of glucose (CMRGlu) with ischemia are becoming clarified by positron emission tomographic (PET) scanning. Cerebral metabolism normally regulates CBF. With a decrease in CBF, $CMRo_2$ and CMRGlu are maintained initially by increased extraction of oxygen and glucose from the blood. This is termed *misery perfusion*. When CBF is inadequate to maintain metabolism, $CMRo_2$ and CMRGlu decline and infarction occurs. The area surrounding the area of infarction shows increased CBF (luxury perfusion) and, for a time, an increase in CMRGlu. Areas functionally connected but remote from the site of infarction show a decline in both CBF and $CMRo_2$. Those cases showing preservation of metabolism and reduced blood flow (misery perfusion) may represent an indication for revascularization, whereas those showing absence of metabolism and luxury perfusion would not be expected to benefit.

One clinical method that gives insight into CBF is measurement of the difference between arterial and venous oxygen saturation. This is measured by arterial O_2 sampling at a peripheral site and sampling of venous blood from the jugular bulb. The latter assumes complete mixing of venous blood from both hemispheres. A fixed relation exists between $AVDo_2$ and CBF at any given $CMRo_2$ (Figure 21.16). High

TABLE 21.1

Glasgow Coma Scale

Eye opening	Verbal response
4 Spontaneous	5 Oriented
3 To sound	4 Confused
2 To pain	3 Words
1 None	2 Sounds
	1 None
Motor response	
6 Follows commands	
5 Localizes stimulus	
4 Withdraws	
3 Flexion posturing	
2 Extension posturing	
1 No movements	

The Glasgow coma scale score is the sum total of responses in each category. Scores range between 3 and 15.

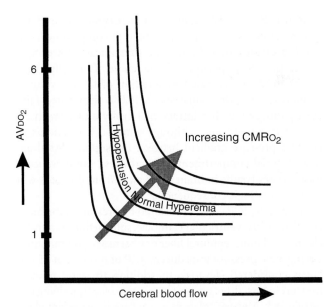

FIGURE 21.16 Graphic representation of the relation between arteriovenous oxygen saturation difference ($AVDO_2$) and cerebral blood flow (CBF) at different levels of metabolic rate of oxygen ($CMRO_2$).

values of 5 or 6 $CMRO_2$ suggest ischemia, whereas low values of 1 suggest relative hyperemia.

Mechanisms leading to ischemic cell death have undergone intensive investigation (3). One of the early biochemical changes in ischemia is the release of arachidonic acid from the cell membrane. This occurs before depletion of adenosine triphosphate (ATP) stores and is, therefore, believed to be an active phenomenon. Arachidonic acid is metabolized further in the presence of oxygen to prostaglandins and leukotrienes, which are involved in vasoactive and inflammatory processes that may propagate tissue damage. Ischemia changes are seen first at synapses with the release of excitatory neurotransmitters, especially glutamate. Depolarization of the postsynaptic membrane allows influx of calcium, and when this is excessive, it can activate phospholipases. These attack the cell membrane to release arachidonic acid. Glutamate receptors, especially the N-methyl-D-aspartate (NMDA) receptor, have been implicated in this process, and selective receptor blockers have been suggested to protect against cerebral ischemia (4).

An important component of these destructive chemical reactions seems to be the generation of oxygen-derived ionic radicals, termed *free radicals*. Oxygen in tissue can undergo several reductions to form superoxide anion. In addition, hydrogen peroxide and its reduced form, the hydroxyl radical, can also be produced. These intermediate radicals are extremely reactive and initiate chemical reactions that are destructive to proteins and phospholipid membranes. Sources for generation of free radicals of oxygen include xanthine oxidase, catecholamine oxidation, mitochondrial electron transport, metabolism of prostaglandins and leukotrienes, peroxidation of lipid membranes, and phagocytosis. Lipid peroxidation is associated with the oxidation of ferrous iron,

which in turn oxidizes the double bonds of fatty acids in the membranes of the cell and its organelles. This perpetuates a cycle of free radical generation. Possible protective compounds include corticosteroids, amino steroids, vitamin E, vitamin C, mannitol, xanthine oxidase inhibitors, dimethyl sulfoxide (DMSO), and the enzyme superoxide dismutase. Another important component of cell membrane damage is the increased entry of calcium into the cell cytoplasm that catalyzes untoward lipid and protein reactions. Calcium channel blockers such as nimodipine may attenuate this effect. Acidosis occurs in ischemic tissue as the metabolism of glucose is converted to anaerobic glycolysis, which results in the production of lactic acid. This effect is potentiated by hypercapnia. This would suggest that glucose- and lactate-containing intravenous fluids may be harmful in cerebral ischemia and emphasizes the importance of preventing hypoxia, hypercapnia, and acidosis in the arterial blood.

In addition to neuronal damage, ischemia also injures the cerebral microcirculation. Reduced blood flow occurs through areas of ischemia after reopening of the circulation (no-reflow phenomenon), which is attributed to endothelial swelling. A few hours after ischemia, the capillaries become permeable to macromolecules, signifying breakdown of the BBB. Associated with this is cerebral edema, which at first involves the glial cells (cytotoxic) and subsequently the extracellular space (vasogenic). The microcirculation either undergoes necrosis or recovers so that after a few weeks the BBB is restored. Damage to the microcirculation may represent a limiting factor to attempted CBF restoration in the clinical setting.

Cerebral Edema

Cerebral edema, or an increase in brain-tissue water content, results from a variety of insults: ischemic, traumatic, neoplastic, and others. Increased water in the brain ultimately derives from the vascular system and is, therefore, related to capillary integrity, the BBB, and the ionic environment of the tissue itself. When pathologic conditions within the tissue increase the ionic or oncotic (protein) osmotic pressure of the extracellular fluid, water moves into the extracellular space and subsequently into glial cells. This is termed *cytotoxic edema*. With damage to the capillary endothelium (ischemia or trauma) or difference in capillary endothelial structure (abscesses or neoplastic processes), solutes and proteins are lost into the extracellular space osmotically carrying water with them. This is termed *vasogenic edema*. Edema fluid moves through the brain by bulk flow and is eventually transferred into the subarachnoid space and ventricles. White matter shows more compliance than gray matter, and edema, therefore, tends to accumulate there.

A variety of biologically active compounds has been implicated in production of cerebral edema. The prostaglandins, leukotrienes, and oxygen-derived free radicals cause cerebral edema when injected directly into brain tissue. Bradykinin and other peptides within the kallikrein-kinin system also have been associated with production of brain edema. Ischemic brain edema shows increased levels of histamine and serotonin in the tissue. A variety of toxins are used experimentally to produce brain edema, but they may act through the earlier mechanisms.

Cerebral edema is important clinically because it raises ICP and induces brain shifts and herniation syndromes. Local compression of the microvasculature has been suggested but is unproven. Also unclear is whether cerebral edema *per se* affects neurologic function by changing the local environment. Experimental studies of controlled focal edema have shown no alteration in neurologic function.

Raised Intracranial Pressure

Pressure–Volume Relations

Mathematical models to describe ICP assume the skull to be an essentially inelastic container with several volume compartments (Monro-Kellie hypothesis): the brain tissue itself (1,500 mL), which is considered incompressible, although it can be distorted or shifted; the cerebral blood volume (CBV, 200 mL), which relates to CBF and vascular diameter; and the cerebrospinal fluid (CSF, 100 mL), which may be displaced from the cranium into the spinal canal and CN foramina or resorbed into the venous circulation. Of the CBV, only approximately 50 mL (3.5% of brain volume) is intraparenchymal; the rest is in the larger arteries, veins, and sinuses. CBV, rather than CBF, is a determinant of ICP. ICP varies with uncompensated changes in one or more of these volume compartments.

The pressure–volume relation describes a curve that is relatively flat to pressure increases over additions of volume until a point at which the curve rapidly steepens to become almost vertical (Figure 21.17). The flat area of the curve is presumed to demonstrate compensatory mechanisms such as movement of blood or CSF out of the cranial cavity, and the steep portion represents exhaustion of these compensatory mechanisms. The ability of the intracranial space to accommodate increases in volume is termed *compliance* (dV/dP), and the resistance to increases in volume is termed *elastance* (dP/dV). The actual curve generated by addition of volume depends on the compliance and elastance of the system and, therefore, varies between patients and pathologic processes. The important consequences of these pressure–volume relations are that, depending where

a given ICP is on the curve, small increases in volume may give precipitous rises in ICP or be well compensated, and small decreases in volume may dramatically lower ICP, as on the steep portion of the curve. Clinically, these curves must be generated by addition of known volumes of fluid to the intracranial space. ICP is distributed fairly evenly throughout the intracranial cavity and from tissue to ventricular pressure, although tentorial herniation may create a pressure gradient between the supratentorial and infratentorial compartments. Nevertheless, the presence of focal masses results in brain shifts away from the mass with severe physiologic consequences.

Clinically, ICP can be measured by pressure transducers coupled to intraventricular cannulae, subarachnoid cannulae (Richmond bolt), epidural fiber optic sensors, and miniature strain gauge pressure transducers. ICP of more than 15 mm Hg is considered elevated. In addition to static pressure measurements, three types of pressure waves (Lundberg) are recognized. A waves (plateau waves) are intermittent elevations of ICP from 50 to 100 mm Hg, lasting several minutes and probably related to vasodilation. These are associated with elevated ICP and herald clinical deterioration. B waves are 1-per-minute rhythmic fluctuations to 50 mm Hg associated with period respirations and a decreased level of consciousness. C waves are 4- to 8-per-minute waves to 20 mm Hg related to periodic fluctuations in ABP (Traube-Hering-Meyer) waves. Fourier waveform analysis has shown that the component frequencies of an ICP waveform shift toward higher frequencies with reduced compliance, but this observation also depends on heart rate and venous outflow resistance. ICP monitoring is used so that physicians may initiate treatment for raised ICP before clinical deterioration ensues.

Cerebral Blood Flow and Intracranial Pressure

To quantify a relation between CBF and ICP, an equation similar to Ohm law can be used with cerebral perfusion pressure (CPP)—the difference between SAP and ICP—representing the potential or voltage, the CBF representing the current flow, and their quotient representing the resistance. CPP = CBF × CVR, where CPP is expressed in mm Hg, CBF in mL/100 g/min, and cerebrovascular resistance (CVR) in mm Hg/mL/100 g/min. With generalized increase in ICP, CBF is maintained until CPP drops below 50 mm Hg. However, CBF is better maintained at the same CPP reached by elevation of ICP than by lowering of SAP. After a period of reduced CPP, lowering ICP to improve CPP causes hyperemia associated with decreased CVR (vasodilation).

Finally, with repeated lowering of CPP, CBF eventually begins to decline even when CPP is restored, suggesting an increase in CVR consistent with capillary endothelial swelling or microcirculatory sludging. With a focal lateralized mass, CBF decreases at the site of the lesion, and with herniations, there are widespread areas of ischemia not directly correlated to elevation of ICP and decrease in CPP. These do not occur with decreases in CPP caused by cisternal infusion when lateralized mass effect is not present. Therefore, the

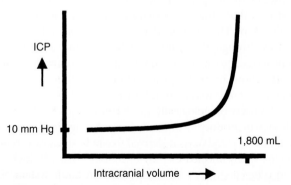

FIGURE 21.17 Relation between intracranial volume and intracranial pressure. ICP, intracranial pressure.

relation between ICP and CBF is complex, with CBF in individual areas of the brain dependent not only on a given ICP (CPP) but on anatomic location, vascular anatomy, preservation of autoregulation, rapidity of ICP increase, neuronal metabolism, and a host of other factors.

Herniation Syndromes

The most important consequence of increased ICP, especially in relation to lateralized mass effect, is brain herniation. Two dural folds, the falx cerebri and the tentorium cerebelli, divide the intracranial space into compartments. The falx separates the two hemispheres as deep as the corpus callosum, and the tentorium separates the cerebrum from the cerebellum with an opening, the tentorial notch or hiatus, to allow the brainstem to pass through. At the foramen magnum, the medulla passes through to spinal cord. Because these structures are essentially unyielding, pressure effects will cause the brain to move through these openings, creating pressure and vascular effects on vital structures.

With a supratentorial mass, especially frontal, subfalcial herniation occurs with the cingulate gyrus and anterior cerebral arteries herniated beneath the falx to the opposite side. More important is herniation of the uncus of the temporal lobe through the tentorial notch. This causes downward displacement of the upper brainstem with associated pressure effects. Two syndromes are recognized, which differ in their earliest presentation. However, both exhibit a rostrocaudal pattern of neurologic deterioration with recognizable brainstem levels of dysfunction. The central type with bilateral temporal lobe herniation begins as agitation, decreasing level of consciousness, small reactive pupils, bilateral increased tone and Babinski sign, and Cheyne-Stokes respirations. The lateral type begins with decreased level of consciousness, ipsilateral oculomotor paresis, generally beginning with a dilated nonreactive pupil and later involving lid elevation and extraocular movements, contralateral hemiparesis, and a sustained hyperventilation. Frequently, an initial hemiparesis ipsilateral to the lesion occurs, explained by compression of the opposite cerebral peduncle against the tentorial edge (Kernohan notch syndrome). Both syndromes progress to decreased responsiveness, decorticate posturing (arm flexed, leg extended) to decerebrate posturing (all extremities extended), midrange nonreactive pupils, loss of oculocephalic and oculovestibular reflexes, loss of corneal reflexes, and ataxic breathing patterns. Progression leads to herniation of the cerebellar tonsils through the foramen magnum with medullary compression, resulting in loss of motor tone, loss of gag and cough reflexes, apnea, and eventually cardiovascular collapse and death. Early signs of tentorial herniation may evolve over minutes, although full progression to death generally takes hours to days, especially if respiration is supported. If herniation cannot be reversed rapidly, hemorrhages appear in the brainstem, leading to a poor prognosis, even if pressure is subsequently relieved.

Increased ICP is managed by head elevation, which improves venous return to the heart; hyperventilation, which causes cerebral vasoconstriction and reduces CBV; mannitol, an osmotic diuretic, which decreases the brain tissue compartment by shrinking the extracellular and perhaps the intracellular space; and in some situations, barbiturates, which decrease CMR_{O_2} and consequently CBF and CBV. Corticosteroids have a beneficial effect with tumors, abscess, and inflammatory diseases and are thought to improve vasogenic edema, although a reduction in ICP is difficult to demonstrate. In many situations, removing a mass lesion or damaged brain is necessary, especially in the frontal and temporal lobes, to control ICP.

Brain Tumors

Brain tumors generally are categorized as: (i) primary, meaning tumors originating from neuroglial tissues, the meninges, reticuloendothelial cells, and vascular cells intrinsic to the brain; and (ii) secondary, or metastatic from tumors elsewhere in the body. Intrinsic brain tumors arise most commonly from glial cells. Astrocytomas, ependymomas, and oligodendrogliomas are seen in decreasing order of frequency and commonly show characteristics of more than one glial type. Poorly differentiated glial tumors—glioblastoma multiforme—are the most common glial tumors in adults. Brain tumors are the second most common form of neoplasia in children and are usually malignant, whereas some cystic astrocytomas in the cerebellum are compatible with decades of survival. Primitive embryonic cells give rise to a variety of tumors—medulloblastoma, germinoma, neuroblastoma, and others in this age group. Protein markers, especially nerve growth factor (NGF) and glial fibrillary acidic protein (GFAP), have been better used to classify these tumors types. In children, tumors arise most commonly in the posterior fossa and around the ventricular system, although in adults they are more common in the cerebral hemispheres, basal ganglia, and thalamus.

Extrinsic brain tumors arise most often from the coverings of the brain (meningioma, acoustic neuroma, and epidermoid) and are usually not invasive into brain tissue. Pituitary adenomas are usually included in this group because they grow into the intracranial cavity. Despite the histologically benign nature of these extra-axial tumors, their typical locations at the base of the skull, around the brainstem, from CNs, and along the dural sinuses can pose considerable problems for complete removal.

Malignant tumors outside the nervous system commonly metastasize to the brain, in both the supratentorial and infratentorial compartments. Lung and breast tumors are the most common metastatic lesions, followed by kidney, melanoma, and gastrointestinal malignancies. Lesions commonly present at the gray-white matter junction, a site were there is a significant reduction in the arteriolar density. Metastatic tumors can be associated with considerable edema of the surrounding brain. Although multiplicity is common, solitary metastases occur and may be the first presenting symptoms of the disease.

The terms *benign* and *malignant* are applied less easily to brain tumors. Primary brain tumors, even histologically poorly differentiated, rarely metastasize outside the nervous

TABLE 21.2

Tumor Syndromes Associated with Neural Involvement and Chromosome Location

Tumor Syndrome	Typical Tumor Types	Chromosome Location
Hereditary cutaneous malignant melanoma/dysplastic nevus syndrome	Dysplastic nevi, melanoma	1p
von Hippel-Lindau syndrome	Hemangioblastoma, pheochromocytoma, renal cell carcinoma	3p
Multiple endocrine neoplasia, type 1	Pituitary tumor, parathyroid adenoma, endocrine pancreatic tumors	11p
Multiple endocrine neoplasia, type 2	Pheochromocytoma, medullary thyroid carcinoma	10
Familial retinoblastoma	Retinoblastoma, osteosarcoma	13q
Neurofibromatosis (NF1)	Neurofibroma, optic glioma, neurofibrosarcoma	17q
Neurofibromatosis (NF2)	Vestibular schwannoma, meningioma, spinal nerve root neurofibroma	22q
Tuberous sclerosis	Subependymal giant cell astrocytomas hamartomas	16q

system, and death is caused by progressive brain involvement. However, histologically well-differentiated tumors are frequently not resectable, and if they are intrinsic to the brain, they generally lead to death. Pathologic criteria for increased aggressiveness in gliomas include hypercellularity, mitoses, pleomorphism, necrosis surrounded by pseudopalisading cells, and hypervascularity. Necrosis seems best correlated to prognosis.

Kinetic studies of tumor growth rates have been proposed to define malignancy better and to aid in prognosis. The cell cycle time, the time between successive mitoses, has been divided into four phases: (i) a mitotic (M) phase during which the cell is dividing, (ii) a postmitotic phase (G_1) of RNA synthesis, (iii) a phase of deoxyribonucleic acid (DNA) synthesis (S), and (iv) a premitotic (G_2) phase before cell division. Cells not actively proliferating are considered to be in the G_0 phase. The proportion of proliferating cells to the total cell population is termed the *growth fraction* (GF). GF is approximated by the number of cells in S phase that can be labeled. The GF has been measured by autoradiography with [³H] thymidine, DNA flow cytometry, and monoclonal antibody directed against bromodeoxyuridine-labeled nuclei or against the nuclear antigen Ki-67. It is not surprising that glioblastoma and medulloblastoma show a much higher GF than astrocytoma and meningioma, and some subgroups of biologic activity are beginning to emerge.

Neurofibromatosis, an autosomal dominant inherited disease, is associated with a marked increase in the incidence of several of the most common brain tumors—gliomas, schwannomas, and meningiomas. Sixteen percent of patients with primary brain tumors have a family history of cancer. With glioblastoma multiforme, primary CNS lymphoma, and neuroblastoma, the number nearly doubles. Many hereditary disorders are associated with neural tumors (Table 21.2). Current theory postulates the presence of tumor-promoting genes (oncogenes) and tumor-suppressing genes (antioncogenes). Genetic abnormalities in this condition may be acquired environmentally, accounting for spontaneously occurring brain tumors. Nitrosourea compounds are especially effective in inducing gliomas experimentally. Epidermal growth factor and platelet-derived growth factor have been considered oncogenic expressions in malignant gliomas. Heterozygosity or nonsymmetric alleles have been demonstrated in glioblastoma on chromosomes 7, 10, and 22. Meningiomas show an estrogen or progesterone receptor in approximately one half of cases, and abnormalities on chromosomes of 22 have been noted.

The failure of surgery and, for the most part, radiation therapy to alter significantly the course of intrinsic brain tumors has prompted increased investigation into molecular biologic and immunologic areas.

Neurotrauma

Head Injury

Brain trauma includes a spectrum of pathophysiologic consequences: synaptic impairment, neuronal disruption, ischemia, increased ICP, edema, bleeding, and herniation syndromes. With cerebral concussion, there is transient loss of consciousness attributed to traction on the upper brainstem and reversible synaptic impairment in the reticular-activating system. Persistent mild impairment of higher cortical functions has been recognized in more severe cases of cerebral concussion. Boxers subjected to repeated concussion may later show a degenerative-type dementia.

With more severe closed head injury, prolonged unconscious may occur, and amnesia, both retrograde and posttraumatic (antegrade), is common. Immediately after injury, there is a marked increase in CBF attributed to vasoparalysis, which is not blocked by sympathectomy or vagotomy and is believed to be brainstem mediated. Afterward, there is a period of decreased CBF, owing either to reduced metabolic demand or to vasospasm. Both decreases in CMRo2 and angiographic vasospasm have been demonstrated after head injury.

Cerebral contusions commonly result from head injury. A contusion may develop beneath the site of impact (coup contusion) but more commonly develops where the brain has struck the internal aspect of the skull on the contralateral side (contrecoup contusion). The irregular surface of the skull base over the orbits and at the sphenoid and petrous ridges makes frontal and temporal lobe contusions more common. Brain contusions initially show small ecchymoses, often at the crowns of the gyri. Edema develops around the areas of contusion and, although it is maximal between 48 and 96 hours, it may persist for weeks. In some cases, sizable intracerebral hematomas occur at the time of injury and, in still others, small areas of contusion coalesce over a few days into sizable clots (delayed traumatic intracerebral hematoma).

Extra-axial hematomas are well recognized complications of head injury. Epidural hematoma usually is associated with skull fracture and bleeding from the meningeal arteries or sinuses. Such hematomas are typically temporoparietal but may occur anywhere, including the posterior fossa. Subdural hematoma results from shearing of bridging veins to the sinuses and from brain lacerations. They are often holoconvex, extending from front to occiput. Skull fractures are present in approximately 50% of subdural hematomas and are often on the contralateral side. If not fatal, a subdural membrane can envelop the clot, and a chronic subdural hematoma may form, which may gradually increase in size. Subdural hematomas present as a variety of neurologic syndromes.

Untreated brain mass lesions, whether contusions or hematomas, may progress rapidly to brain herniations as described previously. Early diagnosis and treatment are mandatory to preserve neurologic function in these cases. Some patients with severe closed head injury will show no abnormalities on imaging studies and are considered to have diffuse axonal shearing injuries. Some of these patients make remarkable recoveries, but others are left in a permanent vegetative state.

Spinal Cord Injury

Trauma to the spinal cord may occur biomechanically, with or without spinal column fracture, or by penetrating injuries. Except for penetrating injuries, most spinal cord injuries are contusive in nature, and complete severance of the spinal cord is uncommon. Experimentally, the earliest finding in a contusive cord lesion is hemorrhage of the gray matter, with subsequent necrosis of the white matter. This occurs within days. Nevertheless, functional impairment is often complete from the time of injury, and pharmacologic strategies to prevent delayed necrosis of the white matter are controversial.

At present, only one randomized controlled study has shown that the administration of methylprednisolone within 8 hours of spinal cord injury results in improved recovery (5).

Approximately half of spinal injuries are cervical and half are thoracolumbar. In addition, approximately half of spinal cord injuries are complete and half are incomplete. Clinical syndromes depend on the level of injury—cervical, thoracolumbar, conus, cauda equina—but syndromes relating to the cross-sectional anatomy of the cord are recognized. Hemisection of the cord (Brown-Séquard syndrome) causes ipsilateral paralysis and position/vibration sense loss, and contralateral pain and temperature loss. Ipsilateral segmental sensory loss completes the syndrome. Anterior cord syndrome describes loss of motor, pain, and temperature sensation bilaterally with preservation of position and vibration sense (posterior column function). This syndrome may have a vascular basis. Central cord syndrome describes an injury for which weakness in the arms, especially distally, is out of proportion to leg weakness, and sensory functions are preserved partially or completely. It is the most common incomplete injury and is associated with preexisting cervical spondylosis. Finally, a central cyst (syringomyelia) can cause loss of pain and temperature sensation, with preservation of other sensory modalities in the upper extremities before motor involvement that is of the central cord type. Most incomplete spinal cord injuries represent a mixture of the above syndromes, but one type often predominates.

In the initial phase of a complete spinal cord injury, the muscles below the injury are flaccid, reflexes are absent, and the autonomics are impaired. This is termed *spinal shock*, which does not denote decreased blood pressure, although mild hypotension is common. Over a period of weeks, tone and reflexes return and eventually become hyperactive with associated pathologic reflexes. The mechanisms underlying spinal shock and subsequent development of spasticity are unknown. Perhaps a mechanism similar to wallerian degeneration in peripheral nerves occurs in descending corticospinal inhibitory pathways with initial release of excessive neurotransmitter, then gradual degeneration of the axon and disinhibition of local reflex arcs. During spinal shock, the bladder is atonic, ileus is common, and the skin is prone to pressure necrosis, all requiring immediate attention in the injured patient.

Peripheral Nerve Injury

Peripheral nerve injury can be graded according to the type of injury a nerve fiber has sustained (Seddon) or from the injury a peripheral nerve has sustained (Sunderland). Both systems are useful conceptually and clinically.

In the Seddon system, neuropraxia is the mildest injury a fiber can receive and is associated physiologically with loss of conduction. The axon is in continuity but is focally demyelinated at the injury site. The endoneurium or connective tissue sheath is intact, and restoration of function occurs with remyelination usually within weeks to months. This type of injury is seen in positioning palsies or after prolonged periods of immobilization. Axonotmesis is a more severe injury in which axonal continuity is lost in addition to demyelination, but the connective tissue sheath is intact. Recovery will depend on axonal regeneration. The fidelity of regeneration is expected to be excellent. Neurotmesis adds to axonotmesis the disruption of the connective tissue support of the axon. This type of injury can range from internal disruption of the connective tissue to nerve transection. With axonotmetic and neurotmetic injuries, wallerian degeneration occurs. The axon degenerates toward the motor endplate, and Schwann cells form tubules to receive regenerating axons.

Many nerve injuries leave the nerve in gross continuity with varying degrees of intraneural damage. The Sunderland-grading method is based on the anatomic structure of the nerve, with progressive grades reflecting more severe damage.

Grade 1 is disruption of the myelin sheath, which manifests as a conduction block.

Grade 2 is the loss of axon continuity with preservation of all layers of connective tissue framework. The endoneurial, perineurial, and epineurial layers all remain intact.

Grade 3 is loss of axon continuity with loss of endoneurial integrity. In this setting, internal endoneurial scarring can prevent reinnervation, and disruption of the endoneurial sheath may allow mismatched reinnervation as regenerating axons stray from their proper endoneurial sheaths.

Grade 4 is loss of perineural integrity and thereby disruption of the fascicle. This is associated with more intraneural scarring and consequently less-effective nerve regeneration. As in grade 3 injuries, the connective tissue disruption will allow mismatch to occur with regeneration, potentially degrading functional recovery.

Grade 5 is loss of epineurial continuity and thereby transection of the nerve.

Most clinical nerve injuries result from of four basic types of trauma: laceration, compression, stretch, and high-velocity missile injury.

Laceration to nerve may be caused by knife wounds, shattered glass, or by more blunt mechanisms such as chain saws, propeller blades, auto metal, and animal bites. Up to 20% of suspected transection injuries actually leave the nerve in continuity, and some of these may recover without surgery. However, most laceration injuries are Sunderland grade 4 or 5 and consequently will require surgical intervention. Direct end-to-end repair, with proper fascicular alignment using either epineurial or fascicular suture, is the mainstay of treatment.

Acute compression injuries are identified by a characteristic history of prolonged immobility. In patients previously well, this immobility usually is associated with extreme fatigue, alcohol intoxication, drug-abuse, or general anesthesia. The type of injury is usually neuropraxic and/or axonotmetic, but on occasion, endoneurial damage does occur. The recovery time will be the major indicator of degree of injury, as these injuries usually do not require surgical intervention. Motor fibers are the most susceptible to compression. They are the first to fail, the last to recover and, in mild injuries, may be the only ones to suffer.

As a nerve is stretched more than 6% to 20% of its length, nerve function starts to fail, cross-sectional area decreases, and intraneural pressure increases. Nerve injury proceeds, starting at Sunderland grade 1 and progressing grade by grade until the upper 30% limit is reached. At this point, the perineurium and then the epineurium give way and the nerve ruptures. In mixed motor sensory nerves, stretching may affect all function, or sensation alone, but seldom affects motor disability without sensory impairment. Given the lengths over which the stretching forces may take place, the damage tends to be spread over a length of nerve rather that at a precise point. Consequently, surgical repair often requires the use of grafts. Because the perineurium provides significant strength to peripheral nerve, the absence of this layer at the spinal rootlet level contributes significantly to the propensity for nerve root avulsion from the spinal cord.

High-velocity missiles generate forces, which take the form of shock waves, with high pressure regions in front of and lateral to the moving body and pressure associated with the formation of a temporary explosive cavity in the track of the missile. Consequently, structures adjacent to and also distant from the missile path may be stretched abruptly and deformed. Nerves directly in the path may be severed or torn, but most are injured secondarily as the result of sudden stretch, with all grades of injury being observed afterwards.

Nerve recovery passes through several stages. After an initial period of retrograde demyelination of the axon and chromatolysis of the cell nucleus, wherein new RNA is manufactured, the axons begin sprouting and will grow into the distal nerve sheath unless inhibited by distance or scar. Once neurotization of the distal stump is achieved, the nerve fibers grow toward the motor endplates and sensory terminals. A period of time is required for these connections to be reestablished. This process continues until the active fiber pool is numerous enough to elicit muscle activity or provide sensation. This process takes months to years to complete. The presence of regenerating unmyelinated fibers may be ascertained by tapping over the course of a nerve. Elicited paresthesias (Tinel sign) are indicative of the forward advance of these axons but are no guarantee of useful functional return.

A useful clinical approximation for recovery of motor function is an overall growth rate of 1 in. per month. The regenerative rate for axons is faster in the proximal limb than in the distal limb. When an axon is lacerated, the time for retrograde degeneration, sprouting, and spanning the injury reduces the expected rate of recovery. This delay may be 2 weeks with axonotmetic injuries and up to 4 weeks with sutured neurotmetic injuries. In stretch injuries, the growth rate is slower.

The time course of nerve recovery will ultimately indicate the degree of injury. Lack of clinical recovery 16 weeks after nerve injury usually indicates a grade 3 or higher injury. The functional potential of nerve recovery decreases with the passage of time. Although variation exists in the intrinsic recoverability of nerves and in the percentage of strength necessary for useful function in associated muscles, most muscles are subject to a 24-month limit of denervation, after which no useful motor recovery is expected from reconnection. The exceptions to this rule are large proximal muscles such as biceps, gastrocnemius-soleus, quadriceps, and, surprisingly, the facial muscle. When sensory function is considered, the period of effective repair may be increased by several years.

Electromyography may further clarify the pattern of neuronal injury and recovery. By 3 weeks after axonotmetic or neurotmetic injury, denervational changes of increased insertional activity, fibrillation potentials, and positive sharp waves may be identified. Later with reinnervation of at least 200 to 400 fibers, motor units under volitional control may be identified.

At least 3,000 to 4,000 myelinated fibers must be present for significant reinnervation to occur. This forms the basis for direct operative evaluation of injured nerve with NAP recordings in those patients with proximal injuries that show no spontaneous recovery in the initial months after nerve injury. The absence of an NAP after adequate time for axonal regrowth to have crossed the damaged segment is an indication that no useful recovery can be anticipated. In such a case, the damaged area is resected and grafts from sensory nerves, such as the sural, can be used as substitute conduit for regenerating axons.

Seizures and Epilepsy

Seizures result from excessive and/or hypersynchronous, usually self-limited abnormal activity of neurons predominately located in the cerebral cortex. A seizure may occur in the normal human brain from a variety of noxious stimuli depending on individual thresholds. In some, mild sleep deprivation, alcohol withdrawal, and in children, fever, can provoke a seizure. In contradistinction, epilepsy is a condition wherein the disturbance of the brain, either microscopic or macroscopic, is responsible for the seizure endures and is responsible for repetitive events. Seizures result in a variety of symptoms, depending upon the area of brain involved. Seizures occurring in childhood and adolescence often have no radiologic abnormalities and may have a genetic basis, whereas seizures in adults are more likely to have associated structural abnormalities.

Seizures are classified as generalized when a loss of consciousness occurs and partial when consciousness is preserved. Complex partial seizures (CPSs) have some alteration in consciousness and are associated with foci in the temporal and frontal lobes. Partial seizures may become generalized. Generalized seizures include tonic-clonic (grand mal) and absence (petit mal) and are believed to be generated with participation of the brainstem reticular formation and thalamic nuclei because of the observed symmetric electrocortical activity. Partial seizures are associated more commonly with a focal brain lesion. Simple partial seizures may be motor (jacksonian) where progressive involvement of one side of the body, sensory or other, exists. CPSs (temporal lobe seizures) frequently have automatism and visceral components.

The spike and wave discharge is the EEG signature of a seizure; this reflects abnormal depolarization and

TABLE 21.3

Sites of Action of Seizure Medications

	Use-Dependant Inhibition of Sodium Channels	Enhanced GABA-Receptor Chloride Current	Inhibition of T-Type Calcium Current
Phenytoin	++	−	−
Carbamazepine	++	−	−
Valproate	++	+/?	−
Ethosuximide	−	−	++
Barbiturates	+	++	−
Primidone	+	−	−
Benzodiazepines	+	++	−

GABA, γ-aminobutyric acid.

hyperpolarization events that occur synchronously in the abnormal region. The spike of the EEG is formed by the summation of the excitatory depolarization, whereas the wave represents the summation of the inhibitory after-hyperpolarizing potentials.

Seizures tend to be self-limited but are often repetitive and at times continuous (status epilepticus). $CRMO_2$ and CBF increases considerably in the involved areas, often with CBF unable to meet metabolic demand, creating a relative ischemia. Interictally, metabolism and CBF may be reduced significantly in 70% to 80% of patients. This finding has been used in PET to localize seizure foci.

Ion channel physiology is important in understanding the mechanisms by which anticonvulsant medications work (Table 21.3). Drugs such as phenytoin, carbamazepine, and valproate bind to activated sodium channels from the inside of the cell membrane and maintain the channel in an inactive form temporarily. Its short duration of blockage will, therefore, minimally affect the normal functioning of the sodium channels but will greatly impede the rapid repetitive firing of neurons characteristic of a seizure.

The chloride channel complex is regulated by GABA, a major inhibitory neurotransmitter of the brain. Opening of the chloride channel by GABA allows chloride ions to enter the neuron and hyperpolarize the cell, thereby making the neuron more difficult to fire. GABA is synthesized in gabaergic nerve terminals by the enzyme glutamic acid decarboxylase (GAD). After its release, it is taken up into neurons and glia by specific transporters γ aminobutyric acid transporter (GAT). GABA is metabolized by GABA transaminase as part of the GABA shunt. The GABA receptor is divided into two types: A and B. The A receptor is formed from five peptide subunits which surround a channel permeable to chloride ion.

Chloride channel activity can be enhanced by three mechanisms: (i) by prolonging the channel's opening time, (ii) by increasing its opening frequency, and (iii) by increasing the channel's conductance. Benzodiazepines act by increasing the frequency of channel openings and barbiturates act by prolonging the channel's opening time. New antiepileptic drugs (AEDs) have been developed to exploit the understanding of GABA functioning. Tigabine (TGB) binds to GAT, thereby inhibiting neuronal reuptake of GABA in the synaptic cleft and has shown efficacy in the treatment of partial complex seizures. Vigabatrin is an irreversible inhibitor of GABA transaminase and has been shown to increase CSF GABA content and reduce seizure frequency in AED-resistant CPS.

Calcium channel physiology is also important in seizure understanding. Ethosuximide, an anticonvulsant effective only in absence seizures, has been shown to block a voltage-dependent calcium channel in thalamocortical relay neurons.

Another focus of AED control is the excitatory amino acids (EAAs). Glutamate coupled with glycine is the major excitatory neurotransmitter of the cortex. Substantial evidence points to the role of abnormal expression or enhanced function in various acquired forms of epilepsy. Three receptor types are recognized currently: the α-amino-3-hyddroxy-5-methyl-4-isoxazolepropionate (AMPA) receptor, the kainic acid receptor, and the NMDA receptor. The NMDA receptor, when activated, allows flow of calcium and sodium ions. It has multiple regulatory sites and is a main focus for AED development. The ion channel is affected by magnesium and the dissociative anesthetics such as ketamine. The sedative effects of drugs developed to block this receptor may limit their usefulness in epilepsy, but the potentially toxic effects of EAAs in trauma and stroke suggests that this class of drugs may have neuroprotective functions.

Seizures are terminated by an active inhibitory process. Adenosine is thought to be involved with seizure termination, which explains why toxic levels of aminophylline may induce seizures that are extremely difficult to control. Second messengers, such as cyclic nucleotides, calcium, and G proteins, offer potential sites of pharmacologic manipulation.

After a seizure, a period of drowsiness and confusion (postictal state) occurs that clears over a few hours. With partial and generalized seizures, a postictal neurologic deficit, such as hemiparesis, commonly occurs and clears over 24 to 48 hours (Todd paralysis).

Surgical excision of the seizure focus is being considered more often in chronic seizure disorders that have not responded favorably to AED therapy. Accurate localization of the seizure focus can be obtained with depth electrodes; continuous recordings, including video monitoring to correlate seizures to EEG events; and PET/MR scanning.

Brain Death

The advent of artificial ventilation has created medical conditions wherein the brain may be completely and irreversibly damaged and the cardiac function maintained. As a consequence, the concept of brain death has been developed to apply to the situations in which the prior standard of death, that is, the cessation of heartbeat, is not a useful criterion of an organism's ability to recover. Understanding the criteria

for brain death is important because the increased availability of organs for transplantation has been allowed by the general acceptance of this concept. The definition of brain death involves legal, ethical, and clinical considerations. Universal criteria for brain death and the acceptance of brain death as equivalent to cardiorespiratory arrest do not exist for every state and country. In making the determination of brain death, therefore, it is important to be familiar with hospital, community, and state guidelines regarding this important question.

The most commonly applied criteria in the United States use the guidelines of the President's Commission, which considers a patient to have died when cerebral and brainstem functions are absent and when the situation is deemed irreversible based on a known cause for brain dysfunction, when no known therapy will promote recovery, and after an adequate period of observation.

Brain death determination rests primarily on the clinical examination. The patient is unresponsive to command or pain and shows no spontaneous movements. Limited limb withdrawal is considered a spinal reflex and not relevant. Brainstem reflexes are not elicitable, including pupillary reaction, oculocephalic reflexes (doll eyes), oculovestibular reflexes (cold calorics), and corneal, gag, and cough reflexes. The patient is apneic with endotracheal oxygen, and the $PaCO_2$ is allowed to rise above 60 mm Hg. The clinical examination is conducted in the absence of sedative drugs, with the temperature higher than 95°C and the systolic blood pressure above 95 mm Hg. Ancillary tests include an isoelectric (flat) EEG and absence of CBF on angiography or radioisotope scan. When ancillary testing is used as an adjunct to clinical examination, brain death may not be declared until the adjunctive test fully supports the clinical diagnosis. Appropriate periods of observation between two examinations range from 6 to 24 hours, and some hospitals require examinations by two independent examiners, especially in cases of transplantation.

The declaration of brain death in children poses additional challenges. The report of the President's Commission outlines criteria valid in children older than 5 years of age. The supposition of increased resistance to injury in the child's brain is controversial and lacks good clinical support. As a consequence, a task force of pediatricians and neurologists developed guidelines to deal with the problem of pediatric brain death (Table 21.4).

The time of death is generally considered when cardiac arrest occurs in cases for which life support is withdrawn. Time of death is at the time of brain death determination in cases of transplantation.

FUTURE DIRECTIONS

Despite the wealth of information that has contributed to the understanding of the nervous system, many of the most fundamental questions remain unanswered or are understood at only a superficial level: How does the nervous

TABLE 21.4

Modification of Brain Death Criteria for Children and Infants Less Than 5 Years Old

Infants 7 d to 2 mo
Two examinations and two confirmatory EEGs separated by at least 48 h

Infants 2 mo to 1 yr
Two examinations and EEGs separated by at least 24 h unless CBG studies document no cerebral perfusion

Children 1–5 yr
When an irreversible cause exists, a 12-h interval between examinations is recommended. In cases of hypoxia-ischemia, a 24-h interval is recommended. If an EEG shows electrical silence or a CBF study demonstrates no cerebral perfusion, the time interval between examinations may be reduced

EEG, electroencephalogram, CBG, coronary bypass graft; CBF, cerebral blood flow.

Recent years have seen the introduction of imaging modalities such as MRI and PET and single proton emission computed tomography (SPECT) scanning that create both physiologic and anatomic maps of the nervous system and help clarify the interrelation of various brain areas in normal and abnormal functional activities. Nervous tissue is being transplanted in degenerative diseases and spinal cord injuries, and in-dwelling pumps and slow-release polymer capsules containing neurotransmitters are being evaluated. Genetic abnormalities associated with brain tumors have been described, and the role of oncogenes and suppressor genes in neoplasia is being elucidated. Plasticity within the nervous system to recover lost functions is under intense scrutiny. Familiarity with the basic concepts of neuroscience will benefit all physicians in understanding developments relevant to their own specialties and keeping abreast of advances in this important area.

system develop? What are the underlying mechanisms for learning and memory? Can the nervous system regenerate and, if so, how? Can neuronal cell death in trauma and ischemia be prevented? Why does the nervous system age and degenerate? Are the genetic changes in neoplasia reversible or preventable? Why do patients with stroke show gradual recovery over months? Can consciousness and behavior be understood completely in electrochemical terms? Many additional basic questions could be posed.

A major area of research effort in the neurosciences is currently in the fields of molecular biology and genetics. The search for neurotransmitters, the structure of their receptors, and the genes regulating them dominates much of the neuroscience literature. The discovery of NGFs has raised hope for promoting regeneration in the nervous system and perhaps elucidating mechanisms underlying neoplasia. Ischemic cell death is considered to be, at least partially, a receptor-mediated phenomenon. Learning and memory may relate to the upregulation of receptors in given neuronal circuits in response to repeated sensory experiences and input. In general, emphasis has shifted from the "hard-wiring" of the nervous system to chemical neurotransmitter relations. Both are essential to proper function of the nervous system, but the neurochemical relations might lend themselves more easily to therapeutic manipulation.

REFERENCES
1. Hodgkin AL, Huxley AF. Quantitative description of membrane current and its application to conduction excitation in nerve. *J Physiol* 1952;117:500.
2. Rexed B. The cytoarchitectonic organization of the spinal cord in the cat. *J Comp Neurol* 1952;96:415.
3. Nordstrom CH, Rehncrona S, Siesjo BK. Cerebral metabolism. In: Youmans JR, ed. *Neurological surgery*. Philadelphia: WB Saunders, 1990:623–661.
4. Meldrum BS, ed. *Frontiers in pharmacology and therapeutics: excitatory amino acid antagonists*. Oxford: Blackwell Science, 1991.
5. Bracken MB, Shepard MJ, Collins WF, et al. A randomized, controlled trial of methylprednisolone or naloxone in the treatment of acute spinal cord injury. *N Engl J Med* 1990;322:1405–1411.

SUGGESTED READINGS
Carpenter MB, Sutin J. *Human neuroanatomy*, 8th ed. Baltimore: Williams & Wilkins, 1983.
Kandel ER, Schwartz JH. *Principles of neuroscience*, 3rd ed. New York: Elsevier Science, 1992.
Kline DG, Hudson AR. *Nerve injuries*. Philadelphia: WB Saunders, 1995.
Salcman M, ed. *Neurobiology of brain tumors. Concepts in neurosurgery*. Baltimore: Williams & Wilkins, 1991.
Schmidt RF, ed. *Fundamentals of neurophysiology*, 3rd ed. New York: Springer-Verlag New York, 1985.
Yasargil MG. *Microneurosurgery*, Vols. 1–2. Stuttgart: Georg Thieme, 1984.
Youmans JR, ed. *Neurological surgery*, Vols. 1–6. Philadelphia: WB Saunders, 1990.

CHAPTER 22

Skin and Subcutaneous Tissue

Colin D. Goodier, Hugo St. Hilaire, and M. Whitten Wise

ANATOMY AND PHYSIOLOGY

The skin and its derivatives constitute the integumentary system, the largest organ of the body, which comprises approximately 15% to 20% of its total mass (1). It is a highly specialized bilaminate organ that provides a number of critical functions. These functions include barrier protection against physical, chemical, and biologic agents, homeostasis through temperature regulation, sensory function, secretory function in the conversion of precursor molecules into vitamin D, as well as an excretory function through sweat glands (1). Each function of the skin directly reflects a cell or area within the skin.

The thickness of the skin varies over the surface of the body from less than 0.5 mm to greater than 6 mm and consists of two main layers, the epidermis and the dermis. In addition, there is a layer referred to as the "hypodermis," the subcutaneous connective tissue under the dermis that contains variable amounts of adipose tissue and vasculature (1).

The outer, highly cellular epidermal layer measures 0.06 mm to 0.8 mm in thickness and is in contact with the dermis through interpapillary ridges and grooves (2). The outer epidermis is composed of stratified squamous epithelium, with four to five layers identified (four layers in thin skin and five in thick skin). The innermost layer is termed the *stratum germinativum*, or *stratum basale*, and is a single layer of cuboidal to low columnar cells that rest on the basal lamina. It contains melanocytes and stem cells that are destined to become keratinocytes. These cells then shift and migrate into subsequent more outward layers until they become a mature keratinized cell on the skin surface. The second layer is the stratum spinosum, which is several cells thick and is larger than the stratum germinativum. These cells exhibit numerous cytoplasmic processes, "spines," which give the cell layer its name. This layer contains most of the viable cells producing keratin and precursor proteins for the granular cell layer. The stratum granulosum is the next layer and is the most superficial layer

of cells that are nonkeratinized. This cell layer is usually relatively thin and contains keratohyalin granules, which give the layer its characteristic name. This layer primarily produces proteins related to the fully keratinized layers. The next layer is a variable layer that is only present in thick skin (palms and soles). This layer is called the *stratum lucidum* and is often considered part of the more superficial stratum corneum, the most superficial cell layer. The stratum corneum is composed of flattened, desiccated, anuclate cells that provide protection and prevent water, electrolyte, and plasma protein loss. This is the layer that varies the most in thickness.

The dermal–epidermal junction undulates in most areas of the body, providing an uneven boundary in all areas except for the thinnest skin. Sections of the skin cut in cross-section reveal numerous finger-like connective tissue protrusions that project into the epidermis called *papillae*. These dermal papillae are complemented by what appear to be similar epidermal papillae projecting into the dermis called *rete ridges*. Between these layers lies the basement membrane. These numerous ridges and papillae vastly increase the surface contact between the two layers to provide resistance of the normal skin to shearing.

The dermis is the deeper layer of skin and is 20 to 30 times thicker than the epidermis. It contains the nervous, vascular, lymphatic, and supporting structures for the epidermis and harbors the epidermal appendages. There are two main zones to the dermis, the papillary and reticular dermis. The papillary layer is the more superficial layer, is relatively thin, and consists of loose connective tissue. The collagen fibers in this layer are not as thick as in the lower reticular dermis, and they contain the substance of the dermal papillae and ridges. Directly under the papillary dermis, separating it from the reticular dermis is a horizontal plexus of vessels that provide the overlying dermis with a rich blood supply. Under this plexus lies the reticular layer. Although it varies in thickness throughout the body, it is always considerably thicker and less cellular than the papillary layer (1). It is characterized by thicker bundles of collagen and elastin than the papillary layer and is oriented to form lines of tension called *Langer's lines.* Incisions that are made parallel to these lines of minimal tension tend to heal with less scarring (1).

The human epidermal appendages include nails, hair, sebaceous glands, and eccrine and apocrine sweat glands. These structures all have unique distributions and functions that involve homeostasis, protection, and thermoregulation.

MALIGNANT TUMORS OF THE SKIN

Basal Cell Carcinoma

Basal cell carcinoma is the most common cutaneous malignancy (77%) and the most common malignant tumor in incidence and prevalence. It outnumbers all other skin cancers combined, and the incidence is on the rise. New cases of basal cell carcinoma arise at a rate of close to 550,000 per year (3). However, the vast majority is of an innocuous nature, and basal cell carcinoma is responsible for only small percentage of deaths per year. These lesions are overwhelmingly more common in fair complected individuals, especially those with a Fitzpatrick skin type of 1 or 2, with a decreasing incidence per higher skin type (4) (Table 22.1 (5)) Skin cancer overall is much less common in darker skinned individuals with a dramatically lower incidence than in the Caucasian population.

Ultra violet B (UVB) in the form of solar ultraviolet light remains the most consistent causative agents of basal cell carcinoma. Despite aggressive campaigns by dermatologic groups, sun bathing and tanning salons remain prevalent pastimes of a significant portion of the American population, especially younger women. Additionally, a substantial proportion of the population works in outdoor environments and sustains ongoing exposure to UVB radiation. Protective clothing and sunscreens are effective in limiting exposure. However, they are far too commonly worn regularly only after adolescence. At this point, many individuals have reached their threshold doses of UVB radiation and are already at significant risk of subsequent development of basal cell carcinoma. The lag time between sunburns and the development of basal cell carcinoma is commonly 20 to 40 years. Recently, ultraviolet A (UVA) has been shown to be an additional risk factor and potentiates the carcinogenic effects of UVB (6). Current recommendations are for sunscreens with a UVA/UVB sun protection factor of 30 or greater.

Similar to their relatives, squamous cell carcinomas, basal cell carcinomas may arise in chronic wounds and burn scars. However, as opposed to squamous carcinomas, basal lesions arising in these chronic wounds do not appear to be more biologically aggressive.

Several carcinogenic compounds are associated with later development of basal cell carcinomas. These include arsenic, radiation in most forms, immunosuppression in all forms, and some medications such as psoralens. Arsenic, as previously used in welding and foundries, and other arsenic compounds contribute to the later development of multiple basal cell carcinomas. In the setting of arsenic exposure, the cutaneous malignancies are often associated with other malignancies, including lung and visceral malignancies. Multiple, scaly, red, plaque-like lesions typically characterize tumors resulting from arsenic exposure.

Several genetic syndromes (genodermatoses) exist, with basal cell carcinoma playing a prominent role. Xeroderma pigmentosum is an autosomal recessive disease, and one of the more well known. Afflicted patients have a defect in the deoxyribonucleic acid (DNA) repair mechanism for ionizing radiation damage to fibroblast DNA. This results in the formation of unrepairable thymidine dimers. Affected individuals begin to develop ichthyotic skin in late childhood, followed by the appearance of basal and squamous cell carcinomas and melanomas. The disease is usually fatal in the third decade of life, often from metastatic melanoma.

An X-linked dominant genodermatosis known as *Bazex syndrome* is characterized by follicular atrophoderma, hypotrichosis, hypohidrosis, and multiple basal cell carcinomas. Albinism is an autosomal recessive disease with a genetic fault in melanin production. These patients are photosensitive and develop multiple and recurrent basal and squamous cell carcinomas. This relates to ethnicity as well, as darker skinned individuals have a larger amount of melanin production and protection from skin cancers. However, across some similar complected groups of individuals there exist significant differences in the rates of development of basal cell carcinomas that is most easily accounted for by differences in genetic background.

Gorlin syndrome, or basal cell nevus syndrome, is an autosomal dominant genodermatosis that has the characteristic findings of jaw cysts, palmar pits, and multifocal basal cell carcinoma. These patients develop multiple and recurrent basal cell carcinomas arising from basal cell carcinoma *in situ* lesions. The genetic defect is believed to be in the patched (*PTCH*) gene (7).

TABLE 22.1

Fitzpatrick Skin Types

Fitzpatrick Skin Type	Color	Reaction to First Sun Exposure
1	White	Always burn/never tan
2	White	Usually burn/tan with difficulty
3	White	Sometimes mild burn/tan average
4	Medium brown	Rarely burn/tan with ease
5	Dark brown	Rarely burn/tan with ease
6	Black	Rarely burn/tan with ease

Basal cell carcinomas arise in the basilar layer of the epidermis from basilar keratinocytes. The proposed mechanism for carcinogenesis from solar UVB and ionizing radiation is damage to the DNA of the basal keratinocyte. If this damage goes unrepaired, the mutation undergoes replication and expression. UVB is responsible for mutations in the *p53* tumor suppressor gene, and the presence of the p53 protein predicts tumor aggressivity (8). UVB radiation is also believed to cause defects in the *PTCH* gene similar to the defects found in Gorlin syndrome, and is therefore responsible for some sporadic basal cell carcinomas (7). Additionally, ultraviolet radiation is proposed to act as an immunosuppressant causing macrophage depletion and stimulation of T-suppressor cells, and is therefore systemically effective (9).

Basal cell carcinoma develops in several distinct subtypes. The most common type arises at the dermal and epidermal interface, and is termed the *nodular type*. Histologically, these lesions are characterized by peripheral palisading, stromal retraction, and dermal fibrosis. These tumors are slow growing and slow spreading and are more easily treated. Other subtypes include the superficial spreading, adenoid, cystic, keratotic, and pigmented subtypes. Of the more difficult subtypes to treat, morpheaform, or fibrosing/sclerosing as it is also known, is much more aggressive. These tumors produce collagenase that allows them to grow and spread rapidly along tissue planes. This makes these lesions difficult to treat, and they are likely to recur following typical treatments.

Most basal cell carcinomas grow slowly. They can also grow deeply until they encounter a fascial plane, such as the galea, or vessels, nervefs or muscle fascia. At this point, they begin to track along these fascial planes and can extend into deeper structures such as skull and orbit along the foramen that pierce them. Regional metastases rarely occur. However, the tumors can be very destructive if undertreated, causing extensive local destruction and infiltrating adjacent and vital structures along tissue planes. When nodal disease does occur, it should be treated similarly to a squamous cell cancer arising in a similar location as described later.

Most basal cell carcinomas are asymptomatic. However, occasionally they can itch, bleed, ulcerate, or produce some type of open sore. They often appear on the sun-exposed areas of the body as pearly white lesions, often with a rodent ulcer or hollowed out central portion and a keratin plug in the center. The superficial spreading subtype often appears as large scaly plaques mimicking psoriasis. They often go for a long time with steroidal treatment before being biopsied. The morpheaform subtype often appears as a waxy, yellow, plaque-like lesion with obscure clinical borders and depth. Pigmented basal cell carcinomas can be readily confused with melanoma. Clinically, they often appear more symmetric and with a more even color distribution than melanoma. This often results in a prolonged history before biopsy. Fibroepithelioma is another type of basal cell carcinoma that appears as a pink papule on the nonsun exposed areas of the body.

These lesions can also be waxy and plaque-like but are adequately treated with local excision and have a lower risk of recurrence.

Secondary to the prevalence of these lesions, much attention has focused on prevention. Specific campaigns encouraging sunscreens and clothing have not made significant improvements. Other attention has focused on the population already exposed to the UVB radiation. This population has shown with some success with retinoid compounds in the prevention of these and squamous lesions.

The first step in treatment of these lesions is diagnosis. Diagnosis can be made with shave, punch, incisional and excisional biopsies. The mainstay of treatment following diagnosis is excision/ablation. Ablative options are reserved for smaller lesions and include curettage, cryosurgery, and electrodesiccation. They are most commonly excised with no more than 0.2 cm to 0.5 cm margins depending on tumor type and size, in the subcutaneous fat below the lesion. For most lesions, the risk of recurrence is low at approximately 5%. Certain lesions require tighter margin control and have been shown to have lower recurrence rates when treated with Mohs micrographic surgery. These include lesions with morpheaform subtype as well as recurrent lesions, and those prone to recurrence such as lesions in cosmetically sensitive or difficult to treat areas such as the medial canthus, the alar base and the pre- and postauricular areas.

Recurrence is more common in several distinct groups, including morpheaform tumors, large tumors, those with prior radiation failure, previously recurrent tumors, tumors with perineural or perivascular invasion, and tumors in difficult to treat areas. Most importantly, patients with a history of basal cell carcinoma should be followed regularly because they carry a significant risk (20%–40% in 2 years) of developing new primary lesions.

Squamous Cell Carcinoma

Squamous cell carcinoma is the second most common cutaneous malignancy (20%). New cases of squamous cell carcinoma arise at a rate of 100,000 to150,000 per year. In contrast to basal cancers, squamous cell carcinomas are much more biologically aggressive, resulting in close to 2,500 deaths per year in the United States (10). As with basal carcinomas, squamous tumors are much more commonly encountered in fair-complected individuals. Incidence of squamous cell carcinoma is higher in men and increases with age.

As with basal cell carcinomas, UVB in the form of solar ultraviolet light is the most consistent causative agent of squamous cell carcinoma. Additionally individuals appear to possess a genetic sensitivity to sun exposure, mostly related to their Fitzpatrick skin type. The distribution of squamous cell carcinomas on sun exposed areas correlates more directly than the distribution of basal cell lesions. Several chemical compounds including arsenic, psoralens, pesticides, aromatic hydrocarbons, soot, pitch, creosote oil, anthracene oil and others have been shown to be risk factors for the development of squamous cell carcinomas. Chronic wounds are also well-known risk factors for squamous carcinomas of an aggressive variety. Those cancers arising in burn scars, osteomyelitis tracts, pressure sores, hidradenitis, and any other chronic wounds are often referred to as Marjolin ulcers, and may have latency periods of 20 to 30 years. Both immunosuppression and radiation are well-known risk factors for squamous carcinomas. Additionally, squamous cell carcinomas often arise out of *in situ* lesions. These *in situ* lesions can be extensive, and several have names based on their location such as Erythroplasia of Queyrat (glans of penis) and Bowen disease. Squamous cell carcinomas can also arise from several benign lesions including leukoplakia, actinic keratoses, and cutaneous horns.

Squamous cell carcinomas often originate from DNA damage suffered by the cell in the malphigian (squamous) layer of the epidermis from the offending agent (UVB, chemicals, etc.) Immunosuppression in all forms plays an even more common role in the development of squamous cell carcinoma than it does in basal lesions (11).

Squamous cell carcinomas are graded by their appearance histologically and clinically. They are graded as well, moderately, or poorly differentiated relating to their histologic appearance and corresponding biological aggressiveness. Clinically more aggressive lesions are ulcerative, infiltrative, and exophytic. Squamous cell carcinomas can present as very aggressive subtypes such as the spindle cell tumor that resembles soft tissue sarcomas. There are also several less aggressive subtypes including verrucous carcinoma (arising in a condyloma) or keratoacanthomas (which can mimic squamous carcinomas with very rapid growth, but are typically characterized by eventual involution). Other varieties include adenoid (acantholytic) and adenosquamous squamous cell carcinomas.

In contrast to basal cell carcinomas, squamous cell carcinomas are much more aggressive and have a significantly higher propensity toward regional and systemic metastases. This risk correlates directly with tumor diameter and depth. Other tumor characteristics predicting both spread and recurrence include perineural and perivascular invasion, rapid growth, and previous recurrence. Regional metastases follow lymphatic spread to the lymphatic basins of the neck, axillae, and groins. A unique nodal basin for the head, cephalad and anterior to the ear, is the parotid nodal basin, which should be examined clinically and histologically when indicated. The overall incidence of regional and systemic metastases is 2% to 6% (12).

Most squamous cell carcinomas are also asymptomatic. However, they occasionally itch, bleed, ulcerate, or produce some type of open sore. They often appear on the sun-exposed areas of the body as a raised pink papule or plaque. Lesions can also be scaly, eroded, crusted, or ulcerated. They can vary tremendously; from flat lesions with ill-defined borders to large ulcerated and invasive lesions. They can resemble cutaneous horns, ill-defined sclerotic plaques, or deep penetrating cystic lesions.

As with basal cell carcinomas, much attention has been given to prevention with little improvement. And as with basal cell lesions, this population has shown some limited success with retinoid compounds in the prevention of these lesions.

The first step in treatment of these lesions remains accurate diagnosis that can be made with shave, punch, incisional, or excisional biopsy. The mainstay of treatment following diagnosis is excision/ablation. As with basal cell carcinoma, small lesions may be adequately treated with cryotherapy or curettage with electrodessication. They are most commonly excised with 0.4- to 1-cm margins (depending on size and grade), in the subcutaneous fat below the lesion. For most lesions, the risk of recurrence is low at 3% to 5%. However, for higher-risk areas and certain histologic criteria, recurrence may be as high as 11% to 53% (10). As with basal cell cancers, lesions prone to recurrence and lesions in cosmetically sensitive areas may be treated with Mohs micrographic surgery with significantly lower recurrence rates. Additionally, both squamous and basal cell cancers can be treated with radiation therapy with equivalent results, but often with significantly more morbidity including xerostomia, epilation, lacrimal duct scarring and skin necrosis (13).

Lymph node basins can be examined clinically, radiographically, and surgically/histologically. Clinically positive nodes are easily confirmed with fine needle aspiration (FNA). The advent of sentinel lymph node biopsy has made evaluation of the lymph node beds easier and with significantly less morbidity. Sentinel lymph node biopsy should be reserved for those lesions showing a higher propensity for spread (larger lesions) and a clinically negative nodal examination. Regional lymphadenectomy should be reserved for those with clinically positive nodes confirmed by FNA or those with a positive sentinel lymph node. Regional lymphadenectomy is but one part of the treatment, and certain groups may need additional or alternative regimens including chemotherapy and radiotherapy.

Recurrence is more common than with basal cell carcinomas, but does tend to occur in similar areas. Treatment should consist of adequate resections with good margin control or Mohs surgery. Additionally, attention should be directed to the lymphatic basins to evaluate for spread.

Malignant Melanoma

Melanoma is the third most common skin malignancy (3%) after basal and squamous cell carcinoma, but is clearly the most aggressive. New cases of melanoma arise at a rate of approximately 45,000 new cases per year in the United States, and result in close to 7,300 deaths per year or close to 65% of all skin cancer deaths. Additionally, melanoma rates in the United States continue to rise. It has become the sixth most common malignancy and the cancer with the fastest rate of increase in men, and its rise is second only to lung cancer in women (14). As with other skin cancers, melanomas are much more commonly encountered in fair-complected individuals and have a slight male predominance.

Sun exposure and a genetic susceptibility play the dominant role in the development of melanoma as they do in all skin cancers. Melanoma is found in an increasing incidence based on latitude, with higher rates closer to the equator. However, sun exposure does not tell the whole story. Sun exposure at an early age increases risk, as does blistering sunburns. Several idiosyncrasies exist, including abnormal distributions within a country or stable incidences with higher altitudes, and having close to 50% of melanomas occurring on non sun-exposed areas of the body. Additionally, melanoma is more closely linked to intermittent and not constant sun exposure (15). Melanoma is a frequent finding in several genodermatoses including xeroderma pigmentosum and dysplastic nevus syndrome. Dysplastic nevus syndrome has been the subject of several genetic evaluations with the mapping of the responsible gene to chromosomes 1 and 9 (16) (17) These and other genetic disorders account for close to 10% of melanomas, with the other 90% arising sporadically (18).

Some skin nevi are at higher risk of malignant degeneration. Congenital nevi carry approximately a 5% risk of malignant degeneration, with most of those becoming malignant in childhood (19). Dysplastic nevi are commonly encountered and are recommended for excision because of the risk of malignant degeneration.

These tumors arise from epidermal melanocytes in distribution in the skin (70%–80%) or from melanocytes concentrated in nevi (20%–30%). The offending agent is DNA damage from solar radiation, immunosuppression, repetitive trauma, or various other methods. This results in a fairly predictable pattern of progression to malignancy. Hormonal stimulation from estrogen is a well-known stimulant of the melanocyte with darkening of nevi and exacerbation of melanoma during pregnancy (20).

Melanomas are divided into four common types based on growth patterns. Superficial spreading melanoma is the most common type (70%–80%), and is recognized commonly as a flat appearing lesion with variations in color and possible nodular components. It can develop in an existing lesion or *de novo*. They are typically slow growing and grow horizontally before a vertical growth phase.

Nodular melanoma compromises approximately 20% of melanomas. They are more aggressive, with an earlier vertical growth phase and a higher incidence of ulceration and metastases. They appear blue-black and rarely arise from an existing nevus.

Acrolentiginous melanomas are significantly less common lesions. They occur in all ethnicities, but are the more common type of melanoma in blacks and other darker-complected individuals. These tumors are always found on the extremities, such as the palms of the hands, soles of the feet, and subungually. They grow rapidly with an early vertical growth phase. Because of their aggressivity and location they are often diagnosed in advanced stages.

Lentigo maligna melanomas are an unusual variant. They are classically described as melanoma *in situ*, but on resection frequently have areas of invasive disease. Lentigo maligna melanomas commonly occur on the face and hands with the appearance of a brownish-red patch. They can be quite large and have very indistinct margins often leading to incomplete resection.

As described earlier, melanomas follow a pattern of growth beginning radially and then becoming vertical. Once the tumor has progressed beyond the *in situ* stage, it is capable of regional and distant metastases. Two distinct staging systems have become extremely useful in determination of the depth of the melanoma, and therefore its propensity to spread. The Clark system describes the depth of the tumor in relation to skin/dermal histology. The second staging system, as described by Breslow, measures only the absolute depth of the tumor. Surprisingly, it has proved to be the more accurate and consistent predictor of regional and distant disease. Additionally, it is more consistently reproduced between pathologists and therefore easily used in investigational studies.

Melanomas often appear as new, pigmented lesions, or alternatively as changes in existing nevi. The classic diagnostic pneumonic is **ABCDE**; relating to the **A**symmetry, **B**order irregularity, **B**leeding, **C**olor change and irregularity, **D**iameter increase (especially >6 mm,) and **E**levation typical of melanomas. One of the earliest symptoms is pruritus; later symptoms include ulceration and bleeding.

As with all skin cancers, accurate treatment requires accurate diagnosis. Melanoma differs from the others in that the biopsy should also provide a means to measure depth. The most common biopsy for melanoma is usually an excisional biopsy with 1 mm to 2 mm margins. This allows for the entire specimen to be examined to determine the maximal depth of invasion and to guide re-excisional margins and further therapy. Alternate means of biopsy include incisional and punch biopsies, occasionally from multiple areas in the tumor, to determine maximal depth of invasion. Under no circumstances should a shave biopsy be contemplated because of the inability to estimate depth in these or subsequent specimens.

After establishing diagnosis, treatment usually involves re-excision to acceptable margins. The definition of acceptable margins has changed tremendously. Previously surgeons would resect up to 5 cm of margins on all sides of the tumor to capture so called in transit metastases and reduce local recurrence. These margins have been gradually reduced over time. Current recommendations are usually for 1 cm margins for thin tumors (<1 mm thick) and 2 cm margins for all others.

Concurrent with re-excision is an evaluation of the lymph nodes. The first evaluation is clinical. Patients with enlarged nodes should undergo FNA. Tumor depth will direct the therapy of patients without clinically enlarged nodes. For individuals with thin melanomas (<1 mm thick) and a negative clinical examination, the risk of regional and distant metastases is small, and recommendations are usually for observation with serial exams, chest x-ray and laboratory evaluation. Patients with intermediate thickness melanomas and a negative clinical examination represent a diagnostic dilemma. Some surgeons have recommended prophylactic regional lymph node dissections to identify occult metastases and hopefully prolong survival. And in certain subgroups, this is a viable option. However, in most centers, the prophylactic lymph node dissection has been replaced by the sentinel lymph node biopsy.

Sentinel lymph node biopsy is performed by injection of radio labeled colloid around the lesion the morning of surgery. This can then be mapped by lymphoscintigraphy to identify the draining nodal basin if it is uncertain (e.g., trunk melanomas that may metastasize to either left or right axillary or inguinal nodal basins benefit greatly from lymphoscintigraphy). This technique is supplemented by an injection of blue dye around the lesion immediately before surgery. Then using a handheld gamma probe, the sentinel lymph nodes (usually multiple) are identified and resected. This results in a major reduction in morbidity by eliminating many unnecessary lymph node dissections. Regional lymphadenectomy is reserved for those with clinically positive nodes confirmed by FNA and for those with positive sentinel lymph node biopsies. This remains true even in the face of distant metastases, as there is no other reasonable method to control potentially morbid nodal disease.

Metastatic melanoma has remained one of the most difficult tumors to treat. It has proved to be resistant to standard chemotherapy and radiation therapy has had only limited success. The most promising adjuvant treatment has been interferon-α-2b that has shown improvements in disease-free and overall survival in node positive patients without evidence of systemic metastases. Systemic metastases are common in deep tumors and some tumor types. They are often symptomatic with the most common sites being lung, liver, brain, bone, and gastrointestinal tract. Treatment guidelines in patients with stage IV disease should be tailored to the individual and the metastases. Some isolated metastases should be considered for resection, but most patients will have diffuse occult visceral metastases at the time of surgery.

Recurrence is uncommon with most melanomas, but is still seen in up to 25% of stage I melanomas. Additionally, tumor characteristics such as ulceration, thick lesions, and microsatellitosis are associated with higher rates of local recurrence. Regional nodes are the most common sites of initial recurrence in those who have not undergone lymphadenectomy. These should by managed by regional lymph node dissection that can be curative in approximately 25%. Local recurrence is defined as recurrence within 2 cm of an excision scar and is often a result of inadequate original margins. Treatment for local recurrence is wide excision, usually with a poor prognosis.

BITES AND STINGS

Spider Bites

There are approximately 30,000 known species of spiders worldwide and all but two are known to contain venom glands. Only two species are a common public health problem in the United States, the brown recluse and the black widow

spiders. One of the difficulties in managing these patients is that it is unusual for a patient to identify the type of spider that bit them.

Loxoscelism

Loxoscelism is a reaction to enovenation by brown recluse spiders in the genus Loxosceles. This spider is found throughout the midwestern and southern United States. These spiders are commonly found in old homes, barns, and woodpiles. They are medium-sized, with a body length between 8 and 15 mm and a leg length between 18 and 30 mm. Typically, they have a small, brown cephalothorax, and a fawn to dark brown abdominal color depending on the habitat. In addition, Loxosceles species contain a violin-shaped figure on the anterior surface of the cephalothorax—giving them the name "fiddle back" (21). Magnification is required to identify the fiddle, and, therefore, patients cannot use this feature as an identifying marker.

Clinical loxoscelism can present with a broad spectrum of cutaneous reactions and various systemic symptoms. Sometimes the bite causes no more than a transient skin irritation and follows a benign course. Other times, severe local cutaneous skin necrosis results, requiring debridement and skin grafts. Systemic symptoms include hemolysis, hemoglobinuria, disseminated intravascular coagulation, renal failure, and possibly death.

In a typical case, a red cutaneous lesion with a central area of necrosis develops 24 hours after envenomation. The pain is intense, localized, and associated with pruritus and a vesiculobullous eruption. The wound can be edematous, mottled, and violaceous with irregular borders surrounded by a large area of erythema. It usually has a dependent, gravitational spread especially when it is on the lower extremities (22).

Biopsies and histologic analysis demonstrate an intense neutrophilic vasculitis that is the hallmark of the lesion and that persists until the wound is healed. Current treatment includes the neutrophil inhibitor dapsone, broad-spectrum antibiotics, ice, and elevation of the affected extremity (23). Treatment should be conservative unless skin necrosis occurs. Immediate surgical excision of these lesions should not be performed as it commonly leads to a chronic nonhealing wound.

Black Widow Spider

The black widow spider of the genus Latrodectus is the most notorious spider in North America. The most common species in the United States is *Latrodectus mactans*. Typically the female, or black widow, has shiny black sepia with an underlying red marking that resembles an hourglass in the mature spider. These spiders are found in undisturbed areas under stones, logs and pieces of bark, as well as around vegetation, barns, outhouses, stone walls, and trash heaps.

The bite of the black widow occurs when its web is disturbed, and it is usually painless without a cutaneous lesion. After 1 to 6 hours, the patient develops intense pain accompanied by anxiety and a variety of symptoms related to the potent neurotoxin in the venom. Paresthesia, described as a burning sensation, may affect the whole body. The patient's pain is often most intense on the soles of the feet. Associated symptoms frequently include a thready pulse, diaphoresis, slurred speech, headache, dizziness, dysphagia, nausea, vomiting, edema, ptosis, and fever. Severe and uncontrolled hypertension with seizures is a dreaded complication of black widow bites.

Treatment begins with a local cleansing of the wound site, application of ice, and sedation of the patient. Muscle spasms, headache, vomiting, and paresthesia may be treated with a solution of 10% calcium gluconate. This may need to be repeated every 2 to 4 hours. Intravenous diazepam or narcotics are helpful for muscle spasm. Usually, the symptoms are self-limited; but the neurotoxin is virulent and envenomination should be treated aggressively.

Hobo Spider

The hobo spider, *Tegenaria agrestis*, is also referred to as the northwestern brown spider because of its geographic distribution in the United States (Alaska, Oregon, Idaho, Montana, and Washington). Generalized constitutional symptoms and intense headaches that are nonresponsive to analgesics are common following envenomation. The site of the bite usually becomes erythematous within 36 hours followed by blistering and, in approximately half the number of the patients, tissue necrosis. Local wound care is the mainstay of therapy. Surgical debridement is occasionally needed in cases of extensive tissue necrosis (24).

Tick Bites

Tick bites are common in spring and summer when people spend a significant amount of time outdoors. The most clinically important tick bites produce a local reaction with an erythematous papule that can develop into a nodular pruritic area. Removing the tick and leaving the hypostome and capitulum within the wound may exacerbate this. Residual tick parts in the skin may be responsible for some of the post bite nodularity.

The major concern of tick bites in the United States is from *Ixodes dammini*, which may be infected with a spirochete responsible for Lyme disease. In this illness, there is chronic migratory arthritis associated with the formation of diffuse erythematous halo patches over the patient's body. Patients may develop nausea, delirium, fever, and must be treated to prevent persistent arthritis. Before beginning treatment with tetracycline, blood should be drawn to confirm the diagnosis.

In addition to Lyme disease, Colorado tick fever and Rocky Mountain spotted fever, are also transmitted through tick bites. Colorado tick fever is an acute viral illness producing fever, malaise, and headache and is caused by the tick *Dermacentor andersoni*, or the dog tick. The tick is common throughout western United States, and the illness is self-limited. Rocky Mountain spotted fever is caused by a spirochete and can produce multiple erythematous spots over the body. It can be fatal if not treated with appropriate antibiotics. The surgeon may be called on to remove the tick parts, and therefore, it is important for him to recognize these illnesses (25).

PRESSURE SORES

In 1873, Paget wrote that "bed sores may be defined as the sloughing and mortification or death of a part produced by pressure." This insightful comment forms the basis for treatment of all pressure sores. They commonly occur in patients with disrupted sensory input in the affected area. Therapeutic interventions for the treatment of pressure sores were initiated during World War II when increasing reports of excision and closure were reported in young veterans. Treatment of this disorder with pedicle flaps and improved nutrition has complemented the advent of modern antibacterial therapy to improve outcome in this patient population.

Pressure sores are often erroneously referred to as *decubitus ulcer*. Although most pressure sores may occur in the lying down, or in Latin *decumbere*, position, pressure sores can occur from the top of the head to the bottom of the foot corresponding to bony prominences (26). In patients with paraplegia, the most common location of pressure sores is the ischium followed by the sacrum and the femoral trochanter. Ulceration over the heel and malleolus are less likely (27). Approximately two thirds of pressure sores are treated in acute care hospitals. Approximately 60% of these pressure sores are hospital acquired and 70% of these occur during the first 2 weeks of hospitalization. This underscores the importance of preventative measures.

The development of pressure sores is not only related to pressure but also shearing forces, friction, and moisture. The single most important factor is pressure on the skin, subcutaneous fat, and muscle. In healthy tissue, the normal capillary arteriolar pressure is 32 mm Hg (28). Experimental model has shown that constant pressure of 70 mm Hg over an area impairs the microcirculation with irreversible tissue damage occurring in 2 hours (29). With increasing pressure, less time is needed to cause irreversible tissue damage.

Shearing forces are also important factors in the etiopathogenesis of pressure sores. In immobilized, bedridden patients with the head raised, the deeper tissues such as muscle and bone tend to slide down whereas the skin and subcutaneous tissues remain adherent to the bed. These two opposing forces can disrupt the blood vessels between the two planes, causing ischemia of the overlying skin. The shearing forces coupled with the constant friction of the skin on the sheets cause skin breakdown. Incontinence, which is common in affected patients, increases moisture and bacterial colonization over the compromised skin, exacerbating the ulceration. Patients most vulnerable to these insults are those with underlying diseases affecting their sensory perception and/or their level of consciousness (spinal cord injuries, cerebral vascular accidents, and central nervous system diseases).

Pressure sores are classified in four stages (30). Stage I is described as an injury limited to the epidermis with superficial induration and erythema. Stage II is an ulceration extending through the dermis but not to the underlying fat. Stage I and II are reversible injuries with good chance for spontaneous healing if appropriate measures are taken. Stage III is an ulceration extending into subcutaneous fat and muscle. Stage IV is an ulceration penetrating into the underlying bone or joint. The appearance of the ulcer may be deceptive, and often a small ulceration may mask a large undermined crater.

A multidisciplinary approach is mandatory to ensure optimal outcome in the management of patients with pressure sores (31). Development of pressure sores occurs through a complex interplay among the patient's underlying disease and various mechanical insults. Appropriate treatment necessitates input from surgical, medical, psychiatric, and rehabilitation disciplines. The best treatment for pressure sores is prevention. All efforts must be made to identify high-risk patients so that appropriate preventive measures can be undertaken. Standardized measures involve placing the patient on a well padded and pressure reducing bed and repositioning the patient from side-to-side frequently to avoid prolonged pressure in one position. Shearing forces can be minimized by keeping the head of the bed in neutral position. Friction can be avoided by lifting instead of dragging the sheets under the patients. Finally, the patient must be maintained in a clean and dry environment. These preventive measures have been shown to be much more cost effective than the treatment of an established pressure sore.

Sheepskin overlying the sheets is an effective method to reduce sheer force against patient's skin. These sheets are dry, absorb moisture, and are capable of dispersing pressure over a large area. Unfortunately, clinical effectiveness has not been achieved in controlled studies. Alternating pressure devices, consisting of a mattress with air cells designed to inflate and deflate and thereby reduce pressure on pressure points have been used extensively, but they can be noisy, expensive, and bulky.

Preoperative Management

Many pressure sores may heal without surgical intervention. Implementation of meticulous wound care, intense nursing efforts, and improved nutrition of the patient are imperative in the management of pressure sores. Nonsurgical conservative therapy is often the preferred treatment if the patient's long-term prognosis is poor. In the initial management of patients with pressure sores, appropriate attention to wound infection and sepsis is required. Bacteremia has been documented in approximately 50% of patients with pressure sores, with half involving anaerobes. A localized infected bursa requires drainage and debridement of necrotic tissue.

The preoperative management should include the correction of any nutritional deficiency. A prealbumin level between 16 and 35 mg/dL should be reached before any surgical intervention to optimize wound healing. Furthermore, when possible, anemia should be corrected. Other preoperative measures include the evaluation of the bony skeleton for the possibility of osteomyelitis as well as determination of joint involvement. Laboratory information such as C-reactive protein and erythrocyte sedimentation rate (ESR) help predict osteomyelitis. Appropriate imaging using computed tomography or magnetic resonance imaging often provides additional information regarding bony involvement.

Finally, an indwelling catheter should provide urinary drainage and mechanical bowel preparation should be performed when indicated. In instances where muscle spasm needs to be controlled, oral diazepam or dantrolene as well as intrathecal baclofen should be considered.

Surgery of the Pressure Sore

In cases of small pressure sores, anesthesia may be unnecessary; however, it is preferred for debridement and closure of larger pressure sores. Appropriate positioning of the patient on the operating table depends on the anatomic location of the lesion. The surgical management of pressure sores should follow several important principles that can be applied to all patients with pressure sores.

The first step should include debridement of necrotic tissue to allow for the development of an appropriate recipient site for eventual reconstruction. Compromised skin, muscle, and bone should be excised. Bleeding tissue should be found at all surfaces of the wound. A bone biopsy will provide the definitive diagnosis of osteomyelitis. Multiple debridements are often required to achieve an appropriate wound bed. In cases where a bursa is present, such as in an ischial or sacral pressure sore, it needs to be completely excised. This is facilitated by using methylene blue to stain the bursa. Great care should be taken to ensure hemostasis, because loss of sympathetic tone in spinal cord injury patients often impedes hemostasis.

Another principle in the management of pressure sores is reconstruction of the defect with well-vascularized tissue, which is best performed by a plastic and reconstructive surgeon. Local and regional tissue in the form of a musculocutaneous or fasciocutaneous flap should be used. They should be inset in a manner to provide a tension-free closure; and the flaps should be designed to allow for readvancement, as recurrence is common.

Extensive Pressure Ulcers

The surgical techniques used in the treatment of decubitus ulcers have improved over the last two decades. However, there are some patients who have severe ulcers that are not amenable to conventional procedures. Large trochanteric ulcers with pyoarthrosis of the hip, osteomyelitis of the pelvis, and flexion contracture have been treated by amputation, hip disarticulation, or resection of the proximal femur. For extensive pressure sores of the sacrum and ischium, high thigh amputations and fillet of leg flaps are effective. This technique is superior to bilateral hip disarticulation as it provides four point pressure instead of two.

A total thigh flap and hip disarticulation can be used for treatment of trochanteric ulcers. These patients often have osteomyelitis of the femur and pyoarthrosis of the hip. The disadvantage of this procedure is that the acetabulum provides an extensive dead space prone to hematomas, seromas, and infection. In contrast, postoperative bony stability is improved if the proximal one third of the femur is preserved.

Postoperative Care

Routine postoperative care includes wound suction, urinary drainage, and avoidance of fecal soiling. Meticulous attention must be paid to patient positioning. Air fluidized beds not only reduce the chance of a second pressure sore but also reduce pressure on the healing flap. If healing of the flap is complete, the patient is allowed out of bed by the third week.

Complications

Because hematoma is a frequent complication, prevention of surgical dead space is important. Multiple large drains should be used. Wound separation usually reflects poor surgical planning, inadequate nutritional status, or persistent spasms. Flap necrosis can be disastrous as it causes recurrence of the ulcer. Other complications include infections, pneumonia, thrombophlebitis, and pulmonary embolism.

BURNS

Thermal, chemical, and electrical burns are a major cause of disability and death in the United States each year. According to the Centers for Disease Control and Prevention (CDC), approximately 1.1 to 1.2 million people are burned seriously enough to seek medical treatment yearly; 50,000 require hospitalization with 4,000 dying of injury or complications annually. Burn deaths occur in a bimodal distribution, either immediately after the initial insult or several days to weeks later due to sepsis and multiorgan failure. Burns typically occur in children younger than age 15, young male adults, and the elderly with approximately two thirds of burn injury occurring in the home (32). In children younger than 4 years of age, 65% of burns are related to scalds due to the spillage of hot liquids. In those children aged 4 to 14, approximately two thirds are due to thermal injury with only one fourth attributable to scald injury (33). In young adults and the elderly, the cause of burn trauma is usually related to thermal injury (due to house fires) or are smoking or alcohol related (34).

Burns have become such a recognized cause of morbidity and mortality, beginning in the 1960s and 1970s burn centers began to be introduced. These centers provide a multidisciplinary approach to burn care including surgeons, nutritionists, wound care specialists, pulmonary/critical care physicians, and others to effectively treat major burn injuries. The treatment of burns is an evolving process with significantly more than simple debridement and skin coverage needed for major injury. The pathophysiology behind this process involves numerous mediators and organ systems.

To understand the pathophysiology of burn injuries, it is important to review clinical burn classification. Burns are classified by the degree of tissue damage: injury to the epidermis, dermis, subcutaneous fat, and underlying organs and structures. First-degree burns are burns that are limited to the epidermis. These burns result in erythema, pain, and edema formation. Examples of these burns are sunburns and minor scalds and heal without scarring. Second-degree burns are divided into superficial and deep burns. Superficial second-degree burns involve the epidermis and the superficial (papillary) dermis. Most of the dermal appendages (hair and glands) are spared. These burns are painful, blisters occur, and the burn sites blanch with pressure. These wounds are edematous and slippery due to the abundance of proteinaceous exudate and typically heal in 7 to 10 days without requiring debridement or grafting. Deep second-degree burns involve the full dermis (papillary and reticular) including most of the dermal appendages. These wounds are white, blistered, edematous, usually painless, and will likely result in severe scarring. Due to progressive ischemia, these burns may convert to third-degree burns and as such remain a diagnostic and therapeutic dilemma. Third-degree burns are full thickness and show disruption of all dermal and epidermal elements. These wounds are leathery, insensate, and nonedematous due to the complete lack of vascularity. These wounds will not undergo spontaneous re-epithelization and require excision and grafting. Fourth-degree burns involve tissues deep to the skin such as muscle and bone.

Thermal Injury

The skin is an impressive and multifunctional organ maintaining fluid regulation and providing an excellent barrier to the transfer of energy, both cold and heat, to deeper tissues. Therefore, much of the injury due to direct contact of flame, hot liquids (scald), and hot objects is confined to this superficial area. However, after this direct injury, the resultant inflammatory response of local tissues and cells, including progressive dermal ischemia, can lead to a deeper injury. Human skin can tolerate temperatures up to 40°C for relatively long periods; however, at temperatures greater than this, tissue destruction increases logarithmically (35). Tissue damage is related not only to the time of exposure and temperature, but also to the specific heat of the causative agent. For example, the specific heat of fat is higher than water; therefore a grease burn would cause a deeper burn than a water burn of the same temperature for the same duration.

In 1953, Jackson described thermal injury in burn wounds as three zones: the zone of coagulation, the zone of stasis, and the zone of hyperemia (36). The central area of burn, that area of necrosis closest to the heat source, is characterized by the coagulation of cells. Therefore, it is called the *zone of coagulation* and is irreversibly injured from contact with the heat source. Extending concentrically from the central zone of coagulation lays a labile zone of injured cells called the *zone of stasis*. At this level, circulation is impaired and if progressive vasoconstriction and thrombosis occur, this potentially salvageable zone will progress to coagulative necrosis. Finally, peripheral to the zone of stasis lies an area that has only sustained minimal injury and is characterized by vasodilation of blood vessels due to inflammatory mediators. This is termed the *zone of hyperemia* and cells in this zone will typically recover over a period of 7 to 10 days unless they are subjected to some additional insult (37).

The initial cytologic evidence of thermal injury is a redistribution of the fluid and solid components of the cell nuclei. Cytoskeletal components are disrupted and changes in membrane permeability lead to an increase in intracellular sodium, hydrogen, and calcium. DNA synthesis and transcription are halted, as is ribonucleic acid (RNA) processing and translation. Progression through the cell cycle is disrupted as proteins denature and disaggregate and are finally degraded through lysosomal and proteasomal pathways (38).

Not all proteins and organelles are equally susceptible to thermal injury due to the unique makeup of each structure. Research evaluating proteins, DNA, RNA, and cell membrane structures exposed to excessive heat found that the lipid bilayer and membrane-bound ATPases are the least stable cell components when subjected to heat and are therefore the most responsible agents for the tissue necrosis (39).

The increase in cell membrane breakdown and permeability allows for the imbibition of fluid, causing nuclear swelling, membrane rupture, and ultimate pyknosis. The cell cytoplasm turns from fluid to granular and then homogenously coagulated. Progressive denaturation of the cell protein continues as the temperature rises. The decrease in enzyme activity of the cell to less than 50% of normal results in irreversible cell death (39).

The theory that the progressive changes in the burn wound may be related to inflammation suggests that inflammatory mediators may play a role in wound progression; specifically, prostaglandins, histamine, oxygen-free radicals, and interleukins. It is well established that there is a massive release of potent vasodilator prostanoids, mainly prostacyclin (PGI_2), and vasoconstrictor prostanoids, such as thromboxane (TXA_2), in edema fluid and plasma following burns (40). The vasodilatory properties of prostacyclin serve to increase local blood flow to the area of injury and thereby increase mediator-induced vascular leak. Thromboxane, on the other hand, increases both platelet aggregation and neutrophil margination in the burn microcirculation, potentiating burn edema and ischemia (41). Inhibition of both of these prostanoids has been studied individually. Topical ibuprofen applied to partial thickness burns has been shown to decrease edema and improve local blood flow (42,43) When the thromboxane response was prevented pharmacologically, platelet adherence was reduced, leukocytes and erythrocytes were prevented from sticking to vessel walls, and vasoconstriction was mediated (44).

Thromboxane synthetase inhibition with imidazole, dipyridamole, and methimazole improved the integrity of the dermal microcirculation.

Vasoactive amines such as histamine are also found in increased concentrations after thermal injury. Histamine is released either as a direct result of heat or by stimulation of mast cells. It is associated with vasodilation and increased permeability (45). This increased protein permeability from capillaries and venules potentiate the edema in tissues following injury (46). However, the increase in histamine levels is transient, showing that this agent may be involved only in the early increase in permeability, and there has been limited success with the use of histamine receptor blockers (H_1, H_2, H_3) in decreasing post burn edema (43,47).

Oxygen-free radicals, or oxidants, are released in large quantities after burn injury and may actually initiate the progressive damage of the burn injury. However, their short half-life makes them difficult to study in humans. Free radicals are produced whenever the energy charge of a cell drops below a critical level, limiting the oxygen availability necessary to produce adenosine 5-triphosphate (ATP). They are also produced as part of the leukocyte respiratory burst to help prevent bacterial invasion when skin integrity is broached. In burns, oxidants are produced secondary to the local tissue hypoxia present in the wounds and increasing levels of xanthine oxidase following reperfusion. These free oxygen radicals then cause endothelial damage which further increases capillary permeability and edema. In addition to increasing edema, the oxidants are also known to denature proteins and structural elements of cells. There have been few trials regarding the use of antioxidants to combat the damaging effects of oxygen-free radicals. Ward proved that free radical scavengers such as catalase or superoxide dismutase could decrease the amount of post burn edema if given before injury, a concept not feasible in clinical practice (48).

In acute burns, the complement system is activated by an undefined mechanism (49). Among the activated products in the complement cascade, C5a appears to be the initiating factor in the inflammatory response. C5a activates the secretion of histamine by intravascular neutrophils. In addition, C5a catalyzes the conversion of xanthine dehydrogenase to xanthine oxidase by interacting with endothelial cells. Elevated levels of xanthine oxidase lead to the production of oxygen free radicals (O_2, HO, H_2O_2), which cause increased vascular permeability as previously discussed. Furthermore, C5a may be a cofactor in the production of cytokines such as tumor necrosis factor α (TNF-α), which are active in the inflammatory reaction in burn patients (50).

The multisystemic responses of the burn patient, and the patient's death or survival, are closely related to the successful management of the burn wound. The first response to evaluate and manage is the vascular response. There is a local and generalized fluid flux, a generalized impairment in cell membrane function, and an increase in burn-tissue osmotic pressure (51). These all lead to fluid entering the interstitial space from the capillary as is described by Starling who published his original equation in 1896 (52). In this theorem, he describes forces in capillaries and interstitium (hydrostatic and osmotic) that counterbalance each other to maintain fluid homeostasis. These forces, along with the state of capillary protein permeability and interstitial compliance are described in the modern version of the Starling equation:

$$Q = K_f(P_{cap} - P_i) + \sigma(\pi p - \pi i)$$

where Q is the fluid filtration rate, or the net rate of fluid crossing the capillary membrane into the interstitium; K_f is the fluid filtration coefficient (composed of the surface area of the capillary bed and the hydraulic conductivity) or ease of fluid accumulation; P_{cap} is the capillary hydrostatic pressure (mm Hg); P_i is the interstitial hydrostatic pressure (mm Hg); σ is the reflection coefficient (a marker of capillary permeability); πp is the plasma colloid osmotic or oncotic pressure; and πi is the interstitial osmotic or oncotic pressure. As has been discussed, in burned tissue there is a massive denaturization of protein, vasoconstriction and venodilation, and increased capillary leak causing both a hydrostatic as well as an osmotic (oncotic) gradient favoring a fluid flux into the interstitial space. This edema, depending on the size of the burn, can be localized to the injured area or become a generalized systemic response.

The hypovolemia due to the massive movement of fluid into the interstitium is accentuated by the increased evaporative loss due to the lack of skin coverage. If the intravascular volume is not restored, perfusion to all organs will be compromised, followed by shock and eventual cell death. To assure adequate fluid resuscitation in burn patients, several formulas can be used to guide fluid requirements (Table 22.2). The most commonly used formula is the Parkland formula (53). Total fluid requirement for the first 24 hours is estimated by multiplying the percentage of body surface area with second-degree burns or greater by the weight of the patient in kilograms and a factor of 4.

$$\text{Volume} = \text{weight (kg)} \times \% \text{ burn} \times 4$$

Lactated Ringers solution is the fluid of choice for the first 24 hours. The percentage of total body surface area (TBSA) burned can be estimated from the Lund and Browder chart, which divides the body into regions, with each region consisting of 9% body surface area (Fig. 22.1) (54). Alternatively, one can use the palmar surface of the patient's hand to estimate the size of the burn with the palmar surface representing 1% body surface area (34). Half of the calculated

TABLE 22.2

Formulas Used for Fluid Replacement in Burn Patients

Formula	Electrolyte	Colloid	Glucose in Water
First 24 h			
Burn budget of FD Moore	Lactated Ringer, 1,000–4,000 mL 0.5N saline, 1,200 mL	7.5% of body weight	1,500–5,000 mL
Evans	Normal saline, 1.0 mL/kg/% burn	1.0 mL/kg/% burn	2,000 mL
Brooke	Lactated Ringer, 1.5 mL/kg/% burn	0.5 mL/kg/% burn	2,000 mL
Parkland	Lactated Ringer, 4 mL/kg/% burn		
Hypertonic sodium solution	Volume to maintain urine output at 30 mL/h (fluid contains 250 mEq Na/L)		
Modified Brooke	Lactated Ringer 2 mL/kg/% burn		
Second 24 h			
Burn budget of FD Moore	Lactated Ringer 1,000–4,000 mL 0.5N saline, 1,200 mL	2.5% of body weight	1,500–5,000 mL
Evans ½ of first 24-h requirement	½ of first 24-h requirement	½ of first 24-h requirement	2,000 mL
Brooke	½ to ¾ of first 24-h requirement	½ to ¾ of first 24-h requirement	2,000 mL
Parkland		20% to 60% of calculated plasma volume	To maintain adequate urine output
Hypertonic sodium solution	⅓ isotonic salt solution orally up to 3,500 mL limit		
Modified Brooke		0.3–0.5 mL/kg/% burn	To maintain adequate urine output

From Ruitt BA. Fluid resuscitation for extensively burned patients. *J Trauma* 1981;21(suppl):690, © by Williams & Wilkins, 1981.

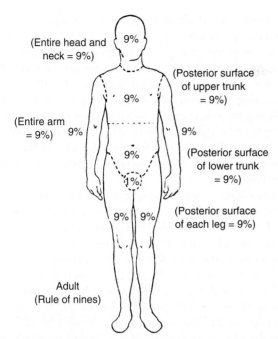

FIGURE 22.1 Estimation of body surface area in burns. (From Shroeder SA, Krupp MA, Tierney LM Jr, et al. *Current medical diaganosis and treatment.* Norwalk, CT: Apppleton & Lange, 1990, with permission.)

fluid is given during the first 8 hours following the burn with the remaining half infused over the next 16 hours. One must be cautioned that these calculations are only estimates of fluid requirements, and more precise intravascular replacement should be based on urine output, which reflects end organ perfusion. If the urine output is low, despite having given the estimated fluid requirement, additional information can be obtained by measuring hemodynamic parameters with a Swan-Ganz catheter. Adequate tissue perfusion is usually assured if urine output is 0.5 to 1 mL/kg/hr in an adult or 1 mL/kg/hr in an infant.

Renal function is altered in the burn patient, similar to that seen in other trauma patients. The normal stress response occurs along with the additional marked loss of intracellular volume. The posterior pituitary releases antidiuretic hormone (ADH), causing increased reabsorption of water in the renal tubules. Simultaneously, maximal sodium reabsorption occurs because of aldosterone release from the adrenals. Under this influence, oliguria ensues as the kidney will only excrete the amount of urine necessary to handle the solute load. The result is a small amount of concentrated urine with a decreased urine sodium concentration (55). Left untreated, acute tubular necrosis and potential renal failure can occur.

The pulmonary response to burns is the result of both the direct injury and circulating inflammatory mediators from distant burned regions. The lungs may be exposed to decreased oxygen secondary to combustion and may be further compromised if smoke inhalation occurs. Although the trachea and bronchi dissipate heat rapidly, the oropharynx and upper airway may be burned. This causes

edema, leading to possible obstruction, and further hypoxia. The hypoxia causes a release of mediators resulting in further constriction of the bronchioles, and can lead to a ventilation-perfusion imbalance. The consequences are inadequate peripheral perfusion, lactic acidosis, and further cellular injury. As resuscitation occurs, the products of the peripheral ischemia are recirculated and must be cleared by the already damaged lungs (39).

Originally, the lung was thought to be compromised further as resuscitation began secondary to an increase in total body capillary permeability; however, the lungs may be spared this added insult (39). The normal respiratory response to burning is hyperventilation, a common stress response. Ventilation is about twice normal with minute volumes of up to 14 L at a ventilatory rate of 20+/minute (56). This is caused by the increased oxygen needs and the ventilatory-perfusion imbalance. In patients with burns greater than 40% of their TBSA, a restrictive process with a decreased lung volume, decreased vital capacity, and an increase in pulmonary resistance can be seen (55).

Thermal injury can also alter the gastrointestinal tract function. The initial response is severe splanchnic vasoconstriction associated with an ileus. If not recognized, acute gastric dilation can occur, leading to regurgitation and aspiration. Gastroduodenal ulceration, a frequent occurrence in burn patients, is not always clinically evident and is not a result of an absolute hyperacidity (57). However, patients developing gastroduodenal injury within 72 hours of the burn do have higher basal outputs than those without gastrointestinal injury (58). Gastrin levels are not increased in thermal trauma and no correlation exists between serum gastrin levels and gastric acid output in burn patients. Additionally, atrophy of small bowel mucosa occurs within 12 hours of injury in proportion to the size of the burn injury and is related to increased epithelial death by apoptosis (59). Intestinal permeability to macromolecules also increases after burn (60). Therefore, the pathophysiology appears to be a relative hyperacidity combined with increased mucosal barrier permeability and primary cytotoxicity with apoptosis of cells.

Burns also alter the hepatobiliary system. These changes may be the result of hypovolemia, hypoxia, or circulating mediators requiring clearance. Liver function tests all show some abnormalities during the course of a severe burn (61). Liver biopsies have shown cloudy swelling as early as 3 hours postburn (39). This can progress to hepatocellular necrosis, vacuolization, and fatty degeneration (2). However, repair and regeneration occur with time. Biliary tract stasis also occurs, as do changes in the normal bile-salt ratios, and sludge frequently forms in the gallbladder (39).

Numerous metabolic and neuroendocrine changes occur throughout the course of injury and recovery. Some of these are due primarily to hypovolemia. However, others occur when perfusion and tissue oxygenation are adequate (62). Hypermetabolism develops with increased oxygen consumption above the basal predicted level in burn patients. This increase in oxygen consumption is linear in patients with up to 40% TBSA burns and can reach a heat production of twice normal levels in 50% to 100% TBSA burns (63). Although the exact cause of this hypermetabolism is not fully elucidated, the metabolic rate gradually falls toward normal with wound healing or burn wound closure (39).

The skin is another organ obviously involved. The fluid-holding lipid in the skin is destroyed by burning so that up to four times the normal amount of body fluids can be lost through burned skin (62). Increased evaporative water loss causes cooling of the body, shivering, and additional heat expenditure. Increasing the environmental temperature and humidity can decrease the energy loss caused by evaporation and shivering. The critical temperature appears to be 32°C to 34°C (39,63).

The hypermetabolic state after thermal trauma causes protein catabolism, hyperglycemia, decreased glucagon-insulin ratios, and extreme intracellular cation alterations. Intracellular sodium concentrations can rise dramatically and will remain elevated unless daily caloric intake is adequate (64). The negative nitrogen balance accompanying hypermetabolism can cause a nitrogen requirement of up to 20 g/m^2/body surface area burn per day during the first month post burn. This nitrogen need is a result of both increased catabolism and decreased protein synthesis (65).

Levels of counter regulatory hormones, glucagons, cortisol, and catecholamines are elevated in burn patients and are thought to play a major role in mediating the catabolic response to injury (66). It appears that these endocrine mediators, working with various inflammatory mediators, are in large part responsible for the various metabolic responses seen after a major burn (39).

Another series of systemic responses to the burn injury involve the immune system. Burn injury induces a state of immunosuppression that predisposes the patient to infection by both endogenous and exogenous bacteria. The immune system can be divided into three units: the skin, which is the first barrier of defense, the nonspecific immune response (innate), and the specific host response (adaptive). All of these are impaired as a result of thermal injury (67). The dryness of the skin and keratin layer provide the first barrier to bacterial invasion. Its normal secretion of sebum further provides bactericidal properties. Burning removes the outer layer, and the local inflammatory response leads to an increase in PGE$_2$ and fluid into the wound. Although the fluid fibrin and thrombin help to localize the bacteria, the fluid also tends to neutralize the bactericidal properties of the sebum (39,66,68). The innate host response is the second line of defense and involves stimulating both localized and systemic inflammatory reactions. In addition to the natural barriers that comprise the integument, there are cellular (leukocyte, natural killer cell, and macrophage) and humoral (complement) elements. Following burns, there is a dysfunction of the cellular elements with both decreased activation and altered function of both natural killer cells and macrophages (69). Neutrophil dysfunction follows a significant thermal injury, with deficits in endothelial adherence, chemotaxis, and intracellular killing (70–72). The complement cascade is an important humoral component of the innate immune system. Following a burn injury, the alternate pathway of the complement system is depressed whereas there is little effect on the classical pathway (73). Circulating complement is decreased by as much as 50% including the ever important C3a, a major element in both alternate and classical pathways (68). These malfunctions of the innate system lead to not only a decrease in the host's natural defenses but also an increased exposure of the host to pathogens.

The adaptive immune system is likewise affected during thermal trauma. There seems to be a decreased production and function of T lymphocytes along with a decrease in T cell–dependent immune functions (69). Decreases in immunoglobulins and inflammatory mediators further the host's predisposition to infection and potential sepsis.

Burn wound sepsis may result from the quantitative disturbance between the host's resistance and the bacterial load (74). Locally, the thermal injury destroys the skin, and alters the balance between competing endogenous flora and skin. Bacteria readily colonize the open burn sites after the thermal insult. The initial colonizing bacteria are the patient's own endogenous gram-positive skin flora. These organisms reside in the hair follicles and the orifices of sebaceous glands in the concentration of 10^3 bacteria per gram of tissue. In the days following injury, endogenous flora from the patient's gastrointestinal tract also colonize the burn wound (75). As the bacteria count reaches 10^5 bacteria per gram of tissue, invasion can occur into the dermal–subcutaneous junction. Deeper incursion into the vascular structures leads to thrombosis of vessels and destruction of surrounding viable tissues. As consequence, burn wound infection may convert a partial thickness burn into a full thickness burn by virtue of ischemia and bacterial autolysis (76).

Before the discovery of penicillin, a 30% of TBSA burn had a mortality rate of 50%, with streptococcal infection responsible for most deaths (75). Penicillin use drastically reduced the mortality from streptococcal infection. After the discovery of penicillin and the virtual elimination of streptococcal mortality, *Staphylococcus aureus* became a principal agent in burn wound infections and remains so to the present. In the 1960s, burn wound sepsis accounted for 70% of all hospital burn deaths, and *Pseudomonas aeruginosa,* either from the patient's gastrointestinal flora and/or from the environment, was the dominant organism (76). Although the incidence of burn wound sepsis from pseudomonas has decreased dramatically because of topical antimicrobials, colonization of the wound with high concentrations of pseudomonas (>10^5) remains potentially lethal. The circulation of byproducts or endotoxin from high Pseudomonas concentration can produce gram-negative sepsis with shock and death. Another organism of interest is *Clostridium tetani*. Because tetanus can occur even in superficial burns, coverage and prophylaxis with tetanus immunoglobulin or tetanus toxoid needs to be instituted based on the patient's immunization history.

Electrical Injury

Electrical injuries are a unique form of thermal trauma. They can be divided arbitrarily into high-tension (>1,000 V) and low-tension (<1,000 V) injuries (39). The passage of the injurious electrical current through tissue is capable of causing injury through one or multiple distinct biophysical energy transduction mechanisms. These mechanisms include the direct action of electrical forces on proteins, membranes, and other biomolecular structures, as well as the indirect action mediated by the generation of heat (77). Additionally, electrical current can disrupt electrically mediated functions such as cardiac rhythm, leading to potentially fatal arrhythmias.

The first method to be discussed is the direct contact of a high voltage injury causing essentially a thermal injury. Passage of electric current through a solid conductor causes the conversion of electric energy into heat (Joule effect) (78). The amount of heat can be determined by Ohm law and the Joule effect. The extent of the injury depends on the type of current, the pathway of flow, the local tissue resistance, and the duration of contact. The electrical forces themselves also further mediate tissue damage through cell membrane electroporation and electroconformational protein denaturation (79).

Several theories to explain the pathologic changes seen after electrical injury have been postulated. The first emphasizes the difference in tissue resistance to current flow. Tissue resistance progressively increases from nerve to blood vessels, muscle, skin, fat, and finally to bone (79). Bone, which has the greatest resistance, generates the most heat and would cause greater necrosis in the deep periosseous tissues (39).

Alternate theories contest the existence of progressive muscle necrosis. Other research has found that the internal body acts as a volume conductor of a single resistance and not as though it was composed of tissues of varying resistances (80). With the onset of current, flow, amperage, and temperature all rose in parallel throughout the limb. By the time of current arching, both muscle and bone temperatures were equal. However, the same research observed that it took bone longer to dissipate heat and postulated that this prolonged elevation in temperature accounted for the periosseous "core" of necrotic muscle seen clinically. Additionally, this study proposed that involved muscle and vessels sustain irreversible damage at the time of current passage with immediate microscopic muscular coagulation necrosis and small nutrient artery thrombosis.

A third theory postulates that inflammatory mediators are responsible for the progressive necrosis that follows electrical injury. By using a rat model, increasing levels of arachidonic acid metabolites, chiefly thromboxane, have been demonstrated in the deep periosseous tissues beneath what appeared to be uninjured skin. With time, the thromboxane increased progressively toward the limb surface until apparently uninjured skin necrosed, just as in the clinical situation (80).

The first step in managing the victim of an electrical injury is to choose among the planning options. As stated, controversy exists whether the hidden damage of tissue beneath apparently uninjured skin is a slow manifestation of irreversible muscle damage secondary to the original insult, or whether it is actually progressive ischemic necrosis secondary to ongoing vascular compromise. Proponents of the pathophysiologic scheme of immediate irreversible cell damage and necrosis advise early aggressive debridement to decrease the septic risk of unexcised nonviable tissue. Proponents of the progressive ischemic necrosis accept the inability to discern the full extent of the injury initially, and they advocate cautious initial debridement followed by periodic debridement as demarcation proceeds. Premature closure over partially necrotic tissue is thereby avoided. If the progressive necrosis is because of cellular injury secondary to mediators released by the heat generated, then pharmacologic means to block or inhibit these mediators may become useful (81,82).

Chemical Injury

Chemical burns occur when a toxic substance comes in direct contact with skin. Chemical burns are usually the result of accidents with household cleaning supplies or industrial injuries. Although chemical burns account for only 3% of all burns, they account for up to 30% of all burn deaths (83). Chemicals burn through oxidation, reduction, corrosion, protoplasmic poisoning, or the ischemic concomitants of vesicant activity. The degree of damage is related to the chemical nature of the agent, the duration of skin exposure, and the specific concentration of the agent. Owing to penetration, injury can continue even after the agent is washed away.

Oxidizing agents cause burn injury when they become oxidized on contact with the skin. The reaction and its by-products account for further toxicity with continued absorption. Commonly encountered oxidizing agents are chromic acid, sodium hypochlorite (bleach), and potassium permanganate. Reducing agents act somewhat similarly and produce protein denaturation by binding free electrons in tissue proteins. Examples of reducing agents include alkyl mercuric agents, hydrochloric acid, and nitric acid.

Corrosive agents act in a variety of ways and are so named due to the degree of denaturation exerted on tissue protein. Their net effect is eschar formation and a shallow, indolent ulcer. Corrosive agents include phenols and cresols, white phosphorous, dichromate salts, sodium metals, and the lyes. Additionally, many chemical agents can produce potentially lethal reactions secondary to systemic absorption as seen with phenol.

Protoplasmic poisons produce their effect by forming salts with proteins or by binding or inhibiting calcium or other inorganic ions necessary for tissue viability and function. Examples include "alkaloidal" acids; acetic acids; formic acid; and metabolic competitors/inhibitors, including oxalic and hydrofluoric acids.

Vesicant agents produce ischemia with anoxic necrosis at the site of contact. Examples are cantharides (Spanish fly), dimethyl sulfoxide, mustard gas, and lewisite. There is also a subgroup of agents that are desiccants and produce their deleterious effects by causing dehydration damage through the production of excessive heat in the tissues. Examples include sulfuric and muriatic acid (39).

Although not as accurate as describing burns by their mechanism of action, burns can also be classified as either acid or alkali. Although the wounds produced from individual acids or alkalis share similarities, their mechanism of action possess enough distinctions to warrant consideration as two separate groups (84). A better predictor than pH alone for acids is the amount of base needed to raise the pH to neutrality (85). As for bases, a pH greater than 11.5 is usually needed to produce severe tissue damage. On a per volume basis, alkalis tend to cause more local tissue damage than acids. This is due to the fact that acids cause coagulation necrosis with the precipitation of proteins through hydrolysis and eschar formation preventing future penetration, whereas alkalis produce liquefactive necrosis and saponification of fat thereby allowing diffusion of the alkali deeper into the tissue.

Whatever the chemical agent, first aid consists of removing the saturated clothing and irrigating the involved area with copious amounts of water. The volume of water will dissipate the heat generated by the dilution of the offending agent. In addition, water hydrotherapy will effectively cleanse the wound of unreacted surface chemicals and may restore tissue water lost to the hygroscopic effect of certain agents. Water constitutes immediate first aid and should continue at the scene of the injury for 30 minutes and thereafter anywhere from 2 to 12 hours. Up to 48 hours of continuous irrigation may be necessary for chemical burns involving the eye. No agent has been found superior to water. The one exception is with hydrofluoric acid. It has been shown that the administration of topical calcium (as in calcium gluconate gel) and intravenous calcium, after copious irrigation, will help prevent further injury and stop pain as well as help correct the hypocalcemia that results from such an injury (84).

Cold Injury

Human skin can also be injured by cold, either by direct cellular injury or by indirect cellular effects. The indirect effects are from microvascular changes that lead to thrombosis and ischemia (39). Some of the recognized and documented changes from direct cellular injury include (i) development of extracellular ice formation, (ii) development of intracellular ice, (iii) cell dehydration and crenation, (iv) abnormal concentrations of electrolytes with in the cell, (v) thermal shock, and (vi) denaturation of lipid–protein complexes.

The rate of freezing is crucial to the location of ice crystal formation. Slow cooling causes extracellular ice crystals whereas rapid freezing causes the more lethal intracellular ice formation. Extracellular crystals are not completely innocuous, as they cause the withdrawal of water across the cell membrane and contribute to cell dehydration and ultimate death.

An incompletely understood concept is the manner in which subzero temperatures can produce denaturation of lipid–protein complexes. Part of the lipid membrane breakup may be caused by the solvent action of the toxic electrolyte

concentration within the cell that has resulted from the cellular dehydration.

Indirect cellular damage appears to result from progressive microvascular insult and is usually more severe than the direct cellular effects. This is emphasized by the fact that skin subjected to a standard freezing and thawing injury that consistently produced necrosis can survive as a full-thickness skin graft when transplanted to an uninjured recipient site (86). Conversely, uninjured full-thickness skin did not survive when transferred to a recipient bed pretreated with the same freezing injury. Therefore direct skin injury appears reversible, and the progressive nature of the injury is most likely caused by microvascular change.

The primary site of injury seems to be the vascular endothelium. By 72 hours postinjury and thawing, there is a loss of vascular endothelium in the capillary walls and substantial fibrin deposition. The endothelium may be totally destroyed and the fibrin may saturate the arteriole walls. It is interesting to note, however, that the injury appears greatest in the venules where the circulation is slower.

Frostbite is defined as the superficial or deep freezing of some part of the body. This can occur rapidly after exposure to freezing temperatures. Clinically, this temperature is 20°F or less for 1 or more hours (87). The skin becomes blanched and a stinging sensation ensues. The affected part eventually becomes numb with a sensation of clumsiness. The most common system of classifying frostbite injuries is based on the actual physical findings after cold exposure and rewarming. The injuries are classified according to degree of injury. First-degree injury is characterized by a white or yellowish firm plaque in the area of the injury, sometimes surrounded by erythema and edema. Tissue necrosis or loss does not usually occur. However, a causalgia-like pain frequently develops, indicating that some degree of nervous damage has occurred. Second-degree injury consists of superficial blisters surrounded by erythema and edema, and containing clear or milky fluid. These injuries usually heal spontaneously unless the initial injury was deep enough to progress to tissue loss. Injury to the blister may cause desiccation of the underlying tissue and subsequent necrosis. Third-degree injury consists of deeper blisters containing red or purple fluid or areas of darkly discolored skin without blisters. Partial-thickness injury is associated more commonly with areas of blister formation whereas full-thickness injury is associated with deeply discolored areas. Prognosis for these injuries has been poor, with tissue loss common. Fourth-degree injury consists of deep cyanosis of the injured part without vesicle formation or local erythema. In these injuries, gangrene is often evident within hours of injury.

Treatment of frostbite is aimed at blocking direct cellular damage, preventing microvascular thrombosis and tissue loss, or correcting the residual defect. It is important to avoid refreezing after the part has been thawed. Direct cellular damage is minimized by thawing rapidly with immersion in water warmed between 104°F and 108°F. The narrow temperature range should be closely observed as rewarming at lower temperatures is less beneficial for tissue survival and higher temperatures may produce a burn injury and further compound the problem.

REFERENCES

1. Ross MH, Romrell LJ, Kaye GI. Integumentary system. In: Coryell Pa, ed. *Histology a text and atlas*. Baltimore: Williams & Wilkins, 1995:370.
2. Robson MC, Krizek TJ, Wray RC. Care of the thermally injured patient. In: Zuidema GD, Rutherford RB, Ballinger A, eds. *Management of trauma*. Philadelphia: WB Saunders, 1979:666–736.
3. Netscher DT, Spira M. Basal cell carcinoma: an overview of tumor biology and treatment. *Plast Reconstr Surg* 2004;113:5.
4. Emmett AJJ, Austin W, Page G. *The bare fact: the effect of sun on skin*. Sydney, Baltimore: Williams & Wilkins, 1988.
5. Fitzpatrick RE, Goldman MP, Satur NM, et al. Pulsed carbon dioxide laser resurfacing of photo-aged facial skin. *Arch Dermatol* 1996;132:395.
6. Buzzell RA. Carcinogenesis of cutaneous malignancies. *Dermatol Surg* 1996;22:209.
7. Lancou JP. Carcinogenesis of basal cell carcinomas: genetics and molecular mechanisms. *Br J Dermatol* 2002;146(Suppl 61):17.
8. De Rosa G, Staibano S, Barra E, et al. p53 protein in aggressive and nonaggressive basal cell carcinoma. *J Cutan Pathol* 1993;20:429.
9. Kripke ML. Immunology and photocarcinogenesis: new Light on an old problem. *J Am Acad Dermatol* 1986;14:149.
10. Rudolph R, Zelac DE. Squamous cell carcinoma of the skin. *Plast Reconstr Surg* 2004;114:6.
11. Hardie IR, Strong FW, Hartley LCJ, et al. Skin cancer in Caucasian renal allograft recipients living in a subtropical climate. *Surgery* 1980;87:177.
12. Goldman GD. Squamous cell cancer: a practical approach. *Semin Cutan Med Surg* 1998;17:80.
13. Netscher DT, Spira M. Basal cell carcinoma: an overview of tumor biology and treatment. *Plast Reconstr Surg* 2004;113:5.
14. Wagner JD, Gordon MS, Chuang T, et al. Current therapy of cutaneous melanoma. *Plast Reconstr Surg* 2000;105:5.
15. Macht SD. Melanoma. In: Achauer BM, Eriksson E, eds. *Plastic surgery indications, operations, and outcomes*. St. Louis: Mosby, 2000:325–355.
16. Bale SJ, Dracopoli NC, Tucker MA, et al. Mapping the gene for hereditary cutaneous malignant melanoma-dysplastic nevus to chromosome 1P. *N Engl J Med* 1989;320:1367–1372.
17. Cannon-Albright LA, Goldgar DE, Meyer LJ, et al. Assignment of a locus for familial melanoma MLM to chromosome 9p 13–22. *Science* 1992;258:1148–1152.
18. Greene MH, Fraumeni JF Jr. The hereditary variant of malignant melanoma. In: Clark WH Jr, Goldman LI, Mastrangelo MJ, eds. *Human malignant melanoma*. New York: Grune & Stratton, 1979.
19. Kaplan EK. The risk of malignancy in large congenital nevi. *Plast Reconstr Surg* 1974;53:421.
20. Evans RN, Kopf AW, Lew RA, et al. Risk factors for the development of malignant melanoma. I. Review of case control study. *J Dermatol Surg Oncol* 1988;14:393.
21. Williams HE, Breene RG, Rees R. The brown recluse spider. *University of Tennessee institute of agriculture PB 1191*. Knoxville: University of Tennessee Press 1988.
22. Dyachenko P, Ziv M, Rozenman D. Epidemiological and clinical manifestations of patients hospitalized with brown recluse spider bite. *J Eur Acad Dermatol Venereol* 2006;20:1121.
23. King LE, Rees RS. Dapsone treatment of a brown recluse spider bite. *JAMA* 1983;250:648.
24. Centers for Disease Control and Prevention. Necrotic arachnidism-Pacific Northwest, 1988–1996. *MMWR Morb Mortal Wkly Rep* 1996;31:433.
25. Bratton RL, Core R. Tick-borne disease. *Am Fam Physician* 2005;12:2323.
26. Rees R, Reilley A, Nanney LB, et al. Sacral pressure sores: treatment with gluteus maximus musculocutaneous flaps. *South Med J* 1985;78:1147.
27. Colen RS. Pressure sores. In: McCarthy JG, ed. *Plastic surgery*. Philadelphia: WB Saunders, 1990:3806–3807.
28. Landis EM. Micro-injection studies of capillary blood pressure in human skin. *Heart* 1930;15:209.
29. Dinsdale SM. Decubitus ulcers: role of pressure and friction in causation. *Arch Phys Med Rehabil* 1974;55:147.
30. Shea JD. Pressure sores-classification and management. *Clin Orthop* 1975;112:89–100.
31. Young JB, Dobrzanski S. Pressure sores: epidemiology and current management concepts. *Drugs Aging* 1992;2:42–57.
32. Barillo DJ, Goode R. Fire fatality study: demographics of fire victims. *Burns* 1996;22:85–88.
33. Roth Jeffrey J, Hughes William B. *The essential burn unit handbook*. St. Louis: Quality Medical Publishing, 2004.
34. Munster AM. Burns of the world. *J Burn Care Rehabil* 1996;17:477.
35. Moritz AR, Henrique FC Jr. Studies of thermal injury: the relative importance of time and surface temperature in the causation of cutaneous burns. *Am J Pathol* 1947;23:695.
36. Jackson DM. The diagnosis of the depth of burning. *Br J Surg* 1953;40:388.
37. Robinson MC, Smith DJ Jr. Management of thermal injuries. In: Jurkiewicz MJ, Kriziek TJ, eds. *Plastic surgery: principles and practice*, Vol 2. St. Louis, 1990:1355–1420.
38. Orgill, Dennis P, Porter, Sacey A, Taylor Helena O. Heat injuries to cells in a perfused system. *Ann N Y Acad Sci* 2005;1066: 106–118.
39. Despa F, Orgill DP, Neuwalder J, Lee RC. The relative thermal stability of tissue macromolecular and cellular structure in burn injury [Review]. *Burns* 2005;31:568–577.
40. Harms B, Bodai B, Fleming R. Prostaglandin release and altered microvascular integrity after burn injury. *J Surg Res* 1981;31:274–280.
41. Demling, RH. The burn edema process: current concepts. *J Burn Care Rehabil* 2005:207–227.
42. Barrow R, Ranwiez R, Zhang X. Ibuprofen modulates tissue perfusion in partial thickness burns. *Burns* 2000;26:341–346.
43. Demling R, LaLonde C. Topical ibuprofen decreases post burn edema. *Surgery* 1987;102:857–861.
44. Raine TJ, Heggers JP, Robson MC, et al. Cooling the burn wound to maintain microcirculation. *J Trauma* 1981;21:394.
45. Robson MC, Smith DJ, Heggers JP. Innovations in burn wound management. *Adv Ophthalmic Plast Reconstr Surg* 1987;4:149.
46. Boykin JV, Eriksson E, Shelley MM, et al. Histamine mediated delayed permeability response after scald burn inhibited by cimetidine or cold water treatment. *Science* 1980;209:815.
47. Rantfors Johanna, Cassuto Jean. Role of histamine receptors in the regulation of edema and circulation postburn. *Burns* 2003;29:769–777.
48. Ward PA. How does the local inflammatory response affect the wound healing process? *J Trauma* 1984;24(Suppl):S18.
49. Ward PA, Till GO. Pathophysiologic events related to thermal injury of skin. *J Trauma* 1990;30(12):75–79.
50. Solomkin JS. Neutrophil disorders in burn injury: complement, cytokines, and organ injury. *J Trauma* 1990;30(12):80–85.
51. Demling RH. Fluid resuscitation. In Boswick JA, ed. *The art and science of burn care*. Rockville: Aspen, 1987:196.
52. Starling E. On the absorption of fluids from the connective tissue spaces. *J Physiol (London)* 1986;19:312–326.
53. Warden, G, Heinbach, DM. Burns. In: Schwartz SI, Shires GT, Spencer FC, et al. *Principles in surgery*, 7th ed. New York: McGraw-Hill, 1984:234–238.
54. Wright HK, Gann DS, Drucker WR. Current concept of therapy for derangements of extracellular fluid. In: Davis JH, ed. *Current concepts in surgery*. New York: McGraw-Hill, 1965:295–320.

55. Robson MC, Parsons RW. Respiratory problems in thermal injury. In: Rattenborg CC, Via-Regue E, eds. *Clinical use of mechanical ventilation.* Chicago: Mosby-Year Book, 1981:156–164.

56. Robson MC. Treatment in burn victims. In: Cushieri A, Gilers GR, Moossa AR, eds. *Essential surgical practice,* 2nd ed. London: John Wright, 1988:312–327.

57. O'Neill JA Jr. The influence of burns on gastric acid secretion. *Surgery* 1970;67:267–271.

58. Rosenthal A, Czaja AJ, Pruitt BA. Gastrin levels and gastric acidity in the pathogenesis of acute gastroduodenal disease after burns. *Surg Gynecol Obstet* 1977;144:232.

59. Wolf SE, Ikeda H, Martin S, et al. Cutaneous burn increases apoptosis in the gut epithelium of mice. *J Am Coll Surg* 1999;188:10–16.

60. Deitch EA, Rutan R, Waymack JP. Trauma, shock, and gut translocation. *New Horiz* 1996;4:289–299.

61. Stenburg T, Hogman KE. Experimental and clinical investigations on liver functions in burns. In: Artz, CP, ed. *Research in burns.* Philadelphia: FA Davis, 1962:171.

62. Jelenko C III, Ginsburg JM. Water holding lipid and water transmission through homeothermic and poikilothermic skin. *Proc Soc Exp Biol Med* 1971;136:1059.

63. Arturson G. Evaporation and fluid replacement: research in burns. In: Matter P, Barclay TL, Konickova Z, eds. *Transaction of the third international congress on the research in burns.* Berne: Hans Huber, 1971:520.

64. Curreri PW. Metabolic and nutritional aspects of thermal injury. *Burns* 1976;2:16.

65. Wilmore DW. Metabolic changes after thermal injury. In: Boswick JA, ed. *The art and science of burn care.* Rockville: Aspen, 1987:137–144.

66. McCutcheon M. Inflammation. In: Anderson WAD, ed. *Pathology.* St. Louis: Mosby, 1948:14–66.

67. Heggers JP, Heggers R, Robson MC. The immunological deficit encountered in thermal injury. *J Am Med Technol* 1982;44:99.

68. Ricketts LR, Squire JR, Topley E, et al. Human skin lipids with particular reference to the self-sterilizing power of the skin. *Clin Sci Mol Med* 1951;10:89.

69. Church D, Elsayed S, Reid O, et al. Burn wound infections. *Clin Microbiol Rev* 2006:403–434.

70. Bjornson AB, Bjornson HS, Altemeier WA. Serum-mediated inhibition of polymorphonuclear leukocyte function following burn injury. *Ann Surg* 1981;194:568–575.

71. Fikrig SM, Karl SC, Suntharalingam K. Neutrophil chemotaxis in patients with burns. *Ann Surg* 1977;186:746–748.

72. Warner GF, Dobson EL. Disturbances in the reticuloendothelial system following thermal injury. *Am J Physiol* 1954;179:93.

73. Gallinaro RW, Cheadle WG, Applegate K, et al. The role of the complement system in trauma and infection. *Surg Gynecol Obstet* 1992;174:435–440.

74. Robson MC, Smith DJ, Jr. Burned hand. In: Jurkwiewicz MJ, Krizek TJ, Mathes SJ, et al. eds. *Plastic surgery, principles and practice,* 1st ed. St Louis, Mosby, 1990:781–802.

75. Krizek TJ. Topical therapy of burns-problems in wound healing. *J Trauma* 1968;8:276.

76. Moncreif JA, Teplitz C. Changing concepts in burn sepsis. *J Trauma* 1964;4:233.

77. Lee RC. Cell injury by electric forces. *Ann N Y Acad Sci* 2005;1066:85–91.

78. Robson MC, Murphy RC, Heggers JP. A new explanation for the progressive tissue loss in electrical injuries. *Plast Reconstr Surg* 1984;73:431.

79. Solem L, Fisher RP, Strate RG. Natural history of electrical injury. *J Trauma* 1977;17:487.

80. Hunt JL, Mason AD, Masterson TS, et al. Pathophysiology of acute electrical injuries. *J Trauma* 1976;16:335.

81. Hunt JL, Sato RM, Baxter CR. Acute electrical burns. *Arch Surg* 1980;115:434.

82. Quinby WC, Burke JF, Trelstad RL, et al. The use of microscopy as a guide to primary excision of electrical burns. *J Trauma* 1978;18:423.

83. Luterman A, Curreri PW. Chemical burn injury. In: Jurkiewcz MJ, Krizek TJ, Mathes SJ, et al. eds. *Plastic surgery: principles and practice.* St. Louis: Mosby, 1990:1355–1440.

84. Wedler V, Guggenheim M, Moron M, et al. Extensive hydrofluoric acid injuries: a serious problem. *J Trauma* 2005;58:852–857.

85. Moriarty RW. Corrosive chemicals: acids and alkalis. *Drug ther* 1979;3:89.

86. Weatherly-White RCA, Sjostrom B, Paton BC. Experimental studies in cold injury. *J Surg Res* 1964;4:17.

87. Knize DM, Weatherly-White RC, Paton BC, et al. Prognostic factors in the management of frostbite. *J Trauma* 1969;9:749.

SUGGESTED READINGS

Netscher DT, Spira M. Basal cell carcinoma: an overview of tumor biology and treatment. *Plast Reconstr Surg* 2004;113;5, 74e–94e.

Robinson MC, Smith DJ Jr. Management of thermal injuries. In: Jurkiewicz MJ, Kriziek TJ, eds. *Plastic surgery: principles and practice,* Vol 2. St. Louis, 1990:1355–1420.

Roth Jeffrey J, Hughes William B. *The essential burn unit handbook.* 2004.

Rudolph R, Zelac DE. Squamous cell carcinoma of the skin. *Plast Reconstr Surg.* 2004;114:6,82e–93e.

Wagner JD, Gordon MS, Chuang T, et al. Current therapy of cutaneous melanoma. *Plast Reconstr Surg* 2000;105:5,1774–1799.

CHAPTER 23

Urology/Urinary System

Donald F. Lynch, Jr., Ann Y. Becker, Victor M. Brugh, John W. Davis, Gregg R. Eure,
Michael D. Fabrizio, Jean G. Hollowell, Charles E. Horton, Jr., Gerald H. Jordan, Peter O. Kwong,
Kurt A. McCammon, Timothy J. Redden, Edwin L. Robey, Paul F. Schellammer, C. William Schwab, II,
Sarah C. Shaves, Jonathan R. Taylor, and Thomas V. Whelan

UROLOGY

Urology is the surgical subspecialty which deals with diseases and disorders of the male and female urinary tract as well as disorders of the male reproductive system. General urologists are trained to deal with all areas of the specialty, but in the last two decades there has been a trend toward further subspecialization, with postresidency fellowships offered in pediatrics, oncology, male infertility, trauma, reconstructive urology, laparoendoscopic urologic surgery, urogynecology, and transplantation, among others.

EMBRYOLOGY

A thorough working knowledge of embryology is essential to understand many of the pathologic conditions of the genitourinary (GU) system. Disordered embryologic differentiation may result in a broad spectrum of clinical problems, ranging from those with relatively minimal clinical impact, such as partial duplication of the ureter, to severe conditions—as in exstrophy of the bladder or renal agenesis. Because many of these conditions are compatible with life, they may be frequently encountered in both pediatric and adult patients, and should be recognized by the astute surgeon.

The kidneys and gonads are derived from a mesodermal structure, the Müllerian ridge. The ridge develops into the metanephros, which matures into the adult renal parenchymal tissues. The Müllerian and mesonephric (Wolffian) ducts differentiate, through different stimuli, into portions of the internal genitalia and the urinary tract. The ureteral bud emanates from the distal Wolffian duct, becomes a tubular structure, and migrates rostrally to impact the metanephros. On impacting the metanephros, it stimulates definitive nephrogenic development, causing the metanephros to divide to form the structures of the renal pelvis, infundibula, and calyces. In the female, the Wolffian duct eventually involutes, although and its vestiges may persist as the Gartner duct cysts. In the male, the Wolffian duct persists and becomes the vas deferens. Agenesis of the Wolffian duct in the male causes aplasia of the vas deferens. Other abnormal conditions in renal development often associated with ureteral anomalies include the multicystic dysplastic kidney, renal agenesis, and horseshoe kidney.

In the female, the Müllerian ducts persist to form the fallopian tubes, uterus, and proximal third of the vagina. Aplasia of the Müllerian system in the female leads to the Meyer-Rokitansky-Kuster complex, manifested by agenesis of fallopian tubes and/or agenesis of the proximal vagina, uterus, and fallopian tubes. In the male, the Müllerian duct regresses under the influence of the Müllerian inhibition factor (MIF). The vestiges become the prostatic utricle (termed *Müllerian cysts* when enlarged) and the appendix testis.

The bladder and proximal urethra are derived from the urogenital sinus, of endodermal origin. After the urogenital sinus arises from the cloaca, it is divided by the transverse rectal folds into the anorectal canal and the anterior urogenital sinus. The urogenital sinus then divides proximally into the bladder, and caudally into the posterior (proximal) urethra in the male and into the entire urethra in the female. Abnormalities in the development of the urogenital sinus and cloaca lead to cloacal malformations, cloacal exstrophy, or the classic exstrophy–epispadias complex.

The anterior urethra is derived from mesodermal structures associated with the genital tubercle. The mesoderm develops into the corpus spongiosum and urethral epithelium and forms the anterior (distal) urethra through a process of progressive tubularization. Failure of the proper progression of anterior urethral development may result in hypospadias and may also be a component of the epispadias complex.

In the male, the gonadal ridge differentiates into the testis under the influence of a locus on the Y chromosome. In the absence of that locus, the gonadal ridge differentiates into the ovary. In those anomalies, such as Turner syndrome, in which abnormal development of the second X chromosome (XO conditions) occurs, ovarian maldifferentiation frequently leads to a streak gonad.

RENAL PHYSIOLOGY AND ANATOMY FOR SURGEONS

The kidney's primary function is regulation of fluid volume. Other crucial homeostatic mechanisms carried out by the kidneys include insulin degradation, erythropoietin production, vitamin D synthesis and activation, secretion of organic ions, ammonia genesis, and bicarbonate reabsorption.

The human kidney is composed of approximately 1 million functional units termed *nephrons*. The nephron consists of the corpuscle (glomerulus), the proximal convoluted tubule, the thin loop of Henle, the distal tubule, and the collecting duct (Fig. 23.1).

Initial ultrafiltration occurs at the level of the renal corpuscle. This filtration is affected by many factors, including renal blood flow; vascular and tubular oncotic and hydrostatic pressure; size, shape, and electric charge of molecular substances; and mechanical forces associated with the capillary wall (Fig. 23.2). Filtration fluid progresses from the glomerular capillary, into the Bowman space, and into the proximal tubular lumen. Most of the filtered solute is reabsorbed in the proximal tubule. Approximately 25% to 40% of the reabsorption of filtered sodium occurs in the thin limb of the loop of Henle. In man, some nephrons have a long loop of Henle, whereas others have a short one. The quantity of each determines the concentrating ability of

the kidney. Because of the relative impermeability to water, the filtrate is diluted in the thin limb of the loop of Henle. Approximately 10% of filtered sodium is reabsorbed in the distal tubule.

Potassium and acid balances are regulated primarily in the collecting duct under the influence of aldosterone. Antidiuretic hormone (vasopressin) also exerts its action at the collecting duct, rendering the duct more permeable to water transport, and further concentrating urine.

The juxtaglomerular apparatus plays a pivotal role in the tubuloglomerular feedback apparatus by contributing to renal blood flow auto regulation. It consists of an intricate complex of cells and blood vessels that are responsible for monitoring a decline in extracellular fluid volume and releasing renin, which converts renin substrate (angiotensinogen) to angiotensin I.

The kidneys receive approximately 20% of cardiac output, a disproportionately high percentage compared to other organs. Regulation of renal blood flow is critical to maintaining normal glomerular filtration rate over a wide range of systemic pressures. Most individuals require a mean arterial pressure of more than 60 mm Hg to maintain a normal glomerular filtration rate.

Although many congenital variants exist, in most individuals, the renovascular network consists of a single renal artery and vein. In the renal hilum, the artery divides into an anterior division and a posterior division each with five branches. These branches become the interlobar arteries, with the sequence of blood flow as follows (i) Quillain arcuate arteries to interlobular arteries; (ii) interlobular arteries to afferent arcuate arteries; (iii) afferent arcuate arterioles to glomerular capillaries; (iv) glomerular capillaries to the efferent arterioles; (v) efferent arterioles to the vasa rectae; and (vi) vasa rectae to the venous return (Fig. 23.3).

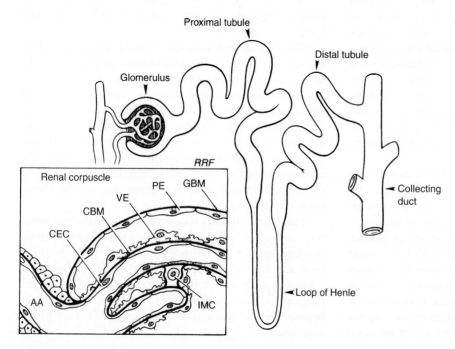

FIGURE 23.1 Illustration of renal corpuscle. AA, afferent arteriole; CEC, capillary endothelial cell; CBM, capillary basement membrane; VE, visceral epithelium; PE, parietal epithelium; GBM, glomerular basement membrane; IMC, intraglomerular mesangial cell.

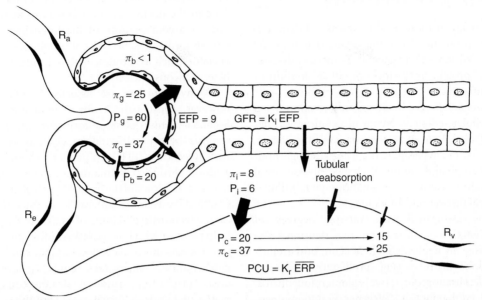

FIGURE 23.2   Forces responsible for filtration of fluid from the glomerular capillaries and reabsorption of fluid into the peritubular capillaries. The values are considered representative of forces in humans. R_a, afferent arteriole resistance; π_b, colloid osmotic pressure of filtrate; π_g, plasma colloid osmotic pressure; P_g, glomerular capillary pressure; P_b = Bowman space pressure; EFP, effective filtration pressure; GFR, glomerular filtration coefficient; π_i, interstitial colloid osmotic pressure; P_i, interstitial space hydrostatic pressure; R_e, efferent arteriole resistance; P_c, capillary hydrostatic pressure; π_c, capillary colloid osmotic pressure; PCU, peritubular capillary uptake; K_r, reabsorption coefficient; ERP, effective reabsorption pressure; R_v, venous resistance. (From: Arends, Horst WJ, Navar LG. Renal circulation and hemodynamics. In Schrier RW, Gottschalk CW, eds. *Diseases of the kidney*, 4th ed. Boston: Little, Brown and Company, 1988.)

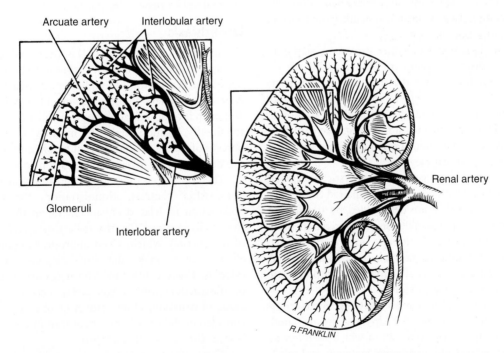

FIGURE 23.3   The macroarterial renal circulation. (From: Pitts RF. *Physiology of the kidney and body fluids*, 3rd ed. Chicago: Year Book Medical Publishers, 1994:1–9.)

NEPHROLOGY FOR SURGEONS

The pathophysiology of most renal parenchymal disease is explained through our understanding of the structure and function of the nephron unit. In general, glomerular diseases lead to a loss of protein in the form of either albumin or larger protein molecules.

Nephrosis is characterized by significant proteinuria and scant, if any, cellular sediment. Nephrotic syndrome is defined as more than 3.5 g/d of proteinuria, systemic edema, hypoalbuminemia, and hyperlipidemia. The pathologic findings for nephrosis include minimal change disease, focal segmental glomerulosclerosis, membranous glomerulopathy, diabetic renal disease, and amyloidosis.

Nephritis is associated with varying degrees of proteinuria, edema, hematuria, and hypertension. The pathologic findings in nephritis include acute poststreptococcal glomerulonephritis, mesangioproliferative glomerulonephritis, membranoproliferative glomerulonephritis, systemic lupus erythematosus, Wegener granulomatosis, Goodpasture syndrome, polyarteritis nodosa, and other vascular diseases.

Tubulointerstitial disease states affect solute, water, acid–base, and electrolyte abnormalities. Examples of tubulointerstitial diseases include infectious, toxic, and systemic processes, such as Fanconi syndrome, lithium nephrotoxicity, and cyclosporine nephrotoxicity.

Vascular insult typically presents as acute tubular necrosis, and is seen in the setting of ischemia. Examples of other diseases affecting the renal vasculature include vasculitis, atheroembolic disease, abnormal renal blood flow associated with dissecting aneurysm, systemic embolization, and renal vein thrombosis.

Renal cystic disease can be either genetic or acquired. Acquired cystic disease develops in patients who are on renal replacement therapy for the treatment of end-stage renal disease. Although infrequent, there is a possibility that these cysts will develop into renal cell adenocarcinoma. Imaging has demonstrated that simple cysts are found in a large percentage of the population and are not generally associated with clinical pathology.

The three categories of genetic renal cystic disease all represent a genetic mutation leading to impaired connective tissue formation, and they are determined by the size of the affected kidney. Nephronophthisis (cystic renal medulla complex) is seen in small kidneys; medullary sponge kidney disease is found in normal sized kidneys; and either autosomal dominant or autosomal recessive polycystic kidney disease is noted in large kidneys.

Other hereditary renal diseases are a heterogeneous group of disorders. The most well known is Alport syndrome. There are six types of Alport syndrome, all of which manifest as microscopic hematuria and progressive azotemia, and most, but not all, are associated with deafness.

Nephrolithiasis, or renal stone disease, is the third most common affliction of the urinary tract. A number of situations can precipitate crystal formation in the urine,

but most are related to an imbalance of the physiochemical state of the urine. This imbalance can be the result of any one, or a combination, of the following: supersaturation, pH abnormalities, a lack of inhibitory substances (i.e., chelators such as citrate), matrix production, infection, or heterogeneous nucleation.

Many disorders are associated with nephrolithiasis; however, most patients have idiopathic hypercalciuria. Secondary causes of stone formation include renal tubular acidosis, hyperparathyroidism, gout, and recurrent urinary tract infections (UTIs). In patients who have renal tubular acidosis, chronic acidemia induces bone resorption, leading to hypercalciuria and the formation of calcium oxalate stones. Crohn disease/colitis patients form calcium oxalate stones caused by impaired binding of oxalate in the gut, which leads to hyperoxaluria. Hyperparathyroidism also causes patients to form calcium oxalate stones. Gout can lead to uric acid nephrolithiasis. Finally, recurrent UTIs, especially those with urease production, cause an alkaline urine and infection matrix that leads to formation of triple phosphate stones.

RADIOGRAPHIC IMAGING FOR GENITOURINARY DISEASES

A variety of imaging modalities can be used to investigate the GU tract, with the appropriate choice dictated by the clinical situation. Uroradiologic studies should be ordered after consideration of indications and clinical need for the information provided by the study with attention to the optimal test to answer the question.

Urolithiasis

The intravenous urogram (IVU) is often used to evaluate the GU system. The IVU is most commonly chosen to evaluate patients with symptoms thought to be caused by urolithiasis. A precontrast view [kidneys, ureters, bladder (KUB)] of the abdomen is critical if radiopaque calculi are to be visualized, to identify location, size and number of stones. Fifteen percent of calculi are radiolucent by plain film, however, or can be obscured by overlying bowel contents.

The IVU detects most stones and almost all symptomatic ones. After contrast administration, the first sign of obstruction is delayed enhancement on the affected side. Eventually contrast fills the collecting system to the level of obstruction, which, given appropriate clinical scenario, allows one to make definitive diagnosis of obstructive calculus. Delayed films may be necessary to identify level of obstruction with longer delay necessary for higher-grade obstruction. Other causes of obstruction should be considered when a column of contrast in obstructed system is seen without radiopaque stone.

Noncontrast computed tomography (CT KUB) is now commonly used to rapidly evaluate patients with suspected stones to determine size of stone and level of obstruction. Almost all stones are radiopaque on CT, even those not visible on plain film, affording noncontrast CT the advantage of making a diagnosis without the use of intravenous contrast. Size and location of the obstructing stone can be seen with sensitivity reaching 100%; associated findings of ureteral dilatation and perinephric/periureteral stranding together give positive predictive value (PPV) of 99% and negative predictive value (NPV) of 95% for ureterolithiasis.

Ultrasonography is commonly used to determine the presence of hydronephrosis. In patients with early obstruction, potential exists for false negative examination as hydronephrosis may not have had time to develop. Ultrasonography usually identifies intrarenal stones, but symptomatic ureteral stones may be missed due to the presence of obscuring bowel gas. Ultrasonography is also not specific with many other causes existing for collecting system dilatation.

Trauma

Because CT has been proved to be more sensitive and specific for identification of injury to the GU tract, IVU is now only used in specific settings such as the one-shot IVU in the emergency department to demonstrate whether both kidneys are present and functioning or if there is contrast extravasation such as with penetrating injury and when the patient will be transferred to the operating room before formal imaging. The CT is the test of choice for the evaluation of most trauma patients with ability to evaluate pedicle or parenchymal injuries on initial scan or collecting system injuries on delayed images.

Trauma patients who have pelvic fractures must undergo urethral evaluation with retrograde urethrography. Any trauma patient with pelvic fracture and hematuria should have bladder evaluation by CT cystogram which must be performed by retrograde filling of the urinary bladder with dilute contrast to voiding pressures. Nonstress CT cystogram (e.g., clamping the bladder catheter) may miss some ruptures.

Masses

IVU is useful in evaluation of the upper urinary tract to identify large parenchymal masses or urothelial lesions. CT urogram including parenchymal and excretory phases is commonly used in patients with hematuria for its added sensitivity (95%–98%) for small renal parenchymal masses. It is often the first-line test chosen and should be used in patients for whom diagnosis remains unclear despite IVU or ultrasonnography as both tests can miss a small percentage of masses. Magnetic resonance imaging (MRI) or ultrasonography may be used in patients who cannot receive iodinated contrast because of allergy or renal insufficiency as gadolinium does not have cross-reactivity with iodinated contrast and does not cause contrast-induced nephropathy. MRI can also aid in tissue characterization.

Ultrasonography is the most operator-dependent and patient-dependent procedure used in the GU tract. It detects most solid renal masses with exception of very small or isodense ones and in most cases can differentiate cystic from solid lesions. Increasing patient size can, however, contribute to limited visualization of the kidneys. Ultrasonography can provide intraoperative guidance for localization or cryoablation of renal masses. Ultrasonography with Doppler evaluation is the test of choice for scrotal pathology from masses or inflammatory processes to torsion, with MRI useful for further characterization of some masses as well as congenital abnormalities.

CT usually adequately evaluates adrenal masses with multiphase examinations assessing density, enhancement, and washout. CT density measurements characterize masses as adenomas with greater than 95% sensitivity and specificity. MRI with opposed phase imaging also evaluates for intracellular lipid in adenomas; myelolipomas may be confirmed with fat saturation sequences.

Other

Renal scintigraphy allows an estimate relative function of each kidney. Renal blood flow and function can be evaluated in patients with renal failure. The functional significance of apparent renal obstruction can also be determined. In renal transplant patients, it can evaluate blood flow to and function of the allograft.

Positron emission tomography (PET) CT (PET fused with CT images) as an evolving modality enhances staging, evaluation of recurrence versus residual disease and response to therapy in patients with testicular carcinoma. In bladder cancer, its utility is limited to evaluation of metastatic disease because excreted tracer obscures urinary bladder. Utility in prostate cancer and renal cell carcinoma are still being developed.

PHYSIOLOGY OF VOIDING/VOIDING DYSFUNCTION

Voiding Anatomy and Physiology

For a complete understanding of voiding dysfunction, it is important to review key aspects of the anatomy and physiology of the lower urinary tract. The lower urinary tract is composed of the bladder, urethra, and their supporting structures and has two main functions: bladder filling (urine storage) and bladder emptying. The neural coordination and integration necessary to accomplish these functions is complex. Storage requires the low-pressure accommodation of increasing volumes of urine and the ability to sense fullness. During the storage phase, the bladder outlet is closed to maintain continence. The vesicoelastic properties of the bladder wall allow for minimal intravesical pressure changes despite increases in volume during filling. The ability of the bladder to accommodate changes in volume while maintaining a low-pressure environment is termed *compliance*. The emptying phase begins with relaxation of the urethral sphincter to open the bladder outlet. This is followed by a coordinated detrusor contraction, which results in increase in bladder pressure and the subsequent expulsion of urine.

The muscle layers of the bladder wall are composed of detrusor smooth muscle fibers that have the ability to exert maximal effective tension over a wide range of fiber lengths. With contraction, the bladder is able to empty continuously and forcefully throughout the voiding phase. On the basis of the formation of the smooth muscle fibers, the bladder is divided into two parts: the body which lies above the ureteral orifices and the base which is composed of the trigone and bladder neck. The body of the bladder is composed of a mass of randomly arranged muscle fibers that allows the bladder to expand and contract. At the trigone, the muscle fibers are arranged into three distinct muscle layers: an inner longitudinal layer, a middle circular layer, and an outer longitudinal layer. These layers form a proximal physiologic sphincter mechanism which is responsible for continence at the level of the bladder neck. It is important to realize that the muscular composition of the bladder neck and urethra differ somewhat between males and females. The outer longitudinal layer extends the entire length of the female urethra, whereas it ends near the membranous urethra in males. Besides, in males the middle smooth muscle layer is well developed and heavily innervated by adrenergic fibers, whereas the middle layer in females is poorly developed and retains very little adrenergic innervation. This differential distribution of adrenergic receptors between males and females explains the more pronounced effect that α-adrenergic receptor blockers have on men in the treatment of bladder outlet obstruction. Collectively, these smooth muscle fibers are oriented in a circular manner, allowing variations in urethral resistance, and are called the *intrinsic portion of the distal sphincter mechanism*. The bladder neck and intrinsic distal sphincter provide involuntary (passive) mechanisms for continence and are not true anatomic sphincters.

The voluntary or external sphincter is composed of striated muscle fibers and comprises the extrinsic portion of the distal sphincteric mechanism. In the female, these fibers form a sphincter around the middle third of the urethra. In males, the external sphincter has fibers surrounding the distal portion of the prostate and the membranous urethra. The external sphincter is also composed of striated muscles of the pelvic floor, including the levator ani and pubococcygeus muscles. The proximal or distal sphincteric mechanisms can provide passive continence in the male, even if one or the other is dysfunctional.

Adequate function of the lower urinary tract requires the coordination and integration of peripheral, spinal, brainstem and cerebral signals to control the storage and emptying of urine. The most fundamental micturition reflex occurs in the spinal cord and is activated by stretching of the bladder wall. This results in the passage of urine, and may be stimulated or inhibited by higher brain centers, thereby allowing for voluntary control. Central nervous control above the level of the spinal cord occurs predominantly in the pons, the basal ganglia, and cerebral cortex. The pontine micturition center (PMC) is the most important motor center in voiding physiology, as it is ultimately responsible for coordinating the activity of the detrusor and the sphincter during voiding. Therefore, lesions below the PMC tend to result in uncoordinated voiding, whereas

lesions above the level of the pons allow for the maintenance of coordinated voiding. Centers located in the basal ganglia appear to be primarily inhibitory to the detrusor muscle. Parkinson disease and other neurologic diseases that affect the basal ganglia thereby usually result in detrusor overactivity. Likewise, the cerebral cortex exerts a primarily inhibitory influence to the micturition reflex, and cerebral lesions such as cerebrovascular accident will result in detrusor overactivity with a coordinated sphincter mechanism.

Urine storage is principally controlled by the sympathetic nervous system, whereas the parasympathetic nervous system controls bladder emptying. Both somatic and parasympathetic neurons originate in the spinal cord at the level of S2-4; sympathetic neurons originate in the spinal cord at the level of T11-L2. Parasympathetic motor neurons travel in the hypogastric and pelvic nerves, which meet and form the pelvic plexus, lateral to the rectum and internal genitalia. Branches of the pelvis plexus innervate all of the pelvic organs, including the detrusor muscle of the urinary bladder. Sympathetic neurons travel through the superior hypogastric plexus, and converge in the pelvic plexus, before branching to innervate the proximal sphincter mechanism and the intrinsic portion of the distal sphincter mechanism. The extrinsic portion of the distal sphincter mechanism and the pelvic floor (levator) muscles receive somatic motor innervation from the spinal cord through the pudendal nerve.

Sensory neurons from the bladder are divided into pain, temperature, and proprioceptive sensation. The sensory afferent neurons of the bladder neck and trigone travel through the pelvic and hypogastric nerves, whereas the sensory innervation of the external sphincter and urethra returns by way of the pudendal nerve.

Infantile voiding patterns well demonstrate the involuntary micturition reflex. In childhood, as the connections between the cerebrum and the brainstem mature, volitional control of micturition occurs. Afferent sensory neurons carry impulses to signal bladder distension, and the cortical acknowledgement of these impulses result in the voluntary ability to initiate micturition. The sympathetic reflex is blocked, allowing the bladder neck and urethra to relax and open the outlet while the parasympathetic micturition reflex contracts the distended bladder. Stimulation of voluntary sphincters is also inhibited. Once the bladder is empty, it returns to the storage phase.

The Neurourologic Evaluation

The evaluation of voiding dysfunction begins with a thorough voiding history. Voiding symptoms can be characterized as either irritative or obstructive; irritative symptoms include urgency, frequency, and incontinence whereas poor urinary stream, hesitancy, and straining are more obstructive-type symptoms. In addition, a complete history of medical problems, neurologic disorders, surgical and obstetrical procedures, and trauma may be important. In most cases, a voiding diary should be included in the initial evaluation.

Physical examination consists of a complete examination with emphasis on the neurologic and GU systems. Adequate neurologic examination includes assessment of gait, mental status, strength, sensation and reflexes. Anal sphincter tone reflects the state of the perineal striated musculature. Deep tendon reflex evaluation provides an indication of segmental and suprasegmental spinal cord function. The bulbocavernosal reflex provides specific information about the S-2 to S-4 region of the spinal cord. It is elicited in females by gently pulling on a Foley catheter or by stroking the labia majora/clitoris with a cotton tip applicator while monitoring for perineal muscle contraction. In the male, it is elicited by squeezing the glans penis. Because infection is the most common cause of changes in voiding function, urinalysis and a urine culture should be included in the initial evaluation.

Evaluation of the lower urinary tract can be augmented by cystoscopy. Direct visualization of the urinary bladder will rule out bladder anomalies or lesions that could contribute to voiding symptoms. If upper tract pathology is suspected, particularly if the patient has gross or microscopic hematuria, radiographic evaluation with modalities such as CT, intravenous pyelogram, or sonography is also warranted. Urodynamic studies reproduce clinical symptoms while yielding objective data. The goals of urodynamic studies are to evaluate capacity, accommodation, intravesical pressure during storage, intravesical pressure during voiding, the presence and quality of detrusor contraction, the presence of uninhibited contractions, the perception of fullness, the ability to inhibit or initiate voiding, and the presence of residual urine.

As a minimum requirement, the initial urodynamic evaluation should include flow cystometry and quantification of emptying with a postvoid residual urine. Normal flow rates are 20 to 25 mL/sec in males, and 20 to 30 mL/sec in females. Normal postvoid residual urine is minimal. The cystometrogram measures bladder pressure during filling and voiding. This is measured by placing small pressure transducing catheters in the bladder and the rectum, and deducing the detrusor pressure by subtracting the abdominal pressure from the vesical pressure. Leak point pressures are measured during urodynamic studies and used as tools to objectively measure bladder compliance and severity of incontinence. The abdominal leak point pressure (ALPP) is defined as the vesical pressure at which the patient leaks during coughing or Valsalva maneuvers. The ALPP has been used to measure the severity of stress urinary incontinence. Another leak point pressure, the detrusor leak point pressure (DLPP) is measured to be the detrusor pressure at which urinary leakage occurs in the absence of abdominal straining or detrusor contraction, and is more a measure of bladder compliance. This is important in the assessment of the neurogenic bladder, as patients with DLPPs of greater than 40 cm H_2O are at greater risk of upper tract deterioration.

Videourodynamic studies are performed with fluoroscopy to allow for real-time imaging of the lower urinary tract during filling and voiding. The bladder is filled with radiopaque contrast and images are taken throughout the study. Normal urodynamic parameters include a bladder capacity of 400 to 500 mL, a storage bladder pressure of less than 15 cm H_2O pressure (the point of voiding), a first sensation of fullness at approximately 150 to 250 mL of urine, and a voiding pressure of less than 30 mL H_2O pressure.

Classification of Voiding Dysfunction

Patients with voiding dysfunction fall into one of three functional categories: failure to store, failure to empty, or a combination of both. Incontinence can occur in any of these circumstances. A thorough history and physical examination can often distinguish among the types of incontinence. Stress urinary incontinence is defined as involuntary leakage of urine during exertion, coughing, or sneezing; whereas urge incontinence is defined as involuntary leakage of urine immediately preceded by urgency. Overflow incontinence is associated with leakage of small amounts of urine in patients with urinary retention.

Failure to store implies an inappropriate loss of urine, and may be related to decreased outlet resistance, bladder overactivity, or poor compliance. Decreased outlet resistance manifests as stress urinary incontinence, and occurs commonly in women and in men who have undergone prostate surgery. The incidence of stress urinary incontinence in females is much higher than in males because the female urethra is shorter, lacks the external support of the male urethra, and lacks the resistive forces of the prostate. Stress urinary incontinence results from the failure of urethral resistance to compensate for transient increases in intra-abdominal pressure, and can occur because of urethral hypermobility and/or intrinsic sphincter deficiency (ISD). Urethral hypermobility results from laxity of the pelvic floor muscles in conjunction with weakening of the pelvic ligaments. Loss of the normal urethral position in the pelvis leads to stress incontinence because of a decreased ability to maintain urethral closure during increases in abdominal pressure.

Patients with ISD typically have more severe stress incontinence. ISD is often a sequela of neurogenic bladder, multiple urethral procedures, radiation, or chronic indwelling foley catheterization. The effects of estrogen on the lower urinary tract are well documented, and urogenital atrophy has been postulated to play a role in the increased prevalence of both stress and urge incontinence in the postmenopausal population. Estrogen deficiency has been demonstrated to decrease collagen content, vascularity, and epithelial maturity of the female urethra, leading to poor coaptation of the urethral walls and a higher prevalence of incontinence in the aging population.

The treatment for stress urinary incontinence varies depending on the severity of the problem. Nonsurgical interventions include α-agonist or sympathomimetic pharmacotherapy, biofeedback, and pessaries, but reported success rates vary significantly with these interventions. Stress incontinence may be surgically managed in females with a variety of procedures, including transvaginal and transobturator sling procedures, pubovaginal slings, intraurethral collagen injections, and rarely, artificial urethral sphincters. In men, surgical intervention after radical prostatectomy is usually delayed for a year to allow for a period of time for continence to be regained; good success rates have been reported with artificial urinary sphincters and male slings.

Detrusor overactivity is the term used to describe urodynamically observed involuntary bladder contractions occurring during the storage phase. This may be neurogenic or non-neurogenic in etiology; infection, inflammation, bladder calculi, tumors, and neurologic disease are common causes, but idiopathic detrusor overactivity may also occur. Symptoms include urgency, frequency, and urge incontinence. Lesions above the brainstem, such as cerebrovascular accident, dementia, closed head injury, brain tumor, cerebral palsy, and Parkinson disease produce a spastic neuropathy that results in decreased bladder capacity, uninhibited bladder contractions, increased intravesical pressure, and hypertrophy of the bladder wall. These suprapontine lesions usually cause detrusor overactivity while maintaining synergy with the smooth and striated sphincter because the PMC is intact.

The primary treatments for detrusor overactivity are removal of the underlying cause and the use of anticholinergic drugs. Behavior modification, exercises to strengthen the pelvic floor musculature, biofeedback, and postmenopausal estrogen replacement therapy can be helpful. Surgical intervention for detrusor overactivity includes sacral nerve stimulation, bladder augmentation, and in rare cases, urinary diversion.

In the initial period after spinal cord injury, the most common pattern of voiding dysfunction is urinary retention and detrusor areflexia secondary to spinal shock. The spinal shock period typically lasts 6 to 12 weeks, and is followed by the development of detrusor overactivity, manifested by frequency, urgency, and urge incontinence. Because the PMC is responsible for the coordination of the detrusor and the sphincter during micturition, injuries below this level result in poorly coordinated voiding, known as *detrusor sphincter dyssynergia* (DSD). In this situation, the detrusor may contract during attempted voiding against a closed sphincter, resulting in a high pressure, hostile bladder environment. Commonly seen in multiple sclerosis, spinal cord injury, tethered cord syndrome, and myelomeningocele, DSD predisposes patients to elevated bladder pressures and the risk of upper tract deterioration, warranting long-term urodynamic follow-up.

A dangerous phenomenon in the population with spinal cord injuries that warrants mention is autonomic dysreflexia. Autonomic dysreflexia classically occurs in patients with complete spinal cord injuries above level T6-8, and results from an uncontrolled sympathetic response to noxious stimulation such as constipation or bladder fullness. The symptoms include a precipitous rise in blood pressure, headache, and diaphoresis. Treatment is removal of the inciting stimulus, and administration of antihypertensive agents such as nifedipine, hydralazine, or nitroprusside.

Prophylaxis of dysreflexia in susceptible patients can include sublingual nifedipine before anticipated procedures such as cystoscopy or urodynamics.

Another cause of failure to store urine is low compliance of the bladder wall. In this circumstance, the ability of the bladder to store urine at low, constant pressures decreases. Overflow incontinence results because the high intravesical pressure exceeds the outlet resistance pressure. Anatomic causes of low bladder wall compliance include detrusor hypertrophy secondary to long-standing outlet obstruction, bladder wall fibrosis secondary to irradiation, tuberculosis, recurrent infections, chronic catheterization, and multiple bladder procedures. Injury to the pelvic plexus caused by pelvic trauma or surgery also may result in a bladder wall with low compliance. Sacral lesions below level S-2 such as sacral agenesis result in poorly compliant, acontractile bladders with open sphincters and loss of voluntary control.

Failure to empty urine can also be attributed to pathology of the bladder itself or of the bladder outlet. The most common pathology associated with failure to empty in the adult male is bladder outlet obstruction secondary to benign prostatic hyperplasia (BPH). The pathophysiology and treatment of BPH are discussed later in this chapter. Bladder outlet obstruction is uncommon in females and primarily results from surgery to correct incontinence.

Failure to empty can also be attributed to a poorly contractile detrusor. Over time, chronic retention from outlet obstruction may result in decompensation of the bladder wall and decreased bladder contractile force. Even after removal of the obstruction, the bladder may not recover its ability to empty completely. Sensory neuropathic disorders, such as diabetes mellitus, tabes dorsalis, and pernicious anemia, can result in reduced bladder sensation. Genital herpes can produce transient urinary retention that may resolve in weeks to months. Lower motor neuron lesions caused by pelvic surgery or trauma can leave a weak or a contractile bladder. With the inability to effectively empty, overflow incontinence can arise once maximum bladder capacity is exceeded. The treatment for these conditions is clean intermittent catheterization. Although cholinergic agonists (i.e., Urecholine) were used in the past, the results have been inconsistent, and these drugs are no longer considered a primary treatment modality for failure to empty. Sacral nerve stimulation has been reported as a possible treatment modality for neurogenic urinary retention, but long-term results are controversial.

Postoperative retention is usually the result of inhibition of the bladder reflex by opioid mediated mechanisms. Transient overdistension of the bladder under anesthesia or analgesic medications can also exacerbate postoperative retention. In these situations, the bladder becomes stretched past normal capacity because of a lack of sensation, and detrusor muscle contractility is diminished temporarily. The primary treatment is bladder rest with an indwelling catheter or the initiation of a clean intermittent catheterization protocol. In some cases, bladder outlet obstruction will coexist and require correction as well.

ADULT URINARY TRACT INFECTIONS

UTIs are characterized by urothelial inflammation secondary to microbial invasion. The term *urinary tract infection* (UTI) is a generalized term used to cover multiple clinical entities such as bacteriuria, cystitis, and pyelonephritis. Although they occasionally result from viral or fungal infections, the majority are caused by bacteria, most commonly *Escherichia* coli.

The prevalence of UTI varies with age and sex. In male infants, there is a higher UTI rate due to redundant preputial skin related to phimosis with bacterial colonization, as well as due to a greater incidence of congenital urologic abnormalities. Beyond that peak, infection in the male is uncommon until the sixth decade of life, at which time prostate-related urinary issues arise.

Other than infants and those older than 50 years of age, females account for most UTIs, primarily due to an anatomically shorter urethra. In females, the incidence also increases with advancing age with school age girls experiencing an incidence of 1% to 5%, and sexually active postmenopausal women experiencing an incidence of 20% to 30%. In the elderly population, a relation exists between the place of residence and the prevalence of infection. Approximately 20% of elderly women and 10% of elderly men living at home have bacteriuria. These figures increase to 25% to 30% of elderly people who reside in a nursing home environment. Furthermore, the figures continue to rise for these patients when hospitalized, with a direct relation to the length of hospitalization.

Bacteriuria is defined as the presence of bacteria in the urine. If asymptomatic, this bacterial colonization does not require treatment. However, antibiotics should be administered in patients who need the urine to be sterile for a procedure. At times, colonization of the urine can progress to microbial invasion of the tissues and cause symptoms, which is defined as a true infection.

In UTIs, bacteria usually gain access to the urinary system by an ascending route (through the urethra), although hematogenous spread is seen occasionally. Host defenses and normal voiding habits as well as the inherent properties of urine will usually keep bacteria from being able to establish a true infection. Alterations in the vaginal environment with subsequent changes in normal flora (lactobacillus) and decreased acidity may lead to increased vaginal bacteria, which then ascend into the urinary system to cause infection. This is seen in females who use spermicidal agents or who are in an estrogen-deficient status (postmenopausal). There are also a number of genetic host defenses as well as virulence factors of the bacteria that make an individual more or less susceptible to UTIs. The risk of UTI is also increased with anatomic or functional abnormalities such as vesicoureteral reflux, obstruction or the presence of a foreign body, such as catheters which allow bacteria to easily migrate to the bladder.

UTIs can involve all parts of the urinary tract, either individually or in combination. Clinical symptoms are useful in distinguishing the site of involvement, and diagnosis is confirmed by urine culture.

Lower Urinary Tract Infection

Lower tract infection involves the urethra, bladder, and/or the prostate or epididymis in males. Urethritis (infection of the urethra) is seen most often in males, with symptoms of dysuria, itch, and a purulent urethral discharge. Urethritis is usually due to sexually transmitted organisms, such as gonorrhea, chlamydia or ureaplasma. Cystitis (infection of the bladder) typically has symptoms of urinary frequency, urgency, suprapubic discomfort, and dysuria.

Infection of the prostate, termed *prostatitis*, can be either acute or chronic. Acute bacterial prostatitis is often associated with a more dramatic presentation, which may include dysuria, difficulty voiding, urgency, fever, and perineal or lower back discomfort. Chronic prostatitis is thought to be the result of incomplete treatment of the acute condition.

Epididymitis usually results from bacterial migration through the vas deferens and has increased incidence with long-term urethral catheterization and with urethral strictures. Epididymitis usually presents with scrotal pain, swelling, and tenderness. In young males, the diagnosis of epididymitis must be distinguished from the diagnosis of testicular torsion, which has a similar presentation. In men younger than 35, epididymitis is often due to a sexually transmitted organism. In the older population, gram-negative organisms (especially *E. coli*) predominate. If left untreated, epididymitis can involve the testicle, a condition termed *epididymoorchitis*.

Upper Urinary Tract Infection

Upper UTI refers to the involvement of the kidney or collecting system. Termed *pyelonephritis*, it is usually accompanied by fever, chills, and flank pain. Bacteremia may also be present and may lead to sepsis. In the young population, the association of pyelonephritis with vesicoureteral reflux is well established. Patients who do not show a prompt initial response to antibiotic therapy when suspected of having pyelonephritis should be suspected of having an upper urinary tract obstruction, which may also lead to sepsis and be fatal. Emphysematous pyelonephritis is a severe form of pyelonephritis associated with gas-forming organisms within the tissue of the renal parenchyma and is mostly seen in diabetic patients.

Evaluation

Collection of a urine specimen is critical to the diagnosis of UTIs. In males, collection of urine specimens is accomplished easily by cleaning the glans and retracting the preputial skin. In females, obtaining a sterile specimen through a "clean catch" may be difficult due to the potential for vaginal contamination and thereby the gold standard would be a catheterized specimen. Traditionally, colony counts of greater than 10^5 organisms per milliliter was required to diagnose a UTI. However, recent data suggest that urine cultures in symptomatic patients may require only 10^2 and

10^3 colony counts of bacteria to be diagnostic of UTI. This may be due to the frequent urinations mechanically clearing the bacteria and the slow growth of bacteria in urine.

UTIs during pregnancy pose additional risks and warrant special considerations. Hormonal changes in pregnancy lead to decreased bladder tone, diminished ureteral peristalsis, and dilation of the collecting system, all increasing the risk of upper UTI (i.e., pyelonephritis), which may lead to premature delivery. Symptomatic or not, bacteriuria in pregnancy needs to be treated because it may lead to pyelonephritis in approximately a fourth of cases. After completion of a course of antibiotics, a follow-up urine culture is recommended to document sterile urine. Patients who do not show a prompt response to antibiotic therapy or who have evidence of sepsis need to be evaluated for obstruction, which would require appropriate drainage.

Treatment

As a general rule, symptomatic UTIs should be treated with antimicrobial therapy. The site and presence of complicating factors, as well as culture sensitivities will dictate the antibiotic agent and duration of therapy needed to eradicate the organism. Complete treatment guidelines are beyond the scope of this text, but several caveats should be addressed. First, for uncomplicated cystitis in women, a 3-day course of antibiotic therapy is adequate. An "uncomplicated" UTI is defined as a UTI occurring in a healthy person with a structurally and functionally normal urinary tract. A "complicated" UTI is defined as a UTI occurring in a person who has a urinary tract abnormality, or occurring in a compromised host or is a nosocomial UTI. For a complicated UTI, a 7- to 14-day course is recommended. UTIs in males are usually considered to be complicated UTIs. Prostatic sources of infection may require treatment for 4 to 6 weeks. Second, some data support the use of topical estrogen therapy to help eradicate UTI in postmenopausal women. Third, recurrent UTIs in young females (ages 15–50) may be addressed in a number of ways. Cranberry juice, avoidance of contraceptive diaphragms with spermicides, low-dose antimicrobial prophylaxis and self-medication are all regimens that have been successful. Fourth, pyelonephritis and small renal abscesses should be aggressively treated with systemic antibiotic therapy. Renal or perirenal abscesses greater than 3 cm should be considered for drainage and or surgical therapy.

UROLITHIASIS

In industrialized countries, urolithiasis occurs in 1% to 5% of the population. The highest incidence is in middle-aged white males. It is estimated that 50% of patients will have recurrent symptoms during the 8 years following the initial diagnosis. The increase in obesity in industrialized countries appears to have increased the occurrence of calculi. An understanding of the physiology of stone formation is necessary to prevent such recurrence.

Seventy-five percent of kidney and ureteral calculi are composed of calcium oxalate and/or phosphate. The remaining 25% are uric acid, struvite (infectious calculi), or cystine calculi. Calcium oxalate stones are more common than calcium phosphate stones. In addition, medications such as crixivan and triamterene can cause calculi to form.

Calcium Calculi

Risk factors for calcium oxalate lithiasis include low urine output (<1,500 mL/d), hypercalciuria, elevated sodium or oxalate excretion, increased protein intake, and low urinary citrate excretion. Maintaining a urine output of greater than 2 L/d is important for preventing all forms of renal calculi. Hypercalciuria is related to either increased absorption of calcium from the bowel, or increased renal excretion of calcium. Increased renal excretion can be related to primary tubular defects or hypercalcemia related to hyperparathyroidism. Increased sodium intake and excretion increases the amount of calcium excreted in the urine, causing hypercalciuria. Hyperoxaluria usually occurs in short gut syndrome and is characterized by increased oxalate absorption from the colon. It can also be seen in patients who have had a jejunoileal bypass that has excluded most of the small intestine. An intact colon is required for increased absorption from the bowel.

Urinary citrate inhibits most stone formation and is excreted in very low levels in the renal tubular defect of distal renal tubular acidosis. The resulting stone type in this setting is often calcium phosphate.

The factors that identify an individual at risk for development of urinary calculi are detected by measurement of serum chemistries and a 24-hour urine collection that quantitates volumes, calcium, oxalate, citrate, and sodium. The foundation of treatment to reverse these factors that place the patient at risk include increasing fluid intake, particularly water, and avoiding excessive intake of meats, calcium, oxalate, and sodium. Severe restriction of calcium intake, however, is thought to possibly increase the likelihood of stone formation because calcium binds oxalate in the gut and thereby prevents absorption of oxalate. Diets high in meat result in high acid load, high sodium excretion, and increased uric acid in the urine, which acts as an initiator for calcium calculi to form so-called heterogeneous nucleation. In some patients, the addition of thiazide diuretics is used to decrease calcium excretion, and the addition of citrate containing alkalinizing medications may further decrease the likelihood of stone formation.

Infection Calculi

Infection stones are typically composed of struvite or magnesium ammonium phosphate. The pathophysiology is initiated by the enzyme urease, which converts urea to ammonia. Ammonia irritates the epithelium of the collecting system. Proteinaceous material and glycosaminoglycans are secreted in response to mucosal irritation, which creates a substance called *matrix*. This substance hardens capturing crystals of magnesium ammonium phosphate and calcium, forming struvite. In some patients, these stones fill the entire collecting system and are then referred to as *staghorn calculi*.

Prevention of infectious calculi involves eradication of chronic UTIs. Treatment of these stones requires removal of all stone material, followed by diligent efforts to maintain a sterile urine. A 24-hour urine collection for measurement of calcium, citrate, oxalate, and uric acid is therefore essential to guide management of these patients.

Uric Acid Calculi

Uric acid calculi occur in approximately 5% of patients with nephrolithiasis. Increased uric acid excretion is related to increased intake or turnover of protein. With an increased intake of protein, there is an increased breakdown of amino acids to uric acid through the enzyme xanthine oxidase. Increased uric acid excretion is also seen during chemotherapy of lymphoproliferative diseases. Uric acid calculi also occur in patients with ileostomies because of high volume fluid loss from the gut along with loss of bicarbonate and resultant metabolic acidosis and low urinary pH.

Hyperuricemia from gout or other inherited disorders of uric acid metabolism can also result in hyperuricosuria and uric acid stone formation. Because uric acid is soluble at a urinary pH of greater than 6.5, once these patients are identified, their stones generally can be prevented by hydration (>2 L output per day) and by the use of urinary alkalinizing medications. In patients with hyperuricemia (if renal function is normal) or if the urinary excretion of uric acid is greater than 800 mg daily, allopurinol can be given at a dose of 150 to 300 mg daily.

Cystine Calculi

Cystine stones result from a defect in renal tubular handling of the amino acids cystine, ornithine, lysine and arginine (COLA). Only cystine is insoluble at high concentrations in the urine and thereby calculi can form. Treatment requires more attention to volume intake and requires urine output at levels of 3 or more L/d. If the cystine excretion can be lowered to less than 250 mg/L of urine then often the formation of cystine calculi will decrease. In addition, urinary alkalinization to pH of 6.5 or greater will improve solubility of cystine in the urine. If these measures are not successful in preventing further calculus formation, then the addition of cystine binding medications such as α-mercaptipropoinylglycine or d-penicillamine will be necessary. These medications have frequent significant side effects such as nephritic syndrome, dermatitis, and jaundice.

MALE INFERTILITY

The testes are responsible for spermatogenesis and the secretion of hormones (primarily testosterone). Both functions are controlled by feedback through the hypothalamic-pituitary-gonadal axis (Fig. 23.4). The initiation of sperm production at puberty requires the presence of both normal luteinizing hormone (LH) and follicle-stimulating hormone (FSH)

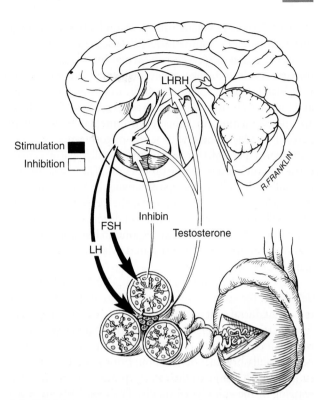

FIGURE 23.4 The pituitary gonadal axis. LHRH, luteinizing hormone-releasing hormone; FSH, follicle-stimulating hormone.

(Fig. 23.4). Gonadotropin-releasing hormone (GnRH) from the hypothalamus stimulates secretion of LH and FSH from the pituitary. LH then stimulates the Leydig cells of the testicle to produce testosterone. Intratesticular concentrations of testosterone are up to 80 times greater than serum concentrations and these high concentrations of testosterone are necessary for normal spermatogenesis. Serum testosterone reduces the secretion of pituitary LH through negative feedback. Therefore, exogenous testosterone (androgen replacement or anabolic steroid abuse) suppresses testicular testosterone production and spermatogenesis. FSH acts on the Sertoli cells of the seminiferous tubules to produce proteins necessary for spermatogenesis. In combination with other factors, a polypeptide secreted by the Sertoli cell, inhibin B, suppresses FSH secretion by negative feedback. The measurement of FSH and testosterone, as well as LH and prolactin (PrL), helps to define the etiology of low (oligo-) or absent (azo-) spermia in the semen analysis.

Factors that result in male infertility are divided into pretesticular, testicular, and post-testicular. Assignment to one of these groups is made on the basis of history, physical examination, semen analysis, and hormone evaluation.

Pretesticular infertility is the result of abnormal hormone production adversely affecting spermatogenesis. Isolated gonadotropin deficiency (Kallman syndrome) or increased production of PrL (prolactinoma) can result in abnormal spermatogenesis. High levels of FSH in an azoospermic postpubertal male suggest a poor prognosis for fertility.

Testicular causes of infertility account for the bulk of male infertility patients. Approximately 40% of these patients have a varicocele, and surgical correction may increase sperm production and lead to subsequent pregnancy. Other causes of testicular infertility include orchitis, undescended testicles, and toxic effects from exposure to agents such as chemotherapeutics, radiation, or other environmental toxins. Eight percent to 12% of men with severe oligospermia (<5 million sperm per mL) or azoospermia will have a genetic cause for their poor sperm production. These genetic abnormalities include karyotype anomalies or Y-chromosome microdeletions. For some patients, the cause for the infertility will not be obvious. Their condition is described as idiopathic. These patients may respond to hormonal manipulation [clomiphene citrate (Clomid, Marion Merrell Dow, Kansas City, MO)].

Post-testicular causes of infertility include problems with delivery of the sperm. They are related to obstruction of the excurrent ductal system (epididymis, vas deferens or ejaculatory ducts) or disorders of ejaculation (retrograde ejaculation or spinal cord injury). Obstructed patients have vasal agenesis, ejaculatory duct obstruction, prior scrotal or inguinal surgery that has injured the vas, or epididymitis resulting in scarring of the epididymal tubule. These patients are often severely oligospermic, with poor sperm motility or azoospermic. Most men with obstructive disorders will have normal spermatogenesis. Therefore, some of these men can be reconstructed. Those patients who cannot be reconstructed may have sperm retrieved from the testis or epididymis and used in an *in vitro* fertilization with intracytoplasmic sperm injection (IVF-ICSI) cycle. If their testicles exhibit active spermatogenesis, sperm can be retrieved by microaspiration of the epididymis or testicular biopsy and used in association with an *in vitro* fertilization program.

ERECTILE DYSFUNCTION

Erectile dysfunction (ED) is defined as the persistent or recurrent inability to achieve and maintain an erection of the penis sufficient for satisfactory sexual performance. The prevalence of ED increases with age. The Massachusetts Male Aging Study reveals ED in approximately 50% of men at age 50 and 70% at age 70. ED is strongly associated with cardiovascular risk factors and lower urinary tract symptoms (LUTSs) and management of these conditions may improve symptoms.

Normal Erectile Physiology

The sexual response cycle in humans includes four phases: (i) sexual desire or libido, which is maintained by testosterone. (ii) Arousal: during which penile erection occurs. The physiologic mechanism of erection begins with parasympathetic outflow and release of nitric oxide from local nerve terminals and vascular endothelial cells. Nitric oxide increases cyclic guanosine monophophate (cGMP) in penile vasculature causing vasodilatation of penile arterioles and arteries, thereby increasing penile blood flow. The expansion of the cavernosal sinusoids with blood compresses emissary veins in the tunica albuginea. This impedes venous outflow and produces erection. (iii) Orgasm/ejaculation: sympathetic signals control ejaculation at the time of orgasm. (iv) Resolution: tumescence. Interruptions in the sexual cycle cause sexual dysfunction including ED.

Etiology of Erectile Dysfunction

Historically, ED was viewed as a mainly psychiatric disorder. Psychogenic causes still persist in the minority (depression, interpersonal or social stressors); however, recent epidemiologic studies demonstrate that organic causes predominate. Vascular disease (atherosclerosis, often accelerated by hypertension, dyslipidemia, and diabetes mellitus) represents 40% of all ED presentations. Medications [diuretics, β blockers, H2-blockers, antiandrogens, protease inhibitors, cytotoxic agents, and selective serotonin reuptake inhibitors (SSRIs)] are responsible for 25% of all cases. Pelvic and penile trauma, extensive bicycle riding, neurologic illness and anatomic abnormalities such as Peyronie and fibrosis from recurrent priapism account for another 5% to 10%. Low testosterone or hypogonadism cause 3% of those presenting with ED. Other endocrine causes include hyperthyroidism and prolactinemia.

Evaluation

Diagnosis is based on history and physical examination with occasional adjunctive laboratory and radiologic testing. History should elicit presence and time course of ED. Psychogenic causes are usually sudden and complete and frequently do not affect nocturnal or morning erections. Organic ED is typically gradual except when of traumatic etiology. One must evaluate cardiovascular risk factors, medications, alcohol history, indices of depression, illicit drug use, sexual history, psychosocial issues involving partners and social stressors. Physical examination includes cardiovascular examination for bruits, evaluation for signs of endocrine abnormalities (gynecomastia, visual field defects, thyromegaly or nodularity) and a thorough neurologic examination (including evaluation of anal tone, bulbar cavernous reflex, and sacral dermatomes). The genital examination must inspect the penis on stretch for Peyronie plaques, fibrosis, and curvature. Testicles are assessed for size, symmetry, and presence of masses. Testosterone should be tested in patients with a suggestive clinical picture: (i) decreased libido, poor erectile quality, decreased nocturnal erections; (ii) changes in mood, intellectual acuity; (iii) decrease in lean body mass; (iv) decrease in body hair; or (vi) decreased bone mineral density or osteoporosis. This represents a small portion of patients. If hypogonadism is present the PrL and LH should be assessed and if PrL is elevated and/or LH is low then a pituitary prolactinoma should be ruled out with MRI.

Management

Initial therapy includes lifestyle modifications (smoking cessation, moderation of alcohol, control of diabetes, etc.), treatment of hypogonadism, medication changes, counseling, assessment of patient/partner expectations and phosphodiesterase 5 (PDE-5) inhibitors. PDE-5 inhibitors are contraindicated in those for whom sexual activity is contraindicated due to cardiovascular disease and those taking nitrates. Nitrates in combination PDE-5 inhibitors can cause profound hypotension. The α blockers can be used concomitantly with precaution (see package inserts for full details side effects and other warnings). PDE-5 inhibitors work by inhibiting the breakdown of cGMP by PDE type 5, thereby prolonging the arterial vasodilatory effect during erection. There are three available PDE-5 inhibitors: sildenafil, vardenafil and tadalafil. Sexual stimulation is required to provoke erection. Efficacy between these agents is similar when taken appropriately, for example, 1 hour before sexual activity and sildenafil should be taken on an empty stomach.

The practice of administering exogenous testosterone without proven hypogonadism is condemned. Unfortunately, in the elderly male, what actually is hypogonadism is difficult to determine. In the past, the comparison to menopause has been made. However, in the aging male, this comparison is not usually an accurate one and the concept of relative gonadal insufficiency is considered a real one. As with all therapy, the administration of exogenous testosterone should be for the treatment of symptoms and must be closely monitored. In addition, it must be remembered that testosterone normal values are based on morning collection values. It is clear that not all testosterone is "bioavailable." Unfortunately, the currently available laboratory testing does not necessarily address and define the patient's true gonadal state, and total testosterone is therefore probably as good a laboratory value as any on which to base therapy.

The introduction of oral agents for addressing ED has revolutionized treatment. PDE-5 inhibitor's mechanism of action is the enhancement of smooth muscle relaxation in the corpus cavernosum. Sildenafil is prescribed in 25-, 50-, or 100-mg doses, and should be taken on an empty stomach. Patients should be instructed to take it 45 minutes before sexual activity. Vardenafil's pharmacokinetics is similar to those of sildenafil. Therefore the instructions for use are similar to those for sildenafil. Vardenafil comes in a 5-, 10-, and 20-mg dose. Tadalafil has quite different pharmacokinetics. Patients using tadalafil take their medication approximately 2 hours before planned intercourse; although, efficacy has been seen in as early as 30 to 40 minutes. The prolonged half-life, however, allows efficacy for as long as 36 hours. Tadalafil comes in a 5-, 10-, and 20-mg dose. Additionally, the food limitations which apply to sildenafil and vardenafil are of much less concern with tadalafil. They must also be reminded that these drugs are facilitating medications and that stimulation is necessary for optimum results. This class of drugs is contraindicated in all patients taking nitrates.

In patients who fail treatment with PDE-5 inhibitors or for whom they are contraindicated, there are alternatives. Intracavernosal injections (prostaglandin E$_1$, phentolamine, papaverine) allow patients to self-inject vasodilators directly into the corporal bodies, but carry the increased small risk of priapism and painful erections. Intraurethral suppositories contain prostaglandin E$_1$ and cause erections by diffusing from the urethra into the corporal bodies and exerting a vasodilatory effect. Side effects include painful erections, bloody urethral discharge, and urethral burning. Vacuum pump devices are least expensive and safest with relatively few contraindications. Vacuum pump devices mechanically cause an erection by creating negative pressure and engorging the penis with blood; then a venous constriction band is used to hold the erection. The constriction band should be removed after 30 minutes.

Surgical therapy would include penile prosthesis and surgical revascularization. Penile implants have been used for 30 years and improvements in the devices have decreased the complications and need for revisions. Revascularization is reserved for young patients with traumatic or congenital etiologies.

PEDIATRIC UROLOGY

Antenatal sonographic imaging has significantly changed management of the fetus with urinary tract abnormalities, allowing many neonates to be identified before birth so early diagnosis and treatment can be instituted. The developing urinary tract is well visualized by modern sonographic surveillance from approximately 12 weeks of gestation.

Masses

The most common cases of abdominal masses in the neonate are actually retroperitoneal in origin, consisting of hydronephrosis and multicystic dysplastic kidney. Neoplastic masses involving the kidney in newborns include Wilms tumor and congenital mesoblastic nephroma. After appropriate evaluation, both masses should be managed with surgical resection.

Urinary Tract Obstruction

Obstruction of the developing urinary tract can have serious consequences. It is classified as supravesical or infravesical in origin. Posterior urethral valves (PUVs) are the most common cause of intravesical obstruction, and if severe can result in bilateral dysplastic kidneys and renal failure. PUVs are frequently detected by antenatal sonography, and if associated with oligohydramnios can lead to stillbirth or neonatal respiratory failure. Transurethral ablation of the valve is recommended unless the neonatal urethra is too small for instrumentation, and a temporary diverting vesicostomy can be performed.

Congenital fetal hydronephrosis should be evaluated postnatally with an ultrasonographic and voiding cystourethrogram. Most cases of ureteropelvic junction obstruction or ureteral vesical junction obstruction can be followed nonoperatively unless associated with renal failure or a severe decrease in differential function on nuclear renogram.

Vesicoureteral Reflux

The neonatal management of vesicoureteral reflux usually consists of an assessment of renal function with radionucleotide imaging and selection of an appropriate course of prophylactic antibiotics. Prevention of an infection allows time for observation of the patient. The indications for surgical management or vesicoureteral reflux are the inability to keep the urinary tract sterile (i.e., breakthrough infections and/or development of new renal scarring on prophylaxis).

Recent studies show that the greatest predictor of vesicoureteral reflux resolution is the grade at discovery. Grading of reflux is generally after the Dwoskin/Perlmutter classification. Grade I is low volume reflux that goes into the ureter. Grade II is reflux of a higher volume, with contrast outlining the entire urinary tract without dilation. Grade III reflux is associated with grade II findings plus some clubbing of the calyces. Grade IV reflux clearly demonstrates hydronephrosis. In grade V reflux, the ureters are markedly tortuous and the architecture of the upper tracts is virtually destroyed. Most children with grade III or less at the time of discovery will resolve their reflux in slightly greater than 3 years. In grade IV and V, reflux resolution is far less predictable. Untreated severe reflux and infections can result in reflux nephropathy and renal failure.

Antireflux surgery is well established and based on a "flap-valve" mechanism. Newer surgical approaches include extravesical reimplantation and endoscopic periureteral injection of dextraisomeryl hyaluronic acid (deflux) in order to minimize morbidity.

Spinal Dysraphism

Spinal dysraphism with neurogenic bladder can be diagnosed on antenatal studies. After birth, these infants require immediate assessment with ultrasonography and a voiding cystourethrogram. These should be scheduled in cooperation with the closure of the myelomeningocele. An important concern in the management of spinal dysraphism is the constantly changing neurologic status. A child without hydronephrosis or evidence of reflux at birth can rapidly become a child with marked hydronephrosis, severe neurogenic bladder, and secondary vesicoureteral reflux. If the initial voiding cystourethrogram demonstrates reflux, with or without poor bladder emptying, it may be necessary to initiate intermittent catheterization. These children should also be maintained on prophylactic antibiotics.

In children with spina bifida, regular studies should be done to assess bladder emptying, renal growth, and to monitor the development of hydronephrosis (ultrasonography and/or radionucleotide scan). Voiding cystourethrogram should also be done to assess reflux.

PEDIATRIC UROLOGIC SURGERY

Circumcision

Circumcision is the most common surgical procedure performed in the United States, with approximately 1.2 million newborns circumcised each year. Routine neonatal circumcision remains controversial, with various groups vigorously advocating both for and against it. The most recent policy statement from the American Academy of Pediatrics, adopted in 1999, states that, "existing scientific evidence demonstrates potential medical benefits; however, these data are not sufficient to recommend routine neonatal circumcision." Very briefly, benefits of circumcision include a decreased risk of UTIs, elimination of the potential for penile problems such as phimosis and paraphimosis, decreased risk for acquiring various sexually transmitted diseases, and protection against penile cancer. Potential disadvantages of circumcision include subjecting the child to a painful, unnecessary procedure, the risk of complications (0.2%–0.5%) and decreased penile sensation and sexual satisfaction related to absence of the prepuce. There are three methods of circumcision that are commonly used in the newborn male: the Gompco clamp, the Mogen clamp, and the Plastibell device. If circumcision is chosen by the parents, local anesthesia such as a penile nerve block should be used. If a boy is born with any type of penile abnormality, then neonatal circumcision is contraindicated.

Hypospadias

Development of the external genitalia is a complex embryologic phenomenon, and failure at any point during the sequence can cause a variety of abnormalities. Hypospadias is one of the most common anomalies, said to occur in approximately 1 in 300 live male births in the United States. Interestingly, the incidence of hypospadias seems to be rising, probably related to environmental toxins in developed countries. Hypospadias results from the incomplete fusion of the urethral folds so that the urethral opening is somewhere on the ventral aspect of the penis or in the scrotum or perineum. Significant downward curvature of the penis, or chordee, is often present. Reconstructive surgery for hypospadias is best done between the ages of 6 to 18 months. The goals of surgery are to achieve a straight penis with a normal urethral meatus at the tip of the glans. Although hypospadias repair remains technically challenging, the results of modern surgery are successful with a single operation in 90% to 95% of cases.

Cryptorchidism

Maldescent of the testicle may be noted at birth. The testes develop intra-abdominally, and normally descend into the scrotum near the end of the seventh month of gestation. Cryptorchidism may be unilateral or bilateral. It is more common in premature boys and occurs in 3% of full term males. Some undescended testes descend spontaneously during the first year of life, so that by age 12 months, the incidence is 0.8%. Cryptorchidism is associated with an increased rate of infertility as well as increased risk of testicular cancer. Most undescended testes are palpable in the groin, and inguinal orchidopexy is successful in achieving the intrascrotal position in 95% of cases. Surgery should be done as soon as practical after the boy becomes a year old. If the testicle is impalpable on physical examination, preoperative imaging studies are usually not reliable in establishing the presence or absence of an intra-abdominal testicle. These cases should be approached with diagnostic laparoscopy and if an abdominal testis is found, laparoscopic orchidopexy can be done.

Testicular Torsion

Testicular torsion is a surgical emergency. This happens when an abnormally mobile testis twists on its vascular pedicle, resulting in ischemia of the gonad. Testicular torsion can occur prenatally, but the most common type of torsion occurs in boys 10 to 18 years of age. Boys with torsion experience onset of severe testicular pain. On physical examination, the testis and scrotum are usually exquisitely tender, erythematous and swollen. A scrotal Doppler ultrasonography will show diminished or absent perfusion of the testis. Emergent scrotal exploration should be done; and if the torsed testicle appears to be viable, it is untwisted and fixed to the scrotal wall, as is the contralateral testis. If testicular torsion is not corrected within 6 to 8 hours of onset, then the testis will infarct and become necrotic.

Ambiguous Genitalia

The most common cause of ambiguous genitalia is congenital adrenal hyperplasia (CAH). CAH results in virilization of the external genitalia in females. The internal reproductive organs are normal and functional. In CAH, there is an enzymatic defect in the way the adrenal glands metabolize cholesterol into cortisol. This results in accumulation of androgens and a deficit of glucocorticoids and mineral corticoids. Severe cases can be life threatening due to salt wasting. Morphologically, these 46XX female infants have various degrees of clitoral hypertrophy and labial fusion and can be easily mistaken for males. An infant with a male phenotype and bilaterally nonpalpable gonads should be evaluated for CAH. Reconstructive surgery is usually undertaken within the first year of life. Feminizing genitoplasty consists of clitoral reduction, creation of labia, and exteriorization of the vagina. The place of genital surgery for ambiguous genitalia continues to be a topic of significant controversy among pediatricians, pediatric surgeons, and pediatric urologists.

Exstrophy–Epispadias

Another dramatic condition affecting both the genitalia and the urinary tract is the exstrophy–epispadias complex Classical bladder exstrophy is rare, occurring in 1:30,000 infants. There is a failure of fusion of the midline structures, so that the pubic bones are separated and the bladder is open and exposed. Unlike other anomalies, exstrophy–epispadias does not represent an arrest of normal fetal development, but rather a completely abnormal departure from normal development. Male exstrophy patients have complete epispadias as well.

The surgical reconstruction of the infant born with exstrophy is one of the most challenging in pediatric urology and can be undertaken in stages. However, the penile disassembly technique allows for some cases to be closed in single stage. It must be realized that even with single stage closure, other surgeries may be needed to completely bring the urethra to the tip of the glans, improve continence, and in many cases to improve cosmetics. Typically, shortly after birth the open bladder and abdominal wall defect are closed. In boys, the penile defect is repaired between ages 1 to 2. These children have no urinary sphincter muscle and require bladder neck reconstruction to achieve continence, which is usually done between 4 to 6 years of age. Because of the complex nature of this surgery, exstrophy is best managed at specialized centers that have considerable experience with this difficult condition.

Pediatric Urinary Tract Infection

All anomalies of the urinary tract are heralded by UTIs. Therefore, when a male or nonsexually active female child presents with a UTI, he or she by definition should be evaluated for other abnormalities. Early intervention unquestionably preserves renal function. A very common cause of UTI in children which does not involve anatomic abnormality is dysfunctional elimination syndrome (DES).

GENITOURINARY TRAUMA

Renal injuries are the most common of all urologic injuries. They can be the result of either penetrating or blunt trauma, and they occur in approximately 10% of all blunt injuries to the abdomen. Laceration injuries of the kidney resulting from blunt trauma are usually associated with lower rib fractures or fractures of the lumbar transverse processes. Although the kidney's retroperitoneal location protects it in most circumstances, deceleration injuries can produce enough motion to stretch or even avulse the main renal vessels, particularly in the pediatric or very slender patients. Stretching injuries cause disruption of the vascular intima, with subsequent subintimal dissection and secondary thrombosis in the renal artery. Penetrating injuries cause a wide range of injuries of varying severity.

Renal injuries have been divided into five classifications by the American Association for Surgery of Trauma: (i) Minor laceration limited to the cortex. Grade I, a renal contusion or bruise. (ii) Grade II, a minor laceration less than 1 cm in length limited to the cortex. (iii) Grade III, injuries involve a major laceration, greater than 1 cm in length, avoiding the collecting system. (iv) Grade IV, injuries represent a major laceration of the kidney involving the collecting system with urinary extravasation. Vascular injuries of the segmental or main renal vessels are classified as grade IV when the hemorrhage is contained in the retroperitoneum. (v) Grade V, injuries are life-threatening emergencies and include the shattered kidney or avulsion of the renal hilum.

This staging system relies on a complete evaluation of the urinary tract, consisting of a three-tiered approach: clinical evaluation with urinalysis and blood pressure monitoring, image evaluation, and (when indicated) surgical evaluation and management. The imaging modalities used most often in this situation are the CT scan and/or IVU. Arteriography and ultrasonography are used much less frequently.

The indications for radiographic assessment in the adult trauma patient include gross hematuria, microscopic hematuria associated with shock, clinical suspicion of injury (i.e., fracture of the transverse processes of lumbar vertebra and/or fractures of T-11 or T-12 rib), splenic injury, and penetrating injuries with any degree of hematuria. Multiple studies have demonstrated that patients with microhematuria alone do not require imaging. In the pediatric population, the parameters become better defined. Although it is true that the anatomy of children can potentially make renal injury more likely, recent analysis shows that the child who is hemodynamically stable, from the time of the accident to the time of being seen, and who has only microhematuria, in most cases does not require imaging. All of the protocols are tempered by suspicion on the part of the physician, however, for example, a child who has had a history of significant deceleration who has suffered significant other trauma does warrant imaging. The same *caveat* is equally applicable to the adult. In the pediatric population, the parameters are less well defined, as the child differs in two important ways: the kidneys are larger and more mobile; and the coexistence of a renal anomaly can make the kidney more easily traumatized. Children with microhematuria, therefore, deserve imaging for both blunt and penetrating trauma.

The treatment of renal injuries is mediated by the stage of the injury and stability of the patient. Grade I through grade III injuries are self-limiting and usually resolve with conservative treatment. Major renal trauma associated with uncontrolled bleeding, major renovascular injury, a large area of devitalized tissue, or significant urinary extravasation as seen in grade VI and V injuries, may require renal exploration. There is increasing enthusiasm for observing many of these severe injuries.

Ureteral injuries account for approximately 1% of GU trauma, and most are the result of penetrating trauma. Blunt trauma is rarely the cause of ureteral injury, and when it does occur, it is usually in the form of traumatic disruption of the ureteropelvic junction. Traumatic disruption of the ureteropelvic junction is seen far more often in the pediatric population than in the adult population.

Ureteral injuries are often missed, resulting in significant morbidity, and unlike renal injuries, are not suited for conservative management. No single radiographic assessment is reliable in the assessment of ureteral injuries, and the best evaluation is provided by direct examination of the ureter's full course while the patient is being explored for other purposes. Intraoperative ureteral canalization and use of methylene blue may help identify a more subtle site of urine extravasation. IVU and CT will often, but not always, show extravasation. Retrograde pyelography provides excellent visualization, but it is frequently impractical in patients with penetrating trauma and other associated injuries. If the

patient has no other reason for exploration, cystoscopy with retrograde pyelography is the imaging modality of choice.

Bladder injuries can occur as a result of either penetrating or blunt trauma. Bladder injuries are classified as extraperitoneal (60%), intraperitoneal (30%), or both (10%). Eighty-five percent of bladder injuries are associated with pelvic fracture, and 10% of pelvic fractures are associated with bladder injury. Therefore, bladder injuries should be suspected in all patients with pelvic fracture, all patients with gross hematuria, or any patient with a mechanism of injury that suggests the potential for bladder or urethral injury.

The diagnostic study of choice for evaluation of bladder injury is the trauma cystogram. A trauma cystogram involves instillation of at least 300 mL of contrast with multiple projections and complete drainage films. The plain cystogram on CT scan has not been shown to be a reliable alternative to the trauma cystogram. However, studies show that CT imaging in concert with a trauma cystogram protocol is very accurate in detecting bladder injuries and, with the current practice of evaluating all trauma patients with CT, have the additional benefit of allowing complete evaluation, all within the CT suite.

Posterior urethral distraction injuries occur almost exclusively with pelvic fracture, with 5% to 10% of pelvic fractures resulting in posterior urethral distraction injuries. In pelvic fracture, the bladder and prostate tend to travel with the bones as they are displaced, whereas the anterior urethra remains relatively fixed, distracting the relatively weak membranous urethra. Long-term sequelae of pelvic fracture and posterior urethral distraction are: urethral stricture, ED, and, in some patients, incontinence. Signs associated with posterior urethral distraction include the presence of blood at the urethral meatus and an impalpable or "high-riding" prostate on rectal examination and perineal ecchymosis.

The treatment of posterior urethral distraction injury typically consists of placement of suprapubic urinary diversion and delayed reconstruction. Placement of the suprapubic tube in the midline facilitates future reconstruction. In addition, with the advent of flexible endoscopic techniques, the placement of an aligning catheter is much easier and has proved beneficial. Neither an aligning catheter nor a suprapubic diversion prevents obliteration of the urethra. However, in many patients, distraction injury does not completely disrupt the continuity of the urethra, and in those patients, an aligning catheter can make the difference between a stricture that is readily manageable by conservative techniques and one that needs complex open reconstruction. Catheterization, in the case of incomplete disruption, should be performed cautiously to prevent additional urethral trauma.

Anterior urethral injuries can be classified as either contusions or disruptions. The location depends on the angle of the patient as the perineum impacts an immovable object. The immovable object acts as a hammer and the pubis acts as an anvil, resulting in injury to the tissues that lie in between. Patients who have sustained straddle perineal trauma should be evaluated with retrograde urethrography just as in the case of suspected posterior urethral distraction. Many of these injuries can be managed initially with placement of an indwelling urethral catheter. In most cases, anterior urethral injuries resulting from penetrating trauma mandate exploration, debridement, and immediate reconstruction. However, mechanism of injury, potential for blast effect, and the condition of the adjacent tissue, all influence the decision to primarily reconstruct or divert and delay reconstruction.

Trauma to the external genitalia has been classified by Culp as nonpenetrating, penetrating, avulsion, burns, or radiation injuries. The most common nonpenetrating injuries are penile or scrotal contusion. Testicular fracture occurs from nonpenetrating trauma, and scrotal ultrasonography differentiates a scrotal contusion from a fractured testicle. Testicular fracture warrants surgical exploration and repair of the tunica albuginea when possible.

A unique nonpenetrating injury in the male is the corporal or penile fracture. This occurs with buckling of the penis during intercourse. When the injury disrupts the tunica albuginea of the corpora along with Buck fascia, findings of immediate detumescence associated with ecchymosis and a hematoma collection in the penis are noted. Most recommend early surgical exploration. Hematoma evacuation and closure of the disrupted tunica albuginea of the corpora is recommended in these cases. Many patients, however, disrupt only one layer of the tunica albuginea or both layers of the tunica without disrupting Buck fascia. Although these patients do not have the dramatic findings of the classic patient with penile fracture, the unfortunate sequelae of penile indentation and curvature of the penis can be seen. Because urethral injury can be associated with injury to the corpora cavernosa, this possibility should be evaluated.

Penetrating injuries to the external genitalia can range from simple injuries to amputation of the penis and/or scrotum and testicles. In simpler penetrating injuries, debridement and anatomic reconstruction are the preferred treatment approach. Microsurgical replantation is the treatment of choice for amputation injuries.

Avulsion injuries can be dramatic in appearance. Unique to the male genitalia, the tissues of the scrotum, penis, and underlying elastic fascial structures are integral to this injury. Avulsion injuries occur when these tissues become entangled, usually in clothing, and are torn off with the clothing, leaving behind the deep structures of the penis and often the denuded testicles. After an avulsion injury, there should be a period of observation to clarify the extent of the injury. Urethral and rectal examination should be accomplished. Reconstruction can be undertaken approximately 12 to 24 hours after presentation.

Burn injuries to the genitalia are treated the same as burn injuries to the rest of the body. Debridement of the penis should be executed carefully. Aggressive debridement of the penis is usually not needed due to its unique vascular characteristics. Urethral injuries must be dealt with later after healing of the burn. Diversion of urine during the acute phase may be indicated. A suprapubic tube can be placed through burned tissue without concern. Chemical burns rarely involve structures deep to the skin. Electrical burns, however, may have extensive and delayed deep tissue destruction. Often, however, the burns to the genitalia that are seen with electrical burns are actually thermal burns that inevitably accompany electrical burns.

Fortunately, as enthusiasm for treatment of genital neoplasm with radiation has waned, direct radiation injuries to the genitalia are no longer seen. However, the genitalia can be involved with "malignant" edema associated with radiotherapy of the pelvis. These patients' injuries are reconstructible with excision of the edematous tissues and with grafting to the deep structures of the penis and testicles with a split-thickness skin graft (STSG). Full thickness skin is associated with significant reaccumulation of edema in these tissues. Because STSGs will not become edematous, they are the graft of choice for reconstruction of radiation edema. In many situations, where the edema is not associated with a "systemic problem," the skin of the lateral scrotum and the posterior scrotum is spared and can be used as local flaps. Scrotal reconstruction using these flaps yields excellent results. However, experience has shown that these areas are seldom spared if the edematous process also involves the lower extremities. In these cases, STSGs are the best choice.

Congenital Bent Penis

Curvature of the penis can be either congenital or acquired. The most frequent cause of congenital curvature of the penis is hypospadias. The constellation of congenital curvatures associated with hyperdistensibility of the corporal bodies is the second most frequent cause of congenital curvature of the penis. These curvatures can be ventral, lateral (left), dorsal, or complex. The least common congenital curvature of the penis is the dorsal curvature associated with epispadias/exstrophy.

The curvature of hypospadias is believed to be caused by the presence of dysgenic tethering tissue on the ventrum of the penis and/or symmetric development of the ventral and dorsal surfaces. Correction of curvature of the penis caused by hypospadias involves resection of the dysgenetic tissue. If resection proves inadequate, shortening of the opposite dorsal side allows for straightening.

In congenital curvatures of the penis associated with hyperdistensibility of the corpora, the flaccid penis is of average size, but the erect penis becomes impressively large. Curvature results in this congenital defect if dys-symmetry exists in the expansion of one aspect of the corpora compared to another corporal disproportion. Techniques to lengthen the short side of the penis have involved grafting of a corporotomy defect, which potentially has ill effects on the erectile mechanism. Therefore, because length of penis is usually not a problem with these patients, techniques to shorten the longer, opposite side are favored over techniques that lengthen the shorter side.

Concerns about length are common among patients with dorsal curvature caused by exstrophy/epispadias complex. For these patients, the curvature is treated by excision of the dysgenetic dorsal tissues, and lengthening of the dorsal aspect with the creation of a corporotomy defect and grafting.

These curvatures can also be corrected by rolling the corpora laterally, resulting in cancellation of the curvature and relative straightening of the penis.

Acquired Bent Penis

Acquired curvature of the penis is usually a result of buckling trauma. In the young individual, buckling trauma leads either to true or subclinical fracture of the corporal body. In the bilaminar tunica albuginea, there is an inner circular and an outer longitudinal layer of fibers. With buckling, the outer layer can be disrupted, whereas the blood tight integrity of the corpus is maintained by the intact inner circular layer. These patients do not experience the classic symptoms of pain, snapping, and immediate detumescence with hematoma. However, within days to weeks, they notice a bend and indentation at the site of the trauma.

With true fracture of the corpus, both layers of the tunica, and often Buck fascia, are disrupted. These patients also notice curvature with indentation at the site of trauma within days to weeks. Preexisting lateral curvature of the penis is thought to be a predisposing cause of fracture or subclinical fracture of the penis. Although the injury actually serves to straighten the penis in these patients, the indentation at the site of injury may be disabling in that it leads to easy buckling of the penis with intercourse.

In the older man, buckling trauma leads to Peyronie disease. In these men, buckling trauma tends to occur in a dorsal, ventral direction as opposed to a lateral one. This places stress at the site of the implantation of the septal fibers, leading to disruption of the fibers as they interweave with the tunica albuginea, and/or a delamination injury at the site of the dorsal or ventral interweaving of the septal fibers of the inner lamina of the tunica albuginea. In the predisposed individual, the inflammatory phase that follows leads to scarring and functional tethering of the involved aspect of the penis. Subtle ED may add to penile instability during penetration, increasing the risk of penile buckling during intercourse.

Acute treatment for acquired curvatures involves reassurance and medical therapy. Although a number of oral agents have been used, none have been demonstrated to be effective through good double-blind drug studies. The most frequently used oral agents are vitamin E, Potaba, antihistamines, nonsteroidal inflammatory agents, colchicines, tamoxifen, esters of carnitine, and PDE-5 inhibitors. A number of intralesional injection protocols have been used, including injection of steroid, injection of collagenase, and injection of calcium channel blockers. The injection of steroids is ineffective. The effects of intralesional injection with collagenase, interferon, and calcium channel blockers are currently the topic of study protocols. Ultrasonographic therapy with steroids (iontophoresis) has enjoyed some enthusiasm, but its efficacy has also not been proved in well-designed clinical trials. Recently the use of topical verapamil has been heavily advertised. It has been suggested that electromotive delivery serves as an adjuvant. Thus far, however, the literature fails to support either as effective.

Radiotherapy has been used at some centers during the inflammatory phase of the acquired curvatures of the penis. Used as a means of delivering anti-inflammatory therapy, it may be effective in shortening the painful stage of acquired curvature, but it has no effect on the curvature itself.

The surgical management of acquired curvatures involves either shortening the long side or lengthening the short side of the penis. Synthetic graft materials have also been used to fill the corporotomy defect, but their use is discouraged without concomitant use of a prosthesis. However, if ED coincides with a disabling curvature, it is acceptable to place a prosthesis, incising the area of scar, and filling the defect with either autologous or synthetic graft material. In some cases, when a prosthesis is to be placed (with Peyronie disease in particular), the penis can be straightened by a technique termed *corporal modeling*. Corporal modeling involves cracking or stretching of the scarred area after the prosthesis is placed, with the inherent straightening characteristics of the prosthesis then serving to splint the straightened penis.

EVALUATION AND MANAGEMENT OF BENIGN PROSTATIC DISEASE

BPH, or proliferation of the epithelium and stromal components of the prostate, afflicts most men after the age of 50 . Although histologic evidence of BPH is found in 90% of men older than 50, the clinical manifestations are found in only 50%. The clinical symptoms are referred to as *LUTS* or lower urinary tract symptoms and include frequency, urgency, hesitancy, and nocturia to name a few.

Although approximately 20% of men receive some form of intervention for the symptoms of LUTS, with the development of medical therapy for these symptoms, the incidence of surgical intervention has decreased. However, the number of patients treated overall will most likely continue to increase because of the availability of less invasive means to get symptomatic relief as well as the increasingly aging population.

Clinical BPH is believed to be secondary to two factors—one static and the other dynamic. The dynamic factor has been recognized more recently; it is descriptive of increased tone at the area of the bladder neck and base, which leads to obstructive symptoms. There is a predominance of α receptors at the bladder base and neck, and an increase in either the number or sensitivity of these receptors leads to an increase in the resistance to urinary flow. One of the current therapies for LUTS is the administration of α blockers. The α blockers, developed as antihypertensive medications, are clinically useful for bladder neck relaxation.

The static component of LUTS results from epithelial and stromal hypertrophy, causing an increase in the volume of the prostate that impinges on the prostatic urethral lumen, producing mechanical obstruction. Although epithelial and stromal hypertrophy that occurs with aging are undoubtedly related to an alteration in the hormonal milieu, the precise alteration and its relative effects have not been defined. 5-α-Reductase is an enzyme that converts testosterone to dihydrotestosterone. Dihydrotestosterone is 50 times more potent than testosterone and is the dominant hormone in prostatic development. Males who are 5-α-reductase deficient, a genetic defect recognized in families in the Dominican Republic, do not develop prostatic enlargement with aging, and blockade of the conversion of testosterone to dihydrotestosterone is believed to reverse the process of prostatic hypertrophy in some individuals without adverse effects. Randomized trials with finasteride and dutasteride, 5-α-reductase inhibitors, have shown it to be safe and effective for the pharmacologic treatment of the static component of LUTS. In fact it is the combination of an α blocker and a 5-α-reductase inhibitor that provide the best relief of symptoms and the slowest progression of the disease state.

Mandatory surgical indications for treatment of BPH include azotemia, recurrent UTIs, recurrent hematuria, bladder calculi, and refractory urinary retention. However, these findings occur infrequently, and the indications for treatment of LUTS generally involve evaluation of the degree to which symptoms interfere with the patient's lifestyle. For those who do not meet the above criteria for surgery, medical management with selective α blockers constitutes a durable, nonsurgical alternative with less morbidity.

The number of treatment options for BPH continues to expand. Most patients who seek treatment choose medical therapy. Many take various herbal therapies with, as yet, unproven benefit. The more severe cases should undergo transurethral resection of the prostate (TURP). A number of minimally invasive techniques are evolving and include thermal therapy, laser and radial frequency ablation, transurethral incision of the prostate, insertion of implantable prostatic stents, and high-intensity focused ultrasonography. The rMatrix is a type of thermal therapy that shows promise from randomized trials to be a safe, effective, office-based treatment option. A high-powered potassium-titanyl-phosphate (KTP) laser has evolved to perform photoselective vaporization of the prostate (PVP). This is an outpatient surgical procedure that is rapidly replacing TURP as the "Gold Standard." It is important that both the patient and physician discuss the lifestyle impact of LUTS and the various treatment modalities so that an informed treatment decision can be made.

EVALUATION AND TREATMENT OF GENITOURINARY TUMORS

Adrenal Malignancies

Adrenocortical carcinoma is a rare and highly aggressive tumor. Its annual incidence is 0.5 to 2 per 1 million. Though is has been reported at all ages, it most often occurs in the fifth to seventh decade and in children younger than 5 years. Tumors occur more commonly on the left than the right. It has been linked to MEN 1, Beckwith-Wideman, and Li-Fraumeni syndromes. Sixty percent of adrenocortical carcinomas demonstrate endocrinologic activity. Approximately 40% will produce Cushing syndrome (excess cortisol production causing central obesity, moon shaped facies, hirsutism, acne, etc.), 25% will produce Cushing syndrome with virilization, and 25% will result in virilization alone. Serum testosterone, dehydroepiandrosterone (DHEA), DHEA-S and urinary 17-ketosteroids are frequently elevated. Feminization and hyperaldosteronism are rare. Adrenocortical carcinomas may become quite large before detection. Most tumors are greater than 6 cm at diagnosis and findings of metastatic disease to the liver, lungs, lymph nodes, or bone may be common.

The only treatment shown to impact survival is surgical resection. The role of cytoreductive surgery in the setting of metastatic disease is controversial. The primary chemotherapeutic agent for treating metastatic disease is mitotane (o, p'-DDD). Though its use has demonstrated short-term benefits, it does not affect long-term survival.

Stage is the most important indicator of prognosis. Stage I and stage II tumors (primary tumor $\leq$5 cm or >5 cm with negative nodes respectively) have a 5-year survival of approximately 50%. Stage III and IV tumors (local extension, positive nodes) have 5-year survivals of 5% and 0%. The prognosis for children is generally better.

Several other benign tumor types may arise in the adrenal glands, including adenomas capable of producing a wide variety of hormones and resultant syndromes. These topics are covered in depth in chapter 14. Pheochromocytomas, although typically benign are known to be malignant in 10% of cases. This finding is more common in women and in extra-adrenal primary tumors. Treatment involves a combination of surgery, radiation, and chemotherapy. Five-year survival is 36% to 60%.

Renal Neoplasms

Renal Cell Carcinoma

Renal cell carcinoma arises from the cells of the proximal collecting tubule. There are 39,000 of these tumors diagnosed annually in the United States, and 12,800 patients die of this cancer each year. Although its etiology is unknown, it has been linked to tobacco use, and recent studies have suggested genetic defect. The study of familial and sporadic cases of renal cell carcinoma has linked its etiology to a loss of the short arm of chromosome 3. Von Hippel-Lindau syndrome is an example of familial renal cell carcinoma, which is characterized by multiple tumors, bilateral tumors, and occurrence at a young age.

In the past, the most common presenting signs and symptoms of possible renal cell carcinoma were flank pain, gross hematuria, and a palpable renal mass. This was often referred to as the *too late triad*. Since the advent of CT, however, an increasing number of renal cell carcinomas are found incidentally during evaluation for other symptoms. Patients whose tumors are detected incidentally typically have smaller lesions with lower stage and a greater likelihood for surgical cure.

Renal cell carcinoma may invade the renal vein and can extend to the vena cava and right atrium. It may present with various manifestations of paraneoplastic syndromes, including polycythemia, anemia, hypercalcemia, and liver function abnormalities. These syndromes resolve with surgical extirpation.

The primary treatment for renal cell carcinoma is surgical excision. Because smaller tumors are now being detected by incidental CT imaging, more patients are being considered for partial nephrectomy, and major cancer series provide comparable data for nephron-sparing surgery regarding recurrence-free and long-term survival. Also, under investigation are cryoablation and radio frequency ablation of small (<4 cm) renal tumors. Larger tumors require radical nephrectomy, laparoscopic or open. Unfortunately, options are limited for the treatment of metastatic renal cell carcinoma. Chemotherapy has been unsuccessful in most cases. Because renal cell carcinoma has been associated with spontaneous regression, several biologic therapies have been tested using interleukin 2 (IL-2), interferon, cellular therapy [lymphokine-activated killer (LAK) cells], or tumor infiltrating infiltrates. Debulking of the primary tumor appears to favor survival in some reported series with metastatic disease. In two prospective randomized controlled trials (one from the United States and one from Europe), radical nephrectomy plus interferon improved survival compared to interferon alone. Long-term responses have been achieved in 10% to 20% of patients with metastatic disease. Oral tyrosine kinase inhibitors, sunitinib, and sorafenib, have recently been approved for advanced renal cell carcinoma with response rates of 25% to 36%.

Angiomyolipoma

Angiomyolipoma is a relatively common, benign tumor that does not metastasize. Tuberous sclerosis is associated with bilateral or multiple angiomyolipoma. In the absence of tuberous sclerosis, the lesions are usually solitary, unilateral, and with a female preponderance. Angiomyolipoma presents clinically with hematuria and is often detected by CT scans done for other reasons. The characteristic finding of fat within the mass differentiates it from renal cell carcinoma on CT scan or ultrasonography. If the tumor is less than 4 cm in size and is asymptomatic, it can be followed. Surgery is appropriate if hemorrhage is present or if the size exceeds 4 cm in diameter.

Wilms Tumor

Wilms tumor is a malignant renal tumor that occurs predominantly in children, although it can appear in adolescents and adults. The incidence is the same for males and females with approximately 500 new cases a year. Approximately 5% are bilateral at the time of diagnosis. An abnormality of chromosome 11 has been reported in patients with a Wilms tumor. Histology is associated with a poor prognosis if the predominant cell type is anaplastic, rhabdoid, or clear cell variant.

Chemotherapy has had a dramatic impact on the survival of children with Wilms tumors. The National Wilms Tumor Project has systematically studied the effects of chemotherapy and radiotherapy combined with surgery. Treatment protocols have been modified to produce the least possible morbidity with the best possible cure rate.

Cancer of the Bladder

Each year 50,000 cases of bladder cancer are diagnosed in the United States with 10,000 deaths being attributed to this disease. It is the fourth most common cause of cancer death in the male population. In the United States, more than 90% of bladder tumors are of the transitional cell variety. The etiology of some bladder cancers has been attributed to tobacco use or salicylate abuse. Additionally, in countries with lax regulation of chemical industries, chemical carcinogens may be implicated in a much larger number of cases. Nontransitional bladder cancer is a result of metaplastic dedifferentiation of the multipotential urothelium toward squamous or adenocarcinomatous histology. Squamous cell carcinoma arising from irritative infestation of the bladder with the parasite *Schistosoma haematobium*, is a distinct form of bladder cancer found in the Nile River delta.

The most frequent presenting symptom of bladder cancer is gross hematuria. Other important symptoms are bladder irritability and dysuria. In patients who are older than 40 years with negative urine cultures and no prior history of UTIs, a detailed evaluation of the kidneys, upper tracts, bladder, and urethra should be carried out. This should include evaluation of the upper tract with intravenous pyelogram or computed tomography scan, urinary cytology, and cystoscopy. Microscopic hematuria should be evaluated similarly. The greatest hindrance to the timely diagnosis of bladder cancer is treatment with prolonged courses of antibiotics for presumed UTIs.

The critical staging distinction for the treatment of transitional cell carcinoma of the bladder is invasion of the muscular wall of the bladder. Superficial tumors involve only the mucosa and submucosa. The loss of chromosome 9p has been found in superficial tumors, whereas tumors that invade the muscle are characterized by the additional loss of chromosome 17. These patients also have alterations in the retinoblastoma (RB) suppressor gene, loss of the p53 oncogene, and mutations in epidermal growth factor receptors (EGFRs). Seventy-five percent of bladder tumors are superficial on presentation. Of this group, approximately 50% recur, and approximately 20% progress to disease with muscle invasion.

Superficial tumors are managed initially by transurethral resection and fulguration. In recurrent superficial tumors, a variety of adjuvant intravesical agents may be employed, directed at reducing recurrences and decreasing the possibility of progression of the tumor to muscular invasion. Intravesical agents used in the past have included chemotherapeutic agents (thiotepa, adriamycin, and mitomycin C) as well as immunopotentiators or biologic agents [most commonly bacillus Calmette-Gúerin (BCG)].

Invasion of the bladder muscle by tumor connotes a much more aggressive and possibly lethal cancer. Muscle invasive transitional cell carcinoma may be treated using a variety of options. However, because transitional cell carcinoma usually represents a field change, (with the potential to develop tumors in all areas of the bladder, a total or radical cystectomy (complete removal of the bladder, prostate, and seminal vesicles and pelvic lymph nodes in the male, and removal of the bladder, pelvic nodes, and the female organs in women) is usually recommended in those patients who are fit enough to undergo such a procedure. Partial cystectomy is used infrequently for those tumors that are solitary and are localized to a portion of the bladder that allows extirpation while retaining the remainder of the bladder tumor free. An example might be an adenocarcinoma of the urachus involving only the bladder dome. External beam radiation therapy is reserved for patients who are elderly or in poor health, although some reports of radiation therapy in conjunction with a chemotherapy protocol have been promising.

Until recently, radical cystectomy implied the need for external urinary drainage. Over the last decade, advances in the understanding of the mechanics of reconfigured bowel have permitted reconstruction of continent urinary reservoirs and orthotopic bladders that avoid the need for external appliances. Protocols combining radiation with surgery, chemotherapy with radiation, and chemotherapy with surgery in a neoadjuvant or adjuvant manner are under investigation.

Because patients with transitional cell carcinoma of the bladder are at increased risk for development of tumors of the renal pelvis and ureters, periodic radiologic and cytologic monitoring is mandatory.

Carcinoma of the Prostate

Etiology and Pathogenesis
Carcinoma of the prostate is the most common cancer in men. More than 230,000 new cases of carcinoma of the prostate and 30,000 related deaths occur yearly in the United States. The incidence of prostate cancer is directly proportional to age. Approximately 30% of men in their fifth decade will have the disease. This figure increases to two thirds of men in their eighth decade. As the population ages over the next two decades, the incidence of prostate cancer diagnosis will likely double and because of improved health status these elderly men will be interested in and suitable for therapy. There appears to be a genetic predisposition to development of prostate cancer. A family history of the disease in a first-order relative increases the risk, particularly if the cancer was diagnosed in a relative younger than 65 years. African-American men are at greater risk for prostate cancer and when prostate cancer occurs in African-American men, it tends to occur earlier in life and has a more aggressive course.

In addition to age and genetic predisposition, hormonal factors, diet, environment, and possibly infection and inflammation may play roles in the development of prostate cancers. Prostate cancer has not been observed in eunuchs. The presence of testosterone appears to be required for tumor initiation. Testosterone will stimulate prostate cells *in vitro* and promote the development of prostate cancers in rats. The supposition that environment and/or diet may be causative is supported by the fact that the clinical incidence of prostate cancer in Japan is much lower than that in the United States. However, second- and third-generation Japanese-Americans are known to develop the disease at rates comparable to American Caucasians. Studies suggest that a high-fat diet, high-calorie intake, sedentary lifestyle, exposure to cadmium, or infections with various viral or bacterial agents may predispose the male population to the development of prostate cancer. However, these relationships have been developed as a result of retrospective analyses and they require prospective validation. Prospective studies would need to be large and long term and therefore are unlikely to be performed.

Prostate cancers are adenocarcinomas which arise from the ductal acinar cells. Seventy percent of tumors arise in the peripheral zone of the prostate gland; the remainder arise in the central zone, inner zones. The location in the peripheral zone makes them accessible to diagnosis by transrectal biopsy guided by ultrasonography.

Tumor grading is an important factor in the prognosis of prostate cancer. The Gleason grading system has supplanted older systems. In this system, the pathologist assigns two grades to the cancer based on a major and minor pattern of glandular differentiation and provides a sum score of ascending virulence. The most common patterns identified are 3 and 4. Score 6 (3 + 3) is least aggressive, 7 (3 + 4 or 4 + 3) moderately aggressive, and 8 (4 + 4) and 9 (4 + 5 or 5 + 4) very aggressive. Scores of less than 6 and greater than 9 are rare and represent the poles of the indolent to aggressive continuum. Tumors arising in the prostate spread by local extension and lymphatic metastasis. When spreading locally, they may invade either through the capsule into the extracapsular fat or into the seminal vesicles. Metastases tend to follow a predictable pattern, with early metastases occurring to the internal iliac and obturator nodal chains and progressing to the external iliac and para-aortic and paracaval chains. Subsequent metastases have a predilection to bone and can include the lumbar spine, pelvis, proximal femur, thoracic spine, ribs, sternum, and skull. These are often blastic or mixed lytic, blastic in appearance. Metastatic deposits in the bone set up a tumor cell bone matrix interaction that is self-generating and is the target of novel therapeutic molecules, that is, zoledronic acid. Metastases to the liver, spleen, and brain occur rarely, and generally only very late in the course of disease. Pulmonary metastases are also rare and when a lung nodule is found in conjunction with prostate cancer, it is most likely a primary lung cancer.

Diagnosis and Staging
Prostate-specific antigen (PSA) is a glycoprotein produced by the acinar cells of the prostate whose function is liquefaction of semen. The older marker, prostatic acid phosphatase, has

been supplanted largely by PSA. PSA leaks into the serum in small quantities on a routine basis and is therefore detectable at some level in all men. Prostatic enlargement (benign) and prostate cancer increases the leak and elevates the serum level. PSA is not specific for carcinoma. Elevations are also observed in prostatitis and prostatic infarction where there is disruption of the integrity of the basement membrane. However, PSA is helpful in the diagnosis of prostate cancer and is indispensable for the follow-up of patients who have undergone treatment for prostate cancer. With regard to diagnosis, normal values were originally set at an absolute upper level of 4.0 ng/dL. It is now recognized that PSA levels represent a continuum for risk and there is no level below which a cancer-free state is assured, that is, the incidence of cancer at PSA less than 0.5 ng/mL is 5%. Much more emphasis is now placed on PSA kinetics [slope, velocity, prostate-specific antigen doubling time (PSA DT)]. With regard to posttreatment levels, following surgery PSA should be undetectable (<0.2 ng/mL); after radiation the expected levels are less absolute. A recent consensus conference established nadir (lowest level) +2 as a benchmark.

In selected patients, CT scans of the abdomen and pelvis may be used to demonstrate nodal metastasis.

Treatment

After staging, localized disease may be treated by extirpative surgery (radical prostatectomy), external beam radiotherapy, interstitial implantation (brachytherapy or radioactive seed therapy) with iodine (^{125}I) or palladium (^{103}Pd), a combination of external beam and interstitial implant, or by cryotherapy (freeze–thaw destruction). Radical surgery may be through the retropubic or perineal route. Laparoscopic techniques for radical prostatectomy are commonly used, and robot-assisted surgery is being more frequently employed. In elderly patients with concomitant medical problems and an expected life span of less than 10 years, no treatment may be recommended since risk of death from comorbid disease far exceeds that from prostate cancer. No initial active therapy may also be appropriate for younger patients with low-grade (3 + 3 or lower), low-volume disease and this strategy is being tested in a randomized phase III trial. Patients with symptomatic metastatic disease should be treated with hormonal therapy, most often luteinizing hormone-releasing hormone (LHRH) agonist, with or without concomitant antiandrogens. The exact timing of androgen deprivation or hormonal therapy remains a subject of uncertainty and debate. There is increasing evidence that its use before the radiologic appearance of metastasis or development of symptoms is warranted. However in conjunction with earlier and therefore longer use, a number of side effects have been recognized and include reduction in sexual function, hot flushes, accelerated osteoporosis, dyslipidemia, weight gain, and cognitive impairment. The risk/benefit calculation for androgen deprivation presents a significant challenge to decision making for the urologist and his patient. When acceptable to the patient, surgical castration is also an option. Spot radiotherapy to localized symptomatic

lesions or the use of radiopharmaceuticals (SR89, samarium) is useful for pain control in late stage symptomatic disease.

Two recent, randomized control trials demonstrated a survival benefit with the use of a taxane and docetaxel regimen, when given to men with metastatic disease. Current trials are testing docetaxel in the neoadjuvant and adjuvant setting for men at high risk, that is high PSA, high Gleason score, palpable local disease. Docetaxel is also being combined with a number of biologic agents (i.e., bevacizumab, atrasantin) to determine the benefit and toxicity of combinations versus chemomonotherapy. Additionally, a vaccine-based therapy is also being explored.

Primary Urethral Cancer

Primary urethral cancer is extremely rare. Tumors occur more often in Caucasians than in non-Caucasians, and present most commonly between the ages of 50 and 70 years. The disease is more common in women than in men.

In men, most tumors are squamous cell carcinoma, with transitional cell carcinoma and adenocarcinoma appearing less frequently. The tumor histology generally reflects the site of origin (e.g., transitional cell carcinoma is predominant in the prostatic urethra). In women, squamous cell carcinoma is also the most commonly encountered, with transitional cell, adenocarcinoma, and melanoma next in frequency.

In both men and women, tumors presenting in the distal urethra tend to be of a lower grade and stage than more proximal lesions, and survival is significantly better than in more proximal urethral lesions.

For small superficial lesions, treatment may include excision, laser therapy, or radiotherapy. For larger lesions, partial or total penectomy, or anterior exenteration may be required. Large tumors are unresponsive to radiation. Tumors presenting with nodal involvement have a poor prognosis. Chemotherapy and immunotherapy have been largely ineffective for primary urethral cancer, although several recent studies using chemotherapy and radiation therapy have demonstrated promising responses. Multimodality treatment protocols involving surgery, chemotherapy, and perhaps radiation may be the best option to manage advanced tumors, particularly those involving the proximal urethra. In general, however, prognosis in advanced disease is poor.

Malignant Tumors of the Testis

Malignant tumors of the testis are rare, with only two to three cases per 100,000 men reported each year. They occur most often in young men between the ages of 17 and 30. The etiology of testis tumors is unknown, but a close association exists with cryptorchidism. In the patient with the cryptorchid testicle in the abdomen, the relative risk of developing a neoplasm is 1:20, whereas if the cryptorchid testicle is in the inguinal canal, the relative risk is 1:80. Orchidopexy is not thought to alter the risk of neoplasm, but does make the testis available for examination.

Approximately 95% of testis tumors arise in the germ cells, and the remainder are nongerminal (Sertoli cell, Leydig cell, or gonadoblastoma). There are five histopathologic elements of germinal tumors: seminoma, teratoma, (mature and immature) yolk sac, embryonal cell carcinoma, and choriocarcinoma. Because cell type is an important consideration in treatment, tumors are classified as either seminomas or nonseminomatous germ cell tumors.

Seminoma

Seminoma is the most common tumor type, comprising 35% of all testis tumors. Syncytiotrophoblastic elements are seen in 10% to 15% of classical seminomas, corresponding to the incidence of β-human chorionic gonadotropin (hCG) production in these tumors. Approximately 5% to 10% of seminomas are classified as anaplastic. These tumors tend to present with a higher stage than classic seminomas, but they have a similar stage for stage prognosis. Another 5% to 10% of seminomas are classified as spermatocytic. These tumors occur more commonly in patients older than 50 years of age, and have a very low metastatic potential.

Seminoma is treated with radical (inguinal) orchiectomy, which serves for treatment and staging purposes. Additional staging workup includes chest x-ray and CT abdomen/pelvis, and tumor markers. An elevated α-fetoprotein (AFP) indicates nonseminomatous disease, despite pathology findings at orchiectomy. Seminoma limited to the testis is most often treated with adjuvant radiation to the para-aortic and ipsilateral pelvic lymph nodes, 25 Gy in 20 fractions. Nonbulky stage IIA/B disease is also treated with radiation, whereas IIC bulky disease and stage III disease would be referred for cisplatin-based multiagent chemotherapy. Residual retroperitoneal lymph node disease after radiation or chemotherapy can be extremely difficult to surgically remove. Masses less than 3 cm can be followed up, whereas masses greater than 3 cm have a higher risk of being malignant and may need removal. PET imaging has shown promise in discriminating residual cancer versus fibrosis.

Nonseminomatous Germ Cell Tumors

Embryonal cell carcinoma constitutes 20% of all germinal cell tumors. Two subtypes are seen: adult and the juvenile embryonal cell tumor or yolk sac tumor. Teratomas contain more than one germ cell layer in various stages of maturation. Teratocarcinoma is actually a mixed cell tumor, composed of teratoma and embryonal cell carcinoma. Seminoma may also comprise part of a mixed germ cell tumor. Mixed tumors constitute 35% to 40% of all testis tumors, and treatment is based on the most malignant component.

Testicular ultrasonography is helpful in determining the nature of scrotal masses. β-HCG, elaborated by the syncytiotrophoblastic cells, is commonly elevated in nonseminomatous tumors. It is also elevated in a small percentage of seminomas. α-Fetoprotein is elaborated by yolk sac tissues and is never present in seminoma. Lactate dehydrogenase (LDH) particularly LDH isoenzyme-1, may reflect tumor burden in some nonseminomatous germ cell tumors. After histologic diagnosis has been established by orchiectomy, careful staging with chest radiograph and CT scan in combination with serum tumor markers should be done. A number of staging systems have been proposed. The tumor staging system used at Memorial Sloan-Kettering Cancer Center has been applied most widely, whereas the International Union Against Cancer/American Joint Commission (UICC)/AJC tumor, node, metastasis (TNM) system is now gaining popularity.

Testicular tumors tend to metastasize to the retroperitoneal lymph nodes around the renal hilum. The exception is choriocarcinoma, which often spreads by hematogenous routes.

Initial treatment is inguinal orchiectomy for all stages. Nonseminomatous germ cell tumors limited to the testis (stage I) have approximately a 25% to 30% risk of subsequent microscopic disease that will relapse in the next 2 years. The optimum treatment strategy is controversial and may include immediate retroperitoneal lymph node dissection, two cycles of chemotherapy, or active surveillance. If disease recurs while the patient is on active surveillance, then three to four cycles of chemotherapy are given. If the lymph nodes are removed and limited disease found (N1), then the patient can be observed with greater than 75% success, and any relapses may be salvaged with three to four cycles of chemotherapy. If more lymph node involvement is found (N2-3), then two cycles of chemotherapy will cure greater than 90% of patients.

Limited lymph node disease, IIA, can also be treated with surgery alone, and this option is preferred if there is teratoma in the orchiectomy specimen, which, if present in the nodes will resist chemotherapy. Chemotherapy is the primary treatment for high-stage disease, with surgery reserved for residual masses. The cure rate for low and moderate stage testicular cancer is approximately 90%. Testicular cancer has become a classic paradigm of successful multimodality disciplinary therapeutic approach.

Cancer of the Penis

Cancer of the penis presents most often in the sixth decade and is usually associated with uncircumcised patients with long-standing poor hygiene. The disease is almost unheard of in cultures where infant circumcision is practiced. It is rare in the United States, but in parts of Africa, Asia, and South America it comprises up to 20% of male genital tumors.

Most penile cancers are squamous cell tumors that first appear as raised ulcers with an indurated base. Verrucous carcinomas are a special variant of squamous cell carcinoma, which occur in 10% to 15% of patients. These tumors do not metastasize, but destroy surrounding tissues by local compression and invasion. These tumors predominate on the glans and may be ulcerative or papillary. Squamous carcinomas are associated with human papilloma virus exposure (particularly subtypes 16, 18, 31, 33 and 35), whereas verrucous carcinoma is associated with subtypes 6 and 13. Carcinoma in situof the penile skin, known as *erythroplasia of Queyrat* when it involves the glans or shaft, or Bowen disease when it involves the scrotum or perineum, is a precursor to penile squamous carcinoma.

Treatment of the primary lesion is surgical. This usually involves local excision, laser therapy, or penile amputation. Enlarged inguinal nodes should be treated with a 6-week course of antibiotic therapy and then reassessed. If the enlarged nodes persist, or if the tumor is invasive or of high grade, then bilateral inguinal lymphadenectomy and occasionally pelvic node dissection is required. Such surgery may be curative. There is increasing evidence to suggest that patients with histologic high-grade tumors should undergo inguinal exploration, even if no palpable adenopathy is present.

Tumor metastasis occurs through the superficial and deep inguinal nodes and subsequently the pelvic nodes. Involvement of the pelvic nodes generally implies a worse prognosis, although some of these patients are cured by lymphadenectomy. Distant metastases at presentation are unusual. Death is usually caused by infection and hemorrhage resulting from groin involvement or distant metastatic disease. Response to chemotherapy is not uniformly achieved and no standard regimen is currently advocated. Regimens featuring *cis*-platinum and bleomycin or taxol-gemcytobine have shown some promise to date. Prognosis in advanced disease is poor.

SUMMARY

A brief working summary of urology and significant disease processes affecting the urinary system is presented in this chapter. Because effective imaging and endourologic techniques have been available to the urologic surgeon for a number of years, the GU surgeon is usually able to assess the nature and extent of the disease process with considerable accuracy before approaching the operating table. Purely exploratory surgery has now become quite rare.

SUGGESTED READINGS

Biagiotti G, Cavallini G. Acetyl-L-Carnitine in the oral therapy of Peyronie's disease: a preliminary report. *Brit J Urol Int* 2001;88:63–67.

Bosniak MA. The small (<3.0 cm) renal parenchyma tumor: detection, diagnosis and controversies. *Radiology* 1991;179:307–317.

Bosniak MA, Retik AB. Pediatric urinary tact obstruction. *Urol Clin North Am* 1990;17(2):247–447.

Burnett AL. Erectile dysfunction. *J Urol* 2006;175:s25–s31.

Caoili EM, Korobkin M, Francis IR, et al. Delayed enhanced CT of lipid-poor adrenal adenomas. *AJR Am J Roentgenol* 2000;175(5):1411–1415.

Cavallini G, Biagiotti G, Koverech A, et al. Oral proprionyl-L-carnitine and intraplaque Verapamil in the therapy of advanced and resistant Peyronie's disease. *Brit J Urol Int* 2002;89(9):895–900.

Deck AJ, Shaves S, Talner L, et al. Computerized tomography cystography for the diagnosis of traumatic bladder rupture. *J Urol* 2000;164(1):43–46.

Droller MJ. Urological oncology: bladder, penis, and urethral cancer and basic principles of urologic oncology. *J Urol* 2003;170:22116–22125.

Ehrlich RM, Alter GJ. *Reconstructive and plastic surgery of the external genitalia*. Philadelphia: WB Saunders, 1999.

Elder JS. *Pediatric urology for the general urologist*. New York: Igaku-Shoin Medical Publishers, 1996.

Howards S. Treatment of male infertility. *N Engl J Med* 1995;332(5):312–317.

Jana S, Blaufox MD. Nuclear medicine studies of the prostate, testes, and bladder. *Semin Nucl Med* 2006;36(1):51–52.

Kaplan GW. Common problems in pediatric urology. *Urol Clin North Am* 1995;22(1):xiii–x230.

Kelalis PP, King LR, Belman AB, eds. *Clinical pediatric urology*, Vol. 1,2. Philadelphia: WB Saunders, 1985.

Kim HL, Steinberg GD. Current status of bladder preservation in the treatment of muscle- invasive bladder cancer. *J Urol* 2000;164:627–632.

King LR, ed. *Urologic surgery in neonates and young infants*. Philadelphia: WB Saunders, 1988.

King LR. Pediatric urologic surgery, section XI. In: Walsh PC, Retik AB, Stamey TA, et al. *Campbell's urology*, 6th ed. Philadelphia: WB Saunders, 1992:1687–2002.

King LR. *Urologic surgery in infants and children*. Philadelphia: WB Saunders, 1999.

Lipschultz L, Howards S, eds. *Infertility in the male*, 2nd ed. St. Louis: Mosby–Year Book, 1990.

Malek R, Nahen K. *Laser treatment of benign prostatic hypertrophy Lesson 20*. American Urological Association, Update Series, 2004.

Mitchell DG, Crovello M, Matteuui T. Benign adrenal cortical masses: diagnosis with chemical shift imaging. *Radiology* 1992;185:339–340.

Santucci RA, Wessells H, Bartsch G, et al. Evaluation and management of renal injuries: consensus statement of the renal trauma subcommittee. *Brit J Urol Int* 2004;90(7):937–954.

Sigman M. Assisted reproductive techniques and male infertility. *Urol Clin North Am* 1994;21(3):505–515.

Smith RC, Verga M, Dalrymple N, et al. Acute ureteral obstruction: value of secondary signs of helical unenhanced CT. *Am J Roentgenol* 1996;167(5):1109–1113.

Valente EG, Ferrini MG, Vernet D, et al. PDF L- Arginine and PDE inhibitors counteract fibrosis in the Peyronie's fibrotic plaque and related fibroblast cultures. *Nitric Oxide* 2003;9:229–244.

Walsh PC. Urologic oncology: prostate cancer. *J Urol* 2003;169:1588–1598.

CHAPTER 24

Anesthesia

Kraig S. de Lanzac, Mack A. Thomas, and James M. Riopelle

Obviously, it is impossible to cover the topic of anesthesia and the practice of anesthesiology in a single chapter. Instead, this chapter will serve as an outline of the physiologic principles involved in the delivery of anesthesia that are important to the surgical specialist. Whenever possible, references to specific drugs are avoided to prevent getting bogged down in pharmacologic profiles.

Anesthesia is the loss of sensation in a part of the body or in the entire body, generally induced by the administration of a drug. The choice of anesthetic technique is usually referred to by the terms *general* and *conductive* anesthesia. General anesthesia is associated with the loss of consciousness. Conductive anesthesia refers to the administration of an agent in an anatomically appropriate site so that painful sensation is interrupted. Conductive anesthesia includes regional anesthetic techniques and injections of local anesthetic agents. The goal of an anesthetic is to produce a physiologic state in which the patient exhibits or experiences minimal to no response to normally painful interventions such as surgical trauma. A balance must be achieved between the prevention of perception of painful stimuli and the cardiovascular and respiratory effects of anesthetic agents. Consideration must also be given to protect against potentially harmful autonomic reflexes and responses in the preoperative and postoperative period. The basic physiologic effects of anesthetic agents and techniques will be discussed with clinical applications provided.

PHARMACOLOGY

To appreciate basic concepts, several principles of pharmacology must be reviewed. Pharmacokinetics describes how a drug is absorbed, distributed, and eliminated from the body. Pharmacodynamics refers to the relative potency of a drug and is often related to a blood or tissue concentration necessary to evoke a given response. A receptor is the component of a cell or organ that interacts with a drug

leading to the pharmacologic effect. Receptors determine selectivity and the quantitative relation between dose and effect. An agonist regulates the function of the receptor molecule as a direct result of the drug binding to it. An antagonist binds to the receptor without directly altering the receptor function and prevents an agonist from stimulating the receptor to function. Two types of antagonism are identified. Competitive antagonism occurs when increasing concentrations of the antagonist progressively inhibit the response to a fixed concentration of agonist. Noncompetitive antagonism occurs when, after administration of an antagonist, increasing concentration of agonists cannot overcome antagonism.

Tissue Uptake

The capacity of tissue uptake of drugs is governed by organ blood flow, concentration gradient, and physicochemical properties of the drug. Approximately 70% of cardiac output (CO) is directed to the brain, kidney, liver, lung, and heart, despite the relatively small contribution of these organs to overall body weight. These organs are collectively referred to as the *vessel-rich group*. These highly perfused tissues receive a high concentration of the total dose of drug administered, and do so within a small period of time. This is seen clinically as a rapid onset of hypnosis following an injection of centrally active drugs such as propofol or thiopental. As the plasma concentration decreases, drugs leave these tissues to be delivered to less perfused sites, which will initiate termination of the clinical effects of the drug. The rapid entry and rapid egress of such drugs are related to their lipid solubility and are termed *redistribution*. Redistribution accounts for the short duration of action of certain hypnotic drugs despite the large volume of distribution and slow clearance of drug by metabolism.

Cell membranes are lipid structures and therefore, lipid solubility is an important factor in the ability of a drug to diffuse across cell membranes. Most drugs are weak bases or weak acids and present as ionized and nonionized molecules in solutions. Nonionized drug is usually lipid soluble and is the active portion pharmacologically. The degree of ionization of a given drug is a function of its dissociation constant (K_a) and the pH of surrounding fluid. If the K_a and pH are identical, then 50% of the drug exists in the ionized form. Relatively small pH changes may cause significant changes in ionization. Acidic drugs such as barbiturates tend to be highly ionized at an alkaline pH, as opposed to basic drugs such as local anesthetics and opioids that are highly ionized at an acid pH.

Protein binding has a significant effect on drug action because only free or unbound drug can cross cell membranes. Drug clearance is influenced by the degree of protein binding because it is the unbound portion that is accessible to hepatic metabolism and renal excretion. Acidic drugs tend to bind to albumin, whereas basic drugs bind with α_1-acid glycoprotein. Protein binding generally parallels lipid solubility.

Drug Distribution

The volume of distribution (V_d) is the parameter that governs the extent of drug distribution. Physiologically, the factor that governs the extent of drug distribution is the tissue capacity for a drug versus the capacity of blood for that drug. Tissue capacity is a function of the total tissue volume into which a drug distributes. The following equation presents an arithmetic approach: $V_d =$ total amount of drug per concentration. If a drug is distributed extensively, then the concentration is lower, meaning it has a larger volume of distribution. Clinically, this means if a drug has a large volume of distribution, then a larger loading dose is required to achieve the same concentration as another drug with a smaller volume of distribution.

Drug Clearance

Drug clearance usually depends on hepatic metabolism, renal elimination, or both. In the case of modern inhalational anesthetic agents, the primary means for drug clearance is by exhalation. Most drugs given in therapeutic dose ranges are cleared from plasma at a rate proportional to the amount of drug present. If a constant plasma concentration of drug is desired, the drug must be administered at a rate equal to the clearance.

Drug Response

Drug response is affected not only by hepatic and renal function but also by cardiac function, age, enzyme activity, and genetic differences. Reduction in CO will decrease renal and hepatic blood flow, causing delays in clearance. Lidocaine used to suppress cardiac dysrhythmias may reach toxic levels in patients with cardiac failure if doses are not reduced. Immaturity of the renal and hepatic systems in the newborn may result in toxic levels if conventional doses are administered. Geriatric patients may exhibit decreased renal function, decreased CO, reduced protein binding, and an enlarged fat compartment. Decreased delivery of drug to liver and kidney may prolong the action of drugs dependent on these organs for excretion.

AUTONOMIC NERVOUS SYSTEM

The portion of the central and peripheral nervous system concerned with the involuntary regulation of cardiac muscle, smooth muscle, glandular, and visceral function throughout the body is known as the *autonomic nervous system* (ANS). Most intraoperative anesthetic practice is concerned with manipulation of the ANS. The anesthesiologist must anticipate normal responses by patients to surgical stimulus and anesthetic agents as well as recognize harmful or pathologic responses or reflexes. Knowledge of the ANS and the normal response to stress in the perioperative period is critical before understanding the occasionally paradoxical response to anesthetic agents by patients. The system is exquisitely responsive to changes in somatic motor and sensory activities of the body. Inasmuch as neither somatic nor ANS activity occurs in isolation, the ANS is not as distinct as the term suggests. A review of the anatomy and physiology of the ANS is required to understand the physiologic response to anesthesia.

Traditionally, the ANS has been viewed as a peripheral efferent system. It is now recognized that most ANS efferent fibers are accompanied by sensory fibers now commonly thought of as components of the system. The afferent fibers cannot be divided as distinctively as can the efferent fibers.

Anatomy

Central autonomic organization is principally located in the hypothalamus, with integration occurring at all levels of the cerebrospinal axis. Sympathetic functions are controlled by nuclei in the posterolateral hypothalamus. The medulla and pons are centers of acute ANS organization and together integrate momentary hemodynamic adjustments. Maintenance of vascular tone is a second-by-second activity controlled by the ANS. Regulation of peripheral vascular resistance is a dynamic example of this tonic activity.

Physiologic anatomy consists of the aforementioned central area as well as the peripheral system consisting of the sympathetic nervous system (SNS) and parasympathetic nervous system (PNS) divisions. Most organs receive fibers from both divisions. Efferent ANS is a two-neuron chain from the central nervous system (CNS) to the effector organ. It then relays the impulse to a second station known as the *autonomic ganglion*, which contains the cell body of the second (postganglionic) neuron. Its axon contacts the effector organ. Preganglionic fibers of both divisions are myelinated and postganglionic fibers are unmyelinated. In contrast, somatic motor efferent fibers are composed of a single neuron with its cell body in the spinal cord ventral gray matter. Their axons extend directly to the striated muscle unit.

Sympathetic Nervous System

The preganglionic fibers of the SNS originate in the intermediolateral gray columns of the 12 thoracic and the first 3 lumbar segments of the spinal cord. These myelinated axons leave the spinal cord with motor fibers to form the white myelinated communicating rami. Rami enter the paired 22 sympathetic ganglia at their respective levels. After entry into the paravertebral ganglia, the preganglionic fibers may synapse with postganglionic fibers at the same level, course upward or downward in the trunk of the SNS to synapse in ganglia at different levels, or exit without synapsing to terminate in an outlying collateral ganglion. The exception is the adrenal gland, in which preganglionic fibers pass directly into the adrenal medulla without synapsing in a ganglion. Neuronal cells of the adrenal medulla are analogous to postganglionic neurons.

Activation of the SNS produces a mass reflex response. A single preganglionic fiber influences a large number of postganglionic fibers, which are dispersed to many organs. In addition, release of catecholamines from the adrenal medulla augments the response.

Parasympathetic Nervous System

The PNS, sometimes called the *craniosacral outflow* because preganglionic cell bodies originate in the brainstem and sacral segments of the spinal cord, also has both preganglionic and postganglionic neurons. Preganglionic fibers are found in cranial nerves III, VII, IX, and X. Sacral outflow originates in the intermediolateral gray horns of the second, third, and fourth sacral nerves. The vagus (cranial nerve X) accounts for more than 75% of PNS activity. In contrast to the sympathetic side of the system, parasympathetic preganglionic fibers pass directly to the organ that is innervated. Postganglionic cells are situated within or near the innervated viscera. Postganglionic fibers do not have an extensive secondary distribution from a single preganglionic fiber as does the SNS. This is consistent with the discrete effect of the PNS. For example, vagal bradycardia may occur without concomitant change in intestinal motility or salivation.

Pharmacology of the Autonomic Nervous System

Transmission of excitation in the ANS occurs through the mediation of liberated chemicals. Pharmacologic terminology designates the SNS and PNS as adrenergic and cholinergic, respectively. PNS postganglionic fibers release acetylcholine (ACh). Norepinephrine (NE) is the neurotransmitter at postganglionic sympathetic terminals, with the exception of sweat glands. Preganglionic fibers of both systems secrete ACh.

The entire system is modulated through a system of receptors, which appears to be protein macromolecules located in the cellular plasma membrane. Several thousand receptors have been demonstrated in the membrane of a single cell. Cholinergic receptors found in the ANS may be subdivided into muscarinic and nicotinic because muscarine and nicotine stimulate them selectively. Both respond to ACh stimulation. Muscarinic receptors may be blocked by atropine without effect on nicotinic receptors. Muscarinic receptors are found at PNS junctions of cardiac and smooth muscle. They are also known to exist at other than PNS postganglionic junctions. They are found on the

presynaptic membranes of sympathetic nerve terminals in the myocardium, coronary vessels, and peripheral circulation. These have been referred to as *adrenergic muscarinic receptors* because of their location. Stimulation of these receptors inhibits release of NE.

Nicotinic receptors are found at synaptic junctions of both SNS and PNS ganglia. Inasmuch as both junctions are cholinergic, ACh or ACh-like substances will excite postganglionic fibers of both systems. Especially important in clinical anesthesia are nicotinic receptors found at the neuromuscular junction because pharmacologic blockade of these receptors produces muscular paralysis.

Adrenergic receptors typically are divided into α and β types, and each type can be divided further (α_1, α_2, and β_1, β_2). In addition, dopaminergic (DA) receptors have been identified. Dopamine receptors are located in the CNS, renal, mesenteric, and coronary vessels. These receptors may explain the action of dopamine (DA receptor effect) on renal and mesenteric vasculature.

α-Adrenergic receptors are subdivided into two sets: α_1 and α_2. The α_1 receptors are postsynaptic in location and are found in smooth muscle cells of the peripheral vasculature of the coronary arteries, skin, uterus, intestinal mucosa, and splanchnic beds. Activation results in either decreased or increased tone, depending on the effector organ. Stimulation of α_1 receptors in resistance and capacitance vessels produces vasoconstriction. Stimulation of presynaptic α_2 receptors mediates inhibition of NE release, resulting in a negative-feedback mechanism. Stimulation of presynaptic α_2 receptors results in sedation, decreased heart rate (HR) and decreased peripheral vascular resistance and blood pressure (BP).

β-Adrenergic receptors are also subdivided into two subsets. Receptors of the β_1 type predominate in the myocardium and sinoatrial (SA) node. The β_2 receptors are located in smooth muscle of blood vessels in the skin, muscle, mesentery, and bronchial musculature. These receptors are more sensitive to epinephrine than NE.

Autonomic reflexes are frequently seen in clinical practice. Such reflexes are operative in the moment-to-moment control of CO, BP, and HR. Baroreceptors located in the carotid sinus and the aortic arch respond to alterations in pressure. Increased BP creates stretch of the receptors, causing an increase in impulses to the central vasomotor center, which produces an increase in vagal tone and a decrease in sympathetic firing. This results in vasodilatation and a decreased HR. Venous baroreceptors also exist in the right atrium and great veins. A reduction in venous tone produces an increase in HR. The integration of the autonomic system as a coordinated unit is of critical importance in the mechanics of autoregulation of organ perfusion. Anesthetic agents and adjuvants, especially when combined with other cardiovascularly active medications taken by the patient, may cause an uncoupling of autonomic reflexes leading to a loss of basic protective responses. The volatile anesthetic halothane causes a decrease in contractility and a blockade of baroreceptor responses leading to a decrease in CO.

The addition of medications such as β blockers may also further exacerbate hemodynamic responses. The potential for increases in HR with volatile anesthetics such as isoflurane and desflurane may mitigate decreases in BP but may also raise questions of tachycardia due to inadequate anesthetic level or intravascular volume.

GENERAL ANESTHESIA

Mechanism of Action

The mechanism of action for volatile anesthetics is not entirely known. Several theories have been proposed with a few gaining acceptance based on clinical and laboratory experience. The use of molecular and genetic engineering has assisted recent investigation, but a single mechanism has not been elucidated (1). Therefore, at this time a single theory explaining the effects of anesthetic agents would be fraught with varying deficiencies.

Volatile agents are believed to produce general anesthesia by modulating synaptic function particularly within the reticular activating system, which is responsible for maintaining "wakefulness." Volatile anesthetics depress excitatory transmission regardless of the specific neurotransmitter. There is little evidence to support blockade of transmission at peripheral sites but instead central modulation of transmission of stimuli is believed to occur.

The association between lipid solubility and anesthetic potency led to the Meyer-Overton theory for volatile agent mechanism of action. The Meyer-Overton theory states that lipid soluble anesthetic molecules occupy cell membranes and potentially distort receptor sites and synaptic receptiveness and transmission. Exceptions to the Meyer-Overton theory are demonstrated by the phenomenon that certain highly lipid soluble agents elicit convulsions. In addition, some anesthetic agents with very similar lipid solubility may possess different anesthetic potencies.

The central receptor theory of volatile anesthetic method of action suggests the potential presence of receptors for volatile anesthetics in the CNS. The steep dose–response curve for volatile anesthetic action suggests occupation of a critical percentage of potential receptors. The difference in the structure of various inhaled anesthetics does not suggest a single specific receptor site.

Several mechanisms and sites of action may be necessary to explain anesthetic effects and structure–response relations. Few data exist to support the theory that volatile anesthetics affect synthesis, release, or binding of neurotransmitters. No particular region of the brain is solely responsible for the pharmacologic control of consciousness or all of the CNS elements of general anesthesia.

Drug–receptor interactions have been described for most of the intravenous drugs used in anesthesia. Opioids by definition work by occupying opioid receptors in the brain and spinal cord. Analgesia results from the modulation of the functions of certain peptides (endorphins and enkephalins) that are endogenous ligands for opiate receptors.

Neurotransmitters may have either inhibitory or excitatory properties. γ-aminobutyric acid (GABA) is the major inhibitory neurotransmitter in the brain, and glycine is the major inhibitory neurotransmitter in the spinal cord. Glutamate is the major excitatory neurotransmitter in the brain. Data have accumulated supporting the concept that several aspects of anesthesia may result from modulation of GABA function. Benzodiazepines, barbiturates, and other intravenous drugs such as ketamine have been shown to enhance inhibitory tone mediated by GABA. When benzodiazepines bind to specific GABA receptors ($GABA_A$), inhibitory tone is enhanced. Similar barbiturate receptors are adjacent to GABA receptors, and the barbiturate receptor occupied is thought to enhance the inhibitory tone of GABA. This is believed to account for the sedative and anticonvulsant effects of these drugs.

Choice of Anesthetics

General anesthesia is a constellation of elements, which are measured or assumed by the clinical responses of the patient. Clinically the term *general anesthesia* consists of the following elements: amnesia, hypnosis, analgesia, and immobility. The ideal anesthetic agent would provide these effects with minimal impact on the cardiovascular or respiratory systems. The ideal anesthetic would also have minimal biotransformation with a lack of active metabolites. General anesthetic delivery is in essence a controlled titration that requires constant monitoring and assessment. The route of administration allows us to classify the type of general anesthetic. The most common routes use inhalation or intravenous techniques. A combination of inhalation and intravenous drugs is referred to as *balanced anesthesia*. Balanced anesthetic techniques attempt to capitalize on the desirable effects of drugs while minimizing side effects. For example, volatile anesthetic agents can produce neuromuscular relaxation but at the doses required, hemodynamic effects are significant. Neuromuscular blockade is best achieved with neuromuscular blocking agents such as pancuronium rather than using high concentrations of volatile anesthetics. In a balanced technique, neuromuscular blockers, analgesics such as opioids, and amnestics such as the benzodiazepines are administered for their specific clinical effect. Therefore, provisions for ideal characteristics of general anesthesia such as unconsciousness, amnesia, analgesia and muscle relaxation are achieved through the combined use of relatively selective agents. The length and intensity of the surgical procedure, as well as the underlying medical condition of the patient, figure into the exact combination of anesthetic agents and adjuvants utilized. Narcotics may provide for a very stable cardiovascular anesthetic but when used in isolation, narcotics may not reliably produce unconsciousness. In addition, the duration of the narcotics required may be prohibitive. In order to plan an anesthetic, the surgical procedure and medical condition of the patient as well as the postoperative plan must be considered. Of particular importance is the potential for discharge to home on the day of surgery. Cost considerations for the selection of anesthetic medications must be made with global implications in mind. For example, the use of shorter acting agents with less emetic potential and better analgesia may come at a higher direct cost which may be mitigated by financial and emotional savings to the patient in the postoperative period by better pain relief, fewer side effects, and earlier discharge.

Inhalational Anesthesia

Inhalational agents may be of several chemical classes, but those clinically useful are halogenated ethers and hydrocarbons as well as nitrous oxide. The ideal anesthetic agent would have the desired effects of an anesthetic with minimal cardiovascular side effects, minimal biotransformation and minimal drug interaction. In clinical practice, halothane and sevoflurane are used as inhalational agents particularly during inhalational induction of anesthesia. These two agents may also be used in the maintenance phase of general anesthesia. Isoflurane, desflurane, and occasionally enflurane are used as maintenance inhalational agents, but possess characteristics (e.g., pungency) unfavorable for use in inhalational induction of anesthesia. Nitrous oxide may be used in combination with other agents as part of an inhalational induction or as part of a maintenance regimen. A summary of basic properties of the commonly used inhalational agents is given in Table 24.1.

Uptake and Distribution

Inhaled anesthetics are administered as gases and enter the body through ventilation. The uptake and distribution of volatile anesthetic agents are dependent upon several factors. The goal of administering inhalational anesthetics is to build up a concentration gradient between the alveolus of the lungs and the bloodstream. Off-loading of inhalational agents in the CNS produces the clinical effects and can be predicted by the characteristics of the agent and the gradient established between the alveolus and the circulation (Fig. 24.1).

Inspired Concentration

The rate of rise of alveolar concentration bears a direct relation to the concentration inspired; therefore, the higher the inspired concentration, the more rapid the rise in alveolar concentration. This can be thought of as preloading of a volatile anesthetic. Alveolar tension results from a balance between the rate of delivery and the rate of uptake of

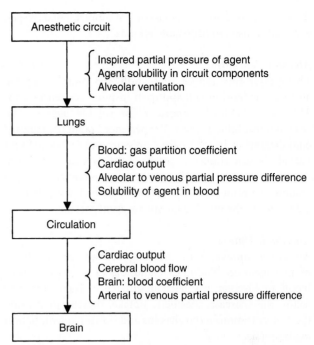

FIGURE 24.1 Several factors influence the transfer of inhalational agent from the anesthetic circuit to the brain during inhalational induction and maintenance of anesthesia.

the anesthetic from the lung by blood and tissues. As the concentration of inhaled anesthetic increases in the alveolus, agent is taken up into circulation and eventually, crosses into the CNS. In time, equilibrium is established between the concentration of agent in the alveolus and the brain. The increasing concentration of agent in the alveolus will increase the rate of rise of the agent in the CNS. In addition to increasing the concentration of inhalational agent inspired, the alveolar concentration of an agent can be increased by the rapid uptake of a second gas from the alveolus. This phenomenon is known as the *second gas effect* and it is most commonly associated with the administration of nitrous oxide with a more potent agent. The rapid diffusion of nitrous oxide into the bloodstream causes a contraction of the volume of the alveolus, thereby increasing the concentration of the volatile agent that remains in the alveolus. The opposite of this effect may be seen at the end of a procedure when the rapid effusion of nitrous oxide out the bloodstream and into the alveolus and cause a decrease in

TABLE 24.1						
Summary of Basic Properties of Inhalational Agents						
	Halothane	Enflurane	Isoflurane	Desflurane	Sevoflurane	Nitrous Oxide
MAC (%)	0.75	1.6	1.2	6.0	1.8	104
Percentage metabolized	20	2	0.2	0.02	2	0.004
Blood: gas partition coefficient	2.4	1.9	1.4	0.42	0.69	0.47

MAC, minimum alveolar concentration.

the alveolar concentration of oxygen if supplemental oxygen is not administered (diffusion hypoxia).

Alveolar Ventilation

The greater the minute ventilation, the more rapid the alveolar gas tension will approach inspired concentrations. This is particularly important for soluble agents. The relatively insoluble agents will experience a rapid rise (toward equilibrium) in alveolar partial pressure and therefore brain partial pressure almost regardless of the alveolar ventilation. Anesthetic agents cause a decreased spontaneous minute volume. Without supplementation or control of ventilation, a decrease in the input of anesthetic agents occurs.

Anesthetic Uptake

Anesthetic uptake from the lung depends on solubility of the agent in blood, CO, and the pulmonary venous blood to alveolar gas tension difference. Increasing any factor will increase anesthetic uptake, thereby decreasing the concentration in the alveolus and slowing the induction of anesthesia.

Solubility

Solubility refers to the extent to which an anesthetic agent dissolves in blood and tissues. Equilibrium exists when the partial pressures of an anesthetic agent in the two phases are equal. If other factors remain stable, the greater the blood/gas solubility coefficient, the greater the uptake of agent, and the slower the increase in alveolar concentration. Upon first consideration it may seem that an increase in the solubility of an agent would increase the amount of drug in circulation and result in a faster onset of anesthesia. It may be useful to think of the partial pressure of the anesthetic agent in the alveolus to be directly related to the partial pressure of the agent in the brain. For a soluble agent, equilibrium between the alveolus and the bloodstream takes time to develop. The bloodstream can be thought to absorb volatile anesthetic, which cannot be released on the brain side until the bloodstream is "saturated." Only then will the alveolar partial pressure rise, leading to a rise in brain partial pressure and clinical effects. On the other end of the spectrum, a hypothetical totally insoluble anesthetic (blood/gas coefficient = 0), would not be taken up into circulation and despite a rapid rise in alveolar partial pressure, no central effects would be achieved. At a fixed concentration of inspired anesthetic agent, alveolar concentration will rise at a rate determined solely by ventilation and functional residual capacity (FRC) and will soon equal the inspired concentration. A rapid rise in alveolar concentration and tension occurs with agents of low solubility due to the small amount of agent taken up into circulation. Tension in arterial blood will rise rapidly although only a small amount is present in the circulation. As distribution to various tissues is accomplished, the anesthetic agent leaves the bloodstream so that venous blood returning to the lung has a reduced tension, creating a gradient. The opposite occurs with soluble agents where a large amount of drug crosses into circulation

resulting in a slow rise in concentration of agent in the alveolus. Low alveolar concentration translates to low blood tension and low brain partial pressure, resulting in slow anesthetic induction.

Cardiac Output

CO carries anesthetic away from the lungs. Again, intuitively one may believe that a high CO would speed the delivery of agent to the brain, as is the case with the administration of intravenous anesthetics. The opposite occurs with inhalational anesthetics. Consider that high CO carries the anesthetic agent away from the lungs, resulting in a slow rate of rise in the alveolar concentration. The magnitude of this effect is related to solubility. Highly soluble agents will be affected more than relatively insoluble agents. CO will have no effect on completely insoluble agents and, therefore, will have no effect on alveolar concentration. Patients with high CO states (i.e., thyrotoxicosis) will demonstrate prolonged inhalational induction times with soluble agents. Low CO states such as cardiac failure or shock lead to rapid rate of induction.

Venous–Alveolar Difference

Mixed venous to alveolar difference is determined by the amount of agent taken up by tissues. During induction, tissues remove nearly all of the anesthetic delivered. The result is a large alveolar-to-venous gradient that causes maximum anesthetic agent uptake. As tissues become saturated, a rise in venous partial pressure occurs, narrowing the venoalveolar gradient, thereby reducing uptake.

Tissues

Anesthetic delivery to tissues depends primarily on blood flow and volume. Tissue:blood partition coefficients vary far less than blood:gas solubility coefficients. Organs that are highly perfused, known as the *vessel-rich group*, include the brain, heart, kidney, splanchnic bed, and endocrine glands. These organs make up only approximately 10% of body mass, but they receive 70% of the CO. The increased perfusion of these organs increases the delivery of anesthetic agent to these tissue sites. The high flow rates result in rapid equilibration to arterial anesthetic partial pressures. Equilibrium is usually established within 5 to 10 minutes of induction. Tissues such as fat and muscle receive less perfusion and are slower to obtain equilibrium. After termination of the administration of anesthetic, the vessel poor group will experience a slow washout of agent and will act as a reservoir of agent for metabolism.

Recovery

Recovery from inhalation anesthesia is governed by the same factors that affect induction with some slight differences. Recovery is mostly due to exhalation of anesthetic gases as most clinically useful agents undergo minimal metabolism. However, small amounts of agent may remain available for metabolism. As described previously, the mechanisms that allow variable absorption of agent by tissue beds result in similarly variable rate of release of the agent back into the bloodstream. Another difference between recovery and induction is the relative lack of a concentration effect. In other words, the partial pressure of agent in the alveolus cannot be lower than zero. This limits the alveolar to venous partial pressure difference during recovery from volatile anesthetics.

Potency

The potency of anesthetic agents is commonly referred to as the *minimum alveolar concentration* (MAC) of the agent. It is the alveolar concentration of anesthesia at 1 atm that prevents a response, in 50% of subjects, to a painful stimulus such as surgical incision. In other words at 1 MAC, 50% of patients will respond to a noxious stimulus. Many factors, both physiologic and pharmacologic, may influence MAC (Table 24.2). Examples of factors that may increase MAC when given concomitantly are chronic ethanol abuse, hyperthermia, and drugs that cause increased central neurotransmitter levels (cocaine, ephedrine, monoamine oxidase inhibitors). Examples of factors that may decrease MAC are hypothermia, metabolic acidosis, hypoxia, induced hypotension, acute ethanol administration, and drugs that cause decreased central neurotransmitter levels (α-methyldopa, reserpine, clonidine). Addition of other drugs, such as barbiturates, benzodiazepines, and opioids, will lower MAC requirements. MAC is not affected by thyroid dysfunction, potassium derangements, and the duration of anesthesia. MAC values are additive, allowing the addition of nitrous oxide to decrease the amount of halogenated volatile agent needed. The MAC for nitrous oxide is 104%, which is obviously not compatible with safe clinical practice. However if 50% nitrous oxide (0.5 MAC) is added to 0.6% isoflurane ($\sim$0.5 MAC) the clinical result is one MAC of anesthetic. Clinical use of volatile anesthetics requires knowledge of the MAC values for the agent and an understanding of the toxicity of the drugs.

Effects of Inhalational Anesthesia on Organs and Systems

Central Nervous System

Inhaled anesthetics produce significant change in mental function, cerebral oxygen requirements, cerebral blood flow, cerebrospinal fluid (CSF) dynamics, and electrophysiology. The obvious effect is an unconscious state with lack of response to painful stimuli. Some studies have alluded to a decrease in intellectual function, psychomotor skills, and driving skills after receiving an anesthetic. These effects of anesthesia and surgery are often referred to as *postoperative cognitive dysfunction* or POCD and they are of particular concern in the elderly. The length and type of surgery as well as the comorbid conditions may play a role in the development of POCD.

All of the potent inhalation agents decrease cerebral metabolic rate (CMR_{O2}) with isoflurane, sevoflurane, and desflurane decreasing CMR_{O2} further than enflurane and halothane. A decrease in CMR_{O2} is linked closely to cerebral electrical activity. Production of an isoelectric electroencephalogram by anesthetic agents produces a 50% percent reduction in cerebral oxygen consumption. Inhalational agents produce an increase in cerebral blood flow while decreasing metabolic rate. This is referred to as *cerebral uncoupling*. In a nonanesthetized state, cerebral blood flow is coupled with the metabolic rate. Under the influences of volatile anesthetic drugs, an increase in cerebral blood flow occurs despite the decrease in cerebral oxygen requirements. This may lead to an increased intracranial pressure especially in patients with intracranial pathology.

All inhalation agents, including nitrous oxide, produce cerebral vasodilatation. The order of potency for this effect is halothane > enflurane > isoflurane $\cong$ desflurane $\cong$ sevoflurane $\gg$ nitrous oxide. This cerebral vasodilatation will cause an increase in cerebral blood flow and cerebral blood volume. This increase in cerebral blood volume leads to an increase in intracranial pressure, which may be attenuated with time. Increases in cerebral blood flow may also be attenuated with prior administration of barbiturates or the presence of hypobaric. There is evidence that the volatile anesthetics may produce some protection against cerebral ischemic effects of hypoperfusion. Electroencephalographic (EEG) evidence of cerebral ischemia as a result of decreased blood flow occurs at lower flow rates with isoflurane than halothane. In humans, the blood flow at which EEG

TABLE 24.2

Factors that Affect Minimum Alveolar Concentration (MAC)

Factors Increasing MAC	Factors Decreasing MAC	Factors with No Effect on MAC
Hyperthermia	Hypothermia	Duration of anesthesia
Hypernatremia	Hyponatremia	Gender
Chronic alcohol abuse	α-2 Agonists	Potassium derangements
Acute amphetamine ingestion	Pregnancy	Blood pressure >40 mm Hg
Cocaine intoxication	Increased age	Thyroid gland dysfunction
Tricyclic antidepressants	Acute alcohol ingestion	Pa_{O2} >40 mm Hg
Monoamine oxidase inhibitors	Intravenous anesthetics and other CNS depressants	Pa_{CO2} 15–95 mm Hg
	Lidocaine	

CNS, central nervous system.
(Modified from: Miller RD. *Anesthesia*, 5th ed. Philadelphia: Churchill Livingstone, 2000.)

evidence of cerebral ischemia occurs is significantly lower with isoflurane than with halothane ($\sim$10 mL/100 g/min and 18–20 mL/100 g/min, respectively). CSF production or reabsorption is essentially unchanged with isoflurane. Halothane decreases the rate of CSF production and also decreases reabsorption. Enflurane increases CSF production and decreases reabsorption. All evidence indicates that enflurane is the least favorable drug regarding control of CSF pressure.

EEG patterns with all inhalation agents are similar in that with increasing concentrations, EEG wave frequency is decreased and voltage is increased. Electrical silence may be produced at high concentrations of volatile anesthetics. Enflurane may produce high-voltage spiking patterns that may be abolished by decreasing the concentration of drug. Owing to the effect of enflurane on CSF production and reabsorption, and the potential for enflurane to produce seizure-like activity, it is the least preferable volatile anesthetic for neurosurgical procedures. Enflurane is rarely used in clinical practice currently.

Sensory-evoked potential monitoring may be complicated by the use of volatile anesthetics. Volatile anesthetics typically increase the latency and decrease the amplitude of the tracing. This appears to be dose related with minimal effects present at less than 0.5 MAC of agent. Somatosensory-evoked potential monitoring is more reliable if the concentration of agent administered remains constant rather than frequent adjustments. Cortical responses such as visual-evoked potentials are more sensitive to the effects of volatile anesthetic agents than subcortical responses such as somatosensory-evoked potentials and brainstem auditory evoked potentials.

Cardiovascular System

Cardiac Physiology

Cardiac performance is determined by the following physiologic parameters: preload, afterload, contractility, rate, and rhythm. The objective of invasive monitoring is to assess each parameter and the interplay among the parameters. CO is determined by the product of stroke volume (SV) and HR.

PRELOAD. Physiologists define preload as actual fiber length at end diastole. Preload from a clinical perspective may be defined as the amount of blood returning to the atria for delivery into the ventricles. In practice, preload is assessed indirectly through right atrial measurement [central venous pressure (CVP)] for the right ventricle and left atrial pressure [pulmonary capillary wedge presssure (PCWP)] for the left ventricle. It must be appreciated that these are mean values and represent estimates of ventricular diastolic pressures. Adequate preload depends on venous return because the heart cannot pump more than it receives. Because 60% to 70% of vascular volume is contained in the venous system, it is important to have a clear understanding of venous return. The arterial system is relatively fixed in its ability to alter volume compared with the venous system. For adequate venous return, a pressure gradient must be created between the peripheral veins and the atrium.

Venous tone is defined as the state of contraction of smooth muscles within venous walls. This is controlled primarily by sympathetic activity and local factors. When venous tone increases, venous capacitance decreases, creating a real decrease in pressure. This is associated with fluid depletion. Atrial filling decreases with a resultant decrease in preload. With maximal venous tonicity, which may occur as a compensatory mechanism in hypovolemia, venous capacitance may be decreased. This may lead to improper interpretation of data.

Increasing driving pressure (venoconstriction) is the common response in the stressed state. Improving conductance (fluid administration) is the most common mechanism used in supportive care. To summarize, optimizing the vascular space in regard to intravascular volume is the primary means to optimize preload.

AFTERLOAD. Afterload is the force opposing ventricular fiber shortening during ejection. Size, shape, radius, and wall thickness are all factors affecting afterload. The principal factors are radius (related to preload) and aortic or pulmonic impedance. Systemic vascular resistance (SVR) and arterial compliance determine aortic impedance. Pulmonary vascular resistance (PVR) and compliance determine pulmonic impedance. Clinically, SVR is used frequently as an estimate of afterload, but it reflects arteriolar tone and not ventricular systolic wall tension. Accurate measurement requires intraventricular measurements combined with echocardiographic studies. Reduction of afterload allows the ventricle to shorten more rapidly and more completely. Increases in afterload decrease the extent and velocity of shortening.

CONTRACTILITY. Contractility is the inherent strength of ventricular muscle when preload and afterload are constant. The ability to quantify contractility remains an illusive entity in the intact system. Such terms as *stroke work indices* and *force velocity measurements* have been used to describe contractility. Certain ions, such as calcium, potassium, sodium, and magnesium, affect contractility.

HEART RATE. HR becomes a critical factor in patients with impairment of coronary blood flow. As rate increases, coronary perfusion is compromised because diastole is shortened to a greater degree than systole and coronary perfusion to the left ventricle occurs only in diastole. It is not surprising that many ischemic episodes occur during periods of tachycardia.

All of these cardiac factors are interrelated and must be understood to properly predict the responses of patients to anesthetic and surgical intervention. Alteration of one factor may affect another determinant, and one must be aware of all these changes to interpret data properly. An example would be vasodilator therapy that may result in a decrease in BP (afterload), venous pooling (preload), and a reflex tachycardia.

Cardiovascular Effects of Anesthetics

The cardiovascular effects of volatile anesthetics are summarized in Table 24.3. Inhalational anesthetics, when studied

TABLE 24.3

Selected Cardiovascular Effects of Inhalational Agents

	Heart Rate	Contractility	Cardiac Output	Systemic Vascular Resistance
Halothane	⇔⇓	⇓⇓	⇓	⇔
Isoflurane	⇔⇑	⇓	⇔⇓	⇓⇓
Enflurane	⇔⇓	⇓⇓	⇓	⇓
Sevoflurane	⇔⇑	⇓	⇔⇓	⇓
Desflurane	⇑	⇓	⇔⇓	⇓
Nitrous oxide	⇔⇑	⇔	⇔⇑	⇔

in vitro (isolated papillary muscle preparations), produce a dose-dependent depression of contractility. *In vivo*, cardiac depression is not observed consistently, probably due to compensatory homeostatic mechanisms. Papillary muscles taken from animals with congestive heart failure are depressed to a greater extent than muscles from normal animals. Patients with impaired contractility as a result of congestive heart failure are known to be particularly sensitive to the direct myocardial depressant effects of inhaled anesthetics. Dose-dependent decreases in systemic BP occur with all of the inhalational anesthetics with the exception of nitrous oxide. SV and myocardial contractility are also decreased by volatile anesthetics. Predicted decreases in CO are mitigated by compensatory increases in HR, which is more significant with isoflurane and desflurane. The combination of volatile anesthetics with drugs that inhibit this reflex such as β blockers, leads to significant decreases in CO. The effects of surgical stimulation lead to an increased sympathetic outflow and a return of the cardiovascular parameters to a near baseline state. This is most apparent after the induction of general anesthesia in a patient. After stimulation by endotracheal intubation and during the initial administration of inhaled volatile anesthetics, patients may experience transient periods of hypotension. This response may be exaggerated in the volume or catecholamine depleted patient. If not anticipated, upon surgical incision, patients may immediately go from a hypotensive and possibly bradycardic state to a state of sympathetic excitation. Communication between surgeon and anesthesiologist may prevent dramatic swings in BP during this initial anesthetic period.

Effects on the myocardial conduction system have been noted with all potent inhalation agents. Atrioventricular junctional rhythms are common with all anesthetics. Volatile anesthetic agents decrease the dose of epinephrine that can be administered before evoking ventricular dysrhythmias. This is clinically important during the injection of local anesthetic agents with epinephrine. Among the volatile anesthetics used clinically, halothane sensitizes the heart to the effects of epinephrine the most. Halothane is also unique in its arrhythmogenic profile in that it causes His–Purkinje conduction depression. HR changes least with halothane and sevoflurane and increases most with desflurane and isoflurane.

Inhalational agents decrease CO and systemic arterial pressure; therefore, myocardial work is decreased. SVR is particularly decreased with administration of isoflurane, leading to a decrease in BP. Replacing equal MAC values of isoflurane with nitrous oxide diminishes the decrease in SVR due to isoflurane administration. Nitrous oxide by itself does not decrease SVR and therefore, BP is maintained.

Respiratory System

The effects of general anesthesia and inhalational anesthetics on respiratory function are due to both central mechanisms and changes in lung mechanics.

Central Effect

All inhaled agents cause a decrease in ventilatory drive in a dose-related manner. Inhaled agents produce a decrease in tidal volume (TV) with an initial increase in ventilatory rate. The characteristic pattern of spontaneous respiration under volatile anesthetics is a rapid, shallow breathing pattern. Volatile anesthetics decrease the sensitivity and reduce the responsiveness of the body to carbon dioxide (CO_2). With time, the responsiveness to CO_2 is improved but the original baseline is usually not achieved. Owing to the combination of volatile and intravenous anesthetics used traditionally in a balanced anesthetic, patients usually require an accumulation of carbon dioxide to reach a threshold necessary to initiate a breath. Response to hypoxia, even with subanesthetic doses of inhalation agents, is significantly depressed. Augmentation of ventilation produced by hypercarbia or hypoxia in the awake state is not observed during anesthesia. As the concentration of inhaled agent increases, a decrease in respiratory rate occurs. The responsiveness of the respiratory center to P_{ACO_2} becomes depressed.

The diaphragm contributes approximately 60% of normal tidal breathing as compared to the 40% by intercostal activity. Depressed intercostal function prohibits stabilization of the rib cage. Diaphragmatic function is also depressed, but phrenic nerve activity is more resistant to the depressive effects of anesthetic agents.

The effect of inhalation agents on hypoxic pulmonary vasoconstriction is controversial. In animal studies, there is general agreement that the response is depressed in a dose-related manner. This factor is important, but it does not preclude the use of inhalation agents. The disease status of the lung and the effects of anesthetic agents are of relatively greater importance in the selection of agents to be used in the clinical setting.

Lung Mechanics and Anesthesia

Pulmonary complications undoubtedly constitute a major source of morbidity and mortality in the postoperative patient. Reported incidences of pulmonary problems vary from 3% to 70%. This discrepancy stems in part from differences in definitions of complications, types of surgery, and patient population. Physicians should have a reasonable grasp of the effects of surgery and anesthesia as they relate to lung function.

UPPER AIRWAY. Stiff hairs in the anterior nasal fossa and the spongy mucous membrane act as important bacterial defense mechanisms. Humidification and warming of inspired gas are probably the most important functions of the nose. The great vascularity of the mucosa helps maintain a constant temperature. Despite wide variations in external temperature, inspired air is warmed to 36°C to 37°C by the time it reaches the mid-tracheal area. The daily production of approximately 1 L of nasal secretions is used in saturating inspired gas. Bronchi and alveoli require 95% humidity for adequate function. Artificial airway placement such as intubation bypasses these mechanisms, allowing relatively dry gases to reach the tracheobronchial tree. The mucosa in this area is then compelled to perform the duties of the nasal mucosa. This process is less efficient and humidification of inhaled gases is recommended even for short periods of intubation. Administration of dry gases leads to cessation of ciliary activity. Cellular degeneration accompanied by mild tracheitis is common after the administration of an endotracheal anesthesia.

The continuous activity of the mucociliary escalator apparatus is probably the most important factor in the prevention of the accumulation of secretions. The coordinated movement of these fine hair-like projections act to move secretions toward the larynx and pharynx. Decrease in temperature, mucus production, and changes in pH decrease ciliary activity. Volatile anesthetics in high concentrations and opiates have a depressant effect on ciliary functions. Inspissated secretions may result from prolonged ventilation through mechanical airway devices without humidification.

The administration of dry volatile anesthetics as well as narcotic premedication adversely affects the humidifying function of the upper airway. The loss of the ability to mobilize secretions produces a viable setting for derangement of pulmonary protective mechanics.

LUNG VOLUMES. Lung volumes commonly used in respiratory physiology generally refer to expired measurements (Fig. 24.2). The amount exhaled during quiet breathing is known as the *TV*. Maximal inhalation followed by maximal exhalation is known as the *vital capacity* (VC). Some gas remains in the lung after a maximal exhalation and is known as the *residual volume* (RV). The combination of the VC and RV is the total lung capacity (TLC). The volume of gas

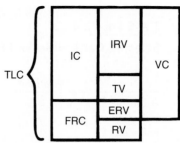

FIGURE 24.2 Lung volumes as a portion of total lung capacity. TLC, total lung capacity; IC, inspiratory capacity; FRC, functional residual capacity; IRV, inspiratory reserve volume; TV, tidal volume; ERV, expiratory reserve volume; RV, residual volume; VC, vital capacity.

in the lung after a normal expiration is the FRC. It is this particular lung capacity that is of critical importance in the surgical patient. Attempts to preserve FRC are important throughout the perioperative period. The administration of 100% oxygen to patients immediately before anesthetic induction is an attempt to denitrogenate the lungs including the FRC. The FRC acts as a reservoir of oxygen in the apneic patient during the period immediately postanesthetic induction and before endotracheal intubation and resumption of ventilation and oxygenation. If arterial oxygen tensions were measured constantly, these values would vary minimally on a minute-to-minute basis, although fresh gas only enters the lung during inspiration. Oxygenation is maintained by gas exchanges occurring in the FRC. Any decrease in the FRC would, therefore, lead to less volume available and hence oxygenation problems. Decreases in FRC, as seen in obese and pregnant patients, predictably decrease the period of apnea that patients may endure before the development of hypoxia. When spontaneous ventilation is allowed to resume at the end of an anesthetic, efforts should be made to preserve TV and FRC in the awakening patient. Inability to preserve FRC leads to atelectasis, which may be difficult to overcome in the postoperative period, especially if the absence of adequate pain control. Because anesthesia and surgery produce restrictive deficits in lung volumes (decreased lung volume), the goal should be to protect and maintain FRC.

Several important factors concerning respiratory physiology must be considered during the perioperative period. To appreciate these, certain other definitions of lung mechanics must be understood. Lung compliance is defined as the volume change per unit of pressure change. In the normal range, the lung is remarkably distensible, or very compliant. Measurement of compliance in normal human lungs is approximately 150 to 200 mL/cm H_2O. At higher volumes, the lung is stiffer and compliance is reduced. Compliance is also reduced at lower lung volumes. This may be of critical importance in maintaining FRC. Engorgement of the lung with blood, increased pulmonary venous pressure, increased unventilated areas of the lung, and interstitial fibrosis may all lead to a decrease in lung compliance. Emphysema, with loss of elastic recoil fibers, leads to more distensible alveoli and causes an increase in lung compliance.

Surfactant produced by alveolar type II cells is a surface tension–reducing agent that allows alveoli to remain distended at smaller volumes. As long as intra-alveolar pressure is greater than pressures in the interstitium of the lung, patency is maintained. The pressure necessary to maintain patent alveoli is, therefore, decreased by the presence of surfactant. Almost all anesthetic techniques using positive pressure ventilation decrease or inhibit surfactant production. This produces a tendency for airway closure to occur at lower lung volumes.

VENTILATORY MECHANICS. Normal spontaneous ventilation occurs because there is a pressure difference between the mouth and the alveolus. The elastic force of the lung and chest wall creates the subatmospheric pressure within the pleural cavity. A gradient of pleural pressures exists in the upright lungs at end expiration varying from 0 to 10 cm of water. Inasmuch as alveoli at the apex of the upright lung are distended to a greater degree because of greater subatmospheric pressure, airflow tends to be distributed to a greater number of alveoli in the lower half of the lung. Gravitational effects and weight of the lung distribute blood to this same area. Hence, during spontaneous ventilation, gas exchange is relatively well-matched. Both blood flow and ventilation are higher at the bases of the lung when compared to the apices. Looking at blood flow and ventilation in relation to gravity, as one moves from superior to inferior in a standing or sitting patient, an increase in blood flow occurs at a faster rate than the increase in ventilation. This produces areas of relative dead space in the superior aspects of the lung and areas of relative shunt in the dependent areas of the lungs. The distribution of blood flow and ventilation is obviously a dynamic process that varies during respiration and changes in body position. In addition, the distribution of blood flow and ventilation varies significantly in the perioperative period depending on the anatomic location of the surgical intervention, adequacy of pain control, use of muscle relaxants, patient positioning and the use of positive pressure ventilation. Blood flow and ventilation relations are particularly critical in intrathoracic surgical procedures performed in the lateral decubitus position with one lung isolation.

Airflow occurs into the lungs due to a pressure gradient that must be developed to overcome the nonelastic or dynamic resistance of the lungs. Orifice size and pattern of airflow affect resistance. Laminar flow occurs down parallel-sided tubes at less than a certain critical velocity. Turbulent flow occurs when flow exceeds a critical velocity. Orifice flow occurs at a constriction such as the larynx. Total cross-sectional area of the airways increases as branching occurs, thereby decreasing the velocity of airflow. Laminar flow is chiefly confined to airways below the main bronchi, orifice flow occurs at the larynx, and turbulent flow occurs in the trachea during most of the respiratory cycle.

EFFECTS OF SURGERY. Position during surgery causes definite decreases in lung volumes. In changing from the upright to the supine position, FRC decreases by 0.5 to 1.0 L with similar decreases in VC. Changes in diaphragmatic function with position have been shown to be of great importance with regard to lung volumes. Excursion of the diaphragm varies from 1 to 2 cm during quiet tidal breathing to as much as 5 to 6 cm during rigorous ventilation. Diaphragmatic motion is restricted in the supine position because of compression by the liver and gravitational changes. Paralysis is accomplished with the use of muscle relaxants and produces a flaccid diaphragm that tends to remain in the end-expiratory state. This position leads to further compression of lung volumes.

Location of the surgical procedure produces a predictable quantitative change in lung volumes. Bedside measurement of VC offers a serial measurement of changes in lung mechanics. With upper abdominal procedures, VC may decrease by 60% to 70%, whereas procedures in the lower abdomen are associated with decreases of 40% to 50%. Chest surgical procedures have not been as well studied, and as a result most data on these type of procedures represent extrapolations from abdominal surgery. Limitation of excursion of the diaphragm, inability to inspire deeply, and lack of an effective cough has been attributed to postoperative pain in the surgical patient. All respiratory care maneuvers in the postoperative patient are aimed at improving inspiration and mobilization of secretions.

DIRECT ANESTHETIC EFFECTS. Anesthesia vapors produce a paralysis of mucociliary function and depress surfactant production. Coupled with the use of positive-pressure ventilation and position problems, it is not difficult to understand why the patient has a decrease in lung compliance and loss of lung volume during anesthesia.

The direct effect on airway caliber of all potent inhalation agents is to decrease airway resistance by producing bronchodilation. Antigens and histamines produce bronchoconstriction that is blocked by potent inhalation agents. If the patient is breathing spontaneously and extubated at the end of the operation, the effect of these agents should disappear within 4 to 6 hours.

Most volatile anesthetics are said to decrease or abolish hypoxic pulmonary vasoconstriction. If the anesthetized patient has normal lungs and is undergoing a nonthoracic procedure, this is probably of little consequence. In the thoracic surgical patient or in the patient with lung disease, the abolition of this reflex may be an important cause of intrapulmonary shunting.

All of the aforementioned factors lead to an intrapulmonary shunt of 10% to 15% in the anesthetized surgical patient with no previous cardiopulmonary disease. Any decrease in ventricular function, excessive fluid administration, or sepsis may cause a decrease in lung compliance and further add to the loss of lung volumes. These problems are additive as far as decreasing FRC.

Carbon Dioxide

CO_2 production in the unstressed patient is in the range of 3 mL/kg body weight. In 1 minute of apnea, CO_2 will raise an

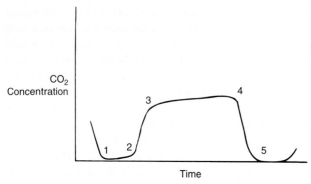

FIGURE 24.3 Normal capnogram. The line represents CO_2 concentration in expired gas through a respiratory cycle. 1–2, anatomic dead space; 2–3, alveolar gas and mixed dead space; 4–3, alveolar gas; 4–5, last portion of alveolar gas.

TABLE 24.4
Table for Capnography

Expired CO_2	Etiology
Rapid decrease to zero	Airway obstruction (kinked ETT)
	Circuit disconnection
	Defective ventilator
	Technical error (sampling line blocked)
Slower decrease (1–3 min)	Decreased cardiac output
	Pulmonary embolism, air embolism
	Hypotension
	Hyperventilation
Increase	Hypoventilation
	Rapid increase in body temperature
	Absorption from external source as CO_2 during laparoscopic surgery
	Increased pulmonary blood flow
	Release of vascular clamps
	Defective CO_2 absorption

ETT, endotracheal tube.

average of 6 mm Hg and will continue to raise an additional 4 mm Hg each minute thereafter. Anesthetic techniques generally decrease CO_2 production due to a decrease in metabolic activity in the anesthetized state. Exhaled CO_2 is an excellent measurement of alveolar ventilation, and assuming reasonable cardiac and normal lung function, values obtained approach arterial CO_2 findings.

CAPNOGRAPHY. The introduction of the continuous measurement of exhaled CO_2 was one of the most important developments toward improving the safety of patients undergoing surgery and anesthesia. The presence of carbon dioxide during exhalation is the gold standard for confirming successful endotracheal tube placement into the trachea. A normal capnogram consists of five basic components as illustrated in Figure 24.3. The waveform can be analyzed for frequency, rhythm, baseline, shape, and height.

Respiratory frequency and rhythm depend on the state of the patient's respiratory center and ventilatory function. Height is a quantitative measure of expired CO_2. Shape depends on expiratory gas flow. A summary of the changes in expired CO_2 and the possible mechanisms is given in Table 24.4.

The value for end tidal carbon dioxide ($ETCO_2$) in normal patients will be approximately 5 mm Hg lower than measured arterial CO_2. A mismatching of ventilation to perfusion causes the discrepancy between $ETCO_2$ and $Paco_2$, which may be diagnostic for certain conditions.

Renal System
Generally, all inhalational anesthetics cause a decrease in urine formation. A decrease in glomerular filtration rate is seen with virtually all anesthetic techniques. This may be caused by direct effects on renal blood flow and changes in renal vascular autoregulation. Some effects seen are undoubtedly due to the effects on the cardiovascular system; however, others are secondary to the stress responses of surgical stimulation and antidiuretic hormone (ADH) secretion. Direct nephrotoxic effects of inhalational agents have not been reported. However, the effects of fluoride-induced nephrotoxicity from the metabolism of certain

anesthetics to fluoride have been described. This has been associated with the use of enflurane and recently with the use of sevoflurane. Fluoride-induced nephrotoxicity causes a clinical picture of nephrogenic diabetes insipidus. A failure in the ability to concentrate urine may lead to an increase in free water loss and eventual dehydration and electrolyte disturbances. Despite the concern over nephrotoxicity, in the concentrations used clinically, fluoride-induced nephrotoxicity is rare. That being said, these agents should be avoided in patients with preexisting renal conditions due to the availability of other anesthetic agents.

Hepatic System
The subject of anesthesia and liver function has been the basis for much controversy and confusion. Different anesthetics affect liver function in various ways. Perioperative hepatic dysfunction may be caused directly by the anesthetic agent or decreased oxygen and blood supply. More complex mechanisms, such as the development of antibodies and involvement of the immune mechanisms, may contribute to hepatic dysfunction. All inhalation agents are metabolized by the liver to some degree (halothane, 18%–20% > enflurane, 2% ≥ sevoflurane, 2% > isoflurane, 0.2% > desflurane, 0.02%).

Blood flow to the liver is normally approximately 25% of the CO. Anesthetic agents may affect hepatic blood flow by changes in CO or through direct effects on hepatic vasculature. Events occurring during the surgical procedure may be stressful enough to cause the release of catecholamines, thereby reducing hepatic blood flow. Surgical procedures and manipulation are probably more significant in reducing hepatic blood flow than the anesthetic agents and techniques utilized (2).

Halothane is the anesthetic studied most regarding possible hepatotoxicity. When the liver is exposed to halothane, histologically a number of changes occur (rounding up of the mitochondria, increased granularity of the rough endoplasmic reticulum, etc.) indicating increased metabolic activity. Strong evidence in the literature indicates certain factors may enhance the risk of halothane hepatotoxicity. They include multiple exposures to halothane, obesity, gender (females > males), advancing age, and ethnic origins (Mexican-Americans seem to be more susceptible than others). Mechanisms proposed for halothane hepatotoxicity are direct hepatotoxic effects of intermediaries of halothane metabolism, hepatic oxygen deprivation secondary to halothane-induced circulatory changes, and immunologically mediated hepatic necrosis.

The frequency of halothane-induced liver necrosis varies from 1 in 6,000 to 1 in 20,000 administrations. The U.S. National Halothane Study analyzed 850,000 anesthetics with 250,000 instances of halothane administration. The incidence in the study was 1:35,000 (3). The incidence of hepatic injury after enflurane and isoflurane is extremely low; therefore an actual estimation of the incidence is impossible. Newer anesthetic agents such as desflurane and sevoflurane have not been clearly associated with hepatic dysfunction.

Neuromuscular System

Potent inhaled anesthetics have inherent muscle relaxant properties. Neuromuscular blockade by inhalation agents may be the result of central upper motor neuron depression or an effect at the myoneural junction. As discussed earlier, the inspired concentration at which significant muscle relaxation occurs is associated with hemodynamic instability. The effects of neuromuscular blocking agents are facilitated by administration of volatile anesthetics in a dose-dependent manner.

Endocrine System

Islet Cell Function and Glucose Metabolism

During anesthesia and surgical stress, blood glucose levels are usually elevated. The plasma insulin response to glucose administration is blunted. Peripheral utilization of glucose is reduced, as is insulin release from pancreatic islet cells.

The metabolic response to stress is characterized by a number of autonomic and neuroendocrine responses. Increased catecholamine and cortisol levels suppress pancreatic insulin release. Glucagon release is stimulated, resulting in glycogenolysis, gluconeogenesis, and hyperglycemia. Release of glycerol and amino acids, which are used by the liver during gluconeogenesis, contributes to the hyperglycemia.

Hyperglycemia, regardless of diabetic status, has been associated with an increase in morbidity and mortality in postoperative patients. This is driving focus toward tight control of glucose during the immediate preoperative, intraoperative, and postoperative periods, even in nondiabetic patients. In addition, hyperglycemia has been associated with increased incidence of surgical site infection. Hyperglycemia affects neutrophil function and alters the immune response and decreases the ability to fight off even a mildly contaminated wound. Tighter control of glucose levels in surgical patients is a rapidly evolving practice which may become standard (4).

Antidiuretic Hormone

Inhalational agents and opioid analgesics are believed to affect ADH or vasopressin release. This augments the massive release of ADH caused by surgical stress. Stimulation of the vasopressin receptor subtype V2 decreases free-water clearance and increases urinary osmolarity. A clinical picture of nephrogenic diabetes insipidus may result from fluoride toxicity related to certain anesthetic agents.

ADH release also acts on the V1 receptor to produce vasoconstriction. This vasoconstriction may assist in the maintenance of BP under general anesthesia when the sympathetic system is blunted. Decreases in ADH and V1 stimulation seen in physiologic states such as sepsis and shock, may explain the exaggerated hypotension when these patients undergo general anesthesia.

Stimulation of V3 receptors by ADH seems to increase plasma cortisol levels by amplifying the effect of corticotrophin-releasing hormone on the anterior pituitary. The presence of V3 receptors in the CNS may also explain the role of ADH in thermoregulation, cognition, and memory (5).

Stress Response

Stress response is the combined result of surgical stimulation and the administration of anesthesia. Induction with inhalational agents has a greater effect than intravenous induction. A general discharge of catecholamines has been quantitatively noted with NE levels elevated within the first 15 minutes of induction of anesthesia. These return to normal within the first hour. An increase in adrenal cortical discharge, renin levels, and aldosterone has been found with surgical stimulation. One of the goals of anesthesia, especially in patients with cardiac disease, is to limit the stress response.

Oxygenation and Oxygen Delivery

Oxygen is the energy source for mammalian cellular metabolism. Organ function represents the unified activity of cells. Any derangement in cellular function results in organ dysfunction. The inability to maintain oxygen delivery is, therefore, the most appropriate definition of circulatory failure. Most information gained in the clinical setting involves use of the senses and invasive and noninvasive techniques. Basic concepts concerning oxygen delivery need to be understood so that clinical observations and interventions are appropriate.

Oxygen delivery may be defined as the amount of oxygen available to tissues each minute. It is a combination of CO and oxygen content. One must be familiar with hemoglobin physiology to gain a clear understanding of oxygen delivery. Hemoglobin combines reversibly with oxygen to form oxyhemoglobin. Oxyhemoglobin is intimately related to arterial oxygen tension but does not exert a partial pressure because it is in the chemically bound state. The bulk of oxygen is bound to hemoglobin and the pressure gradient created by dissolved oxygen is important because diffusion from plasma to cells is a pressure-related process. Therefore, almost all oxygen must first break the bond with hemoglobin so it becomes available to the cells.

The strength with which hemoglobin binds oxygen is referred to as *oxygen-hemoglobin affinity*. An increased affinity will allow fewer molecules to be transferred per unit time, whereas a decreased affinity will result in greater transfer. Each hemoglobin molecule has four O_2 binding sites. Normal O_2 demand is met by release from one binding site, leaving three sites occupied. Therefore, normal mixed venous saturation (Pvo_2) is 75%. Venous oxygen tension represents the lowest oxygen tension in that particular capillary bed. At an arterial O_2 tension of 26 mm Hg, hemoglobin saturation is 50%.

Arterial oxygen content (Cao_2) defines the amount of oxygen available in blood. Because hemoglobin (Hb) is expressed in volume percent (vol %), content values are expressed in terms of O_2/100 mL blood. Oxygen exists as oxyhemoglobin and is dissolved in plasma. When hemoglobin is fully saturated, it will combine with 1.34 mL of oxygen. Arterial hemoglobin saturation (Sao_2) is commonly measured using pulse oximetry or arterial blood gas analysis. The amount of oxygen dissolved can be converted by multiplying the Pao_2 times 0.0031 (solubility coefficient). The sum of the oxygen bound to hemoglobin ($1.34 \times Hb \times Sao_2$) and the amount of oxygen dissolved in blood ($0.0031 \times Pao_2$) determines the oxygen content. Therefore, oxygen content can be expressed mathematically by the equation:

$$Cao_2 = (1.34 \times Hb \times Sao_2) + (0.0031 \times Paov)$$

If one now examines oxygen availability based on the preceding facts, one sees by examining the oxygen-hemoglobin dissociation curve that a change in Pao_2 from 95 to 65 mm Hg (33% decrease) results in a decrease in saturation from 97% to 92%. Therefore, one sees a considerable protection during changes in arterial oxygen tension. As one approaches the venous portion of the curve (Pvo_2 40 mm Hg/75%), small changes in Pa/vo_2 effect greater changes in saturation. Changes in Pvo_2 have important implications with respect to oxygen unloading at the tissue level. The preceding points may be summarized as follows: (i) 98% of oxygen is combined with hemoglobin and less than 2% is dissolved, and (ii) Pao_2 is a major determinant of hemoglobin saturation.

Oxygen transport represents the amount of oxygen delivered by the cardiovascular system per unit of time. Cardiac function now becomes a major determinant of oxygen delivery. Oxygen transport may be calculated by multiplying CO by arterial O_2 content. If arterial oxygen content is 20 mL/100 mL blood and CO is 5 L/min, then 1,000 mL of oxygen is delivered to tissues each minute.

Once oxygen is delivered, tissues use a certain amount and the term *oxygen consumption* is introduced. If the quantity delivered is known and the amount returning through the venous system is calculated, the difference is the amount consumed. In the clinical setting, oxygen content from the arterial and mixed venous samples is collected. CO is available through thermodilution techniques, and oxygen consumption may be calculated as follows: arterial O_2 content = 20.4 mL; mixed venous O_2 content = 15.4 mL/5 mL/100 blood consumed; CO = 5 L/min $\times$ 10 = 50; therefore, O_2 consumed = 50 $\times$ 5 = 250 mL. With an arterial O_2 content of 20.4 mL/100 mL blood and a CO of 5 L, the total oxygen available is 1000 mL; a reserve or safety factor is built into the system.

What factors in the clinical setting may threaten the homeostasis? The major factors are (i) decrease in CO, (ii) decreased hemoglobin, and (iii) decrease in arterial Po_2. One must also be aware of the compensatory mechanism that may be used under stress. Two fundamental steps are to increase CO and to increase extraction from capillary blood, producing a decrease in venous saturation. Most normal individuals can triple CO and also increase extraction by a factor of 3. These mechanisms are seen in the anemic patient.

The common denominator in the shock syndrome is the development of lactic acidosis. Regardless of the etiology of the problem, an elevated blood lactate is associated with an ominous prognosis. The anemic patient who is able to compensate will not develop lactic acidosis in the unstressed state. Decreases in arterial saturation with concomitant increases in CO and maximal extraction will not result in lactic acidosis. Arterial hypoxemia without other complications will not lead to lactic acidosis unless other problems ensue. The chronic lung disease patient exemplifies this axiom.

The final factor regarding oxygen availability is CO. A fall in CO is qualitatively a much greater threat to oxygen consumption. A decreased CO not only threatens the homeostasis in the same way that anemia and arterial desaturation do, but it removes one of the major compensatory mechanisms. Instead of a ninefold increase in the safety factor, there is only a threefold margin. The only mechanism that remains is for the body to extract more oxygen, thereby decreasing venous saturation. Failure of perfusion represents the most common cause of lactic acidosis.

Oxygenation is a complex process. From the clinical viewpoint, by assessment of hemoglobin levels, saturation, and cardiovascular function, an attempt is made to define the defect by using concepts of tissue oxygenation in the context of hemodynamic monitoring.

Temperature
Hypothermia

Hypothermia is the most common temperature disorder resulting from anesthesia and surgery. At least 70% of patients have temperatures of less than 36°C on admission to thepostanesthesia care unit (PACU). Important factors contributing to heat loss are (i) cold operating room (temperature <21°C); (ii) administration of inadequately warmed intravenous fluids; (iii) nonwarmed, unhumidified anesthetic gases; (iv) use of cold irrigating solutions; (v) interference with thermoregulatory mechanism by anesthetic agent(s); (vi) reduction of metabolic rate by anesthetic agent(s); and (vii) vasodilatation induced by anesthetic agent(s). The greatest heat loss usually occurs during the first hour of surgery when the patient's skin is exposed and prepped with a cold prep solution. Heat loss occurs by the following mechanisms: radiation (60%), conduction (5%), convection (10%), and evaporation (25%).

Radiation is the loss of heat by electromagnetic radiation to cooler objects in the room. Covering exposed body parts can diminish most of the losses due to radiation. Convective heat loss is loss of heat to air currents passing over the patient. Covering the patient can also diminish this type of heat loss. Convective heat gain is now commonly employed perioperatively to elevate or maintain patient body temperature through forced air warming devices. Conduction refers to heat that is lost to objects that touch the body. Evaporative heat losses occur through humidification of dry airway gases, sweating and through insensible losses through large wounds. Heating and humidifying ventilatory circuits and airway gases may help to contain evaporative losses.

Certain types of patients are at a particularly high risk for hypothermia. These include elderly patients, infants, trauma patients, and patients that have suffered acute burns. All patients have characteristic changes to hypothermia. Of particular concern are the cardiovascular effects of hypothermia. A shivering patient may have as much as a 400% increase in myocardial oxygen consumption. For this reason, patients with hypothermia or shivering should be given supplemental oxygen until normothermia is achieved. The incidence of surgical site infections is also elevated in patients who are even mildly hypothermic postoperatively (5). Hypothermia may also lead to clotting abnormalities, altered metabolism of drugs, vasoconstriction and diuresis from ADH inhibition.

Infants are at a particularly high risk for the development of hypothermia. Infants, and in particular neonates, have inadequate insulation from subcutaneous fat. These patients also have large surface area related to mass, allowing more heat loss through conductive, convective, and radiant mechanisms. Another reason for the susceptibility of infants to heat loss is the rather inefficient mechanism of nonshivering thermogenesis. Infants and neonates have brown fat stores located between the scapulae and around major thoracic and abdominal blood vessels. Brown fat becomes metabolically active in response to sympathetic discharge. CO is diverted to brown fat so that heat is distributed to the rest of the body.

Elderly patients and burn patients share a similar problem of decreased subcutaneous fat tissue. In addition, elderly patients can have impaired or delayed vasoconstriction in response to hypothermia (6). Trauma victims tend to arrive in the emergency department hypothermic either from exposure to the climate or from large volume resuscitation. Intraoperatively, trauma patients experience further heat loss due to the continued rapid administration of blood products and crystalloid despite use of fluid warmers. Trauma patients also tend to undergo procedures that involve large incisions and the use of large volumes of irrigating fluid. These factors further decrease core body temperature under anesthesia.

Prevention of heat loss during anesthesia and surgery should be a priority for the anesthesiologist and surgical specialist. The potential for significant physiologic side effects due to hypothermia should be understood and respected. Once hypothermia develops, treatment efforts should be viewed as a critical part of the overall perioperative care of the surgical patient.

Hyperthermia

Hyperthermia increases oxygen consumption and carbon dioxide production due to an increase in basal metabolic rate. Myocardial effects of hyperthermia include arrhythmias and tachycardia, which increase myocardial oxygen demand and place patients at risk for ischemia. CNS effects such as altered sensorium and seizures may also occur. The differential diagnosis of intraoperative hyperthermia includes infection, hyperthyroidism, excessive external warming, drug or blood reaction, and malignant hyperthermia (MH). MH should always be considered in a patient developing hyperthermia under anesthesia.

MALIGNANT HYPERTHERMIA. MH is a genetically transmitted syndrome estimated to occur in 1 in 50,000 anesthetized adults and 1 in 15,000 anesthetized children (although there is marked regional variation). MH is a severe, life-threatening condition that must be recognized early and treated aggressively. The pathophysiology of MH remains unclear, but grossly elevated calcium ion (Ca^{2+}) levels in the muscle myoplasm have been found in laboratory studies suggesting a sudden release or decreased reuptake of calcium into the sarcoplasmic reticulum. Drugs that are referred to as *triggering agents* initiate this process. Triggering agents are believed to release large amounts of Ca^{2+} from the sarcoplasmic reticulum. The excess calcium ions within the muscle cell cause extreme muscle tension and increased metabolic activity. Muscle cell membrane disruption leads to huge increases in creatine kinase and myoglobin. Triggering agents include all inhalation agents (except N_2O), depolarizing muscle relaxants (succinylcholine), and potassium salts.

Classic signs of MH are tachypnea (usually not seen in the anesthetized, paralyzed patient), tachycardia, and hypercarbia. If expired CO_2 is measured, hypercarbia will be the first sign noted. Muscle rigidity, temperature elevation (1°C–2°C increases every 3–4 minutes), hypertension, acidosis, hypoxemia, hyperkalemia, and cardiac dysrhythmias may all be seen. Initial management steps are summarized in Table 24.5. Management includes discontinuance of all inhaled agents and succinylcholine (SCh), hyperventilation with 100% oxygen, administration of dantrolene (2.5 mg/kg i.v.), cooling techniques, and $NaHCO_3$ administration. Efforts should be

TABLE 24.5

Initial Management of Malignant Hyperthermia

- Early suspicion and recognition
- Termination of the surgical procedure
- Discontinue anesthetic agents
- Administer 100% oxygen
- Hyperventilation
- Dantrolene 2.5 mg/kg i.v. every 5 minutes up to a total of 10 mg/kg as needed until symptoms abate
- Administration of bicarbonate as guided by blood gases
- Aggressive cooling methods including gastric lavage
- Maintenance of brisk urine output
- Consider central venous access
- Monitor for arrhythmias
- Monitor electrolytes and arterial blood gases
- Monitor coagulation studies

made to induce and continue diuresis through fluid and mannitol administration. Termination of the surgical procedure should be seriously considered until the MH has been treated. Increased heat production from cells and increased metabolic rate increases the production of carbon dioxide and acidosis develops. Significant muscle breakdown and rhabdomyolysis may induce acute tubular necrosis and renal failure.

The mainstay of MH treatment is the administration of dantrolene. Dantrolene is a muscle relaxant that will completely reverse all of the clinical signs of MH. It is unique because it operates within the muscle cell by reducing intracellular calcium levels. This may be the result of reduced sarcoplasmic reticulum calcium release with inhibition of excitation contracture coupling. Dantrolene and supplies for its administration should be maintained wherever general anesthesia is delivered or where SCh is administered.

Once a patient has had either a highly suspicious event or a confirmed episode of MH, they should be considered MH susceptible. A detailed history of the event should be obtained during the preanesthestic evaluation. All patients should be questioned regarding family history of adverse reactions to anesthesia, as the occurrence of an MH episode in a direct relative is an indicator of MH susceptibility. Consideration should be given to contracture testing or possibly genetic testing in patients who have an uncertain clinical picture or family history. The economics involved in these tests in light of safe, accepted nontriggering anesthetic techniques, makes the decision to test for MH more complicated for both the physician and the patient. During future anesthetic interventions, triggering agents should be avoided and a high level of vigilance should be maintained for early signs of MH. Pretreatment of susceptible patients with dantrolene is no longer recommended as it may only mask symptoms of MH until the patients are out of a monitored setting. One very controversial issue regarding MH susceptible patients is outpatient surgery. Decisions and

policies regarding this issue should be made by consultation between the patient, the anesthesiologist, and the surgical specialist. MH-susceptible patients may undergo anesthesia safely if appropriate steps are taken and proper perioperative management is implemented.

Intravenous Agents

The intravenous anesthetics may be classified as hypnotics, dissociative anesthetics, benzodiazepines, and opioids. These drugs are used as induction agents, maintenance agents, and primary anesthetics as well as sedatives to augment regional or general anesthesia.

The goal of anesthetic induction is to provide a physiologically and psychologically stress-free state. Anesthesia management thereby encompasses the proper pharmacologic recipe, which is tailored to the patient's physiologic state and the anticipated surgical procedure. Induction is most commonly accomplished by the inhalational or intravenous route. Clinically useful induction agents are typically drugs with a rapid onset and short duration of action.

Barbiturates

Barbiturates are the classic intravenous induction drugs. Barbiturates are substituted barbituric acid compounds with the sulfur substituted or thiobarbiturates being the most common in clinical anesthesia practice. Thiobarbiturates produce a sleep state with a rapid return to consciousness secondary to redistribution. Thiobarbiturates cause a decrease in BP due to a negative inotropic effect and an increase in venous capacitance. A compensatory increase in HR maintains CO in well-hydrated, healthy patients. In patients unable to produce an increase in HR such as the elderly or patients on β blockers, the decrease in CO and BP may be severe. Barbiturates cause respiratory depression by affecting the medullary ventilatory centers. A large bolus dose of barbiturates, such as thiopental, leads to apnea whereas smaller doses can result in a slow, shallow breathing pattern.

Propofol

Propofol is an isopropyl phenol induction drug that is very popular in anesthetic practice. The sedative-hypnotic effects of propofol are very quick and a return to consciousness reflects not only redistribution but also rapid metabolism by hepatic and extrahepatic sites. The cardiovascular effects of propofol include a decrease in BP due to an increase in venous capacitance and a negative inotropic effect in some patients. Propofol also interferes with compensatory baroreceptor reflexes. Propofol, like thiopental, can cause profound respiratory depression. Owing to rapid metabolism and the lack of a cumulative drug effect, propofol has gained popularity as an intravenous general anesthetic alternative to inhalational agents. It is the drug of choice for maintenance of anesthesia for patients that are susceptible to MH. It is also commonly used for sedation of patients undergoing short procedures not requiring general anesthesia.

Etomidate

Etomidate is an intravenous induction agent with a carboxylated imidazole structure, chemically unrelated to other sedative-hypnotics. Clinically, etomidate is used when there is concern over the negative inotropic effects of thiopental and propofol. Etomidate is considered to be cardiovascularly stable with minimal effects on CO in standard doses. The respiratory effects of etomidate are similar to thiopental. An interesting concern about etomidate is the potential for adrenal suppression. Adrenal suppression is not believed to be clinically important if a single dose of etomidate is used.

Ketamine

Ketamine is a dissociative analgesic and anesthetic which is structurally similar to phencyclidine. *In vitro*, ketamine is a negative inotrope, but due to an *in vivo* release of NE at sympathetic terminals, ketamine has a positive or neutral inotropic effect clinically. The sympathomimetic effects of ketamine may not be expressed in catecholamine-depleted patients such as victims of massive trauma, and therefore the negative inotropic effects may be expressed. Ketamine may cause an increase in PVR, which may not be desirable in certain patients. Ketamine has favorable effects on the respiratory system in that it produces bronchodilation and maintenance of spontaneous respiration. The effect of ketamine on the CNS is a potential towards increased intracranial pressure, although this is not believed to be important in the presence of normocapnia. Ketamine may produce unusual skeletal muscle movements despite a state of unconsciousness. Ketamine is not used commonly as an intravenous induction agent due to associated dysphoria and postoperative hallucinations.

Opioids

Opioids include both synthetic and naturally occurring compounds that exert an effect on opioid receptors. Several opioid receptors have been described with their associated clinical effects. The degree of agonism or antagonism on the various receptors determines the clinical profile of the drug. Narcotics have a relatively stable cardiovascular profile with the exception of the mild negative inotropic and anticholinergic effects of meperidine. The respiratory effects of narcotics are characterized by a slow and deep respiratory pattern and apnea in higher doses. Opioids may be used as induction drugs in patients with cardiovascular instability or as adjuvants in an anesthetic to supplement analgesia or to blunt sympathetic responses. Troublesome side effects of narcotics include diminished bowel function, pruritus, and nausea and vomiting.

Benzodiazepines

Benzodiazepines are rarely used as induction agents in modern anesthetic practice. Benzodiazepines are used extensively as part of a preoperative medication regimen or as a supplemental amnestic during general anesthesia or sedation. Benzodiazepines are relatively cardiovascularly stable and have minimal effects on respiration, except in large dosages or when combined with other CNS depressants.

Neuromuscular Blocking Agents

The use of a drug to produce neuromuscular blockade is a part of the anesthetic plan in the daily administration of general anesthesia. Use of neuromuscular blocking agents allows the patient to be maintained at lighter levels of general anesthesia, which translates to patient safety. Neuromuscular blocking agents do not have sedative or analgesic properties. They exert their effects at the neuromuscular junction and not in the CNS.

Neuromuscular Function

A motor unit consists of a single nerve fiber, with its branches innervating many muscle fibers so that muscular contraction occurs in an organized manner. Electrochemical balance in the resting state is such that a high concentration of extracellular sodium ions (Na^+) and intercellular potassium ions (K^+) exists. Balance is maintained through the Na^+/K^+ pump, so that the resting membrane potential is approximately -90 mV. When stimulation takes place, Na^+ channels open, causing the nerve membrane to become selectively permeable to Na^+. Reversal in polarity of the action potential occurs when Na^+ channels close and K^+ channels open, returning the transmembrane potential to its resting level. During this period, the nerve membrane is refractory to additional excitation.

There is a junctional gap between motor nerve endings and muscle motor endplates of approximately 50 nm. When an action potential reaches a nerve ending, a neurotransmitter is released from vesicles into the junctional gap, carrying the electrical stimulation to nicotinic cholinergic receptors on the motor endplate. Muscle contraction is thereby produced. ACh is synthesized from choline and acetylcoenzyme A (acetyl-CoA) in the axoplasm of the nerve terminal. Choline acetylase catalyzes the reaction. Under normal conditions, the amount of ACh released is approximately five times that required to induce muscular contraction. Calcium ions (Ca^{2+}) must be present to aid in the release of ACh and receptor activation. Cyclic adenosine monophosphate (AMP) serves as a cofactor in the synthesis and storage of ACh in nerve terminals and may play a role in ACh release.

The inactivation of ACh occurs in the junctional cleft between nerve and muscle. Acetylcholinesterase (AChE) inactivates ACh by hydrolyzing it to choline and acetate. Choline is then captured by the nerve terminal for synthesis of new ACh.

Muscle contraction occurs when its nerve is stimulated, allowing movement of Na^+ into the cell. This causes depolarization of the membrane (creating a less negative intracellular atmosphere) and generates the action potential. The action potential is propagated along the muscle membrane, initiating Ca^{2+} release from sarcoplasmic reticulum into the sarcoplasm where myosin ATPase activation leads to excitation contraction coupling of the myofilaments. Potency of the muscular contraction depends on successive, summated, and fused muscular contractions rather than the amplitude of individual action potentials.

Pharmacology

Neuromuscular-blocking drugs are classified as either depolarizing or nondepolarizing, depending on the effect at the motor endplates. The clinical effect of these drugs is to produce muscular weakness, which has allowed the term *muscle relaxants* to be used synonymously in anesthesia.

Neuromuscular blockade occurs so that the muscles of ventilation are the last to be paralyzed but also the first to recover. Small facial and hand muscles, trunk, and extremities are blocked before the ventilatory musculature. This is a relevant clinical observation when recovery from neuromuscular blockade is assessed. Clinically, this is evidenced by the difficulty in achieving total diaphragmatic paralysis despite evidence of profound skeletal muscle paralysis.

Depolarizing Muscle Relaxants

Depolarizing muscle relaxants possess chemical structures similar to ACh, but they are resistant to hydrolysis by AChEs. The only depolarizing muscle relaxant used clinically is succinylcholine. SCh is metabolized quickly by plasma cholinesterase, but as mentioned earlier, it is resistant to AChE present at the neuromuscular junction. Depolarizing muscle relaxants achieve their effects by binding to ACh receptors and causing a depolarization of the endplate. Once SCh is bound, motor endplates remain in a state of persistent depolarization. Repolarization does not occur and clinical weakness of the muscle results. Owing to the relative lack of pseudocholinesterase at the neuromuscular junction, metabolism of depolarizing agents is very slow once the drug is bound to the receptor. The bound muscle relaxant does not allow a further depolarization of the endplate and a contraction of the muscle is not possible. The administration of SCh is associated with several side effects including arrhythmias, hyperkalemia, increased intraocular pressure, increased intracranial pressure, and postoperative myalgias. The elevation of plasma potassium after administration of SCh deserves further discussion.

Hyperkalemia

Hyperkalemia may result after administration of depolarizing muscle relaxants under certain circumstances. In normal individuals, depolarization results in an elevation of serum K^+, averaging 0.5 to 1.0 mEq/L. Traumatized or denervated muscle may extrude sufficient K^+ to result in cardiac arrest after injection. This is believed to be due to an increase in extrajunctional receptors for ACh, which allows a greater shift in potassium. Similar rises in serum K^+ have been observed in patients who have sustained large burn injuries. Explanation of the mechanism involved may be the loss of cellular membrane integrity that might interfere with the return of potassium into its intracellular position.

Denervation-type injuries such as quadriplegia or paraplegia are said to result in a proliferation of extrajunctional

cholinergic receptors in response to lack of neural stimulation. Administration of depolarizing muscle relaxants under these conditions results in a large efflux of potassium, which may prove lethal. Patients suffering from upper motor neuron lesions, recent cerebrovascular accidents, or severe Parkinson disease also must be considered at risk as long as the nerve dysfunction remains unresolved. The elective use of depolarizing neuromuscular blocking agents in patients with the earlier mentioned conditions or in patients with serum potassium levels greater than 5.5 mEq/L should be avoided.

Nondepolarizing Muscle Relaxants

Nondepolarizing muscle relaxants act by competitive inhibition of the neuromuscular junction. They work by binding to the postsynaptic cholinergic receptor. This action prevents ACh from activating Na^+ channels so that initiation of an action potential is inhibited. Blockade of Na^+ channels at presynaptic sites may also occur, resulting in impairment of ACh mobilization from synthesis sites to release sites.

The nondepolarizing neuromuscular blocking agents can be divided according to their duration of action. In the moderately long duration of action group are *d*-tubocurarine (*d*Tc), metocurine, pancuronium, and gallamine. Vecuronium, atracurium, and *cis*-atracurium have an intermediate duration of action. Drugs with a rapid onset such as mivacurium and rocuronium have been developed to obviate the need for depolarizing neuromuscular blockers and to minimize side effects. The duration of these rapid acting drugs varies from the short duration of action of mivacurium to the intermediate to long acting effects of rocuronium depending on the dose administered.

The termination of the effect of nondepolarizing muscle relaxants is by metabolism and by competition for receptor sites by ACh. Pharmacologically, the termination or reversal of the effects of nondepolarizing muscle relaxants can be achieved by administering anticholinesterase drugs such as neostigmine or edrophonium. Administration of anticholinesterase drugs causes a decrease in the metabolism of ACh, thereby increasing available ACh at the neuromuscular junction. The ACh at the neuromuscular junction competes with the neuromuscular blocking agent, allowing the strength of muscle contraction to increase. In addition to the effects at the nicotinic sites such as the neuromuscular junction, ACh also exerts its effects at muscarinic sites causing bradycardia and bronchospasm amongst other side effects. In order to prevent muscarinic side effects, anticholinergic agents such as atropine or more commonly glycopyrrolate are administered with the selected anticholinesterase agents. The effects of depolarizing muscle relaxants are not pharmacologically reversible.

Awareness and Recall under General Anesthesia

The topic of awareness and recall under general anesthesia is a significant concern for patients undergoing surgical procedures as well as for the surgeons and anesthesiologists caring for these patients. Awareness occurs when patients become conscious enough during a surgical procedure to allow recall of events or sensations. The surgical specialist may be the first person that the patient informs after a recall event as these memories may not be present even at the time of discharge from the hospital or surgery center. Additionally, patients may question their surgeon before surgery about awareness under anesthesia as this is a frequently publicized complication and a common fear in the public. Fortunately, we believe the incidence of awareness under anesthesia is low with estimates approximately 0.1% to 0.3% (7). Understanding the types of patients and scenarios that put patients at risk can help prevent recall events and possibly alleviate fear in surgical patients.

Preoperatively the anesthesiologist should evaluate patients for predisposing factors such as previous events of anesthesia awareness, poor hemodynamic reserve, use of chronic pain medication, drug abuse, and potential for difficult intubation. In addition to patient factors, certain procedures should raise the index of suspicion for potential intraoperative awareness. These include cardiac surgery, trauma surgery, cesarean section, emergency surgery, reduced anesthetic doses in the presence of paralysis, planned use of muscle relaxants, and planned use of nitrous oxide-opioid technique.

These patients, and possibly all patients, should be informed of the possibility of awareness under anesthesia. After a thorough preoperative evaluation, decisions should be made about the anesthetic technique and the need for additional monitoring. The best defense against awareness is a vigilant, trained anesthesia provider performing a well-planned anesthetic. Routine monitoring and clinical assessment should be performed as in all anesthetics. All standard hemodynamic monitors should be routinely maintained and in proper working order. Anesthesia delivery systems such as pumps and vaporizers should also be calibrated and maintained appropriately and in working order before use during a procedure. Basic clinical monitoring of reflexes and hemodynamic responses should be followed for any signs of increased levels of consciousness during anesthesia. Postoperatively all patients should be interviewed for any signs or symptoms of anesthetic side effects or complications including awareness. If a patient reports awareness of any type, hospital staff and physicians should reconsult an anesthesiologist so that the patient can be evaluated and appropriately counseled as needed. Development of post-traumatic stress disorder has been described, and without reassurance and treatment, patients who have suffered a recall event may refuse future necessary surgery.

Recently, CNS monitors have been developed and are in use to assess the depth of anesthesia or level of consciousness. The use of these monitors is not standard and research is yet to confirm their effectiveness in preventing awareness under anesthesia (8). The Bispectral Index or BIS by Aspect Medical Systems is a summated frontal nonevoked EEG which is common in clinical use. The BIS utilizes an algorithm to convert EEG informational into a digital representation

of level of consciousness. BIS values are scaled from 1 to 100 with values of less than 60 representing a low level of awareness. The American Society of Anesthesiologists (ASA) states that a brain electrical activity monitor, such as the BIS should be used to assess intraoperative anesthesia depth in cases with patients with conditions or anesthetic techniques used that may place them at higher risk for intraoperative awareness (9). The ASA has not recommended the standard use of CNS monitors such as the BIS.

CONDUCTION ANESTHESIA

Pharmacodynamics

Most of the cells in the human body exhibit electrical potentials across cell membranes. Nerve fiber cells or neurons have the ability to develop and propagate changes in membrane potential down a cell length allowing signals to be carried. Through active and passive processes, a relatively negative ionic state is present within the interior of the cell as opposed to the exterior. Most of this potential may be attributed to potassium ions with smaller contribution from the distribution of sodium and chloride ions. Despite the importance of the potassium ion, it is the sodium ion and its channels that are best understood. When a nerve cell membrane reaches a threshold potential, sodium ion channels open and allow passive movement of the ion down its gradient. The result is a positive membrane potential due to the increase of intracellular sodium ions and the very slow efflux of potassium ions. If the depolarization is significant enough to be transmitted to nearby membrane segments resulting in an action potential propagating down the fiber. If the depolarization is not enough to trigger nearby membrane segments to also depolarize, the potential is not propagated. This is referred to as the *all or none phenomenon*. Drugs with local anesthetic properties exert their effects on the sodium channel by blocking the flux of sodium ions, and if a significant concentration of local anesthetic is present, an action potential does not develop.

The specific characteristics of the nerve fiber including diameter and presence of myelin were believed to influence the susceptibility of the nerve to blockade. It was traditionally asserted that smaller, myelinated fibers are blocked first. This has been challenged by studies involving single isolated nerve preparations (10,11). The differential functional susceptibility of nerve fibers may relate to the anatomic position of the nerve (12). Clinically, it has been noted that blockade of sympathetic and sensory fibers can be achieved with lower concentrations of local anesthetic solutions as opposed to blockade of fibers that carry motor impulses and proprioception. This is demonstrated by noting that patients often report sensing pressure but not pain during procedures performed using local anesthetic agents.

Communication along human peripheral nerves is encoded digitally as a temporal series of transient, localized membrane polarity reversals (depolarization). The depolarization is propagated along axonal membranes at speeds of

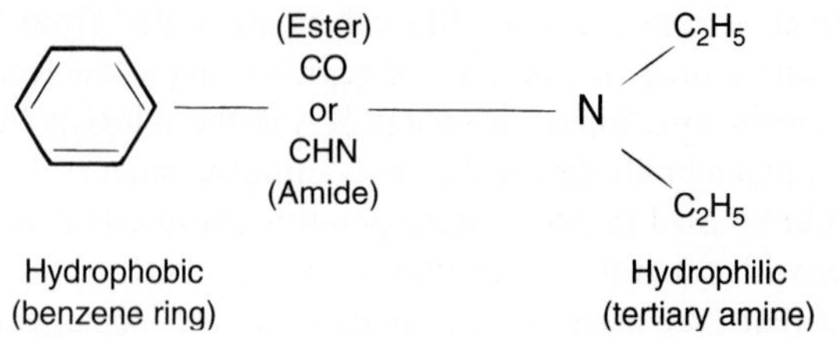

FIGURE 24.4   Chemical structure of a typical local anesthetic.

between 0.5 and 130 m/s. Impulses travel inward from the periphery along sensory nerve axons and outward from the cord along neuroeffector (including motor) axons. At the molecular level, membrane depolarization is linked to the movement of ions, especially sodium, across the nerve membrane through specialized pores, or channels. Local anesthetic drugs block these pores and, when present in sufficient concentration, prevent both propagation of electrical nerve impulses and the messages (including pain) they encode. Catastrophic complications from local anesthetic drug administration result when these drugs exert their membrane-stabilizing effects on the wrong excitable tissues, such as the brain, heart, and cervical spinal cord.

Chemistry

Organic compounds with many different chemical structures exert local anesthetic activity *in vitro* and *in vivo*. Only a few are sufficiently safe and effective to be clinically useful. The chemical structure of most commercially available local anesthetic drugs includes one hydrophilic terminal (usually a tertiary amine) and one hydrophobic terminal (usually a substituted benzene ring) (Fig. 24.4). The two terminals are connected by either an ester or an amide group. The nature of the linkage allows these drugs to be classified as either esters or amides. The amides include lidocaine, bupivacaine, mepivacaine, ropivacaine, etidocaine, and prilocaine. These drugs are metabolized by hepatic enzymes and are not usually associated with allergic reactions. Ester local anesthetics include procaine, chloroprocaine, and tetracaine. These drugs are metabolized by ester hydrolysis in the plasma and to a lesser extent in the liver. Ester metabolism may be associated with the formation of para-aminobenzoic acid (PABA), which acts as an antigen potentially leading to allergic reactions. Owing to the more complex nature of the metabolism of amide local anesthetics, these drugs are metabolized slower and are associated with more systemic side effects.

Pharmacokinetics

Local Diffusion

Several factors influence the pharmacokinetics of local anesthetics. The first factor in local anesthetic activity is getting the local anesthetic to the site of action. Some are active topically whereas others must be injected directly in the area of activity. Once local anesthetic molecules reach the nerve, they must diffuse across nerve membranes. Most local anesthetics are weak bases and exist at physiologic pH

in the ionized nonlipid soluble state. Although this ionized form is the active form of the drug, it cannot diffuse to its site of action. Ideally, the local anesthetics would be injected into an area with a pH higher than 7.4 in order to increase the amount of drug that may diffuse across cell membranes. This has led to the use of bicarbonate solutions in some commercially available local anesthetic preparations. Areas of lower pH such as infected or ischemic tissue are resistant to local anesthetic effects do to the predominance of the ionized form of the compound. Therefore, the onset of local anesthetic activity is dependant on the pK_a of the drug.

Two other principles of local anesthetic activity that are important to the clinician are potency and duration of action. Potency refers to amount of drug necessary to achieve a desired effect. Potency of local anesthetics is directly related to the lipid solubility of the drug. The duration of local anesthetics is related to several factors such as location of injection and use of vasoconstrictors in the solution, but it also appears to be related to the degree of protein binding. Presumably the highly protein-bound molecules of local anesthetic attach themselves to proteins within the cell membrane and lengthen the duration of action. The addition of a vasoconstrictor to local anesthetic injections leads to a decrease in the blood flow available to the affected area and thereby decreases washout of drug from the area. Use of vasoconstrictors increases the mass of drug that can be injected before toxic side effects are noted. Addition of vasoconstrictors also leads to a decrease in surgical blood loss from the affected area.

Termination of drug action results from redistribution away from the relevant nerve membranes. Mass of drug injected, site of injection, physical characteristics of the local anesthetics and the perfusion of the tissue involved influence the absorption of the drug into circulation and metabolism. The following classification of the commonly used agents is based on duration of action: short acting (procaine, chloroprocaine); intermediate acting (lidocaine, mepivacaine); and long acting (bupivacaine, ropivicaine, etidocaine, and tetracaine).

Systemic Absorption and Metabolism

The molecules of all administered local anesthetics (with the possible exception of benzocaine, which is absorbed poorly) eventually reach the systemic circulation. The time interval between local anesthetic administration and peak blood level is highly variable and depends on the anatomic site of application.

Metabolism of commercially available ester-linked local anesthetics occurs predominantly within the bloodstream by plasma cholinesterase. Amide-linked local anesthetics are metabolized primarily in the liver. Large or repeated doses of these drugs must be given with great caution to patients with reduced hepatic function.

Hazards of Local Anesthetic Administration

There are two common misconceptions related to the use of local anesthetics. The first is that the use of local anesthetics and regional anesthesia is safer than general anesthesia. The other is the association of local anesthetics with allergic reactions. Patients will often state that they are allergic to local anesthetics because they had palpitations or tinnitus associated with injection of local anesthetics. This most often results from either an intravascular injection of local anesthetic or an inappropriately high dose of local anesthetic used. The exact toxicity of the individual local anesthetics relates to the potency and lipid solubility of the drug. However, even the safest local anesthetics in the wrong dosage or injected into the wrong location can be potentially lethal. Complications arise from elevated plasma levels as a result of direct intravascular injection or inappropriate dosing. Catastrophic side effects may also result from unexpected and unintended injection of local anesthetic into epidural and subarachnoid spaces producing total spinal anesthesia. Another potential complication to local anesthetic injection is direct needle-induced neurovascular trauma. True allergic reactions to local anesthetics may also occur. These are usually associated with ester anesthetics as previously discussed. Allergic reactions may be due to the presence of methylparaben or preservatives used in local anesthetic packaging. Patients known to be allergic to ester local anesthetics will not necessarily be reactive to amide local anesthetics. However, care should be taken with the use of amide local anesthetics from multidose vials or those containing preservatives, as these may be the culprits. The exact nature of the patient's reaction should also be elicited to determine the presence of a true allergic reaction as noted earlier. Clinically significant methemoglobinemia has been reported after administration of benzocaine, especially in children.

Recognition and Treatment of Systemic Toxicity
Dangerously elevated concentrations of drugs in the blood can occur after inadvertent intravascular injection of local anesthetics. Toxic blood levels can also arise from absolute drug overdose even when proper injection techniques are used. In the former case, symptoms and signs of toxicity occur immediately. In the latter case, symptoms and signs of toxicity may be delayed for 45 minutes.

A grand mal seizure, coma, apnea, or cardiovascular collapse may be the initial manifestation of systemic toxicity. Often patients complain of sudden wooziness or drowsiness, sometimes accompanied by tinnitus, auditory distortions, or a metallic taste. These ominous symptoms and signs should never be discounted, as they may be harbingers of potentially catastrophic side effects such as seizures or cardiac arrest. The presence of symptoms and signs of toxicity should result in the immediate discontinuation of drug administration until the presence of systemic toxic reaction can be excluded conclusively. At higher plasma levels, local anesthetics produce direct myocardial depression and depression of electrical automaticity of the conduction system of the heart. Support of ventilation and the cardiovascular system are required frequently and resuscitative efforts may be prolonged. In addition to

standard resuscitative and supportive measures, intralipid infusions have also been used successfully in humans to treat local anesthetic toxicity (13). Even when drug doses are weighted for intrinsic potency, the longer-acting agents appear to be more cardiotoxic than either intermediate or short-acting agents.

Prevention of systemic toxicity depends on avoiding unintentional intravascular injection and keeping total drug dosages within recommended guidelines. Knowledge of, and adherence to, safe dosing ranges based on patient weight should be integral to the injection of local anesthetics. Staying within these ranges and performing slow injections with frequent aspirations should serve to prevent potential side effects. It should be highlighted that just because the dose of local anesthetic is within the "safe" range, patients may still experience severe side effects. One strategy to prevent systemic toxicity is to monitor patient pulse and use epinephrine-containing solutions with temporal fractionation. An increase in HR of 20 beats per minute or more within 30 to 60 seconds of injection of 3 to 4 mL of local anesthetic with 5 μg/mL epinephrine (1:200,000) strongly suggests the occurrence of intravascular injection. Patients with heart disease, with implanted cardiac pacemakers, or taking β antagonists may not demonstrate HR increase.

Neuraxial Blockade (Spinal and Epidural)
Neuraxial blockade refers to the placement of local anesthetic in the epidural or subarachnoid space. These techniques are not only technically more difficult than subcutaneous blocks, but the potential for side effects is increased. Dosages of local anesthetic used to produce these blocks are significantly different from each other and the placement of an epidural dose in the subarachnoid space will produce serious and potentially lethal consequences. Just as in other injection sites, the effect of the local anesthetic is dependent on the volume and concentration of the drug and ultimately on the mass of the drug administered.

Physiologic Effects
In the setting of surgical anesthesia, blockade of pain and motor fibers are sought from neuraxial anesthesia. A fortuitous side effect is the decreased blood loss and decreased incidence of deep vein thrombosis from the performance of neuraxial blockade in certain types of procedures. Sympathetic fibers are blocked most easily and the dermatomal level of their blockade and blockade of fibers responsible for temperature sensation usually exceeds sensory (pain) blockade by as much as two dermatomes. Sensory (pain) blockade in turn usually exceeds motor blockade by approximately two dermatomes. This is important clinically as the physician must realize that the level of sympathetic blockade may exceed the apparent level of pain control. The blockade of sympathetic fibers causes a decrease in preload to the heart by increasing venous capacitance and to a lesser extent by decreasing SVR. The resulting decrease in CO and BP may be marked in patients with uncorrected hypovolemia and as a result, these patients

are poor candidates for neuraxial blockade. The presence of epinephrine in the injected local anesthetic may lead to a more profound degree of hypotension. This is believed to be due to epinephrine-induced stimulation of β_2-adrenergic receptors, which results in peripheral vascular bed vasodilation. If the level of sympathetic blockade rises into the high thoracic dermatomes, blockade of the cardioaccelerator fibers may occur resulting in bradycardia and resultant further decreases in cardiac BPs.

In order to protect patients against the effects of hypotension from neuraxial blockade, a volume preload is administered before the onset of the block. The exact volume of the preload should be tailored to the patient and the ability to handle an increased intravascular volume. Upon resolution of the sympathetic blockade, the intravascular volume necessary to maintain stable hemodynamics may result in relative volume overload and symptoms of cardiac failure. This need for temporary increased intravascular volume in patients undergoing neuraxial blockade may be a potential drawback to using these techniques in patients with compromised cardiac function. That being said, patients with cardiac failure often have improvement in symptoms as a result of the decreased preload during the effective period of the blockade.

The effects of neuraxial blockade on respiration depend upon the level of blockade and the hemodynamic effects seen. The decrease in BP discussed earlier may result in hypoperfusion of medullary ventilatory centers leading to respiratory distress or apnea. The administration of volume or the use of vasoconstrictors will increase BP and medullary perfusion resolving the respiratory embarrassment. In addition to this phenomenon, a high thoracic or cervical blockade can lead to motor blockade of the intercostal muscles, abdominal musculature, and accessory muscles of respiration. Phrenic nerve blockade may also result from high dermatomal levels of blockade. These effects may be longer lasting than medullary hypoperfusion and may require immediate intubation and positive pressure ventilation. Owing to the very rapid development of problems and the potential for serious complications during the performance of neuraxial blockade, the availability of resuscitation equipment should always be confirmed. This includes all of the necessary equipment for endotracheal intubation.

Regional blood flow depends on the level of blockade and presence of hypotension. Little effect on cerebral, cardiac, renal, or hepatic perfusion is found when sensory levels of blockade do not exceed the T-10 dermatome. At higher dermatomal levels, decreases in blood flow to these organs may occur especially when BP is below the autoregulatory range. Myocardial oxygen demand is decreased because of afterload reduction (arterial vasodilation), preload reduction (decreased venous return), and decreased HR (block of cardiac accelerator fibers). A marked increase in blood flow in the lower extremities occurs with spinal and epidural anesthesia.

The use of neuraxial blockade may produce a decrease in the stress response to surgery. In addition, blockade of afferent pathways may allow better postoperative pain control due to preemptive analgesia. The extent to which this occurs appears to be dependent on the location of the surgical procedure relative to the dermatomal level of the blockade.

PAIN MANAGEMENT

Pain management in the surgical patient is one of the most important tasks a physician accomplishes; yet patients often recall periods of inadequate postoperative pain relief. For many patients, pain and disability postoperatively is more frightening than even mortality. Physicians, nurses, and health care institutions have responded to this by setting a goal of making assessment of pain as common as measurement of vital signs through the use of various pain scale scores. Unlike vital sign measurement, pain assessment is very difficult due to the many psychosocial factors that affect patients' experiences and expectations regarding pain. Medical and nursing education has improved to include effective pain management strategies, but clearly more work has to be done.

Anatomic and Physical Basis of Pain

Tissue damage such as that from surgery causes a release of prostaglandins, histamine, bradykinin, serotonin, and substance P. In addition to the release of these substances, peripheral nociceptors are activated. Nociceptors are unencapsulated nerve endings that discharge when noxious stimuli threaten or produce injury. Information is transmitted to the spinal cord through A delta and C nerve fibers where modulation takes place. These small primary afferents enter the spinal cord primarily in the lateral portion of the dorsal root, and then bifurcate into rostral and caudal branches. The nociceptor signal is then relayed to projection cells for transmission to the brain. Individual pathways in the anterolateral cord presumed to be responsible for pain transmission are the spinothalamic, spinoreticular, and spinomesencephalic tracts.

From the earlier description it should be evident that pain treatment may be geared toward one or more of the steps in the pathway of pain. Nonsteroidal anti-inflammatory drugs such as ketorolac and the newer agents such as cyclooxygenase 2 inhibitors can be used to modulate the release and effects of analgesic substances such as prostaglandins. Local anesthetics may be injected regionally or at the site of the incision to block transmission of pain impulses to the spinal cord. In addition, opioids may be administered for their agonist effect on central opioid receptors. Multimodal approaches utilizing combinations of these agents or techniques has gained acceptance.

Opioids include naturally occurring and synthetic compounds that exert effects on opioid receptors. The nature of the interaction classifies the drugs as agonists, antagonists and mixed agonist/antagonists. Several types of opioid receptors have been identified. The degree of agonism or antagonism of each receptor gives the drug its clinical profile. Opioid receptors include μ, κ, σ, and δ. The μ receptors mediate supraspinal analgesia, miosis, respiratory depression, and opioid withdrawal syndrome. The κ receptors mediate spinal analgesia but not opioid withdrawal. The σ receptors mediate pupillary dilatation, tachypnea, and dysphoria. The δ receptors modulate effects of the μ response. Visceral pain may be more responsive to μ-receptor agonists, whereas cutaneous (somatic) pain responds best to κ-receptor agonists.

Difficulty arises in predicting the response of patients to narcotics and in balancing adequate pain relief with systemic side effects. This has led to the development and utilization of nonopioid pain medications such as nonsteroidal anti-inflammatory agents. The administration of the anti-inflammatory agents through the oral or intravenous route, and the use of local anesthetics either in the epidural space, regionally, or directly into the incision site, has gained acceptance as an alternative to narcotic pain control.

Techniques

Intravenous Narcotics

Individual responses to parenteral narcotics are difficult to predict. Small intravenous doses of narcotics have been shown to provide satisfactory pain relief as opposed to the traditional intramuscular injection. Patient-controlled analgesia (PCA) mechanisms have gained acceptance due to patient satisfaction, as well as staffing time and personnel limitations. Administration of intravenous narcotics by PCA pumps allows the physician to program a prescribed dose of narcotic to be administered on patient demand within the limitations of a lockout time and an hourly maximum. Occasionally, the physician may choose to administer a basal rate of narcotic in addition to the patient controlled doses. This should be reserved for unique cases, as excessive sedation and overdose are potential complications. PCA pumps should be adjusted according to patient input as to adequacy of pain control and use of the pump. Benefits of PCA pain control are that patients require less narcotics and they are also exposed to smaller bolus doses of narcotics.

Intrathecal and Epidural Narcotics

The highly specific opioid receptors (μ) are located in high concentrations in the lamina I and II of the substantia gelatinosa. These areas coincide with termination areas for nociceptive fibers. Most opioids act at these receptor sites to inhibit release of substance P, a neurotransmitter of nociceptive stimuli. Numerous studies have demonstrated the efficacy of both epidural and intrathecal narcotics in the control of pain. For postsurgical control of pain, continuous or intermittent administration of epidural narcotics has gained acceptance. In addition to the complications associated with the technique of epidural placement, administration of epidural narcotics may lead to respiratory depression, pruritus, nausea, and urinary retention. Owing to the relatively small doses of narcotics administered

into the epidural space, sedation is minimized allowing better respiratory function. Additional benefits of epidural or intrathecal pain management are decreased pulmonary complications and reduced intensive care unit and hospital stay.

Epidural narcotics such as morphine may be administered at the lumbar level despite thoracic levels of surgical intervention. This is attributed to the hydrophilic nature of morphine which allows the drug to spread in a cephalad direction. This same phenomenon explains the delayed respiratory depression seen with morphine when given into the epidural space (14). This is the late phase of the biphasic respiratory depression associated with epidural morphine. The first phase is within the first hour and is due to intravascular absorption or injection. Cephalad spread of morphine can produce a second phase of respiratory depression, sometimes severe enough to produce apnea, as late as 12 to 24 hours following injection. Apnea may result from epidural injection of morphine. This phenomenon does not occur with the injection of more lipid soluble narcotics such as fentanyl. Fentanyl injected into the epidural space will not spread cephalad but will remain at the site of injection. In addition to bolus injection or continuous infusion of epidural narcotics, patient-controlled epidural analgesia (PCEA) has gained acceptability. The combination of a narcotic such as morphine and a weak concentration of a local anesthetic can be set up as a continuous infusion with the capability of the patient to administer a small bolus as necessary. PCEA has the same beneficial effects of PCA with regards to staffing needs and patient satisfaction.

Intrathecal analgesia may be accomplished by a variety of drugs, but single-dose morphine or fentanyl is used most commonly. Intrathecal dosing of narcotics is not as predictable as epidural administration. In addition, intrathecal administration of narcotics, unless through an intrathecal catheter, is not useful as a long-term acute pain regimen.

Side effects of both epidural and intrathecal methods include pruritus, nausea, and vomiting, urinary retention, and respiratory depression. Small doses of naloxone or nalbuphine will control these problems without disturbance in pain relief. Epidural or intrathecal narcotics do not disturb motor sensory and sympathetic function. If local anesthetic mixtures are used for pain control, very small concentrations of local anesthetic should be used to minimize muscle weakness and cardiovascular side effects.

Other Pain Management Strategies

Other methods of pain relief include catheters placed through the interscalene or axillary approach for upper extremity analgesia and intercostal nerve block or intrapleural instillation of local anesthetics for thoracic procedures. In patients undergoing hip and lower extremity procedures, lumbar plexus, femoral, and sciatic single shot or continuous nerve blocks can be performed. The advancement of available equipment including the development of nerve stimulating catheters and the use of ultrasonography in peripheral nerve blocks as well as the increased emphasis on training in these techniques during residency programs in anesthesiology, has increased the prevalence of peripheral nerve blockade for postoperative pain control. The availability of relatively inexpensive disposable infusion pumps has also increased the use of continuous peripheral nerve blocks for pain control in outpatient orthopedic procedures. Continuous peripheral nerve blocks offer the benefit of pain control with no sedative effects, minimal cardiovascular side effects, and improved bowel function. Side effects include direct neural trauma during performance of the blockade, complications due to use of local anesthetics, and possibly, injury to the affected area while it is insensate.

REFERENCES

1. Sonner JM, Antognini JF, Dutton RC, et al. Inhaled anesthetics and immobility: mechanisms, mysteries, and minimum alveolar anesthetic concentration. *Anesth Analg* 2003;97(3):718–740.
2. Gelman SI. Disturbances in hepatic blood flow during anesthesia and surgery. *Arch Surg* 1976;111:881–883.3
3. Subcommittee on the National Halothane Study of the Committee on Anesthesia. National Academy of Sciences-National Research Council. Summary of the National Halothane Study. Possible association between halothane anesthesia and postoperative necrosis. *JAMA* 1966;197:775–788.
4. Mauermann WJ, Nemergut EC. The anesthesiologist's role in the prevention of surgical site infections. *Anesthesiology* 2006;105(2):413–421.
5. Treschan TA, Peters J, Warltier DC. The vasopressin system: physiology and clinical strategies. *Anesthesiology* 2006;105(3):599–612.
6. Ozaki M, Sessler DI, Suziki H, et al. The threshold for thermoregulatory vasoconstriction during nitrous oxide/sevoflurane anesthesia is reduced in elderly patients. *Anesth Analg* 1997;84:1029–1033.
7. Sebel PS, Bowdle TA, Ghoneim MM, et al. The incidence of awareness during anesthesia: a multicenter United States study. *Anesth Analg* 2004;99(3):833–839.
8. Rampersad SE, Mulroy MF. A case of awareness despite an "adequate depth of anesthesia" as indicated by a Bispectral Index Monitor. *Anesth Analg* 2005;100(5):1361–1362.
9. American Society of Anesthesiologists Task Force on Intraoperative Awareness. Practice advisory for intraoperative awareness and brain function monitoring. *Anesthesiology* 2006;104:847–864.
10. Fink B, Cairns A. Differential slowing and block of conduction by lidocaine in individual afferent myelinated and unmyelinated axons. *Anesthesiology* 1984;60:111–120.
11. Fink B, Cairns A. Lack of size-related differential sensitivity to equilibrium conduction block along mammalian myelinated axons exposed to lidocaine. *Anesth Analg* 1987;66:948–953.
12. Raymond SA, Steffensen SC, Gugino LD, et al. The role of length of nerve exposed to local anesthetics in impulse blocking action. *Anesth Analg* 1989;68:563–570.
13. Rosenblatt MA, Abel M, Fischer GW, et al. Successful use of a 20% lipid emulsion to resuscitate a patient after a presumed bupivacaine-related cardiac arrest. *Anesthesiology* 2006;105(1):217–218.
14. Kafer ER, Brown J, Scott D, et al. Biphasic depression of ventilatory responses to CO_2 following epidural morphine. *Anesthesiology* 1983;58:418–427.

SUGGESTED READINGS

Barash PG, Cullen BF, Stoelting RK, eds. *Clinical anesthesia*, 5th ed. Philadelphia: Lippincott Williams& Wilkins, 2005.

Miller RD, ed. *Miller's anesthesia*, 6th ed. Philadelphia: Churchill Livingstone, 2000.

Stoelting RK. *Pharmacology and physiology in anesthesia practice*, 4th ed. Philadelphia: Lippincott Williams& Wilkins, 2005.

Stoelting RK, Dierdorf SF. *Anesthesia and co-existing disease*, 4thed. Churchill Livingstone, 2002.

CHAPTER 25

Physiologic Changes Of Aging

Walter E. Pofahl, II and Ronnie A. Rosenthal

Over the last two-and-a-half decades alone, the proportion of the surgical population older than 65 in the United States has nearly doubled (19%–37%), whereas, the general population older than 65 has increased by only a little more than 1% (11.3%–12.4%). This impressive increase is the result of a combination of positive changes; surgery and anesthesia have become safer, and lifestyle modification and medical advances have led to healthier, longer lives. With these changes, referring physicians and patients have become more willing to consider surgery as a therapeutic option. In the next 25 years, thanks in large part to the aging of the baby boomer generation, the older population in the United States is expected to increase dramatically, reaching 20% of the general population, or 69 million persons, by 2030. Of these, approximately 8.5 million will be older than 85. It is very likely that by the middle of the next decade, most patients in most adult surgical practices will be well over 65 years of age.

It is essential, therefore, that surgeons understand the impact of aging on the physiologic parameters that govern the responses to surgical stress. Acquiring this knowledge, however, is made more difficult by the fact that aging clearly progresses at different rates in different individuals. The results of studies of physiologic decline in "healthy aging" may be confounded by subtle changes. Even in the absence of overt disease, alterations attributed to "aging," such as modest cognitive deterioration or changes in blood glucose metabolism may not necessarily be "normal." The impact of aging on an individual's ability to respond to stress is actually determined by the combination of changes directly attributable to aging *per se* and those associated with the diseases that typically accompany aging. Assessing the impact of aging must therefore be determined in each individual rather than using chronologic age alone as the determinant of the degree of decline.

In spite of this difficulty, it is important to understand that aging in general is associated with a progressive loss of those physiologic processes necessary to maintain homeostasis, death being the ultimate failure of these mechanisms. The impact of this loss of function on the outcome of surgery is difficult to quantify. Conceptually, as physiologic reserves decline, whether from "aging" *per se* or from disease, there are

fewer reserves available to meet demand when the individual is stressed. Figure 25.1 is a graphic representation of this concept of "homeostenosis," with the *arrows* representing physiologic stress and the precipice being organ failure or death. In early life, even large physiologic challenges can be met easily without going over the precipice. However, in later life, as physiologic reserves are increasingly employed just to maintain normal homeostasis, a considerably smaller challenge may be sufficient to push a patient over the edge into organ failure or death. The physiologic demands of an uneventful surgical procedure, particularly one designed to improve physiologic function such as coronary artery bypass grafting, can usually be met by all but the most compromised of older persons. However, when demand is increased, either by a long, complicated procedure with extensive tissue injury and excessive blood loss or by a postoperative complication, reserves may well be insufficient.

In the chapter that follows, we will describe some of the physiologic changes that limit reserves in various organ systems and thereby render the older patient at greater risk for poor outcome. A complete discussion of the physiology of aging, including cellular and molecular theories, is beyond the scope of this chapter but interested readers are directed to the annotated references that follow the text.

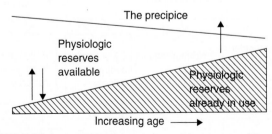

FIGURE 25.1 Graphic representation of the concept of "homeostenosis," with the *arrows* representing physiologic stress and the precipice being organ failure or death. (Reprinted from Taffett, GE. Physiology of aging. In: Cassel CK, Leipzig RM, Cohen HJ, Larson EB, et al. eds. *Geriatric Medicine. An Evidence-Based Approach*, 4th ed. New York: Springer-Verlag, 2003.)

CARDIOVASCULAR

Cardiac complications are the leading postoperative morbidity in elderly patients. This is due to an increased incidence of underlying cardiovascular disease in older patients and the physiologic changes associated with the aging cardiovascular system. The significant changes in the older cardiovascular system include diminished compliance, reduction in maximal heart rate, and diminished early left ventricular early diastolic filling. These changes are summarized in Figure 25.2. Although most older patients adequately compensate for these changes, the physiologic derangements associated with major surgery and any complications can overwhelm the aged cardiovascular system. A thorough understanding of the physiologic changes is important to prevent and treat these complications.

One of the most notable changes associated with aging is an increased resistance to left ventricular ejection (afterload). Changes in aortic and peripheral vascular compliance are due to several factors, including an age-associated decrease in connective tissue compliance and distensibility, primarily due to increasing cross-bridging between elastin and collagen filaments. Other contributing factors include thickening of the aortic intima and media and increased calcification. The resulting aortic dilatation and "stiffening" cause greater resistance to left ventricular ejection, leading to higher peak systolic pressure. This same phenomenon occurs throughout the more distal vascular tree. In addition to systemic vascular resistance, each pulse wave travels through the stiffer vascular tree and is reflected back towards the heart earlier and more strongly than in a young vascular tree. This early and more powerful reflected wave from the periphery, combined with the previously noted structural changes, increases the afterload on the left ventricle. Pulse wave velocity increases twofold to threefold with aging. In young cardiovascular systems, the reflected pulse wave tends to arrive following systole, but in the elderly this component is appended to the end systolic afterload. Standard measurement of blood pressure by forearm sphygmomanometry fails to discern this aspect of pressure as the reflected wave is not retransmitted significantly down the arterial tree.

Structural alterations to the heart and vessels are part of normal aging and affect interpretation of blood pressure and approach to perioperative fluid management. Age-related alteration in aortic-arterial stiffness is one of the most serious normal changes that affect the aging human cardiovascular system. Figure 25.2 depicts the typical alterations of the aging heart as a response to increased afterload. The two primary alterations noted in elderly hearts, *in the absence of disease states and severe deconditioning,* are concentric

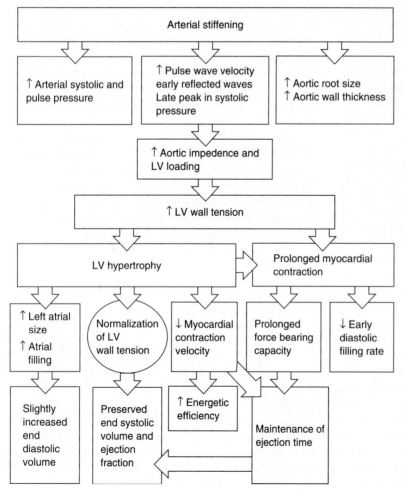

FIGURE 25.2 The essential alterations of the aging heart as a response to increased afterload. LV, left ventricular. (From Abrams WB, Beers MH, Berkow R, eds. *The Merck manual of geriatrics,* 2nd ed. Whitehouse Station: Merck & Co, 1995, with permission.)

left ventricular hypertrophy and a substantial decline in diastolic compliance. The heart appears to be unique in that it does not decrease in size with age as compared to most other organs. Although fewer myocytes are present, there is a general hypertrophy of the cells and a marked increase in connective tissue. Myocardial hypertrophy and increases in connective tissue components, including fibrous tissue, lipids and collagen result in increases in left ventricular wall thickness with age. There is approximately a 30% increase in left ventricle thickness, with intraventricular septal thickness increasing to the greatest extent.

A number of factors, including decreased diastolic compliance, result in a 50% decline in early diastolic ventricular filling in the aged. Myocardial relaxation is dependent on calcium removal from the myocardial cytoplasm into the sarcoplasmic reticulum during diastole, an energy-dependent process that is substantially impaired during aging. There is also a suggestion of decreased mitochondrial oxygen utilization. Finally, a prolonged action potential and isovolemic relaxation time in senescent hearts delays diastolic filling. The importance of atrial contraction to ventricular filling increases from 10% to 30% in elderly subjects. Altered diastolic relaxation causes increased left ventricular end-diastolic pressure, both at rest and during exercise. Higher pressures are generated to achieve the same stroke volume. The aged heart can be exquisitely sensitive to alterations in ventricular preload, particularly loss of the atrial systole, that is, Frank–Starling relations become increasingly important for aged patients. Cardiac output, despite multiple reports of progressive decline with age, is essentially maintained in subjects who are carefully screened for occult disease. Diastolic dysfunction is intrinsic to aging rather than the result of a reduction in aerobic capacity. The nature of the aging cardiac physiology predicts the clinical implications. Diastolic-based cardiac dysfunction has been distinguished from the more commonly recognized systolic dysfunction as a pathophysiology of heart failure.

Although cardiac performance at rest may not be altered, major limitations become obvious during strenuous exercise. Maximum aerobic capacity decreases with age. The presence of even occult coronary artery disease and individual conditioning play important limiting roles. It is possible that age-related alterations in oxidation capacity per unit muscle, ability to shunt blood to exercising muscles, and/or muscle mass could also contribute (Table 25.1).

The basis of adrenergic function is described in detail in chapter 14. As described in the preceding text, in healthy humans in the absence of coronary artery disease, hypertension or severe deconditioning, cardiovascular performance is not significantly altered. However, during significant exercise heart rate increases minimally, whereas stroke volume is maintained or increased. Circulating levels of norepinephrine, but not epinephrine, increase progressively with age without any decrease in β-adrenergic receptor density. β-Adrenergic receptors are G protein–linked and are proposed to exist in at least two states described as high and low affinity states. β-Adrenergic agonist binding affinity

TABLE 25.1

Changes in Healthy Elderly Patients Associated with Vigorous Exercise

Parameter	Change
Oxygen consumption	– –
(A-V)O$_2$	–
Cardiac index	–
Heart rate	–
Stroke volume	0
Preload	+
End diastolic volume	+
Afterload	+
Peripheral vascular resistance	+
End systolic volume	+ + + +
End diastolic volume	+
Contractility	– –
Ejection fraction	–
Plasma catecholamines	+
Cardiovascular responses to catecholamines	–

(A-V)O$_2$, arterial-venous oxygen difference.
Adapted from Lakatta EG. Heart, Lung. *Circulation* 2002;11:76–91.

is significantly decreased with aging in rat myocardium, associated primarily with a decrease in the proportion of receptors in the high-affinity state. However, affinity for β-adrenergic antagonists is not altered with age. Other aspects of the β-adrenergic cascade including G-protein activity and the adenylyl cyclase catalytic unit have also been shown to decrease with aging, but less consistently than the relative affinity alterations of the β-adrenergic receptor changes. Evidence regarding age-related alteration in cyclic adenosine monophosphate (cAMP), stimulated by mechanisms distal to the β-adrenergic, continues to be contradictory. There are data consistent with the notion that β-adrenergic–mediated phosphorylation, but not dephosphorylation of troponin-1, is decreased in aging myocytes. Therefore, the alterations in β-adrenergic function in the aging myocardium are not the result of a single specific alteration but rather of multiple changes that occur at different levels of the β-adrenergic signaling cascade. In contrast to β-adrenergic function, α_1-adrenergic function appears to be preserved in aging whereas α_2-mediated responses appear to be decreased.

Perioperative β-adrenergic blockade in elderly patients is associated with decreased postoperative cardiac events following major noncardiac surgery. The exact mechanism of this effect is unknown. β Blockade leads to decreased heart rate, which increases diastolic filling (and associated coronary perfusion) time. β Blockade also decreases myocardial contractility, which reduces myocardial oxygen consumption. Therefore, it would appear that perioperative β blockade provides myocardial protection by shifting the myocardial oxygen delivery-consumption balance toward greater delivery. Other potential contributing benefits include antiarrythmic effects, coronary plaque stabilization through reduction in mechanical shear forces, inflammatory reduction, and reduced platelet aggregation.

RESPIRATORY

Pulmonary complications are nearly as frequent as cardiac complications in the elderly and in fact may be a more important contributor to postoperative mortality. Changes in structure and function of the respiratory system as well as an increase in diseases of the lung and related organs contribute to the development and severity of these complications. The normal decline in respiratory function that accompanies aging can be attributed to changes in the lung and chest wall, although alteration in control of ventilation and decreased ability to protect against environmental injury are also important. A summary of the changes in the respiratory system with age are found in Table 25.2.

In the lung, there are changes in the type of cells found on bronchoalveolar lavage with an increase in Europhiles and decreased macrophages with age. There is also an increase in several inflammatory substances, such as interleukin 8 (IL-8), which may be important in explaining the increased susceptibility of the elderly to lower respiratory infections. In lung tissue there is an increase in elastin and a decrease in collagen, which may partially explain the increase in lung compliance that accompanies aging. There is also enlargement of the airspaces, which in the past was erroneously referred to as *senile emphysema* although it has no relation to the inflammatory and destructive changes seen true emphysema.

The major change in the lung with age, however, is the loss of elastic recoil in the alveoli which leads an overall increased alveolar compliance. Patency of the small airways is maintained by the elastic properties of the lung. Loss of elasticity leads to collapse of these airways and subsequent

uneven alveolar ventilation and air trapping. Uneven alveolar ventilation leads to mismatches in ventilation-perfusion with increased shunt and dead space ventilation, which then results a decline in arterial oxygen tension. Arterial oxygen tension falls by approximately 5 mm Hg per decade from age 20. The partial pressure of CO_2, however, does not change, in spite of an increase in dead space. The declining production of CO_2 that accompanies falling basal metabolic rates with age, may partially explain this finding. Residual volume (RV), or the volume remaining after maximal expiration, also increases as a result of air trapping. In the chest wall, there is a decrease in mobility of the ribs caused by calcification of the costal cartilage and contractures of the intercostal muscles. Overall, chest wall compliance declines secondary to changes in structure caused by kyphosis and exaggerated by vertebral collapse. The strength of the respiratory muscles progressively decreases leading to a decline in the maximum inspiratory and expiratory force generated, and easy fatigability.

The balance between elastic recoil and chest wall compliance affects lung volumes and ventilatory flow rates. The loss of elastic inward recoil of the lung with aging (increased compliance) is balanced somewhat by the decline in outward forces of chest wall (decreased compliance). Total lung capacity (TLC), therefore, remains unchanged and there is only a mild increase in resting lung volume, or functional residual capacity (FRC). Because TLC remains unchanged, the increase in RV results in a decrease in vital capacity (VC). The loss of support of the small airways further leads to compression during forced expiration, which limits dynamic lung volumes and flow rates. Forced vital capacity (FVC) decreases by 14 to 30 mL/yr and forced expiratory volume in 1 second (FEV_1) decreases by 23 to 32 mL/yr (in men).

The control of ventilation is also affected by aging. Ventilatory responses to hypoxia and hypercapnia fall by 50% and 40% respectively. The exact mechanism of this decline has not been well defined but may be the result of declining chemoreceptor function either at the peripheral or central nervous system level. The subjective feeling of dyspnea in response to bronchoconstriction may also decline with increasing age.

In addition to the intrinsic changes in the respiratory system, pulmonary function is affected by alterations in the ability of the body to protect against infection and environmental injury. With age, there is a progressive decrease in T-cell function (see wound healing/immunology in subsequent text) and a decline in mucociliary clearance of the airways. There is also a significant loss of cough reflex in healthy older subjects, which is further exacerbated by neurologic disorders. This loss of cough reflex may predispose to aspiration, particularly when the older patient is sedated in the perioperative period. In addition to these factors, the increased frequency and severity of postoperative pneumonia in older persons may be attributed to an increased incidence of oropharyngeal colonization with gram-negative and pathogenic gram-positive organisms. This colonization correlates closely with overall health and with the ability

TABLE 25.2

Normative Changes in Respiratory Function with Age

Parameter	Change with Age
Airspace size	Increased
Maximal inspiratory pressure	Decreased
Maximal voluntary ventilation	Decreased
Lung compliance	Increased
Thoracic compliance	Decreased
Total compliance	Decreased
Force vital capacity (FVC)	Decreased
Forced expiratory volume in 1 second (FEV$_1$)	Decreased
Total lung capacity (TLC)	Unchanged
Residual volume	Increased
Dead space ventilation	Increased
Shunt perfusion	Increased
Diffusion capacity	Decreased
Arterial partial pressure of O_2	Decreases
Arterial partial pressure of CO_2	Unchanged
Maximum oxygen consumption	Decreases

Adapted from: Zeleznik J. Normative aging of the respiratory system. *Clin Geriatr Med* 2003;19:1–18.

of the older individual to perform the activities of daily living. Assessing preoperative functional capacity is therefore a critical factor in determining postoperative pneumonia risk in older patients.

NEUROLOGICAL SYSTEMS

Central neurologic changes account for approximately 50% of disability after age 65. Neuronal loss was long thought to be a hallmark of aging based principally upon neuroanatomic studies. A 48% decrease in neuronal density was noted in the visual cortex from the third to the ninth decade of life. Similar losses were reported to occur in the anterior thalamus, cortex, hippocampus, and in the locus ceruleus. This well-accepted concept was brought into question in the late 1990s when advanced screening methods were used to eliminate patients with signs of Alzheimer disease. Although atrophy of cortical neurons occurs in healthy elderly patients, in the absence of neurodegenerative conditions there is little significant change in brain weight or volume with normal aging. The neuronal atrophy and changes in specific anatomic areas are variable in aging subjects. The change in perception of patterns of neuronal loss and reactive gliosis in the brain has yet to be evaluated to the same extent in the spinal cord, particularly with regard to rigorous control for potential pathology. It is reasonable to speculate that aging is associated with more limited anatomic change than previously reported.

Elderly patients are uniquely subject to central nervous system failure that frequently occurs in the perioperative period. Although complaints of subjective memory loss and cognitive deficits are common and neuropsychological evaluation does show slowing of central processing time, acquisition of new information, and a decline in "fluid intelligence," these changes are below the threshold of detection of most clinical mental state examinations. Clear abnormalities in mental state should not be attributed to aging but should lead to consideration of a differential diagnosis. Two major syndromes have been described. Postoperative delirium typically develops 6 to 12 hours following surgery and is characterized by disordered thinking and confusion that waxes and wanes overtime. Postoperative cognitive dysfunction (POCD) describes a deterioration of psychomotor capacities such as memory, ability to sort and order items, etc. POCD may or may not be clinically evident. To date, neither the pathophysiology of postoperative delirium nor POCD has been explained with any degree of certainty. The incidence of these problems is particularly noticeable following cardiac surgery, where cardiopulmonary bypass has been suspected as the culprit, although predisposing factors have been described. Much work remains to determine the nature of elderly brain dysfunction following surgery.

Loss of hearing with age is common in humans, affecting greater than 30% of adults between the ages of 65 and 74 and approximately 50% of individuals between the ages of 75 and 80. Presbycusis is an age-associated bilaterally symmetric,

sensorineural hearing loss. Hearing loss is 2.5 to 5 times more frequent in men than women and likely to be more severe. Presbycusis can be divided into sensory, metabolic, neural, and cochlear conductive defects. High frequencies are much more affected than lower frequencies. Acute sensorineural hearing loss can occur following general anesthesia (not ear surgery) or spinal anesthesia. This 10 to 20 dB hearing loss appears to be more common in the elderly and is generally transient. The cause is still speculative. Postoperative hearing deficits can exacerbate postoperative confusion or simply impair communication. Strategies for overcoming hearing impairment include (i) deliberate and clear speech; (ii) sitting directly in the patient's field of vision; and (iii) reduced speed of speech, but not too slow.

Visual loss is a common component of normal aging. This is due to structural changes in the eye, retinal deterioration, and changes in the central visual pathways. The structural changes associated with aging include changes in the lens (cataract deposition, changes in circumference, and shape) and decreased pupil size. Retinal and central visual pathway changes of aging include loss of rods from the central retina and loss of retinal ganglion cells. These changes lead to reduced visual threshold, increased susceptibility to glare, reduced visual acuity, reduced accommodation, visual field loss, and impaired depth perception.

RENAL

Chronic renal insufficiency is present in approximately one fourth of persons older than 70 years but may be unrecognized in some because creatinine levels remain in the "normal" range. Normal creatinine, however, does not reflect normal renal function in the elderly as changes in body composition, with increased fat and loss of lean muscle mass, lead to the production of less creatinine.

In fact, renal function declines with aging even in the healthy elderly. Between the ages of 30 and 85 there is a progressive sclerosis of up to 40% of nephrons with a compensatory hypertrophy of the remaining functional units. This is accompanied by atrophy of the afferent and efferent arterioles, a decrease in renal tubular cell number, and a decline in renal blood flow of approximately 50%. As a result, there is a decline in glomerular filtration rate (GFR) of approximately 45% by age 80. Creatinine clearance as a function of serum creatinine at ages 30 and 85 is shown in Figure 25.3. Serum creatinine can be estimated by the Cockcroft–Gault equation:

$$\text{Creatinine clearance } (C_{cr}) = (140 - \text{Age})$$
$$\times \ [\text{weight (kg)}/72] \times \text{serum creatinine}$$

Renal tubular function also declines with advancing age. There is a decrease in sodium ion concentration and hydrogen ion excretion, which leads to altered capacity to regulate fluid and acid–base balance. The usual methods of compensation for losses of sodium and water from nonrenal sources, increased renal sodium retention, increased urinary

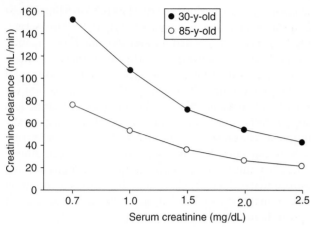

FIGURE 25.3 Differences in creatinine clearance as a function of serum creatinine with age. (Reprinted from Luckey AF, Parsa CJ. Fluids and electrolytes in the aged. *Arch Surg* 2003;138:1055–1060.)

concentration, and increased thirst, are impaired in the aged and dehydration is therefore a common problem. Impaired sodium retention is believed to be secondary to a decrease in the activity of the renin-angiotensin system. Impaired ability to concentrate the urine is related to a decline in end organ responsiveness to antidiuretic hormone. The failure to recognize thirst in spite of significant elevations in serum osmolality is well documented but not yet well understood. Alterations of osmoreceptor function in the hypothalamus may be responsible.

Impaired renal function, as well as alterations in body composition, affects the type, dosage and volume of distribution of drugs used in older patients. Because most changes in renal drug processing parallel GFR, creatinine clearance can be used to adjust dosing for most drugs cleared by the kidney. For some drugs, the concentration of the protein that is its principle binding site determines the free fraction of the drug and therefore the clearance and volume of distribution. These drugs must be considered individually as the relative production of these binding protein changes with advancing age. It is also important to remember that the sensitivity of the kidney to neprhotoxic agents is increased in the elderly.

There are also changes in the lower urinary tract that are important in the perioperative period. Increased collagen in the bladder limits distensibility and impairs emptying, which is further impaired by prostatic hypertrophy in men. These, among other alterations in the local environment combined with declining host defenses, are thought to be responsible for an increased prevalence of asymptomatic bacteriuria in the aged. Gender, mobility, degree of comorbidity, and place of residence influence the prevalence of asymptomatic bacteria, which ranges from 10% to 50%. Urinary tract infections are common in older patients in the postoperative period and cause significant morbidity. Preoperative urinalysis is therefore important to identify those older patients with asymptomatic bacteriuria before instrumentation of the bladder with urethral catheters.

WOUND HEALING/IMMUNITY

The physiology of wound healing is a well-integrated multiphase process that includes phases of hemostasis, inflammation, proliferation, and maturation (see Chapter 5). In elderly patients, wound healing is delayed, but qualitatively is equivalent to younger patients. Additionally, comorbidities that are more common in elderly patients can impair wound healing in this population. In the absence of local tissue ischemia, diabetes, or pressure, elderly patients do not develop chronic wounds. Skin changes associated with aging, most due to a lifetime of sun exposure, increase susceptibility to traumatic wounds. These changes include atrophy, dryness, and diminished cellular content of the dermis. Flattening of the dermal/epidermal junction makes skin more susceptible to shear injury in older patients. The changes that occur in the phases of wound healing may slow the process, but in the absence of the noted comorbidities, wound closure will occur. These changes are summarized in Table 25.3.

The hemostatic phase of wound healing is characterized by formation of a fibrin clot at the site of injury and platelet aggregation. In elderly patients, there is an increase in platelet adherence. There is also an age-associated increase in platelet release of α granules containing a variety of growth factors. The clinical implications of these changes are uncertain.

The inflammatory phase overlaps the hemostatic phase. It is associated with infiltration into the wound of neutrophils, lymphocytes, and macrophages. In elderly patients, vascular permeability is likely reduced by a nitric oxide–mediated mechanism. This leads to a decrease in neutrophil, lymphocyte, and macrophage infiltration. In addition, macrophage function is reduced in elderly patients. However, these

TABLE 25.3

Changes in Wound Healing Associated with Aging

Phase	Change
Hemostasis	Increased platelet adherence
	Increased released platelet-associated growth factors
Inflammatory	Decreased vascular permeability
	Decreased inflammatory cell infiltration
	Decreased macrophage function
	Increased secretion inflammatory mediators
Proliferation	Decreased fibroblast number, size, response to growth factors
	Decreased rate collagen synthesis
	Decreased levels angiogenic growth factors
	Decreased capillary ingrowth
Maturation	Decreased collagen turnover and remodeling

changes are counterbalanced by an increased secretion of inflammatory mediators by these cells in the wound.

The proliferation phase is associated with capillary ingrowth, formation of granulation tissue, and subsequent re-epithelialization. Each of these components is decreased in older patients. Reduced levels of angiogenic factors lead to reduced capillary ingrowth. This has an additional effect of reducing the rate of re-epithelialization. The formation of granulation tissue is slowed by a reduced rate of collagen synthesis in elderly patients. However, the final collagen content is similar to younger patients. Decreased fibroblast numbers, size, and response to growth factors slow the rate of re-epithelialization.

The maturation phase is characterized by remodeling and strengthening of the wound. In elderly patients, this phase is prolonged because of a slower rate of collagen turnover. Studies of the tensile strength of wounds in elderly patients have had a large number of confounding variables including comorbidities that affect wound healing.

Aging is associated with a number of changes in immune function, which are typically only important in the presence of infection, comorbidities, and/or other stressors. The major changes associated with immunosenescence are summarized in Table 25.4.

Thymic involution is a normal component of aging. There are quantitative and qualitative changes in T-cell lymphocytes with aging. There is a reduction in unstimulated (naïve) cells and an increase in primed T-cells. There is a reduced proliferative response to antigens and mitogens possibly due to impaired membrane signal transduction pathways. These changes are evident clinically in the high incidence of anergy to delayed type hypersensitivity skin testing.

There are variable changes in antibody production by B lymphocytes. Many of these changes are related to alterations in T-cell function. Primary and secondary antibody responses are impaired in elderly patients. However, autoantibody production is increased in elderly patients. This is likely a manifestation of increased helper T cell and reduced suppressor T cell responses to nonspecific antibody production. Monocyte function is impaired in elderly patients. As with changes in B cell responses, the impairment is due to defects in the interactions with T cells.

GLUCOSE METABOLISM

Recent evidence strongly supports the importance of blood glucose control for the successful outcome of surgery. Changes in glucose homeostasis are common in the elderly as glucoregulatory mechanisms decline. In the United States, 20% of people older than 60 have type II diabetes and an additional 20% are glucose intolerant. Fasting blood glucose increases 1 to 2 mg/dL per decade of life and postchallenge blood glucose increases 6 to 9 mg/dL per decade. When given a glucose load, even healthy older subjects have a much higher blood glucose response than younger subjects.

Although glucose homeostasis is a complex interaction of several interrelated processes, the question of how aging effects these interactions can be simplified to "Is aging associated with a decrease in insulin secretion or an increase in insulin resistance, or both?" There is now general consensus that β-cell function and insulin secretion decline as a function of age. When the β cell is challenged by hyperglycemia, the insulin response is not augmented sufficiently to maintain euglycemia. This defect in β-cell response may be compounded by comorbidity, medications and genetic factors

The question of whether glucose intolerance is the result of increased insulin resistance caused by aging *per se* is more controversial. Some believe that the increase in insulin resistance observed in the aged is the result of changes in the level of activity and body composition, with increased adipose tissue and decreased lean muscle mass, rather than direct effects of age on insulin action. Others believe that there is a decrease in insulin mediated muscle glucose metabolism and an increase in intracellular lipid accumulation that may be a direct effect of changes in mitochondrial function that accompany aging. These changes may likewise be compounded by comorbidity, medications and genetic factors (Fig. 25.4).

The stress response to injury or surgery creates a hyperglycemic, insulin-resistant state. It should not be surprising that when elderly patients are subjected to these

TABLE 25.4

Summary of Major Immune Changes in Aging

Hematopoiesis	Impaired progenitor cells' proliferative response to stress
Thymus	Thymic involution
	Reduced thymic hormone production
T cells	Increased ratio of memory versus naïve phenotype
	Reduced proliferative response
	Impaired IL-2 production
	Impaired DTH response
	Impaired cytotoxic function
B cells	Impaired humoral responses
	Increased IgA, IgG production
	Decreased IgM, IgD production
	Increased levels of autoantibodies
NK cells	Increased number in peripheral blood
	Decreased/no change in function
Accessory cells	Decreased number of Langerhans cells
	Decreased lymph node accessory cell function
Cytokines	Increased/no change in IL-6, IL-4 production
	Decreased/no change in IL-2, IL-10, IL-12, IFN-γ production

IL, interleukin; DTH, delayed-type hypersensitivity; Ig, immunoglobulin; NK, natural killer; IFN, interferon.

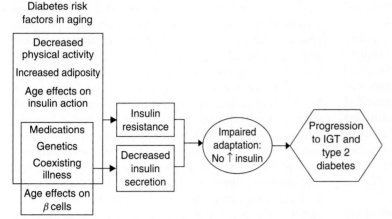

FIGURE 25.4 With aging decreased insulin secretion and increased insulin resistance (whether related to aging *per se* or to changes in body composition and physical activity) combined with comorbid illness, genetic factors and medications lead to a decline in glucoregulatory control. (Reprinted from Chang AM, Halter JB. Aging and insulin secretion. *Am J Physio Endocrinol Metab* 2003; 284:E7–E12.)

stresses, blood glucose levels may increase more than their younger counterparts. It is important that normoglycemia be maintained by exogenous insulin, particularly in the intensive care unit (ICU) setting, even when there is no history of diabetes preoperatively. Patents undergoing a variety of surgeries, particularly cardiac surgery, whose blood glucose levels are maintained in the normal range have better ICU outcomes, few infections and lower overall mortality than those in whom blood glucose is allowed to be even modestly elevated.

CONCLUSION

Aging *per se*, is no longer a contraindication to surgery as it was just a few decades ago. Many of the diseases that require surgical intervention are diseases of aging, such as coronary artery disease, colon cancer, and degenerative joint disease. As the older population increases, surgeons will be treating larger and larger numbers of older patients, including those older than 85 years. Although older patients are in general more fit and better able to tolerate the stress of a well-conducted surgery than older patients were several decades ago, physiologic changes as well as the acquisition of diseases over the years, limits the reserves available to them should a complication occur. By understanding how declines in organ system function may place the older patient at increased risk for a complication, the surgeon can take steps to minimize the impact of these changes. The use of

perioperative β blockade is an excellent example of one such strategy and maintenance of perioperative euglycemia another. Over the next decade, much more work needs to be done to identify other interventions such as those that will allow surgeons to treat even our oldest patients with minimum stress and maximum chances for excellent recovery.

SUGGESTED READINGS

Burns EA, Goodwin JS. Effects of aging on immune function. In: Rosenthal RA, Zenilman ME, Katlic MR, ed. *Principles and practice of geriatric surgery*. New York: Springer-Verlag New York, 2001: 46–63.

Castle SC. Clinical relevance of age-related immune dysfunction. *Clin Infect Dis* 2000;31:578–585.

Gosain A, DiPietro LA. Aging and wound healing. *World J Surg* 2004; 28:321–326.

Lakatta EG. Cardiovascular aging in health sets the stage for cardiovascular disease. *Heart Lung Circ* 2002;11:76–91.

London MJ, Zaugg M, Schaub MC, et al. Perioperative beta-adrenergic receptor blockade: physiologic foundations and clinical controversies. *Anesthesiology* 2004;100:170–175.

Maggio PM, Taheri PA. Perioperative issues: myocardial ischemia and protection—beta-blockade. *Surg Oncol Clin N Am* 2005;85: 1091–1102.

de la Torre JC, Fay LA. Effects of aging on the human nervous system. In: Rosenthal RA, Zenilman ME, Katlic MR, ed. *Principles and practice of geriatric surgery*. New York: Springer-Verlag New York, 2001: 926–948.

Thomas DR. Age-related changes in wound healing. *Drugs Aging* 2001;18:607–620.

CHAPTER 26

Selected Technologies in General Surgery

Seza A. Gulec, Erica N. Hoenie, Navin Bedi, Le Roy D. Weaver, Jr., and Jody M. Barber

PROLOGUE

We need to open our minds to expand the concept of "physical examination" in the 21st century. Just like we accepted the stethoscope 150 years ago, we should include ultrasound (US) examination as part of the physical examination. We should stop scrutinizing the liberal applications of evolving positron emission tomography (PET)/computed tomography (CT), magnetic resonance (MR) technology in daily problems of surgery. It is time to embrace the art and science of imaging as an integral part of the art, science and craft of surgery. "Image-guided surgery" is the imprint of our age.

DIAGNOSTIC TECHNOLOGIES

Ultrasound

Ultrasonography is an imaging modality that generates images from ultrasonic waves reflected at interfaces between different body constituents. To produce a reflected pulse of ultrasonic energy, the interface must separate structures with different acoustic impedances. The acoustic impedance of a medium is defined as the product of the physical density of the medium and the velocity of US through the medium. If the difference in acoustic impedance across an interface is substantial, considerable energy is reflected at the interface, resulting in an intense electronic signal from the detector that produces a bright spot in the image. If the acoustic impedances are similar on opposite sides of the interface, little energy is reflected and the resulting electronic signal furnishes a dim spot in the image. In this manner, a gray-scale image is produced of interfaces between different anatomic structures in the patient.

The US transducer receives a short electrical pulse and generates a corresponding pressure wave pulse. The pulse is only several cycles long. The pulsed wave propagates down through the tissue, away from the transducer. The tissue absorbs, scatters, reflects, and refracts the wavefront. The reflected waves return to the transducer. The transducer switches to receiver mode and, as it receives pressure waves, converts them into electrical pulses. After a fixed period of time, the transducer stops receiving and transmits the next pressure wave.

Echogenecity and Echo Patterns

The brightness corresponds to the strength of the reflected wave. Soft tissue reflects sound to varying degrees and is echogenic; simple fluid reflects little sound and is hypoechoic or anechoic. Calcified structures as well as pockets of air or gas produce strong echoes at the soft tissue–calcified object interface or soft tissue–air interface. Although cysts are generally rounded in shape, they often exhibit irregular shapes, with wrinkles in their walls or lobulated appearances. Blood vessels or ligaments can tether the walls of cysts. These will exert an influence on them, resulting in changes in shape secondary to the external pressure on them. Nevertheless, the appearance of sharp near and deep walls still is seen, and a clearly defined strong back wall remains a hallmark of a cyst. Cysts are often filled with internal echoes that represent particles or debris. When fine internal echoes are seen in a cyst, they are hypoechoic and homogeneous. Inasmuch as a cyst may no longer appear as strictly anechoic, it will usually be represented with the most hypoechoic appearance of any structure in the image. It is helpful to compare a cyst with other known fluid structures in the image, such as the urinary bladder, the gallbladder, or a blood vessel that is seen clearly. Hydroceles, spermatoceles, and endometriomas frequently show internal echoes. Even blood vessels will show moving internal echoes when imaged optimally with modern scanning. Hemangiomas of the liver and a thick secretory endometrium almost always show increased through transmission. It is a nice feature if seen, but by itself it is somewhat of an antique sign. However, although a cyst may not necessarily show posterior acoustic enhancement, it will never attenuate the sound (Fig. 26.1).

The differences in sound transmission between two tissues is a property referred to as the *acoustic impedance* of the tissue, which allows the reflection of echoes from the

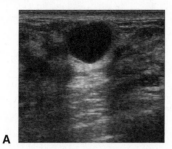
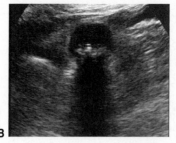
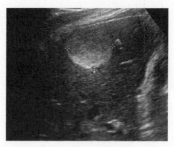

FIGURE 26.1   Sonographic tissue characteristics. **A:** A fluid filled cyst appears as an unechoic structure with sharp near and far walls along with posterior acoustic enhancement. **B:** Gall bladder stones shown with a bright echo from the leading edge and an acoustic shadow deep to this edge. **C:** A solid mass appearing as an hyper-echoic structure in the liver with no acoustic shadow.

different interfaces as sound is transmitted deep into the body. The difference between the speed of transmission of sound in water versus air or bone is great. Bone is too hard and inelastic for transmission, and it serves as too strong a reflector of sound, allowing no transmission deeper into the body. This results in an area behind the bone with no echoes. This is called an *acoustic shadow*. Calcifications also behave like bones. Conversely, the molecules of gas or air are too far apart for effective transmission of a wave front, which also will result in shadowing deep to that area. In other words, US cannot be transmitted through bones, stones, air, or gas, and imaging of structures deep to such areas is impossible. As with air and bone, fat is also a barrier. Adipose tissue has numerous angled interfaces that scatter the sound beam. Fat effectively works as a filter. It scatters the sound being transmitted as well as the echoes returning to the probe. The more adipose tissue that exists between the transducer and at the region of interest, the less information there is that is available. Bones, air, gas, and fat all cause severe limitations to US. They may not be absolute limitations, but it should be recognized that the confidence levels of these scans are severely reduced, and often only the most gross information is obtainable. Looking for an abdominal abscess in an obese postoperative patient with an ileus is generally fruitless.

A water-density window is needed for sound transmission. With all US scanning, a thick, watery gel is used as an acoustic coupler on the body to eliminate the air at the transducer/skin interface. Bandages, ostomies, and open wounds will all trap air and hence interfere with the transmission of diagnostic US waves. The liver and spleen are seen easily against the body wall without any interposing air or gas. Acoustic windows are available in the lower intercostal surfaces. The liver and spleen are good windows for imaging of the kidneys. A full urinary bladder lifts small bowel loops out of the pelvis, which allows imaging of the female organs.

Resolution and Penetration

The resolution of an US transducer is directly related to its frequency. As the frequency of sound increases, its wavelength decreases. A smaller wavelength is capable of discriminating between smaller objects (high spatial resolution). A larger wavelength sound beam, however, may display two small objects as only a single larger object. Hence, to increase the resolution of an US system, higher frequency transducers are used. Unfortunately, a price is paid in penetration. Higher frequency sound waves reflect more echoes more frequently from smaller structures, and they are attenuated more easily than lower frequency transducers. When a lower frequency US probe is used, more penetration into the body can be achieved, but there will be less resolution (Fig. 26.2). With a higher frequency transducer, increased resolution of smaller structures can be achieved, but there will be less penetration. Higher frequency transducers offer superb resolution but are limited to superficial parts scanning. The situation here is similar to playing a stereo system in an apartment building. The music sounds fine in the room where the speakers are and where all the instruments are heard. In the adjacent apartments, the music

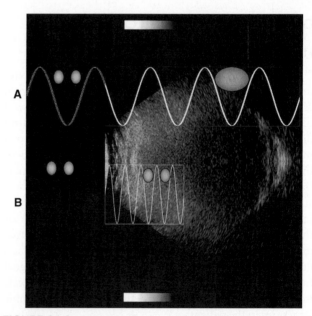

FIGURE 26.2   Ultrasound wave characteristics. **A:** Long wave length corresponds to low frequency with deep penetration in the tissue. **B:** Short wave length corresponds to high frequency with lower penetration. Longer wave length has lower spatial resolution and might display two small objects as a single object on ultrasound images.

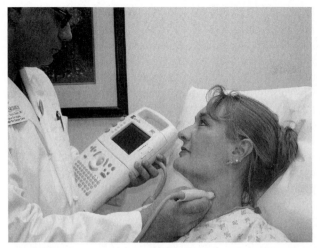

FIGURE 26.3 A compact ultrasound unit, particularly helpful in examining thyroid and breast patients. These units have become part of routine physical examination.

will be muffled with loss of the high-frequency instruments such as violins, and only the annoying booming of low-frequency sounds such as bass drums will be heard through the walls.

Probe Types and Special Clinical Applications

The frequencies of diagnostic US transducers vary from approximately 2 MHz to approximately 10 MHz. The low-frequency probes (2 MHz) are used for imaging large body areas such as the right upper quadrant in an obese person. Midrange probes (3–5 MHz) are used for all-purpose imaging in normal to thin individuals. High-frequency probes (7–10 MHz) are used for superficial parts scanning. Compact units, with variable size and shape probes, have become part of standard physical examination (Fig. 26.3). This particularly applies to breast and thyroid evaluations. The limit of detection of nodules by palpation alone remains to be 1 to 2 cm, whereas a US can detect subcentimeter lesions, and most importantly allows more reliable follow-up evaluations with less interobserver variations.

Intraoperative Ultrasound and Needle Guides

Intraoperative US, by eliminating image degrading anatomic barriers, provides images with improved sensitivity and resolution. Most common applications include liver and pancreas scanning for tumor localization and final staging. Curved array transducers with a larger field of view allow not only detection of lesions that are not seen on preoperative imaging, but also help determine relation with adjacent vasculature and biliary tree. Small, high-frequency linear array transducers can maneuver into smaller spaces and have a clearer near field of view.

Many modern probes are available with needle guides for direct image-guided interventional purposes. If a deep target can be seen from the skin, it can usually be punctured percutaneously from the same window. Brackets are attached to the probe where the needle is held in a fairly rigid manner along a path at an angle to the sound beam and in the plane of the image. Software in the scanner places a target pathway on the image. The target is lined up in the path, and the needle is watched as it enters the target. This tool is very helpful in obtaining fine needle aspiration biopsies, and drainage of abscesses or small fluid collections. Some intraoperative US probes are also equipped with a needle guidance apertures allowing placement of biopsy needles and ablation probes (Fig. 26.4).

Endoluminal Ultrasound

Endoluminal probes have high-frequency transducers and are used on long probes inserted into body openings. This allows superficial parts-type imaging of the rectum, prostate, and the female pelvic organs with high resolution (Fig. 26.5). Transesophageal probes are used in cardiac evaluation and intravascular probes are also currently available. Some endoluminal probes rotate to produce a circular image, with the probe site in the center.

Vascular Ultrasound-Duplex Scan

Duplex scan (US) combines the 2-D gray-scale US with color doppler US. Doppler US detects blood flow and measures its velocity. The principle of this technique is based on the

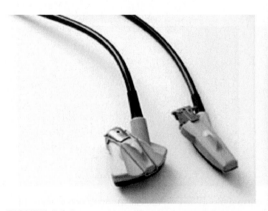
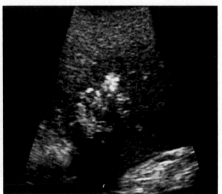

FIGURE 26.4 Intraoperative ultrasound devices ergonomically designed to reach difficult areas during intraoperative exploration. These are particularly useful in the imaging of the liver. Some transducers have an apparatus to allow placement of biopsy needles and ablation probes.

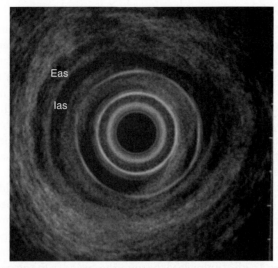

FIGURE 26.5 Endorectal ultrasound showing mucosal, submucosal and muscular layers. Endoscopic ultrasound has become the standard T and N staging of rectal tumors.

exploitation of the *"Doppler phenomenon."* The Doppler effect is the change in the perceived frequency of sound when there is relative motion between the source of the sound and the detector. The classic example of the Doppler effect is the change heard in the pitch of a train whistle by an observer standing on the side of the tracks as the train approaches and then passes. A subject on the moving train hears only a whistle of unchanging frequency, because he or she also is moving along with the train. An observer on the ground first hears the pitch of the whistle increase as the train approaches because the sound wave essentially is chasing itself. Its wavelength effectively shortens as the wave front becomes compressed. When the train passes the observer on the tracks, the frequency of the whistle then decreases as the wave front stretches out because the sound now is running away from itself. When US waves are used in the body, the echoes reflected are the same frequency as those transmitted if there is no motion. Echoes reflected from moving red blood cells (RBCs) return at different frequencies than what was transmitted. Doppler scanners are able to detect and analyze these frequency changes. Therefore, an echo from a red cell in a vessel in which blood is flowing toward the transducer will return at a slightly higher frequency than what was transmitted and would be assigned a positive frequency shift. Conversely, blood cells flowing away from the transducer will produce a negative frequency shift. The changes in frequency of reflected echoes are recorded in individual pixels in the US image.

The entire image is analyzed pixel by pixel, and the average frequency shift in each pixel is determined. The positive and negative shifts are generally displayed in two different colors that are superimposed on the appropriate pixels in the 2-D black-and-white image. If there is no flow, no color will appear in the image. Flow toward the probe will be shown in one of the two colors, and flow away from the probe will be displayed in the other color. Within each color there is also a color scale. Slow flow (low-frequency shifts) will be assigned a deeper color, and higher velocities (high-frequency shifts) will be displayed with brighter intensities of that color. The colors that are used are arbitrary and can be changed with a switch on the scanner. Several different color scales are usually available for different purposes. It must be emphasized that arteries are not necessarily red and veins are not necessarily blue. Only the relative direction of the blood flow in relation to the transducer is shown. A single tortuous vessel changing course up and down relative to the probe will be displayed in two different colors.

The frequency shifts above or below the baseline are also displayed in graphic format which allows quantitative analysis of the flow dynamics at any given site. The velocities of systolic and diastolic flow are measured, resistive indices, pulsatility indices are calculated, and comparisons can be made using spectral doppler (Fig. 26.6).

Computed Tomography

Imaging Principle and Image Contrast

CT is a technique that generates cross-sectional or tomographic images of the body through the use of x-ray beams passed through the patient from multiple angular projections (with a 360-degree range). Complex mathematical

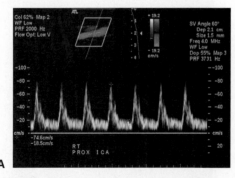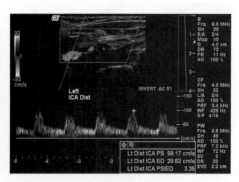

FIGURE 26.6 Duplex scan images. **A:** Shows normal blood flow to the carotid with no evidence of narrowing or hemodynamic compromise. Pulse characteristics are also consistent with normal blood flow. **B:** Shows significantly narrowed carotid with hemodynamically significant stenosis and flat pulse amplitude. WF, wave frequency; PRF, pulse rate frequency; ICA, independent component analysyis.

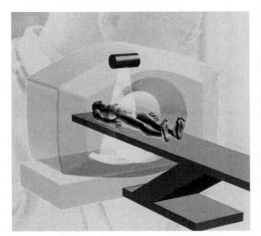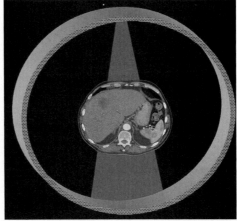

FIGURE 26.7 The basic principle of computed tomography (CT) scanner. An x-ray tube circling the patient produces a beam that passes through the patient and is absorbed by a ring of detectors surrounding the patient. The intensity of the x-ray beam reaching the patient is dependent on the absorption characteristics of tissues it passes through. The amount of x-ray absorption is used as basis of construction of the CT images.

algorithms are used to create the composite CT images, based on degree of x-ray beam attenuation by different density tissue components (Fig. 26.7).

During a CT image acquisition an x-ray tube circling the patient produces a beam that passes through the patient and is absorbed by a ring of detectors surrounding the patient. The intensity of the x-ray beam reaching the detectors is dependent on the absorbtion characteristics of tissues it passes through. Because the beam is moving around the patient, each anatomic structure is exposed from multiple directions. Using a process called *Fourier analysis*, the computer uses the information obtained from different amounts of x-ray absorption to reconstruct the density and position of the different structures contained within each slice. The computer receives a signal in analog form and converts it to a binary digit. The digital signal is stored and the image is reconstructed in a digital format after the scan is over. Each picture is displayed on a matrix, each square in a matrix is called a *pixel*. The reconstructed image anatomy is in a three-dimensional (3-D) digital format composed of unit blocks called *voxel*. The depth of the voxel is determined by the slice thickness.

The Hounsfeld Number and Computed Tomography Windows

The digital value ascribed to each pixel is called the *Hounsfeld number* (HN). The HN corresponds different attenuation values reflecting various densities on CT images. By convention, water has an HN of 0, air has an HN of −1,000, and cortical bone has a measurement of +1,000. Fat is typically −80 to −120 HN. The HN values depend on the mean energy of the entering x-ray beam and are thereforerelative values (Table 26.1). Therefore, rather than relying on absolute HN, characterization of tissues is often best accomplished by using known structures within the body as internal standards (e.g., a patient's subcutaneous fat

as lipid density and muscles as soft tissue density). By using sophisticated image reconstruction algorithms, a gray-scale image is constructed based on each pixel's HN. Air, the largest negative value, appears black, and cortical bone, the largest positive value, appears white.

CT scans are displayed as a monochrome image on a screen. The value of the pixel at a specific point in the image is converted to a grey level. Contemporary CT scanners can assign a scale with 2,000 shades of gray. However, human eye can only distinguish limited hues of gray (32 gray levels at best). To optimize visualization of specific structures of interest, the acquired image data can be manipulated by altering the window width and center. The window width determines the number of attenuation values chosen to represent these shades of gray. The width may be wide, such as 2,000 HN (range −1,000 to +1,000 HN). Alternatively, a narrow width, such as 100 HN (range −50 to +50 HN), may be selected. In the last instance, all CT values of −50 or less will be displayed as black, and all values of +50 or more will be displayed as white. The narrow window width

TABLE 26.1

Hounsfeld Units of Different Tissue Structures

Tissue	HN range
Air	−1,000
Lungs	−900 to −300
Fat	−120 to −80
Water	0
Muscle	10 to 30
Soft tissue	10 to 30
Cortical bone	50 to 100
Trabecular bone	500 to 1,000

HN, Hounsfeld number.

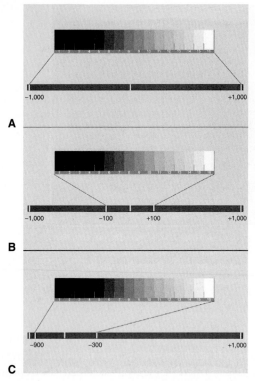

FIGURE 26.8 Window widths describe the Hounsfeld number [or Hounsfeld unit (HU)] over which the shades of gray are distributed. **A:** A wide window (2,000 HU, centered on zero). **B:** A narrow window (200 HU, centered on zero). **C:** A narrow window (200 HU, centered on 600).

maximizes contrast and is, therefore, particularly useful when searching for subtle attenuation differences between tissues. The window center is that HN about which the shades of gray are distributed. The average HN value of the tissue of interest is selected as the window center. Manipulation of both the window width and the center are therefore used to idealize the visualization of various structures and pathologic anatomy (Fig. 26.8).

Image Quality: Resolution and Artifacts
The measure of how closely structures can be discerned in an image is called *spatial resolution*. Spatial resolution is

determined by voxel size which is comprised of pixel size and slice thickness. In general, thinner slices have better spatial resolution.

Contrast resolution is the ability to discern subtle differences in HN. Contrast resolution is directly related to the intensity of the radiation beam and the signal to noise ratio.

CT images occasionally contain some rather typical artifacts that degrade the images. As in standard photography, any motion that takes place during the acquisition of the image will limit its definition. Therefore, motion artifacts are frequently seen secondary to bowel peristalsis, respiration, or cardiac pulsation. Rapid acquisition of image data (1–3 seconds per image) helps to reduce motion artifact.

A second type of artifact is produced by metal joint prostheses, surgical clips, electronic pacing devices, and other high-density structures. In this case, any high-density material acts to stop or attenuate many of the radiographs such that image quality is reduced and information adjacent to the devices is lost.

A third common artifact in CT scan is known as *partial volume artifact*. Partial volume artifacts arise when a voxel contains different type of tissue (different HN). This produces an averaged HN to be assigned to that voxel. Here, the partial inclusion of a structure in an axial slice leads to false attenuation values and therefore alters the final image (Fig. 26.9). The use of thinner slices eliminates or reduces the partial volume artifact.

Contrast
There are two types of contrast administration important to CT images: gastrointestinal (GI) and intravenous. GI (oral, rectal, or both) contrast material usually consists of either a water-soluble iodine compound or a dilute barium solution. The concentration of the barium used for a CT study is typically 2%–3%). rather than the 55% to 85% used for the GI studies. If the higher concentration were used, it would act to attenuate a large percentage of the radiographs and give artifacts similar to those seen with metal joint prosthesis. Therefore, if a patient is to undergo both a CT scan of the abdomen and a GI study, either do the CT scan first or allow all of the barium from the GI study to clear before doing

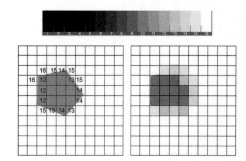

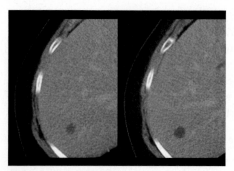

FIGURE 26.9 Partial volume artifact. The borders of a lesion appear rather indistinct due to averaging of Hounsfeld numbers in the marginal pixels. The use of thin slice imaging reduces the partial volume artifacts.

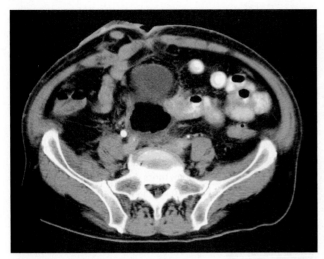

FIGURE 26.10 Computed tomography (CT) scan of a patient with intra-abdominal abscess and free air. The use of gastrointestinal contrast material is essential to discriminate distended bowel loops from intra-abdominal collections. The CT scan is also very sensitive for detection of intra-abdominal air, far superior to plain x-rays.

the CT scan. GI contrast administration is crucial in the evaluation of the abdomen and pelvis when in search of an abscess. Nonopacified loops of bowel may appear identical to an abscess, and differentiation between the two often relies on filling the bowel with contrast material (Fig. 26.10).

The second type of contrast important to CT images is the intravenous type, often called *dye* in lay terms. These materials are various water-soluble solutions containing iodine. Iodine acts to attenuate radiographs, and this appears as a whiter area on the CT images. The liver, spleen, kidneys, pancreas, and major vessels can be seen to enhance (brighten) after intravenous contrast administration. Tissues such as renal cysts, various neoplasms, and infarcted areas often do not enhance to the degree of surrounding tissue and therefore appear relatively dark on the CT image. There are two large categories of intravenous contrast material available: the ionic and the nonionic groups. Both of these types of agents contain iodine, but the carrier molecule to which the iodine is bound is different, as is the osmolality and number of ions in solution. In general, there are less adverse effects associated with the nonionic contrast (although severe reactions are possible). However, the cost of the nonionic material ranges from 10 to 15 times that of ionic contrast. Therefore, each patient must be evaluated individually to determine which type of intravenous contrast is to be used.

The degree of enhancement is a function of the concentration and amount of intravenous contrast given as well as the method in which it is administered. Typically, 100 to 180 mL of a 60% iodine solution are administered. Maximal enhancement is seen when the contrast is given quickly (1.5–2.5 mL/s) and images are acquired rapidly during the inflow of contrast. Once equilibrium between the intravascular and interstitial components of tissue is reached, lesions may become isodense (indistinguishable/same HN)

with the surrounding tissue. Contrast may be administered through an intravenous catheter using an electronically powered injector or manually with a syringe. The power injector allows both a steady delivery of contrast and rapid infusion and requires relatively proximal good venous access (i.e., antecubital veins).

Intravenous contrast material carries some inherent risks to the patient. Mild side effects such as sneezing, nausea, vomiting, hives, or heat sensation are relatively common. More serious reactions, such as cardiac arrhythmia, anaphylaxis, or renal failure, occur in approximately 1/10,000 patients. The overall risk of death from ionic intravenous contrast is estimated at 1/40,000 or roughly the same risk as having a fatal reaction to penicillin. It is generally accepted that nonionic contrast poses less risk to the patient.

Caution should be exercised when contemplating intravenous contrast administration to patients with pheochromocytoma, multiple myeloma, or myasthenia gravis. A hypertensive crisis can be induced in a patient with a pheochromocytoma. Similarly, on rare occasions a myasthenia gravis crisis can be induced after intravenous contrast, ultimately leading to respiratory difficulty or failure. Patients with multiple myeloma are at risk of precipitating abnormal proteins in the renal-collecting tubules and thereby inducing acute renal failure. Recent reports have disputed this argument and maintain that intravenous contrast can be administered safely to patients with multiple myeloma, providing they are well hydrated.

Image acquisition at different stages of contrast flow/distribution allows for more sensitive detection of lesions and evaluation of the anatomic relation of the tumors with adjacent vasculature, therefore assessment for resectability. Specific protocols have been developed for liver and pancreas imaging to optimize the clinical information. Contrast-enhanced liver CT involves acquisition of three sets of images at different phases of contrast distribution in the liver. The first phase is the arterial phase in which contrast enters the liver through the hepatic artery. The second phase is also known as *portal phase*, and this corresponds to the reentry of contrast to the liver through the portal vein. The third phase is the equilibrium phase. Primary and metastatic tumors of the liver derive majority of their flow from the hepatic artery. Most tumors appear as hypodense lesions on contrast-enhanced CT. Hypervascular lesions show rim enhancement in the arterial phase. Lesion to liver contrast is highest in the portal phase (Fig. 26.11).

Helical (Spiral) Computed Tomography and Multislice Scanning

Early generation CT scanners have a fixed gantry position. The bed position is advanced step-wise as the acquisition of each slice is completed. Spiral/helical CT has the ability to simultaneously acquire data and advance gantry position. The radiograph tube rotates around the patient as the patient is moved along the horizontal axis, thereby circumscribing a spiral path (Fig. 26.12). Projection data acquired at selected locations along this spiral path are interpolated to achieve

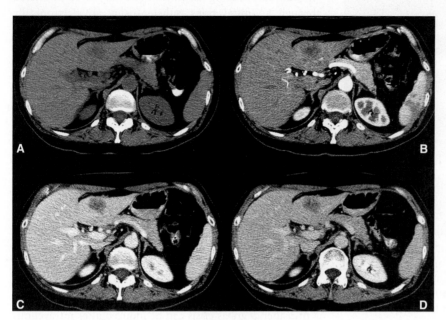

FIGURE 26.11   A three-phase liver scan. **A:** A noncontrast computed tomography (CT) scan (not considered as a separate phase by many radiologists). **B:** Arterial phase as evident from intense contrast in the aorta. This image shows a metastatic lesion in the left lateral segment of the liver. **C:** The portal venous phase when the contrast is in the portal vasculature. It's marked by enhancement of the normal liver parenchyma. The metastatic lesion becomes more distinct with an excellent lesion to liver background ratio. **D:** The equilibrium phase. Three phase liver scan is very helpful in correction of liver lesions, primary or metastatic liver lesions with high vascularity show enhancement in the arterial phase. Colorectal cancer metastases are best demonstrated on portal phase where the image contrast is the highest. Neuro-endocrine tumors might be best visualized on the equilibrium phase images.

image reconstruction. This simultaneous operation of data acquisition and patient translation allows scan time to be significantly reduced. Typical spiral acquisitions of the chest, abdomen, or pelvis, for example, are completed in 30 to 40 seconds, roughly a single breath-hold. In addition to the obvious advantage of shortening scan time, complete imaging during a single breath-hold improves detection of small lesions, previously easily missed because of respiratory variation and misregistration. Furthermore, rapid coverage of large areas allows imaging to be performed at the most optimal stage of contrast enhancement, which again improves lesion detection. Finally, small-lesion conspicuity can be enhanced further by overlapping reconstruction, thereby reducing partial volume effects. For example, 10-mm sections can be reconstructed at 5-mm intervals. Also, high-quality coronal, sagittal, or 3-D reconstruction of images can be obtained, which, unlike conventional CT, does not suffer from motion artifact, assuming the patient was able to hold still for the 30 to 40 seconds.

The total volume of contrast required for certain applications of spiral scanning can be reduced substantially. Contrast-enhanced spiral scans of the chest, for example, can be performed with half the usual dose (60 mL instead of 120 mL of 60% contrast) and yet allow imaging during peak opacification of the major vascular structures. Therefore,

spiral CT has many advantages over conventional CT. Its improved technology can be applied to all the usual CT imaging indications, along with promising strides being made in more innovative fields, such as CT angiography of the cerebrovascular and peripheral circulations and oncologic applications.

The number of row of detectors in the spiral CT determines the efficacy and speed of the image acquisition. The first multislice CT scanners (multiple row of detectors) were introduced in the early 1990s. The 4-slice scanner was introduced in 1998; these scanners were capable of processing scans within 0.5 seconds. Such short scan times translated into shorter examination times (Fig. 26.13). Reduced scan time allows acquisition of images with fewer artifacts caused by movement. Enhanced, visually superb images have been possible with the introduction of the 16-slice scanners, which could collect all data within 20 to 25 seconds. Such reduced scan times allow more patients to hold their breath for the entire duration of the scan period. The introduction of 64-slice cardiac CT allows nearly all patients to be scanned with very high resolution. Scan times are now on the order of several seconds (usually 5–13 seconds); this means that even patients with severe pulmonary disease and congestive heart failure can hold their breath for the required length of time. Reduced time translates to minimal or no motion artifacts. Furthermore, higher number of slices means higher resolution; the current 64-slice scanners are capable of performing 64 slices per rotation at less than 0.4 to 0.7 mm resolution. Such high resolution allows visualization of the entire coronary tree with extremely high accuracy and detail. Individual atheromatous plaques can be detected and characterized. Calcification can be visualized and used as an added variable in disease management. The CT technology continues to be refined. Prototypes for 128-slice and even 256-slice scanners are under development.

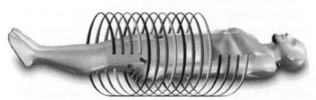

FIGURE 26.12   The spiral movement in helical computed tomography (CT) with both the gantry and the patient in motion.

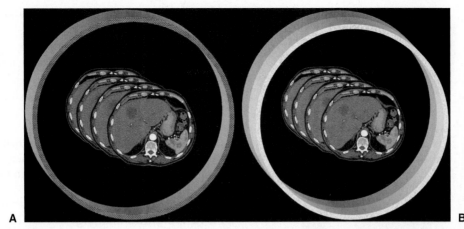

FIGURE 26.13 **A:** Helical computed tomography (CT) unit with a single row of detectors. **B:** Helical CT unit with two rows of detectors. Multidetector design increases the speed of imaging. As the slice number increases, the speed of the scanner increases.

Specialized Computed Tomography Scans
Computed Tomography Angiography

The basic principle of computed tomography angiography (CTA) is a carefully timed helical acquisition during rapid peripheral administration of contrast.

CT is an excellent imaging modality for visualizing blood vessel morphology and lumen patency. Helical multislice CT scanners have allowed the development of sophisticated noninvasive vascular imaging. As discussed earlier, conventional CT scanners imaged one slice at a time, with the table in a stationary position. Imaging with conventional CT was therefore too slow to be used for angiographic studies. Helical CT images continuously as the patient is moved rapidly through the gantry. The scan time is therefore dramatically reduced in comparison to conventional CT, so that a continuous column of intravenous contrast can be followed as it opacifies a vascular bed. Helical CT also allows acquisition of a "volume" of information that can be processed similar to magnetic resonance imaging (MRI) technology. Initial helical scanners were equipped with a single row of detector elements. With the development of

multidetector row technology (MDCT), imaging times have further decreased. With multiple rows of detector elements, interweaving spiral acquisitions can occur simultaneously, resulting in reduction of scan time, reduced volumes of contrast and reduced motion and pulsatility artifacts. Slice thickness is determined by the thickness of the detector elements rather than x-ray beam collimation and may be less than 1 mm providing exquisite spatial resolution.

One of the major advantages of CTA is that the images are single axial slices with intense vascular opacification. All the information regarding the vascular wall and perivascular structures on a CT scan is preserved. The initial data can be processed and reformatted to be displayed in different planes (i.e., coronal slices from axially acquired data). 3-D volume renderings can be created that permit visualization of the vascular lumen (Figs. 26.14 and 26.15).

Computed Tomography Colonoscopy (Virtual Colonoscopy)

Virtual colonoscopy is a technique that utilizes a CT scanner and computer virtual reality software to reconstruct data into

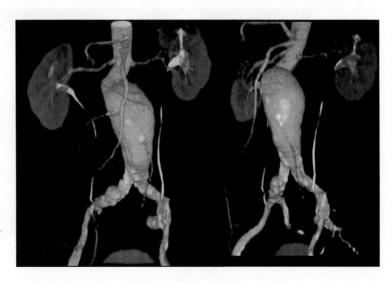

FIGURE 26.14 Computed tomography (CT) angiogram demonstrating an abdominal aortic aneurysm with tortuous iliac vessels. An excellent image detail can be obtained with fast scanners using this technique.

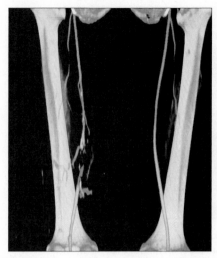

FIGURE 26.15 Computed tomography (CT) angiogram of lower extremities. Complete blockage of left superficial femoral artery with collateralization, normal right superficial femoral artery.

endoscopic-like images. Typically the patient undergoes the same oral preparation before the procedure as conventional endoscopy. The patient is then placed in the supine position on the CT scanner table and a flexible rubber catheter is placed in the rectum, and just before imaging, carbon dioxide is insufflated to distend the entire colon. Manual air insufflation has the advantage of easy administration; however, carbon dioxide has a much faster reabsorption rate with better patient tolerance. A thin-section CT imaging with a multislice scanner (16 or above) is performed.

Two-dimensional (2-D) source images are adequate for primary investigation of the colon in both lung and soft tissue windows. This source information is then processed with volume rendering algorithms to create 3-D shaded surface display images. These images are similar to endoscopic images with exquisite endoluminal detail (Fig. 26.16).

Data indicate that virtual colonoscopy has a very good sensitivity in detecting and characterizing polyps in comparison to barium enema and is nearly as accurate as conventional endoscopy. The clear advantage of this procedure is its noninvasive nature, as compared to conventional endoscopy. Inability to instantly biopsy a positive finding is its major shortcoming. The role of virtual colonoscopy in clinical practice is yet to be determined.

Magnetic Resonance Imaging

MRI is based on the signals created in tissues in response to magnetic field changes imposed upon them. MR signals stem from the interactions of radiowaves with the atomic nuclei. No ionizing radiation is used in MRI.

T1/T2 Weighted Imaging

The first step in the process of MRI generation is placement of the patient in a strong magnetic field in the MR scanner. The hydrogen ions in the body allign with the applied external magnetic field (Fig. 26.17). The second step is the application of short bursts of electromagnetic energy in the form of radiofrequency pulse (Fig. 26.18). When a short burst of radio waves is applied [radio frequency (RF) pulse], the nuclei are disturbed from their alignment with the external magnetic field. As they attempt to realign with the magnetic field, they emit a signal that can be detected and processed to generate an MR image. The relaxation processes that establish equilibrium following RF excitation is associated with two phenomena: (i) realignment with the main magnetic field, and (ii) dephasing of spinning protons, both of which occur in milliseconds but at a different rate. T1 describes the rate at which the protons, disturbed by the RF pulse, realign with the external magnetic field. T2 refers to a process in which spinning protons no longer spin in phase with one another.

The number of available protons (proton density) in a sample of tissue is the first determinant of signal strength. Areas of high proton density such as urine are capable of giving off strong signals. Areas of low proton density (i.e., low water content) such as cortical bone, air, and tendons typically give off weak signals and are seen as black areas in the images. In addition to proton density, the T1 and T2

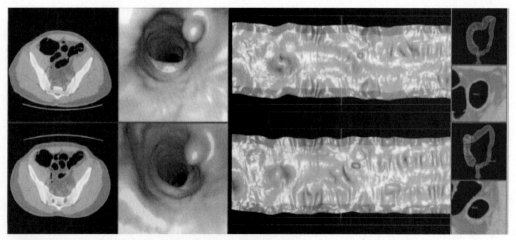

FIGURE 26.16 Appearance of polyps on virtual colonoscopy. Excellent image detail comparable to endoscopy.

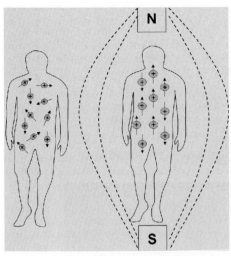

FIGURE 26.17   Hydrogen ions aligning in the line of the main magnetic field.

	High MR Signal (White)	Low MR Signal (Black)
Proton density	High	Low
T1 relaxation	Short	Long
T2 relaxation	Long	Short
Blood flow	Slow/static	Fast

TABLE 26.2

Signal Characteristics of Tissues in Response to Different Pulse Sequences

MR, magnetic resonance.

values of a given tissue determine final signal intensity. T1 and T2 are independent of one another and are distinct for each tissue. Every MR image is composed of T1, T2, proton density, and flow information.

Certain parameters can be adjusted to alter the contribution from each of the previous tissue characteristics. Therefore, a T1-weighted image contains mainly information about the T1 relaxation time, although contributions are also present from T2, proton density, and flow information. In general, tissues with short T1 values (e.g., fat) will be bright on a T1-weighted image (Table 26.2). On the contrary, tissues with long T2 values (e.g., water) will be bright on a T2-weighted image. Many pathologic areas have a longer T1 and T2 than surrounding normal tissue. The effects of flowing blood on the final images are complex and beyond the realm of this discussion. Depending on the parameters chosen, flowing blood may be black or white on the MR image.

Although CT provides good *spatial resolution* (the ability to distinguish two structures an arbitrarily small distance from each other as separate), MRI provides comparable resolution with far better *contrast resolution* (the ability to distinguish the differences between two arbitrarily similar but not identical tissues).

The basis of this ability is the complex library of RF pulse sequences that are used, each of which is optimized to provide unique image details based on the composition of normal and pathologic tissues. The inherent soft tissue contrast of MRI is particularly useful in interpreting musculoskeletal abnormalities. Muscles, tendons, cartilage, and ligaments that are poorly visualized on plain radiographs are seen in exquisite detail by MRI. Bone marrow or medullary bone is well visualized by MRI, and a process that replaces normal marrow is readily detected. MRI has also been useful in the evaluation of the neurologic system. The brain and spinal cord are well imaged without the artifact from overlying bone, which can be problematic on CT. MRI of the abdomen is often limited by motion artifact from breathing, bowel peristalsis, and pulsatile blood flow. Despite these limitations, abdominal MRI can be of use in selected cases. Detection of subtle hepatic metastasis and extent of renal cell carcinoma are two situations for which MRI may be useful.

Tesla: the Unit of Magnetic Field Strength

Magnetic field strength employed in an MRI unit is expressed in Tesla unit. This is an important factor determining image quality. Higher magnetic fields produce higher resolution and faster scanning. An anology can be made to a horsepower of a car. The strength of most clinical magnets in use currently ranges from 1.5 to 3 T (this is approximately 40,000 times the force of gravity on earth!). Obviously, a higher magnetic field increases cost and potential hazards of magnetization.

Safety of Magnetic Resonance Imaging

The magnetic force of the magnet can transform a normally benign object into a potentially lethal projectile. Objects such as scissors, oxygen tanks, "crash carts," intravenous poles, jewelry, and keys have been drawn into the magnet. It is

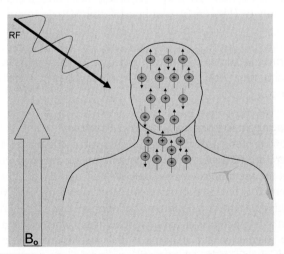

FIGURE 26.18   Additional radio frequency (RF) pulse applied to previously aligned hydrogen ions inline with main magnetic field. The RF pulse destabilizes them for subsequent realignment and emission of characteristic radiofrequency signals.

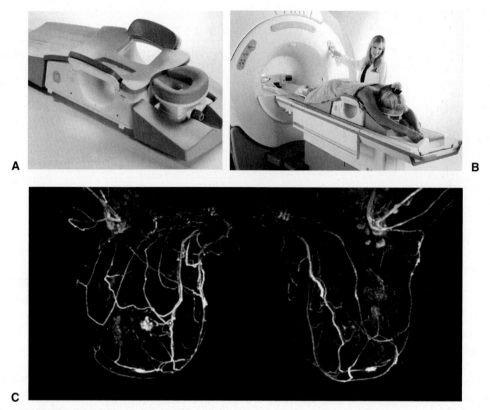

FIGURE 26.19 **A:** The breast coil. **B:** Patient positioning in the magnetic resonance imaging (MRI) unit with breast coil. **C:** Demonstration of a breast lesion with detailed display of vasculature and axillary nodes.

crucial, therefore, that patients and physicians be screened for such objects before entering the MR area. Similarly, patients with certain types of implanted metal, surgical clips, or shrapnel are at risk if the metal is a type that is attracted to the magnetic field. Such objects may then be torqued, moved, or disabled. Not all implanted metals pose a threat to patient safety. Some are not attracted to the external magnetic field and, therefore, do not run the risk of displacement. However, they do cause a distortion of the local magnetic field and thereby image degradation. Examples would include most prosthetic joints, dental braces, and most rods, nails, and screws used in orthopedic hardware. Patients with implanted pacemakers risk pacer malfunction when exposed to high electromagnetic forces. A less common hazard exists as the result of the heating effects of the RF energy generated by the MR systems. This energy can potentially heat the wires and gating devices attached to the patient to the point at which they burn the patient or set fire to combustible material. Electrocardiographic leads, pacing leads, and electrodes should be used and placed with care. The wires should not be excessively long, coiled, or touching the sides of the magnet.

The Magnetic Resonance Imaging Coil

Coil is the component that transmits the RF pulse and receives the returning electromagnetic signal. Body coil is fixed in the MR unit, is oriented in the x, y, and z directions

of the scanner and determine the plane of (transverse, coronal and sagittal) imaging. Although it is possible to scan using the integrated coil for transmitting and receiving, if a small region is being imaged, then better image quality is obtained by using a close-fitting smaller coil. A variety of coils are available which fit around parts of the body, (head, knee, wrist, breast) or internally (rectum). Breast coil allows very high-resolution MR images of breast, increasing detection sensitivity (Fig. 26.19). Endorectal coil MRI is useful for determining the extent of spread and local invasion of cancers of the prostate, rectum, and anus. The coil consists of a probe with an inflatable balloon which helps maintain appropriate positioning. Similar coils may be used vaginally for evaluating cervical cancer.

Magnetic Resonance Imaging Contrast

Flowing blood provides inherent contrast in MR images, and therefore adequate information can often be obtained without the use of intravenous contrast. MRI uses paramagnetic agents for contrast enhancement. Most commonly used MRI contrast agent is gadolinium. Gadolinium, one of the "rare earth" elements is a paramagnetic agent which increases the magnetic field adjacent to the gadolinium molecule. This shortens the T1 relaxation time of any substance in the region of the gadolinium molecule and enhances the MR signal intensity of blood on the T1-weighted postcontrast images. This contrast mechanism creates true anatomic images of vascular lumen, analogous to conventional angiography. There is no detectable toxicity to gadolinium and it can be used in patients with renal failure. Gadolinium is excreted by the kidneys, and its half-life is 1.5 hours. Gadolinium-enhanced tissues and fluids appear extremely bright on T1-weighted images. This provides high sensitivity for detection of vascular tissues (e.g., tumors) and permits assessment of brain perfusion (e.g., in stroke). More recently, superparamagnetic contrast agents such as iron oxide nanoparticles have been introduced for clinical use. These agents appear very dark on T2-weighted images and may be used for liver imaging—normal liver tissue retains the agent, but abnormal areas (e.g., scars, tumors) do not.

Specialized Magnetic Resonance Imaging Scans
Magnetic Resonance Angiography

Contrast-enhanced magnetic resonance angiography (CE-MRA) imaging is obtained after intravenous administration of gadolinium. CE-MRA is a tomographic imaging modality which is a viable alternative to standard angiography in the routine evaluation of patients with vascular disease. The advantages of MR angiography compared to standard angiography include noninvasiveness, avoiding ionizing radiation and a nephrotoxic contrast agent. One of the strengths of CE-MRA is acquired images are thin enough so that 3-D reconstructions can be obtained, and the resolution is high (Fig. 26.20). This allows rotation of the imaging volume in space. CE-MRA is widely used in: (i) screening for vaso-occlusive disease—carotid arteries, arch vessels, renal arteries, peripheral vessels; (ii) evaluating the anatomy of the aortic valve and origin of the coronary arteries; (iii) preoperative planning and postoperative follow-up of

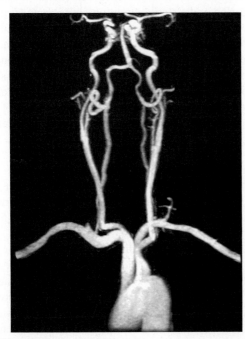

FIGURE 26.20 A magnetic resonance angiogram image of aortic arch and its branches.

abdominal/thoracic aortic aneurysms; (iv) diagnosis of aortic dissection; and (v) diagnosis of vasculitis.

Magnetic Resonance Cholangiopancreatography

Magnetic resonance cholangiopancreatography (MRCP) is a technique that produces images of the pancreaticobiliary tree that are similar in appearance to those obtained by endoscopic retrograde cholangiopancreatography (ERCP)(Fig.26.21). MRCP takes advantage of the inherent contrast-related properties of fluid in the biliary and pancreatic ducts. MRCP does not require an administration of any exogenous contrast material. The technique was initially performed with the use of heavily T2-weighted MR pulse sequences. These had the effect of making stationary or slow-flowing fluid within the bile and pancreatic ducts to appear very bright relative to the low signal intensity produced by adjacent solid tissues. Since its introduction in 1991, technologic refinements have made it an extremely useful modality in the evaluation of the hepatobiliary tree with excellent image resolution. With different pulse sequences and image acquisition protocols, signals from flowing blood are reduced to immeasurable levels; as a result, blood vessels do not interfere with clear identification of bile or pancreatic ducts. The ducts could be visualized from multiple projections, thereby providing multiplanar cholangiographic images noninvasively. With the new rapid acquisition protocols a high-quality MRCP can be performed in a breath-hold period with a scan time of less than 20 seconds.

Unlike conventional ERCP, MRCP does not require contrast material to be administered into the ductal system. Therefore, the morbidity associated with endoscopic procedures and contrast materials is avoided. The main potential problems with MRCP are image artifacts and difficulty in patient compliance. Image artifacts can be produced by a bright signal arising from stationary fluid within the adjacent duodenum, duodenal diverticulae, and ascitic fluid. In addition, local areas of dropout of signal can be caused by metallic clips following cholecystectomy, crossing defects induced by the right hepatic artery, or from severely narrowed ducts, such as occurs with primary sclerosing cholangitis. The presence of metal leads or fragments precludes any MR imaging study.

Conventional Nuclear Imaging

Nuclear medicine images display physiology and pathophysiology. Unlike other radiologic modalities, nuclear scans always require the administration of radioisotopes. These radiotracers or radiopharmaceuticals provide the signal used for imaging. The tracer distribution reflects a combination of blood flow, capillary permeability, and tissue extraction. By selecting radiopharmaceuticals extracted by specific organs and recording images of the activity distribution, one can determine the function and dysfunction of those organs.

Traditional nuclear medicine imaging technology has been built around single photon emitting radioisotopes where a γ-camera collects photons (γ-rays) emitted from the patient's body during decay of the single photon emitting

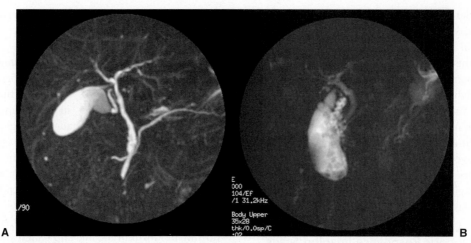

FIGURE 26.21 A magnetic resonance cholangio-pancreatogram (MRCP). **A:** Normal anatomy. **B:** Gall bladder with multiple stones. This modality is extremely helpful in noninvasive assessment of periampullary lesions and pancreatic abnormalities.

radiotracer. Routine 2-D (planar) images are obtained either directly from the γ-camera (analog images) or through an interfaced computer system (digital images). The resolution of nuclear images are improved by utilization of tomographic techniques [single photon emission computed tomography (SPECT)]. This technique creates images oriented in transverse, coronal, and sagittal planes, yielding improved detection and localization of certain disease processes when compared with planar imaging.

Radiopharmaceuticals, Localization Mechanisms, and Clinical Applications

Iodine, gallium, and thallium radioisotopes are examples of natural physiologic substrates that are used in nuclear medicine imaging. Most, however, are complicated radio-pharmaceuticals consisting of a radiolabel (source of γ signal) and a ligand (determines the physiology/pathophysiology of the specific uptake). Technetium-99m (^{99m}Tc) and Indium-111 (^{111}In) are the most common radiolabels used in clinical practice. A list of the most commonly used radiopharmaceuticals, their localization mechanism, and clinical applications are shown in Table 26.3.

Hepatobiliary Imaging

Hepatobiliary imaging uses ^{99m}Tc-labeled iminodiacetic acid (IDA) compounds that are taken up and excreted into bile by the same hepatocellular mechanism as is bilirubin. Diagnostic results could be obtained even with high bilirubin levels. A failure to visualize the gallbladder is diagnostic for cystic duct obstruction, the hallmark of acute cholecystitis. To shorten study time from the conventional 4 hours to 90 minutes and to decrease false-positive results, pharmacologic intervention with intravenous morphine sulfate is often used. Through its physiologic action of increasing the tone of sphincter of Oddi, morphine promotes retrograde filling of the gallbladder with radioactive bile, thereby establishing cystic duct patency. Cholecystokinin (CCK), on the other hand, decreases the sphincter of Oddi tone and

causes increased tone and contraction of the gallbladder. The utilization of this pharmacologic action during a hepatobiliary scan allows assessment of gallbladder ejection fraction, a way of diagnosing biliary dyskinesia.

Infection Localization

Both Gallium-67 (^{67}Ga) and radiolabeled autologous white blood cells (WBCs) accumulate in the regions of infection, and are helpful in localizing occult abdominal infections. Two major limitations to the use of ^{67}Ga, which is available ready for injection, are (i) delay in imaging (typically 48–96 hours after injection), and (ii) prominent physiologic bowel excretion that can obscure abnormal accumulation at sites of intra-abdominal infection. Labeled WBCs require several hours of careful preparation to maintain cell viability and function under sterile conditions, but imaging is usually completed within 24 hours of injection. The abdomen is evaluated more readily with WBCs than with ^{67}Ga because any radioactivity outside the liver, spleen, and bone marrow is abnormal and may represent a site of infection or inflammation. Both chronicity of infection and prior antibiotic therapy may decrease the sensitivity of WBC imaging; despite its limitations, ^{67}Ga may be the preferred imaging agent under these circumstances.

Blood Pool Imaging

^{99m}Tc-labeled RBCs distribute in the cardiovascular compartment. Cinecardiographic images [multigated analysis, multiple-gated acquisition or (MUGA) scan] allows for determination of cardiac ejection fraction.

The site of active GI bleeding in the small bowel or colon may be identified readily by the intraluminal extravasation of ^{99m}Tc-labeled RBCs. When intraluminal, this tracer activity moves and changes configuration over time. The study is less sensitive for localizing gastric and duodenal sites of bleeding. Bleeding rates as low as 0.1 mL/min can be detected; by comparison, standard angiography requires much faster bleeding rates of 0.5 to 1.0 mL/min for detection. The nuclear

TABLE 26.3

Most Commonly Used Radiopharmaceuticals, Their Localization Mechanisms and Clinical Applications

Radiopharmaceutical	Localization	Applications
Iodine-123 or -131 (^{123}I or ^{131}I) (as sodium iodide)	Uptake and organification	Thyroid function
Thallium-201 (^{201}Tl) (as thallium chloride)	Uptake through Na/K ATPase pump	Myocardial perfusion
Gallium-67 (^{67}Ga) (as gallium citrate)	Binding transferrin receptors	Inflammation/tumor imaging
Technetium-99m (^{99m}Tc) radiopharmaceuticals		
^{99m}Tc-Phosphonates	Osteoblastic activity	Bone scanning
^{99m}Tc-Microaggregate albumin	Capillary blocking	Perfusion scanning
^{99m}Tc-Human serum albumin	Albumin distribution	Blood pool imaging
^{99m}Tc-RBC	Blood distribution	Bleeding scan
		Blood pool imaging
^{99m}Tc-Sulfur colloid	Uptake by RES	Liver–spleen scan
		Lymphoscintigraphy
^{99m}Tc-Disofenin (HIDA)	Hepatocyte uptake	Hepatobiliary scan
	Biliary excretion	
^{99m}Tc-Sestamibi	Mitochondrial uptake	Tumor imaging
		Parathyroid imaging
^{99m}Tc-DTPA	Glomerular filtration	Renal scan
^{99m}Tc- and ^{111}I-labeled WBC/antibodies/peptides		Inflammation/tumor imaging

ATPase, adenosine triphosphatase; RBC, red blood cell; RES, reticuloendothelial system; DTPA, diethylenetriamine penta-acetate; WBC, white blood cell.

bleeding scan best serves as a precursor to more definitive therapy by directing the site of surgery, colonoscopy with laser therapy, or selective angiography with intra-arterial vasopressin or embolization.

Another specific application, ^{99m}Tc-labeled RBC blood pool imaging, is the diagnosis of liver hemangiomas, which are common benign liver tumors found in up to 10% of the general population that pose an important diagnostic problem in colon cancer patients with solitary liver lesions. The ^{99m}Tc RBC scan with SPECT imaging can accurately identify a hemangioma as small as 1.4 cm, eliminating the need for more extensive evaluation.

Radioimmunoscintigraphy

Scintigraphic imaging of cancer after administration of radiolabeled monoclonal antibodies (MoAbs) raised against various tumor antigens has been referred to as *radioimmunoscintigraphy* (RIS). The MoAbs tested as RIS immunoconjugates have been used both as the intact immunoglobulin (Ig, most are IgG) and as dimeric F(ab')$_2$, or monomeric (Fab') antigen reactive fragments. Radioisotopes used in RIS include ^{111}In, Iodine 131 (^{131}I), Iodine 123 (^{123}I), and ^{99m}Tc. Intact MoAbs have generally been conjugated to radiolabels with longer half-lives (^{111}In or ^{131}I, with half-lives of 68 hours and 8 days, respectively) so that the radiation signal is still strong after blood pool activity has decreased to levels that allow visualization of the tumor. γ-Camera imaging after injection of radiolabeled MoAbs is highly satisfactory when a short half-life isotope (^{123}I or ^{99m}Tc, with half-lives of 13 hours and 6 hours, respectively) is used. Metabolism of intact MoAb immunoconjugates is predominantly through the liver and spleen, whereas MoAb fragments are eliminated through the kidneys; high radiation background in these organs resulting from immunoconjugate metabolism can pose a challenge in interpretation of RIS scans.

Somatostatin Receptor Imaging

Tumors of neuroendocrine origin (APUDomas) express somatostatin receptors (mostly type 2). Radiolabeled octreotide (^{111}In-pentetreotide) has been used successfully to locate the primary and metastatic tumors expressing sst 2. It has been demonstrated that the angiogenic tumor response is associated with sst two receptor upregulation. Tumors with no intrinsic neuroendocrine differentiation can still be imaged through their angiogenic vessels with radiolabeled somatostatin analogs.

Lymphoscintigraphy and Lymphatic Mapping

Lymphoscintigraphy is the localization and external imaging of the lymph nodes following the interstitial injection of radiolabeled particles. Lymphoscintigraphy is based on the mechanism of the transport of a radioparticle injected into the interstitial space (intracutaneous, subcutaneous, or intraparenchymal). If the radioparticle is injected intravenously, it is localized within the reticuloendothelial system of the liver, spleen, and bone marrow. When radioparticles are injected interstitially they enter lymphatic capillaries and travel to the regional nodes where they are phagocytosed by lymph node macrophages. Successful localization is dependent on patency of the lymphatic channels as well as lymph node integrity.

The transfer of interstitially injected particles across lymphatic endothelial cells begins within seconds of injection. These particles enter the lymphatic capillary lumen through the patent junctions. This passage is accelerated by higher interstitial pressures as the patent junctions between the endothelial leaflets are distended more widely. Particle transport across the lymphatic endothelial cell also occurs by pinocytosis. Particle uptake in the lymph nodes is a function of macrophage phagocytosis. The collagen meshwork in the subcapsular sinus functions as a mechanical filter and plays a role in particle uptake.

The most readily used radioparticle for lymphoscintigraphy is ^{99m}Tc sulfur colloid. Particle size of nonfiltered sulfur colloid ranges from 50 to 1,000 nm (average size, 200 nm). Solutions of smaller particle size can be obtained by different preparation techniques and filtration.

Sentinel Node Localization

The sentinel node is that lymph node in a given lymphatic basin that receives lymphatic flow from a primary tumor site. This node should be the first to become involved by metastasis from this tumor. The concept is based on the evidence that there is an orderly progression of nodal metastases in a lymph node basin. All the nodes in a given lymphatic basin are expected to be free of metastasis when the sentinel node is negative. Sentinel node(s) can be mapped by using a vital dye (isosulfan or blue) or radiolabeled particles. When radiolabeled particles are utilized, a gamma detection probe is used for localization of the radioactive nodes. Lymphoscintigraphy and intraoperative gamma probe detection for lymphatic mapping are now important techniques in the surgeons' armamentarium. Sentinel node biopsy is currently being used in melanoma and breast cancer, and other potential applications are under investigation. Probe detection is a highly sensitive technique. Nodes smaller than 5 mm can be identified by the gamma probe.

^{99m}Tc-labeled sulfur colloid is injected in the dermis for melanoma application. Sentinel node localization in breast cancer patients involves injection of ^{99m}Tc sulfur colloid around the primary tumor site. Intradermal injection in the overlying skin or subareolar injection methods have also been proved to work effectively and accurately. External lymphoscintigraphy is performed using dynamic and static imaging techniques to trace lymphatic channels from the primary site to sentinel lymph nodes (SLNs) in the regional lymphatic basin. Sentinel node localization by the radiocolloid can occur as early as 10 minutes, and could take upto a few hours.

A gamma probe is used at surgery to identify the sentinel node. Sensitivity is adjusted according to the signal intensity. The entire nodal region is then scanned by moving the probe in a grid pattern over the skin. The SLN in the basin is identified by an intense focus of radioactivity (the hot spot), and a small incision is made on the overlying skin. The node is found in situ and excised. The high levels of activity in the removed node and minimal-to-no background activity in the remainder of the basin confirm that the SLN has been removed.

Gamma Probe–Guided Surgery

Intraoperative nuclear probes are special detector systems designed that locate γ emissions in pretargeted tissues. The concept of intraoperative tumor localization by using radiation detection probes started with cylindrical Geiger-Mueller tubes more than 60 years ago, and led eventually to the development of small handheld intraoperative radiation-sensitive probes. The modern era of gamma probe–guided surgery, however, evolved with the radioimmunoguided surgery technique. Development of radiocolloid-directed lymphatic mapping and the sentinel node biopsy technique popularized the use of medium-energy gamma probes. Gamma probes are being successfully used for radioguided minimally invasive parathyroidectomy with ^{99m}Tc sestamibi and localization of occult neuroendocrine tumors by using ^{111}In octreotide. Contemporary gamma probes are sophisticated detector systems ergonomically designed for specific surgical applications, including laparoscopic procedures. Currently, most gamma probe systems are optimized for detection of low-energy (140 keV) ^{99m}Tc-based or medium-energy (174 and 250 keV) ^{111}In-based radiotracers. Recently, gamma probes that are designed to detect and process 511-keV high-energy photons of PET radioisotopes. These probes have different detector design and heavier shielding (Fig. 26.22).

Positron Emission Tomography and Positron Emission Tomography/Computed Tomography

PET is a very high-resolution nuclear imaging system. Radioisotopes used in this technique, the detector design, and image reconstruction algorithms differ fundamentally from those of conventional SPECT. Positrons are the antimatter equivalent of electrons. When ejected from the nucleus, a positron collides with an electron, resulting in the annihilation of both particles and the release of two high-energy (511 keV) γ photons in opposite trajectory (180 degrees apart). For this reason, PET is also referred to as *dual photon emission tomography*. A ring of detectors in the PET scanning device can record the arrival of the photon pair by virtue of a coincidence detection algorithm, and a further computer analysis produces a 3-D map of the radiotracer distribution, revealing a biologic profile.

PET imaging allows a comprehensive tumor/tissue characterization, and an *in vivo* profiling of tumor biology. Tumor metabolism, altered metabolic pathways, blood flow, proliferative activity, and receptor expression can be mapped with precision, and more importantly, quantified. A clinically accepted method for quantification is the determination of the standard uptake value (SUV). SUV is a measure for the preferential uptake for the radiopharmaceutical in a lesion compared with a homogenous distribution in the body. Maximum and median SUV values can be computed in a region of interest. The SUV is clinically most useful for the monitoring of response to treatment evaluation. In order for an SUV to be meaningful, image acquisition parameters have to be kept consistent from one study to another (Fig. 26.23).

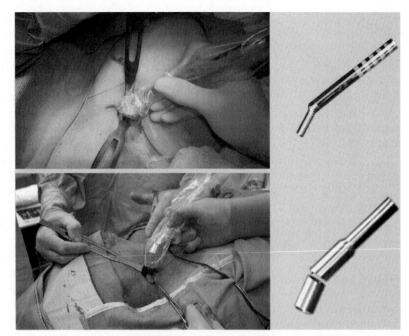

FIGURE 26.22 Intraoperative gamma probes. The upper row shows a standard gamma probe that is designed for ^{99m}Tc based radiopharmaceuticals (sentinel node and parathyroid localization). The lower row demonstrates positron emission tomography (PET) probe which is designed for detection of high-energy (511 keV) γ rays of positron emitting radiopharmaceuticals. Note the thicker collimation on the PET probe.

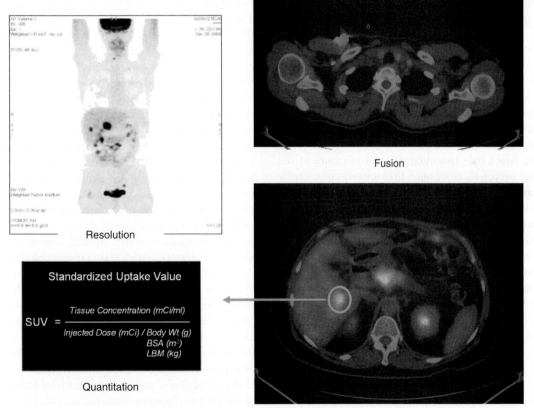

FIGURE 26.23 Positron emission tomography (PET) images offer the highest resolution in the functional imaging field (nuclear medicine). Combining PET images with computed tomography (CT) provides excellent anatomical localization together with quantitation of the biologic function being investigated. BSA, body surface area; LBM, lean body mass.

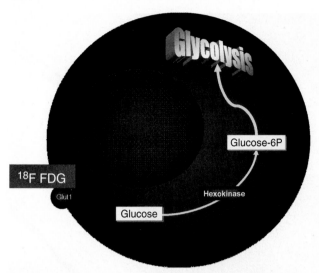

FIGURE 26.24 Flourine-18 fluorodeoxyglucose (FDG) is taken up by the cells using the same mechanism the glucose molecule uses. FDG enters the cells using glucose transport protein 1 (Glut-1). Inside the cell FDG is phosphorylated by the hexokinase enzyme to deoxyglucose-6 phosphate. Deoxyglucose 6-phosphate is not a good substrate for further steps of glycolysis and therefore is retained in the cell; however, it serves as an excellent marker of glycolysis.

Fluorodeoxyglucose Imaging

Fluorodeoxyglucose (FDG), a fluorinated analog of glucose enters into the cells by a facilitated diffusion mechanism using glucose transporters. It is phosphorylated by hexokinase to FDG phosphate which is not a good substrate for the next enzymatic step, and is therefore entrapped in the cell. FDG uptake in the cell correlates with glycolytic activity (Fig. 26.24). Since the pioneering work of Warburg in the 1920s, it has been well established that tumors consistently rely on anaerobic pathways to convert glucose to adenosine triphosphate (ATP) even in the presence of abundant oxygen. Since the anaerobic metabolism of glucose to lactic acid is substantially less efficient than the oxidation to CO_2 and H_2O, tumor cells maintain ATP production by increasing glucose flux. This metabolic alteration forms the basis for tumor imaging with FDG-PET. FDG-PET is now widely applied to human cancers and has confirmed that the vast majority of primary and metastatic tumors demonstrate substantially increased glucose uptake compared to normal tissue.

Diagnostic Performance of Fluorodeoxyglucose-Positron Emission Tomography

A large body of clinical studies and reviews attest to the clinical value of FDG-PET in staging, restaging, evaluation of response to systemic and regional therapies and radiation treatment planning. FDG-PET demonstrates a superior sensitivity in detecting malignant lesions in areas where CT image contrast is less than desired. Recurrent lesions of breast cancer in the axilla, the mediastinal/internal mammary lymph node basins, intramuscular/soft tissue metastatic disease in melanoma, extrahepatic metastases in

colorectal cancer, and the occult, radioactive iodine-negative thyroid cancer lesions are clearly better detected by FDG-PET. Previously unrecognized patterns of nodal involvement such as axillary metastases in lung cancer, and mediastinal metastases in hepatocellular cancer, are becoming more familiar events to oncologic surgeons.

An optimal utilization of any new technology requires a thorough understanding of its inherent limitations as well as its potential. FDG-PET certainly is no exception. Although FDG is an outstanding tumor localizing molecular probe, it is not tumor specific. The FDG uptake indicates high (or heightened) metabolic/glycolytic activity. As such, all metabolically active tissues, including active and chronic-active inflammatory processes are expected to show enhanced FDG uptake. This, by no means, should be regarded as a false positivity, but rather a biologic phenomenon that needs to be taken into account when interpreting FDG images. An analogy can be made to elevations in the WBC count, which could be associated with many well identified altered physiologic states but not necessarily be due to the presence of an infection *per se*.

Fluorodeoxyglucose-Positron Emission Tomography and Tumor Biology

PET literature is beset with reviews citing the relative avidity of different cancer types for FDG. Moderate to high uptake is a common occurrence with lung, esophageal, colorectal, head and neck, and breast cancers, and with melanoma. In contrast, a variable uptake is seen in pancreatic, hepatocellular and renal cancers, sarcomas and neuroendocrine tumors. Although, this information may have some practical clinical value, it is also a pitfall leading to the underappreciation and underutilization of the technology. There is a direct correlation between tumor aggressiveness (and prognosis) and the rate of glucose consumption as demonstrated by FDG-PET imaging and glucose transport proteins (mainly Glut-1) expression by immunohistochemistry studies. The end result of an accelerated glycolysis is increased tumor cell acid production. An acid-mediated tumor invasion hypothesis was developed to explain the clinical correlations between FDG uptake and tumor prognosis. The general concept is that the tumor cells become invasive because they perturb the environment to make it optimal for their proliferation and toxic to the normal cells with which they compete for space and substrate. Through a variety of mechanisms, acidification of the extracellular environment leads to destruction of the normal tissue. These mechanisms include caspase-mediated activation of p53-dependent apoptosis pathways, promotion of angiogenesis through acid-induced release of vascular endothelial growth factor and interleukin 8, and extracellular matrix degradation by proteolytic enzymes such as cathepsin B and inhibition of immune function. FDG-PET imaging data provides substantially more information than merely locating the tumors. A reasonable outlook is to regard FDG uptake as a prognostic marker, analogous to some other markers such as estrogen–progesterone status. Indeed,

FDG-PET is an *in vivo* quantifiable prognostic marker. In this context, false negativity in FDG-PET is an incorrect connotation. Rather, tumor(s) should be denoted as FDG-positive or FDG-negative. Not unique to any particular type of cancer, it is not uncommon to see low or absent uptake in the primary tumor, with its metastases showing enhanced uptake. Similarly, lesions of any given cancer at different anatomic locations could display varying degrees of FDG uptake. Both these observations are the reflections of the phenomenon of synchronous progression of variable clonal expansions with differing biologic activities.

The Limitations of the Positron Emission Tomography Technology

One intrinsic limitation of PET derives from the nature of positron decay and the principle of coincidence detection. A positron must generally travel a certain distance in tissues before being able to collide with an electron. Annihilation often occurs approximately 1 to 2 mm away from the origin of the positron. This phenomenon places a theoretic limit on PETs achievable spatial resolution, which is estimated at 2 to 3 mm. Understanding this limitation of PET has a practical value in the appropriate use of the technology. Numerous studies, particularly those published in surgical literature have demonstrated that the sensitivity of PET for detecting microscopic metastatic disease is low. In general for most lesions less than 1 cm the detection sensitivity of PET is less than 10%.

A second limitation of the technique is associated with the molecular probe currently being used. Although FDG is an outstanding tumor localizing molecular probe, it is not tumor specific. The FDG uptake indicates high (or heightened) metabolic/glycolytic activity. As such, all metabolically active tissues, including active and chronic-active inflammatory processes are expected to show enhanced FDG uptake. Tumors with relatively attenuated glycolytic activity also may not be readily detected using FDG-PET. However, multiple studies have attested that this phenotypic expression is correlated with tumors, biologic behavior, and not necessarily regarded as false negativity.

Positron Emission Tomography/Computed Tomography Technology

Stand-alone PET systems do not provide sufficient anatomical detail. The development of PET-CT integrated units solved this technical shortcoming of PET imaging. The integrated systems house PET and CT components together, and acquire and register respective image data in one session. The integrated technology is different than the fusion technique where PET and CT images are obtained on separate scanners, and coregistered utilizing computer algorithms where the image quality is affected by the differences due to patient positioning. The contemporary integrated scanners use up to a 64-slice CT component and a high-resolution PET device. Special viewing tools are provided with the standard integrative software, which allow the viewer to scroll through any of the individual and combined image sets (Fig. 26.25).

The concept of contrast enhancement in imaging has evolved to a new level with the development of PET/CT technology. The standard iodine-based contrast enhancement, which is the basis of tumor/lesion characterization in anatomic imaging, is merely a reflection of the blood flow/pool in the microvascular compartment, and does not correlate with biologic characteristics of the tumors. However, a PET radiopharmaceutical (molecular probe) essentially serves as a biologic contrast agent enhancing the tissue function being examined. Metabolically active tissues are enhanced with F-18 fluoro deoxyglucose. Similarly, tumors/tissues with a high fraction of cells in a proliferative phase, actively incorporating thymidine in their DNA, are enhanced with F-18 fluoro thymidine (or C-11 thymidine). PET/CT represents a new vision in functional imaging. It combines the superior anatomic definition capability of advanced CT systems with the functional tumor/tissue characterization capability of PET. Most comprehensive staging is obtained by a PET/CT full-contrast study.

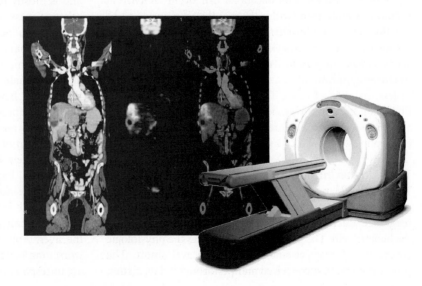

FIGURE 26.25 State of the art positron emission tomography/computed tomography (PET/CT) scanner. CT images are obtained in a few minutes with a multislice spiral CT and then fluorodeoxyglucose positron emission tomography (FDG PET) images are acquired in the next 15 minutes. Image coregistration allows two images to be superimposed for providing anatomic localization for PET images and tissue characterization for CT images.

THERAPEUTIC TECHNOLOGIES

Interventional radiology continues to expand in its applications parallel to the developments in the imaging and instrumentation technology. Many radiologic interventions have become standard aid in surgical management, and a number of techniques have become preferred alternatives to surgical procedures. Transvascular interventions now play significant role in the management of complex surgical problems.

Transvascular and Endovascular Interventions

Transvascular access has proved to be a very effective route to accomplish many surgical objectives much more safely and less invasively. The clinical applications of this technology continue to expand complementing and in many indications replacing standard surgical interventions.

Inferior Vena Cava Filter Placement

Inferior vena cava (IVC) filter was developed to treat patients with deep venous thrombosis (DVT), who present with a contraindication for anticoagulation. An IVC filter is designed to be placed percutaneously in the infrarenal IVC to act as a mechanical barrier to development of pulmonary embolism in patients who are at high risk for development of venous thromboembolic (VTE) disease. Filters do not prevent the formation of thrombus or treat pulmonary embolism that has already occurred.

An IVC filter can be placed from a femoral, internal jugular, or brachial vein approach. Typically a flush catheter is placed into the IVC or common iliac vein and a cavagram is performed. This is done to measure the diameter of the IVC and determine the location of renal veins. If the diameter of the IVC filter is greater than 28 mm (megacava) IVC filter placement could be problematic. The filter is typically placed with its apex below the level of the orifice of the lowest renal vein to minimize the risk for renal vein thrombosis.

Placement of an IVC filter is generally a very safe procedure; however, complications can occur. Recurrent pulmonary embolism (within 16 months) is reported to be less than 5%. Symptomatic IVC occlusion can occur up to 5% of the patients, especially those with hypercoagulable states. Filter migration (renal vein, right atrium) and fracture/significant tilt have also been reported to occur in less than 1% of cases. The long-term outcomes of IVC filters is not well known, because most of the patients that are reported in the literature have been very ill with short life expectancies.

Transjugular Intrahepatic Portosystemic Shunt

The transjugular intrahepatic portosystemic shunt (TIPS) procedure involves the percutaneous creation of a low resistance tract in the liver between the portal vein and the hepatic vein. The TIPS procedure creates the physiologic equivalent of surgical side-to-side portacaval shunt. The procedure was first conceived and performed in late sixties, and has gone through significant evolution in its technique since then. TIPS is of documented benefit in the management of cirrhotic patients with intractible variceal bleeding and refractory ascites.

TIPS is successfully used as a bridge to liver transplantation as a preferred alternative to surgical shunt procedures. Unlike surgical shunts, TIPS generally does not interfere with subsequent liver transplantation. In some studies, pretransplantation TIPS has been shown to improve the nutritional status and general condition of the patient.

The technique of TIPS involves a transjugular access of cava and hepatic veins. A tract is created between the right, middle or left hepatic veins (depending upon size, orientation, and patency) and the intrahepatic portal vein. This tract is then dilated to 10 to 12 mm in size and lined with a stent graft to maintain patency.

Short-term results (6 months) for TIPS procedures are generally very good. The created shunt is usually effective in lowering portal pressures in greater than 95% of cases. This leaves a portosystemic gradient of less than 12 mm Hg, or a reduction of greater than 50% in most cases. In patients treated for variceal hemorrhage, early rebleeding (defined as <6 months time) occurs in up to 15% of patients. This is more effective than sclerotherapy. Approximately 50% to 75% of patients treated for intractable ascites have partial or complete resolution within 1 month of shunt placement.

Without repeated US surveillance and repeated intervention, most TIPS shunts do not remain patent. The current reported primary patency rates for TIPS are 50% to 60% at 1 year and approximately 30% to 40% at 2 years. With the development of newly covered stent grafts, however, primary patency rates are improving. Patients should have routine US surveillance and potential angioplasty to maintain patency. After TIPS is created, a layer of pseudointima forms around the stented segment. Neointimal hyperplasia progresses within the track and most commonly around the outflow hepatic venous end.

The immediate procedure associated mortality rate of TIPS is reported between 1% and 2% in the literature, and is mostly related to the clinical experience. Most cases relate to massive intraperitoneal hemorrhage from capsular perforation, inadvertent hepatic arterial injury/thrombosis with fulminant hepatic failure or acute right heart failure. Major technical complications of TIPS include hemobilia and stent malposition/migration. Complications related to the altered hepatic flow dynamics present with varying degrees of hepatic dysfunction. A major concern after creation of any side to side portosystemic shunt is the development of hepatic encephalopathy. This complication is more likely to occur when the residual portosystemic gradient is less than 10 mm Hg. With diversion of mesenteric venous blood into the shunt, ammonia produced by bacterial action on nitrogen containing compounds enters systemic circulation before being metabolized by the liver. Approximately 25% of patients develop new or worsening hepatic encephalopathy; however, less than 5% are unresponsive to medical therapy.

Portal Vein Embolization

Portal vein embolization (PVE) is a preoperative interventional technique designed to induce hypertrophy in the functional liver remnant (i.e., the liver to remain after hepatectomy), and is intended to minimize the incidence of perioperative complications related to hepatic insufficiency from complex extended hepatic resections.

As advances in hepatobiliary surgical techniques occur, more patients are candidates for surgical resection of hepatobiliary tumors with improved postoperative outcomes. Extended hepatectomy (resection of five or more hepatic segments) is now considered a safe and appropriate treatment option in patients with hepatobiliary malignancies. However, in many patients, complications related to postoperative hepatic insufficiency can occur, including cholestasis, coagulopathy, bleeding, fluid retention, and impaired hepatic synthetic function.

The capability of both diseased and healthy hepatic tissue to regenerate in response to injury or resection provides the functional basis for preoperative PVE. Full recovery of functional liver can occur within as early as 2 weeks of the loss of as much as two thirds of functioning liver tissue. The regenerative response is typically mediated by the proliferation of surviving hepatocytes within the acinar architecture of the remaining liver.

PVE involves the utilization of embolic agents (platinum coils, polyvinyl alcohol particles, absolute ethanol, tris-acryl gelatin microspheres, etc.) to occlude portal vein branches from feeding diseased segments of the liver. It also helps to redirect portal venous flow to the intended future liver remnant. Embolization can be performed through a percutaneous transhepatic approach either through the nondiseased liver (contralateral) or through the diseased liver (ipsilateral). Portal blood flow to nonembolized segments, measured by Doppler US, increases significantly and then decreases near baseline after approximately 11 days. The resultant hypertrophy rates therefore correlate with the changes in portal venous flow rates.

PVE is a safe percutaneous procedure with little postprocedure complications. Hepatocytes undergo apoptosis (programmed cell death), and not necrosis. Patients therefore have very few side effects, such as fever pain or nausea, relating to inflammation.

As advances in oncologic treatments occur, and understanding of the molecular mechanisms mediating hepatocyte regeneration improves, both selection criteria and outcomes of patients undergoing PVE may improve. Currently, at least three major factors should be considered when determining whether a patient will benefit from PVE. First, the presence or absence of underlying liver disease will determine the necessary volume of remnant needed to reduce the risk of inducing postoperative hepatic insufficiency. Second, patient size also needs to be considered as larger patients will require larger functional liver remnants. Third, the extent and complexity of planned surgery and additional procedures must be considered. Currently, PVE is considered in patients with an intended future liver remnant that is 20% or less in the setting of a nondiseased liver, or less than 40% in the setting of a diseased liver.

Currently, there are no absolute contraindications for portal venous embolization. Relative contraindications include uncorrectable coagulopathy, tumor extension into the liver remnant, tumor invasion into the portal vein (which may render the procedure of no significant benefit), tumor precluding safe transhepatic access, or renal failure. Technical complications or PVE relate to the transhepatic approach including subcapsular hematoma, hemoperitoneum, arterial pseudoaneurysm or arteriovenous fistula, portal venous thrombosis, hemobilia, transient liver failure, and sepsis.

Hepatic Arterial Treatment Techniques

Hepatic artery provides more than 95% of the blood flow of the liver tumors (primary or metastatic), whereas most of the nutrient blood flow to the normal liver is supplied by the portal vein. This unique distribution pattern of blood flow allows utilization of hepatic artery as a venue to deliver therapeutic agents.

Hepatic Arterial Infusion Pump

Hepatic arterial infusion pump (HAIP) is designed to administer chemotherapy through hepatic artery. The pump consists of a reservoir with a mechanism that infuses chemotherapeutic agent at a constant rate, and a catheter that is placed surgically inside the gastroduodenal artery to direct the flow towards proper hepatic artery. The reservoir rests in the subcutaneous area in the anterior abdominal wall for easy access. This technique was developed for therapy of colorectal cancer liver metastases. The use of drugs that are largely extracted by the liver during the first pass results in a high local concentration of drug with minimal systemic toxicity. The chemotherapeutic agent of choice is fluorodeoxyuridine (FUDR). Following the injection of FUDR into the hepatic artery of patients, mean concentrations of drug in normal liver tissue do not differ significantly. However, mean tumor FUDR levels are markedly increased (15 times) when the drug is injected through the hepatic artery. This technique was used more extensively before the development of new generation systemic chemotherapeutic agents.

Because the bile ducts derive their blood supply from the hepatic artery, biliary toxicity is the most problematic adverse event seen with hepatic arterial chemotherapy. The studies point to a combined ischemia and inflammatory effect on the bile ducts as the most important etiology of the toxicity.

Chemoembolization

Transarterial chemoembolization (TACE) involves administration of embolic particles along with chemotherapeutic agents. The hypoxic/anoxic effect of embolization leads tumor ischemia and necrosis. The stagnant circulatory state created inside the tumor allows prolonged exposure of the tumor to the chemotherapeutic agent. Chemoembolization has been used mostly for hepatocellular cancer. A variety of embolization agents including polyvinyl alcohol particles, particles of gelatin, ivalon, Gelfoam, or lipiodol have been used. Most commonly used chemotherapeutic agents are Adriamycin, mitomycin-C, and cisplatin.

Postembolization syndrome (abdominal pain, fever, leukocytosis) is common and occurs in more than 50% of cases. Although self-limited in most patients, it does necessitate a period of hospitalization and observation.

Radioembolization

Radioembolization or selective internal radiation treatment (SIRT) is the delivery of radiation treatment through intrahepatic arterial administration of Yttrium-90 (Y-90) microspheres. Y-90 is a high-energy β particle emitting radioisotope. It is incorporated in biocompatible microspheres measuring 30 to 40 μ. Intrahepatic arterially administered Y-90 microspheres are entrapped within the microvasculature, and release β radiation with a maximum energy of 2.27 MeV, and a maximum range of 11 mm in the liver tissue. Owing to the 2.67 days half-life of Y-90, 94% of the radiation dose is delivered over 11 days following the administration of the treatment. The high tumor to liver concentration ratio of Y-90 microspheres results in an effective tumoricidal radiation absorbed dose whilst limiting the radiation injury to the normal liver.

SIRT is frequently referred to as *radioembolization* because of some technical similarities with chemoembolization. In reality, however, both theory and the practice of SIRT are different than chemoembolization. Contrary to chemoembolization, optimal perfusion and blood flow is required to enhance the free radical–dependent cell death in SIRT. Radiation combined with embolization-induced hypoxia is therefore undesirable. The biologic response is optimized by preservation of flow to the target area, and hence oxygenation.

Ablative Therapies

Ablative therapies include cryoablation radiofrequency ablation (RFA) and microwave ablation. Currently RFA is the most commonly employed method for tumor destruction.

Cryoablation

Cryoablation is a technique that uses subzero temperatures to necrose tumor cells. It was developed for the treatment of unresectable liver tumors. The procedure can be performed laparoscopically, percutaneously, or by open surgical procedure. The cryoprobe will be safely guided to the center of the lesion using image guidance. The probe tip then is positioned toward the opposite margin to ensure that the whole lesion will get frozen. The probe itself is vacuum insulated and contains supercooled liquid nitrogen. Depending on the size of the lesion(s), up to four probes can be used simultaneously. For example, two 8-mm probes can be used together to create a 10-cm freeze zone, whereas one 8-mm probe by itself will only produce a 6-cm freeze zone. Once turned on, the probe(s) will reach a temperature of -100°C, but the lesion as a whole will experience a cooling gradient. The cells closest to the probe will be cooled rapidly, approximately 50°C/min. Cells in the mid-zone will experience intermediate

cooling rates (10°C/min), whereas those on the periphery will experience slow cooling rates. For cryoablation to be effective, hypothermia (-40°C) be achieved for all regions. To achieve hypothermia in all cells, two freeze–thaw cycles must be performed. The cells in the rapidly cooling zone are killed because intracellular fluid freezes before dehydration can occur and the ice crystals damage the organelles and cell membranes, causing cell death. Those in the slow cooling zone are killed by cellular dehydration. The extracellular fluid freezes more rapidly than the intracellular fluid, causing an osmotic gradient. The internal fluid flows out of the cells and transmembrane potential becomes abnormal, resulting in a pH change, protein denaturation, and cell death. Cells in the intermediate zone do not die as readily. Their intracellular liquid freezes fast enough that cellular dehydration does not occur. Therefore, freeze–thaw cycles are needed to produce dehydration. Throughout the procedure, freezing of the lesion is monitored in real time by US. The freeze front appears as a hyperechoic ring or edge and has posterior acoustic shadowing. The cooling procedure is completed once the freeze front reaches 1 cm past the tumor margin (approximately 10–15 minutes). After a warming period, the process gets repeated to ensure cell death in all regions of the lesion. The mortality rate is 5% or less, and the morbidity rates range from 10% to 40%. Mechanical complications of cryotherapy include biliary fistula, abscess. Cryoablation may also induce physiologic complications such as hypothermia, coagulopathy, and triggering of systemic immune response syndrome (SIRS).

Radiofrequency Ablation

RFA is a technique that utilizes thermal energy for destruction of tumors. RFA is mostly used for the treatment of hepatic tumors. Safety studies indicate that the technique can also be applied to lung tumors. A RF probe is placed in the tumor tissue. With the activation of the RF energy, a high-frequency alternating current moves from the tip of the probe into the surrounding tumor tissue. As the ions within the tissue attempt to follow the change in the direction of the alternating current their movement results in frictional heating of the tissue. Cellular necrosis begins when the temperature within the tissue rises above 60°C. A typical RFA treatment produces local tissue temperatures that exceed 100°C, resulting in coagulation necrosis of the tumor tissue and surrounding parenchyma. Only the tissue through which radiofrequency electrical current passes directly is heated above a cytotoxic temperature. The geometry of the radiofrequency current pathway around the ablation probe creates a relatively uniform zone of radiant/conductive heat within the first few millimeters of electrode–tissue interface. The conductive heat emitted from the tissue radiates out from the electrode; and if the tissue impedance is relatively low, a dynamic expanding zone of ablated tissue is created. The final size of the region of heat-ablated tissue is proportional to the square of the radiofrequency current, also known as the *radiofrequency power density*. The radiofrequency power/current delivered through a monopolar electrode decreases in proportion to the square of the distance for the electrode. Therefore, the tissue temperature falls rapidly with increasing distance away from the electrode, and reliable production of cytotoxic temperatures can only be expected 5 to 10 mm away from the multiple array hook electrodes.

An RF probe is advanced into the liver tumor to be treated through either a percutaneous, laparoscopic, or open (laparotomy) route. Using transcutaneous or intraoperative ultrasonography to guide placement, the probe is advanced to the targeted area of the tumor. Tumors less than 2.5 cm in their greatest diameter can be ablated with the placement of a needle electrode with an array diameter of 3.5 to 4 cm when the electrode is positioned in the center of the tumor. Tumors larger than 2.5 cm may require multiple placements and repeat applications to completely destroy the tumor. Treatment is planned such that the zones of coagulative necrosis overlap to ensure complete destruction of the tumor.

CT scans performed after RFA of primary or metastatic liver tumors initially demonstrate a cystic-density lesion larger than the original tumor; the size of this cystic area decreases slightly over time. FDG-PET scan is highly sensitive in demonstrating the ablation of viable tumor tissue, and can be used as early as 2 to 4 weeks postablation. The role of RFA in the management of primary and metastatic liver cancer is expanding parallel to the advances in the multimodality, multistage therapeutic strategies.

Microwave Ablation

Tumor ablation is a method of killing or substantially destroying a tumor by thermal or chemical methods. Microwave ablation is a recent advance in tumor ablation technologies. It uses electromagnets, producing frequencies near 1 GHz, to destroy tumors. It is set apart from other thermoablation technologies because it has higher intratumoral temperatures and can destroy larger tumor volumes in less time.

The procedure begins by localizing the tumor using imaging guidance. Then an antenna is placed into the middle of the tumor either percutaneously, laparoscopically, or through open surgical access. This antenna is connected to a microwave generator that, upon activation, will emit microwaves and destroy the surrounding tumor cells. How does this work? Water molecules in the cells are dipoles and are easily influenced by electromagnetic currents. Since the microwaves oscillate from positive to negative, they cause the water molecules to oscillate with them. At a frequency of 1 GHz, they oscillate 1 billion times per second. This motion produces a large quantity of heat and causes cell death by means of coagulation necrosis.

Magnetic Resonance Guided Focused Ultrasound

Magnetic resonance guided focused ultrasound (MRgFUS) therapy is a modality where US beams are focused on a tissue for thermal ablation. Focused US beam, through significant energy deposition at the focus and increasing temperature within the tissue above 65°C, leads ablation of diseased tissue. The MR imaging provides quantitative, real-time, 3-D thermal images of the treated area. This allows precise targeting and monitoring of the temperature generated during each cycle of US energy delivery to ensure ensure effective treatment.

Dissection/Hemostasis Tools

Electrocautery

The principle behind the electrocautery is the generation of heat energy using high-frequency electrical current. Standard electrical current is of relatively slow oscillation (60 cps or 60 Hz) and leads to polarization/depolarization of the neuromuscular junction, manifested clinically as twitching. At 100,000 cps (100 kHz), the effect is one of tetanic contraction. At 200 kHz to 5 MHz, the oscillations are so rapid that tetany never occurs, but rather the high-frequency molecular oscillations generate heat. Most electrosurgical units function in the midrange of 500 kHz. Most electrosurgical units function in the midrange of 500 kHz. At the high end of electrosurgical frequencies, for example, 4 MHz, the energy is similar to the electromagnetic energy of radio waves and difficult to contain within tissue. Because the spectrum of electrical frequencies approaches that of classic radiofrequency, electrical energy is grouped with other forms of radiofrequency electromagnetic energy. The electrical current in the monopolar Bovie unit flows through the patient to the indifferent "ground" plate and back to the electrosurgical unit, completing the circuit.

The tissue response to electrosurgical energy is dependent on (i) power density, (ii) resistance/absorption, and (iii) time of application. Power density refers to watts of energy per square centimeter of tissue. Power or current density is inversely proportional to the cross-sectional area of the affected tissue. Therefore, the identical energy (watts) dispersed over a broad surface has a vastly different biologic effect than pinpoint application. For example, by reducing the area of the electrode (e.g., from surgical clamp to endoscopic wire), the power density and tissue effect is magnified. Conversely, the dispersal of the current over the large surface area of a ground plate greatly reduces the power density. Therefore, the ground plate is felt cold although it is in fact active. Too small a ground plate can result in a localized skin burn by concentrating the current to a small area.

The power and rate (time intervals) at which the energy is applied determines the speed and magnitude of heating, which in turn, determines the surgical effects on the tissue, that is, coagulation versus incision. Intermediate tissue heating (37°C–60°C) results in protein denaturation and slow water evaporation. The most obvious result of this effect is tissue desiccation and blood coagulation. The coagulating current (COAG) of an electrosurgical unit produces this form of intermediary tissue heating by rapid discharge of greater than 400 kHz energy with intermittent pause. This pattern results in a deep, relatively even heating. COAG uses high voltage to drive the current deeper into the tissue as the surface layer dries. Therefore, the current is able to burn or fulgurate the tissue even after much of the water has evaporated from the cell. Water is the main conducting medium in cells. As heating occurs, water evaporates, the tissue begins to desiccate, and resistance increases. Increased resistance leads to decreased observed coagulation effect. If the response to increasing resistance is to increase the power, the higher current creates the potential for electrical arcing to tissues of lower, more normal, resistance and unexpected distant tissue injury. This is the probable mechanism of GI tract injury seen with electrocautery and laparoscopic cholecystectomy. By contrast, instantaneous heating to 100°C results in evaporation, that is, cellular vaporization at the point of contact. This instantaneous tissue lysis produces steam and cellular debris with minimal surrounding tissue damage. Cutting current is a continuous application of low-voltage, higher-frequency, 500-kHz current energy. If COAG settings are high enough, incision can be achieved but with increased local tissue damage compared with cutting current.

BLEND is a combination of the two energy patterns, that is, longer pulses resulting in heating and vaporization. This same phenomenon of cellular microevaporation is seen with the application of continuous cutting laser energy as well. Defocused laser energy results in coagulation similar to the principles of coagulating electrosurgical current.

Monopolar Versus Bipolar Electrosurgical Current

Electricity will flow only when the circuit is completed or grounded. In monopolar current, the active electrode is in contact with the patient's tissue; the current passes through the patient with the ground plate completing the circuit through the electrosurgical unit. Monopolar current has the principal advantage of providing a wide spectrum of energy forms, that is, cutting, coagulation, and blended currents. The primary disadvantage is the arcing phenomenon to nearby tissues as desiccation occurs. In bipolar current, both electrodes are in close proximity. The circuit is completed between the local tissue only. Bipolar current requires greatly reduced power density because the conducting tissue is small. Waveforms similar to monopolar coagulating current are used in bipolar cautery. Bipolar current is typically used through endoscopes and is effective for coagulation.

Argon Beam Coagulation

The argon beam electrocoagulator is an alternative mode of current delivery, not a new technology *per se*. In essence, the jet of argon gas replaces the 3-cm metal tip of the typical electrosurgical unit. Argon gas conducts the electrical current, completing the typical current of a coagulation unit. Because of the gas, small amounts of blood can be blown away from the area to be coagulated, leading to more efficient coagulation with no crusting of the metal tip. Penetration is minimal at usual power density. The argon beam is useful for the coagulation of surface capillaries, for example, in liver and spleen surgery, but is rarely of use in vessels more than 1 mm in size.

Laser

Laser is the acronym for light amplification by stimulated emission of radiation. Normal light energy is dispersed in small packets of electromagnetic waves (photons) when electrons decay from a higher energy to a more stable lower energy state. Normal light is dispersed randomly without synchronicity. Different atoms/molecules release light of different wavelengths; therefore, most natural and artificially produced light is polychromatic. By contrast, laser light is a monochromatic in-phase synchronous parallel beam of light, resulting in amplification, power, and direction.

If high-energy electrons are pumped into a given atomic compound (e.g., carbon dioxide or argon), progressively more atoms are raised to a high-energy level. When the rate of energy input exceeds spontaneous decay, a state defined as population inversion occurs, that is, excessively high-energy atoms. Photons are emitted spontaneously by these high-energy atoms. As the photons strike other nearby hyperexcited atoms, further light energy is released. This phenomenon of population inversion and subsequent stimulated emission of electromagnetic light produces a beam of pure monochromatic light unique to the atomic structure of the excited substance.

In clinical lasers, the excited atoms in their population inversion state are contained within a mirrored resonator. Initially the photons are emitted at directions. As the photons are reflected within the mirrored chamber, the stimulated emissions of photons line themselves in a coherent in-phase beam. In addition to being parallel, the waves are synchronous (i.e., positive and negative amplitudes match). This coherent beam is permitted to exit the calibrated point in their reflective chamber, producing the laser beam that is a coherent monochromatic of a single wavelength. It is the synchronicity of wavelength and phase that confers amplification, power, and direction to laser energy.

Laser energy, like other electromagnetic energy, is measured in watts. Power density is defined as watts per square centimeter, and varies according to the excited substance and the degree of focus. Lasers that can be focused to a very narrow pinpoint, for example, CO_2, can be used to make incisions, whereas others are useful in coagulation (see "Electrosurgery"). Laser light interaction with tissue produces four possible events: (i) reflection, (ii) transmission, (iii) scatter, and (iv) absorption. It is the absorption of laser energy that results in the biologic effect. Reflection, transmission, and scatter are responsible for the complications of laser therapy.

The absorption of laser energy depends on the nature of the monochromatic beam. Like electrosurgery, absorption that results in gradual tissue heating produces coagulation, hemostasis, and even necrosis. Instantaneous heating higher than 100°C results in cellular vaporization, and is useful as a cutting instrument. Ultrasonic effects result in membrane disruption secondary to cavitation.

Clinical lasers depend on the substance exalted (e.g., CO_2, Nd:YAG, and argon) and, therefore, the monochromatic light emitted and the absorption of that specific wavelength by local tissue chromophores. The presence of melanin, hemoglobin and so on, determines which wavelength will be most useful for a given function. Because of the focus and precision of clinical lasers, the area affected is small. In general surgery, the combination of safety precautions, especially in the retina, and small areas leads to longer operating times in most situations.

Carbondioxide Laser

CO_2 laser light is in the midportion of the infrared spectrum and is principally absorbed by water. (Note: infrared radiation is invisible and, therefore, a guiding beam of red light is integrated with the laser only for directional purposes.) Because of the water absorption, the accuracy of focusing determines whether coagulation is achieved (defocused beam) versus an incision (a precisely focused narrow beam leading to vaporization). Although the CO_2 laser has the advantage of broad application in terms of cutting and coagulation, its major disadvantage is the inability to be transmitted along fiber optic bundles, that is, endoscopes.

Nd:YAG Laser

Nd:YAG laser is based on yttrium-aluminum-garnet crystal doped with Nd, leading to laser light in the near-infrared spectrum. Deep tissue penetration is achieved with the Nd:YAG because there is limited chromophore absorption at this wavelength and moderate scatter. The Nd:YAG laser is most effective when high-power heat coagulation is required such as for removing obstructive tumors in the bronchus.

Argon Laser

The argon laser works in the visible light spectrum at approximately 500 nm and is well absorbed by tissue chromophores, particularly melanin and hemoglobin. For these reasons, argon is ideally suited for treating pigmented lesions of the skin and neovascularization of the retina.

Dye Laser

The dye laser group depends on the solution of organic fluorescent compounds in water or alcohol. The different dyes allow for the production of different wavelengths and, therefore, laser beams with different properties. In contrast to more classical continuous wave lasers, dye lasers are typically pulsed (shuttered) at higher peak energy for brief periods. By varying the medium and the exciting source, these pulse dye lasers can result in highly selective tissue damage, depending on the absorbed wavelength. The specific wavelength can be matched to the absorbed property of the tissue chromophore, maximizing laser absorption and minimizing tissue effect.

Excimer Lasers

Excited dimers (halide gases in their excited state) are the basis of the high-energy ultraviolet light excimer lasers. Depths of penetration are extremely shallow ($<100 \mu m$) and can be used for precise cuts (primarily in ophthalmology).

Ultrasonic Dissector

The basic principle underlying the ultrasonic aspirator is the fragmentation of cells by cavitation, that is, the rapid formation and collapse of vapor bubbles in liquids. Sound waves produce a local change in pressure, typically depicted as a positive and negative sine wave. These waves represent regions of relative compression and rarefaction within tissue water as the wave passes through a specific point. Frequency represents the number of peaks (or troughs) passing a particular point per second and is an inverse function of the wavelength.

Sound waves produce local pressure variations in the surrounding cellular fluid. At supersonic speed, the sudden compression and release caused by sound waves encourages submicroscopic bubbles to grow, leading to the phenomenon of cavitation, an effect not unlike the wake seen from high-speed propellers in water. The rapidity of the collapse of the bubble is accelerated by the arrival of the next pressure wave, resulting in magnified pressure changes, molecular motion, heat, and ultimately tissue destruction. It is the cavitation effect, not the sound wave itself, that leads to tissue fragmentation with the ultrasonic scalpel [cavitron ultrasonic aspirator (CUSA)]. The same cavitation is the phenomenon responsible for stone fragmentation with lithotripsy.

At the cellular level, with normal sound waves, cavitation is insignificant. The repetitive release of energy at the cavity expands and collapses at millions of cycles per second; however, it has a cumulative destructive effect. The aggregate effect of cavitation results in rupture of cells when the ultrasonically vibrating probe is brought in contact with living tissue. In addition, water under the action of cavitation decomposes partially into free radicals, producing hydroxy radicals, and causing secondary effects and local tissue death.

These two actions are responsible for the biologic usefulness of the ultrasonic aspirator. Water is injected in a spray with the CUSA to dissipate heat. Local heat production leads to coagulation of blood and cellular proteins. Suction is necessary to remove cellular debris and water.

Harmonic Scalpel

The harmonic scalpel unit is made up of an ultrasonic generator, hand piece, blade extender, and the blade unit. The blade unit is curved and consists of a cutting edge (on bottom) and a grasping edge (on top). It operates by passing and electric current to the hand piece. Inside the hand piece, piezo-electric ceramic disks become excited. These disks convert the electric energy into mechanical energy, which is amplified longitudinally within the shaft. This amplification reaches its maximum at the blade tip; vibrating longitudinally 55,500 cycles per second across a 50 to 100 μ range. As the blade cuts through tissue, it coagulates simultaneously. The coagulation occurs from the transfer of the mechanical energy to the tissue. As the blade contacts the tissue, pressure causes coaptation of blood vessels. Hydrogen bonds are broken and proteins in the cells denature forming a sticky coagulum. The coagulum is what seals the vessels, incredibly, at a temperature under 100°C. Also, because the electrical energy is converted to mechanical energy, no electricity passes through the patient. Therefore, cutting and hemostasis can be achieved with minimal tissue damage and minimal risk to the patient.

EPILOGUE

Technology that applies perioperative and intraoperative management of surgical patients continue to evolve. The current innovations in surgical treatment may soon become obsolete with discoveries of more efficient means of diagnosis and treatment. Our humble duty is to implement the best techniques now available.

SUGGESTED READINGS

Absten CT, Joffee SN. *Lasers in medicine: an introductory guide.* Cambridge, UK: Cambridge University Press, 1985.

Blumgart LH. *Surgery of the liver, biliary tract, and pancreas,* 4th ed. Philadelphia: WB Saunders, 2007.

Curley AS. Radiofrequency ablation of malignant liver tumors. *Ann Surg Oncol* 2003;10:338–347.

Dogra V, Rubens DJ. *Ultrasound secrets.* Philadelphia: Hanley & Belfus, 2004.

Fishman EK, Jeffrey RB Jr. *Spiral CT: principles, techniques, and clinical applications.* New York: Raven Press, 1995.

Fogelman I, Maisey MN, Clarke SEM. *An atlas of clinical nuclear medicine,* 2nd ed. London: Martin Dunitz Ltd, 1994.

Gulec SA, Hoenie E, Hostetter R, Schwartzentruber D. PET probe-guided surgery: applications and clinical protocol. *World J Surg Oncol* 2007;5:65.

Gulec SA, Fong Y. Y-90 microsphere selective internal radiation treatment of hepatic colorectal metastases. *Arch Surg* 2007;142:675–682.

Gulec SA, Moffat FL, Carroll RG, et al. Gamma probe guided sentinel node biopsy in breast cancer. *Q J Nucl Med* 1997;41:251–261.

Haaga JR, Lanzieri CF, Gilkeson RC. *CT and MR imaging of the whole body,* 4th ed. Philadelphia: Mosby, 2003.

Karthikeyan D, Chegu D. *Step by step CT scan.* Kent, UK: Anshan Ltd, 2006.

Kaufman J, Lee M. *Vascular and interventional radiology: the requisites.* 2004:387–400.

Madoff D, Abdalla E, Vauthey J. Portal vein embolization in preparation for major hepatic resection: evolution of a new standard of care. *J Vasc Interv Radiol* 2005;16:779–790.

Mariana G, Gulec SA, Rubello D, et al. Preoperative localization and radioguided parathyroid surgery. *J Nucl Biol Med* 2003;44:1443–1458.

Mettler FA Jr, Guiberteau MJ. *Essentials of nuclear medicine imaging,* 5th ed. Philadelphia: WB Saunders, 2006.

Moffat FL, Gulec SA, Serafini AN, et al. A thousand points of light or just dim light bulbs? Radiolabeled antibodies and colorectal cancer imaging. *Cancer Invest* 1999;17(5):322–334.

Odell RC. Principles of electrosurgery. In: Sivak MV, ed. *Gastroenterologic endoscopy,* Vol. 7. Philadelphia: WB Saunders, 1987:128–142.

Ong JP, Snads M, Younossi ZM. Transjugular intrahepatic portosystemic shunt (TIPS) a decade later. *J Clin Gastroenterol* 2000;30:13–28.

Palmer EL, Scott JA, Strauss HW. *Practical nuclear medicine.* Philadelphia: WB Saunders, 1992.

Reddy J, Prasad V. *Step by step MRI.* New Delhi: Martin Dunitz, 2005.

Simon CJ, Dupuy DE, Mayo-Smith WW. Microwave ablation: principles and applications. *RadioGraphics* 2005;25:S69–S83.

Soares GM, Murphy TP. *Vena cava filters.* Abram's Angiography, 2006:1157–1169.

Strang JG, Dogra V. *Body CT secrets.* Philadelphia: Mosby, 2007.

Weissleder R, Wittenberg J, Harisinghani MG. *Primer of diagnostic imaging,* 3rd ed. Philadelphia: Mosby, 2003.

INDEX

Note: Page numbers followed by *f* indicate figures; those followed by *t* indicate tables.